Kanski's Clinical Ophthalmology

A SYSTEMATIC APPROACH

Dedication

To Jack Kanski, an exceptional teacher and inspirational mentor

Content Strategist: *Rus Gabbedy*
Content Development Specialist: *Louise Cook*
Content Coordinator: *John Leonard*
Project Manager: *Anne Collett*
Design: *Christian Bilbow*
Illustration Manager: *Brett MacNaughton*
Illustrators: *Terry Tarrant, Ian Ramsden, Antbits*
Marketing Manager (USA): *Melissa Fogarty*

Kanski's Clinical Ophthalmology

A SYSTEMATIC APPROACH

EIGHTH EDITION

Brad Bowling
FRCSEd(Ophth), FRCOphth, FRANZCO

Ophthalmologist
Sydney
New South Wales
Australia

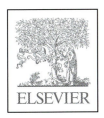

ELSEVIER

For additional online content visit expertconsult

ELSEVIER

First edition 1984
Second edition 1989
Third edition 1994
Fourth edition 1999
Fifth edition 2003
Sixth edition 2007
Seventh edition 2011
Eighth edition 2016

Notices

Knowledge and best practice in this field are constantly changing. As new research and experience broaden our understanding, changes in research methods, professional practices, or medical treatment may become necessary.

Practitioners and researchers must always rely on their own experience and knowledge in evaluating and using any information, methods, compounds, or experiments described herein. In using such information or methods they should be mindful of their own safety and the safety of others, including parties for whom they have a professional responsibility.

With respect to any drug or pharmaceutical products identified, readers are advised to check the most current information provided (i) on procedures featured or (ii) by the manufacturer of each product to be administered, to verify the recommended dose or formula, the method and duration of administration, and contraindications. It is the responsibility of practitioners, relying on their own experience and knowledge of their patients, to make diagnoses, to determine dosages and the best treatment for each individual patient, and to take all appropriate safety precautions.

To the fullest extent of the law, neither the Publisher nor the authors, contributors, or editors, assume any liability for any injury and/or damage to persons or property as a matter of products liability, negligence or otherwise, or from any use or operation of any methods, products, instructions, or ideas contained in the material herein.

ISBN: 978-0-7020-5572-0
978-0-7020-5573-7

ELSEVIER your source for books, journals and multimedia in the health sciences
www.elsevierhealth.com

Working together to grow libraries in developing countries

www.elsevier.com • www.bookaid.org

Printed in China

Last digit is the print number: 9 8 7 6 5 4 3 2 1

The publisher's policy is to use **paper manufactured from sustainable forests**

Contents

Preface to the Eighth Edition

I first met Jack Kanski when I rotated to The Prince Charles Eye Unit in Windsor as part of the Oxford Deanery ophthalmology residency programme. Jack had actually just retired from clinical practice, but continued to attend the unit's weekly education meetings. As the senior registrar, I was responsible for the organization of these sessions, to which Jack brought the same qualities that have facilitated his amazing success as a medical author – his encyclopaedic knowledge of ophthalmology and unerring ability to isolate the critical issues in a topic, not to mention his incisive wit, made the meetings extraordinarily effective as well as hugely enjoyable.

Jack was aware that I had done some textbook writing previously, and after one of the teaching sessions asked me whether I would be interested in writing a basic interactive text with him for medical students and novice ophthalmologists. I was a little daunted at first – Jack had written more than thirty ophthalmology textbooks by this time – but duly proceeded; we worked together extremely well, the book was written to deadline, was critically popular and sold lots of copies.

After I left Windsor, Jack and I worked with each other again on one or two projects and kept in touch socially, and a couple of years later he raised the possibility of collaboration on the next edition of *Clinical Ophthalmology*. I was thrilled. I recall vividly when, just prior to my first ophthalmology post, I contacted two registrars independently to enquire about initial textbook choice, receiving a curt single-word response from both: 'Kanski', with the implication that there was no need to ask. Big shoes to fill.

I have striven to maintain Jack Kanski's approach of presenting core clinical knowledge in a systematic and succinct form; the extent of subject coverage by the later editions of the book is easily underestimated, and it is intended that a thorough acquaintance with its contents will provide a comprehensive basis for general ophthalmic practice. In the present edition every attempt has been made to completely update each chapter, with inclusion of the latest practical evidence-based diagnostic and treatment approaches, and replacement and upgrading of images as appropriate, such as where novel imaging modalities offer an enhanced perspective. The index for this edition has been written by the author to ensure its ease of use and clinical applicability.

I am incredibly indebted to Jack Kanski for the opportunity to contribute to *Clinical Ophthalmology* and other books, and for his ongoing mentoring and support. I have received invaluable help with the eighth edition from colleagues; Simon Chen generously furnished a large number of photographic and other images and gave his time to advise in depth on various posterior segment topics, Chris Barry also kindly provided and edited very numerous images, and many other ophthalmologists, optometrists, ophthalmic photographers and other eyecare professionals contributed one or a small number of figures and are acknowledged in individual legends. Philip Spork was good enough to review the section on macular antioxidant supplements. I am also indebted to the numerous colleagues who contacted Jack Kanski or myself with helpful comments on particular points in the seventh edition. Many individuals have helped substantially with the previous editions of *Clinical Ophthalmology*, the core of which has been brought forward into the present book; Ken Nischal and Andy Pearson both carried out detailed reviews of sections in the seventh edition, Jay Menon made a major contribution to the fifth edition, Anne Bolton and Irina Gout provided photographic expertise over many years and, of course, Terry Tarrant supplied a large number of amazingly authentic ocular paintings. My wife, Suzanne, and sons, Edward and Oliver, supported me unreservedly during the extended revision of the book, tolerating my absence over the course of many months without complaint. Finally, I would like to acknowledge the cheerful and expert support and commitment of the staff at Elsevier, especially Russell Gabbedy, Louise Cook, John Leonard, Anne Collett and Marcela Holmes.

It would be impossible for me to replicate Jack Kanski's style precisely, but I have tried to retain the essence of his approach as faithfully as possible, and hope that this book will prompt in the reader at least some of the enthusiasm for the subject that the second edition of *Clinical Ophthalmology* engendered in me.

B.B.
2015

Abbreviations

AAION	arteritic anterior ischaemic optic neuropathy	CNV	choroidal neovascularization
AAU	acute anterior uveitis	CNVM	choroidal neovascular membrane
AC	anterior chamber	COX-2	cyclo-oxygenase-2
AC/A ratio	accommodative convergence/accommodation ratio	CPEO	chronic progressive external ophthalmoplegia
		CRAO	central retinal artery occlusion
AD	autosomal dominant	CRP	C-reactive protein
AF	autofluorescence	CRVO	central retinal vein occlusion
AHP	abnormal head posture	CSC	central serous chorioretinopathy
AI	accommodative insufficiency	CSMO	clinically significant macular oedema (US = CSME)
AIBSE	acute idiopathic blind spot enlargement syndrome	CSC/CSCR	central serous chorioretinopathy
AIDS	acquired immune deficiency syndrome	CSR	central serous chorioretinopathy
AIM	(unilateral) acute idiopathic maculopathy	CSS	central suppression scotoma
AION	anterior ischaemic optic neuropathy	CT	computed tomography
AIR	autoimmune retinopathies	DCR	dacryocystorhinostomy
AKC	atopic keratoconjunctivitis	DMO	diabetic macular oedema (US = DME)
ALT	argon laser trabeculoplasty	DR	diabetic retinopathy
AMD	age-related macular degeneration	DVD	dissociated vertical deviation
AMN	acute macular neuroretinopathy	ECG	electrocardiogram
ANA	antinuclear antibody	EDTA	ethylenediaminetetraacetic acid
ANCA	antineutrophil cytoplasmic antibodies	EKC	epidemic keratoconjunctivitis
APD	afferent pupillary defect	EOG	electro-oculography/gram
APMPPE	acute posterior multifocal placoid pigment epitheliopathy	ERG	electroretinography/gram
		ESR	erythrocyte sedimentation rate
AR	autosomal recessive	ETDRS	Early Treatment Diabetic Retinopathy Study
AREDS	Age-Related Eye Disease Study	FA	fluorescein angiography (also FFA)
ARN	acute retinal necrosis	FAF	fundus autofluorescence
ARPE	acute retinal pigment epitheliitis	FAP	familial adenomatous polyposis
AZOOR	acute zonal occult outer retinopathy	FAZ	foveal avascular zone
AZOR	acute zonal outer retinopathy	FBA	frosted branch angiitis
BCC	basal cell carcinoma	FBC	full blood count
BCVA	best-corrected visual acuity	FFM	fundus flavimaculatus
BIO	binocular indirect ophthalmoscopy	GA	geographic atrophy
BP	blood pressure	GAT	Goldmann applanation tonometry
BRAO	branch retinal artery occlusion	GCA	giant cell arteritis
BRVO	branch retinal vein occlusion	GPC	giant papillary conjunctivitis
BSV	binocular single vision	HAART	highly active antiretroviral therapy
BUT	breakup time	HIV	human immunodeficiency virus
CAI	carbonic anhydrase inhibitor	HM	hand movements
CCDD	congenital cranial dysinnervation disorders	HRT	Heidelberg retinal tomography
CCT	central corneal thickness	HSV-1	herpes simplex virus type 1
CDCR	canaliculodacryocystorhinostomy	HSV-2	herpes simplex virus type 2
CF	counts (or counting) fingers	HZO	herpes zoster ophthalmicus
CHED	congenital hereditary endothelial dystrophy	ICG	indocyanine green
CHP	compensatory head posture	ICGA	indocyanine green angiography
CHRPE	congenital hypertrophy of the retinal pigment epithelium	Ig	immunoglobulin
		IK	interstitial keratitis
CI	convergence insufficiency	ILM	internal limiting membrane
CMO	cystoid macular oedema (US = CME)	INO	internuclear ophthalmoplegia
CNS	central nervous system	IOFB	intraocular foreign body

IOID	idiopathic orbital inflammatory disease		PP	pars planitis
IOL	intraocular lens		PPCD	posterior polymorphous corneal dystrophy
IOP	intraocular pressure		PPDR	preproliferative diabetic retinopathy
IRMA	intraretinal microvascular abnormality		PPM	persistent placoid maculopathy
IRVAN	idiopathic retinal vasculitis, aneurysms and neuroretinitis syndrome		PPRF	paramedian pontine reticular formation
ITC	iridotrabecular contact		PRK	photorefractive keratectomy
IU	intermediate uveitis		PRP	panretinal photocoagulation
JIA	juvenile idiopathic arthritis		PS	posterior synechiae
KC	keratoconus		PUK	peripheral ulcerative keratitis
KCS	keratoconjunctivitis sicca		PVD	posterior vitreous detachment
KP	keratic precipitate		PVR	proliferative vitreoretinopathy
LA	local anaesthetic		PXF	pseudoexfoliation
LASEK	laser (also laser-assisted) epithelial keratomileusis		RAO	retinal artery occlusion
LASIK	laser-assisted *in situ* keratomileusis		RAPD	relative afferent pupillary defect
LN	latent nystagmus		RD	retinal detachment
MCP	multifocal choroiditis and panuveitis		RNFL	retinal nerve fibre layer
MEWDS	multiple evanescent white dot syndrome		ROP	retinopathy of prematurity
MFC	multifocal choroiditis and panuveitis		RP	retinitis pigmentosa
MLF	medial longitudinal fasciculus		RPC	relentless placoid chorioretinitis
MRI	magnetic resonance imaging		RPE	retinal pigment epithelium
MS	multiple sclerosis		RRD	rhegmatogenous retinal detachment
NF1	neurofibromatosis type I		RVO	retinal vein occlusion
NF2	neurofibromatosis type II		SAP	standard automated perimetry
NPDR	non-proliferative diabetic retinopathy		SCC	squamous cell carcinoma
NRR	neuroretinal rim		SD-OCT	spectral domain optical coherence tomography
NSAID	non-steroidal anti-inflammatory drug		SF	short-term fluctuation
NSR	neurosensory retina		SFU	progressive subretinal fibrosis and uveitis syndrome
NTG	normal-tension glaucoma		SIC	solitary idiopathic choroiditis
NVD	new vessels on the disc		SJS	Stevens–Johnson syndrome
NVE	new vessels elsewhere		SLK	superior limbic keratoconjunctivitis
OCT	optical coherence tomography/gram		SLT	selective laser trabeculoplasty
OHT	ocular hypertension		SRF	subretinal fluid
OKN	optokinetic nystagmus		SS	Sjögren syndrome
PAC	primary angle closure		STIR	short T1 inversion recovery
PACG	primary angle-closure glaucoma		TAL	total axial length
PACS	primary angle-closure suspect		TB	tuberculosis
PAM	primary acquired melanosis		TEN	toxic epidermal necrolysis
PAN	polyarteritis nodosa		TGF	transforming growth factor
PAS	peripheral anterior synechiae		TIA	transient ischaemic attack
PC	posterior chamber		TTT	transpupillary thermotherapy
PCO	posterior capsular opacification		TM	trabecular meshwork
PCR	polymerase chain reaction		TRD	tractional retinal detachment
PCV	polypoidal choroidal vasculopathy		UBM	ultrasonic biomicroscopy
PDR	proliferative diabetic retinopathy		US	ultrasonography
PDS	pigment dispersion syndrome		VA	visual acuity
PDT	photodynamic therapy		VEGF	vascular endothelial growth factor
PED	pigment epithelial detachment		VEP	visual(ly) evoked potential(s)
PIC	punctate inner choroidopathy		VFI	visual field index
PIOL	primary intraocular lymphoma		VHL	von Hippel–Lindau syndrome
PION	posterior ischaemic optic neuropathy		VKC	vernal keratoconjunctivitis
PKP	penetrating keratoplasty		VKH	Vogt–Koyanagi–Harada syndrome
POAG	primary open-angle glaucoma		VZV	varicella zoster virus
POHS	presumed ocular histoplasmosis syndrome		XL	X-linked

Chapter 1

Eyelids

INTRODUCTION

Anatomy

The skin (Fig. 1.1A) consists of the epidermis, dermis and related structures (adnexa).

Epidermis

The epidermis is comprised of four layers of keratin-producing cells (keratinocytes). It also contains melanocytes, Langerhans cells and Merkel cells. The layers of the epidermis around the eye are described below; cells migrate superficially, undergoing maturation and differentiation through successive layers.

- **Keratin layer** (stratum corneum or horny layer) consists of flat cells devoid of nuclei.

- **Granular cell layer** (stratum granulosum) typically consists of one or two layers of flattened cells containing keratohyaline granules.
- **Prickle cell layer** (stratum spinosum) is approximately five cells deep. The cells are polygonal in cross-section and have abundant eosinophilic cytoplasm. Their free borders are united by spiny-appearing desmosomes (cellular junctions).
- **Basal cell layer** (stratum basale) comprises a single row of columnar-shaped proliferating cells containing melanin derived from adjacent melanocytes.

Dermis

The dermis is much thicker than the epidermis. It is composed of connective tissue and contains blood vessels, lymphatics and nerve

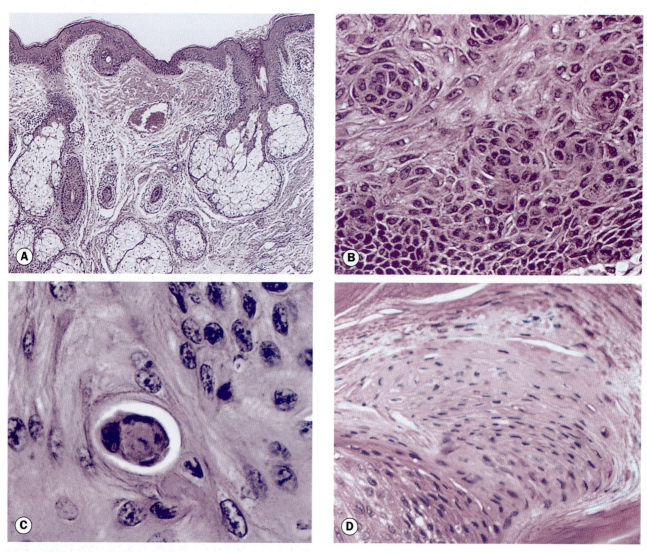

Fig. 1.1 Eyelid skin. **(A)** Normal skin is composed of keratinized stratified epithelium that covers the surface; pilosebaceous elements are conspicuous in the dermis and a few blood vessels and sweat glands are also seen; **(B)** dysplasia with loss of cell polarity; **(C)** dyskeratosis – a non-surface epithelial cell producing keratin; **(D)** parakeratosis – retention of cell nuclei into the surface keratin layer

(Courtesy of J Harry – fig. A; J Harry and G Misson, from Clinical Ophthalmic Pathology, Butterworth-Heinemann, 2001 – figs B–D)

fibres in addition to fibroblasts, macrophages and mast cells; upward dermal extensions (papillae) interdigitate with downward epidermal projections (rete ridges). In the eyelid the dermis lies on the orbicularis muscle. Adnexa lie deep in the dermis or within the tarsal plates.

- **Sebaceous glands** are located in the caruncle and within eyebrow hairs. Tiny sebaceous glands are associated with the thin (vellus) hairs covering periocular skin.
- **Meibomian glands** are modified sebaceous glands found in the tarsal plates. They empty through a single row of 20–30 orifices on each lid. A gland consists of a central duct with multiple acini, the cells of which synthesize lipids (meibum) that form the outer layer of the tear film.
- **Glands of Zeis** are modified sebaceous glands associated with lash follicles.
- **Glands of Moll** are modified apocrine sweat glands opening either into a lash follicle or directly onto the anterior lid margin between lashes; they are more numerous in the lower lid.
- **Eccrine sweat glands** are distributed throughout eyelid skin and are not confined to the lid margin, in contrast to glands of Moll.
- **Pilosebaceous units** comprise hair follicles and their sebaceous glands (see Fig. 1.1A).

Terminology

Clinical

- **Macule.** Localized area of colour change without infiltration, depression or elevation, less than 1 cm in diameter.
- **Papule.** A solid elevation less than 1 cm in diameter.
- **Vesicle.** Circumscribed lesion containing serous fluid; less than 0.5 cm across.
- **Bulla.** A large (more than 0.5 cm) serous fluid-filled lesion; plural – bullae.
- **Pustule.** A pus-filled elevation less than 1 cm in diameter.
- **Crust.** Solidified serous or purulent exudate.
- **Nodule.** A palpable solid area measuring more than 1 cm.
- **Cyst.** A nodule consisting of an epithelial-lined cavity filled with fluid or semi-solid material.
- **Plaque.** A solid elevation of the skin, greater than 1 cm in diameter.
- **Scale.** Readily detached fragments of shed keratin layer.
- **Papilloma.** A benign neoplastic warty or tag-like projection of the skin or mucous membrane.
- **Ulcer.** A circumscribed area of epithelial loss; in skin an ulcer extends through the epidermis into the dermis.

Histological

- **Tumour** strictly refers only to a swelling, though is commonly used to denote a neoplasm.
- **Neoplasia.** Abnormal tissue growth, either benign (localized, non-invasive and non-spreading) or malignant (progressive growth with the potential for distant spread).
- **Atypia** refers to an abnormal appearance of individual cells, e.g. abnormal mitotic figures.
- **Dysplasia** is an alteration of the size, morphology and organization of cellular components of a tissue. There is disturbance of normally structured and recognized layers of tissue (e.g. loss of cell polarity – Fig. 1.1B).
- **Carcinoma *in situ*** (intraepidermal carcinoma, Bowen disease) exhibits dysplastic changes throughout the thickness of the epidermis.
- **Hyperkeratosis.** An increase in thickness of the keratin layer that appears clinically as scaling. Hyperkeratosis can be a feature of benign or malignant epithelial tumours.
- **Acanthosis.** Thickening of the prickle cell layer.
- **Dyskeratosis** is keratinization other than on the epithelial surface (Fig. 1.1C).
- **Parakeratosis** is the retention of nuclei into the keratin layer (Fig. 1.1D).

General considerations

- **Classification.** Epidermal, adnexal or dermal.
- **Diagnosis.** The clinical characteristics of benign lesions are a tendency to a lack of induration and ulceration, uniform colour, limited growth, regular outline and preservation of normal lid margin structures. Biopsy may be required if the appearance is suspicious.
  - Incisional biopsy involves removal of a portion of a lesion for histopathology.
  - Excision biopsy is performed on small tumours and fulfils both diagnostic and treatment objectives.
- **Treatment** options include:
  - Excision of the entire lesion and a small surrounding portion of normal tissue.
  - Marsupialization involves the removal of the top of a cyst allowing drainage of its contents and subsequent epithelialization.
  - Ablation with laser or cryotherapy.

NON-NEOPLASTIC LESIONS

Chalazion

Pathogenesis

A chalazion (meibomian cyst) is a sterile chronic granulomatous inflammatory lesion (lipogranuloma) of the meibomian, or sometimes Zeis, glands caused by retained sebaceous secretions. Histopathology shows a lipogranulomatous chronic inflammatory picture with extracellular fat deposits surrounded by lipid-laden epithelioid cells, multinucleated giant cells and lymphocytes (Fig. 1.2A). Blepharitis is commonly present; rosacea can be associated with multiple and recurrent chalazia. A recurrent chalazion should be biopsied to exclude malignancy.

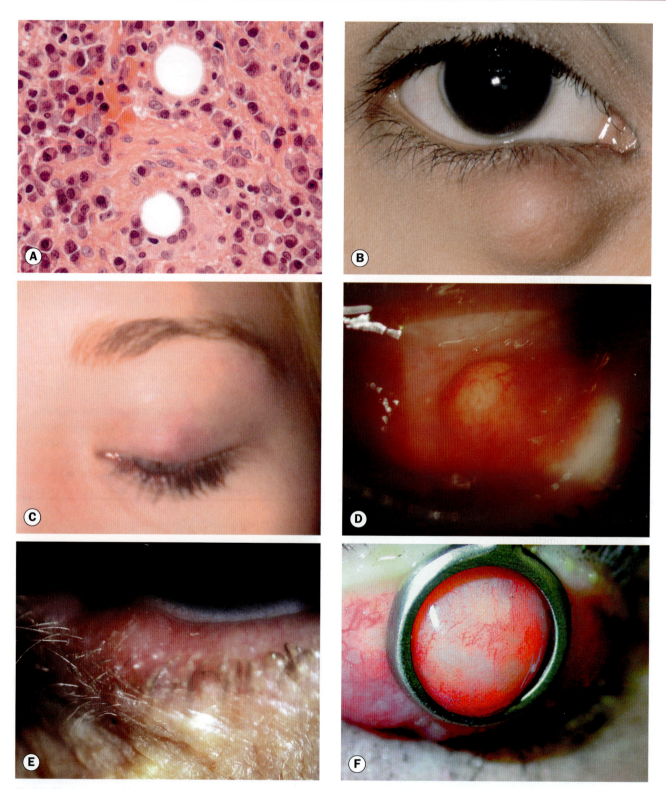

Fig. 1.2 Chalazion. **(A)** Histopathology shows a lipogranuloma; the large pale cells are epithelioid cells and the well-demarcated empty space contained fat dissolved out during processing; **(B)** uninflamed chalazion; **(C)** acutely inflamed lesion; **(D)** conjunctival granuloma; **(E)** marginal chalazion; **(F)** conjunctival view of chalazion clamp in place prior to incision and curettage

(Courtesy of J Harry and G Misson, from Clinical Ophthalmic Pathology, Butterworth-Heinemann 2001 – fig. A; J Nerad, K Carter and M Alford, from 'Oculoplastic and Reconstructive Surgery', in Rapid Diagnosis in Ophthalmology, Mosby 2008 – fig. F)

Diagnosis

- **Symptoms**
  - Subacute/chronic: gradually enlarging painless rounded nodule (Fig. 1.2B).
  - Acute: sterile inflammation or bacterial infection with localized cellulitis (Fig. 1.2C); differentiation may be difficult. A secondarily infected meibomian gland is referred to as an internal hordeolum.
- **Signs**
  - A nodule within the tarsal plate, sometimes with associated inflammation.
  - Bulging inspissated secretions may be visible at the orifice of the involved gland.
  - There may be an associated conjunctival granuloma (Fig. 1.2D).
  - A lesion at the anterior lid margin – a marginal chalazion (Fig. 1.2E) – may be connected to a typical chalazion deeper in the lid or be due to isolated involvement of a gland of Zeis.

Treatment

- **Oral antibiotics** are required for significant bacterial infection, but not for sterile inflammation.
- **Conservative.** At least a third of chalazia resolve spontaneously so observation may be appropriate, especially if the lesion is showing signs of improvement, though early definitive treatment has been reported to lead to higher patient satisfaction.
- **Hot compress** application several times daily may aid resolution, particularly in early lesions.
- **Expression.** Compression between two cotton-tipped applicators is sometimes effective in expressing the contents of a fresh lesion near the lid margin.
- **Steroid injection** into or around the lesion has been reported to give similar resolution rates to incision and curettage (see below). It may be preferred for marginal lesions or lesions close to structures such as the lacrimal punctum because of the risk of surgical damage.
  - Reported regimens include 0.2–2 ml of triamcinolone acetonide aqueous suspension diluted with lidocaine to a concentration of 5 mg/ml, and 0.1–0.2 ml of 40 mg/ml, injected with a 27- or 30-gauge needle.
  - The success rate following one injection is about 80%; a second can be given 1–2 weeks later.
  - Local skin depigmentation and fat atrophy are potential but uncommon complications, the risk of which may be reduced by avoidance of infiltration immediately subcutaneously or by utilizing a conjunctival approach.
  - Retinal vascular occlusion has been described as a complication, probably due to intravascular injection with subsequent embolization.
- **Surgery**
  - Following local anaesthesia infiltration, the eyelid is everted with a specialized clamp (Fig. 1.2F), the cyst is incised vertically through the tarsal plate and its contents curetted.
  - Limited excision of solid inflammatory material (sent for histopathology) with fine scissors may be helpful in some cases, especially if there is no focus of secretions.
  - A suture should not be used.
  - Topical antibiotic ointment is used three times daily for 5–7 days following curettage.
- **Marginal lesions** can be managed by steroid injection, by curettage of an associated deeper chalazion, by shave curettage or by incision and curettage via a horizontal incision on the conjunctival surface or vertically through the grey line.
- **Prophylaxis**
  - Treatment of blepharitis, e.g. daily lid hygiene regimen.
  - Systemic tetracycline may be required as prophylaxis in patients with recurrent chalazia, particularly if associated with acne rosacea.

Other eyelid cysts

- **Cyst of Zeis** is a small, non-translucent cyst on the anterior lid margin arising from obstructed sebaceous glands associated with the eyelash follicle (Fig. 1.3A).
- **Cyst of Moll** (apocrine hidrocystoma) is a small retention cyst of the lid margin apocrine glands. It appears as a round, non-tender, translucent fluid-filled lesion on the anterior lid margin (Fig. 1.3B).
- **Sebaceous (pilar) cyst** is caused by a blocked pilosebaceous follicle and contains sebaceous secretions; the gland orifice will often be visible (Fig. 1.3C). It is only rarely found on the eyelid although it may occasionally occur at the inner canthus.
- **Comedones** are plugs of keratin and sebum within the dilated orifice of hair follicles that often occur in patients with acne vulgaris. They may be either open (blackheads) containing a darkened plug of oxidized material (Fig. 1.3D), or closed (whiteheads).
- **Milia** are caused by occlusion of pilosebaceous units resulting in retention of keratin. They are tiny, white, round, superficial papules that tend to occur in crops (Fig. 1.3E).
- **Epidermal inclusion** cyst is usually caused by implantation of epidermis into the dermis following trauma or surgery. It is a slow-growing, round, firm, superficial or subcutaneous lesion containing keratin (Fig. 1.3F).
- **Epidermoid** cyst is uncommon and usually developmental, occurring along embryonic lines of closure. It is similar in appearance to an epidermal inclusion cyst.
- **Dermoid** cyst is usually subcutaneous or deeper and is typically attached to the periosteum at the lateral end of the brow (Fig. 1.3G). It is caused by skin sequestered during embryonic development.
- **Eccrine hidrocystoma** is less common but similar in appearance to a cyst of Moll except that it is usually located along the medial or lateral aspects of the lid, and is close to but does not involve the lid margin itself (Fig. 1.3H).

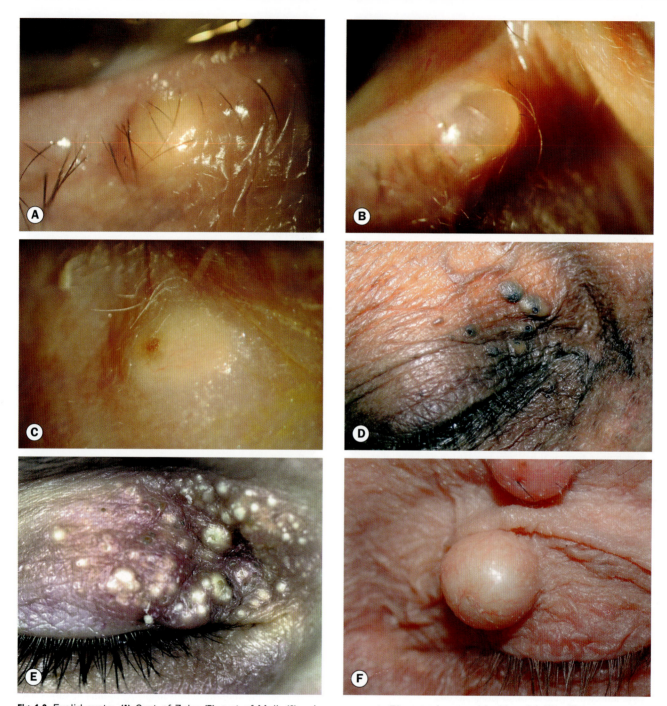

Fig. 1.3 Eyelid cysts. **(A)** Cyst of Zeis; **(B)** cyst of Moll; **(C)** sebaceous cyst; **(D)** comedones – blackheads; **(E)** milia; **(F)** epidermal inclusion cyst;

Xanthelasma

Introduction

Xanthelasma (plural – xanthelasmata) is a common, frequently bilateral condition typically affecting middle-aged and elderly individuals. It is a subtype of xanthoma. Hyperlipidaemia is found in about one-third of patients, in whom corneal arcus may also be present. In contrast to chalazion, fat in xanthelasmata is mainly intracellular, with lipid-laden histiocytes (foam cells) in the dermis (Fig. 1.4A).

Diagnosis

Xanthelasmata are yellowish subcutaneous plaques, usually in the medial aspects of the eyelids (Fig. 1.4B), commonly bilateral and are multiple (Fig. 1.4C).

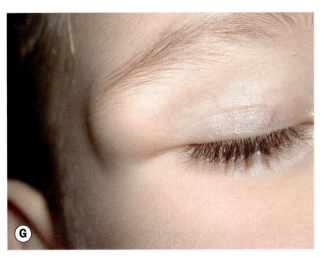

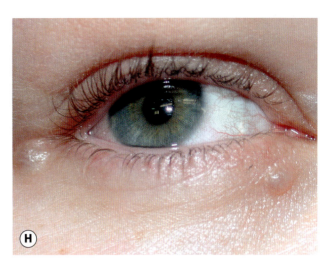

Fig. 1.3, Continued (G) dermoid cyst; **(H)** eccrine hidrocystomas

(Courtesy of A Pearson – figs D, F and H)

Treatment

This is principally for cosmesis. Recurrence occurs in up to 50%, and is most common in patients with hypercholesterolaemia.

- **Simple excision** is commonly performed where adequate excess skin is present.
- **Microdissection.** Larger lesions can be raised in a flap, the fatty deposits dissected from overlying skin under a surgical microscope using microscissors, and the skin replaced.
- **Other methods.** Good results can be obtained using chemical peeling with bi- or trichloroacetic acid. Laser

ablation and cryotherapy have advantages but may be more prone to scarring, including pigmentary changes.

BENIGN EPIDERMAL TUMOURS

Squamous cell papilloma

Squamous cell papilloma is a very common benign epithelial tumour with a variable clinical appearance, including narrow-based (pedunculated or 'skin tag' – Fig. 1.5A), pink broad-based

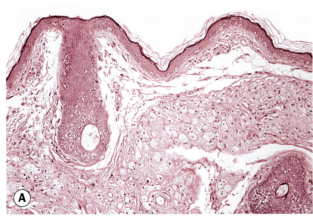

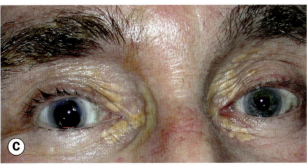

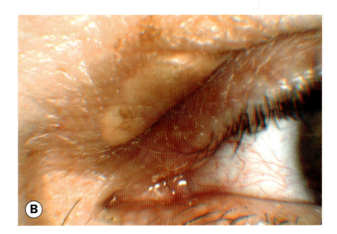

Fig. 1.4 Xanthelasma. **(A)** Histopathology showing foamy histiocytes within the dermis; **(B)** large isolated lesion; **(C)** multiple bilateral smaller lesions

(Courtesy of J Harry – fig. A; S Chen – fig. C)

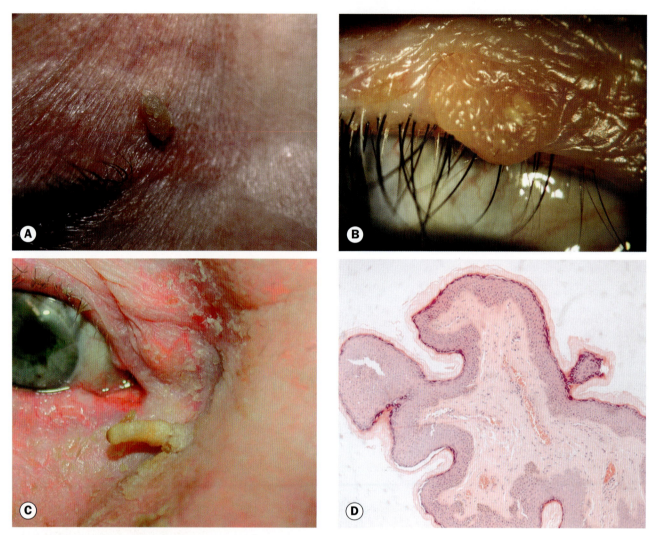

Fig. 1.5 Squamous cell papilloma. **(A)** Pedunculated 'skin tag'; **(B)** sessile lesion; **(C)** hyperkeratotic filiform lesion; **(D)** histopathology shows finger-like projections of fibrovascular connective tissue covered by irregular acanthotic and hyperkeratotic squamous epithelium

(Courtesy of A Pearson – fig. C; J Harry – fig. D)

(sessile – Fig. 1.5B) and whitish thread-like (filiform) hyperkeratotic lesions similar to a cutaneous horn (Fig. 1.5C). Histopathology in all clinical types is similar, showing finger-like projections of fibrovascular connective tissue covered by irregular acanthotic and hyperkeratotic squamous epithelium (Fig. 1.5D). The incidence increases with age; at least some cases result from human papilloma virus infection. Treatment usually involves simple excision, but other options include cryotherapy and laser or chemical ablation.

Seborrhoeic keratosis

Seborrhoeic keratosis (basal cell papilloma) is an extremely common slowly growing lesion found on the face, trunk and extremities of elderly individuals as a discrete light- to dark-brown plaque with a friable, greasy, verrucous surface and a 'stuck-on' appearance (Fig. 1.6A). They are frequently numerous. The differential diagnosis includes pigmented basal cell carcinoma,

naevus and melanoma. Histopathology shows expansion of the squamous epithelium of the epidermis by proliferating basal cells, sometimes with keratin-filled horns or cystic inclusions (Fig. 1.6B). Treatment involves shave biopsy (occasionally simple excision), electrodesiccation with curettage, laser ablation, cryotherapy with liquid nitrogen, and chemical peeling.

Actinic keratosis

Actinic (solar, senile) keratosis is a common slowly growing lesion that rarely develops on the eyelids. It typically affects elderly, fair-skinned individuals on areas of sun-damaged skin such as the forehead and backs of the hands, and appears as a hyperkeratotic plaque with distinct borders and a scaly surface that may become fissured (Fig. 1.7A). Occasionally the lesion is nodular or wart-like and may give rise to a cutaneous horn. Histopathology shows irregular dysplastic epidermis with hyperkeratosis, parakeratosis and cutaneous horn formation (Fig. 1.7B). It has potential, though

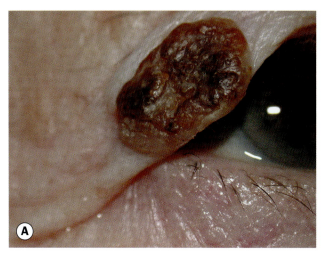

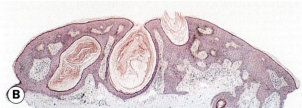

Fig. 1.6 Basal cell papilloma. **(A)** Typical 'stuck-on' appearance; **(B)** histopathology showing an elevated expansion of the epidermis with proliferation from basal cells – horn cysts and pseudohorn cysts are present
(Courtesy of A Pearson – fig. A; J Harry – fig. B)

low, for transformation into squamous cell carcinoma. Treatment involves biopsy followed by excision or cryotherapy.

BENIGN PIGMENTED LESIONS

Freckle

A freckle (ephelis, plural ephelides) is a small (generally 1–5 mm) brown macule due to increased melanin in the epidermal basal layer, typically in sun-exposed skin (Fig. 1.8); numbers vary with the level of sun exposure and can sometimes regress completely. Histopathology shows hyperpigmentation of the basal layer of the epidermis, with a normal melanocyte population.

Congenital melanocytic naevus

Congenital naevi are uncommon and histologically resemble their acquired counterparts (see below). They are usually small and of uniform colour. Rare variants include a 'kissing' or split naevus that involves the upper and lower eyelid (Fig. 1.9A) and may occasionally contain numerous hairs (Fig. 1.9B), and a very large lesion covering an extensive area of the body ('giant hairy naevus' – Fig. 1.9C). Large lesions have the potential for malignant transformation (up to 15%). Treatment, if necessary, involves complete surgical excision.

Acquired melanocytic naevus

Diagnosis

The clinical appearance and potential for malignant transformation of naevi are determined by their histological location within the skin.

- **Junctional** naevus occurs in young individuals as a uniformly brown macule or plaque (Fig. 1.10A). The naevus cells are located at the junction of the epidermis and dermis and have a low potential for malignant transformation (Fig. 1.10B).
- **Compound** naevus occurs in middle age as a raised papular lesion. The shade of pigment varies from light tan to dark

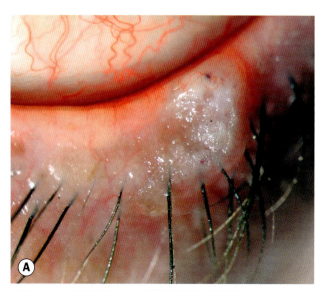

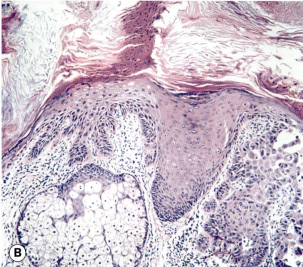

Fig. 1.7 Actinic keratosis. **(A)** Clinical appearance; **(B)** histopathology shows irregular dysplastic epidermis with hyperkeratosis, parakeratosis and cutaneous horn formation
(Courtesy of M Jager – fig. A; J Harry and G Misson, from Clinical Ophthalmic Pathology, *Butterworth-Heinemann 2001 – fig. B)*

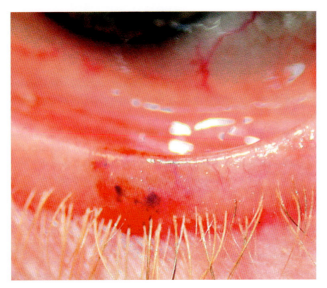

Fig. 1.8 Freckle (ephelis)

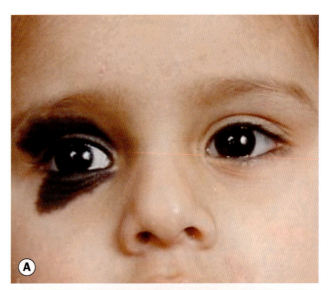

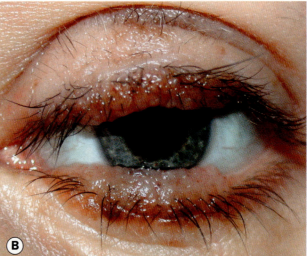

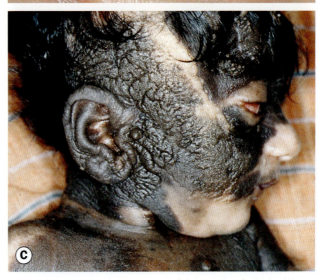

Fig. 1.9 Congenital melanocytic naevus. **(A)** Split naevus; **(B)** split naevus containing hair; **(C)** extensive cutaneous involvement

(Courtesy of A Pearson – fig. B; U Raina – fig. C)

brown but tends to be relatively uniform throughout (Fig. 1.10C). The naevus cells extend from the epidermis into the dermis (Fig. 1.10D). It has a low malignant potential related to the junctional component.

- **Intradermal** naevus, the most common, typically occurs in older patients. It is a papillomatous lesion, with little or no pigmentation (Fig. 1.10E). Histologically, naevus cells are confined to the dermis and have essentially no malignant potential (Fig. 1.10F).
- **Variants** of naevi include balloon cell naevi, halo naevi, Spitz naevi (juvenile melanomas) and dysplastic naevi (atypical moles). Multiple dysplastic naevi constitute the dysplastic naevus syndrome (atypical mole syndrome – AMS). Individuals with AMS are at increased risk of developing conjunctival and uveal naevi and cutaneous, conjunctival and uveal melanomas.

Treatment

Treatment is indicated for cosmesis or for concern about malignancy. Excision should be complete in most cases, with at least a 3 mm margin if melanoma is strongly suspected.

BENIGN ADNEXAL TUMOURS

Syringoma

Syringomas are benign proliferations arising from eccrine sweat glands. They are characterized by small papules that are often multiple and bilateral (Fig. 1.11).

Pilomatricoma

Pilomatricoma (pilomatrixoma, calcifying epithelioma of Malherbe) is derived from the germinal matrix cells of the hair bulb and is the commonest hair follicle proliferation seen by

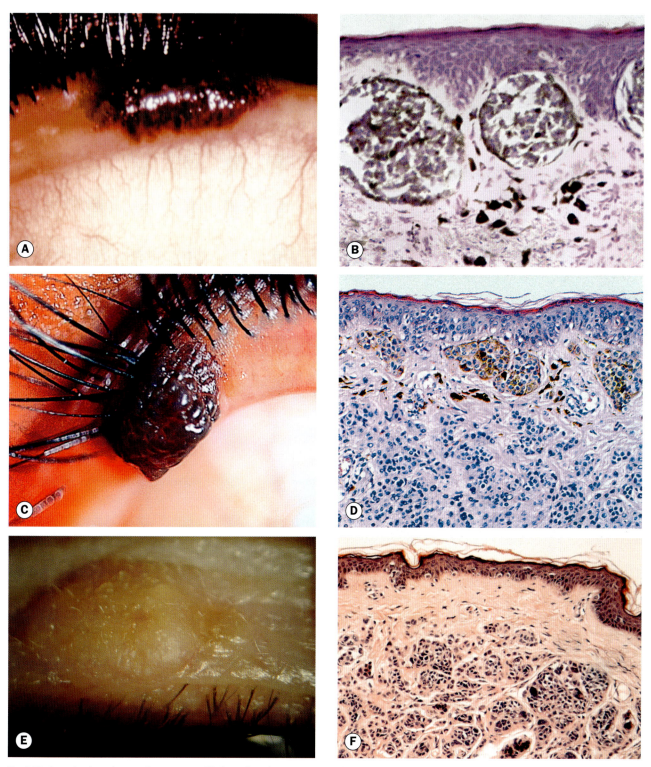

Fig. 1.10 Acquired melanocytic naevus. **(A)** Junctional naevus; **(B)** histopathology shows heavily pigmented naevus cells at the epidermal/dermal junction; **(C)** compound naevus; **(D)** histopathology shows naevus cells both at the epidermal/dermal junction and within the dermis; **(E)** intradermal naevus; **(F)** histopathology shows naevus cells within the dermis separated from the epidermis by a clear zone

(Courtesy of J Harry – figs B, D and F)

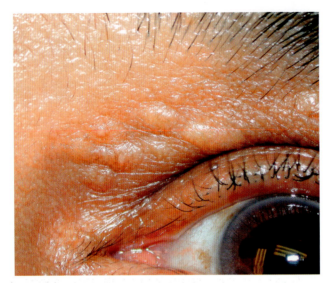

Fig. 1.11 Syringomas
(Courtesy of A Pearson)

ophthalmologists. It affects children and young adults and is more common in females. Clinically it appears as a mobile purplish dermal nodule that may have a hard consistency due to calcification (Fig. 1.12A). Histopathology shows irregular epithelial islands exhibiting viable basophilic cells at the periphery and degenerate 'shadow' cells more centrally (Fig. 1.12B). Calcification is frequently present and there is often a foreign body giant cell reaction. Treatment involves excision. Malignant change is rare. Other, less common, hair follicle proliferations include trichofolliculoma, trichoepithelioma and trichilemmoma.

MISCELLANEOUS BENIGN TUMOURS

Capillary haemangioma

Capillary haemangioma (strawberry naevus) is one of the most common tumours of infancy; it is three times as common in boys as girls. It presents shortly after birth as a unilateral, raised bright red lesion (Fig. 1.13A), usually in the upper lid; a deeper lesion appears purplish (Fig. 1.13B and see also Fig. 3.31). Ptosis is frequent. The lesion blanches on pressure and may swell on crying. There may be orbital extension (see Ch. 3). Occasionally the lesion may involve the skin of the face and some patients have strawberry naevi on other parts of the body. Histopathology shows proliferation of varying-sized vascular channels in the dermis and subcutaneous tissue (Fig. 1.13C). It is important to be aware of an association between multiple cutaneous lesions and visceral haemangiomas, and to consider systemic assessment in appropriate cases. Treatment is described in Ch. 3.

Port-wine stain

Introduction

Port-wine stain (naevus flammeus) is a congenital malformation of vessels within the superficial dermis, consisting histopathologically

of vascular spaces of varying calibre separated by thin fibrous septa (Fig. 1.14A). About 10% have associated ocular or CNS involvement, including Sturge–Weber (see below) and other defined syndromes.

Diagnosis

Port-wine stain manifests clinically as a sharply demarcated soft pink patch that does not blanch with pressure, most frequently located on the face. It is usually unilateral and tends to be aligned with the skin area supplied by one or more divisions of the trigeminal nerve (Figs 1.14B and C). Darkening to red or purple takes place with age, and there is commonly associated soft tissue hypertrophy (Figs 1.14D–F). Bleeding may occur from focal overlying lobulations (pyogenic granulomas – see below).

Treatment

Treatment with laser (e.g. pulsed-dye) is effective in decreasing skin discoloration; cosmetically superior results are usually

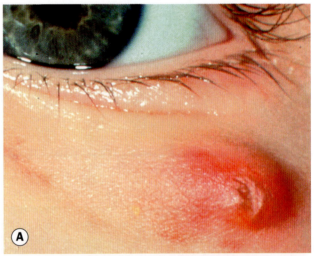

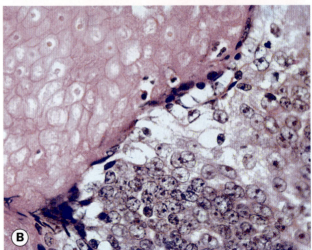

Fig. 1.12 Pilomatricoma. **(A)** Clinical appearance; **(B)** histopathology shows viable basophilic cells to the right and degenerate 'shadow' cells to the left

(Courtesy of J Krachmer, M Mannis and E Holland, from Cornea, Elsevier 2005 – fig. A; J Harry and G Misson, from Clinical Ophthalmic Pathology, Butterworth-Heinemann 2001 – fig. B)

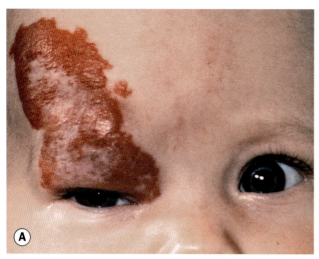

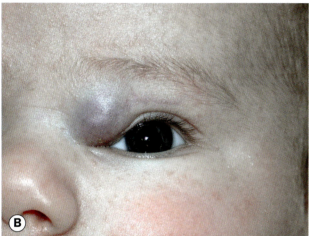

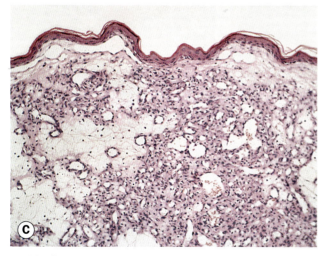

Fig. 1.13 Capillary haemangioma. **(A)** Medium-sized haemangioma; **(B)** mechanical ptosis due to a large lesion; **(C)** histopathology shows vascular channels of varying size within the dermis and subcutaneous tissue

(Courtesy of S Chen – fig. A; J Harry – fig. C)

achieved by early treatment. Topical preparations such as imiquimod and rapamycin, alone or with adjuvant laser, show promise. Soft tissue debulking is used in a small number of cases. Screening for glaucoma should begin in infancy. Systemic investigation is considered in some patients, particularly those with a lesion of the lumbar area.

Sturge–Weber syndrome

Sturge–Weber syndrome (encephalotrigeminal angiomatosis) is a congenital, sporadic phacomatosis.
- **Port-wine stain**, extending over the area corresponding to the distribution of one or more branches of the trigeminal nerve.
- **Leptomeningeal haemangioma** involving the ipsilateral parietal or occipital region may cause contralateral focal or generalized seizures, hemiparesis or hemianopia.
- **Ocular** features may include ipsilateral glaucoma, episcleral haemangioma, iris heterochromia and diffuse choroidal haemangioma (see Ch. 12).

Pyogenic granuloma

Pyogenic granuloma is a rapidly growing vascularized proliferation of granulation tissue that is usually antedated by surgery, trauma or infection, although some cases are idiopathic. Clinically there is a painful, rapidly growing, vascular granulating polypoidal lesion (Fig. 1.15) that may bleed following relatively trivial trauma. Treatment of cutaneous lesions involves excision; conjunctival pyogenic granuloma is discussed in Ch. 5.

Neurofibroma

Cutaneous neurofibromas are benign nerve tumours, usually nodular or pedunculated, that can be found anywhere on the skin. Isolated neurofibromas are common in normal individuals, but if multiple lesions are present neurofibromatosis (see Ch. 19) should be excluded. Plexiform neurofibromas typically present in childhood as a manifestation of neurofibromatosis type 1 with a characteristic S-shaped deformity of the upper eyelid (Fig. 1.16). Treatment of solitary lesions involves simple excision but removal of the more diffuse plexiform lesions may be difficult.

MALIGNANT TUMOURS

The treatment of malignant eyelid tumours in general is discussed at the end of this section.

Rare predisposing conditions

Young patients who suffer from one of the following conditions may develop eyelid malignancies.
- **Xeroderma pigmentosum** is characterized by skin damage on exposure to sunlight, leading to progressive cutaneous abnormalities (Fig. 1.17A). It is inherited in an autosomal recessive (AR) fashion. Affected patients have a bird-like facies and a great propensity to the development of basal cell carcinoma (BCC), squamous cell carcinoma (SCC)

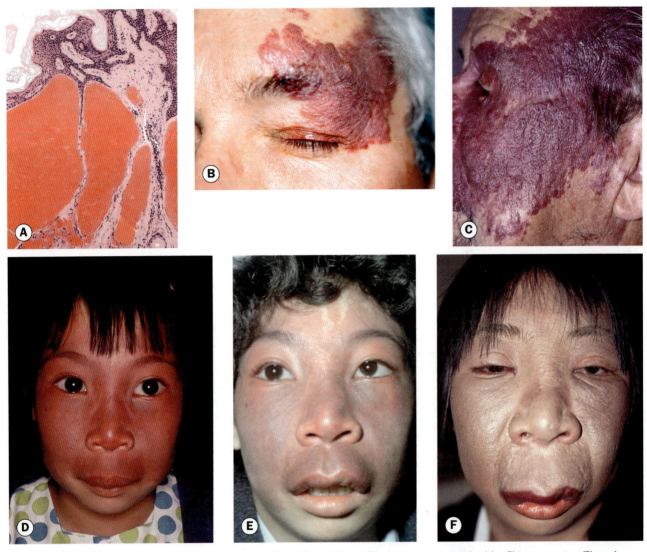

Fig. 1.14 Port-wine stain. **(A)** Histopathology shows widely dilated blood-filled spaces separated by fibrous septa; **(B)** and **(C)** clinical appearance; **(D–F)** progression of port-wine stain over time, with associated underlying soft tissue hypertrophy

(Courtesy of L Horton – fig. A)

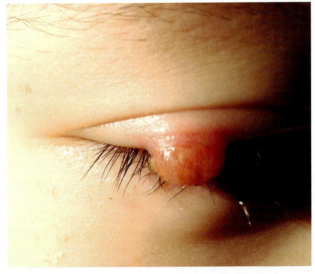

Fig. 1.15 Pyogenic granuloma

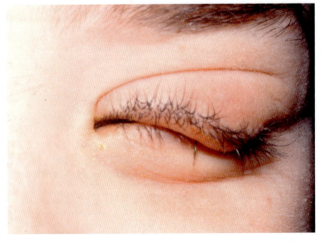

Fig. 1.16 Plexiform neurofibroma – characteristic S-shaped upper lid

(Courtesy of J Harry)

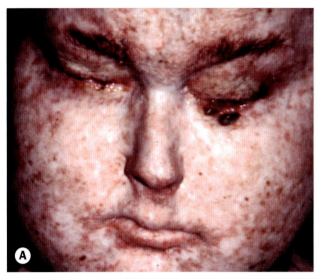

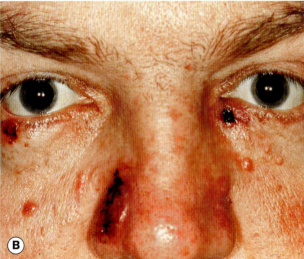

Fig. 1.17 Predispositions to eyelid malignancies.
(A) Xeroderma pigmentosum; **(B)** Gorlin–Goltz syndrome
(Courtesy of J Krachmer, M Mannis and E Holland, from Cornea, Mosby 2005 – fig. B)

and melanoma, which are commonly multiple. Conjunctival malignancies have also been reported.

- **Gorlin–Goltz syndrome** (naevoid basal cell carcinoma syndrome) is a rare autosomal dominant (AD) disorder characterized by extensive congenital deformities of the eye, face, bone and central nervous system. Many patients develop multiple small BCC during the second decade of life (Fig. 1.17B) and are also predisposed to medulloblastoma, breast carcinoma and Hodgkin lymphoma.
- **Muir–Torre syndrome** is a rare AD condition that predisposes to cutaneous and internal malignancies. Cutaneous tumours include BCC, sebaceous gland carcinoma and keratoacanthoma. Colorectal and genitourinary carcinomas are the most common systemic tumours.
- **Bazex syndrome** can be used to describe two distinct conditions: (i) Bazex–Dupré–Christol syndrome, an

X-linked dominant condition characterized by multiple BCCs, commonly facial including the eyelids, associated with skin changes including follicular indentations without hairs on extensor surfaces (follicular atrophoderma), hypohidrosis and hypotrichosis; (ii) acrokeratosis paraneoplastica of Bazex, in which eczema-like and psoriatiform lesions are associated with an underlying malignancy of the upper respiratory or digestive tract.

- **Other predispositions** include immunosuppression, prior retinoblastoma and albinism.

Basal cell carcinoma

Introduction

BCC is the most common human malignancy and typically affects older age groups. The most important risk factors are fair skin, inability to tan and chronic exposure to sunlight. Ninety per cent of cases occur in the head and neck and about 10% of these involve the eyelid. BCC is by far the most common malignant eyelid tumour, accounting for 90% of all cases. It most frequently arises from the lower eyelid, followed in relative frequency by the medial canthus, upper eyelid and lateral canthus. The tumour is slowly growing and locally invasive but non-metastasizing. Tumours located near the medial canthus are more prone to invade the orbit and sinuses, are more difficult to manage than those arising elsewhere and carry the greatest risk of recurrence. Tumours that recur following incomplete treatment tend to be more aggressive.

Histopathology

The tumour arises from the cells that form the basal layer of the epidermis. The cells proliferate downwards (Fig. 1.18A) and characteristically exhibit palisading at the periphery of a tumour lobule of cells (Fig. 1.18B). Squamous differentiation with the production of keratin results in a hyperkeratotic type of BCC. There can also be sebaceous and adenoid differentiation while the growth of elongated strands and islands of cells embedded in a dense fibrous stroma results in a sclerosing (morphoeic) type of tumour.

Clinical features

Eyelid BCC generally conforms to one of the morphological patterns below.

- **Nodular BCC** is a shiny, firm, pearly nodule with small overlying dilated blood vessels. Initially, growth is slow and it may take the tumour 1–2 years to reach a diameter of 0.5 cm (Figs 1.19A and B).
- **Noduloulcerative BCC (rodent ulcer)** is centrally ulcerated with pearly raised rolled edges and dilated and irregular blood vessels (telangiectasis) over its lateral margins (Fig. 1.19C); with time it may erode a large portion of the eyelid (Fig. 1.19D).
- **Sclerosing (morphoeic) BCC** is less common and may be difficult to diagnose because it infiltrates laterally beneath

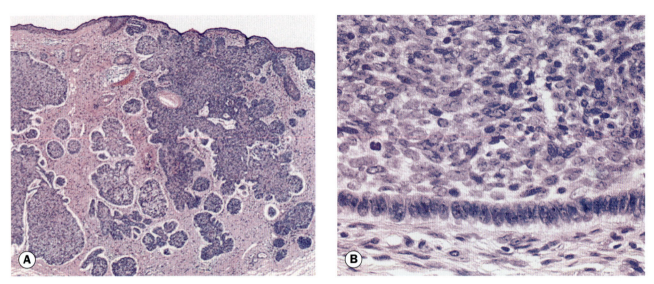

Fig. 1.18 Histopathology of basal cell carcinoma. **(A)** Histopathology shows downward proliferation of lobules of basophilic (purple) cells; **(B)** palisading of cells at the periphery of a tumour lobule

(Courtesy of J Harry)

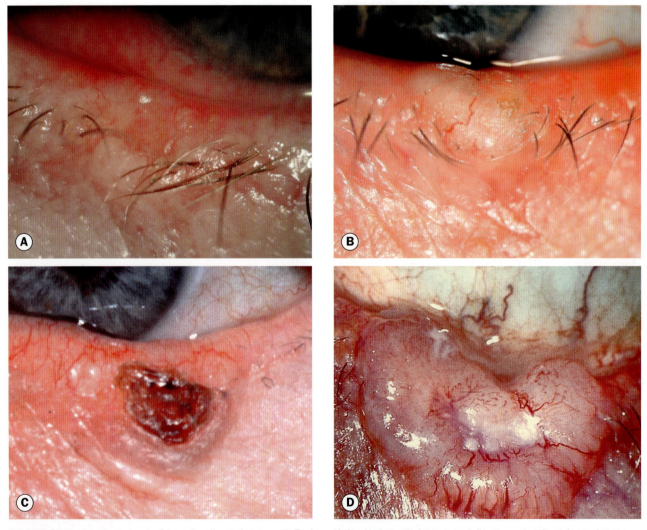

Fig. 1.19 Clinical appearance of basal cell carcinoma. **(A)** Early nodular lesion; **(B)** larger nodular tumour; **(C)** rodent ulcer; **(D)** large rodent tulcer;

Continued

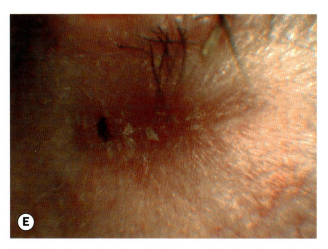 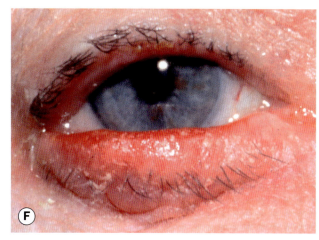

Fig. 1.19, Continued **(E)** sclerosing tumour; **(F)** extensive sclerosing tumour

the epidermis as an indurated plaque (Figs 1.19E and F). The margins of the tumour may be impossible to delineate clinically and the lesion tends to be much more extensive on palpation than inspection. On cursory examination a sclerosing BCC may simulate a localized area of chronic blepharitis.

- **Other types** not usually found on the lid are cystic, adenoid, pigmented and multiple superficial.

Squamous cell carcinoma

Introduction

SCC is a much less common, but typically more aggressive tumour than BCC with metastasis to regional lymph nodes in about 20% of cases. Careful surveillance of regional lymph nodes is therefore an important aspect of initial management. The tumour may also exhibit perineural spread to the intracranial cavity via the orbit. SCC accounts for 5–10% of eyelid malignancies and may arise *de novo* or from pre-existing actinic keratosis or carcinoma *in situ* (Bowen disease, intraepidermal carcinoma – Fig. 1.20). Immuno-compromised patients, such as those with acquired immunodeficiency syndrome (AIDS) or following renal transplantation are at increased risk, as are those with a predisposing syndrome such as xeroderma pigmentosum. The tumour has a predilection for the lower eyelid and the lid margin. It occurs most commonly in older individuals with a fair complexion and a history of chronic sun exposure. The diagnosis of SCC may be difficult because certain ostensibly benign lesions such as keratoacanthoma and cutaneous horn may reveal histological evidence of invasive SCC at deeper levels of sectioning.

Histopathology

The tumour arises from the squamous cell layer of the epidermis. It is composed of variably sized groups of atypical epithelial cells with prominent nuclei and abundant eosinophilic cytoplasm within the dermis (Fig. 1.21A). Well-differentiated tumours may show characteristic keratin 'pearls' and intercellular bridges (desmosomes).

Clinical features

The clinical types are variable and there are no pathognomonic characteristics. The tumour may be indistinguishable clinically from a BCC but surface vascularization is usually absent, growth is more rapid and hyperkeratosis is more common.

- **Nodular SCC** is characterized by a hyperkeratotic nodule that may develop crusting, erosions and fissures (Fig. 1.21B).
- **Ulcerating SCC** has a red base and sharply defined, indurated and everted borders, but pearly margins and telangiectasia are not usually present (Fig. 1.21C).
- **Cutaneous horn** with underlying invasive SCC (Fig. 1.21D).

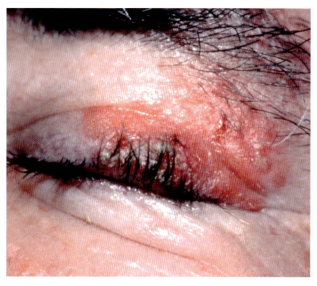

Fig. 1.20 Carcinoma *in situ*
(Courtesy of H Frank)

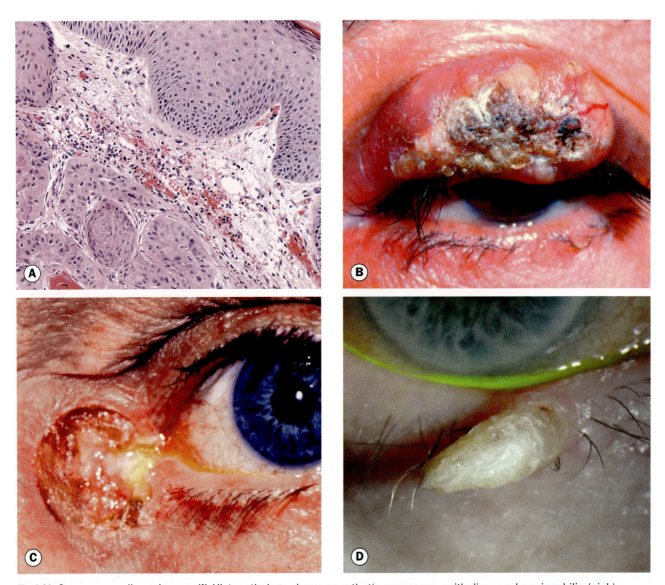

Fig. 1.21 Squamous cell carcinoma. **(A)** Histopathology shows acanthotic squamous epithelium and eosinophilic (pink) islands of dysplastic squamous epithelium within the dermis; **(B)** nodular tumour with surface keratosis; **(C)** ulcerating tumour; **(D)** cutaneous horn

(Courtesy of L Horton – fig. A; A Singh, from Clinical Ophthalmic Oncology, Saunders 2007 – fig. B; H Frank – fig. C; S Farley, T Cole and L Rimmer – fig. D)

Keratoacanthoma

Introduction

Keratoacanthoma is a rare, rapidly growing but subsequently regressing tumour that usually occurs in fair-skinned individuals with a history of chronic sun exposure. Immunosuppressive therapy is also a predisposing factor. It is regarded as falling within the spectrum of SCC, and although invasion and metastasis are rare, definitive treatment is usually indicated. Histopathologically, irregular thickened epidermis is surrounded by acanthotic squamous epithelium; a sharp transition from the thickened involved area to normal adjacent epidermis is referred to as shoulder formation (Fig. 1.22A); a keratin-filled crater may be seen.

Diagnosis

A pink dome-shaped hyperkeratotic lesion develops, often on the lower lid (Fig. 1.22B), and may double or treble in size within weeks (Fig. 1.22C). Growth then ceases for 2–3 months, after which spontaneous involution occurs, when a keratin-filled crater may develop (Fig. 1.22D). Complete involution may take up to a year and usually leaves an unsightly scar.

Treatment

Treatment generally involves complete surgical excision with a margin of at least 3 mm, or utilizing Mohs surgery; radiotherapy, cryotherapy or local chemotherapy are sometimes used. Observation is now regarded as inappropriate.

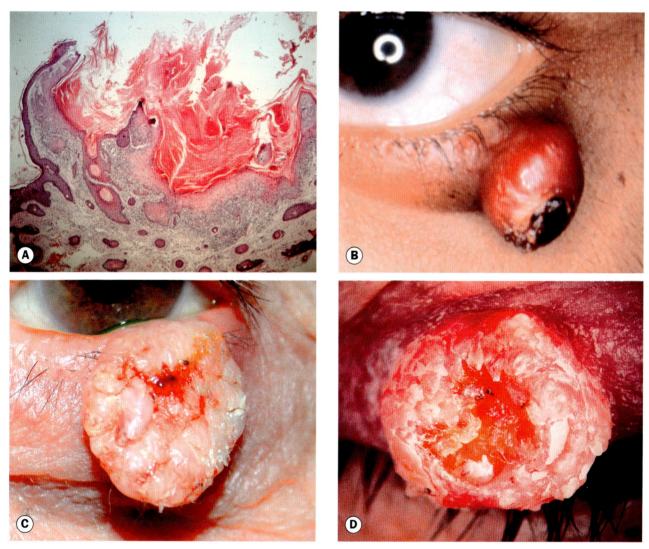

Fig. 1.22 Keratoacanthoma. **(A)** Histopathology shows irregularly thickened eosinophilic epidermis with a keratin-containing cup and well-marked shoulder formation; **(B)** hyperkeratotic nodule; **(C)** large tumour; **(D)** keratin-filled crater during involution

Sebaceous gland carcinoma

Introduction

Sebaceous gland carcinoma (SGC) is a very rare, slowly growing tumour that most frequently affects the elderly, with a predisposition for females. It usually arises from the meibomian glands, although on occasion it may arise from the glands of Zeis or elsewhere. The tumour consists histopathologically of lobules of cells with pale foamy vacuolated lipid-containing cytoplasm and large hyperchromatic nuclei (Fig. 1.23A). Pagetoid spread refers to extension of a tumour within the epithelium, and is not uncommon. Overall mortality is 5–10%; adverse prognostic features include upper lid involvement, tumour size of 10 mm or more and duration of symptoms of more than 6 months.

Clinical features

In contrast to BCC and SCC, SGC occurs more commonly on the upper eyelid where meibomian glands are more numerous;

there may be simultaneous involvement of both lids on one side (5%).

- **Yellowish material** within the tumour is highly suggestive of SGC.
- **Nodular SGC** presents as a discrete, hard nodule, most commonly within the upper tarsal plate (Fig. 1.23B), and may exhibit yellow discoloration due to the presence of lipid; it can be mistaken for a chalazion.
- **Spreading SGC** infiltrates into the dermis and causes a diffuse thickening of the lid margin (Fig. 1.23C) often with eyelash distortion and loss, and can be mistaken for blepharitis.

Lentigo maligna and melanoma

Introduction

Melanoma rarely develops on the eyelids but is potentially lethal. Although pigmentation is a hallmark of skin melanomas, half of

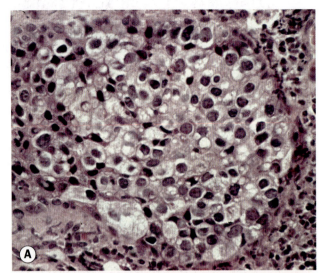

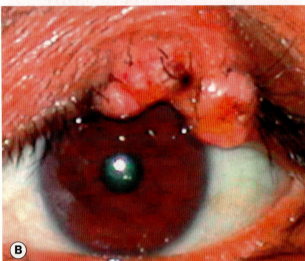

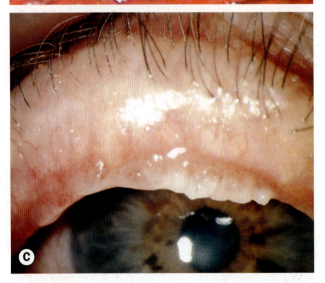

Fig. 1.23 Sebaceous gland carcinoma. **(A)** Histopathology shows cells with large hyperchromatic nuclei and vacuolated cytoplasm; **(B)** nodular tumour; **(C)** spreading tumour

(Courtesy of A Garner – fig. A; A Singh, from Clinical Ophthalmic Oncology, *Saunders 2007 – fig. B; S Tuft – fig. C)*

lid melanomas are non-pigmented and this may give rise to diagnostic difficulty. Features suggestive of melanoma include recent onset of a pigmented lesion, change in an existing pigmented lesion, irregular margins, asymmetrical shape, colour change or presence of multiple colours, and diameter greater than 6 mm.

Lentigo maligna

Lentigo maligna (melanoma *in situ*, intraepidermal melanoma, Hutchinson freckle) is an uncommon condition that develops in sun-damaged skin in elderly individuals. Malignant change may occur, with infiltration of the dermis. Histopathology shows intraepidermal proliferation of spindle-shaped atypical melanocytes replacing the basal layer of the epidermis (Fig. 1.24A). Clinically lentigo maligna presents as a slowly expanding pigmented macule with an irregular border (Fig. 1.24B). Treatment is usually by excision. Nodular thickening and areas of irregular pigmentation are highly suggestive of malignant transformation (Fig. 1.24C).

Melanoma

Histopathology shows large atypical melanocytes invading the dermis (Fig. 1.25A). Superficial spreading melanoma is characterized by a plaque with an irregular outline and variable pigmentation (Fig. 1.25B). Nodular melanoma is typically a blue – black nodule surrounded by normal skin (Fig. 1.25C). Treatment is usually by wide excision and may include local lymph node removal. Radiotherapy, chemotherapy, biological and 'targeted' therapy may also be used, generally as adjuvants.

Merkel cell carcinoma

Merkel cells are a form of sensory receptor concerned with light touch. Merkel cell carcinoma is a rapidly growing, highly malignant tumour that typically affects older adults. Its rarity may lead to difficulty in diagnosis and delay in treatment, and 50% of patients have metastatic spread by presentation. A violaceous, well-demarcated nodule with intact overlying skin is seen, most frequently involving the upper eyelid (Fig. 1.26). Treatment is by excision, often with adjuvant therapy.

Kaposi sarcoma

Kaposi sarcoma is a vascular tumour that typically affects patients with AIDS. Many patients have advanced systemic disease although in some instances the tumour may be the only clinical manifestation of human immunodeficiency virus (HIV) infection. Histopathology shows proliferating spindle cells, vascular channels and inflammatory cells within the dermis (Fig. 1.27A). Clinically a pink, red-violet to brown lesion (Fig. 1.27B) develops, which may be mistaken for a haematoma or naevus. Treatment is by radiotherapy or excision, and by optimal control of AIDS where relevant.

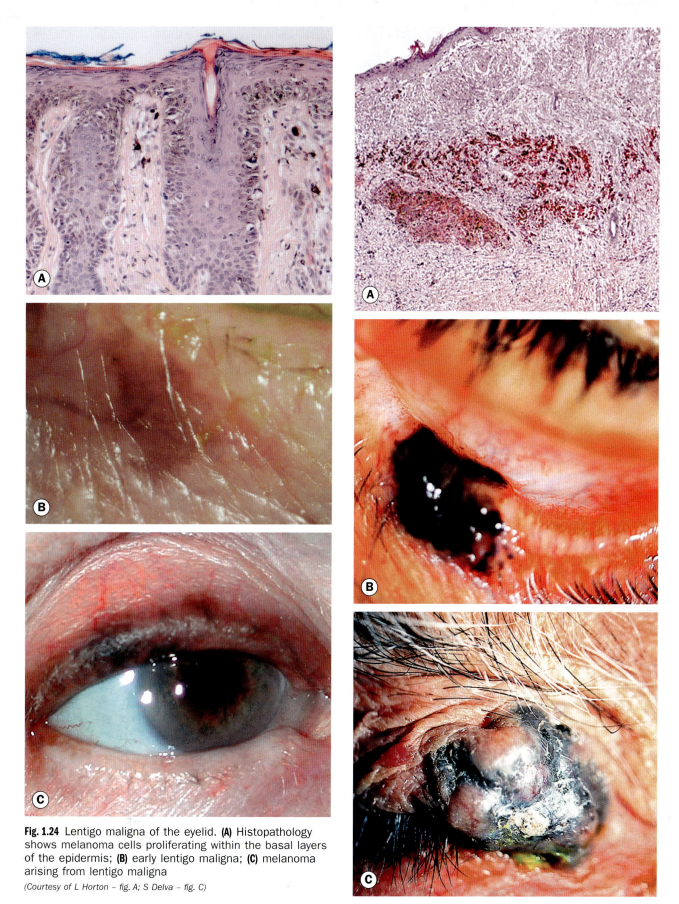

Fig. 1.24 Lentigo maligna of the eyelid. **(A)** Histopathology shows melanoma cells proliferating within the basal layers of the epidermis; **(B)** early lentigo maligna; **(C)** melanoma arising from lentigo maligna

(Courtesy of L Horton – fig. A; S Delva – fig. C)

Fig. 1.25 Melanoma. **(A)** Histopathology shows melanoma cells within the dermis; **(B)** superficial spreading melanoma; **(C)** nodular melanoma

(Courtesy of J Harry – fig. A)

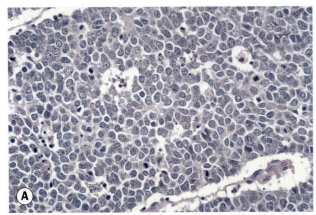

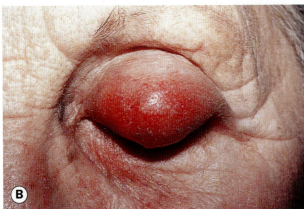

Fig. 1.26 Merkel cell carcinoma. **(A)** Histopathology shows a sheet of Merkel cells; **(B)** clinical appearance

(Courtesy of J Harry and G Misson, from Clinical Ophthalmic Pathology, *Butterworth-Heinemann 2001 – fig. A)*

Treatment of malignant tumours

Biopsy

Biopsy can be (i) *incisional*, using a blade or a biopsy punch, in which only part of the lesion is removed for histological diagnosis, or (ii) *excisional*, in which the entire lesion is removed; the latter may consist of shave excision using a blade to remove shallow epithelial tumours, such as papillomas and seborrhoeic keratosis, or full-thickness skin excision for tumours that are not confined to the epidermis.

Surgical excision

Surgical excision aims to remove the entire tumour with preservation of as much normal tissue as possible. Smaller tumours can be removed via an excision biopsy and the defect closed directly, whilst awaiting histological confirmation of complete clearance. Most small BCCs can be cured by excision of the tumour together with a 2–4 mm margin of clinically normal tissue. More radical surgical excision is required for large BCCs and aggressive tumours such as SCC, SGC and melanoma. It may not be possible to close all defects at the time of initial removal, but it is necessary to ensure complete clearance of tumour prior to undertaking any

reconstruction. There are several options for the coordination of histopathological diagnosis and tumour clearance with excision.

- **Conventional paraffin-embedded specimen.** Rapid processing can reduce the interval to confirmation of histological clearance but still requires that reconstruction be performed as a separate procedure. Faster confirmation can be achieved using either frozen-section control or micrographic surgery (see next), and reconstruction can then take place on the same day.

- **Standard frozen section** involves histological examination of the margins of the excised specimen at the time of surgery to ensure they are tumour-free. If no tumour cells are detected, the eyelid is reconstructed on the same day; if residual tumour is present, further excision is performed at the appropriate edge of the surgical site until no tumour is detected.

- **Mohs micrographic surgery** involves layered excision of the tumour; specimens are usually examined frozen. Processing of each layer enables a map of the edges of the tumour to be

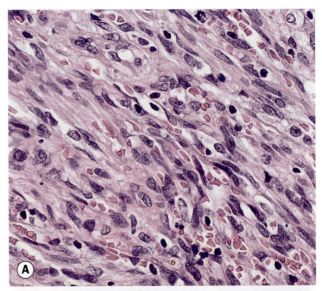

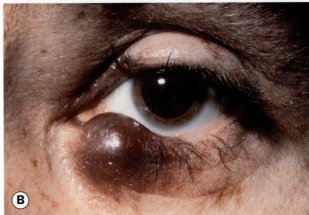

Fig. 1.27 Kaposi sarcoma. **(A)** Histopathology shows a proliferation of predominantly spindle-shaped cells; vascular channels are evident; **(B)** clinical appearance

(Courtesy of J Harry – fig. A)

developed. Further tissue is taken in any area where tumour is still present until clearance is achieved. Although time-consuming, this technique maximizes the chances of total tumour excision whilst minimizing sacrifice of normal tissue. This is a particularly useful technique for tumours that grow diffusely and have indefinite margins with finger-like extensions, such as sclerosing BCC, SCC, recurrent tumours and those involving the medial or lateral canthi. The irregular contours around the eyelids and extension of tumours into orbital fat can make interpretation difficult.

Reconstruction

The technique of reconstruction depends on the extent of tissue removed. It is important to reconstruct both anterior and posterior lamellae, each of which must be reconstructed with similar tissue. Anterior lamellar defects may be closed directly or with a local flap or skin graft. Options for the repair of full-thickness defects are set out below.

- **Small defects** involving less than one-third of the eyelid can usually be closed directly, provided the surrounding tissue is sufficiently elastic to allow approximation of the cut edges (Fig. 1.28). If necessary, a lateral cantholysis can be performed for increased mobilization.
- **Moderate size defects** involving up to half of the eyelid may require a flap (e.g. Tenzel semicircular) for closure (Fig. 1.29).
- **Large defects** involving over half of the eyelid may be closed by one of the following techniques:
  - Posterior lamellar reconstruction may involve an upper lid frcc tarsal graft, buccal mucous membrane or hard palate graft, or a Hughes tarsoconjunctival flap from the upper lid, which is left attached for 4–6 weeks before transection (Fig. 1.30).
  - Anterior lamellar reconstruction may involve skin advancement, a local skin flap or a free skin graft (Fig. 1.31); the patient must be made aware that grafted skin is unlikely to be a perfect match. At least one reconstructed lamella requires its own blood supply to maximize the viability of a free graft component.

Laissez-faire

Full reconstruction of the defect created by tumour removal may not always be required. In the *laissez-faire* approach the wound edges are approximated as far as possible and the defect is allowed to granulate and heal by secondary intention. Even large defects can often achieve a satisfactory outcome with time.

Radiotherapy

The recurrence rate following irradiation alone is higher than after surgery, and radiotherapy does not allow histological confirmation of tumour eradication. Recurrences following radiotherapy are difficult to treat surgically because of the poor healing properties of irradiated tissue. However, it still has utility in some circumstances.

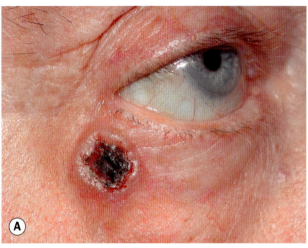

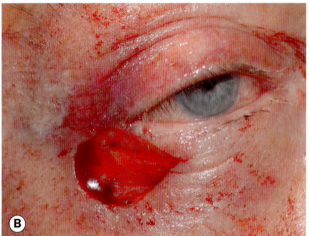

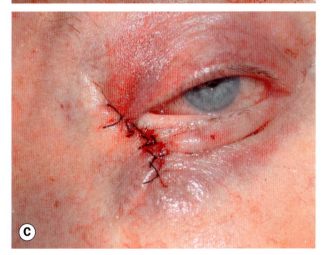

Fig. 1.28 Direct closure. **(A)** Preoperative appearance of a basal cell carcinoma; **(B)** appearance following excision; **(C)** direct closure of defect
(Courtesy of A Pearson)

- **Indications**
  - Patients who are either unsuitable for or refuse surgery.
  - Highly radiosensitive tumours, such as Kaposi sarcoma.
  - Adjunctive therapy in some cases.
  - Palliative treatment.

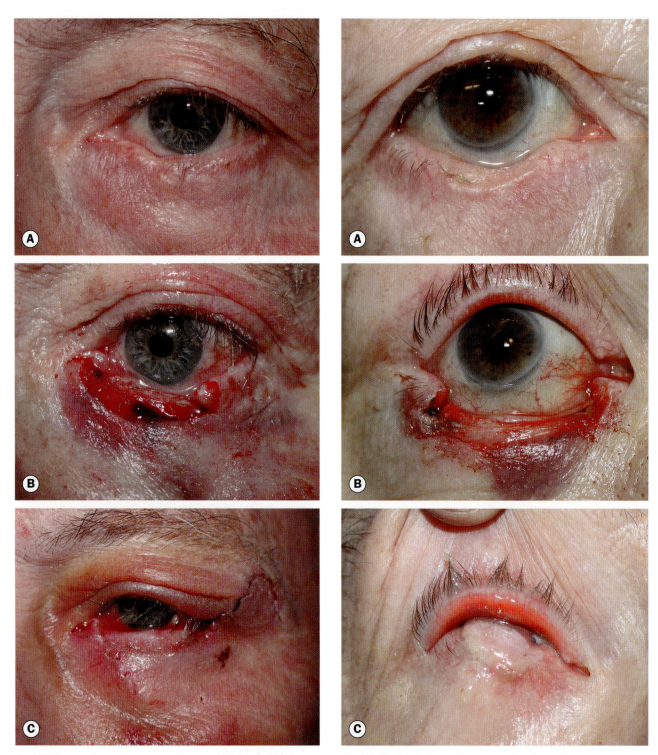

Fig. 1.29 Tenzel flap. **(A)** Preoperative appearance; **(B)** appearance following excision; **(C)** appearance following closure of the flap

(Courtesy of A Pearson)

Fig. 1.30 Posterior lamellar reconstruction with a Hughes upper lid flap. **(A)** Preoperative appearance; **(B)** appearance following excision; **(C)** postoperative appearance with the flap yet to be divided

(Courtesy of A Pearson)

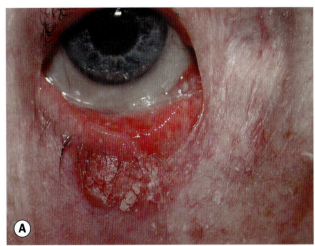

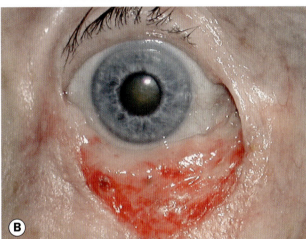

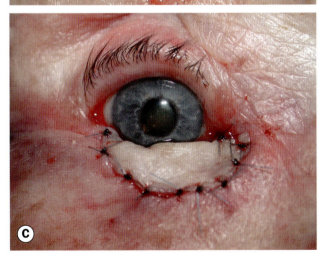

Fig. 1.31 Anterior lamellar reconstruction with a free skin graft. **(A)** Preoperative appearance; **(B)** appearance following excision; **(C)** skin graft in place
(Courtesy of A Pearson)

- **Relative contraindications**
  - Medial canthal lesions due to the high probability of lacrimal canalicular damage.
  - Upper eyelid tumours – conjunctival keratinization is common and difficult to manage.

- Aggressive tumours such as SGC are relatively radio-resistant, but higher-dose treatment may be effective.
- **Complications.** Many of these can be minimized by appropriate shielding.
  - Skin damage and madarosis (eyelash loss).
  - Nasolacrimal duct stenosis following irradiation to the medial canthal area.
  - Conjunctival keratinization, dry eye, keratopathy and cataract.
  - Retinopathy and optic neuropathy.

Cryotherapy

Cryotherapy may be considered for small superficial BCCs; it can be a useful adjunct to surgery in some patients. Complications include skin depigmentation, madarosis and conjunctival overgrowth.

DISORDERS OF THE EYELASHES

Misdirected lashes

Introduction

The roots of the eyelashes (cilia) lie against the anterior surface of the tarsal plate. The cilia pass between the main part of the orbicularis oculi and its more superficial part (Riolan muscle), exiting the skin at the anterior lid margin and curving away from the globe. It is particularly important to be familiar with the normal anatomical appearance of the lid margin in order to be able to identify the cause of eyelash misdirection. From anterior to posterior:
- **Eyelashes** (cilia).
- **The grey line,** by definition the border between the anterior (lashes, skin and orbicularis) and posterior (tarsal plate and conjunctiva) lamellae.
- **The meibomian gland orifices** are located just anterior to the mucocutaneous junction. The edge of the tarsal plate is deep to the gland orifices; the glands themselves run vertically within the plate.
- **The mucocutaneous junction** is where keratinized epithelium of the skin merges with conjunctival mucous membrane.
- **Conjunctiva** lines the posterior margin of the lid.

Clinical features

Trauma to the corneal epithelium may cause punctate epithelial erosions, with ocular irritation often worsened by blinking. Corneal ulceration and pannus formation may occur in severe cases. The clinical appearance varies with the cause.
- **Trichiasis** refers to misdirection of growth from individual follicles (Fig. 1.32A), rather than a more extensive inversion of the lid or lid margin. The follicles are at anatomically normal sites. It is commonly due to inflammation such as chronic blepharitis or herpes zoster ophthalmicus, but can

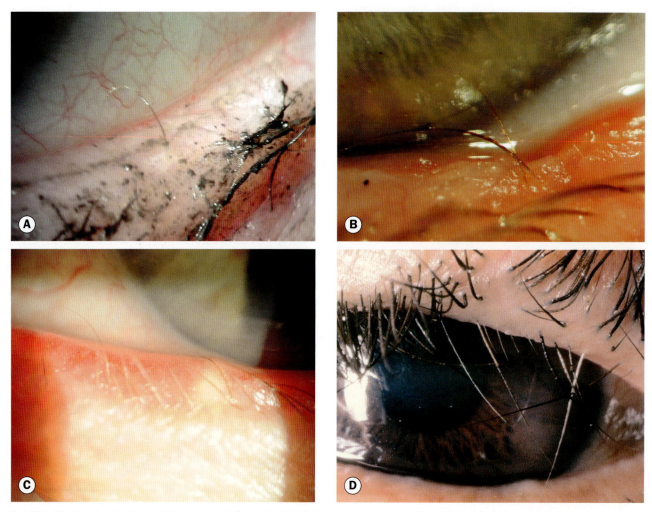

Fig. 1.32 Misdirected lashes. **(A)** Single trichiatic lash; **(B)** trichiasis associated with a lid notch following chalazion surgery; **(C)** marginal entropion showing rows of misdirected lashes, anterior migration of the mucocutaneous junction, and a rounded posterior lid margin; **(D)** acquired distichiasis
(Courtesy of S Chen – fig. A; R Bates – fig. D)

also be caused by trauma, including surgery such as incision and curettage of a chalazion (Fig. 1.32B).

- **Marginal entropion** has increasingly been recognized as a very common cause of eyelash misdirection, the mechanism of which is thought to be subtle cicatricial posterior lamellar shortening that rotates a segment of the lid margin towards the eye. The mucocutaneous junction migrates anteriorly and the posterior lid margin becomes rounded rather than physiologically square. Typically, numerous aligned lashes are involved (Fig. 1.32C).

- **Congenital distichiasis** is a rare condition that occurs when a primary epithelial germ cell destined to differentiate into a meibomian gland develops instead into a complete pilosebaceous unit. The condition is frequently inherited in an autosomal dominant manner with high penetrance but variable expressivity. The majority of patients also manifest primary lymphoedema of the legs (lymphoedema–distichiasis syndrome). A partial or complete second row of lashes is seen to emerge at or slightly behind the meibomian gland orifices. The aberrant lashes tend to be thinner and

shorter than normal cilia and are often directed posteriorly. They are usually well tolerated during infancy and may not become symptomatic until the age of about 5 years.

- **Acquired distichiasis** is caused by metaplasia of the meibomian glands into hair follicles such that a variable number of lashes grow from meibomian gland openings. The most important cause is intense conjunctival inflammation (e.g. chemical injury, Stevens–Johnson syndrome, ocular cicatricial pemphigoid). In contrast to congenital distichiasis, the cilia tend to be non-pigmented and stunted (Fig. 1.32D), and are usually symptomatic.

- **Epiblepharon** – see later.

- **Entropion.** In contrast to marginal entropion, profound inversion of a substantial width of the lid is readily identified – see later.

Treatment

- **Epilation** with forceps is simple and effective but recurrence within a few weeks is essentially invariable. It can be used as a temporizing measure or in the occasional patient who refuses or cannot tolerate surgery.

- **Electrolysis** or electrocautery (hyfrecation) are broadly similar electrosurgical techniques in which, under local anaesthesia, a fine wire is passed down the hair follicle to ablate the lash. It is generally useful for a limited number of lashes; scarring can occur. Frequently multiple treatments are required to obtain a satisfactory result.
- **Laser ablation** is also useful for the treatment of limited aberrant eyelashes, and is performed using a spot size of 50 μm, duration of 0.1–0.2 s and power of 800–1000 mW. The base of the lash is targeted and shots are applied to create a crater that follows the axis of the follicle (Fig. 1.33). Success is broadly comparable to that achieved with electrosurgery.
- **Surgery**
  ○ Tarsal facture (transverse tarsotomy) is performed for marginal entropion. After placing a 4-0 traction suture, a horizontal incision is made through the tarsal plate via the conjunctiva, at least halfway down the plate, along the affected length of the lid and extended to 2–3 mm either side of the involved region. Depending on the extent of lid involvement, either two or three double-armed absorbable sutures are passed through the upper edge of the lower section of the tarsal plate to emerge just anterior to the lashes, leaving the lid margin very slightly everted (Fig. 1.34). The sutures are left in place following the surgery; occasionally short-term use of a bandage contact lens is required to prevent corneal abrading.
  ○ A full-thickness eyelid pentagon resection can be used for a focal group of aberrant lashes, typically after trauma, or for localized marginal entropion.
  ○ Other options include lid splitting (see next) with follicle excision, and anterior lamellar rotation surgery.
- **Cryotherapy** applied externally to the skin just inferior to the base of the abnormal lashes or – especially in distichiasis – to the internal aspect of the anterior lamella of the lid following splitting of the margin at the grey line (Fig. 1.35), can be used for numerous lashes. A double freeze–thaw cycle at −20 °C is applied under local anaesthesia (including adrenaline) with a plastic eye protector in place; suturing of the lid margin is not usually necessary following limited splitting. The method is effective but carries a high rate of local adverse effects, and is less commonly performed than previously.

Eyelash ptosis

Eyelash ptosis refers to a downward sagging of the upper lid lashes (Fig. 1.36A). The condition may be idiopathic or associated with floppy eyelid syndrome, dermatochalasis with anterior lamellar slip or long-standing facial palsy.

Trichomegaly

Trichomegaly is excessive eyelash growth (Fig. 1.36B); the main causes are listed in Table 1.1.

Madarosis

Madarosis is the term used for the loss of lashes (Fig. 1.36C). The main causes are shown in Table 1.2.

Poliosis

Poliosis is a premature localized whitening of hair, which may involve the lashes and eyebrows (Fig. 1.36D); the main causes are shown in Table 1.3.

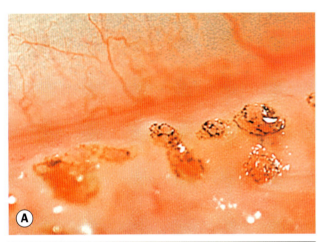
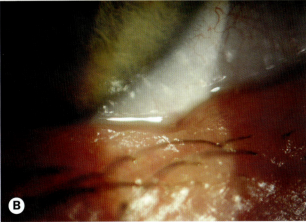

Fig. 1.33 Laser for trichiasis. **(A)** Appearance following ablation of multiple lashes; **(B)** the eye in Fig. 1.32B 6 weeks after laser ablation

Table 1.1 Causes of trichomegaly

Drug-induced – topical prostaglandin analogues, phenytoin and ciclosporin
Malnutrition
AIDS
Porphyria
Hypothyroidism
Familial
Congenital: Oliver–McFarlane, Cornelia de Lange, Goldstein–Hutt, Hermansky–Pudlak syndromes

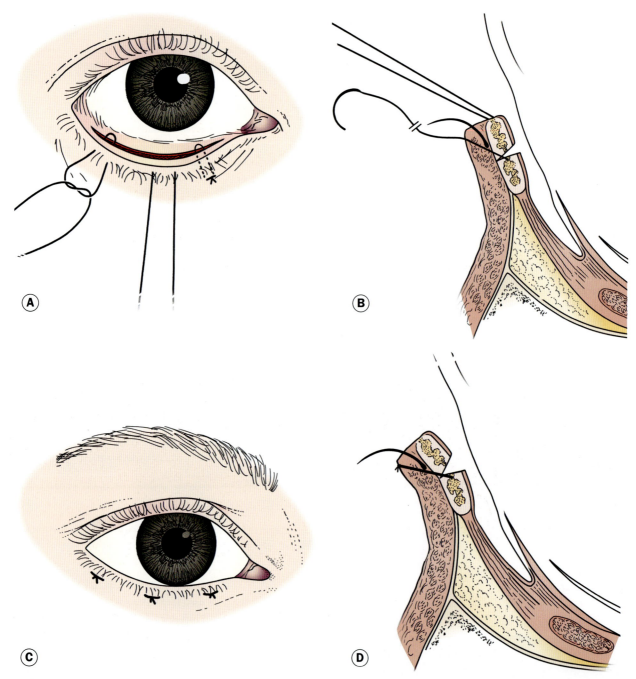

Fig. 1.34 Tarsal fracture for repair of marginal entropion. **(A)** and **(B)** insertion of everting sutures following traction suture emplacement and horizontal tarsal plate incision; **(C)** and **(D)** everting sutures in place

(Courtesy of JA Nerad, from Techniques in Ophthalmic Plastic Surgery, Saunders 2010)

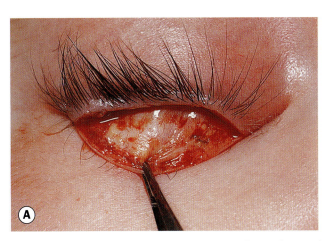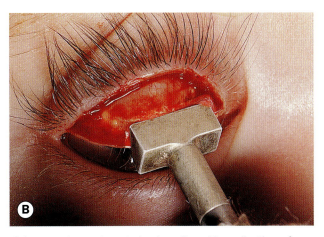

Fig. 1.35 Cryotherapy to the eyelid in distichiasis. **(A)** Separation of the anterior and posterior lamellae; **(B)** application of cryoprobe to the posterior lamella

(Courtesy of AG Tyers and JRO Collin, from Colour Atlas of Ophthalmic Plastic Surgery, *Butterworth-Heinemann 2001)*

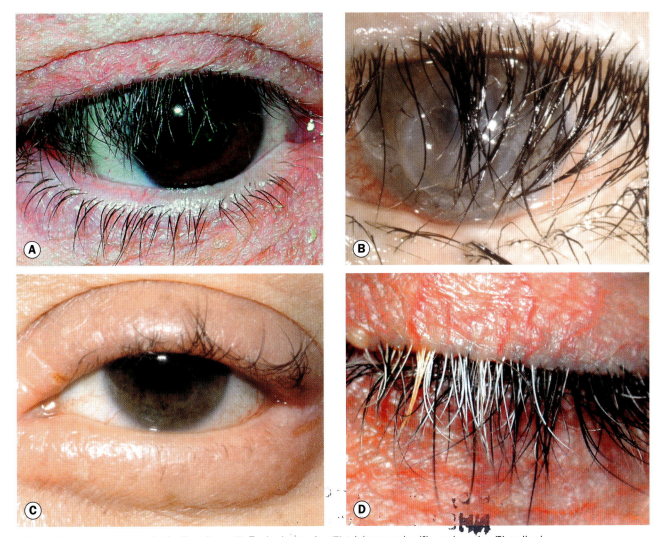

Fig. 1.36 Miscellaneous eyelash disorders. **(A)** Eyelash ptosis; **(B)** trichomegaly; **(C)** madarosis; **(D)** poliosis

(Courtesy of A Pearson – fig. A; L Merin – fig. B; S Tuft – fig. C)

Table 1.2 Cause of madarosis

1. Local
   Chronic anterior lid margin disease
   Infiltrating lid tumours
   Burns
   Radiotherapy or cryotherapy of lid tumours
2. Skin disorders
   Generalized alopecia
   Psoriasis
3. Systemic diseases
   Myxoedema
   Systemic lupus erythematosus
   Acquired syphilis
   Lepromatous leprosy
4. Following removal
   Procedures for trichiasis
   Trichotillomania – psychiatric disorder of hair removal

Table 1.3 Causes of poliosis

1. Ocular
   Chronic anterior blepharitis
   Sympathetic ophthalmitis
   Idiopathic uveitis
2. Systemic
   Vogt–Koyanagi–Harada syndrome
   Waardenburg syndrome
   Vitiligo
   Marfan syndrome
   Tuberous sclerosis

ALLERGIC DISORDERS

Acute allergic oedema

Acute allergic oedema is usually caused by exposure to pollen or by insect bites, and manifests with the sudden onset of bilateral boggy periocular oedema (Fig. 1.37A), often accompanied by conjunctival swelling (chemosis – see Ch. 5). Treatment is often unnecessary, but systemic antihistamines are sometimes given.

Contact dermatitis

Contact dermatitis is an inflammatory response that usually follows exposure to a medication such as eye drops (often preservative-containing), cosmetics or metals. An irritant can also cause a non-allergic toxic dermatitis. The individual is sensitized on first exposure and develops an immune reaction on further exposure; the mediating reaction is type IV (delayed type) hypersensitivity. Signs consist of lid skin scaling, angular fissuring, oedema and tightness (Fig. 1.37B); there may be chemosis, redness and papillary conjunctivitis. Corneal involvement is usually limited to punctate epithelial erosions. Treatment consists primarily of avoidance of allergen exposure, provided it can be identified. Cold compresses provide symptomatic relief. Topical

steroids and oral antihistamines can be used, but are rarely required.

Atopic dermatitis

Atopic dermatitis (eczema) is a very common idiopathic condition, typically occurring in patients who also suffer from asthma and hay fever. Eyelid involvement is relatively infrequent but when present is invariably associated with generalized dermatitis. Thickening, crusting and fissuring of the lids (Fig. 1.37C) is typical, and staphylococcal blepharitis, vernal or atopic keratoconjunctivitis are also commonly present. Herpetic blepharitis and keratoconjunctivitis is more common and more severe in patients with atopy (eczema herpeticum). Treatment of the lid features is with emollients to hydrate the skin and the judicious use of mild topical steroid such as hydrocortisone 1%. Uncommon ocular associations include keratoconus, cataract and retinal detachment (see also Ch. 5).

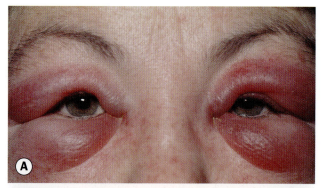

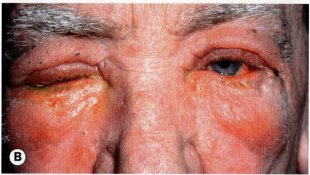

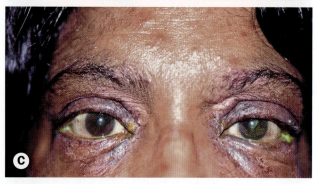

Fig. 1.37 Allergic disorders. **(A)** Acute allergic oedema; **(B)** contact dermatitis; **(C)** atopic dermatitis

BACTERIAL INFECTIONS

External hordeolum

An external hordeolum (stye) is an acute staphylococcal abscess of a lash follicle and its associated gland of Zeis that is common in children and young adults. A stye presents as a tender swelling in the lid margin pointing anteriorly through the skin, usually with a lash at its apex (Fig. 1.38A). Multiple lesions may be present and occasionally abscesses may involve the entire lid margin. Treatment involves topical (occasionally oral) antibiotics, hot compresses and epilation of the associated lash.

Impetigo

Impetigo is an superficial skin infection caused by *Staphylococcus aureus* or *Streptococcus pyogenes*; it typically affects children. Involvement of the eyelids is usually associated with infection of the face. Painful erythematous macules rapidly develop into thin-walled blisters, which develop golden-yellow crusts on rupturing (Fig. 1.38B). There may be fever, malaise and local lymphadenopathy. Treatment is with topical and sometimes oral antibiotics (beta-lactamase resistant), and preventative measures to reduce transmission as the condition is highly contagious; it is particularly dangerous to neonates, contact with whom should be avoided.

Erysipelas

Erysipelas (St Anthony's fire) is an uncommon acute, potentially severe, dermal and superficial lymphatic infection usually caused by *S. pyogenes*. Diabetes, obesity and alcohol abuse are predisposing. An inflamed erythematous plaque develops (Fig. 1.38C); a well-defined raised border distinguishes erysipelas from other forms of cellulitis. Complications such as metastatic infection are rare. Treatment is with oral antibiotics, but recurrence is common.

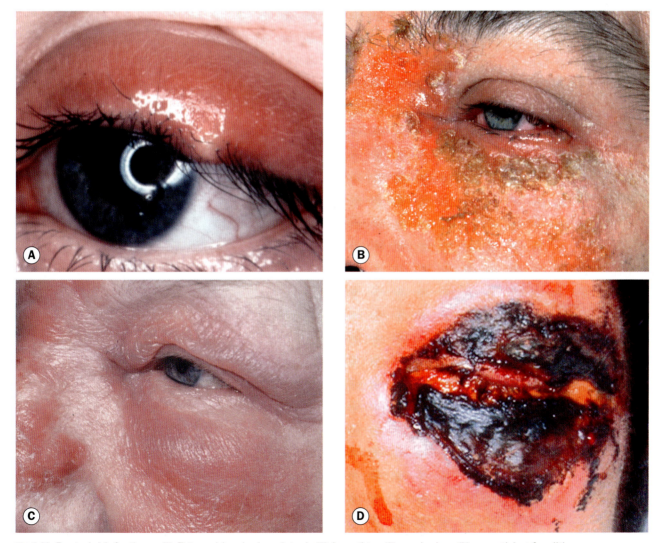

Fig. 1.38 Bacterial infections. **(A)** External hordeolum (stye); **(B)** impetigo; **(C)** erysipelas; **(D)** necrotizing fasciitis

Necrotizing fasciitis

Necrotizing fasciitis is a rare but commonly very severe infection involving subcutaneous soft tissue and the skin, with associated rapidly progressive necrosis. It is usually caused by *S. pyogenes* and occasionally *S. aureus*. The most frequent sites of involvement are the extremities, trunk and perineum, as well as postoperative wound sites. Unless early aggressive treatment is instituted, in the form of surgical debridement and high-dose intravenous antibiotics, death may result. Periocular infection is rare; redness and oedema are followed by the formation of large bullae and black discoloration of the skin due to necrosis (Fig. 1.38D).

VIRAL INFECTIONS

Molluscum contagiosum

Introduction

Molluscum contagiosum is a skin infection caused by a human-specific double-stranded DNA poxvirus that typically affects otherwise healthy children, with a peak incidence between 2 and 4 years of age. Transmission is by contact and subsequently by autoinoculation. Multiple, and occasionally confluent, lesions may develop in immunocompromised patients. Histopathology shows a central pit and lobules of hyperplastic epidermis with intracytoplasmic (Henderson–Patterson) inclusion bodies that displace the nuclear remnant to the edge of the cell. The bodies are small and eosinophilic near the surface, and large and basophilic deeper down (Fig. 1.39A).

Diagnosis

Single or multiple pale, waxy, umbilicated nodules develop (Fig. 1.39B); white cheesy material consisting of infected degenerate cells can be expressed from the lesion. Lesions on the lid margin (Fig. 1.39C) may shed virus into the tear film and give rise to a secondary ipsilateral chronic follicular conjunctivitis. Unless the lid margin is examined carefully the causative molluscum lesion may be overlooked.

Treatment

Spontaneous resolution will usually occur within a few months so treatment may not be necessary, particularly in children, unless complications such as a significant secondary conjunctivitis are problematic. Options include shave excision, cauterization, chemical ablation, cryotherapy and pulsed dye laser.

Herpes zoster ophthalmicus

Herpes zoster ophthalmicus (HZO – Fig. 1.40) is a common, generally unilateral infection caused by varicella-zoster virus. It is discussed in detail in Ch. 6.

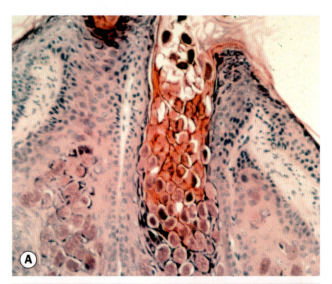

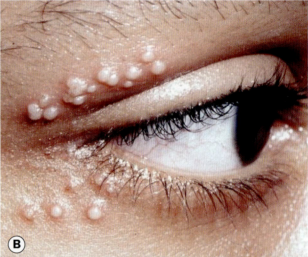

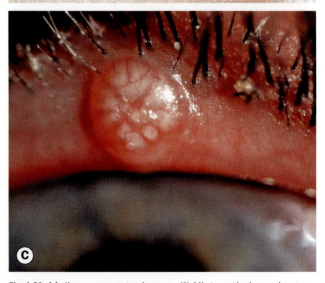

Fig. 1.39 Molluscum contagiosum. **(A)** Histopathology shows lobules of hyperplastic epidermis and a pit containing intracytoplasmic inclusion bodies; **(B)** multiple molluscum nodules; **(C)** lid margin nodule
(Courtesy of A Garner – fig. A; N Rogers – fig. B)

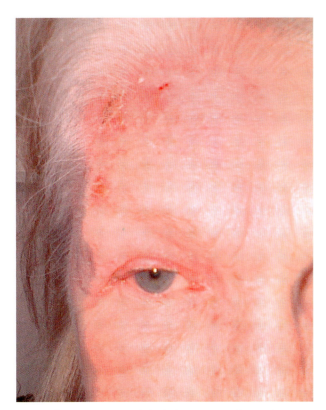

Fig. 1.40 Herpes zoster ophthalmicus – maculopapular crusting rash with periocular oedema, showing clear midline delineation

Herpes simplex

Introduction

Herpes simplex skin rash results from either primary infection or reactivation of herpes simplex virus previously dormant in the trigeminal ganglion. Prodromal facial and lid tingling lasting about 24 hours is followed by the development of eyelid and periocular skin vesicles (Fig. 1.41A) that break down over 48 hours (Fig. 1.41B). Although typically still confined to a single dermatome and with individual lesions that are often similar in appearance, the distribution of the herpes simplex skin rash contrasts with the sharply delineated unilateral involvement in HZO (see Fig. 1.40). There is commonly associated papillary conjunctivitis, discharge and lid swelling; dendritic corneal ulcers can develop, especially in atopic patients, in whom skin involvement can be extensive and very severe (eczema herpeticum – Fig. 1.41C).

Treatment

In many patients things will gradually settle without treatment over about a week. If treatment is necessary, a topical (aciclovir cream five times daily for 5 days) or oral (oral aciclovir, famciclovir or valaciclovir) antiviral agent can be used. Antibiotics (e.g. co-amoxiclav, erythromycin) may also be required in patients with secondary bacterial infection; this is particularly common in eczema herpeticum.

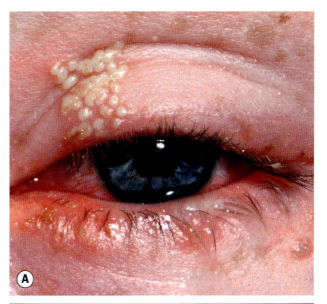

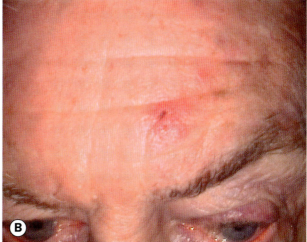

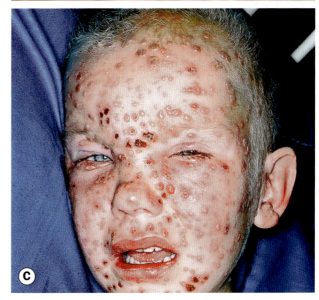

Fig. 1.41 Herpes simplex. **(A)** Vesicles; **(B)** progression to crusting; **(C)** eczema herpeticum

BLEPHARITIS

Chronic blepharitis

Introduction

Chronic blepharitis (chronic marginal blepharitis) is a very common cause of ocular discomfort and irritation. The poor correlation between symptoms and signs, the uncertain aetiology and mechanisms of the disease process all combine to make management difficult. Blepharitis may be subdivided into anterior and posterior, although there is considerable overlap and both types are often present (mixed blepharitis).

- Anterior blepharitis affects the area surrounding the bases of the eyelashes and may be staphylococcal or seborrhoeic. It is sometimes regarded as related more to chronic infective elements and hence more amenable to treatment and remission than the posterior form. An aetiological factor in staphylococcal blepharitis may be an abnormal cell-mediated response to components of the cell wall of *S. aureus*, which may also be responsible for the red eyes and peripheral corneal infiltrates seen in some patients; it is more common and more marked in patients with atopic dermatitis. Seborrhoeic blepharitis is strongly associated with generalized seborrhoeic dermatitis that characteristically involves the scalp, nasolabial folds, skin behind the ears and the sternum.
- Posterior blepharitis is caused by meibomian gland dysfunction and alterations in meibomian gland secretions. Bacterial lipases may result in the formation of free fatty acids. This increases the melting point of the meibum, preventing its expression from the glands, contributing to ocular surface irritation and possibly enabling growth of *S.*

aureus. Loss of the tear film phospholipids that act as surfactants results in increased tear evaporation and osmolarity, and an unstable tear film. Posterior blepharitis is commonly thought of as a more persistent and chronic inflammatory condition than anterior blepharitis; there is an association with acne rosacea.

- A reaction to the extremely common hair follicle and sebaceous gland-dwelling mite *Demodex* and other microorganisms may play a causative role in some patients – *Demodex folliculorum longus* in anterior blepharitis and *Demodex folliculorum brevis* in posterior blepharitis – though the mite can be found normally in a majority of older patients, most of whom do not develop symptomatic blepharitis. It has been proposed that circumstances such as overpopulation or hypersensitivity (perhaps to a bacillus carried symbiotically by *Demodex*) may lead to symptoms. *Demodex* mites are a major cause of the animal disease mange.

The characteristics of the different forms of blepharitis are set out in Table 1.4.

Diagnosis

Involvement is usually bilateral and symmetrical.

- **Symptoms** are caused by disruption of normal ocular surface function and reduction in tear stability, and are similar in all forms of blepharitis, though stinging may be more common in posterior disease. Because of poor correlation between the severity of symptoms and signs it can be difficult to objectively assess the benefit of treatment. Burning, grittiness, mild photophobia, and crusting and redness of the lid margins with remissions and exacerbations are characteristic. Symptoms are usually worse in the mornings although in patients with associated dry eye they

Table 1.4 Summary of characteristics of chronic blepharitis

	Feature	Anterior blepharitis		Posterior blepharitis
		Staphylococcal	Seborrhoeic	
Lashes	Deposit Loss Distorted or trichiasis	Hard ++ ++	Soft + +	
Lid margin	Ulceration Notching	+ +		 ++
Cyst	Hordeolum Meibomian	++		 ++
Conjunctiva	Phlyctenule	+		
Tear film	Foaming Dry eye	 +	 +	++ ++
Cornea	Punctate erosions Vascularization Infiltrates	+ + +	+ + +	++ ++ ++
Commonly associated skin disease		Atopic dermatitis	Seborrhoeic dermatitis	Acne rosacea

may increase during the day. Contact lens wear may be poorly tolerated.

- **Signs – staphylococcal blepharitis**
  - ○ Hard scales and crusting mainly located around the bases of the lashes; collarettes are cylindrical collections around lash bases (Fig. 1.42A).
  - ○ Mild papillary conjunctivitis and chronic conjunctival hyperaemia are common.
  - ○ Long-standing cases may develop scarring and notching (tylosis) of the lid margin, madarosis, trichiasis and poliosis.
  - ○ Associated tear film instability and dry eye syndrome are common.
  - ○ Atopic keratoconjunctivitis may be present in patients with atopic dermatitis.
- **Signs – seborrhoeic blepharitis**
  - ○ Hyperaemic and greasy anterior lid margins with soft scales and adherence of lashes to each other (Fig. 1.42B).

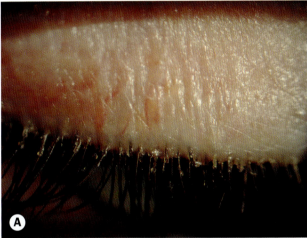

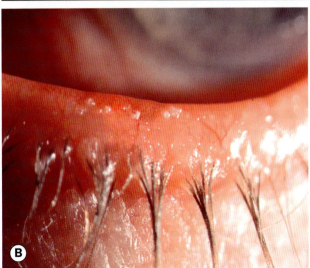

Fig. 1.42 Chronic anterior blepharitis. **(A)** Scales and crusting including collarettes in staphylococcal; **(B)** greasy lid margin with sticky lashes in seborrhoeic

- **Signs – posterior blepharitis** (meibomian gland disease)
  - ○ Excessive and abnormal meibomian gland secretion, manifesting as capping of meibomian gland orifices with oil globules (Fig. 1.43A).
  - ○ Pouting, recession, or plugging of meibomian gland orifices (Fig. 1.43B).
  - ○ Hyperaemia and telangiectasis of the posterior lid margin.
  - ○ Pressure on the lid margin results in expression of meibomian fluid that may be turbid or toothpaste-like (Fig. 1.43C); in severe cases the secretions become so inspissated that expression is impossible.
  - ○ Lid transillumination may show gland loss and cystic dilatation of meibomian ducts.
  - ○ The tear film is oily and foamy and often unstable, and froth may accumulate on the lid margins (Fig. 1.43D) or inner canthi.
- ***Demodex* infestation** may lead to cylindrical dandruff-like scaling (collarettes) around the base of eyelashes, though this is not always present. The mites can be demonstrated under ×16 slit lamp magnification by first manually clearing around the base of an eyelash then with fine forceps gently rotating the lash or moving it from side to side for 5–10 seconds, when if one or more mites (0.2–0.4 mm long – Fig. 1.44) does not emerge the lash should be gently epilated; slide microscopy can be performed on the mites or lashes if necessary.
- **Secondary changes** include papillary conjunctivitis, inferior corneal punctate epithelial erosions, corneal scarring and vascularization including Salzmann nodular degeneration and advancing wave-like epitheliopathy-type changes, stye formation, marginal keratitis, and occasionally bacterial keratitis (especially in contact lens wearers) and phlyctenulosis.

Treatment

There is limited evidence to support any particular treatment protocol for blepharitis. Patients should be advised that a permanent cure is unlikely, but control of symptoms is usually possible. The treatment of anterior and posterior disease is broadly similar for both types, particular given that they commonly co-exist, but some treatments are fairly specific for one or the other.

- **Lid hygiene** can be carried out once or twice daily initially; compliance and technique is highly variable.
  - ○ A warm compress should first be applied for several minutes to soften crusts at the bases of the lashes.
  - ○ Lid cleaning is subsequently performed to mechanically remove crusts and other debris, scrubbing the lid margins with a cotton bud or clean facecloth dipped in a warm dilute solution of baby shampoo or sodium bicarbonate.
  - ○ Commercially produced soap/alcohol impregnated pads for lid scrubbing are available and are often highly effective, but care should be taken not to induce mechanical irritation.

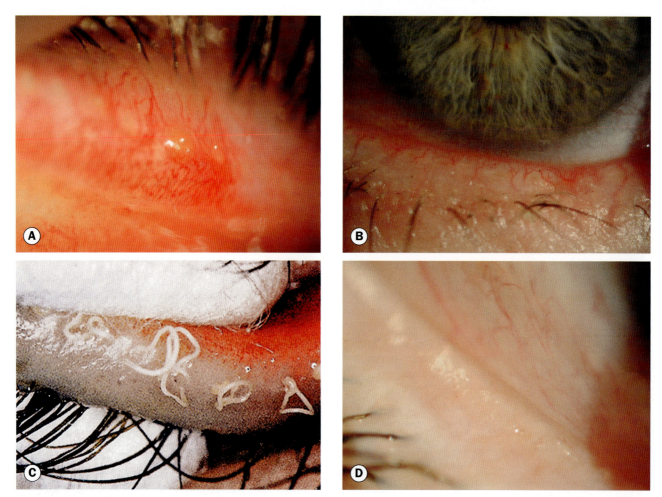

Fig. 1.43 Chronic posterior blepharitis. **(A)** Capping of meibomian gland orifices by oil globules; **(B)** hyperaemic, telangiectatic lid margin; **(C)** expressed toothpaste-like material; **(D)** froth on the eyelid margin

(Courtesy of J Silbert, from Anterior Segment Complications of Contact Lens Wear, *Butterworth-Heinemann 1999 – fig. C)*

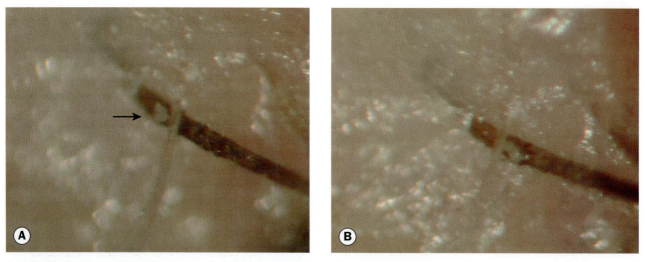

Fig. 1.44 *Demodex* mite. **(A)** Mite visible at eyelash base as a whitish lesion (arrow) after lash manipulation following clearance of collarette; **(B)** photograph taken two seconds later showing rapid migration

○ When substantial meibomian gland disease is present, the regimen may include expression of accumulated meibum by rolling the finger anteriorly over the margin.

○ The putative action of lid hygiene against *Demodex* is via prevention of reproduction.

○ Lid hygiene can be performed less frequently as the condition is brought under control.

● **Antibiotics**

○ Topical sodium fusidic acid, erythromycin, bacitracin, azithromycin or chloramphenicol is used to treat active folliculitis in anterior disease and is occasionally used for an extended period. Following lid hygiene the ointment should be rubbed onto the anterior lid margin with a cotton bud or clean finger.

○ Oral antibiotic regimens include doxycycline (50–100 mg twice daily for 1 week and then daily for 6–24 weeks), other tetracyclines, or azithromycin (500 mg daily for 3 days for three cycles at 1-week intervals); antibiotics are thought to reduce bacterial colonization and may also exert other effects such as a reduction in staphylococcal lipase production with tetracyclines. Tetracyclines may be more effective in the treatment of posterior disease, and azithromycin in anterior. Tetracyclines should not be used in children under the age of 12 years or in pregnant or breast-feeding women because they are deposited in growing bone and teeth; patients should also be aware of the possibility of increased sun sensitivity. Erythromycin 250 mg once or twice daily is an alternative.

● **Plant and fish oil supplements** have been shown to be of substantial benefit in some cases.

● **Topical steroid.** A low potency preparation such as fluorometholone 0.1% or loteprednol four times daily for 1 week is useful in patients with substantial active inflammation, especially papillary conjunctivitis; occasionally a higher strength preparation is used.

● **Tear substitutes** and other dry eye treatments are typically helpful for associated tear insufficiency and instability.

● **Tea tree oil** has been suggested as a treatment, based primarily on its likely activity against *Demodex* infestation; the optimal vehicle and regimen has not been established but lid, eyebrow and periocular skin cleansing once daily with a 50% scrub and application of 5% ointment has been described. Topical permethrin and topical (1% cream) or oral (two doses of 200 μg/kg 1 week apart) ivermectin have also been used by some practitioners. High temperature cleaning of bedding, the use of tea tree shampoo and facial soap, and treating the patient's partner may all help to reduce recurrences.

● **Novel therapies** include topical ciclosporin, pulsed light application, and purpose-designed devices to probe, heat and/or express the meibomian glands (e.g. Lipiflow ™) in posterior disease.

● **Complications** are treated specifically.

Phthiriasis palpebrarum

The crab louse *Phthirus pubis* is adapted to living in pubic hair, but is also commonly found in other hair-covered body areas such as the chest, axillae and eyelids (phthiriasis palpebrarum). Symptoms consist of chronic irritation and itching of the lids, but the lice are often an incidental discovery. Conjunctivitis is uncommon. The lice are readily visible anchored to lashes (Fig. 1.45A); lice have six legs rather than the eight possessed by ticks (see next). Ova and their empty shells appear as oval, brownish, opalescent pearls adherent to the base of the cilia (Fig. 1.45B). Treatment consists of mechanical removal of the lice and their attached lashes with fine forceps. If necessary, topical yellow mercuric oxide 1% or petroleum jelly can be applied to the lashes and lids twice a day for 10 days. Delousing of the patient, family members, clothing and bedding is important to prevent recurrence.

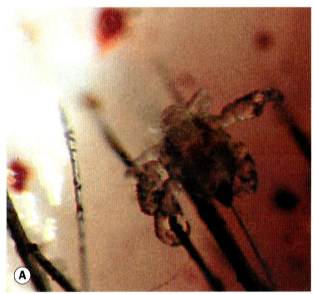

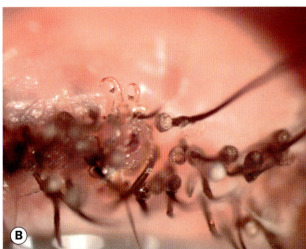

Fig. 1.45 Phthiriasis palpebrarum. **(A)** Louse anchored to lashes; **(B)** louse, ova and shells
(Courtesy of D Smit – fig. B)

Tick infestation of the eyelid

Ticks (see Fig. 11.69B) can attach themselves to the eyelid and should be removed at the earliest opportunity in order to minimize the risk of contracting a tick-borne zoonosis such as Lyme disease, Rocky Mountain fever or tularaemia. If the tick is attached some distance from the eye such that spray can safely be applied, an insect repellent containing pyrethrin or a pyrethroid should be sprayed on the tick twice at intervals of a minute; alternatively a scabies cream containing permethrin can be applied. These have a toxic effect that prevents the tick from injecting saliva, and after 24 hours it should drop off or can be removed with fine-tipped forceps at the slit lamp (blunt-tipped needle-holders are an alternative in restrained small children). It is critical that the tick is detached as close to its skin attachment as possible in order to remove its head and mouthparts, following which it might be retained in sealed packaging to permit identification if necessary. In areas endemic for Lyme disease, some authorities suggest routine antibiotic prophylaxis with doxycycline (in the absence of contraindications) following a confirmed deer tick bite, but as a minimum patients should be told to seek medical advice urgently at the onset of suspicious symptoms, particularly erythema migrans, over the subsequent few weeks. Lyme disease transmission is thought to require attachment of the tick for at least 36 hours.

Angular blepharitis

The infection is usually caused by *Moraxella lacunata* or *S. aureus* although other bacteria, and rarely herpes simplex, have also been implicated. Red, scaly, macerated and fissured skin is seen at the lateral and/or medial canthi of one or both eyes (Fig. 1.46A). Skin chafing secondary to tear overflow, especially at the lateral canthus, can cause a similar clinical picture, and may also predispose to infection (Fig. 1.46B). Associated papillary and follicular conjunctivitis may occur. Treatment involves topical chloramphenicol, bacitracin or erythromycin.

Childhood blepharokeratoconjunctivitis

Childhood blepharokeratoconjunctivitis is a poorly defined condition that tends to be more severe in Asian and Middle Eastern populations. Presentation is usually at about 6 years of age with recurrent episodes of anterior or posterior blepharitis, sometimes associated with recurrent styes or chalazia. Constant eye rubbing and photophobia may lead to misdiagnosis as allergic eye disease. Conjunctival changes include diffuse hyperaemia, bulbar phlyctens and follicular or papillary hyperplasia.

Corneal changes include superficial punctate keratopathy, marginal keratitis, peripheral vascularization and axial subepithelial haze. Treatment is with lid hygiene and topical antibiotic ointment at bedtime. Topical low-dose steroids (prednisolone 0.1% or fluorometholone 0.1%) and erythromycin syrup 125 mg daily for 4–6 weeks may also be used.

PTOSIS

Classification

Ptosis is an abnormally low position of the upper lid; it may be congenital or acquired.

- **Neurogenic** ptosis is caused by an innervational defect such as third nerve paresis and Horner syndrome (see Ch. 19).
- **Myogenic** ptosis is caused by a myopathy of the levator muscle itself, or by impairment of transmission of impulses at the neuromuscular junction (neuromyopathic). Acquired myogenic ptosis occurs in myasthenia gravis, myotonic dystrophy and progressive external ophthalmoplegia (see Ch. 19).
- **Aponeurotic** or involutional ptosis is caused by a defect in the levator aponeurosis.
- **Mechanical** ptosis is caused by the gravitational effect of a mass or by scarring.

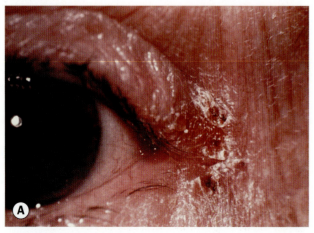
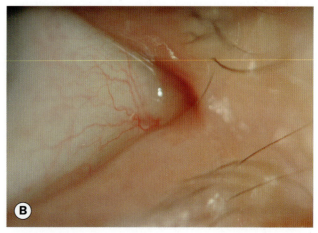

Fig. 1.46 (A) Angular blepharitis; **(B)** tear overflow from a lax and rounded lateral canthus

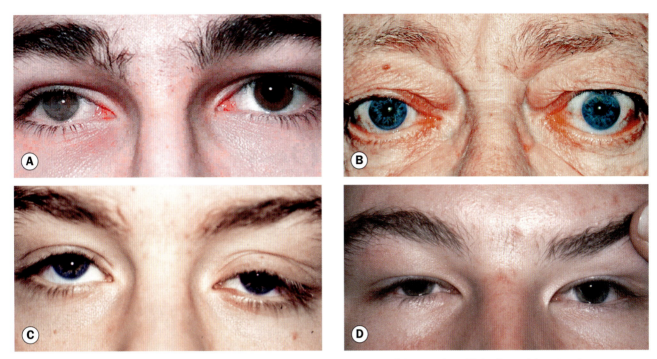

Fig. 1.47 Causes of pseudoptosis. **(A)** Right phthisis bulbi; **(B)** contralateral lid retraction; **(C)** ipsilateral hypotropia; **(D)** bilateral brow ptosis
(Courtesy of S Webber – figs C and D)

Clinical evaluation

General

The age at onset of ptosis and its duration will usually distinguish congenital from acquired cases. If the history is ambiguous, old photographs may be helpful. It is also important to enquire about symptoms of possible underlying systemic disease, such as associated diplopia, variability of ptosis during the day and excessive fatigue.

Pseudoptosis

A false impression of ptosis may be caused by the following:
- **Lack of support** of the lids by the globe may be due to an orbital volume deficit associated with an artificial eye, microphthalmos, phthisis bulbi (Fig. 1.47A), or enophthalmos.
- **Contralateral lid retraction**, which is detected by comparing the levels of the upper lids, remembering that the margin of the upper lid normally covers the superior 2 mm of the cornea (Fig. 1.47B).
- **Ipsilateral hypotropia** causes pseudoptosis because the upper lid follows the globe downwards (Fig. 1.47C). It disappears when the hypotropic eye assumes fixation on covering the normal eye.
- **Brow ptosis** due to excessive skin on the brow, or seventh nerve palsy, which is diagnosed by manually elevating the eyebrow (Fig. 1.47D).

- **Dermatochalasis.** Overhanging skin on the upper lids (Fig. 1.48) may be mistaken for ptosis, but may also cause mechanical ptosis.

Measurements

- **Margin–reflex distance** is the distance between the upper lid margin and the corneal reflection of a pen torch held by the

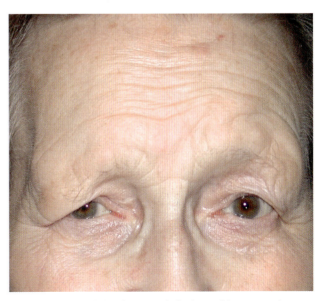

Fig. 1.48 Marked right dermatochalasis and brow ptosis
(Courtesy of S Chen)

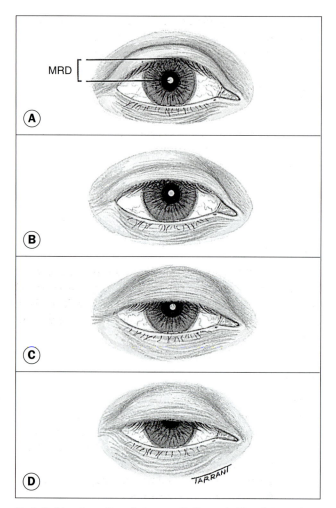

Fig. 1.49 Margin–reflex distance. **(A)** Normal; **(B)** mild ptosis; **(C)** moderate ptosis; **(D)** severe ptosis

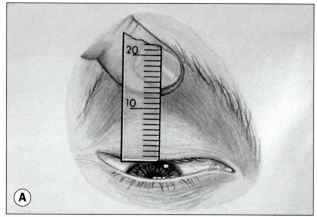

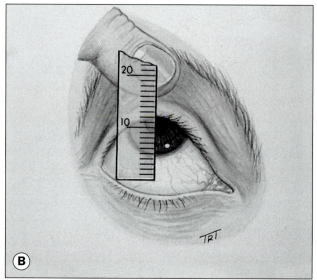

Fig. 1.51 Measurement of levator function

examiner on which the patient fixates (Fig. 1.49); the normal measurement is 4–5 mm.

- **Palpebral fissure height** is the distance between the upper and lower lid margins, measured in the pupillary plane (Fig. 1.50). The upper lid margin normally rests about 2 mm below the upper limbus and the lower 1 mm above the lower limbus. This measurement is shorter in males (7–10 mm) than in females (8–12 mm). Unilateral ptosis can be

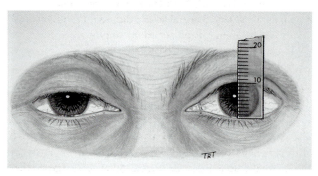

Fig. 1.50 Measurement of palpebral fissure height

quantified by comparison with the contralateral side. Ptosis may be graded as mild (up to 2 mm), moderate (3 mm) and severe (4 mm or more).

- **Levator function** (upper lid excursion) is measured by placing a thumb firmly against the patient's brow to negate the action of the frontalis muscle, with the eyes in downgaze (Fig. 1.51A). The patient then looks up as far as possible and the amount of excursion is measured with a rule (Fig. 1.51B). Levator function is graded as normal (15 mm or more), good (12–14 mm), fair (5–11 mm) and poor (4 mm or less).
- **Upper lid crease** is taken as the vertical distance between the lid margin and the lid crease in downgaze. In females it measures about 10 mm and in males 8 mm. Absence of the crease in a patient with congenital ptosis is evidence of poor levator function, whereas a high crease suggests an aponeurotic defect (usually involutional). The skin crease is also used as a guide to the initial incision in some surgical procedures.
- **Pretarsal show** is the distance between the lid margin and the skin fold with the eyes in the primary position.

Associated signs

- **The pupils** should be examined to exclude Horner syndrome and a subtle pupil-involving third nerve palsy – the latter is an unlikely acute clinical presentation (see Ch. 19).
- **Increased innervation** may flow to the levator muscle of a unilateral ptosis, particularly in upgaze. Associated increased innervation to the contralateral normal levator will result in lid retraction. The examiner should therefore manually elevate the ptotic lid and look for drooping of the opposite lid. If this occurs, the patient should be warned that surgical correction may induce a lower position in the opposite lid.
- **Fatigability** is tested by asking the patient to look up without blinking for 30–60 seconds. Progressive drooping of one or both lids, or an inability to maintain upgaze, is suggestive of myasthenia gravis (see Ch. 19). Myasthenic ptosis may show an overshoot of the upper lid on saccade from downgaze to the primary position (Cogan twitch sign) and a 'hop' on side-gaze.
- **Ocular motility defects**, particularly of the superior rectus, must be evaluated in patients with congenital ptosis. Correction of an ipsilateral hypotropia may improve the degree of ptosis. Deficits consistent with a subtle or partial third nerve paresis should be identified.
- **Jaw-winking** can be identified by asking the patient to chew and move the jaws from side to side (see below).
- **The Bell phenomenon** is tested by manually holding the lids open, asking the patient to try to shut the eyes and observing upward and outward rotation of the globe. A weak Bell phenomenon carries a variable risk of postoperative exposure keratopathy, particularly following large levator resections or suspension procedures.
- **The tear film** should be inspected – a poor volume or unstable film may be worsened by ptosis surgery and should be addressed preoperatively as far as possible.

Simple congenital ptosis

Diagnosis

Congenital ptosis probably results from a failure of neuronal migration or development with muscular sequelae secondary to this; a minority of patients have a family history.

- **Signs** (Fig. 1.52)
  - Unilateral or bilateral ptosis of variable severity.
  - Absent upper lid crease and poor levator function.
  - In downgaze the ptotic lid is higher than the normal because of poor relaxation of the levator muscle. This is in contrast to acquired ptosis, in which the affected lid is either level with or lower than the normal lid on downgaze.
  - Following surgical correction the lid lag in downgaze may worsen.
- **Associations**
  - Superior rectus weakness may be present because of its close embryological association with the levator.

  - Compensatory chin elevation in severe bilateral cases.
  - Refractive errors are common and more frequently responsible for amblyopia than the ptosis itself.

Treatment

Treatment should be carried out during the preschool years once accurate measurements can be obtained, but may be considered earlier in severe cases to prevent amblyopia. Levator resection (see below) is usually required.

Marcus Gunn jaw-winking syndrome

Introduction

About 5% of all cases of congenital ptosis are associated with the Marcus Gunn jaw-winking phenomenon. The vast majority are unilateral. Although the exact aetiology is unclear, it has been postulated that a branch of the mandibular division of the fifth cranial nerve is misdirected to the levator muscle.

Diagnosis

- **Signs**
  - Retraction of the ptotic lid in conjunction with stimulation of the ipsilateral pterygoid muscles by chewing, sucking, opening the mouth (Figs 1.53A and B) or contralateral jaw movement.
  - Less common stimuli to winking include jaw protrusion, smiling, swallowing and clenching of teeth.
  - Jaw-winking does not improve with age (Figs 1.53C and D), although patients may learn to mask it.

Treatment

Surgery should be considered if jaw-winking or ptosis represents a significant functional or cosmetic problem.
- **Mild cases** with reasonable levator function of 5 mm or better, and little synkinetic movement may be treated with unilateral levator advancement.
- **Moderate cases.** Unilateral levator disinsertion can be performed to address the synkinetic winking component, with ipsilateral brow (frontalis) suspension so that lid elevation is due solely to frontalis muscle elevation.
- **Bilateral surgery.** Bilateral levator disinsertion with bilateral brow suspension may be carried out to produce a symmetrical result.

Third nerve misdirection syndromes

Third nerve misdirection syndromes may be congenital, but more frequently follow acquired third nerve palsy. Bizarre movements of the upper lid accompany various eye movements (Fig. 1.54). Ptosis may also occur following aberrant facial nerve regeneration. Treatment is by levator disinsertion and brow suspension.

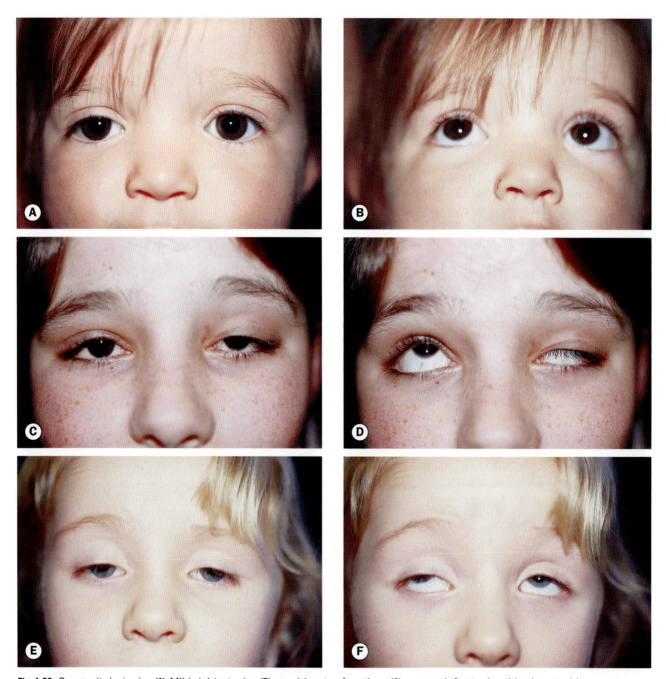

Fig. 1.52 Congenital ptosis. **(A)** Mild right ptosis; **(B)** good levator function; **(C)** severe left ptosis with absent skin crease; **(D)** very poor levator function; **(E)** severe bilateral ptosis; **(F)** very poor levator function

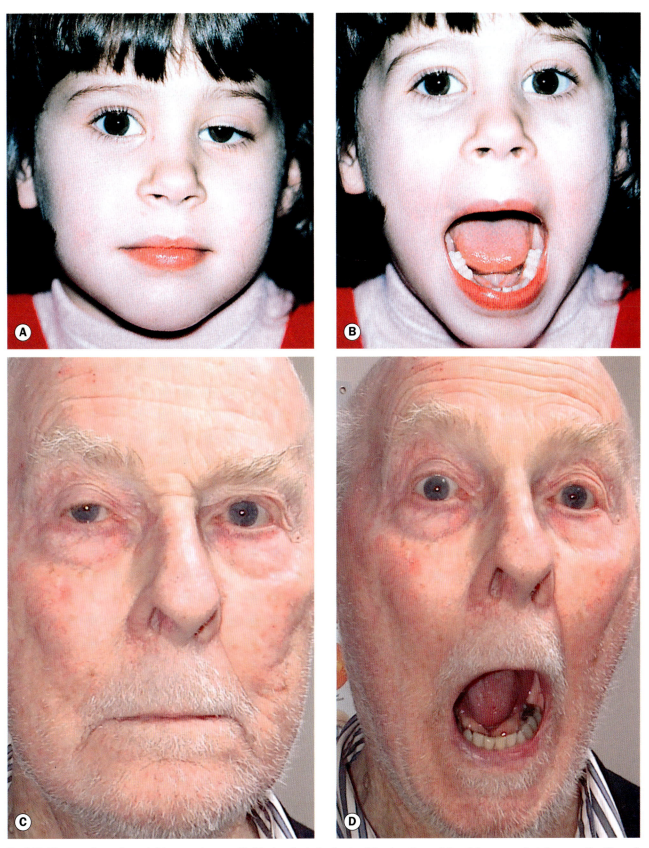

Fig. 1.53 Marcus Gunn jaw-winking syndrome. **(A)** Moderate left ptosis; **(B)** retraction of the lid on opening the mouth; **(C)** and **(D)** similar phenomenon in an older patient

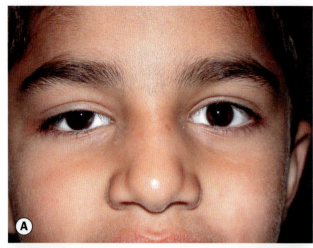

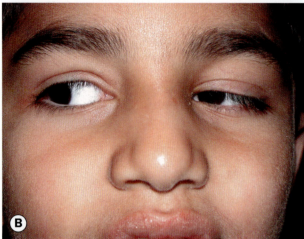

Fig. 1.54 Third nerve redirection. **(A)** Moderate right ptosis; **(B)** retraction of the lid on right gaze
(Courtesy of A Pearson)

Involutional ptosis

Involutional (aponeurotic) ptosis is an age-related condition caused by dehiscence, disinsertion or stretching of the levator aponeurosis, limiting the transmission of force from a normal levator muscle to the upper lid. Due to fatigue of the Müller muscle it frequently worsens towards the end of the day, so that it can sometimes be confused with myasthenic ptosis. There is a variable, usually bilateral, ptosis with a high upper lid crease and good levator function. In severe cases the upper lid crease may be absent, the eyelid above the tarsal plate very thin and the upper sulcus deep (Fig. 1.55). Treatment options include levator resection, advancement with reinsertion or anterior levator repair.

Mechanical ptosis

Mechanical ptosis is the result of impaired mobility of the upper lid. It may be caused by dermatochalasis, large tumours such as neurofibromas (Fig. 1.56), heavy scar tissue, severe oedema and anterior orbital lesions.

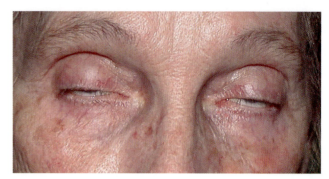

Fig. 1.55 Severe bilateral involutional ptosis with absent skin creases and deep sulci

Surgery

Anatomy

- **The levator aponeurosis** fuses with the orbital septum about 4 mm above the superior border of the tarsal plate (Fig. 1.57). Its posterior fibres insert into the lower third of the anterior surface of the tarsal plate. The medial and lateral horns are expansions that act as check ligaments. Surgically, the aponeurosis can be approached through the skin or conjunctiva.
- **Müller muscle** is inserted into the upper border of the tarsal plate and can be approached transconjunctivally.
- **The inferior tarsal aponeurosis** consists of the capsulopalpebral expansion of the inferior rectus muscle and is analogous to the levator aponeurosis.
- **The inferior tarsal muscle** is analogous to Müller muscle.

Conjunctiva–Müller resection

This involves excision of Müller muscle and overlying conjunctiva (Fig. 1.58A) with reattachment of the resected edges (Fig. 1.58B).

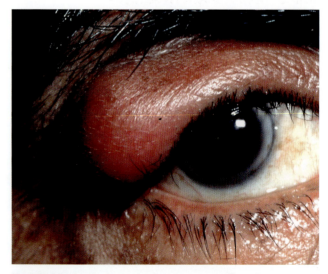

Fig. 1.56 Mechanical ptosis due to a neurofibroma

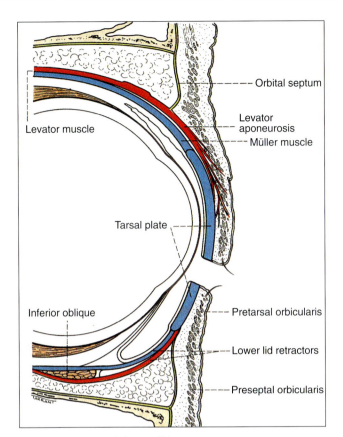

Fig. 1.57 Anatomy of the eyelid

Labels: Orbital septum · Levator aponeurosis · Müller muscle · Levator muscle · Tarsal plate · Inferior oblique · Pretarsal orbicularis · Lower lid retractors · Preseptal orbicularis

The maximal elevation achievable is 2–3 mm, so it is used in cases of mild ptosis with good (at least 10 mm) levator function, which includes most cases of Horner syndrome and mild congenital ptosis.

Levator advancement (resection)

In this technique the levator complex is shortened through either an anterior – skin (Fig. 1.59) – or posterior – conjunctival – approach. Indications include ptosis of any cause, provided residual levator function is at least 5 mm. The extent of resection is determined by the severity of the ptosis and the amount of levator function.

Brow (frontalis) suspension

Brow (frontalis) suspension is used for severe ptosis (>4 mm) with very poor levator function (<4 mm) from a variety of causes, typical indications being ptosis associated with third nerve palsy, blepharophimosis syndrome and following an unsatisfactory result from previous levator resection. The tarsal plate is suspended from the frontalis muscle with a sling consisting of autologous fascia lata (Fig. 1.60) or non-absorbable material such as prolene or silicone.

ECTROPION

Involutional ectropion

Introduction

Involutional (age-related) ectropion affects the lower lid of elderly patients. It causes epiphora (tear overflow) and may exacerbate ocular surface disease. The red appearance of the exposed conjunctiva is cosmetically poor. In long-standing cases the tarsal conjunctiva may become chronically inflamed, thickened and keratinized (Fig. 1.61). Aetiological factors include:

- **Horizontal lid laxity** can be demonstrated by pulling the central part of the lid 8 mm or more from the globe, with a failure to snap back to its normal position on release without the patient first blinking.

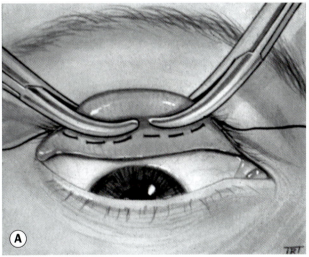

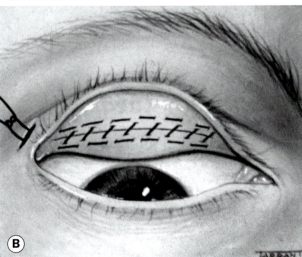

Fig. 1.58 Conjunctiva–Müller resection. **(A)** Clamping of conjunctiva and Müller muscle; **(B)** appearance after excision and suturing

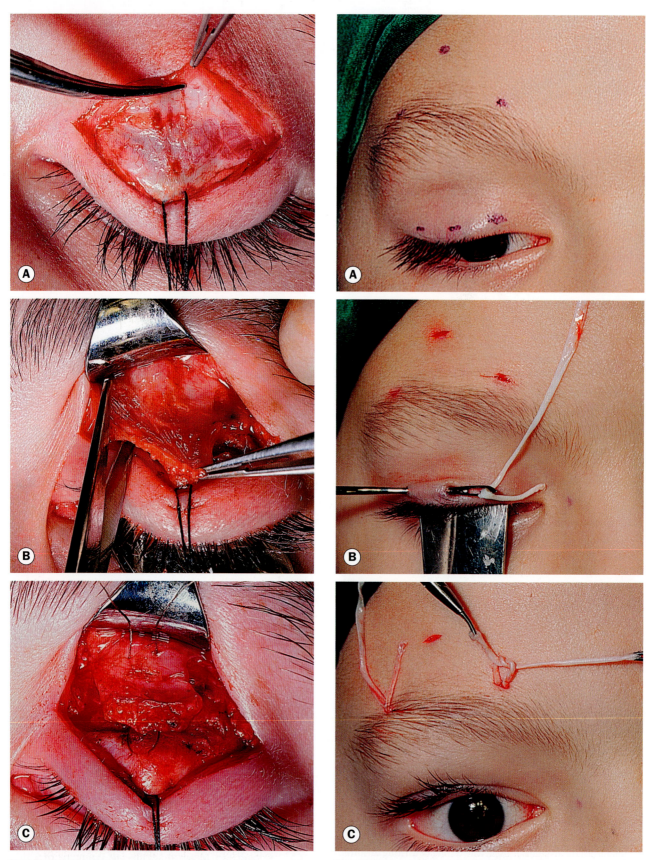

Fig. 1.59 Anterior levator resection. **(A)** Skin incision;
(B) dissection and resection of levator aponeurosis;
(C) levator reattachment to the tarsal plate

(Courtesy of AG Tyers and JRO Collin, from Colour Atlas of Ophthalmic Plastic
Surgery, *Butterworth-Heinemann 2001)*

Fig. 1.60 Brow suspension. **(A)** Site of incisions marked;
(B) threading of fascia lata strips; **(C)** tightening and tying
of strips

(Courtesy of AG Tyers and JRO Collin, from Colour Atlas of Ophthalmic Plastic
Surgery, *Butterworth-Heinemann 2001)*

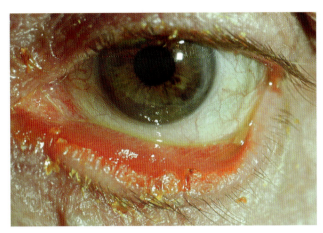

Fig. 1.61 Severe long-standing involutional ectropion with keratinization of the marginal conjunctiva
(Courtesy of C Barry)

- **Lateral canthal tendon laxity**, characterized by a rounded appearance of the lateral canthus (see Fig. 1.46B) and the ability to pull the lower lid medially more than 2 mm.
- **Medial canthal tendon laxity**, demonstrated by pulling the lower lid laterally and observing the position of the inferior punctum. If the lid is normal the punctum should not be displaced more than 1–2 mm. If laxity is mild the punctum reaches the limbus, and if severe it may reach the pupil.

Treatment

The approach to repair depends on apparent causation and the predominant location of the ectropion.

- **Generalized** ectropion is treated with repair of horizontal lid laxity. This is achieved with a lateral tarsal strip procedure, in which the lower canthal tendon is tightened by shortening and reattachment to the lateral orbital rim (Fig. 1.62); this is particularly helpful if the lateral canthus is rounded and lax, with associated tear overflow. Excision of a tarsoconjunctival pentagon (Fig. 1.63) is an alternative that can be placed to excise an area of misdirected lashes or keratinized conjunctiva.
- **Medial** ectropion, if mild, may be treated with a medial conjunctival diamond excision (medial spindle procedure), though must often be combined with a tarsal strip or lateral canthal sling (see 'Treatment'), or pentagon excision as significant horizontal laxity frequently co-exists.
- **Medial canthal tendon laxity**, if marked, requires stabilization prior to horizontal shortening to avoid excessive dragging of the punctum laterally.
- **Punctal ectropion** without more extensive lid involvement is considered in Ch. 2.

Cicatricial ectropion

Cicatricial ectropion is caused by scarring or contracture of the skin and underlying tissues, which pulls the eyelid away from the globe (Fig. 1.64). If the skin is pushed up over the orbital margin

with a finger the ectropion will be relieved. Opening the mouth tends to accentuate the eversion. Depending on the cause, both lids may be involved and the defect may be local (e.g. trauma) or general (e.g. burns, dermatitis, ichthyosis). Mild localized cases are treated by excision of the offending scar tissue combined with a procedure that lengthens vertical skin deficiency, such as Z-plasty. Severe generalized cases require transposition flaps or free skin grafts; sources of skin include the upper lids, posterior auricular, preauricular and supraclavicular areas.

Paralytic ectropion/facial nerve palsy

Introduction

Paralytic ectropion is caused by ipsilateral facial nerve palsy (Fig. 1.65) and is associated with retraction of the upper and lower lids and brow ptosis; the latter may mimic narrowing of the palpebral aperture.

Complications include exposure keratopathy due to lagophthalmos, and watering caused by malposition of the inferior lacrimal punctum, failure of the lacrimal pump mechanism and an increase in tear production resulting from corneal exposure.

Treatment

- **Temporary** measures may be instituted to protect the cornea in anticipation of spontaneous recovery of facial nerve function.
  - Lubrication with higher viscosity tear substitutes during the day, with instillation of ointment and taping shut of the lids during sleep, are usually adequate in mild cases.
  - Botulinum toxin injection into the levator to induce temporary ptosis.
  - Temporary tarsorrhaphy may be necessary, particularly in patients with a poor Bell phenomenon with the cornea remaining exposed when the patient attempts to blink; the lateral aspects of the upper and lower lids are sutured together.
- **Permanent** treatment should be considered when there is irreversible damage to the facial nerve as may occur following removal of an acoustic neuroma, or when no further improvement has occurred for 6-12 months in a Bell palsy.
  - Medial canthoplasty may be performed if the medial canthal tendon is intact. The eyelids are sutured together medial to the lacrimal puncta (Fig. 1.66A) so that the puncta become inverted and the fissure between the inner canthus and puncta is shortened.
  - A lateral canthal sling or tarsal strip may be used to correct residual ectropion and raise the lateral canthus (Fig. 1.66B).
  - Upper eyelid lowering by levator disinsertion.
  - Gold weight implantation in the upper lid can assist closure.
  - A small lateral tarsorrhaphy is usually cosmetically acceptable.

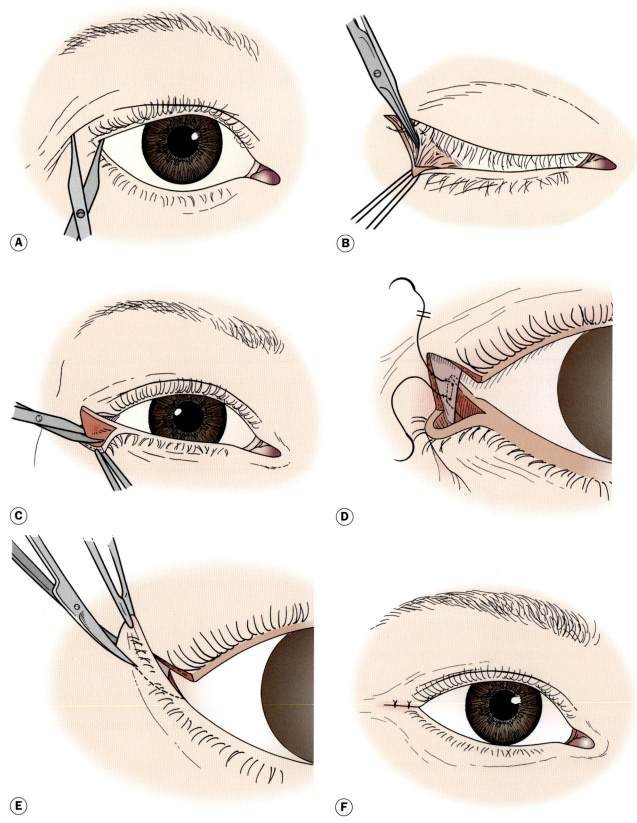

Fig. 1.62 Lateral tarsal strip procedure. **(A)** Lateral canthotomy; **(B)** cantholysis – the lower limb of the lateral canthal tendon is cut away from the inferior orbital rim; **(C)** the anterior and posterior lid lamellae are divided, and a 'strip' of tendon/ lateral tarsal plate dissected out; **(D)** the strip is shortened and then reattached to the inner aspect of the orbital rim periosteum with 4-0 absorbable suture; **(E)** excess lid margin is trimmed; **(F)** the skin incision (canthotomy) is closed

(Courtesy of JA Nerad, from Techniques in Ophthalmic Plastic Surgery, Saunders 2010)

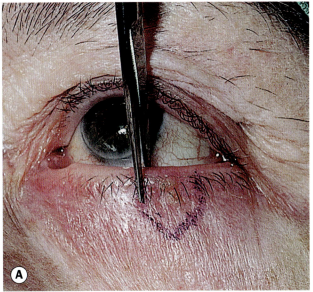

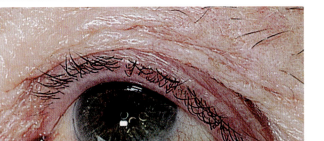

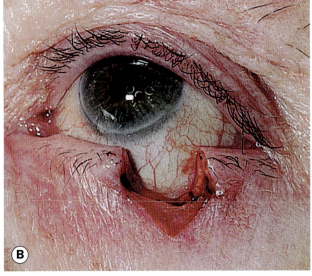

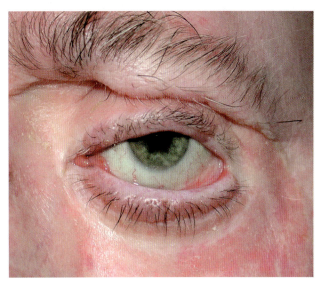

Fig. 1.64 Cicatricial ectropion
(Courtesy of A Pearson)

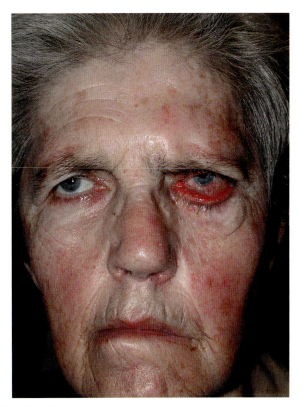

Fig. 1.65 Left facial palsy and severe paralytic ectropion
(Courtesy of A Pearson)

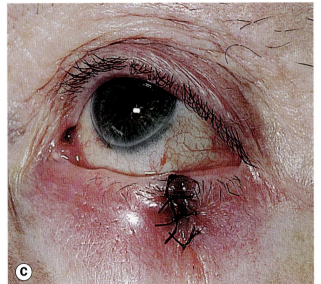

Fig. 1.63 Horizontal lid shortening to correct ectropion.
(A) Marking; **(B)** excision of a pentagon; **(C)** closure

(Courtesy of AG Tyers and JRO Collin, from Colour Atlas of Ophthalmic Plastic Surgery, Butterworth-Heinemann 2001)

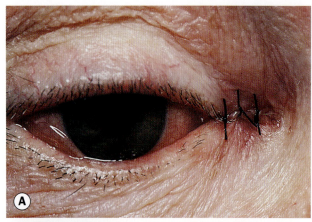

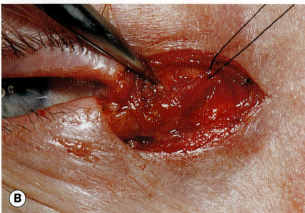

Fig. 1.66 Permanent treatment of paralytic ectropion. **(A)** Medial canthoplasty; **(B)** lateral canthal sling – refashioned canthal tendon from the lower lid is passed through a buttonhole in the tendon from the upper lid

(Courtesy of AG Tyers and JRO Collin, from Colour Atlas of Ophthalmic Plastic Surgery, *Butterworth-Heinemann 2001)*

Mechanical ectropion

Mechanical ectropion is caused by tumours on or near the lid margin that mechanically evert the lid. Treatment involves removal of the cause if possible, and correction of significant horizontal lid laxity.

ENTROPION

Involutional entropion

Introduction

Involutional (age-related) entropion affects mainly the lower lid. The constant rubbing of the lashes on the cornea in long-standing entropion (pseudotrichiasis – Fig. 1.67A) may cause irritation, corneal punctate epithelial erosions and, in severe cases, pannus formation and ulceration. Aetiological factors include:

- **Horizontal lid laxity** caused by stretching of the canthal tendons and tarsal plate.

- **Vertical lid instability** caused by attenuation, dehiscence or disinsertion of the lower lid retractors. Weakness of the latter is recognized by decreased excursion of the lower lid in downgaze.
- **Over-riding of the pretarsal** by the preseptal orbicularis during lid closure tends to move the lower border of the tarsal plate anteriorly, away from the globe, and the upper border towards the globe, thus tipping the lid inwards (Fig. 1.67B).
- **Orbital septum laxity** with prolapse of orbital fat into the lower lid.

Treatment

Temporary protection must be as short-term as possible; options include lubricants, taping, soft bandage contact lenses and orbicularis chemodenervation with botulinum toxin injection.

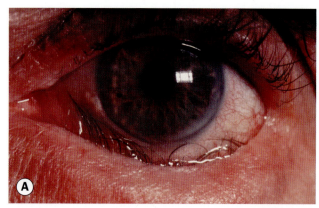

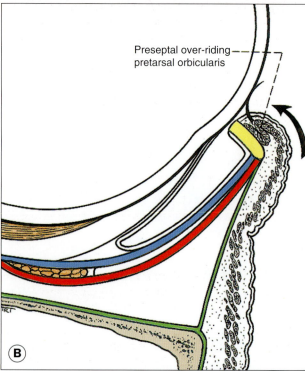

Preseptal over-riding pretarsal orbicularis

Fig. 1.67 (A) Involutional entropion and pseudotrichiasis; **(B)** preseptal orbicularis over-riding the pretarsal orbicularis

Surgical treatment aims to correct the underlying problems as follows:

- **Over-riding** and disinsertion
  - Transverse everting sutures prevent over-riding of the preseptal orbicularis. They are quick and easy to insert (Fig. 1.68), providing a correction typically lasting several months, and may be used in circumstances (e.g. a confused patient) where a more intricate procedure is not likely to be tolerated.
  - The Wies procedure gives a durable correction. It consists of full-thickness horizontal lid-splitting and insertion of everting sutures (Fig. 1.69). The scar creates a barrier between the preseptal and pretarsal orbicularis, and the everting suture fairly effectively transfers the pull of the lower lid retractors from the tarsal plate to the skin and orbicularis.
  - Lower lid retractor reinsertion (Fig. 1.70) involves direct exposure and advancement of the retractors as opposed to the less precise approach used in the Wies procedure. The subciliary skin incision used, and its repair, also create a barrier to over-riding of the preseptal orbicularis muscle. It can be performed as a primary treatment but may be reserved for recurrence.
- **Horizontal lid laxity** is usually present and can be corrected with a lateral canthal sling (tarsal strip – see Fig. 1.62) or, less commonly, a full-thickness lateral pentagon excision (see Fig. 1.63). Tightening serves also to retain the lid in apposition against the globe, preventing over-correction.

Cicatricial entropion

Scarring of the palpebral conjunctiva can rotate the upper or lower lid margin towards the globe. Causes include cicatrizing conjunctivitis, trachoma, trauma and chemical injuries. Temporary measures are similar to those listed for involutional entropion. Definitive surgical treatment of mild cases is by tarsal fracture (transverse tarsotomy) with anterior rotation of the lid margin, as for marginal entropion of the lower lid. Treatment of severe cases is difficult and is directed at replacing deficient or keratinized conjunctiva and replacing the scarred and contracted tarsal plate with composite grafts.

MISCELLANEOUS ACQUIRED DISORDERS

Varix

An eyelid varix (plural – varices) is a common lesion that may be mistaken for a naevus or haemangioma. A varix is commonly an

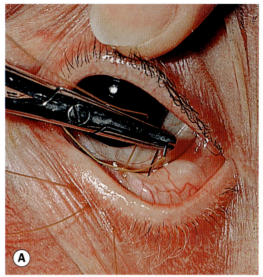

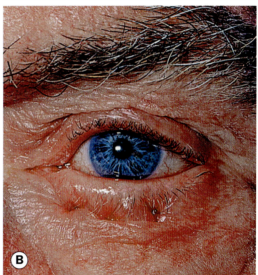

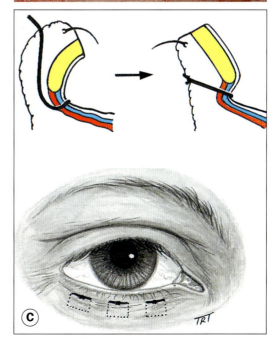

Fig. 1.68 Lid-everting sutures for entropion. **(A)** Three double-armed sutures are passed as shown; **(B)** sutures are tied; **(C)** schematic

(Courtesy of AG Tyers and JRO Collin, from Colour Atlas of Ophthalmic Plastic Surgery, *Butterworth-Heinemann 2001)*

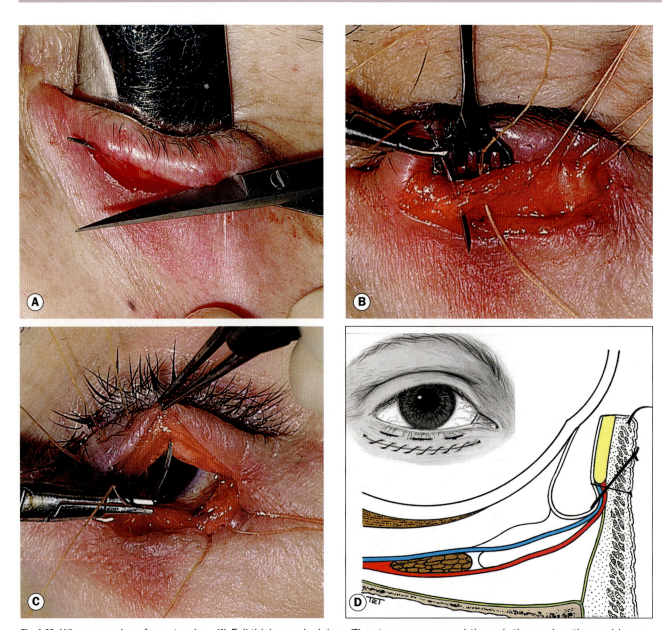

Fig. 1.69 Wies procedure for entropion. **(A)** Full-thickness incision; **(B)** sutures are passed through the conjunctiva and lower lid retractors; **(C)** sutures are passed anterior to the tarsal plate to exit inferior to the lashes; **(D)** schematic
(Courtesy of AG Tyers and JRO Collin, from Colour Atlas of Ophthalmic Plastic Surgery, Butterworth-Heinemann 2001 – figs A–C)

isolated lesion, but may be associated with orbital involvement (see Ch. 3). It appears as a dark red or purple subcutaneous compressible (unless thrombosed) lesion (Figs 1.71A and B), which in some cases becomes apparent only with a Valsalva manoeuvre (Figs 1.71C and D). It is clinically and histologically similar to a lymphangioma. Simple excision may be performed for diagnostic or cosmetic reasons; the possibility of orbital communication should be borne in mind during surgery.

Dermatochalasis

This is described in the discussion of pseudoptosis (above) and upper lid blepharoplasty (below).

Floppy eyelid syndrome

Introduction

Floppy eyelid syndrome (FES) is an uncommon unilateral or bilateral condition that is often overlooked as a cause of persistent ocular surface symptoms. It typically affects obese middle-aged and older men who sleep with one or both eyelids against the pillow, leading to pulling of the lid away from the globe; consequent nocturnal exposure and poor contact with the globe, often exacerbated by other ocular surface disease such as dry eye and blepharitis, result in chronic keratoconjunctivitis. Obstructive sleep apnoea (OSA) is strongly associated; OSA is linked to

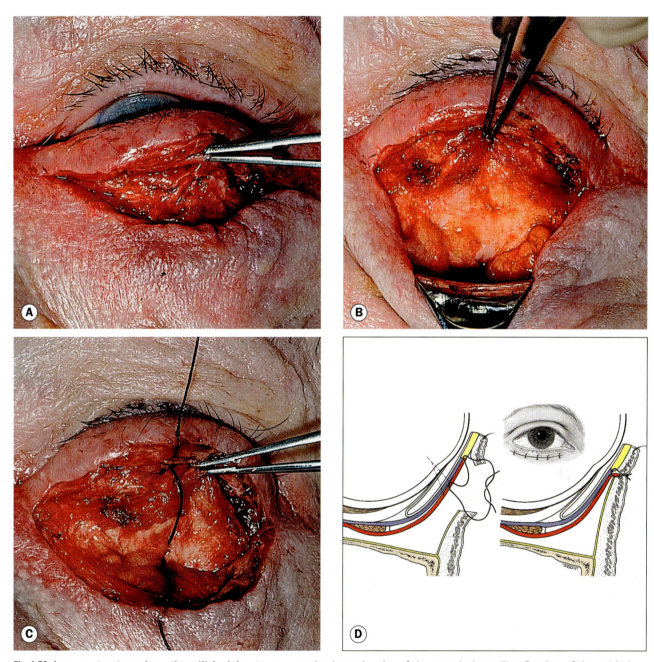

Fig. 1.70 Lower retractor reinsertion. **(A)** Incision to expose the lower border of the tarsal plate; **(B)** reflection of the orbital septum and fat pad to expose the lower lid retractors; **(C)** tightening of retractors by plication; **(D)** schematic
(Courtesy of AG Tyers and JRO Collin, from Colour Atlas of Ophthalmic Plastic Surgery, Butterworth-Heinemann 2001)

significant morbidity, including cardiopulmonary disease and subtle but irreversible mental dysfunction.

Diagnosis

- **The upper eyelid** is typically extremely lax, often with substantial excess loose upper lid skin (Fig. 1.72A). The tarsal plate has a rubbery consistency (Fig. 1.72B); the lid is very easy to evert (Fig. 1.72C), to fold and to pull away from the eye.

- **Papillary conjunctivitis** of the superior tarsal conjunctiva may be intense (Fig. 1.72D).
- **Keratopathy.** Punctate keratopathy, filamentary keratitis and superior superficial vascularization may be present.
- **Other findings** may include eyelash ptosis, lacrimal gland prolapse, ectropion and aponeurotic ptosis. Patients with both FES and OSA seem to have a considerably higher than average prevalence of glaucoma.
- **Investigation for OSA** should be considered in most cases of FES, particularly if the patient reports substantial snoring and/or excessive daytime sleepiness.

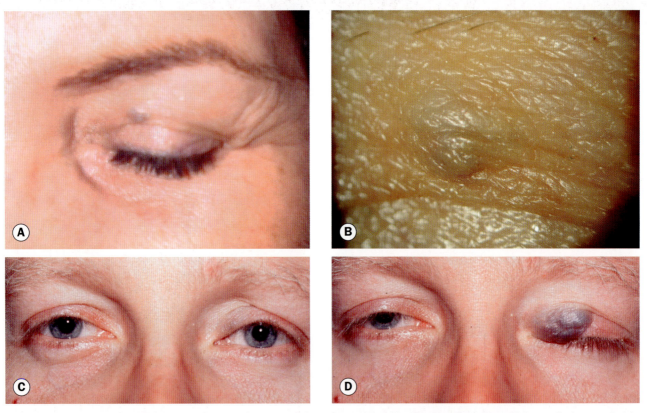

Fig. 1.71 Eyelid varices. **(A)** Typical appearance of a commonly seen small varix; **(B)** magnified view; **(C)** larger lesion, probably with orbital involvement, before Valsalva manoeuvre; **(D)** during Valsalva

(Courtesy of G Rose – figs C and D)

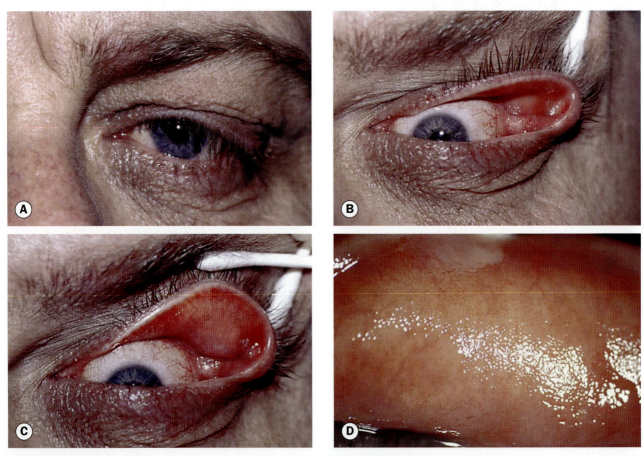

Fig. 1.72 Floppy eyelid syndrome. **(A)** Redundant upper lid skin; **(B)** loose and rubbery tarsal plates; **(C)** very easily everted eyelid; **(D)** superior tarsal papillary conjunctivitis

(Courtesy of C Barry)

Treatment

- Treatment of associated OSA is likely to be of benefit; overweight patients should be encouraged to lose weight.
- Mild cases may respond to lubrication together with nocturnal eye shield wear or taping of the lids.
- Moderate to severe cases require horizontal shortening to stabilize the lid and ocular surface and prevent nocturnal lagophthalmos; a pentagonal excision of 10 mm or more is taken from the junction of the lateral third and medial two-thirds of the upper lid.

Blepharochalasis

Blepharochalasis is an uncommon condition characterized by recurrent episodes of painless, non-pitting oedema of both upper lids which usually resolves spontaneously after a few days. Presentation is usually around puberty, episodes becoming less frequent with time. Eyelid skin becomes stretched and atrophic, characteristically said to resemble wrinkled cigarette paper; severe cases may give rise to stretching of the canthal tendons and levator aponeurosis resulting in ptosis (Fig. 1.73), and lacrimal gland prolapse may occur. A hypertrophic form with orbital fat herniation and an atrophic form with absorption of orbital fat have been described. The differential diagnosis includes similarly episodic conditions, particularly drug-induced urticaria and angioedema. Treatment involves blepharoplasty for redundant upper lid skin, and correction of ptosis.

Eyelid imbrication syndrome

Eyelid imbrication syndrome is an uncommon and frequently unrecognized disorder in which the upper lid overlaps the lower on closure so that the lower lashes irritate the superior marginal tarsal conjunctiva.

It may be unilateral or bilateral and the major symptom is ocular irritation. It can be acquired, commonly associated with floppy eyelid syndrome, or – very rarely – congenital; occasionally

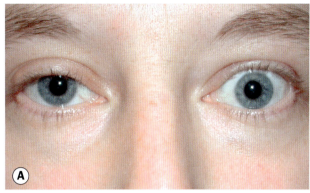
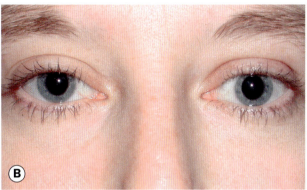

Fig. 1.74 (A) Left lid retraction in thyroid eye disease; **(B)** following Müller muscle recession
(Courtesy of A Pearson)

it may follow lower lid tarsal strip surgery. Associated signs include superior tarsal papillary conjunctivitis and rose Bengal staining of the superior marginal conjunctiva. Definitive treatment consists of upper lid pentagon resection and/or lateral canthal tightening.

Upper lid retraction

Upper lid retraction is suspected when the upper lid margin is either level with or above the superior limbus (Fig. 1.74A); the causes are listed in Table 1.5. Where there is no loss or tightness of the upper eyelid skin, retraction is corrected by surgical release of the eyelid retractors, usually via a transconjunctival posterior approach. Mild retraction may be treated with Müller muscle recession (Fig. 1.74B). Moderate to severe retraction may require levator aponeurosis recession.

Lower lid retraction

Inferior scleral show may be physiological in patients with large eyes or shallow orbits, but is commonly involutional or secondary to some of the conditions in Table 1.5. It may follow lower lid blepharoplasty, when aggressive upward massage of the lid for 2 or 3 months may be curative for minor degrees. In other cases, a tarsal strip operation may raise the lid slightly, but when moderate elevation is required inferior retractor recession with a posterior lamellar spacer is likely to be necessary; more aggressive procedures have been described for severe cases.

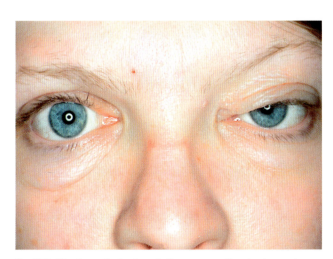

Fig. 1.73 Blepharochalasis – left aponeurotic ptosis and thinned upper lid skin

Table 1.5 Causes of lid retraction

1. Thyroid eye disease
2. Neurogenic • Contralateral unilateral ptosis (Fig. 1.75A) • Unopposed levator action due to facial palsy • Third nerve misdirection • Marcus Gunn jaw-winking syndrome • Collier sign of the dorsal midbrain (Parinaud syndrome – Fig. 1.75B) • Infantile hydrocephalus (setting sun sign – Fig. 1.75C) • Parkinsonism (Fig. 1.75D) • Sympathomimetic drops
3. Mechanical • Surgical over-correction of ptosis • Scarring of upper lid skin
4. Congenital • Isolated • Duane retraction syndrome • Down syndrome • Transient 'eye popping' reflex in normal infants
5. Miscellaneous • Prominent globe (pseudo-lid retraction) • Uraemia (Summerskill sign) • Idiopathic

COSMETIC EYELID AND PERIOCULAR SURGERY

Involutional changes

Involutional (age-related) changes around the eyes can lead to functional and cosmetic concerns that may require treatment.

- Reduction in cutaneous elasticity and thickness results in loose, wrinkled skin.
- Weakening of the orbital septum may lead to orbital fat prolapse.
- Thinning and stretching of the canthal tendons, levator aponeurosis and lower lid retractors may cause eyelid laxity and ptosis.
- Atrophy of orbital and eyebrow fat pads can give enophthalmos and eyebrow sagging.
- Weakening of the frontalis muscle and epicranial aponeurosis may cause descent of the eyebrows and increasing looseness of upper eyelid skin.
- Thinning and stretching of midfacial support leads to descent with formation of a tear trough depression and exacerbation of lower eyelid changes.
- Thinning and resorption of periorbital bone exacerbates the appearance of surplus overlying tissues.

Non-surgical techniques

Botulinum toxin injection to periocular muscles

Botulinum toxin injection can be used to reduce wrinkling, particularly for 'crows' feet' at the lateral canthus and for glabellar frown lines, and 'brow lift' by a reduction in the action of brow depressors. Complications include temporary ptosis, lagophthalmos, ectropion and diplopia.

Tissue fillers

These are used to address age-related wrinkles, and less commonly defects from other causes such as trauma. Complications include hypersensitivity reactions.

- **Hyaluronic acid** is the most commonly used tissue filler, and can be used to temporarily fill in hollows and replace lost volume. They are injected deep to orbicularis and the effects generally last 3–12 months depending on the agent used.
- **Autologous fat** gives a more permanent replacement.
- **Others** include collagen, microspheres of calcium hydroxyapatite and synthetic fillers.

Skin resurfacing

Removal of the superficial layers of the skin, by chemical peels or laser, can lead to a reduction in wrinkling, increased evenness of pigmentation, removal of blemishes and improved texture by generating new epidermis and increasing collagen production in the dermis.

Surgical techniques

Upper eyelid blepharoplasty

Upper eyelid involutional changes are characterized by surplus upper eyelid skin (dermatochalasis) that leads to baggy lids with indistinct creases and pseudo- or mechanical ptosis. It may cause a heavy sensation around the eyes, brow ache and, in more advanced cases, obstruction of the superior visual field (Fig. 1.76A). Upper lid blepharoplasty (Fig. 1.76B) is effective for the removal of surplus skin and can be combined with reduction of the superior orbital fat pads. Care must be taken prior to surgery to look for ptosis of the eyelid or eyebrow and ocular surface dryness. Complications include removal of excess skin leading to lagophthalmos and corneal drying, and removal of excess orbital fat leading to an unattractive hollowed out upper eyelid sulcus.

Lower eyelid blepharoplasty

Lower lid involutional changes are characterized by excess skin and/or prolapsed orbital fat (Fig. 1.77A); blepharoplasty can address these (Fig. 1.77B).

- **Anterior approach.** Where there is excess skin an anterior approach is used to raise a skin/muscle flap that can be lifted and re-draped on the lid with the surplus removed. At the same time the inferior orbital fat pads can be reduced by a small incision through the septum.
- **Posterior approach.** Bulging of the lower eyelid fat pads without eyelid laxity or surplus skin is best reduced by a

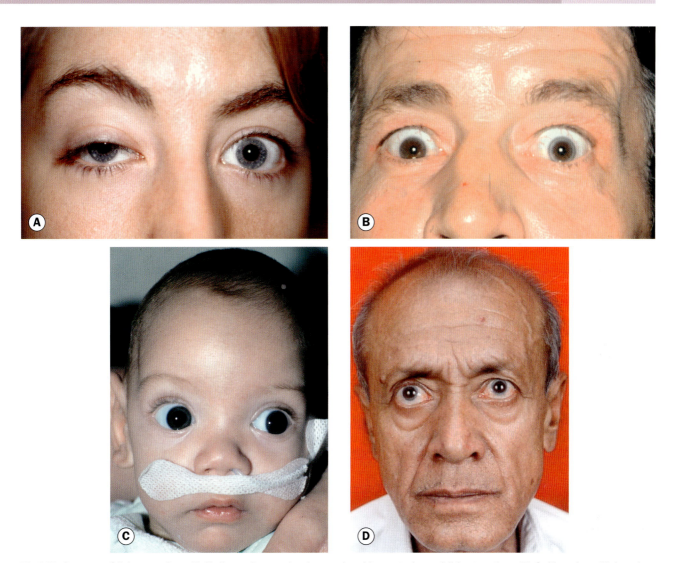

Fig. 1.75 Causes of lid retraction. **(A)** Unilateral myasthenic ptosis with contralateral lid retraction; **(B)** Collier sign; **(C)** 'setting sun' sign in infantile hydrocephalus; **(D)** parkinsonism

(Courtesy of R Bates – fig. C)

posterior, transconjunctival approach. Complications include lower eyelid retraction, contour abnormalities (particularly lateral drooping), and frank ectropion.

Brow ptosis correction

Brow ptosis frequently accompanies dermatochalasis (Fig. 1.78A) and may also follow facial nerve palsy or localized trauma. Lifting of the brow needs to precede or occasionally be combined with upper lid blepharoplasty.

- **Direct brow lift.** An incision is made above the eyebrow hairs and an ellipse of skin removed (Fig. 1.78B).
- **Endoscopic brow lift.** Small incisions within the hair-line enable endoscopic elevation of the whole forehead tissues and release at the eyebrow periosteum to allow lifting of the eyebrows through sutures supported on frontal bone anchors within the hair-line.

CONGENITAL MALFORMATIONS

Epicanthic folds

Epicanthic folds are bilateral vertical folds of skin that extend from the upper or lower lids towards the medial canthi. They may give rise to a pseudoexotropia. The folds may involve the upper or lower lids or both; lower lid folds extending upwards to the medial canthal area (epicanthus inversus – Fig. 1.79A) are associated with the blepharophimosis syndrome. Treatment is by V–Y (Fig. 1.79B) or Z-plasty.

Telecanthus

Telecanthus is an uncommon condition that may occur in isolation or in association with blepharophimosis and some systemic

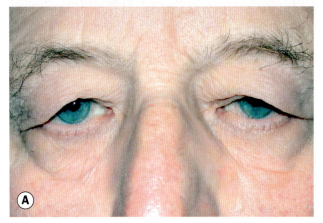

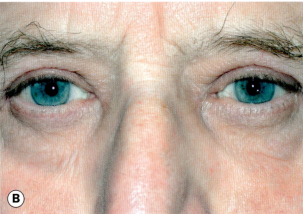

Fig. 1.76 (A) Severe dermatochalasis causing reduction of upper visual field; **(B)** appearance following surgery

(Courtesy of A Pearson)

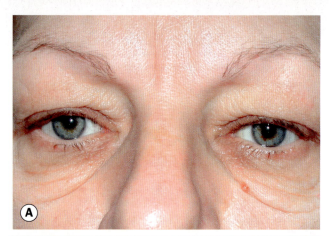

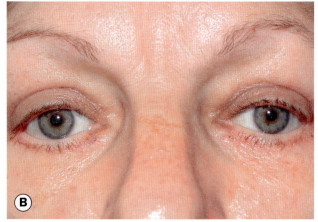

Fig. 1.77 (A) Mild dermatochalasis and excess lower lid skin; **(B)** appearance following upper and lower lid blepharoplasty

(Courtesy of A Pearson)

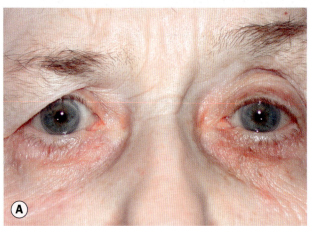

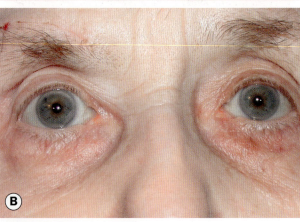

Fig. 1.78 (A) Right brow ptosis and dermatochalasis; **(B)** following direct brow-lift

(Courtesy of A Pearson)

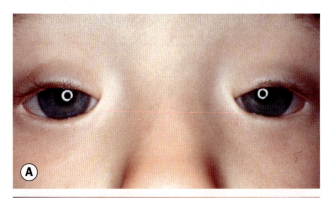

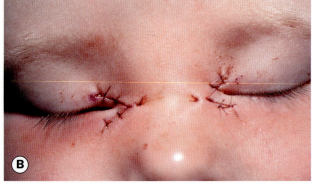

Fig. 1.79 Epicanthus inversus. **(A)** Preoperative appearance; **(B)** immediately after V–Y plasty

(Courtesy of R Bates – fig. B)

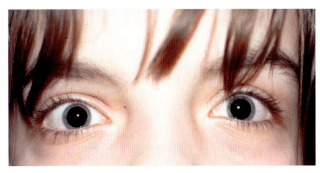

Fig. 1.80 Telecanthus

syndromes. It consists of increased distance between the medial canthi due to abnormally long medial canthal tendons (Fig. 1.80). It should not be confused with hypertelorism in which there is wide bony separation of the orbits. Treatment involves shortening and refixation of the medial canthal tendons to the anterior lacrimal crest, or insertion of a trans-nasal suture.

Blepharophimosis, ptosis and epicanthus inversus syndrome

Blepharophimosis, ptosis and epicanthus inversus syndrome (BPES) is a complex of eyelid malformations consisting of moderate to severe symmetrical ptosis with poor levator function, telecanthus, epicanthus inversus (see Fig. 1.79A), manifesting with small palpebral fissures (Fig. 1.81). Other minor facial anomalies

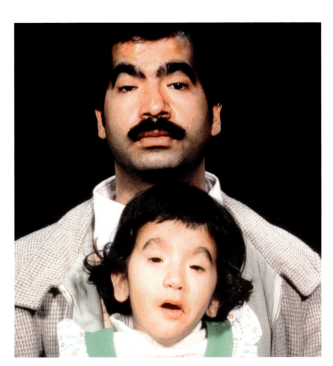

Fig. 1.81 Blepharophimosis ptosis and epicanthus inversus syndrome

are commonly present. Inheritance is usually autosomal dominant; both BPES type I (with premature ovarian failure) and BPES type II (without premature ovarian failure) are caused by mutations in the *FOXL2* gene on chromosome 3. Treatment initially involves correction of epicanthus and telecanthus, followed later by bilateral frontalis suspension. It is also important to treat amblyopia, which is present in about 50%.

Epiblepharon

Epiblepharon comprises an extra horizontal fold of skin stretching across the anterior lid margin; it is very common in individuals of Eastern Asian ethnicity. The lashes are directed vertically, especially in the medial part of the lid (Figs 1.82A and B). When the fold of skin is pulled down the lashes turn out and the normal location of the lid becomes apparent (Fig. 1.82C); it should not be confused with the much less common congenital entropion (see next). Treatment is not required in the majority of Caucasians because spontaneous resolution with age is usual. Persistent cases may be treated surgically.

Congenital entropion

Upper lid entropion is usually secondary to the mechanical effects of microphthalmos, which cause variable degrees of upper lid inversion. Lower lid entropion (Fig. 1.83) is generally caused by maldevelopment of the inferior retractor aponeurosis. Treatment involves the excision of a strip of skin and muscle, and fixation of the skin crease to the tarsal plate (Hotz procedure).

Coloboma

A congenital coloboma is an uncommon, unilateral or bilateral, partial- or full-thickness eyelid defect. It occurs when eyelid development is incomplete, due to either failure of migration of lid ectoderm to fuse the lid folds or to mechanical forces such as amniotic bands. Colobomata elsewhere in the eye, as well as a range of other associations, may be present. The treatment of small defects involves primary closure, while large defects require skin grafts and rotation flaps.

- **Upper lid colobomas** occur at the junction of the middle and inner thirds (Fig. 1.84A); relatively strong associations include cryptophthalmos (see below), facial abnormalities and Goldenhar syndrome.
- **Lower lid colobomas** occur at the junction of the middle and outer thirds (Fig. 1.84B) and are frequently associated with systemic conditions.
- **Treacher Collins syndrome** (mandibulofacial dysostosis) is a genetically heterogeneous condition characterized by malformation of derivatives of the first and second branchial arches, principally mandibular and ear anomalies. Lower eyelid coloboma is a feature; ocular anomalies also described include slanted palpebral apertures, cataract, microphthalmos and lacrimal atresia.

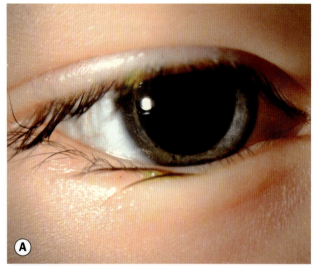

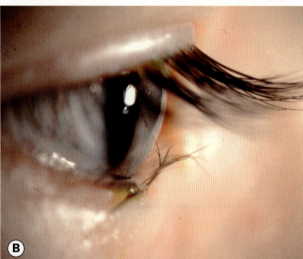

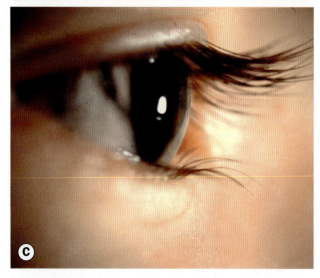

Fig. 1.82 (A) Epiblepharon; **(B)** lashes pointing upwards; **(C)** normal position of lashes following manual correction

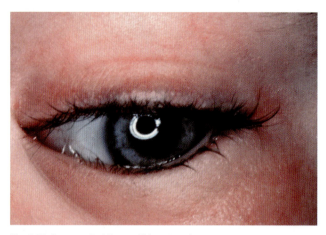

Fig. 1.83 Congenital lower lid entropion

Cryptophthalmos

Cryptophthalmos is a rare congenital anomaly in which the eyelids are absent, replaced by a continuous layer of skin.

- **Complete cryptophthalmos.** A microphthalmic eye (Fig. 1.85A) is covered by a fused layer of skin with no separation between the lids.
- **Incomplete cryptophthalmos** is characterized by rudimentary lids and microphthalmos (Fig. 1.85B).
- **Fraser syndrome** is a dominantly inherited condition in which cryptophthalmos is a common finding; other features can include syndactyly, urogenital and craniofacial anomalies.

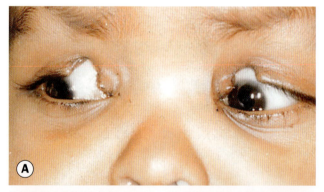

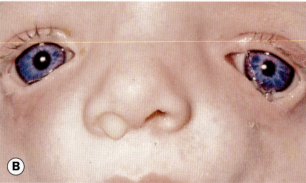

Fig. 1.84 (A) Upper lid colobomas; **(B)** lower lid colobomas in Treacher Collins syndrome

(Courtesy of U Raina – fig. A)

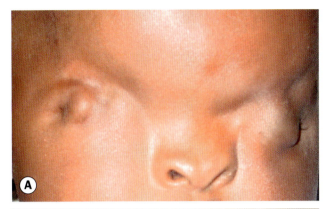

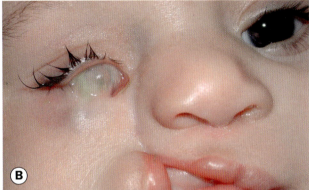

Fig. 1.85 Cryptophthalmos. **(A)** Complete; **(B)** incomplete
(Courtesy of D Meyer – fig. A)

Euryblepharon

Euryblepharon refers to horizontal enlargement of the palpebral fissure with associated lateral canthal malposition and lateral ectropion (Fig. 1.86); lagophthalmos and exposure keratopathy may result.

Microblepharon

Microblepharon is characterized by small eyelids, often associated with anophthalmos (Fig. 1.87).

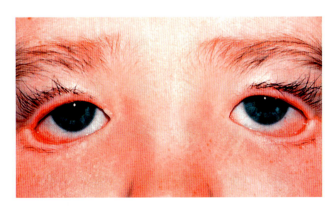

Fig. 1.86 Euryblepharon

(Courtesy of D Taylor and C Hoyt, from Pediatric Ophthalmology and Strabismus, *Elsevier 2005)*

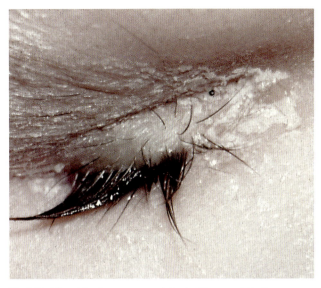

Fig. 1.87 Microblepharon associated with anophthalmos

Ablepharon

Ablepharon consists of deficiency of the anterior lamellae of the eyelids (Fig. 1.88A); treatment involves reconstructive skin grafting. Ablepharon-macrostomia syndrome is characterized by an enlarged fish-like mouth (Fig. 1.88B), ear, skin and genital anomalies.

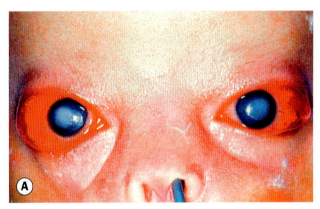

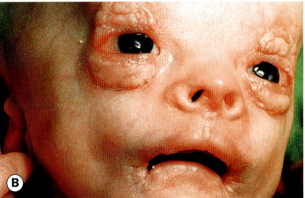

Fig. 1.88 (A) Ablepharon; **(B)** following reconstruction – note enlarged fish-like mouth

(Courtesy of D Taylor and C Hoyt, from Pediatric Ophthalmology and Strabismus, *Elsevier 2005 – fig. A; H Mroczkowska – fig. B)*

Congenital upper lid eversion

Congenital upper lid eversion is a rare condition more frequently seen in infants of Afro-Caribbean origin, in Down syndrome and in congenital ichthyosis (collodion skin disease – Fig. 1.89). It is typically bilateral and symmetrical. It may resolve spontaneously with conservative treatment or require surgery.

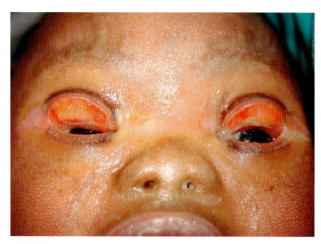

Fig. 1.89 Congenital upper lid eversion in a patient with ichthyosis

(Courtesy of D Meyer)

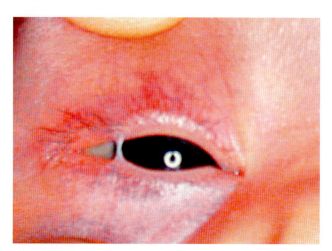

Fig. 1.90 Ankyloblepharon filiforme adnatum

(Courtesy of D Taylor and C Hoyt, from Pediatric Ophthalmology and Strabismus, *Elsevier 2005)*

Ankyloblepharon filiforme adnatum

In ankyloblepharon filiforme adnatum the upper and lower eyelids are joined by thin tags (Fig. 1.90); most cases are sporadic. Treatment involves transection with scissors; anaesthesia is not required.

Lacrimal drainage system

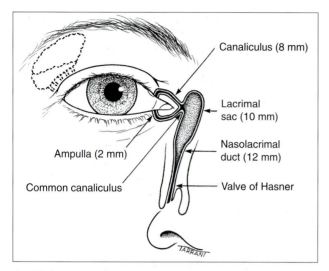

Fig. 2.1 Anatomy of the lacrimal drainage system

INTRODUCTION

Anatomy

The lacrimal drainage system consists of the following structures (Fig. 2.1):

- **The puncta** are located at the posterior edge of the lid margin, at the junction of the lash-bearing lateral five-sixths (pars ciliaris) and the medial non-ciliated one-sixth (pars lacrimalis). Normally they face slightly posteriorly and can be inspected by everting the medial aspect of the lids. Treatment of watering caused by punctal stenosis or malposition is relatively straightforward.
- **The canaliculi** pass vertically from the lid margin for about 2 mm (ampullae). They then turn medially and run horizontally for about 8 mm to reach the lacrimal sac. The superior and inferior canaliculi usually (>90%) unite to form the common canaliculus, which opens into the lateral wall of the lacrimal sac. Uncommonly, each canaliculus

opens separately into the sac. A small flap of mucosa (Rosenmüller valve) overhangs the junction of the common canaliculus and the lacrimal sac (the internal punctum) and prevents reflux of tears into the canaliculi. Treatment of canalicular obstruction may be complex.

- **The lacrimal sac** is 10–12 mm long and lies in the lacrimal fossa between the anterior and posterior lacrimal crests. The lacrimal bone and the frontal process of the maxilla separate the lacrimal sac from the middle meatus of the nasal cavity. In a dacryocystorhinostomy (DCR) an anastomosis is created between the sac and the nasal mucosa to bypass an obstruction in the nasolacrimal duct.
- **The nasolacrimal duct** is 12–18 mm long and is the inferior continuation of the lacrimal sac. It descends and angles slightly laterally and posteriorly to open into the inferior nasal meatus, lateral to and below the inferior turbinate. The opening of the duct is partially covered by a mucosal fold (valve of Hasner).

Physiology

Tears secreted by the main and accessory lacrimal glands pass across the ocular surface. A variable amount of the aqueous component of the tear film is lost by evaporation, with the remainder of the tears hypothesized to drain substantially as follows (Fig. 2.2):

- Tears flow along the upper and lower marginal strips (Fig. 2.2A), pooling in the lacus lacrimalis medial to the lower puncta, then entering the upper and lower canaliculi by a combination of capillarity and suction.
- With each blink, the pretarsal orbicularis oculi muscle compresses the ampullae, shortens and compresses the horizontal canaliculi, and closes and moves the puncta medially, resisting reflux. Simultaneously, contraction of the lacrimal part of the orbicularis oculi creates a positive pressure that forces tears down the nasolacrimal duct and into the nose, mediated by helically arranged connective tissue fibres around the lacrimal sac (Fig. 2.2B).
- When the eyes open, the canaliculi and sac expand, creating negative pressure that draws tears from the canaliculi into the sac (Fig. 2.2C).

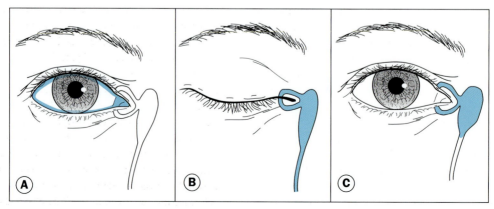

Fig. 2.2 Physiology of the lacrimal drainage system

CHAPTER 2

Causes of a watering eye

Epiphora is the overflow of tears at the eyelid margin; strictly, it is a sign rather than a symptom. There are two mechanisms:

- **Hypersecretion** secondary to anterior segment disease such as dry eye ('paradoxical watering') or inflammation. In these cases watering is associated with symptoms of the underlying cause, and treatment is usually medical.
- **Defective drainage** due to a compromised lacrimal drainage system; this may be caused by:
  - Malposition (e.g. ectropion) of the lacrimal puncta.
  - Obstruction at any point along the drainage system, from the punctal region to the valve of Hasner.
  - Lacrimal pump failure, which may occur secondarily to lower lid laxity or weakness of the orbicularis muscle (e.g. facial nerve palsy).

Evaluation

History

Enquiry should be made about ocular discomfort and redness to aid in excluding hypersecretion. Drainage failure tends to be exacerbated by a cold and windy environment, and to be least evident in a warm dry room; a complaint of the tears overflowing onto the cheek is likely to indicate drainage failure rather than hypersecretion.

External examination

Punctal abnormality is the most common cause of lacrimal drainage failure.

- **The puncta and eyelids** should be examined using a slit lamp. It is critical that examination of the puncta is performed prior to cannulation for diagnostic irrigation, which temporarily dilates the punctal opening and masks stenosis.
  - There will often be obvious tear overflow from the medial, or less commonly the lateral, canthal region; this is more likely to indicate defective drainage than an irritative cause.
  - Visible mucopurulent discharge is more likely to occur with nasolacrimal duct obstruction than a blockage more proximally.
  - Punctal stenosis (Fig. 2.3A). This is extremely common, and has been reported as present in up to about half of the general population; over half of patients with evident stenosis are asymptomatic, in many cases due to insufficiency of tear production or increased evaporation.
  - Ectropion, either localised to the punctal region or involving the wider lid, is often associated with secondary stenosis (Fig. 2.3B).
  - Punctal obstruction, usually partial, by a fold of redundant conjunctiva (conjunctivochalasis – Fig. 2.3C) is common but underdiagnosed.
  - Occasionally an eyelash may lodge in the ampulla (Fig. 2.3D).
  - A large caruncle may displace the punctum away from the globe (Fig. 2.3E).
  - In the presence of substantial lid laxity, the puncta may rarely over-ride each other.
  - A pouting punctum (Fig. 2.3F) is typical of canaliculitis.
  - The eyelid skin will often be moderately scaly and erythematous in chronic epiphora.
- **The lacrimal sac** should be palpated. Punctal reflux of mucopurulent material on compression is indicative of a mucocoele (a dilated mucus-filled sac; US spelling – mucocele) with a patent canalicular system, but with an obstruction either at or distal to the lower end of the lacrimal sac. In acute dacryocystitis palpation is painful and should be avoided. Rarely, palpation of the sac will reveal a stone or tumour.

Fluorescein disappearance test

The marginal tear strip of both eyes should be examined on the slit lamp prior to any manipulation of the eyelids or instillation of topical medication. Many patients with watering do not have obvious overflow of tears but merely show a high meniscus (marginal tear strip) of 0.6 mm or more (Fig. 2.4) versus 0.2–0.4 mm normally. The fluorescein disappearance test is performed by instilling fluorescein 1 or 2% drops into both conjunctival fornices; normally, little or no dye remains after 5–10 minutes. Prolonged retention is indicative of inadequate lacrimal drainage. This should be distinguished from the 'fluorescein clearance test' used to assess tear turnover in dry eye, in which retained stain is measured in the meniscus 15 minutes after instillation of 5 μl of fluorescein.

Lacrimal irrigation

Lacrimal irrigation should be performed only after ascertaining punctal patency; if absent or severely stenosed, surgical enlargement of the punctum may be needed before canalicular and nasolacrimal duct patency can be confirmed. It is contraindicated in acute infection.

- Local anaesthetic is instilled into the conjunctival sac.
- A punctum dilator is used to enlarge the punctal orifice (Fig. 2.5A), entering vertically and then tilting the instrument horizontally whilst exerting lateral tension on the lid (Fig. 2.5B,C).
- A gently curved, blunt-tipped 26- or 27-gauge lacrimal cannula on a 3 ml saline-filled syringe is inserted into the lower punctum and, whilst keeping a gentle stretch laterally on the eyelid, advanced a few millimetres, following the contour of the canaliculus (Fig. 2.5D).
- **A hard stop** occurs if the cannula enters the lacrimal sac, coming to a stop at the medial wall of the sac, through which can be felt the rigid lacrimal bone (Fig. 2.6A). This excludes complete obstruction of the canalicular system. Gentle saline irrigation is then attempted. If saline passes into the nose and throat, when it will be tasted by the patient, a patent lacrimal system is present, although there may still be stenosis; alternatively, symptoms may be due to subtle lacrimal pump failure. Failure of saline to reach the throat is indicative of total obstruction of the nasolacrimal

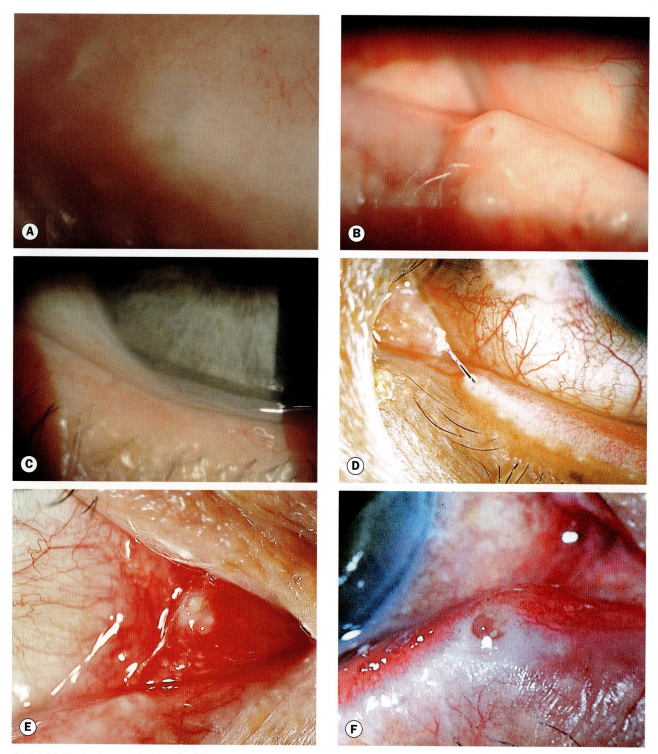

Fig. 2.3 (A) Marked punctal stenosis; **(B)** punctal ectropion and stenosis; **(C)** conjunctivochalasis; **(D)** punctal obstruction by an eyelash; **(E)** large caruncle; **(F)** pouting punctum

duct. In this situation, the lacrimal sac will distend slightly during irrigation and there will be reflux, usually through both the upper and lower puncta. The regurgitated material may be clear, mucoid or mucopurulent, depending on the contents of the lacrimal sac.

- **A soft stop** is experienced if the cannula stops at or proximal to the junction of the common canaliculus and the lacrimal sac. The sac is thus not entered – a spongy feeling is experienced as the cannula presses the soft tissue of the common canaliculus and the lateral wall against the medial

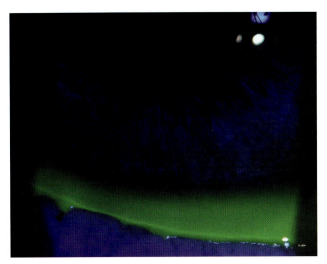

Fig. 2.4 High marginal tear strip stained with fluorescein

wall of the sac and the lacrimal bone behind it (Fig. 2.6B). As a crimped canaliculus with occlusion of the cannula tip against the canalicular wall can also give this impression, it is worthwhile slightly retracting the tip, increasing the lateral tension on the lid, and gently repeating the attempt to advance the probe. In the case of lower canalicular obstruction, a soft stop will be associated with reflux of saline through the lower punctum. Reflux through the upper punctum indicates patency of both upper and lower canaliculi, but obstruction of the common canaliculus.

Jones dye testing

Dye testing is indicated only in patients with suspected partial obstruction of the drainage system. Epiphora is present, but there is no punctal abnormality and the patient tastes saline in his or her throat on irrigation.

- **The primary test** (Fig. 2.7A) differentiates partial obstruction of the lacrimal passages and lacrimal pump failure from primary hypersecretion of tears. A drop of 2% fluorescein is instilled into the conjunctival sac of one eye only. After about 5 minutes, a cotton-tipped bud moistened in local anaesthetic is inserted under the inferior turbinate at the nasolacrimal duct opening. The results are interpreted as follows:
  - ○ Positive: fluorescein recovered from the nose indicates patency of the drainage system. Watering is due to primary hypersecretion and no further tests are necessary.
  - ○ Negative: no dye recovered from the nose indicates a partial obstruction (site unknown) or failure of the lacrimal pump mechanism. In this situation the secondary dye test is performed immediately. There is a high false-negative rate – that is, dye is commonly not recovered even in the presence of a functionally patent drainage system. Modifications involving direct observation of the oropharynx using cobalt blue light for up to an hour may reduce the false-negative rate almost to zero.

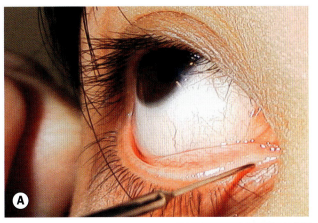

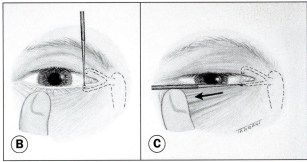

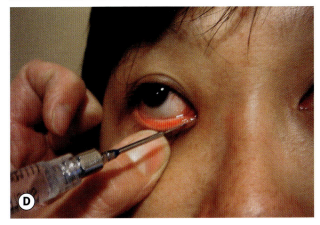

Fig. 2.5 (A) Dilatation of the inferior punctum; **(B,C)** dilatation technique; **(D)** irrigation
(Courtesy of K Nischal – figs A and D)

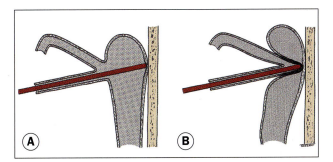

Fig. 2.6 Possible results of probing. **(A)** Hard stop; **(B)** soft stop

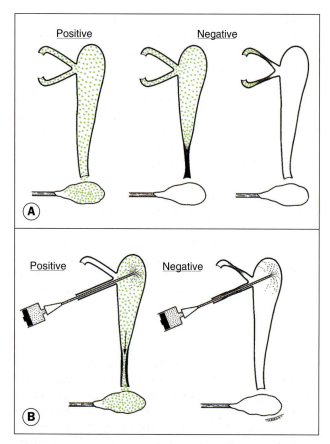

Fig. 2.7 Jones dye testing. **(A)** Primary; **(B)** secondary

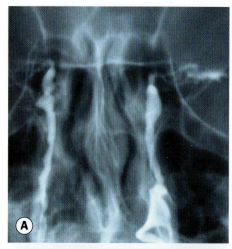

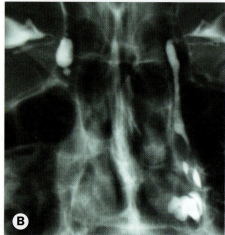

- **The secondary (irrigation) test** (Fig. 2.7B) identifies lacrimal pump failure or the probable site of partial obstruction, on the basis of whether the topical fluorescein instilled for the primary test entered the lacrimal sac. Topical anaesthetic is instilled and any residual fluorescein washed out from the conjunctival fornix. The drainage system is then irrigated with a cotton bud under the inferior turbinate.
  - Positive: fluorescein-stained saline recovered from the nose indicates that fluorescein entered the lacrimal sac, thus confirming functional patency of the upper lacrimal passages. Partial obstruction of the nasolacrimal duct distal to the sac is inferred.
  - Negative: unstained saline recovered from the nose indicates that fluorescein did not enter the lacrimal sac. This implies upper lacrimal (punctal or canalicular) dysfunction, which may be due to partial physical occlusion and/or pump failure.

Contrast dacryocystography

Dacryocystography (DCG – Fig. 2.8) involves the injection of radio-opaque contrast medium (ethiodized oil) into the canaliculi followed by the capture of magnified images. Indications include confirmation of the precise site of lacrimal drainage obstruction to guide surgery, and the diagnosis of diverticuli, fistulae and filling defects (e.g. stones, tumours). It should not be performed

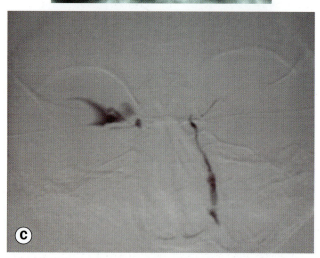

Fig. 2.8 Dacryocystography (DCG). **(A)** Conventional DCG without subtraction shows normal filling on both sides; **(B)** normal left filling and obstruction at the junction of the right sac and nasolacrimal duct; **(C)** digital subtraction DCG showing similar findings to **(B)**

(Courtesy of A Pearson)

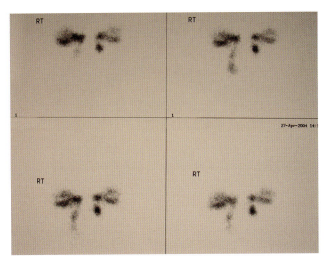

Fig. 2.9 Nuclear lacrimal scintigraphy showing passage of tracer via the right lacrimal system but obstructed drainage in the left nasolacrimal duct
(Courtesy of A Pearson)

in the presence of acute infection. A DCG is unnecessary if the site of obstruction is obvious (e.g. regurgitating mucocoele). A normal dacryocystogram in the presence of subjective and objective epiphora suggests failure of the lacrimal pump, though this is more readily demonstrated by simple irrigation.

Nuclear lacrimal scintigraphy

Scintigraphy (Fig. 2.9) assesses tear drainage under more physiological conditions than DCG, by labelling the tears with a radioactive substance and tracking their progress. Although it does not provide the same detailed anatomical visualization as DCG, it may be used to identify the location of a partial or functional block (e.g. indicating the absence of significant tear entry to the canaliculi, localizing the site of physiological obstruction to the eyelids), to confirm functional obstruction, or sometimes to confirm the presence of normal drainage such that surgery is not indicated.

CT and MRI

Computed tomography (CT) and magnetic resonance imaging (MRI) are occasionally employed in the assessment of lacrimal obstruction, for instance in the investigation of paranasal sinus or suspected lacrimal sac pathology.

Internal nasal examination

Assessment of the nasal cavity, especially with endoscopy, can be invaluable in the detection of obstructions such as nasal polyps or a deviated septum.

ACQUIRED OBSTRUCTION

Conjunctivochalasis

Conjunctivochalasis is characterized by one or more folds of redundant conjunctiva prolapsing over the lower eyelid margin

(see Fig. 2.3C). It can exacerbate the symptoms of dry eye and commonly contributes to epiphora, of which it can be an under-recognized cause. It is thought to be predominantly an involutional process involving the loss of conjunctival adhesion to underlying Tenon capsule and episclera and may be analogous to the conjunctival abnormalities leading to superior limbic keratoconjunctivitis (see Ch. 5). Chronic low-grade ocular surface inflammation (e.g. dry eye, blepharitis) is likely to play a role. If severe, exposure of a redundant fold can occur (Fig. 2.10).

- **Observation or lubricants** alone may be appropriate in mild cases.
- **Topical steroids** or other anti-inflammatories.
- **Surgical options** include securing the bulbar conjunctiva to the sclera with three absorbable sutures (e.g. 6-0 polyglactin) placed 6–8 mm from the limbus, or excision of a crescent-shaped area of excess bulbar conjunctiva, with an anterior limit of around 6 mm from the limbus; suturing the edges of the excised patch together, or replacement with amniotic membrane have been described.

Primary punctal stenosis

Primary stenosis (see Fig. 2.3A) occurs in the absence of punctal eversion. The most common causes are chronic blepharitis and idiopathic stenosis; others include herpes simplex and herpes zoster lid infection, local radiotherapy, cicatrizing conjunctivitis, chronic topical glaucoma treatment, systemic cytotoxic drugs such as 5-fluorouracil, and rare systemic conditions such as porphyria cutanea tarda.

- **Dilatation** of the punctum alone can be tried but rarely gives sustained benefit.
- **Punctoplasty** is usually required. A number of techniques have been described, including one-, two- (Fig. 2.11) or three-snip enlargement with removal of the posterior ampulla wall, and procedures using a mechanical punch, laser or microsurgery; a temporary stent can be used.

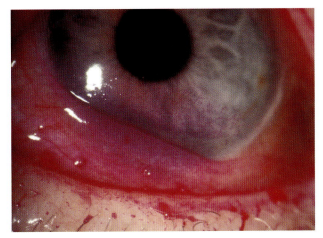

Fig. 2.10 Conjunctivochalasis. Substantial exposed fold with conjunctival and corneal rose Bengal staining
(Courtesy of S Tuft)

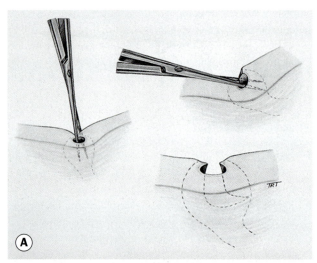

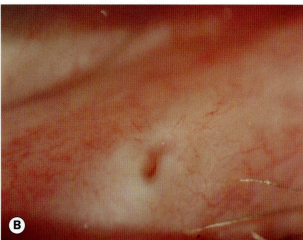

Fig. 2.11 Two-snip punctoplasty. **(A)** Technique; **(B)** postoperative appearance

Secondary punctal stenosis

Secondary stenosis occurs after punctal eversion leads to chronic failure of tear entry, and punctoplasty is usually performed in conjunction with correction of the eversion.

- *Retropunctal (Ziegler) cautery* can be used for pure punctal eversion. Burns are applied to the palpebral conjunctiva at approximately 5 mm below the punctum. Subsequent tissue shrinkage should invert the punctum.
- *Medial conjunctivoplasty* can be used in medial ectropion of a larger area of lid if there is no substantial horizontal laxity. A diamond-shaped piece of tarsoconjunctiva is excised, about 4 mm high and 8 mm wide, parallel with and inferolateral to the canaliculus and punctum, followed by approximation of the superior and inferior wound margins with sutures (Fig. 2.12). Incorporation of the lower lid retractors in the sutures further aids repositioning.
- *Lower lid tightening*, usually with a tarsal strip, is used to correct lower lid laxity and may be combined with medial conjunctivoplasty where there is a significant medial ectropion component.

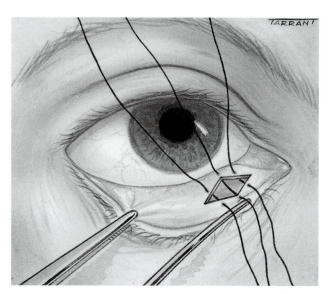

Fig. 2.12 Medial conjunctivoplasty

Canalicular obstruction

Causes include congenital, trauma, herpes simplex infection, drugs and irradiation. Chronic dacryocystitis can cause a membrane to form in the common canaliculus. The initial surgical approach has tended over recent years to attempt to preserve the physiological anatomy.

- **Partial obstruction** of the common or individual canaliculi, or anywhere in the lacrimal drainage system, may be treated by simple intubation of one or both canaliculi with silicone stents. These are left *in situ* for 6 weeks to 6 months (Fig. 2.13).
- **Total individual canalicular obstruction**
  - Canalicular trephination using a purpose-made minitrephine (Sisler), followed by intubation; trephination has also been described using an intravenous catheter with a retracted introducer needle used as a stent and then advanced to overcome the obstruction. Balloon canaliculoplasty and endoscopic laser techniques are

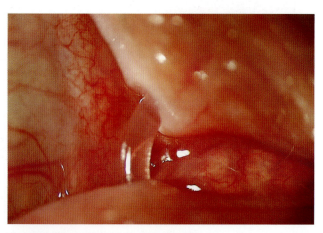

Fig. 2.13 Silicone lacrimal stent *in situ*

available. These less invasive options may have lower success rates than more aggressive surgery.

○ With 6–8 mm of patent normal canaliculus between the punctum and the obstruction, anastomosis of the patent part of the canaliculus into the lacrimal sac, with intubation, can be performed (canaliculodacryocystorhinostomy – CDCR).

○ Where obstruction is severe or it is not possible to anastomose functioning canaliculi to the lacrimal sac, conventional surgery consists of conjunctivodacryocystorhinostomy and the insertion of a toughened glass (Lester Jones) tube (Fig. 2.14); this may also be used when the lacrimal system is intact but non-functioning due to failure of the physiological pump (e.g. facial nerve palsy). The surgery is performed as for an external approach dacryocystorhinostomy (DCR – see below) but the caruncle is excised and a track for the tube created between the lacus lacrimalis and the lacrimal sac. Patient satisfaction is variable.

Nasolacrimal duct obstruction

- **Causes**
  ○ Idiopathic stenosis – by far the most common.
  ○ Naso-orbital trauma, including nasal and sinus surgery.
  ○ Granulomatous disease such as Wegener granulomatosis and sarcoidosis.
  ○ Infiltration by nasopharyngeal tumours.
- **Treatment**
  ○ Conventional (external approach) dacryocystorhinostomy (DCR) is indicated for obstruction distal to the medial opening of the common canaliculus, and consists of anastomosis of the lacrimal sac to the mucosa of the middle nasal meatus. The procedure is usually performed under hypotensive general anaesthesia. A vertical skin incision is made 10 mm medial to the inner canthus, the

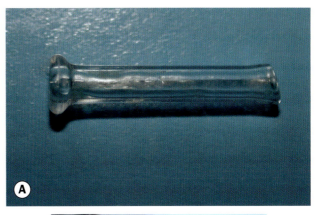

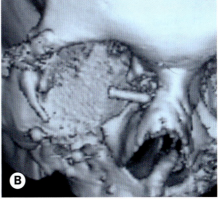

Fig. 2.14 (A) Lester Jones tube; **(B)** CT scan 3D reconstruction of tube *in situ*

medial canthal tendon and lacrimal sac exposed and reflected, and after removal of the intervening bone the sac is incised and attached to an opening created in the nasal mucosa (Fig. 2.15). The success rate is over 90%; causes of failure include inadequate size and position of the ostium, unrecognized common canalicular

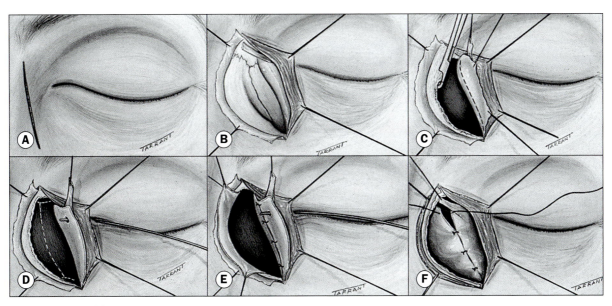

Fig. 2.15 Dacryocystorhinostomy

obstruction, scarring and the 'sump syndrome', in which the surgical opening in the lacrimal bone is too small and too high. Complications include cutaneous scarring, injury to medial canthal structures, haemorrhage, infection and cerebrospinal fluid rhinorrhoea if the subarachnoid space is inadvertently entered.

○ Endoscopic DCR encompasses several techniques. A light pipe can be passed through the canalicular system into the lacrimal sac to guide an endoscopic approach from within the nose, or a microendoscopic transcanalicular procedure can be performed using a drill or laser to establish communication with the nasal cavity. Advantages over conventional DCR include less marked systemic disturbance with minimal blood loss and a lower risk of cerebrospinal fluid leakage, the avoidance of a skin incision and generally a shorter operating time. Disadvantages include generally a slightly lower success rate and visualization difficulties, meaning that additional procedures are sometimes needed.

○ Other procedures, often reserved for partial nasolacrimal duct obstruction, include probing and intubation, stent insertion and balloon dacryocystoplasty.

Dacryolithiasis

Dacryoliths (lacrimal stones) may occur in any part of the lacrimal system. They are more common in males. Although the pathogenesis is unclear, it has been proposed that tear stagnation secondary to inflammatory obstruction may precipitate stone formation, which tends to be associated with squamous metaplasia of the lacrimal sac epithelium. Presentation is often in late adulthood; symptoms may include intermittent epiphora, recurrent attacks of acute dacryocystitis and lacrimal sac distension.

The lacrimal sac is distended and relatively firm, but is not inflamed and tender as in acute dacryocystitis.

Mucus reflux on pressure may or may not be present. Treatment involves a DCR.

CONGENITAL OBSTRUCTION

Nasolacrimal duct obstruction

The lower end of the nasolacrimal duct, in the region of the valve of Hasner, is the last portion of the lacrimal drainage system to canalize, with complete patency most commonly occurring soon after birth. Epiphora affects at least 20% of neonates, but spontaneous resolution occurs in over 95% within the first year; it has been suggested that early epiphora with resolution may be regarded as a normal variant.

- **Signs**
  ○ Epiphora and matting of eyelashes may be constant or intermittent, and may be particularly noticeable when the child has an upper respiratory tract infection; intercurrent frank bacterial conjunctivitis may be treated with a broad-spectrum topical antibiotic.

○ Gentle pressure over the lacrimal sac may cause mucopurulent reflux.
○ Acute dacryocystitis is very rare.
○ Normal visual function should be confirmed as far as possible, and an anterior segment examination with assessment of the red reflex performed.
○ The fluorescein disappearance test (see above) is highly specific in this setting; only a fine line of dye, at most, should remain at 5–10 minutes under inspection with a blue light in a darkened room.

- **Differential diagnosis** includes other congenital causes of a watering eye, such as punctal atresia; it is important to exclude congenital glaucoma, chronic conjunctivitis (e.g. chlamydial), keratitis and uveitis.

- **Treatment**
  ○ Massage of the lacrimal sac has been suggested as a means of rupturing a membranous obstruction by hydrostatic pressure. The index finger is initially placed over the common canaliculus to block reflux, and then rolled over the sac, massaging downwards. The likelihood of success and the optimal regimen is undetermined.
  ○ Probing. Passage of a fine wire via the canalicular system and nasolacrimal duct (Fig. 2.16) to disrupt the obstructive membrane at the valve of Hasner is usually regarded as the definitive treatment, and may be preceded and followed by irrigation to confirm the site of obstruction and subsequent patency respectively. Probing can be repeated if a first procedure is unsuccessful. Nasal endoscopic guidance may enhance success, and should be considered at least for repeat procedures. If symptoms are mild–moderate, probing may be delayed until the age of 12–18, or even 24, months and is carried out under general anaesthesia. For more marked symptoms, early probing may be appropriate and in young children is sometimes performed under topical anaesthesia in an outpatient setting. Risks include the induction of canalicular stenosis due to probe trauma, which may be relatively common. It should be noted that there is little

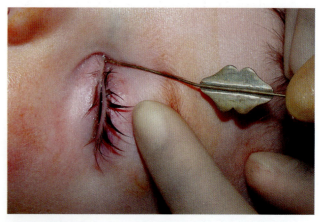

Fig. 2.16 Probing of the nasolacrimal duct
(Courtesy of K Nischal)

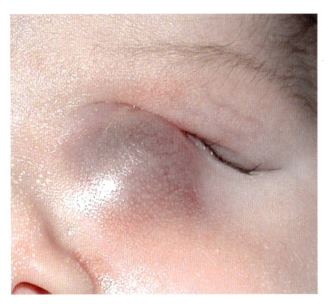

Fig. 2.17 Congenital dacryocoele
(Courtesy of A Pearson)

evidence of a difference in final outcome at 24 months conferred by intervention versus non-intervention. Failure of probing may result from abnormal anatomy, which can usually be recognized by difficulty in passing the probe and subsequent non-patency of the drainage system on irrigation.

○ Options after probing failure include intubation with silastic tubing with or without balloon dilatation of the nasolacrimal duct, endoscopic procedures, and dacryocystorhinostomy.

Congenital dacryocoele

A congenital dacryocoele (amniontocoele) is a collection of amniotic fluid or mucus in the lacrimal sac caused by an imperforate Hasner valve. Presentation is perinatal with a bluish cystic swelling at or below the medial canthus (Fig. 2.17), accompanied by epiphora. If an intranasal component is large it can cause respiratory distress. It should not be mistaken for an encephalocoele, the latter being characterized by a pulsatile swelling above the medial canthal tendon. Resolution is common with only conservative treatment, but if this fails, probing is usually adequate.

CHRONIC CANALICULITIS

Chronic canaliculitis is an uncommon condition, frequently caused by *Actinomyces israelii*, anaerobic Gram-positive bacteria. Occasionally scarring and canalicular obstruction may result. Presentation is with unilateral epiphora associated with chronic mucopurulent conjunctivitis refractory to conventional treatment. There is pericanalicular redness and oedema, and mucopurulent discharge on pressure over the canaliculus (Fig. 2.18A). A 'pouting' punctum (see Fig. 2.3F) may be a diagnostic clue in mild cases. In contrast to dacryocystitis, there is no lacrimal sac

involvement. Concretions (sulfur granules) are metabolic products of *Actinomyces* and other hydrogen sulfide-utilizing bacteria, and classically are expressed on canalicular compression or following canaliculotomy (Fig. 2.18B). A topical antibiotic such as a fluoroquinolone four times daily for 10 days may be tried initially but is rarely curative unless combined with canaliculotomy (a linear incision into the conjunctival side of the canaliculus) and curettage of concretions. Giant fornix syndrome (see Ch. 5), dacryolithiasis and lacrimal diverticulum may give a similar clinical picture. Herpes simplex is a classic cause of acute – as opposed to chronic – canaliculitis.

DACRYOCYSTITIS

Infection of the lacrimal sac is usually secondary to obstruction of the nasolacrimal duct. It may be acute or chronic and is most commonly staphylococcal or streptococcal.

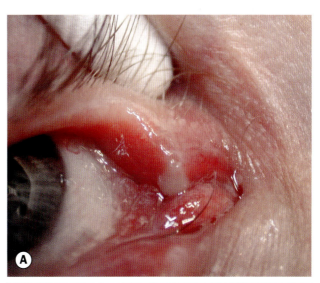

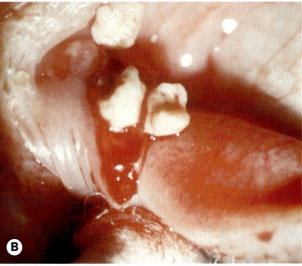

Fig. 2.18 Chronic canaliculitis. **(A)** Mucopurulent discharge on pressure over an inflamed upper canaliculus; **(B)** sulfur concretions released by canaliculotomy
(Courtesy of S Tuft – fig. B)

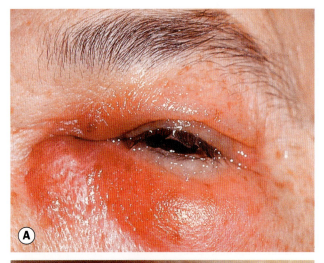

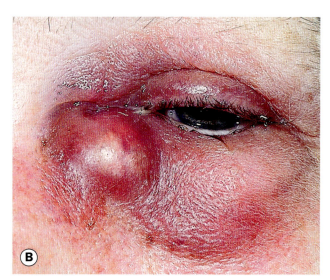

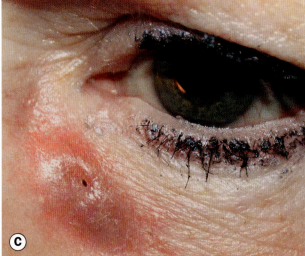

Fig. 2.19 (A) Acute dacryocystitis; **(B)** lacrimal abscess and preseptal cellulitis; **(C)** lacrimal fistula

(Courtesy of A Pearson – figs B and C)

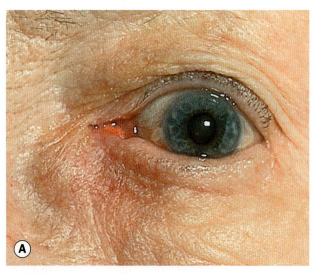

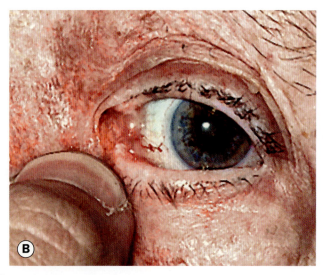

Fig. 2.20 (A) Mucocoele; **(B)** expression of mucopurulent material

Acute dacryocystitis

Presentation is with the subacute onset of pain in the medial canthal area, associated with epiphora. A very tender, tense red swelling develops at the medial canthus (Fig. 2.19A), commonly progressing to abscess formation (Fig. 2.19B); there may be associated preseptal cellulitis.

- **Treatment**
  - Initial treatment involves the application of warm compresses and oral antibiotics such as flucloxacillin or co-amoxiclav; irrigation and probing should not be performed.
  - Incision and drainage may be considered if pus points and an abscess is about to drain spontaneously. However, this carries the risk of a persistent sac–skin fistula (Fig. 2.19C).
  - Dacryocystorhinostomy is commonly required after the acute infection has been controlled, and may reduce the risk of recurrent infection.

Chronic dacryocystitis

Presentation is with chronic epiphora, which may be associated with a chronic or recurrent unilateral conjunctivitis. A mucocoele is usually evident as a painless swelling at the inner canthus (Fig. 2.20A), but if an obvious swelling is absent pressure over the sac commonly still results in mucopurulent canalicular reflux (Fig. 2.20B). Treatment is with a dacryocystorhinostomy; the enlarged sac often makes this technically easier.

Chapter 3

Orbit

INTRODUCTION

Anatomy

The orbit is a pear-shaped cavity, the stalk of which is the optic canal (Fig. 3.1).

- **The roof** consists of two bones: the lesser wing of the sphenoid and the orbital plate of the frontal bone. It is located subjacent to the anterior cranial fossa and the frontal sinus. A defect in the orbital roof may cause pulsatile proptosis due to transmission of cerebrospinal fluid pulsation to the orbit.
- **The lateral wall** also consists of two bones: the greater wing of the sphenoid and the zygomatic. The anterior half of the globe is vulnerable to lateral trauma since it protrudes beyond the lateral orbital margin.
- **The floor** consists of three bones: the zygomatic, maxillary and palatine. The posteromedial portion of the maxillary bone is relatively weak and may be involved in a 'blowout' fracture (see Ch. 21). The orbital floor also forms the roof of the maxillary sinus so that maxillary carcinoma invading the orbit may displace the globe upwards.
- **The medial wall** consists of four bones: maxillary, lacrimal, ethmoid and sphenoid. The lamina papyracea, which forms part of the medial wall, is paper-thin and perforated by numerous foramina for nerves and blood vessels. Orbital cellulitis is therefore frequently secondary to ethmoidal sinusitis.
- **The superior orbital fissure** is a slit linking the cranium and the orbit, between the greater and lesser wings of the sphenoid bone; through it pass numerous important structures.
  - o The superior portion contains the lacrimal, frontal and trochlear nerves, and the superior ophthalmic vein.
  - o The inferior portion contains the superior and inferior divisions of the oculomotor nerve, the abducens and nasociliary nerves, and sympathetic fibres from the cavernous plexus.
  - o Inflammation of the superior orbital fissure and apex (Tolosa–Hunt syndrome) may therefore result in a multitude of signs including ophthalmoplegia and venous outflow obstruction.
- **The inferior orbital fissure** lies between the greater wing of the sphenoid and the maxilla, connecting the orbit to the pterygopalatine and infratemporal fossae. Through it run the maxillary nerve, the zygomatic nerve and branches of the pterygopalatine ganglion, as well as the inferior ophthalmic vein.

Clinical features

Symptoms

Symptoms of orbital disease include eyelid and conjunctival swelling, redness, watering, pain (sometimes on, or exacerbated by, eye movement), increasing ocular prominence, displacement or a sunken impression of the eye, double vision and blurring, and sometimes a pulsing sensation or audible bruit.

Soft tissue involvement

Eyelid and periocular oedema, skin discoloration, ptosis, chemosis (oedema of the conjunctiva, which may involve the plica and caruncle) and epibulbar injection (Fig. 3.2) may be seen; causes include thyroid eye disease, orbital inflammatory diseases and obstruction to venous drainage.

Proptosis

Proptosis (Fig. 3.3) describes an abnormal protrusion of an organ, but is generally applied to the eyeball; exophthalmos refers

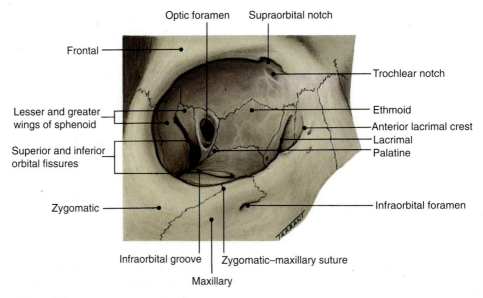

Fig. 3.1 Anatomy of the orbit

Frontal

Optic foramen

Supraorbital notch

Trochlear notch

Lesser and greater wings of sphenoid

Ethmoid

Anterior lacrimal crest

Lacrimal

Palatine

Superior and inferior orbital fissures

Zygomatic

Infraorbital foramen

Infraorbital groove

Zygomatic–maxillary suture

Maxillary

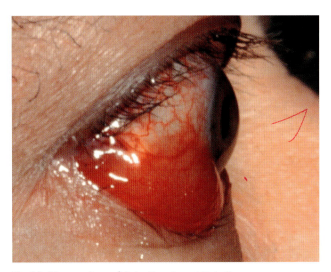

Fig. 3.2 Chemosis and injection in orbital disease

specifically to the eyeball only. Proptosis may be caused by retro-bulbar lesions or, less frequently, a shallow orbit. The intraorbital portion of the optic nerve is longer (25 mm) than the distance between the back of the globe and the optic canal (18 mm). This allows for significant forward displacement of the globe (proptosis) without excessive stretching of the nerve.

- **Asymmetrical proptosis** is readily detected by looking down at the patient from above and behind (Fig. 3.4A).
- **The direction** of proptosis may indicate the likely pathology. For example, space-occupying lesions within the muscle cone such as a cavernous haemangioma or optic nerve tumours cause axial proptosis, whereas extraconal lesions usually give rise to combined proptosis and dystopia (see next).
- **Dystopia** implies displacement of the globe in the coronal plane, usually due to an extraconal orbital mass such as a lacrimal gland tumour (Fig. 3.4B). Horizontal displacement is measured from the midline (nose) to the centre of the pupil while vertical dystopia is read on a vertical scale perpendicular to a horizontal rule placed over the bridge of the nose. The measured eye should fixate straight ahead, if necessary facilitating this by occluding the fellow eye.
- **The severity** of proptosis can be measured with a plastic rule resting on the lateral orbital margin, or with the Luedde™ exophthalmometer using a similar principle. Commonly, a binocular exophthalmometer (e.g. Hertel) is employed, using visualization of the corneal apices to determine the

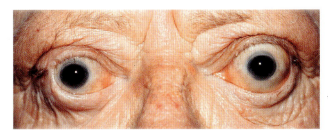

Fig. 3.3 Bilateral proptosis
(Courtesy of C Barry)

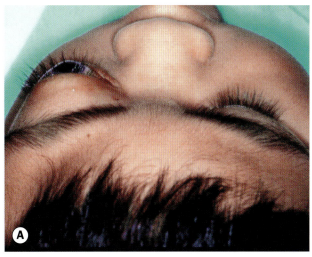

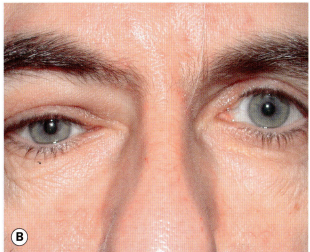

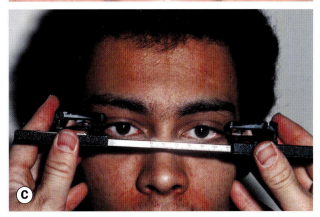

Fig. 3.4 General signs of orbital disease. **(A)** Left proptosis visualized from above; **(B)** right inferior dystopia; **(C)** measurement of proptosis with an exophthalmometer

degree of ocular protrusion from a scale (Fig. 3.4C). Measurements can be taken both relaxed and with the Valsalva manoeuvre. Readings greater than 20 mm are indicative of proptosis and a difference of 2–3 mm or more between the two eyes is suspicious regardless of the absolute values. The dimensions of the palpebral apertures and any lagophthalmos should also be noted.

- **Pseudoproptosis** (the false impression of proptosis) may be due to facial asymmetry, enlargement of the globe (e.g. high myopia or buphthalmos), lid retraction or contralateral enophthalmos.

Enophthalmos

Enophthalmos implies recession of the globe within the orbit. Causes include congenital and traumatic orbital wall abnormalities, atrophy of the orbital contents (e.g. radiotherapy, scleroderma, chronic eye poking in blind infants – the 'oculodigital' sign) or sclerosis (e.g. metastatic scirrhous carcinoma, sclerosing orbital inflammatory disease). Pseudoenophthalmos may be caused by a small or shrunken eye (microphthalmos or phthisis bulbi), by ptosis, or by contralateral proptosis or pseudoproptosis.

Ophthalmoplegia

Defective ocular motility is very common in orbital disease. Causes include an orbital mass, restrictive myopathy (e.g. thyroid eye disease – Fig. 3.5, orbital myositis, tethering of muscles or tissue after orbital wall fracture), ocular motor nerve involvement associated with lesions in the cavernous sinus, orbital fissures or posterior orbit (e.g. carotid–cavernous fistula, Tolosa–Hunt syndrome, malignant lacrimal gland tumours). The following tests may be used to differentiate a restrictive from a neurological motility defect:

- **Forced duction test.** Under topical anaesthesia, the insertion of the muscle in an involved eye is grasped with forceps and the globe rotated in the direction of reduced mobility; checked movement of the globe indicates a restrictive problem; no resistance will be encountered with a neurological lesion.
- **Differential intraocular pressure (IOP) test** involves less discomfort than forced duction and an objective rather than subjective endpoint. The IOP is measured in the primary position of gaze and then with the patient attempting to look in the direction of limited mobility; an increase of 6 mmHg or more denotes resistance transmitted to the globe by muscle restriction (the Braley sign).
- **Saccadic eye movements** in neurological lesions are reduced in velocity, while restrictive defects manifest normal saccadic velocity with sudden halting of ocular movement.

Dynamic properties

- **Increasing venous pressure** by dependent head position, the Valsalva manoeuvre or jugular compression may induce or exacerbate proptosis in patients with orbital venous anomalies or infants with orbital capillary haemangioma.
- **Pulsation** is caused either by an arteriovenous communication or a defect in the orbital roof. In the former, pulsation may be associated with a bruit depending on the size of the communication. In the latter the pulsation is transmitted from the brain by the cerebrospinal fluid and there is no associated bruit. Mild pulsation is best detected on the slit lamp, particularly by applanation tonometry.
- **A bruit** is a sign found with a larger carotid–cavernous fistula. It is best heard with the bell of the stethoscope and is lessened or abolished by gently compressing the ipsilateral carotid artery in the neck.

Fundus changes

- **Optic disc swelling** may be the initial feature of compressive optic neuropathy (Fig. 3.6A).
- **Optic atrophy** (Fig. 3.6B), which may be preceded by swelling, is a feature of severe compressive optic neuropathy. Important causes include thyroid eye disease and optic nerve tumours.

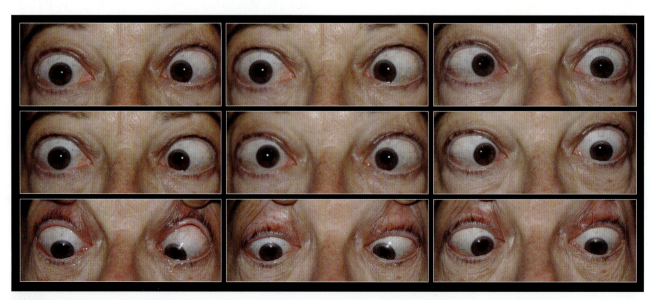

Fig. 3.5 Restrictive myopathy and bilateral lid retraction and proptosis in thyroid eye disease – nine positions of gaze
(Courtesy of C Barry)

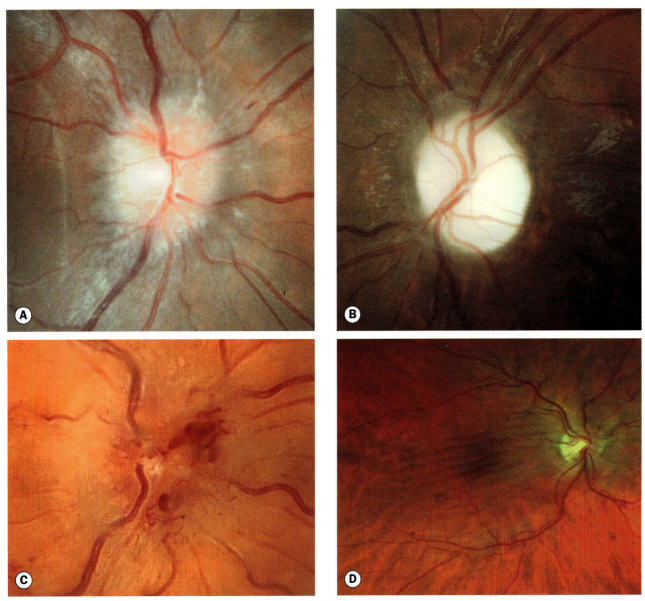

Fig. 3.6 Fundus changes in orbital disease. **(A)** Disc swelling; **(B)** optic atrophy; **(C)** opticociliary vessels on a chronically swollen disc; **(D)** choroidal folds

(Courtesy of S Chen – fig. D)

- **Opticociliary collaterals** consist of enlarged pre-existing peripapillary capillaries that divert blood from the central retinal venous circulation to the peripapillary choroidal circulation when there is obstruction of the normal drainage channels. On ophthalmoscopy the vessels appear as large tortuous channels most frequently sited temporally, which disappear at the disc margin (Fig. 3.6C). The collaterals may be associated with any orbital or optic nerve tumour that compresses the intraorbital optic nerve and impairs blood flow through the central retinal vein. The most common tumour associated with shunts is an optic nerve sheath meningioma but they may also occur with optic nerve glioma, central retinal vein occlusion, idiopathic intracranial hypertension and glaucoma.

- **Choroidal folds** (Fig. 3.6D) are discussed in detail in Ch. 14; they may occur in a wide variety of orbital lesions. Although tending to be more common with greater amounts of proptosis and anteriorly located tumours, in some cases their presence can precede the onset of proptosis.

Investigation

- **Computed tomography (CT)** is useful for depicting bony structures and the location and size of space-occupying lesions. It is of particular value in patients with orbital trauma because it can detect small fractures, foreign bodies, blood, herniation of extraocular muscle and emphysema (see Ch. 21). It is, however, unable to distinguish different pathological soft tissue masses that are radiologically isodense. Confirmation of an orbital abscess in cellulitis is a relatively common indication.

- **Magnetic resonance imaging (MRI)** can demonstrate orbital apex lesions and intracranial extension of orbital tumours, and is useful for imaging orbital inflammatory disease. Serial short T1 inversion recovery (STIR) scans are valuable in assessing inflammatory activity in thyroid eye disease (see Ch. 19).
- **Plain X-rays** are little used except for the initial diagnosis of traumatic bony injury.
- **Ultrasonography** can provide useful information, particularly with high-grade apparatus and an experienced operator, but does not image the orbital apex well.
- **Fine needle biopsy** is sometimes performed, particularly in suspected neoplastic disease. Potential problems include haemorrhage and ocular penetration.

THYROID EYE DISEASE

Introduction

Thyroid eye disease (TED), also known as thyroid-associated orbitopathy and Graves ophthalmopathy, is a very common orbital disorder, and is the most common cause of both bilateral and unilateral proptosis in an adult.

Thyrotoxicosis

Thyrotoxicosis (hyperthyroidism) is a condition involving excessive secretion of thyroid hormones. Graves disease, the most common form of hyperthyroidism, is an autoimmune disorder in which IgG antibodies bind to thyroid stimulating hormone (TSH) receptors in the thyroid gland and stimulate secretion of thyroid hormones. It is more common in females and may be associated with other autoimmune disorders. Presentation is often in the fourth or fifth decades with symptoms including weight loss despite good appetite, increased bowel frequency, sweating, heat intolerance, nervousness, irritability, palpitations, weakness and fatigue. There may be enlargement of the thyroid gland, tremor, palmar erythema, and warm and sweaty skin. Thyroid acropachy is a phenomenon similar to clubbing of the fingers, occurring in 1%; pretibial myxoedema (1–5%) is indurated thickening of the skin of the shins. Cardiac manifestations may include sinus tachycardia and other arrhythmias. Other autoimmune disorders can be associated. Thyroid function is commonly tested initially with a TSH level; if this is low, or normal but thyroid disease is still suspected, a range of additional investigations can be carried out. Treatment options include carbimazole, propylthiouracil, propranolol, thyroid ablation with radioactive iodine, and partial thyroidectomy.

Risk factors for ophthalmopathy

Once a patient has Graves disease, the major clinical risk factor for developing TED is smoking. The greater the number of cigarettes smoked per day, the greater the risk, and giving up smoking seems to reduce the risk. Women are five times more likely to be affected by TED than men, but this largely reflects the increased incidence of Graves disease in women. Radioactive iodine used to treat hyperthyroidism can worsen TED. TED can also, though less commonly, occur in euthyroid and hypothyroid (including treated hyperthyroid) patients. It can sometimes be the presenting manifestation of thyroid-related disease.

Pathogenesis of ophthalmopathy

Thyroid ophthalmopathy involves an organ-specific autoimmune reaction in which an antibody that reacts against thyroid gland cells and orbital fibroblasts leads to inflammation of extraocular muscles, interstitial tissues, orbital fat and lacrimal glands characterized by pleomorphic cellular infiltration, associated with increased secretion of glycosaminoglycans and osmotic imbibition of water. There is an increase in the volume of the orbital contents, particularly the muscles, which can swell to eight times their normal size. There may be a secondary elevation of intraorbital pressure, and the optic nerve may be compressed. Subsequent degeneration of muscle fibres eventually leads to fibrosis, which exerts a tethering effect on the involved muscle, resulting in restrictive myopathy and diplopia.

Clinical features

Introduction

TED typically proceeds through a congestive (inflammatory) stage in which the eyes are red and painful; this tends to remit within 1–3 years and only about 10% of patients develop serious long-term ocular problems. A fibrotic (quiescent) stage follows in which the eyes are white, although a painless motility defect may be present. Clinical features broadly can be categorized into (i) soft tissue involvement, (ii) lid retraction, (iii) proptosis, (iv) optic neuropathy and (v) restrictive myopathy. A commonly used classification for the severity of TED has been issued by the European Group on Graves Orbitopathy (EUGOGO): (i) sight-threatening due to optic neuropathy or corneal breakdown; (ii) moderate–severe, with one of moderate–severe soft tissue involvement, lid retraction of 2 mm or more, diplopia and proptosis of 3 mm or more; (iii) mild, with only a minor impact on daily life.

Soft tissue involvement

- **Symptoms.** Grittiness, red eyes, lacrimation, photophobia, puffy lids and retrobulbar discomfort.
- **Signs** may include:
  - Epibulbar hyperaemia. This is a sensitive sign of inflammatory activity. Intense focal hyperaemia may outline the insertions of the horizontal recti (Fig. 3.7A).
  - Periorbital swelling is caused by oedema and infiltration behind the orbital septum; this may be associated with chemosis and prolapse of retroseptal fat into the eyelids (Fig. 3.7B).

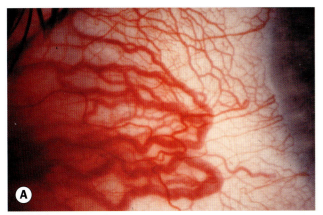

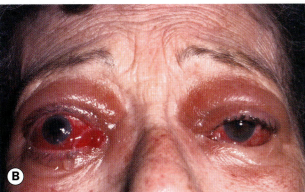

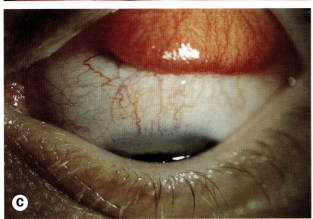

Fig. 3.7 Soft tissue involvement in thyroid eye disease. **(A)** Epibulbar hyperaemia overlying a horizontal rectus muscle; **(B)** periorbital oedema, chemosis and prolapse of fat into the eyelids; **(C)** superior limbic keratoconjunctivitis

○ Tear insufficiency and instability is common.
○ Corneal signs are exacerbated by lid retraction (see next) and can include punctate epithelial erosions, superior limbic keratoconjunctivitis (Fig. 3.7C and see Ch. 5), and occasionally bacterial keratitis, thinning and scarring.

Lid retraction

Retraction of upper and lower lids occurs in about 50% of patients with Graves disease. Humorally induced overaction of Müller muscle is postulated to occur as a result of sympathetic overstimulation secondary to high levels of thyroid hormones. Fibrotic contracture of the levator palpebrae and inferior rectus muscles associated with adhesion to overlying orbital tissues is another probable mechanism, together with secondary overaction in response to hypo- or hypertropia produced by fibrosis.

- **Symptoms.** Patients may complain of a staring or bulging-eyed appearance, difficulty closing the eyes and ocular surface symptoms.
- **Signs**
  ○ The upper lid margin normally rests 2 mm below the limbus (Fig. 3.8A, right eye). Lid retraction is suspected when the margin is either level with or above the superior limbus, allowing sclera to be visible ('scleral show'; Fig. 3.8A, left eye).
  ○ The lower eyelid margin normally rests at the inferior limbus; retraction is suspected when sclera shows below the limbus. Lid retraction may occur in isolation or in association with proptosis, which exaggerates its severity.
  ○ The Dalrymple sign is lid retraction in primary gaze (Fig. 3.8B).
  ○ The Kocher sign describes a staring and frightened appearance of the eyes which is particularly marked on attentive fixation (Fig. 3.8C).
  ○ The von Graefe sign signifies retarded descent of the upper lid on downgaze (lid lag – Fig. 3.8D).

Proptosis

- **Symptoms** are similar to those of lid retraction.
- **Signs.** Proptosis is axial, unilateral or bilateral, symmetrical (Fig. 3.9A) or asymmetrical (Fig. 3.9B), and frequently permanent. Severe proptosis may compromise lid closure and along with lid retraction and tear dysfunction can lead to exposure keratopathy, corneal ulceration and infection (Fig. 3.9C).

Restrictive myopathy

Between 30% and 50% of patients with TED develop ophthalmoplegia and this may be permanent. Ocular motility is restricted initially by inflammatory oedema, and later by fibrosis.

- **Symptoms.** Double vision, and often discomfort in some positions of gaze.
- **Signs,** in approximate order of frequency:
  ○ Elevation defect (Fig. 3.10A) caused by fibrotic contracture of the inferior rectus, may mimic superior rectus palsy and is the most common motility deficit.
  ○ Abduction defect due to fibrosis of the medial rectus, which may simulate sixth nerve palsy.
  ○ Depression defect (Fig. 3.10B) secondary to fibrosis of the superior rectus.
  ○ Adduction defect caused by fibrosis of the lateral rectus.

Optic neuropathy

Optic neuropathy is a fairly common (up to 6%) serious complication caused by compression of the optic nerve or its blood supply at the orbital apex by the congested and enlarged recti (Fig. 3.11) and swollen orbital tissue. Such compression, which may

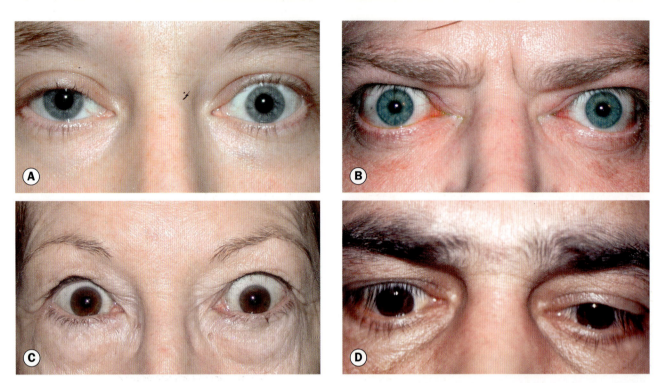

Fig. 3.8 Lid signs in thyroid eye disease. **(A)** Mild left lid retraction; **(B)** moderate bilateral symmetrical lid retraction – Dalrymple sign; **(C)** severe bilateral lid retraction – Kocher sign; **(D)** right lid lag on downgaze – von Graefe sign
(Courtesy of G Rose – fig. B; S Chen – fig. C)

occur in the absence of significant proptosis, may lead to severe visual impairment if adequate and timely treatment is not instituted.

- **Symptoms.** Impairment of central vision occurs in conjunction with other symptoms of TED. In order to detect early involvement, patients should be advised to monitor their own visual function by alternately occluding each eye, reading small print and assessing the intensity of colours, for example on a television screen.
- **Signs.** A high index of suspicion should be maintained for optic neuropathy, and it is important not to mistakenly attribute disproportionate visual loss to minor disease.
  - ○ Visual acuity (VA) is usually reduced, but not invariably.
  - ○ Colour desaturation is a sensitive feature.
  - ○ There may be diminished light brightness appreciation.
  - ○ A relative afferent pupillary defect, if present, should give cause for marked concern.
  - ○ Visual field defects can be central or paracentral and may be combined with nerve fibre bundle defects. These findings, in concert with elevated IOP, may be confused with primary open-angle glaucoma.
  - ○ The optic disc may be normal, swollen or, rarely, atrophic.

Investigation

Investigations other than blood tests for thyroid disease are not necessary if the diagnosis is evident clinically, but the exclusion of other conditions is sometimes indicated. Visual field testing is carried out if there is a suspicion of optic nerve compromise, and

may be performed as part of a baseline evaluation even if there is no apparent visual impairment. MRI, CT and ultrasonographic imaging of the orbits are indicated in some circumstances, such as helping to confirm an equivocal diagnosis by identification of the typical pattern of extraocular muscle involvement in TED, consisting of muscle belly enlargement with tendon sparing. Imaging is also used in the assessment of optic nerve compression and prior to orbital wall surgery. Visual evoked potentials are sometimes utilized in optic neuropathy.

Treatment

Treatment can be classified into that of mild disease (most patients), moderate to severe active disease, and treatment of post-inflammatory complications. The first measure taken in all cases should be the cessation of smoking. Thyroid dysfunction should also be managed adequately; if radioiodine treatment is administered in patients with pre-existing TED, a short course of oral steroids should be given in concert.

- **Mild disease**
  - ○ Lubricants for superior limbic keratoconjunctivitis, corneal exposure and dryness.
  - ○ Topical anti-inflammatory agents (steroids, non-steroidal anti-inflammatory drugs (NSAIDs), ciclosporin) are advocated by some authorities.
  - ○ Head elevation with three pillows during sleep to reduce periorbital oedema.
  - ○ Eyelid taping during sleep may alleviate mild exposure keratopathy.

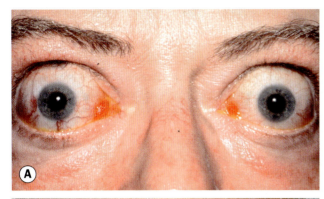

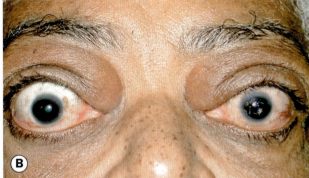

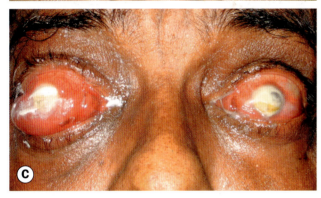

Fig. 3.9 Proptosis in thyroid eye disease. **(A)** Symmetrical; **(B)** asymmetrical; **(C)** bacterial keratitis due to severe exposure

(Courtesy of A Pearson – figs A and B; S Kumar Puri – fig. C)

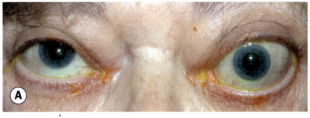

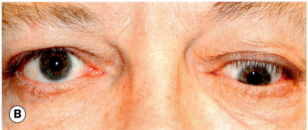

Fig. 3.10 Restrictive thyroid myopathy. **(A)** Defective elevation of the left eye; **(B)** defective depression of the right eye

6. Chemosis.

7. Inflammation of caruncle or plica.

During subsequent review, a point is allocated for an increase in proptosis of 2 mm or more, a decrease in uniocular excursion in any one direction of 8° or more, or a decrease in Snellen acuity of one line.

○ Systemic steroids are the mainstay of treatment for moderate to severe disease. Oral prednisolone 60–80 mg/day may be given initially, and tapered depending on response. Intravenous methylprednisolone is often reserved for acute compressive optic neuropathy (see below), but tolerability is better and outcomes may be superior compared with oral treatment; a lower-intensity regimen in the absence of acute sight-threatening disease is 0.5 g once weekly for 6 weeks followed by 0.25 g once weekly for 6 weeks. A reduction in discomfort, chemosis and periorbital oedema usually occurs within 24 hours, with a maximal response within 2–8 weeks. Ideally, oral steroid therapy should be discontinued after several months, but long-term low-dose maintenance may be necessary.

○ Orbital steroid injections are occasionally used in selected cases to minimize systemic side effects, but are typically considerably less effective than systemic treatment.

○ Low-dose fractionated radiotherapy may be used in addition to steroids or when steroids are contraindicated or ineffective, but because of the delayed effect is not used as the sole treatment of acute optic nerve compression. A positive response is usually evident within 6 weeks, with maximal improvement by 4 months; around 40% will not respond. Adverse effects include cataract, radiation retinopathy, optic neuropathy and an increased risk of local cancer; the threshold for its use should be higher in younger patients and diabetics, the latter because of a possibly increased risk of retinopathy.

• **Moderate to severe active disease**

○ Clinical activity score. EUGOGO suggests calculating a 'clinical activity score' to aid in determining a threshold for the use of immunosuppressives, assigning one point for each feature present from the following list and considering treatment for a score of 3 or more out of 7.

1. Spontaneous orbital pain.

2. Gaze-evoked orbital pain.

3. Eyelid swelling considered to be due to active (inflammatory phase) TED.

4. Eyelid erythema.

5. Conjunctival redness considered to be due to active (inflammatory phase) TED.

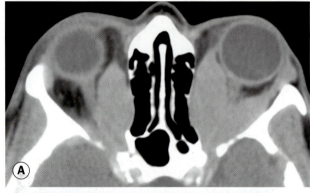

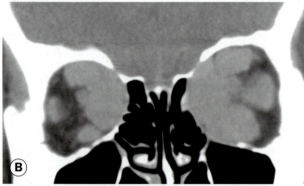

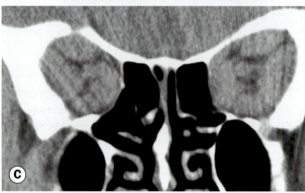

Fig. 3.11 CT shows muscle enlargement in thyroid eye disease. **(A)** Axial view; **(B)** coronal view – note sparing of the right lateral rectus muscle; **(C)** coronal view shows crowding at the orbital apex

(Courtesy of N Sibtain – figs A and B; J Nerad, K Carter and M Alford, from 'Oculoplastic and Reconstructive Surgery', in Rapid Diagnosis in Ophthalmology, Mosby 2008 – fig. C)

- ○ Combined therapy with irradiation, azathioprine and low-dose prednisolone may be more effective than steroids or radiotherapy alone.
- ○ Optic neuropathy, and less commonly intractable corneal exposure, requires aggressive treatment. Pulsed intravenous methylprednisolone is commonly used, regimens including 0.5–1 g on three successive days with conversion to oral treatment (e.g. 40 mg/day prednisolone) or 0.5–1 g on alternate days, 3–6 times, keeping the maximum dose below 8 g to reduce the risk of liver compromise, followed by oral prednisolone; appropriate monitoring should be instituted, including

liver function tests, as well as gastric protective treatment and osteoporosis prophylaxis if necessary. Orbital wall decompression (see below) and/or orbital apex decompression may be considered if steroids are ineffective (20% receiving intravenous treatment) or contraindicated. Orbital radiotherapy may also be administered, but is generally only used as an adjunct to other modalities.

- ○ Several drugs targeting specific aspects of the immune response in TED are under investigation, notably monoclonal antibody treatment with rituximab.

- **Post-inflammatory complications.** Eyelid surgery should be performed only after any necessary orbital and then strabismus procedures have been undertaken, as orbital decompression may impact both ocular motility and eyelid position, and extraocular muscle surgery may affect eyelid position.

- ○ Proptosis. After active inflammation has remitted, the patient can be left with cosmetically and functionally significant proptosis, the treatment of which is essentially surgical. Surgical decompression increases the volume of the orbit by removing the bony walls and may be combined with removal of orbital fat. Most surgery is undertaken via an external approach, though the medial wall and the medial part of the floor can be reached endoscopically. One-wall (deep lateral) decompression is effective (approximately 4–5 mm reduction in proptosis) and may reduce the risk of postoperative diplopia; two-wall (balanced medial and lateral – Fig. 3.12) decompression provides a greater effect but with a significant risk of inducing diplopia; three-wall decompression includes the floor with a reduction in proptosis of 6–10 mm but may lead to hypoglobus and carries a higher risk of infraorbital nerve damage and diplopia; very severe proptosis may require removal of part of the orbital roof in addition (four-wall decompression).

- ○ Restrictive myopathy. Surgery is required in most cases experiencing persistent diplopia in the primary or reading

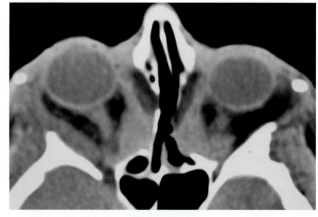

Fig. 3.12 Axial CT following bilateral lateral and medial wall decompression

(Courtesy of A Pearson)

positions of gaze, provided the inflammatory stage has subsided and the angle of deviation has been stable for at least 6–12 months. Until these criteria are met, diplopia may be alleviated, if possible, with prisms or sometimes botulinum toxin. The goal of operative treatment is to achieve binocular single vision in the primary and reading positions; restrictive myopathy often precludes binocularity in all positions of gaze, though with time the field of binocular single vision may enlarge as a result of increasing fusional vergence. Recession of the inferior and/or medial recti is the most commonly indicated surgery (a rectus muscle is never resected, only recessed in TED), generally utilizing adjustable sutures (see Ch. 18). The suture is adjusted later the same day or on the first postoperative day to achieve optimal alignment, and the patient is encouraged subsequently to practise achieving single vision with a consistently accessible target such as a television.

o Lid retraction. Mild lid retraction frequently improves spontaneously so does not require treatment. Control of hyperthyroidism may also be beneficial. Botulinum toxin injection to the levator aponeurosis and Müller muscle may be used as a temporary measure in patients awaiting definitive correction. Müllerotomy (disinsertion of Müller muscle) is effective for mild lid retraction, but more severe cases may also require recession/disinsertion of the levator aponeurosis and the suspensory ligament of the superior conjunctival fornix. Recession of the lower lid retractors, with or without a hard palate graft, can be used when retraction of the lower lid is 2 mm or more (see also Ch. 1).

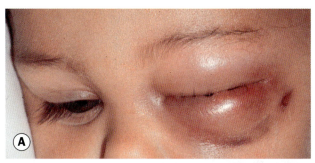

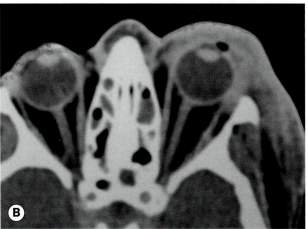

Fig. 3.13 Preseptal cellulitis. **(A)** Left preseptal cellulitis resulting from an infected eyelid abrasion; **(B)** axial CT shows opacification anterior to the orbital septum
(Courtesy of C Barry – fig. A)

INFECTIONS

Preseptal cellulitis

Introduction

Preseptal cellulitis is an infection of the subcutaneous tissues anterior to the orbital septum. It is considerably more common than orbital cellulitis, and though regarded as less serious, can still be associated with severe complications such as abscess formation, meningitis and cavernous sinus thrombosis. Rapid progression to orbital cellulitis may occasionally occur. Organisms typically responsible are *Staphylococcus aureus* and *Streptococcus pyogenes*, with causes including skin trauma such as laceration or insect bites, spread from focal ocular or periocular infection such as an acute hordeolum, dacryocystitis, conjunctivitis or sinusitis, and haematogenous spread from remote infection such as the upper respiratory tract or middle ear.

Diagnosis

The condition manifests with a swollen, often firm, tender red eyelid that may be very severe (Fig. 3.13A); however, in contrast to

orbital cellulitis, proptosis and chemosis are absent, and visual acuity, pupillary reactions and ocular motility are unimpaired. The patient is often pyrexial. Imaging with MRI or CT (Fig. 3.13B) is not indicated unless orbital cellulitis or a lid abscess is suspected, or there is a failure to respond to therapy.

Treatment

Treatment is with oral antibiotics such as co-amoxiclav 250–500 mg/125 mg 2–3 times daily or 875/125 mg twice daily, depending on severity. Severe infection may require intravenous antibiotics. The patient's tetanus status should be ascertained in cases following trauma.

Bacterial orbital cellulitis

Introduction

Bacterial orbital cellulitis is a serious infection of the soft tissues behind the orbital septum, which can be sight- and life-threatening. It can occur at any age but is more common in children. *Streptococcus pneumoniae*, *Staphylococcus aureus*, *Streptococcus pyogenes* and *Haemophilus influenzae* are common causative organisms, with infection originating typically from the paranasal (especially ethmoid) sinuses. Infection can also spread from preseptal cellulitis, dacryocystitis, midfacial skin or dental infection, and can follow trauma, including any form of ocular surgery. Blood-borne spread from infection elsewhere in the body may occur.

Clinical features

- **Symptoms** consist of the rapid onset of pain exacerbated by eye movement, swelling of the eye, malaise, and frequently visual impairment and double vision. There is commonly a recent history of nasal, sinus or respiratory symptoms.
- **Signs**
  - Pyrexia, often marked.
  - VA may be reduced and colour vision impaired, raising the possibility of optic nerve compression; the presence of a relative afferent pupillary defect in a previously normal eye makes this almost certain.
  - Tender, firm, erythematous and warm eyelids, with periocular and conjunctival (chemosis) oedema, conjunctival injection and sometimes subconjunctival haemorrhage; the signs are usually unilateral, though oedema may spread to the contralateral eyelids.
  - Proptosis is common in established infection, but is often obscured by lid swelling; it may be non-axial (dystopia), particularly if an abscess is present.
  - Painful ophthalmoplegia (Fig. 3.14A).

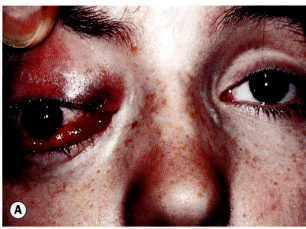
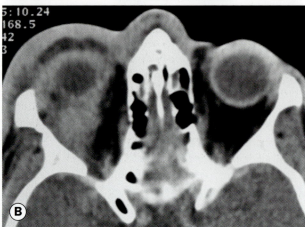

Fig. 3.14 (A) Right orbital cellulitis with ophthalmoplegia; **(B)** axial CT shows both preseptal and orbital opacification

Table 3.1 Differential diagnosis of an acutely inflamed orbit

Infection
• Bacterial orbital cellulitis
• Fungal orbital infection
• Dacryocystitis
• Infective dacryoadenitis
Vascular lesions
• Acute orbital haemorrhage
• Cavernous sinus thrombosis
• Carotid–cavernous fistula
Neoplasia
• Rapidly progressive retinoblastoma
• Lacrimal gland tumour
• Other neoplasm, e.g. metastatic lesion with inflammation, lymphoma, Waldenström macroglobulinaemia
• Rhabdomyosarcoma, leukaemia, lymphangioma or neuroblastoma in children
Endocrine
• Thyroid eye disease of rapid onset
Non-neoplastic inflammation
• Idiopathic orbital inflammatory disease
• Tolosa–Hunt syndrome
• Orbital myositis
• Acute allergic conjunctivitis with lid swelling
• Herpes zoster ophthalmicus
• Herpes simplex skin rash
• Sarcoidosis
• Vasculitides: Wegener granulomatosis, polyarteritis nodosa
• Scleritis, including posterior scleritis
• Ruptured dermoid cyst

  - Choroidal folds and optic disc swelling may be present on fundus examination.
- **Differential diagnosis.** Major diagnostic alternatives are listed in Table 3.1.
- **Complications**
  - Ocular complications include optic neuropathy, exposure keratopathy, raised IOP, endophthalmitis and occlusion of the central retinal artery or vein.
  - Subperiosteal abscess, most frequently located along the medial orbital wall.
  - Intracranial complications, which are uncommon (3–4%) but extremely serious, include meningitis, brain abscess and cavernous sinus thrombosis.

Investigation

Investigations may include:
- Ascertainment of tetanus immunization status in cases of trauma.
- White cell count.
- Blood cultures.
- Culture of nasal discharge.
- High-resolution CT of the orbit, sinuses and brain (Fig. 3.14B) is vital to confirm the diagnosis and exclude a

subperiosteal or intracranial abscess. MRI is also sometimes performed.

- Lumbar puncture if meningeal or cerebral signs develop.

Treatment

- **Hospital admission** is mandatory, with urgent otolaryngological assessment and frequent ophthalmic review. Paediatric specialist advice should be sought in the management of a child, and a low threshold should be adopted for infectious disease specialist consultation.
- **Delineation** of the extent of erythema on the skin using a surgical marker may help in judging progress.
- **Antibiotics** are given intravenously, with the specific drug depending on local sensitivities; ceftazidime is a typical choice, supplemented by oral metronidazole to cover anaerobes. Intravenous antibiotics should be continued until the patient has been apyrexial for 4 days, followed by 1–3 weeks of oral treatment.
- **Monitoring of optic nerve function** is performed at least every 4 hours initially by testing VA, colour vision, light brightness appreciation and pupillary reactions. Deterioration should prompt the consideration of surgical intervention.
- **Surgery.** Drainage of an orbital abscess should be considered at an early stage; drainage of infected sinuses should be considered if there is a lack of response to antibiotics, or if there is very severe sinus disease. Biopsy of inflammatory tissue may be performed for an atypical clinical picture. Severe optic nerve compression may warrant an emergency canthotomy/cantholysis (see Ch. 21).

Rhino-orbital mucormycosis

Introduction

Mucormycosis is a rare aggressive and often fatal infection caused by fungi of the family Mucoraceae. It typically affects patients with diabetic ketoacidosis or immunosuppression and is extremely rare in the immunocompetent. Infection is acquired by the inhalation of spores, which give rise to an upper respiratory infection. Spread then occurs to the contiguous sinuses and subsequently to the orbit and brain. Invasion of blood vessels by the hyphae results in occlusive vasculitis with infarction of orbital tissues.

Diagnosis

- **Symptoms.** Gradual onset facial and periorbital swelling, diplopia and visual loss.
- **Signs** are similar to bacterial orbital cellulitis, but tend to be less acute and with slower progression. Infarction superimposed on septic necrosis is responsible for the classic black eschar that may develop on the palate, turbinates, nasal septum, skin and eyelids (Fig. 3.15).
- **Complications** include retinal vascular occlusion, multiple cranial nerve palsies and cerebrovascular occlusion.
- **Differential diagnosis** is listed in Table 3.1.

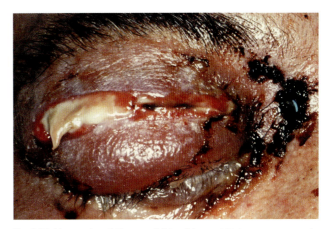

Fig. 3.15 Necrosis of the eyelid in rhino-orbital mucormycosis

- **Investigation** is much the same as for bacterial orbital cellulitis.

Treatment

- Correction of the underlying metabolic defect should be instituted if possible.
- Intravenous antifungal treatment.
- Daily packing and irrigation of the involved areas with antifungal agent.
- Wide excision of devitalized and necrotic tissues; exenteration may be required in unresponsive cases in order to reduce the risk of death.
- Adjunctive hyperbaric oxygen may be helpful.

NON-INFECTIVE INFLAMMATORY DISEASE

Idiopathic orbital inflammatory disease

Idiopathic orbital inflammatory disease (IOID; also non-specific orbital inflammation or orbital pseudotumour) is an uncommon disorder characterized by non-neoplastic, non-infective, space-occupying orbital infiltration with inflammatory features. The process may preferentially involve any or all of the orbital soft tissues. Histopathological analysis reveals pleomorphic inflammatory cellular infiltration followed by reactive fibrosis. Unilateral disease is typical in adults, although in children bilateral involvement may occur. Intracranial extension is rare; simultaneous orbital and sinus involvement is also rare, and may be a distinct entity.

Diagnosis

- **Symptoms** typically consist of acute or subacute ocular and periocular redness, swelling and pain (Fig. 3.16A). systemic symptoms are common in children.

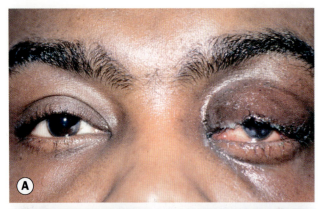

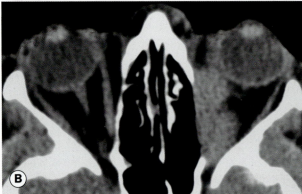

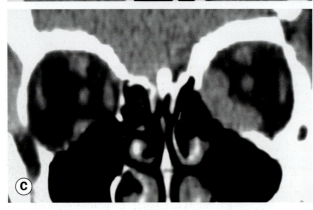

Fig. 3.16 (A) Left idiopathic orbital inflammatory disease; **(B)** CT axial view shows ill-defined orbital opacification; **(C)** coronal view

(Courtesy of R Bates – fig. A; A Pearson – figs B and C)

- **Signs**
  - Pyrexia is present in up to 50% of children, but is rare in adults.
  - Congestive proptosis.
  - Mild to severe ophthalmoplegia may occur.
  - Features of optic nerve dysfunction, particularly if the inflammation involves the posterior orbit; there may be optic disc swelling.
  - Choroidal folds, if present, may be associated with reduced vision but optic neuropathy must always be suspected.

- **Course.** The natural history of the inflammatory process is very variable.
  - Spontaneous remission after a few weeks without sequelae.
  - Intermittent episodes of activity, usually with eventual remission.
  - Severe prolonged inflammation eventually leading to progressive fibrosis of orbital tissues, resulting in a 'frozen orbit' characterized by ophthalmoplegia, which may be associated with ptosis and visual impairment caused by optic nerve involvement.
- **Investigation**
  - CT shows ill-defined orbital opacification and loss of definition of contents (Figs 3.16B and C).
  - Biopsy is generally required in persistent cases to confirm the diagnosis, and particularly to rule out neoplasia and systemic inflammatory conditions.
  - A wide range of other investigations may be considered to aid in the exclusion of alternative diagnoses, particularly infection, lymphoma and non-neoplastic infiltrative disorders such as sarcoidosis and Wegener granulomatosis.

Treatment

- **Observation**, for relatively mild disease, in anticipation of spontaneous remission.
- **NSAIDs** alone (e.g. ibuprofen) are often effective and may be tried in mild disease prior to steroid therapy. Co-prescription of a proton pump inhibitor should be considered.
- **Systemic steroids** should be administered only after the diagnosis has been confirmed, as they may mask other pathology such as infection and Wegener granulomatosis. Oral prednisolone is initially given at a dose of 1.0–1.5 mg/kg/day, subsequently being tapered and discontinued over a number of weeks depending on clinical response; further treatment may be needed in the event of recurrence.
- **Orbital depot steroid** injection may be useful in some cases.
- **Radiotherapy** may be considered if there has been no improvement after 2 weeks of adequate steroid therapy. Even low-dose treatment (e.g. 10 Gy) may produce remission, though much higher total doses may be necessary.
- **Other options**, usually as supplementary treatments or in resistant cases, include cytotoxic drugs (e.g. methotrexate, azathioprine), calcineurin inhibitors (e.g. ciclosporin, tacrolimus) and biological blockers.
- **Surgical resection** of an inflammatory focus may be contemplated in highly resistant cases.

Orbital myositis

Introduction

Orbital myositis is an idiopathic, non-specific inflammation of one or more extraocular muscles and is considered a subtype of

IOID. Histology shows a chronic inflammatory cellular infiltrate associated with the muscle fibres (Fig. 3.17A).

Diagnosis

- **Symptoms.** Acute pain, exacerbated by eye movement, and diplopia; onset is usually in early adulthood.
- **Signs** are generally more subtle than IOID.
  - Lid oedema, ptosis and chemosis.
  - Pain and diplopia associated with eye movements.
  - Vascular injection over the involved muscle (Fig. 3.17B).
  - In chronic cases the affected muscle may become fibrosed, with permanent restrictive myopathy.
- **Course**
  - Acute non-recurrent involvement that resolves spontaneously within 6 weeks.
  - Chronic disease characterized by either a single episode persisting for longer than 2 months (often for years) or recurrent attacks.
- **Investigation** consists primarily of MRI or CT, which show enlargement of the affected muscles (Fig. 3.17C), with or without involvement of the tendons of insertion; this is in contrast to TED-related muscle enlargement, in which the tendon is always spared. Additional investigations may be required in some cases.

Treatment

Treatment is aimed at relieving discomfort and dysfunction, shortening the course and preventing recurrences. NSAIDs may be adequate in mild disease, but systemic steroids are generally required and usually produce dramatic improvement, although recurrence is seen in 50%. Radiotherapy is also effective, particularly in limiting recurrence.

Acute dacryoadenitis

Acute dacryoadenitis may be idiopathic or due to viral (e.g. mumps, Epstein–Barr, cytomegalovirus) or – rarely – bacterial infection; the lacrimal gland is often involved in IOID. Chronic conditions such as sarcoidosis, Sjögren syndrome, thyroid disease and some chronic infections usually give a less acute onset, and involvement can be bilateral. Presentation in acute disease is with the rapid onset of discomfort in the region of the gland. Lacrimal secretion may be reduced or increased, and discharge may be reported. Swelling of the lateral aspect of the eyelid overlying the palpebral lobe leads to a characteristic S-shaped ptosis, and enlargement of the orbital lobe may give a slight downward and inward dystopia (Fig. 3.18A) and occasionally proptosis and other signs of orbital disease. There is tenderness over the lacrimal gland, and injection of the conjunctiva overlying the palpebral lobe may be seen on upper lid eversion (Fig. 3.18B). Chemosis may be present. There may be local (e.g. pre-auricular) lymph node enlargement. CT shows enlargement of the gland and involvement of adjacent tissues (Fig. 3.18C) without bony erosion; the latter suggests a tumour. Biopsy is sometimes indicated, particularly to

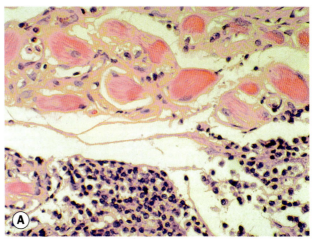

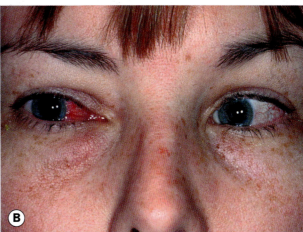

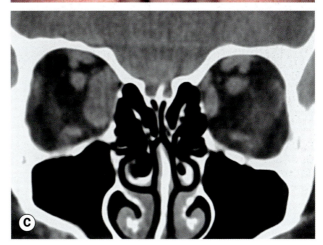

Fig. 3.17 Orbital myositis. **(A)** Histology shows a chronic inflammatory cellular infiltrate in relation to muscle fibres; **(B)** vascular injection over the insertion of the right medial rectus; **(C)** coronal CT shows enlargement of the right medial rectus

(Courtesy of J Harry and G Misson, from Clinical Ophthalmic Pathology, *Butterworth-Heinemann 2001 – fig. A; J Nerad, K Carter and M Alford, from 'Oculoplastic and Reconstructive Surgery', in* Rapid Diagnosis in Ophthalmology, *Mosby 2008 – figs B and C)*

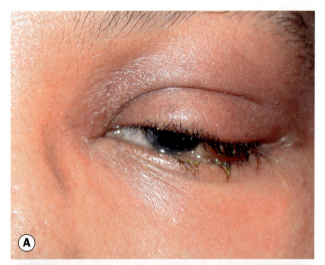

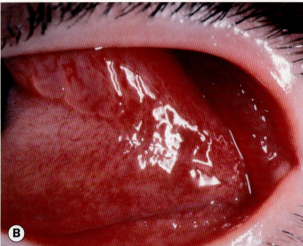

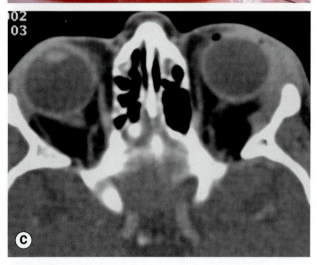

Fig. 3.18 Left acute dacryoadenitis. **(A)** Swelling on the lateral aspect of the eyelid and an S-shaped ptosis; **(B)** injection of the palpebral portion of the lacrimal gland and adjacent conjunctiva; **(C)** axial CT shows enlargement of the gland and opacification of adjacent tissues

(Courtesy of R Bates – fig. B; A Pearson – fig. C)

exclude a tumour. Treatment varies according to the cause, but in many cases is not required.

Tolosa–Hunt syndrome

Tolosa–Hunt syndrome is a rare idiopathic condition caused by non-specific granulomatous inflammation of the cavernous sinus, superior orbital fissure and/or orbital apex. It is a diagnosis of exclusion and should be investigated fully. Presentation is with ipsilateral periorbital or hemicranial pain, and diplopia due to one or more ocular motor pareses, with pupillary and eyelid involvement in many cases. Proptosis, if present, is usually mild. Sensory loss along the distribution of the first and second divisions of the trigeminal nerve is common. The patient may be pyrexial. Diagnosis is with imaging, together with other investigations to rule out identifiable causes, including neoplasia. Treatment is with systemic steroids and other immunosuppressants as necessary; the clinical course is characterized by remissions and recurrences.

Wegener granulomatosis

Wegener granulomatosis (see Ch. 8), an idiopathic multisystem granulomatous disorder that may involve the orbit, often bilaterally, usually by contiguous spread from the paranasal sinuses or nasopharynx. Primary orbital involvement is less common. The possibility of Wegener granulomatosis should be considered in any patient with bilateral orbital inflammation, particularly if associated with sinus pathology. Antineutrophilic cytoplasmic antibody (cANCA variant) is a useful serological test. Other ocular features include scleritis, peripheral ulcerative keratitis, intraocular inflammation and retinal vascular occlusions. Treatment is with cyclophosphamide and steroids, which are usually effective. In resistant cases ciclosporin, azathioprine, antithymocyte globulin or plasmapheresis may be useful. Surgical decompression may be required for severe orbital involvement.

NON-NEOPLASTIC VASCULAR ABNORMALITIES

Cavernous sinus thrombosis

This refers to clotting within the cavernous sinus, usually resulting from infection such as sinusitis, orbital or preseptal cellulitis or otitis. There is a high mortality rate: 20% treated and up to 100% untreated. Features are of rapid onset and may include severe headache, malaise, nausea and vomiting, unilateral or often bilateral proptosis, chemosis, congestion of the facial, conjunctival and retinal veins, reduced vision, and signs resulting from compromised function of the third to sixth cranial nerves, which run through the cavernous sinus. Diagnosis is with imaging, especially MRI and MRI venography; systemic investigation for infection is also performed, including lumbar puncture. Treatment consists of intravenous antibiotics and sometimes surgical drainage.

Carotid–cavernous fistula

Introduction

A carotid–cavernous fistula involves the development of an arteriovenous fistula between the carotid artery and the venous cavernous sinus (see Fig. 19.60) with a rise in venous pressure in the sinus and structures draining to it. Ocular manifestations occur because of venous and arterial stasis around the eye and orbit, increased episcleral venous pressure and a decrease in arterial blood flow to the cranial nerves within the cavernous sinus. Carotid–cavernous fistulae are classified into 'direct' and 'indirect' forms.

- Direct fistulae are high-flow shunts in which carotid artery blood passes directly into the cavernous sinus through a defect in the wall of the intracavernous portion of the internal carotid artery as a result of trauma (75%), including surgery, spontaneous rupture of an intracavernous carotid aneurysm or an atherosclerotic artery, the latter frequently in a middle-aged hypertensive woman; spontaneous fistulae usually have lower flow.
- In an indirect fistula ('dural shunt'), the intracavernous portion of the internal carotid artery remains intact. Arterial blood flows through the meningeal branches of the external or internal carotid arteries indirectly into the cavernous sinus, and the clinical features are more subtle than in a direct fistula such that the condition may be overlooked. Spontaneous rupture of an atherosclerotic artery or of a congenital malformation is the usual cause, and may be precipitated by minor trauma or straining. Connective tissue and collagen vascular disorders can be associated.

Diagnosis

- **Symptoms – direct.** Presentation may be days or weeks after head injury with a classic triad of pulsatile proptosis, conjunctival chemosis and a whooshing noise in the head.
- **Symptoms – indirect.** Gradual onset of redness of one or both eyes is a typical presentation, caused by conjunctival vascular engorgement.
- **Signs – direct**
  - Immediate visual loss may be due to ocular or optic nerve damage at the time of head trauma.
  - Delayed visual loss may occur as a result of exposure keratopathy, secondary glaucoma, central retinal vein occlusion, anterior segment ischaemia or ischaemic optic neuropathy.
  - Signs are usually ipsilateral to the fistula but may be bilateral, or even contralateral, because of midline connections between the two cavernous sinuses.
  - Marked epibulbar vascular dilatation (Fig. 3.19A).
  - Chemosis, commonly haemorrhagic, particularly in the early stages (Fig. 3.19B).
  - Pulsatile proptosis associated with a bruit and a thrill, both of which can be abolished by ipsilateral carotid compression in the neck.
  - Increased IOP due to elevated episcleral venous pressure and orbital congestion, and sometimes angle-closure glaucoma.
  - Anterior segment ischaemia, characterized by corneal epithelial oedema, aqueous cells and flare, and in severe cases iris atrophy, cataract and rubeosis iridis.
  - Ptosis due to third nerve involvement.
  - Ophthalmoplegia (60–70%) due to the ocular motor nerve damage from initial trauma, an intracavernous aneurysm or the fistula itself. The sixth cranial nerve is most frequently affected because of its free-floating location within the cavernous sinus. The third and fourth nerves, situated in the lateral wall of the sinus, are less frequently involved. Engorgement and swelling of extraocular muscles may also contribute to defective ocular motility.
  - Fundus examination may show optic disc swelling, venous dilatation and intraretinal haemorrhages (Fig. 3.19C) from venous stasis and impaired retinal blood flow. Vitreous haemorrhage is rare.
- **Signs – indirect**
  - Milder epibulbar vascular dilatation than with a direct fistula (Fig. 3.19D).
  - Exaggerated ocular pulsation; this is readily detected on slit lamp applanation tonometry.
  - The presence of 'corkscrew' epibulbar vessels (Fig. 3.19E) is a common subtle later sign; these are not pathognomonic and can be found in normal eyes.
  - Raised IOP, often bilateral but higher on the side of the fistula.
  - Proptosis and bruit are mild if present.
  - Ophthalmoplegia caused by sixth nerve palsy or swelling of extraocular muscles in marked cases.
  - Fundus may be normal or manifest moderate venous dilatation, with later tortuosity (Fig. 3.19F); as with corkscrew conjunctival vessels, this is not pathognomonic (see Ch. 13).
- **Investigation.** CT and MRI may demonstrate prominence of the superior ophthalmic vein (Fig. 3.20A) and diffuse enlargement of extraocular muscles (Fig. 3.20B), though these may only be visible with a direct fistula. Orbital Doppler imaging may show abnormal flow patterns, particularly in the superior orbital vein. Definitive diagnosis may involve selective catheter digital subtraction angiography, especially in mild dural fistulae, though CT and MRI angiography can be useful.

Treatment

Ocular complications may require specific measures in addition to treatment of the fistula itself. Neurological subspecialist opinion should be sought at an early stage, even if features are mild, as some fistula patterns (e.g. cortical venous drainage) carry a high risk of stroke.

- **Direct.** Most carotid–cavernous fistulae are not life-threatening; the organ at major risk is the eye. Surgery is indicated if spontaneous closure does not occur. A

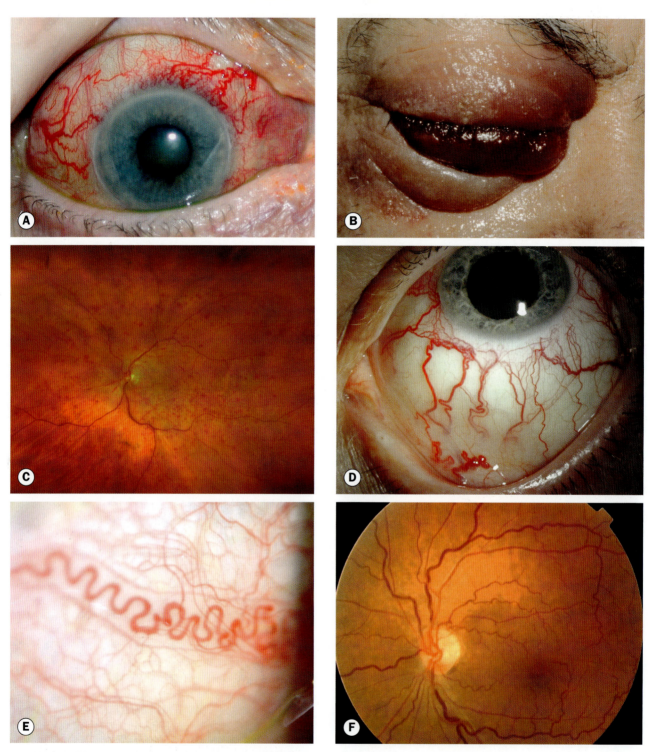

Fig. 3.19 Carotid–cavernous fistula. **(A)** Marked epibulbar vascular dilatation in an established direct fistula; **(B)** haemorrhagic chemosis in an acute direct fistula; **(C)** acute fundus appearance in a moderate direct fistula; **(D)** mild epibulbar vascular dilatation in an indirect fistula; **(E)** corkscrew conjunctival vessel; **(F)** retinal venous tortuosity

(Courtesy of S Chen – figs A and F; C Barry – figs C and D)

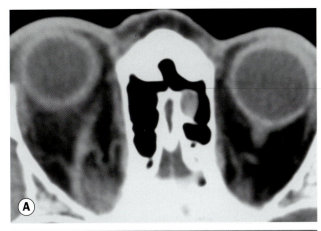

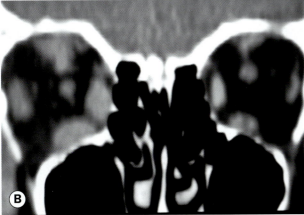

Fig. 3.20 CT in direct carotid–cavernous fistula. **(A)** Axial image shows enlargement of the right superior ophthalmic vein; **(B)** coronal view shows enlargement of extraocular muscles on the right

post-traumatic fistula is much less likely to close on its own than a spontaneous fistula because of higher blood flow. Treatment is likely to consist of a transarterial approach to repair the artery (e.g. coil – Fig. 3.21, other) or occlude the involved sinus (e.g. coil, balloon, other). Craniotomy for arterial repair is occasionally needed.

- **Indirect.** If required, treatment usually involves transvenous occlusion of the involved sinus. Spontaneous closure or occluding thrombosis sometimes (up to 50%) occurs; intermittent carotid compression under specialist supervision has been reported to increase the likelihood that this will take place.

CYSTIC LESIONS

Dacryops

A dacryops is a frequently bilateral cyst of the lacrimal gland that is thought to develop from a dilated obstructed duct. A round cystic lesion protrudes into the superior fornix from the palpebral lobe of the gland (Fig. 3.22), and may present with inflammation. The possibility of a malignant tumour should always be considered. Treatment involves excision or marsupialization, with histopathological analysis.

Dermoid cyst

Introduction

An orbital dermoid cyst is a choristoma (a mass of histologically normal tissue in an abnormal location) derived from displacement of ectoderm to a subcutaneous location along embryonic lines of closure. Dermoids are lined by keratinized stratified squamous epithelium (like skin), have a fibrous wall and contain dermal

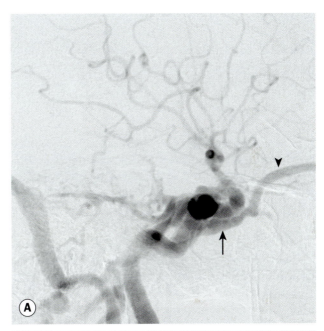

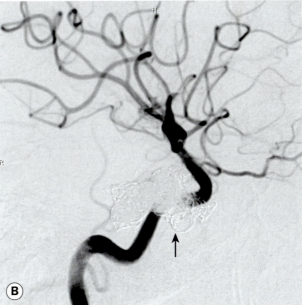

Fig. 3.21 Coil embolization of a direct carotid–cavernous fistula. **(A)** Early arterial phase catheter angiogram shows filling of the cavernous sinus (arrow) and superior ophthalmic vein (arrowhead); **(B)** following deposition of coils in the cavernous sinus – the fistula is closed and there is no retrograde flow in the superior ophthalmic vein
(Courtesy of J Trobe, from 'Neuro-ophthalmology', in Rapid Diagnosis in Ophthalmology, *Mosby 2008)*

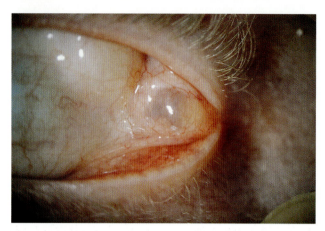

Fig. 3.22 Dacryops

appendages such as sweat glands, sebaceous glands and hair follicles; epidermoid cysts do not contain adnexal structures. Dermoids may be 'superficial' or 'deep', located anterior or posterior to the orbital septum respectively. Epibulbar dermoids and dermolipomas are related lesions (see Ch. 12).

Diagnosis

Dermoid cysts are one of the most frequently encountered orbital tumours in children.

- **Symptoms**
  - A superficial orbital dermoid cyst presents in infancy with a painless nodule, most commonly located in the superotemporal and occasionally the superonasal part of the orbit.
  - A deep dermoid cyst presents in adolescence or adult life with a gradually increasing protruding eye, or acutely with an inflamed orbit due to rupture.
- **Signs**
  - Superficial: a firm round smooth non-tender mass 1–2 cm in diameter (Fig. 3.23A), mobile under the skin but usually tethered to the adjacent periosteum. The posterior margins are easily palpable, denoting a lack of deeper origin or extension.
  - Deep: proptosis, dystopia or a mass lesion with indistinct posterior margins (Fig. 3.23B).
- **Investigation**
  - Superficial: imaging shows a well-circumscribed heterogeneous cystic lesion (Fig. 3.24A).
  - Deep: imaging again shows a well-circumscribed lesion (Fig. 3.24B). Some deep dermoids, associated with bony defects, may extend into the inferotemporal fossa or intracranially.

Treatment

Small lesions may be observed, bearing in mind the possibility of rupture, particularly from trauma; the inflammation can be addressed with oral steroids.

- **Superficial dermoid.** Treatment is by excision *in toto* (Fig. 3.25), taking care not to rupture the lesion, since leaking of keratin into the surrounding tissue typically results in severe granulomatous inflammation.
- **Deep dermoid.** Excision *in toto* is advisable because deep dermoids enlarge and may leak into adjacent tissues inducing inflammation, often followed by fibrosis. If incompletely excised, dermoids may recur with persistent low-grade inflammation.

Sinus mucocoele

A mucocoele (US spelling – mucocele) develops when the drainage of normal paranasal sinus secretions is obstructed due to infection, allergy, trauma, tumour or congenital narrowing. A slowly expanding cystic accumulation of mucoid secretions and epithelial debris develops and gradually erodes the bony walls of the sinus, causing symptoms by encroachment upon surrounding tissues. Orbital invasion occurs usually from a frontal or ethmoidal

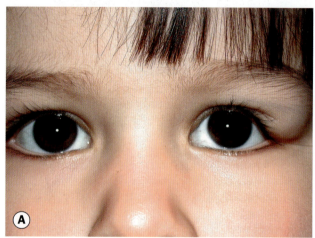

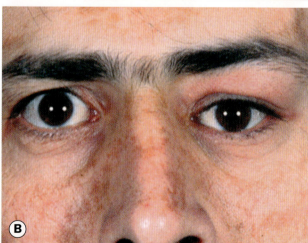

Fig. 3.23 Orbital dermoid cysts. **(A)** Superficial cyst left eye; **(B)** left deep cyst causing mild dystopia
(Courtesy of A Pearson – fig. B)

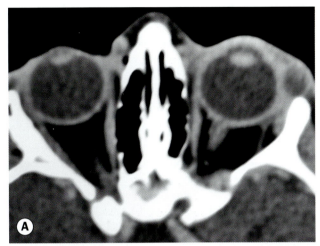

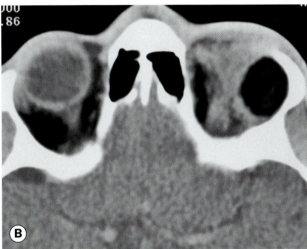

Fig. 3.24 Orbital dermoid cysts – imaging. **(A)** Axial CT image showing a well-circumscribed heterogeneous superficial lesion; **(B)** deep dermoid – CT showing a well-circumscribed cystic lesion and bone remodelling

(Courtesy of K Nischal – fig. A; A Pearson – fig. B)

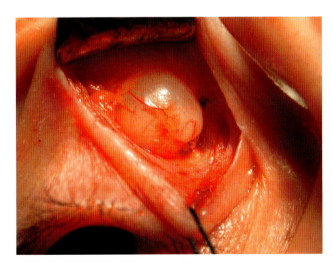

Fig. 3.25 Superficial orbital dermoid cyst – appearance at surgery (orbitotomy)

(Courtesy of A Pearson)

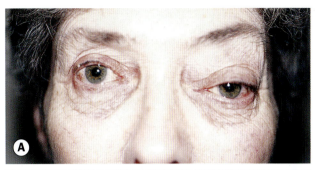

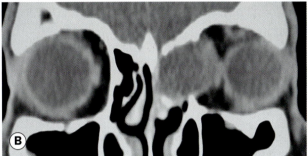

Fig. 3.26 (A) Left ethmoidal sinus mucocoele causing dystopia; **(B)** coronal CT shows orbital involvement and indentation of the medial rectus

mucocoele, but rarely from those arising in the maxillary sinus. Presentation is in adult life with proptosis or dystopia (Fig. 3.26A), diplopia or epiphora. Pain is uncommon unless secondary infection develops (mucopyocoele). CT shows a soft tissue mass with thinning or erosion of the bony walls of the sinus (Fig. 3.26B). Treatment involves complete excision.

Encephalocoele

An encephalocoele (US spelling – encephalocele) is formed by herniation of intracranial contents through a congenital defect of the base of the skull, and can be located at the front or back of the head. A meningocoele contains only dura whilst a meningo-encephalocoele also contains brain tissue. Presentation is usually during infancy. Anterior orbital encephalocoeles involve the superomedial part of the orbit and displace the globe forwards and laterally (Fig. 3.27A), whereas posterior orbital encephalocoeles (frequently associated with neurofibromatosis type I) displace the globe forwards and downwards (Fig. 3.27B). The displacement increases on straining or crying and may be reduced by manual pressure. Pulsating proptosis may occur due to communication with the subarachnoid space but, because the communication is not vascular, there is neither a thrill nor a bruit. CT shows the bony defect responsible for the herniation (Fig. 3.27C). The differential diagnosis of anterior encephalocoele includes other causes of medial canthal swelling such as dermoid cyst and amniontocoele, and of posterior encephalocoele includes other orbital lesions that present during early life such as capillary haemangioma, juvenile xanthogranuloma, teratoma and microphthalmos with cyst.

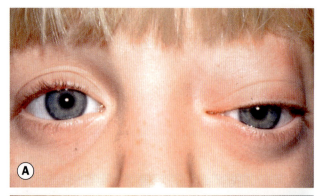

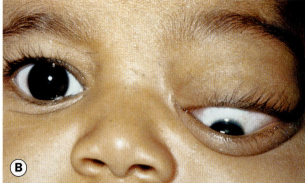

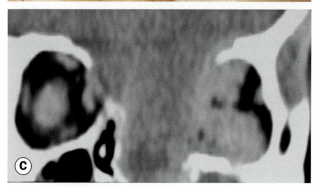

Fig. 3.27 Encephalocoele. **(A)** Anterior superomedial encephalocoele causing proptosis and down and out dystopia; **(B)** posterior encephalocoele causing proptosis and inferior dystopia; **(C)** coronal CT of posterior encephalocoele showing a large bony defect

(Courtesy of A Pearson – fig. C)

VASCULAR TUMOURS

Varices

Introduction

Primary orbital varices (combined venous–lymphatic malformations of the orbit – see also next topic) consist of a plexus of thin-walled distensible low-flow vein-like vessels that are commonly, though not always, intrinsic to the normal circulation. They are probably hamartomatous (hamartoma – a disorganized overgrowth of mature tissues normally present in the involved area). Associations include varices of the eyelids (Fig. 3.28A and see Fig. 1.71) and conjunctiva (Fig. 3.28B). They commonly present at any time from early childhood to late middle age, but occasionally can be acquired later secondary to a local high-flow vascular lesion or trauma.

Diagnosis

Most cases are unilateral and the most frequent site is upper nasal. Intermittent non-pulsatile proptosis without a bruit is reported. If there is free communication with the normal circulation, reversible proptosis may be precipitated or accentuated by increasing venous pressure through coughing, straining, the Valsalva manoeuvre (Figs 3.28C and D), assuming a head-down position or external compression of the jugular veins. Imaging (e.g. MRI and magnetic resonance venography (MRV), CT, ultrasound, venography) shows a lobulated mass with variable contrast enhancement, and may demonstrate phleboliths (Fig. 3.28E) and sometimes orbital expansion (particularly in childhood) or an associated orbital wall defect. Complications include acute orbital haemorrhage, thrombosis (pain, proptosis, decreased vision) and optic nerve compression. Patients with long-standing lesions may develop atrophy of surrounding fat, giving enophthalmos with a deepened superior sulcus (Fig. 3.28F).

Treatment

Small lesions generally do not require treatment. Surgical excision is technically difficult and often incomplete because the lesions are friable and bleed easily; it can be complicated by severe orbital haemorrhage and vascular optic nerve compromise. Specialized techniques such as embolization and carbon dioxide laser surgery may be helpful adjuncts. Indications include recurrent thrombosis, pain, severe proptosis and optic nerve compression.

Lymphangioma

Introduction

Lymphangioma is a rare hamartomatous vascular tumour that tends to enlarge and infiltrate diffusely with time. Some authorities believe lymphangiomas to be a variant of venous orbital anomaly (varices) across a single spectrum, and the term combined venous–lymphatic malformations of the orbit has been suggested. Although usually isolated from the main circulation, bleeding into the lumen may occur with subsequent formation of blood-filled 'chocolate cysts' that may regress spontaneously with time. Presentation is usually in early childhood. Differential diagnosis is principally from orbital venous anomalies and haemangiomas. Intracranial vascular malformations can be present in association.

Diagnosis

Anterior lesions typically manifest as several soft bluish masses in the upper nasal quadrant (Fig. 3.29).

Posterior lesions may cause slowly progressive proptosis, or initially may lie dormant and later present with the sudden onset

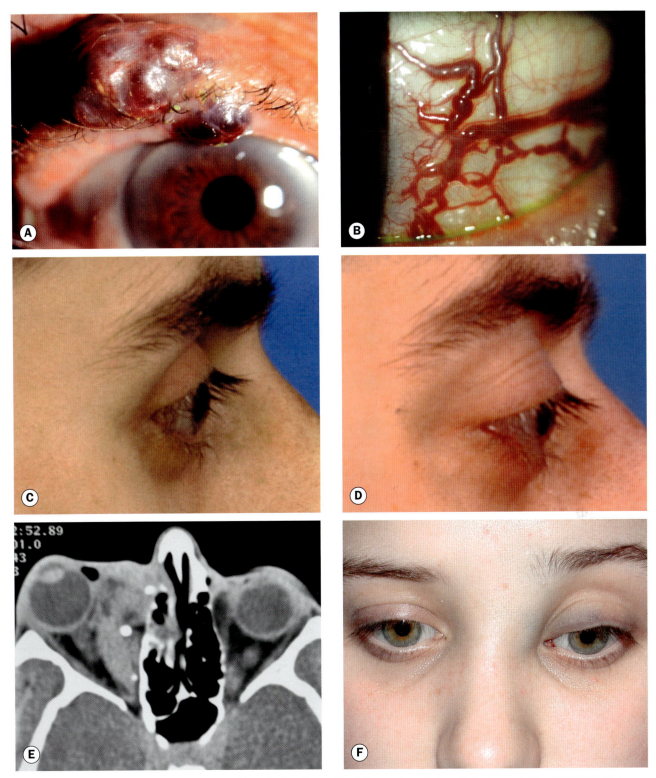

Fig. 3.28 (A) Substantial eyelid varices; **(B)** conjunctival varices; **(C)** orbital varices before Valsalva and **(D)** with Valsalva; **(E)** axial CT shows medial opacification and phleboliths; **(F)** left fat atrophy resulting in enophthalmos and deep superior sulcus

(Courtesy of G Rose – figs C and D; A Pearson – figs E and F)

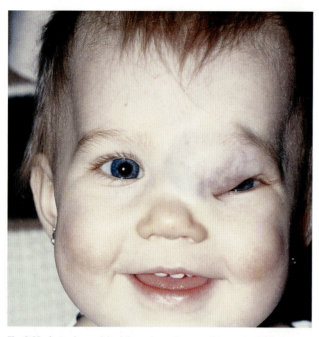

Fig. 3.29 Anterior orbital lymphangioma with typical bluish discoloration

of painful proptosis (Figs 3.30A and B) secondary to spontaneous haemorrhage, which may be associated with optic nerve compression. Involvement of the lids, conjunctiva (Fig. 3.30C) and oropharynx (Fig. 3.30D) may be seen; intracranial lesions may also be present.

Treatment

In many cases the visual prognosis is good without treatment. Surgical excision is difficult because lesions are unencapsulated, friable, bleed easily and commonly infiltrate normal orbital tissues; repeated subtotal excision may be necessary. Persistent sight-threatening chocolate cysts can be drained or removed sub-totally by controlled vaporization using a carbon dioxide laser.

Capillary haemangioma

Introduction

Capillary haemangioma is the most common tumour of the orbit and periorbital area in childhood. Girls are affected more commonly than boys (3:1). It may present as a small isolated lesion of

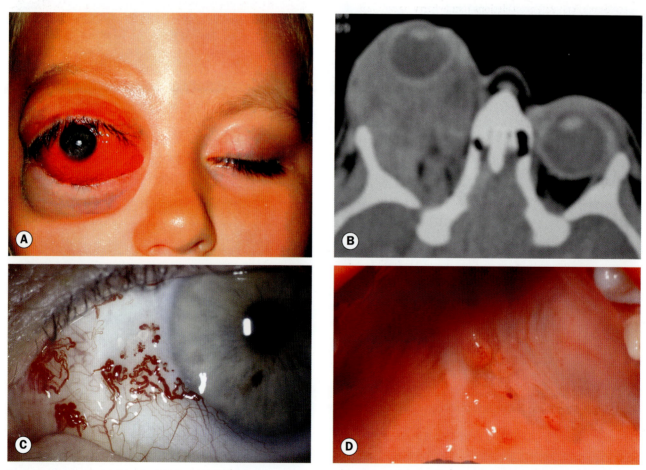

Fig. 3.30 (A) Severe proptosis due to bleeding from a posterior lymphangioma; **(B)** axial CT shows proptosis and orbital opacification; **(C)** conjunctival involvement; **(D)** oral lesions

(Courtesy of A Pearson – figs A and B; C Barry – fig. C)

minimal clinical significance, or as a large disfiguring mass that can cause visual impairment and systemic complications. An established tumour is composed of anastomosing small vascular channels without true encapsulation (see Fig. 1.13C); it is a hamartoma – a disorganized overgrowth of mature tissues normally present in the involved area – and believed to be due principally to endothelial cell proliferation. Large or multiple lesions may have associated visceral involvement, which can lead to serious complications such as thrombocytopenia (Kasabach–Merritt syndrome, with up to 50% mortality) and high-output cardiac failure, and systemic investigation should be considered. The incidence of infantile haemangioma in the general population is around 5%, and a small proportion of these, especially if a large facial haemangioma is present, will have PHACE (PHACES) syndrome, which includes a range of possible systemic features including eye involvement.

Diagnosis

- **Symptoms.** The lesion is usually noticed by the parent, usually in the first few months of life; approximately 30% are present at birth.
- **Signs.** Extensive underlying orbital involvement should always be ruled out in a seemingly purely superficial lesion.
  - ○ Superficial cutaneous lesions ('strawberry naevi') are bright red (Fig. 3.31A and see Fig. 1.13A).
  - ○ Preseptal (deeper) tumours appear dark blue or purple through the overlying skin (Fig. 3.31B and see Fig. 3.31A) and are most frequently located superiorly.
  - ○ A large tumour may enlarge and change in colour to a deep blue during crying or straining, but both pulsation and a bruit are absent.
  - ○ Deep orbital tumours give rise to unilateral proptosis without skin discoloration.
  - ○ Haemangiomatous involvement of the palpebral or forniceal conjunctiva is common (Fig. 3.31C).
  - ○ Additional haemangiomas on the eyelids (see Ch. 1) or elsewhere are common.
- **Investigation.** Imaging is generally performed for other than very small lesions, mainly to rule out more extensive orbital disease. Ultrasound shows medium internal reflectivity (Fig. 3.32A), and on MRI or CT the lesion appears as a soft tissue mass in the anterior orbit or as an extraconal mass with finger-like posterior expansions (Fig. 3.32B). The orbital cavity may show enlargement but there is no bony erosion.

Treatment

The natural course is characterized by rapid growth 3–6 months after diagnosis (Fig. 3.33), followed by a slower phase of natural resolution in which 30% of lesions resolve by the age of 3 years and about 75% by the age of 7. Treatment is indicated principally for amblyopia secondary to induced astigmatism, anisometropia, occlusion or strabismus, and less commonly for cosmesis, optic nerve compression or exposure keratopathy.

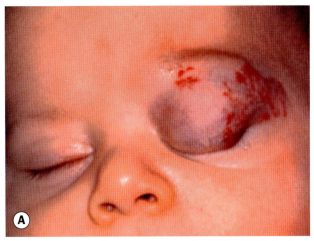

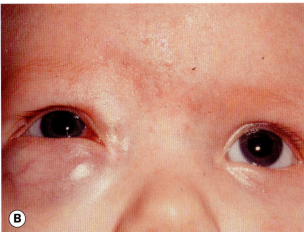

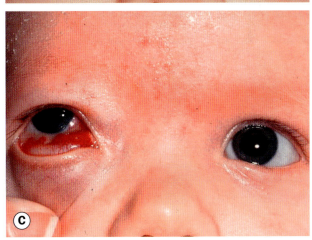

Fig. 3.31 Capillary haemangioma. **(A)** Large preseptal tumour causing ptosis and purple cutaneous discoloration – there is a superficial component (strawberry naevus); **(B)** inferior preseptal tumour; **(C)** involvement of forniceal conjunctiva
(Courtesy of K Nischal – figs B and C)

- **Beta-blockers.** Oral propranolol is now widely used, and seems most effective in the proliferative stage; prescription and monitoring should generally be carried out by a paediatrician. Topical preparations including timolol are also under investigation, with initially favourable results.

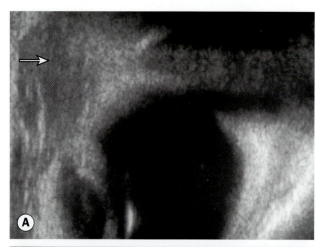

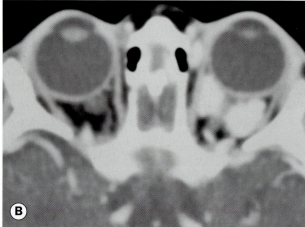

Fig. 3.32 Imaging of capillary haemangioma. **(A)** Ultrasound of a preseptal lesion with an intraorbital component; **(B)** axial enhanced CT shows a homogeneous intraconal orbital soft tissue mass

(Courtesy of K Nischal – fig. A; A Pearson – fig. B)

- **Steroids**
  - ○ Injection of triamcinolone acetonide (1–2 ml total of 40 mg/ml over several injection sites) or betamethasone (4 mg/ml) into a cutaneous or preseptal tumour is usually effective in early lesions. Regression usually begins within 2 weeks but, if necessary, second and third injections can be given after about 2 months. It is advisable not to inject deeply into the orbit for fear of causing occlusion of the central retinal artery due to retrograde introduction of the suspension. Other complications include skin depigmentation and necrosis, fat atrophy and systemic effects such as adrenal suppression.
  - ○ Topical high-potency steroids (e.g. clobetasol propionate cream) are sometimes appropriate but are slow to exert their effect.
  - ○ Systemic steroids administered daily over several weeks may be used, particularly if there is a large orbital component or a rapid onset of action is required.

- **Laser** may be used to close blood vessels in superficial skin lesions less than 2 mm in thickness.
- **Interferon alfa-2a** and **vincristine** may be used for some steroid-resistant sight-threatening lesions.
- **Local resection** with cutting cautery or carbon dioxide laser may reduce the bulk of an anterior circumscribed tumour, but is usually reserved for the late inactive stage unless a resistant tumour is sight- or life-threatening.

Cavernous haemangioma

Introduction

Cavernous haemangioma occurs in middle-aged adults, with a female preponderance of 70%; growth may be accelerated by pregnancy. It is the most common orbital tumour in adults, and is probably a vascular malformation rather than a neoplastic lesion. Although it may develop anywhere in the orbit, it most frequently occurs within the lateral part of the muscle cone just behind the globe, and behaves like a low-flow arteriovenous malformation.

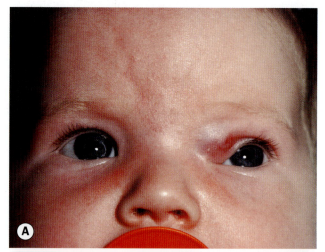

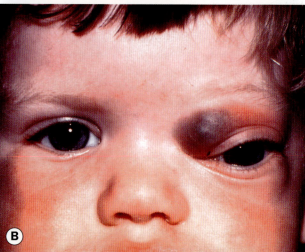

Fig. 3.33 Growth of capillary haemangioma. **(A)** At presentation; **(B)** several months later

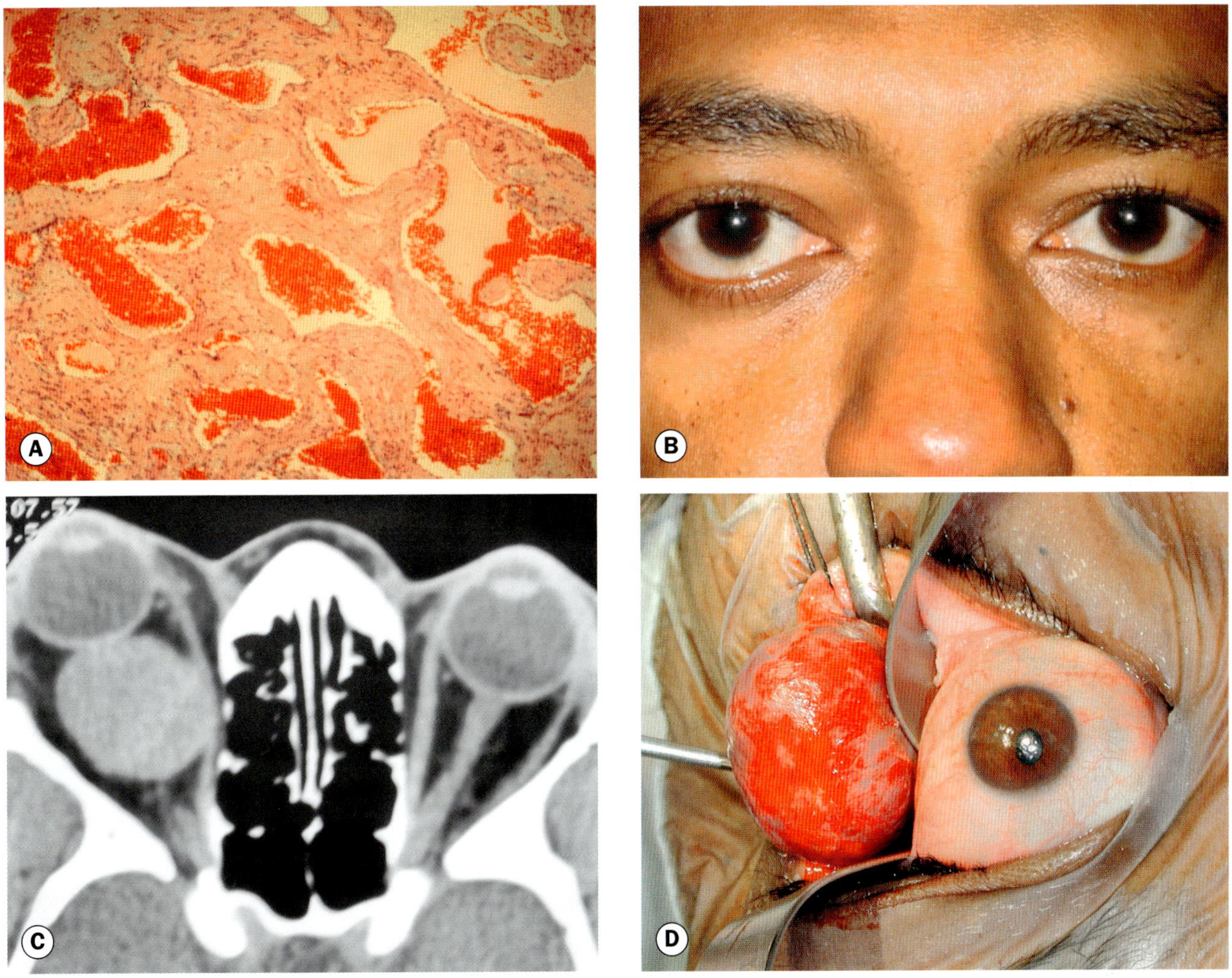

Fig. 3.34 Cavernous haemangioma. **(A)** Histology shows congested variably sized endothelial-lined vascular channels separated by fibrous septa; **(B)** right axial proptosis; **(C)** axial CT shows a well-circumscribed retrobulbar oval lesion and proptosis; **(D)** the tumour is encapsulated and relatively easy to remove
(Courtesy of A Pearson – figs B, C and D)

Histology shows endothelial-lined vascular channels of varying size separated by fibrous septa (Fig. 3.34A).

Diagnosis

- **Symptoms.** Slowly progressive unilateral proptosis; bilateral cases are very rare.
- **Signs**
  - Axial proptosis (Fig. 3.34B), which may be associated with optic disc oedema and choroidal folds.
  - A lesion at the orbital apex may compress the optic nerve without causing significant proptosis; gaze-evoked transient blurring of vision may occur.
  - There may be impairment of extraocular muscle excursion.
- **Investigation.** CT (Fig. 3.34C) and MRI show a well-circumscribed oval lesion, usually within the muscle cone. There is only slow contrast enhancement. Ultrasound is also useful.

Treatment

Many cavernous haemangiomas are detected by chance on scans performed for unrelated reasons and observation alone is often appropriate. Symptomatic lesions require surgical excision in most cases because they gradually enlarge. The cavernous haemangioma, unlike its capillary counterpart, is usually well-encapsulated and relatively easy to remove (Fig. 3.34D).

LACRIMAL GLAND TUMOURS

Pleomorphic lacrimal gland adenoma

Introduction

Pleomorphic adenoma (benign mixed-cell tumour) is the most common epithelial tumour of the lacrimal gland and is derived

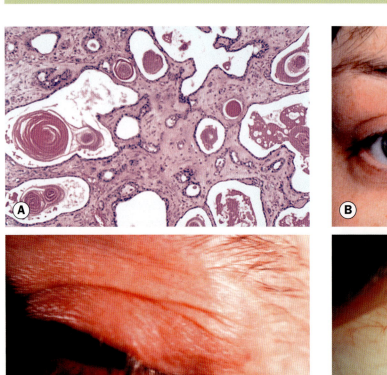

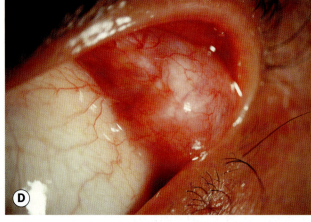

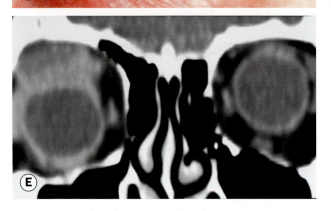

Fig. 3.35 Pleomorphic lacrimal gland adenoma. **(A)** Histology shows glandular tissue and squamous differentiation with keratin formation; **(B)** inferonasal dystopia due to a tumour arising from the orbital lobe; **(C)** eyelid swelling without dystopia; **(D)** eversion of the upper eyelid reveals the tumour; **(E)** coronal CT showing an orbital lobe lesion

(Courtesy of J Harry and G Misson, from Clinical Ophthalmic Pathology, *Butterworth-Heinemann 2001 – fig. A; A Pearson – figs B and E)*

from the ducts and secretory elements including myoepithelial cells. On histopathology, the inner layer of cells forms glandular tissue that may be associated with squamous differentiation and keratin production (Fig. 3.35A); the outer cells undergo metaplastic change leading to the formation of myxoid tissue. Young to middle-aged adults are the predominantly affected group.

Diagnosis

- **Symptoms.** Painless slowly progressive proptosis or swelling in the superolateral eyelid, usually of more than a year's duration. Old photographs may reveal an abnormality many years prior to presentation.
- **Signs**
  - ○ Orbital lobe tumour presents as a smooth, firm, non-tender mass in the lacrimal gland fossa with inferonasal dystopia (Fig. 3.35B); posterior extension may cause proptosis, ophthalmoplegia and choroidal folds.
  - ○ Palpebral lobe tumour is less common and tends to grow anteriorly causing upper lid swelling without dystopia (Fig. 3.35C); it may be visible to inspection (Fig. 3.35D).
- **Investigation.** CT shows a round or oval mass, with a smooth outline and indentation but not destruction of the lacrimal gland fossa (Fig. 3.35E). The lesion may indent the globe, and calcification may be shown.

Treatment

Treatment involves surgical excision. If the diagnosis is strongly suspected, it is wise to avoid prior biopsy to prevent tumour seeding into adjacent orbital tissue, although this may not always

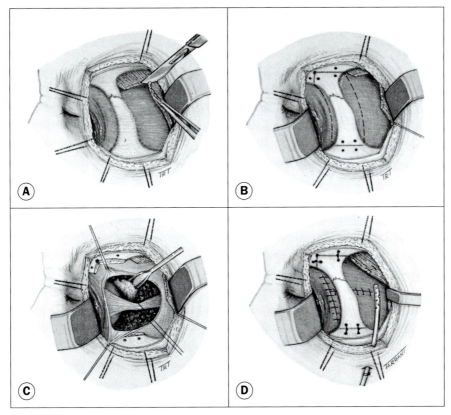

Fig. 3.36 Lateral orbitotomy. **(A)** Incision of temporalis muscle; **(B)** drilling of underlying bone for subsequent wiring; **(C)** removal of the lateral orbital wall and the tumour; **(D)** repair of the lateral orbital wall

be possible in the context of diagnostic uncertainty. Tumours of the palpebral lobe are usually resected, along with a margin of normal tissue, through an anterior (trans-septal) orbitotomy. Those of the orbital portion are excised through a lateral orbitotomy:

1. The temporalis muscle is incised (Fig. 3.36A).
2. The underlying bone is drilled for subsequent wiring (Fig. 3.36B).
3. The lateral orbital wall is removed and the tumour excised including a margin of adjacent tissue and periorbita (Fig. 3.36C).
4. The lateral orbital wall (Fig. 3.36D) and temporalis are repaired. The prognosis is excellent provided excision is complete and without disruption of the capsule. Incomplete excision or preliminary incisional biopsy may result in seeding of the tumour into adjacent tissues, with recurrence and occasionally malignant change.

Lacrimal gland carcinoma

Lacrimal gland carcinoma is a rare tumour that carries a high morbidity and mortality. In order of frequency the main histological types are adenoid cystic (50%), pleomorphic adenocarcinoma, mucoepidermoid and squamous cell. Histopathology shows nests of basaloid cells with numerous mitoses (Fig. 3.37A). The peak incidence is in middle-aged adults.

Diagnosis

- **Symptoms.** A malignant mixed-cell tumour presents in three main clinical settings:

  - After incomplete or piecemeal excision of a benign pleomorphic adenoma, followed by one or more recurrences over a period of several years with eventual malignant transformation.
  - As a long-standing proptosis or swollen upper lid that suddenly starts to increase.
  - Without a previous history of a pleomorphic adenoma as a rapidly growing lacrimal gland mass, usually of several months' duration.
  - The history is shorter than that of a benign tumour.
  - Pain is a frequent feature of malignancy but may also occur with inflammatory lesions.

- **Signs**
  - A mass in the lacrimal area causing inferonasal dystopia.
  - Posterior extension, with involvement of the superior orbital fissure, may give rise to epibulbar congestion, proptosis, periorbital oedema and ophthalmoplegia (Fig. 3.37B).
  - Hypoaesthesia in the region supplied by the lacrimal nerve.
  - Optic disc swelling and choroidal folds.

- **Investigation**
  - CT shows a globular lesion with irregular serrated edges, often with contiguous erosion or invasion of bone (Fig. 3.37C). Calcification is commonly seen within the tumour.

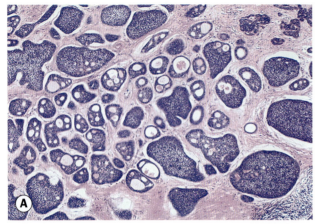

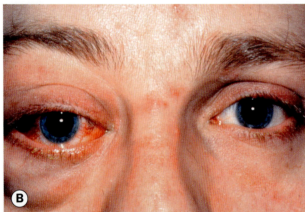

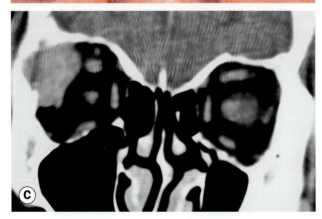

Fig. 3.37 Lacrimal gland carcinoma. **(A)** Histology of adenoid cystic carcinoma shows nests of basaloid cells with solid and cribriform areas; **(B)** dystopia, proptosis, periorbital oedema and epibulbar congestion due to extension involving the superior orbital fissure; **(C)** coronal CT shows contiguous erosion of bone and spotty calcification in the tumour

(Courtesy of J Harry and G Misson, from Clinical Ophthalmic Pathology, Butterworth-Heinemann 2001 – fig. A; A Pearson – fig. C)

- ○ Biopsy is necessary to establish the histological diagnosis. Subsequent management depends on the extent of tumour invasion of adjacent structures as seen on imaging.
- ○ Neurological assessment is mandatory because adenoid-cystic carcinoma exhibits perineural spread and may extend into the cavernous sinus.

Treatment

Treatment involves excision of the tumour and adjacent tissues. Extensive tumours may require orbital exenteration or midfacial resection, but the prognosis for life is frequently poor. Radiotherapy combined with local resection may prolong life and reduce pain. Adjuvant intra-arterial chemotherapy and/or brachy-therapy may be utilized in some cases.

NEURAL TUMOURS

Optic nerve glioma

Introduction

Optic nerve glioma is a slowly growing, pilocytic astrocytoma that typically affects children (median age 6.5 years); histopathology shows spindle-shaped pilocytic (hair-like) astrocytes and glial filaments (Fig. 3.38A). The prognosis is variable; some have an indolent course with little growth, while others may extend intracranially and threaten life. Approximately 30% of patients have associated neurofibromatosis type I (NF1 – see Ch. 19) and in these patients the prognosis is generally superior. Malignant glioma (glioblastoma) is rare, has a very poor prognosis, and usually occurs in adult males.

Diagnosis

- **Symptoms**
  - ○ Slowly progressive visual loss, followed later by proptosis, although this sequence may occasionally be reversed.
  - ○ Acute loss of vision due to haemorrhage into the tumour can occur, but is uncommon.
- **Signs**
  - ○ Proptosis is often non-axial, with temporal or inferior dystopia (Fig. 3.38B).
  - ○ The optic nerve head, initially swollen, subsequently becomes atrophic.
  - ○ Opticociliary collaterals (see Fig. 3.6C) and other fundus signs such as central retinal vein occlusion are occasionally seen.
  - ○ Intracranial spread to the chiasm and hypothalamus may develop.
- **Investigation**
  - ○ MRI effectively demonstrates the tumour, and may show intracranial extension if present.
  - ○ CT in patients with associated NF1 shows a fusiform enlargement of the optic nerve with a clear-cut margin produced by the intact dural sheath (Fig. 3.38C). In patients without NF1 the nerve is more irregular and shows low-density areas.

Treatment

As the tumour is intrinsic to the optic nerve, resection means that all vision will be lost in the operated eye.

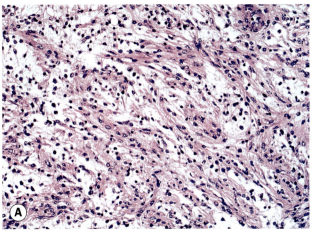

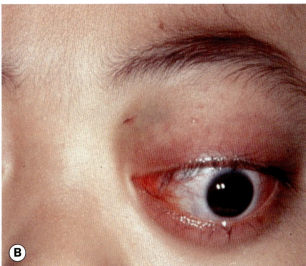

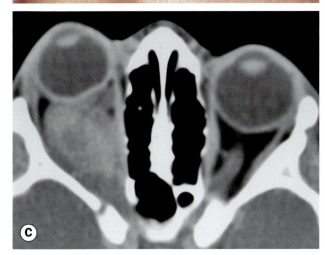

Fig. 3.38 Optic nerve glioma. **(A)** Histopathology – spindle-shaped pilocytic astrocytes and glial filaments; **(B)** proptosis with inferior dystopia; **(C)** axial CT showing fusiform optic nerve enlargement

(Courtesy of J Harry – fig. A; K Nischal – fig. B; A Pearson – fig. C)

- **Observation** may be considered in patients with a typical pilocytic astrocytoma on imaging in whom the tumour is confined to the orbit, especially if there is good vision and no significant cosmetic impairment; serial MRI is important if this option is chosen. Spontaneous regression has been reported, usually in NF1, but is very rare.
- **Surgical excision** with preservation of the globe is indicated in those with large or growing tumours where complete resection of the tumour can be achieved, particularly if vision is poor and proptosis significant. A key goal is to prevent chiasmal involvement, and an intracranial approach may be necessary to achieve adequate resection.
- **Radiotherapy** may be combined with chemotherapy for tumours with extension that precludes complete surgical excision.

Optic nerve sheath meningioma

Introduction

Optic nerve sheath meningioma is a benign tumour arising from meningothelial cells of the arachnoid villi surrounding the intraorbital, or less commonly the intracanalicular, portion of the optic nerve. In some cases the tumour merely encircles the optic nerve whilst in others it invades the nerve, growing along the fibrovascular pial septa. However, about two-thirds of all meningiomas affecting the optic nerve arise from extension of primarily intracranial lesions. Primary optic nerve sheath meningiomas are less common than optic nerve gliomas and, as with other meningiomas, typically affect middle-aged women. Histopathologically, meningothelial (irregular lobules of meningothelial cells separated by fibrovascular strands – Fig. 3.39A) and psammomatous (psammoma bodies among proliferating meningothelial cells – Fig. 3.39B) types are distinguished. The prognosis for life is good in adults, although the tumour may be more aggressive in children, in whom 25% occur. They are more common in neurofibromatosis type II (NF2).

Diagnosis

- **Symptoms** typically consist of gradual visual impairment in one eye. Transient obscurations of vision may occur.
- **Signs.** The classic (Hoyt–Spencer) triad consists of progressive visual loss, optic atrophy and opticociliary shunt vessels, although the simultaneous occurrence of all three signs in one individual is actually uncommon. The usual sequence of involvement is the opposite of that seen in tumours that develop outside the dural sheath:
  1. Optic nerve dysfunction and chronic disc swelling followed by atrophy.
  2. Opticociliary collaterals (30%); these regress as optic atrophy supervenes.
  3. Restrictive motility defects, particularly in upgaze (Fig. 3.39C).
  4. Proptosis.

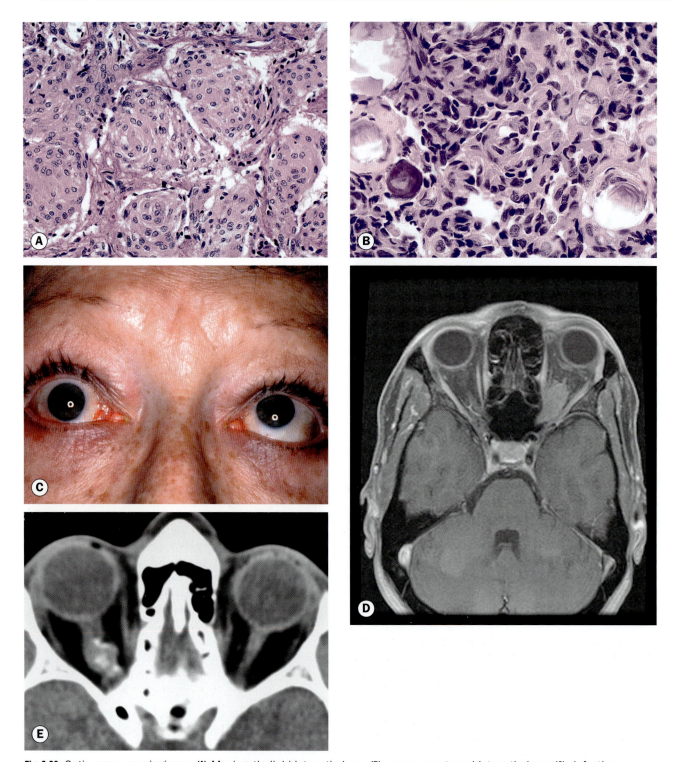

Fig. 3.39 Optic nerve meningioma. **(A)** Meningothelial histopathology; **(B)** psammomatous histopathology; **(C)** defective elevation of the right eye; **(D)** MRI showing lesion associated with left optic nerve; **(E)** axial CT of a small tumour showing calcification

(Courtesy of J Harry and G Misson, from Clinical Ophthalmic Pathology, *Butterworth-Heinemann 2001 – figs A and B; A Pearson – fig. E)*

- **Investigation**
  - ○ MRI is the investigation of choice (Fig. 3.39D).
  - ○ CT shows thickening and calcification of the optic nerve (Fig. 3.39E).
  - ○ Ultrasonography (especially coronal) may be useful.

Treatment

Treatment may not be indicated in a middle-aged patient with a slowly growing lesion, but excision is required for an aggressive tumour, particularly if the eye is blind or there is a risk of intracranial extension. Attempts at optic nerve-sparing surgery commonly fail but may be considered on a case basis. Fractionated stereotactic radiotherapy may be appropriate as a vision-sparing approach, or as adjunctive treatment following surgery.

Plexiform neurofibroma

Plexiform neurofibroma is the most common peripheral neural tumour of the orbit. It occurs almost exclusively in association with NF1. Presentation is in early childhood with periorbital swelling; classically, involvement of the eyelids causes mechanical ptosis with a characteristic S-shaped deformity (see Fig. 1.16), but diffuse involvement of the orbit with disfiguring hypertrophy of periocular tissues may occur. On palpation the involved tissues are said to resemble a 'bag of worms'. Malignant change can occur, and should be suspected if there is rapid change; radiotherapy may promote this. Treatment is often unsatisfactory and complete surgical removal is extremely difficult. Orbital surgery should be avoided when possible because of the intricate relationship between the tumour and important structures.

Isolated neurofibroma

Isolated (localized) neurofibroma is less common than plexiform neurofibroma; about 10% of patients have NF1. Presentation is in the third or fourth decades with insidious mildly painful proptosis, usually not associated with visual impairment or ocular motility dysfunction. Excision is commonly straightforward because the tumour is well-circumscribed and relatively avascular.

LYMPHOMA

Introduction

Lymphomas of the ocular adnexa constitute approximately 8% of all extranodal lymphomas. The majority of orbital lymphomas are non-Hodgkin, and most of these (80%) are of B-cell origin. Those affected are typically older individuals. The condition may be primary, involving one or both orbits only, or secondary if there are one or more identical foci elsewhere in the body; a substantial proportion of apparently primary lesions will develop disease elsewhere within a few years. The course is variable and relatively unpredictable. In some patients histological features raise suspicion of malignancy and yet the lesion resolves spontaneously or with steroid treatment. Conversely, what appears to be reactive lymphoid hyperplasia may be followed by the development of lymphoma. Small lesions and those involving only the conjunctiva have the best prognosis. Conjunctival and intraocular lymphomas are discussed in Chapter 12.

Diagnosis

The onset is characteristically insidious.
- **Symptoms.** An absence of symptoms is common, but may include discomfort, double vision, a bulging eye or a visible mass.

- **Signs**
  - Any part of the orbit may be affected (Fig. 3.40A); anterior lesions may be palpated, and generally have a rubbery consistency (Fig. 3.40B).
  - Occasionally the lymphoma may be confined to the conjunctiva or lacrimal glands, sparing the orbit.
  - Local lymph nodes should be palpated, but systemic evaluation by an appropriate specialist is required.
- **Investigation**
  - Orbital imaging, usually with MRI (Fig. 3.40C).
  - Biopsy is usually performed to establish the diagnosis.
  - Systemic investigation to establish the extent of disease.

Treatment

Radiotherapy is used for localized lesions, and chemotherapy for disseminated disease and some subtypes. Immunotherapy (e.g. rituximab) is a newer modality that may assume a dominant role in the future. Occasionally a well-defined orbital lesion may be resected.

RHABDOMYOSARCOMA

Introduction

Rhabdomyosarcoma (RMS) is the most common soft tissue sarcoma of childhood: 40% develop in the head and neck, and it is the most common primary orbital malignancy in children but is still a rare condition; 90% occur in children under 16 and the average age of onset is 7 years. The tumour is derived from undifferentiated mesenchymal cells that have the potential to differentiate into striated muscle. Various genetic predispositions have been identified, including variants of the *RB1* gene responsible for retinoblastoma. Four subtypes are recognized:
- **Embryonal** constitutes the majority (85%) of orbital lesions. Cells may show light microscopic features of striated muscle differentiation. Embryonal usually carries a good prognosis.
- **Alveolar** makes up most of the balance of orbital RMS. Fewer cells show skeletal muscle differentiation than embryonal, and the prognosis is worse. Particular chromosomal translocations are characteristic on cytogenetic analysis of biopsy material.
- **Botyroid** (4%) and **pleomorphic** RMS are much less common in the orbit.

Diagnosis

- **Symptoms.** Rapidly progressive unilateral proptosis is usual, and may mimic an inflammatory condition such as orbital cellulitis.
- **Signs**
  - The tumour is most commonly superonasal or superior, but may arise anywhere in the orbit, including inferiorly (Figs 3.41A and B). It can also arise in other tissues, such as conjunctiva and uvea.

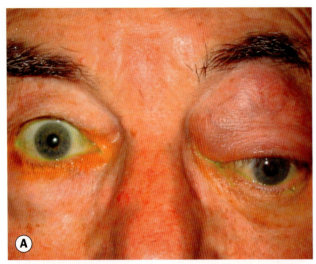

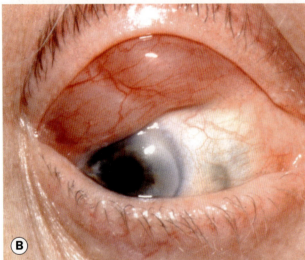

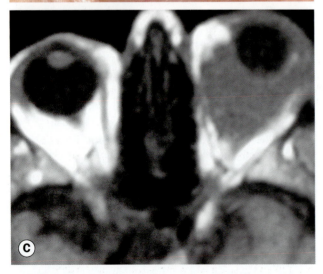

Fig. 3.40 Orbital lymphoma. **(A)** Involvement of the superior orbit causing proptosis and inferior dystopia; **(B)** anterior lesion; **(C)** axial T1-weighted MR of the patient in **(A)** shows a large orbital soft tissue mass and proptosis

(Courtesy of A Pearson – figs A and C)

○ Swelling and redness of overlying skin develop but the skin is not warm (see Fig. 3.41A).
○ Diplopia is frequent, but pain is less common.
● **Investigation**
○ MRI shows a poorly defined mass (Fig. 3.41C).
○ CT shows a poorly defined mass of homogeneous density, often with adjacent bony destruction (Fig. 3.41D).
○ Incisional biopsy is performed to confirm the diagnosis and establish the histopathological subtype and cytogenetic characteristics.
○ Systemic investigation for metastasis should be performed; the most common sites are lung and bone.

Treatment

Commonly used guidelines for staging and a corresponding treatment protocol were produced by the Intergroup Rhabdomyosarcoma Study Group (IRSG); treatment encompasses a combination of radiotherapy, chemotherapy and sometimes surgical debulking. The prognosis for patients with disease confined to the orbit is good.

METASTATIC TUMOURS

Adult metastatic tumours

Introduction

Orbital metastases are an infrequent cause of proptosis, and are much less common than metastases to the choroid. If the orbit is the site of initial manifestation of the tumour, the ophthalmologist may be the first specialist to see the patient. In approximate order of frequency the most common primary sites are breast (up to 70%), bronchus, prostate, skin (melanoma), gastrointestinal tract and kidney.

Diagnosis

● **Signs.** Associated with the range of tumours that can spread to the orbit, presentation can take a variety of forms.
○ Dystopia and proptosis (Fig. 3.42A) are the most common features.
○ Infiltration of orbital tissues characterized by ptosis, diplopia, brawny indurated periorbital skin and a firm orbit, with resistance to manual retropulsion of the globe.
○ Enophthalmos with scirrhous tumours.
○ Chronic inflammation.
○ Primarily with cranial nerve involvement (II, III, IV, V, VI) and only mild proptosis with orbital apex lesions.
● **Investigation**
○ Imaging: CT (Fig. 3.42B) and MRI typically show a non-encapsulated mass.
○ Fine needle biopsy is useful for histological confirmation. If this fails, open biopsy may be required.
○ A search for a primary must be carried out if the patient was not previously known to have cancer.

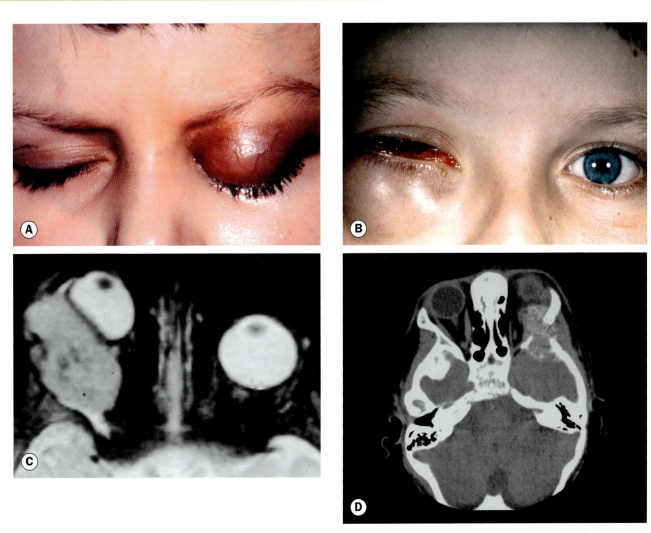

Fig. 3.41 Rhabdomyosarcoma. **(A)** Superiorly and **(B)** anteroinferiorly located lesions; **(C)** axial T2-weighted MR showing a large retrobulbar mass with indentation of the globe and proptosis; **(D)** CT showing bony destruction and intracranial spread
(Courtesy of M Szreter – fig. A; A Pearson – fig. B; S Chen – fig. D)

Treatment

Treatment is aimed at preserving vision and relieving pain, because most patients die within a year (average 4 months). Radiotherapy is the mainstay of local treatment, but systemic therapy may also be of benefit. Surgical excision of the focus is occasionally carried out. Orbital exenteration is usually only performed if other modalities fail to control intolerable symptoms.

Childhood metastatic tumours

Neuroblastoma

Neuroblastoma is one of the most common childhood malignancies. It arises from neural crest-derived tissue of the sympathetic nervous system, most commonly in the abdomen (Fig. 3.43A). Presentation is usually in early childhood; in almost half of all cases the tumour is disseminated at diagnosis, when it carries a very poor prognosis. Orbital metastases may be bilateral and

typically present with the abrupt onset of proptosis accompanied by a superior orbital mass and lid ecchymosis (Fig. 3.43B).

Myeloid sarcoma

Myeloid sarcoma (granulocytic sarcoma) is a solid tumour composed of malignant cells of myeloid origin. Because the tumour may exhibit a characteristic green colour it was formerly referred to as chloroma. Myeloid sarcoma may occur as a manifestation of established myeloid leukaemia, or it may precede the disease. Orbital involvement usually presents at about age 7 years with the rapid onset of proptosis, sometimes bilateral, and can be associated with ecchymosis and lid oedema. When orbital involvement precedes systemic leukaemia, the diagnosis may be difficult.

Langerhans cell histiocytosis

Langerhans cell histiocytosis is a rare group of disorders due to clonal proliferations of histiocytes. Presentation ranges from localized disease, usually with bone destruction (eosinophilic granuloma), through multifocal bone involvement to a fulminant

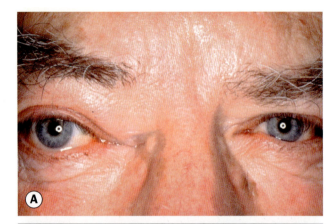

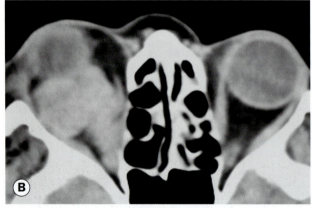

Fig. 3.42 Metastatic renal carcinoma. **(A)** Proptosis; **(B)** axial CT showing a non-encapsulated retrobulbar mass

(Courtesy of A Pearson – fig. B)

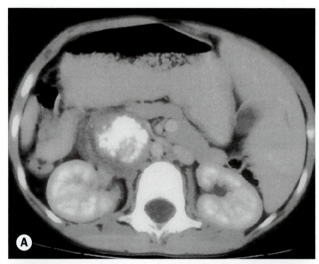

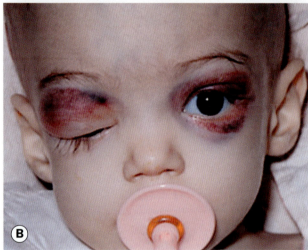

Fig. 3.43 Neuroblastoma. **(A)** Axial CT shows a tumour adjacent to the kidney; **(B)** bilateral orbital metastases

(Courtesy of B Zitelli and H Davis, from Atlas of Pediatric Physical Diagnosis, *Mosby 2002)*

systemic disease. Soft tissues are less commonly involved, but cutaneous and visceral lesions may occur. Orbital involvement consists of unilateral or bilateral osteolytic lesions and soft tissue involvement, typically in the superotemporal quadrant (Fig. 3.44). Patients with solitary lesions tend to have a more benign course, and respond well to treatment with local curettage and intralesional steroid injection or radiotherapy. Systemic disease has a worse prognosis.

Orbital invasion from adjacent structures

Sinus tumours

Malignant tumours of the paranasal sinuses, although rare, may invade the orbit and carry a poor prognosis unless diagnosed early. It is therefore important to be aware of both their otorhinolaryngological and ophthalmic features.

- **Maxillary carcinoma** is by far the most common sinus tumour to invade the orbit (Fig. 3.45).
  - o Otorhinolaryngological manifestations include facial pain and swelling, epistaxis and nasal discharge.
  - o Ophthalmic features include upward dystopia, diplopia and epiphora.

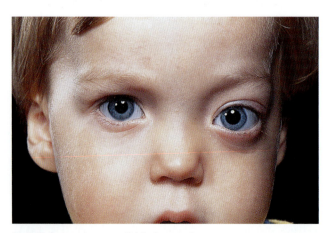

Fig 3.44 Langerhans cell histiocytosis

(Courtesy of D Taylor)

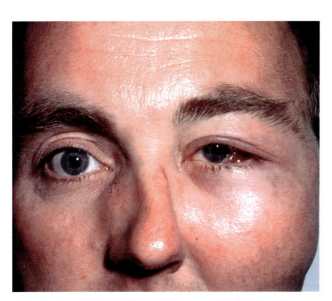

Fig. 3.45 Advanced maxillary carcinoma showing facial swelling and upward dystopia

- **Ethmoidal carcinoma** may cause lateral dystopia.
- **Nasopharyngeal carcinoma** may spread to the orbit through the inferior orbital fissure; proptosis is a late finding.

Bony invasion

- **Intracranial meningioma** arising from the sphenoid ridge may invade the orbit by direct spread and cause proptosis (see Fig. 19.54). Occasionally tumours arising from the tuberculum sellae or olfactory groove may invade the orbit through the superior orbital fissure or optic canal.
- **Fibrous dysplasia** is a disorder in which fibrous tissue develops instead of normal bone, leading to weakening and a mass effect (Fig. 3.46A), usually in childhood or early adulthood. Within the orbital region this may cause facial asymmetry, proptosis, dystopia (Fig. 3.46B) and visual loss. Most orbital disease is due to the monostotic form; polyostotic disease is associated with endocrine disorders and cutaneous pigmentation (McCune–Albright syndrome – 10% of cases).

Orbital invasion from eyelid, conjunctival and intraocular tumours

- Orbital invasion may occur from eyelid malignancies such as basal cell carcinoma, squamous cell carcinoma or sebaceous gland carcinoma, from conjunctival tumours (e.g. melanoma – Fig. 3.47A), and from intraocular tumours such as choroidal melanoma or retinoblastoma (Fig. 3.47B).

THE ANOPHTHALMIC SOCKET

Surgical procedures

Removal of an eye or the contents of the orbit may be indicated for intraocular or orbital malignancy or where the eye is blind and painful or unsightly. A number of different surgical and rehabilitation techniques are available.

Enucleation

Enucleation (removal of the globe) is indicated in the following circumstances:

- **Primary intraocular malignancies** where other treatment modalities are not appropriate. The tumour is left intact within the eye for histopathological examination.
- **After severe trauma** where the risk of sympathetic ophthalmitis may outweigh any prospect of visual recovery; a rare indication (see Ch. 21).
- **Blind painful or unsightly eyes** can also be managed by enucleation, although evisceration is generally considered the procedure of choice.

Evisceration

Evisceration refers to removal of the entire contents of the globe, whilst the sclera and extraocular muscles remain intact. Generally the cornea is removed (Fig. 3.48) to provide access to the ocular contents. Retention of the sclera and lack of disruption of the

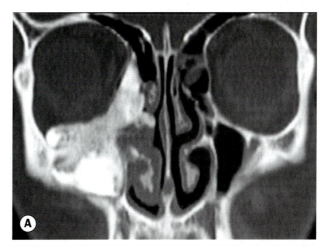

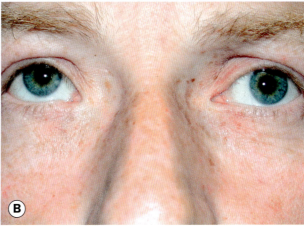

Fig. 3.46 Fibrous dysplasia of the orbit. **(A)** Coronal CT scan showing involvement of the floor and medial wall of the right orbit; **(B)** upward dystopia of the right eye
(Courtesy of A Pearson)

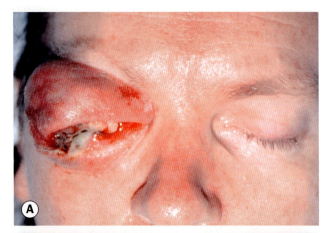

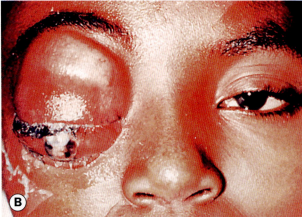

Fig. 3.47 (A) Orbital invasion by conjunctival melanoma; **(B)** orbital invasion by retinoblastoma

extraocular muscles is considered to provide somewhat better motility than is achieved after enucleation. Evisceration provides disrupted and incomplete material for histology and should not be undertaken in the presence of suspected intraocular malignancy.

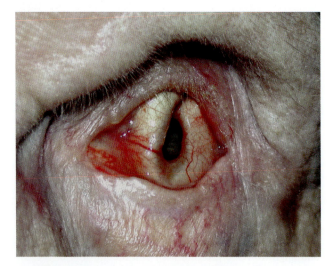

Fig. 3.48 Appearance following evisceration
(Courtesy of S Chen)

Exenteration

Exenteration involves removal of the globe together with the soft tissues of the orbit (Figs 3.49A and B). Indications include:

- **Orbital malignancy**, either primary or where a tumour has invaded the orbit from the eyelids, conjunctiva, globe or adnexa, when other forms of treatment have a very poor chance of success. Anteriorly sited tumours may allow relative sparing of posterior orbital tissue, and posterior tumours may allow sparing of eyelid skin to line the socket (Fig. 3.49C). Following exenteration, prostheses can be attached to the surrounding skin with adhesive, mounted on glasses (Fig. 3.50), or secured with osseo-integrated magnets mounted on the orbital rim bones. The socket may be lined with skin or a split-skin graft, or left to heal by secondary intention.
- **Non-malignant disease** such as orbital mucormycosis is a rare indication.

Rehabilitation

Cosmetic shell

A cosmetic shell is an ocular prosthesis that is used to cover a phthisical or unsightly eye. The shell can restore volume, and often provides a good cosmetic appearance, with reasonable motility as a result of transmitted movements from the globe.

Orbital implants

Enucleation or evisceration leads to a reduction in volume of the orbital contents. A large prosthetic eye without an underlying orbital implant does not provide a satisfactory solution, due to stretching of the lower lid under its weight and to poor motility. An implant is usually inserted during the surgery at which the eye is removed, though secondary placement can be performed later or a previously inserted implant exchanged. Implant materials may be solid ('non-integrated', e.g. silicone, acrylic) or porous ('integrated', e.g. polyethylene, hydroxyapatite). Fibrovascular ingrowth into the latter facilitates motility of an overlying prosthesis; a peg can also be inserted into porous implants to improve later motility, though the peg must be covered *in situ* by socket tissue and cannot attach directly to the overlying prosthesis. The motility of unpegged implants is also usually good, particularly if donor sclera or a mesh wrap is used and the extraocular muscles secured to the surface.

- **Post-enucleation socket syndrome** (PESS) is caused by failure to correct the volume deficit adequately. It is characterized by a deep upper lid sulcus, ptosis, enophthalmos (Fig. 3.51) and backwards rotation of the top of the prosthesis.
- **Extrusion** (Fig. 3.52) is a significant concern with all implants. Careful placement of an implant, ensuring it is sufficiently deep and is well covered with vascularized tissue, is more important than the choice of implant material.

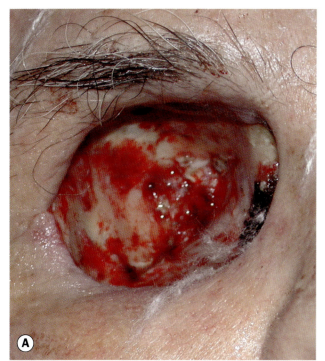

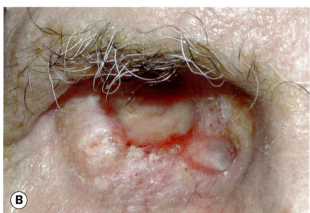

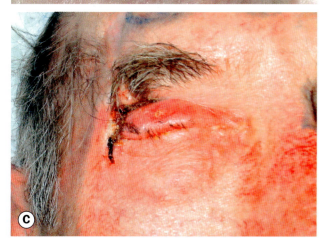

Fig. 3.49 Exenteration. **(A)** Including eyelid removal, 2 days postoperatively; **(B)** patient in (A) 6 months later; **(C)** with sparing of the eyelids

(Courtesy of S Chen – figs A and B; A Pearson – fig. C)

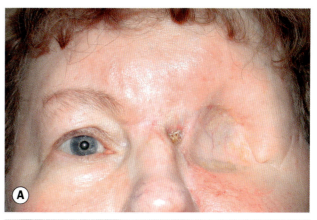

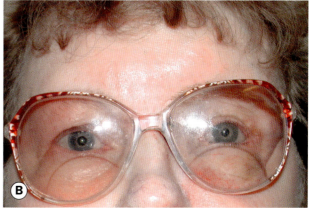

Fig. 3.50 (A) Healed exenteration; **(B)** prosthesis attached to glasses

(Courtesy of A Pearson)

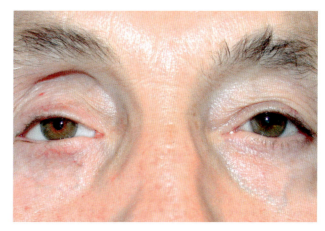

Fig. 3.51 Right post-enucleation socket syndrome (PESS)

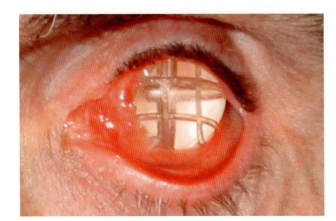

Fig. 3.52 Extruding orbital implant

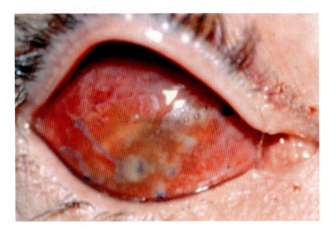

Fig. 3.53 Conformer in place

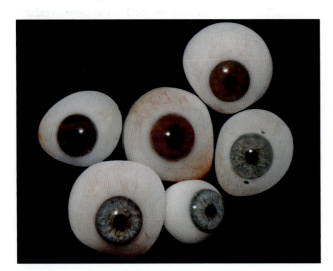

Fig. 3.54 A selection of artificial eyes
(Courtesy of C Barry)

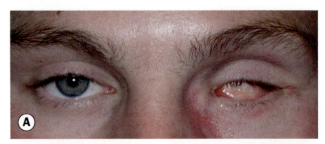

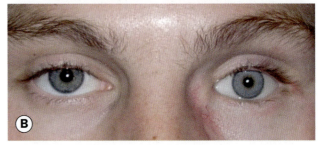

Fig. 3.55 Prosthetic eye. **(A)** Empty socket; **(B)** matching prosthesis in place
(Courtesy of S Chen)

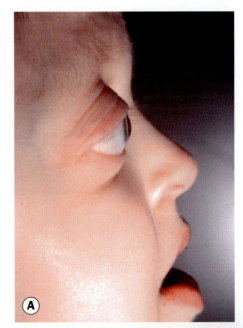

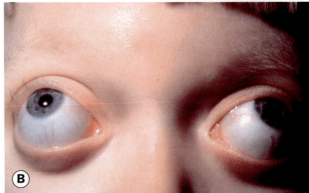

Fig. 3.56 Crouzon syndrome. **(A)** Proptosis, midfacial hypoplasia and mandibular prognathism; **(B)** proptosis and hypertelorism – a 'V' exotropia is also shown

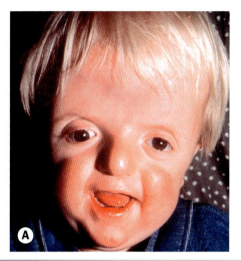

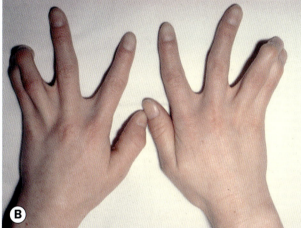

Fig. 3.57 Apert syndrome. **(A)** Mild shallow orbits, midfacial hypoplasia and 'parrot-beak' nose; **(B)** syndactyly

Ocular prosthesis

After enucleation or evisceration a conformer (Fig. 3.53) made of silicone or acrylic material is placed to support the conjunctival fornices and remains in place until the socket is fitted with an artificial eye (Fig. 3.54). Initial socket impression moulds can usually be taken at around 6–8 weeks postoperatively and a temporary artificial eye placed whilst waiting for manufacture of a prosthesis shaped to fit the individual socket and matched to the fellow eye (Fig. 3.55).

CRANIOSYNOSTOSES

The craniosynostoses are a group of rare congenital conditions in which an abnormally shaped skull results from premature closure of skull sutures.

- **Crouzon syndrome** features a short anteroposterior skull diameter, with midfacial hypoplasia giving a prominent lower jaw (Fig. 3.56A); proptosis due to shallow orbits and hypertelorism (wide orbital separation) are the most conspicuous ocular features (Fig. 3.56B). Vision-threatening complications include exposure keratopathy and optic atrophy, mechanisms including chronic papilloedema and cerebral hypoperfusion secondary to sleep apnoea. Strabismus ('V' exotropia – see Fig. 3.56B), ametropia and amblyopia can occur, and other ocular associations have been reported. Inheritance is usually autosomal dominant (AD); allelic variants in the gene *FGFR2* are responsible.
- **Apert syndrome** is the most severe of the craniosynostoses. Oxycephaly (conical skull), midfacial hypoplasia with a beaked nose and low-set ears (Fig. 3.57A), syndactyly (Fig. 3.57B) and developmental delay (30%) may be present. Shallow orbits, proptosis and hypertelorism are generally less pronounced than in Crouzon syndrome, but the same vision-threatening complications occur. Inheritance can be AD, but in the majority of cases the condition is sporadic and associated with older parental age. As with Crouzon syndrome, it is frequently the result of mutations in *FGFR2*.
- **Pfeiffer syndrome** features midfacial hypoplasia and down-slanting palpebral fissures. Ocular features are similar to Apert syndrome. Inheritance is AD with genetic heterogeneity.

Chapter

Dry eye

4

INTRODUCTION

Definitions

Dry eye occurs when there is inadequate tear volume or function, resulting in an unstable tear film and ocular surface disease. It is an extremely common condition, particularly in postmenopausal women and the elderly.

- **Keratoconjunctivitis sicca** (KCS) refers to any eye with some degree of dryness.
- **Xerophthalmia** describes a dry eye associated with vitamin A deficiency.
- **Xerosis** refers to the extreme ocular dryness and keratinization that occurs in eyes with severe conjunctival cicatrization.
- **Sjögren syndrome** is an autoimmune inflammatory disease of which dry eyes is a feature.

Physiology

Tear film constituents

The tear film has three layers (Fig. 4.1):
- **Lipid** layer secreted by the meibomian glands.
- **Aqueous** layer secreted by the lacrimal glands.
- **Mucous** layer secreted principally by conjunctival goblet cells.

The constituents are complex, with as many as a hundred distinct proteins identified.

Spread of the tear film

The tear film is mechanically distributed over the ocular surface through a neuronally controlled blinking mechanism. Three factors are required for effective resurfacing of the tear film:
- Normal blink reflex.
- Contact between the external ocular surface and the eyelids.
- Normal corneal epithelium.

Lipid layer

- **Composition**
  - The outer lipid layer is composed of a polar phase containing phospholipids adjacent to the aqueous-mucin phase and a non-polar phase containing waxes, cholesterol esters and triglycerides.
  - The polar lipids are bound to lipocalins within the aqueous layer. These are small secreted proteins that have the ability to bind hydrophobic molecules and may also contribute to tear viscosity.
  - Lid movement during blinking is important in releasing lipids from glands. The thickness of the layer can be increased by forced blinking, and conversely reduced by infrequent blinking.
- **Functions**
  - To prevent evaporation of the aqueous layer and maintain tear film thickness.
  - To act as a surfactant allowing spread of the tear film.
  - Deficiency results in evaporative dry eye.

Aqueous layer

- **Secretion**
  - The main lacrimal glands produce about 95% of the aqueous component of tears and the accessory lacrimal glands of Krause and Wolfring produce the remainder.
  - Secretion of tears has basic (resting) and much greater reflex components. The latter occurs in response to corneal and conjunctival sensory stimulation, tear break-up and ocular inflammation, and is mediated via the fifth cranial nerve. It is reduced by topical anaesthesia and falls during sleep. Secretion can increase 500% in response to injury.
- **Composition**
  - Water, electrolytes, dissolved mucins and proteins.
  - Growth factors derived from the lacrimal gland, the production of which increases in response to injury.

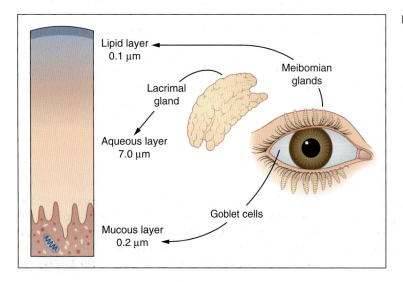

Fig. 4.1 The three layers of the tear film

Lipid layer
0.1 μm

Lacrimal gland

Meibomian glands

Aqueous layer
7.0 μm

Goblet cells

Mucous layer
0.2 μm

o Pro-inflammatory interleukin cytokines that accumulate during sleep when tear production is reduced.

- **Functions**
  - o To provide atmospheric oxygen to the corneal epithelium.
  - o Antibacterial activity due to proteins such as IgA, lysozyme and lactoferrin.
  - o To wash away debris and noxious stimuli and facilitate the transport of leukocytes after injury.
  - o To optically enhance the corneal surface by abolishing minute irregularities.

Mucous layer

- **Composition**
  - o Mucins are high molecular weight glycoproteins that may be transmembrane or secretory in type.
  - o Secretory mucins are further classified as gel-forming or soluble. They are produced mainly by conjunctival goblet cells but also by the lacrimal glands.
  - o The superficial epithelial cells of the cornea and conjunctiva produce transmembrane mucins that form their glycocalyx (extracellular coating).
  - o Staining of diseased epithelium with rose Bengal indicates that the transmembrane and gel mucous layers are absent and the cell surface exposed. Damage to the epithelial cells will prevent normal tear film adherence.
- **Functions**
  - o To permit wetting by converting the corneal epithelium from a hydrophobic to a hydrophilic surface.
  - o Lubrication.
  - o Deficiency of the mucous layer may be a feature of both aqueous deficiency and evaporative states. Goblet cell loss occurs with cicatrizing conjunctivitis, vitamin A deficiency, chemical burns and toxicity from medications.

Regulation of tear film components

- **Hormonal**
  - o Androgens are the prime hormones responsible for regulation of lipid production.
  - o Oestrogens and progesterone receptors in the conjunctiva and the lacrimal glands are essential for the normal function of these tissues.
- **Neural** via fibres adjacent to the lacrimal glands and goblet cells that stimulate aqueous and mucus secretion.

Mechanism of disease

The four core inter-related mechanisms thought to be responsible for the manifestations of dry eye are tear instability, tear hyperosmolarity, inflammation and ocular surface damage. Inflammation in the conjunctiva and accessory glands as well as the ocular surface is present in 80% of patients with KCS and may be both a cause and consequence of dry eye, amplifying and perpetuating disease; the presence of inflammation is the rationale for specific anti-inflammatory measures such as steroid therapy.

Classification

The classification of dry eye usually applied is that of the 2007 International Dry Eye Workshop (DEWS), with a basic division into aqueous-deficient and evaporative types. Most individuals have considerable overlap between mechanisms, and it is important to be aware during patient assessment of the likely presence of multiple contributory factors.

Aqueous-deficient

- **Sjögren syndrome** dry eye (primary or secondary).
- **Non-Sjögren syndrome** dry eye.
  - o Lacrimal deficiency: primary (e.g. age-related dry eye, congenital alacrima, familial dysautonomia) or secondary (e.g. inflammatory and neoplastic lacrimal gland infiltration, acquired immunodeficiency syndrome (AIDS), graft-versus-host disease, lacrimal gland or nerve ablation).
  - o Lacrimal gland duct obstruction, e.g. trachoma, cicatricial pemphigoid, chemical injury, Stevens–Johnson syndrome.
  - o Reflex hyposecretion: sensory (e.g. contact lens wear, diabetes, refractive surgery, neurotrophic keratitis) or motor block (e.g. seventh cranial nerve damage, systemic drugs).

Evaporative

- **Intrinsic**
  - o Meibomian gland deficiency, e.g. posterior blepharitis, rosacea.
  - o Disorders of lid aperture, e.g. excessive scleral show, lid retraction, proptosis, facial nerve palsy.
  - o Low blink rate, e.g. Parkinson disease, prolonged computer monitor use, reading, watching television.
  - o Drug action, e.g. antihistamines, beta-blockers, antispasmodics, diuretics.
- **Extrinsic**
  - o Vitamin A deficiency.
  - o Topical drugs including the effect of preservatives.
  - o Contact lens wear.
  - o Ocular surface disease such as allergic conjunctivitis.

Effect of environmental factors

As well as the basic classification, DEWS draws attention to the effect of the environment on the type of dry eye with which a patient presents. These can be both internal, such as age, hormonal status and behaviour patterns, and external, such as the exacerbation of evaporative factors in an atmosphere with low relative humidity.

SJÖGREN SYNDROME

Sjögren syndrome (SS) is an autoimmune disorder characterized by lymphocytic inflammation and destruction of lacrimal and salivary glands (Fig. 4.2A) and other exocrine organs. The classic clinical triad consists of dry eyes, dry mouth (Fig. 4.2B) and parotid gland enlargement (Fig. 4.2C), but other features are

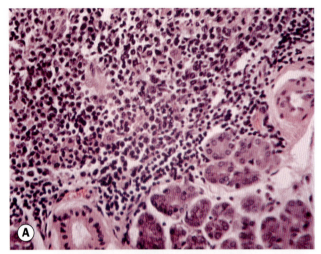

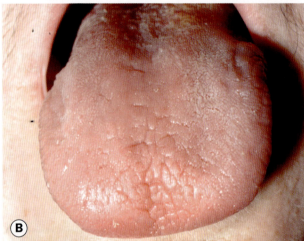

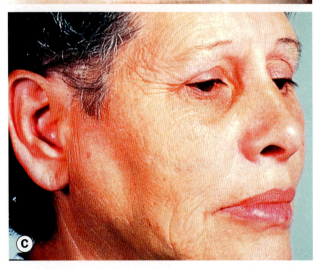

Fig. 4.2 Sjögren syndrome. **(A)** Histology of the lacrimal gland shows lymphocytic infiltration; **(B)** dry fissured tongue; **(C)** parotid gland enlargement
(Courtesy of MA Mir, from Atlas of Clinical Diagnosis, Saunders 2003 – fig. C)

common and can affect all organ systems. The condition is classified as primary when it exists in isolation, and secondary when associated with another disease, commonly rheumatoid arthritis or systemic lupus erythematosus. Primary SS affects females more frequently than males. Although in clinical practice the diagnosis may be made on less stringent grounds, the American College of Rheumatology (ACR) criteria for diagnosis specify, in patients with a clinical picture suggestive of SS:

- Positivity for anti-SSA or anti-SSB antibodies, or positive rheumatoid factor together with significantly positive antinuclear antibody.
- Ocular surface staining above a certain grade.
- Focal lymphocytic sialadenitis to a specified extent on salivary gland biopsy (see Fig. 4.2A).

Widely used but older American-European Consensus Group criteria are more extensive and include more clinical findings, but give results substantially consistent with the ACR criteria.

Treatment options for SS include a range of symptomatic treatments for dry eye, as discussed below, dry mouth and other manifestations, salivary stimulants (e.g. oral pilocarpine) and in some cases immunosuppression and biological blockers such as rituximab.

CLINICAL FEATURES

Symptoms

The most common ocular symptoms are feelings of dryness, grittiness and burning that characteristically worsen over the course of the day. Stringy discharge, transient blurring of vision, redness and crusting of the lids are also common. Lack of emotional or reflex tearing is unusual. The symptoms of KCS are frequently exacerbated on exposure to conditions associated with increased tear evaporation (e.g. air-conditioning, wind and central heating) or prolonged reading or video display unit use, when blink frequency is reduced.

Signs

- **Posterior (seborrhoeic) blepharitis** with meibomian gland dysfunction is often present (Figs 4.3A and B).
- **Conjunctiva**
  - Redness.
  - Staining with fluorescein (Fig. 4.4A) and rose Bengal (Fig. 4.4B).
  - Keratinization.
  - Conjunctivochalasis is a common response to, and exacerbating factor for, the chronic irritation of dry eye, such that a self-sustaining cycle is maintained. It also commonly occurs in other ocular surface disease (see Ch. 5).
- **Tear film**
  - In the normal eye, as the tear film breaks down the mucin layer becomes contaminated with lipid but is washed away.
  - In the dry eye, the lipid-contaminated mucin accumulates in the tear film as particles and debris that move with each blink (Fig. 4.5A).

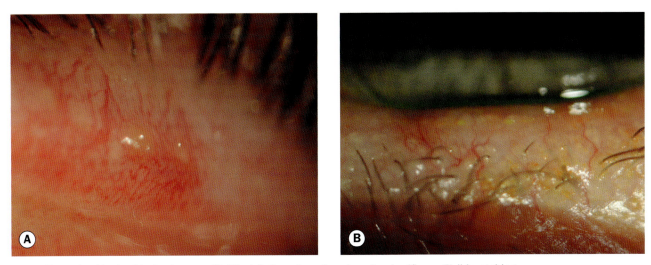

Fig. 4.3 Posterior blepharitis in dry eye. **(A)** Oil globules at meibomian gland orifices; **(B)** lid notching

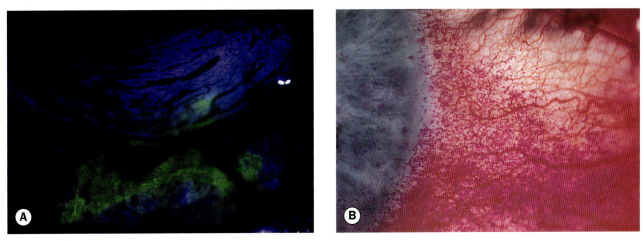

Fig. 4.4 Conjunctival staining in dry eye. **(A)** Fluorescein; **(B)** rose Bengal

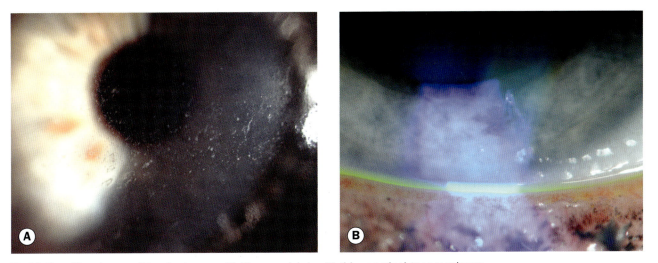

Fig. 4.5 Tear film abnormalities in dry eye. **(A)** Mucous debris; **(B)** thin marginal tear meniscus

○ The marginal tear meniscus (strip) is a crude measure of the volume of aqueous in the tear film. In the normal eye the meniscus is 0.2–0.4 mm in height, but in dry eye becomes thin or absent (Fig. 4.5B).

- **Cornea**
  ○ Punctate epithelial erosions that stain well with fluorescein (Figs 4.6A and B).
  ○ Filaments consist of strands of mucus and debris such as shed epithelial cells, and are typically attached at one end to the corneal surface (Fig. 4.6C); they stain well with rose Bengal but less so with fluorescein.
  ○ Mucous plaques with similar constituents may occur in severe dry eye. They consist of semi-transparent, white-to-grey, often slightly elevated lesions of varying size (Figs 4.6D and E).
- **Complications** can be vision-threatening and include epithelial breakdown, melting (Fig. 4.7A), perforation (Fig. 4.7B) and bacterial keratitis (Fig. 4.7C).

INVESTIGATION

The aim of investigation is to confirm and quantify a clinical diagnosis of dry eye. Unfortunately, although the repeatability of symptoms is good, that of clinical tests is poor, as is the correlation between symptoms and tests. The reliability of tests improves as the severity of dry eye increases. The tests measure the following parameters:

- Stability of the tear film as related to its break-up time (BUT).
- Tear production (Schirmer, fluorescein clearance and tear osmolarity).
- Ocular surface disease (corneal stains and impression cytology).

There is no clinical test to confirm the diagnosis of evaporative dry eye. It is therefore a presumptive diagnosis based on the presence of associated clinical findings. It is suggested the tests are performed in the following order because the Schirmer strip paper can damage the ocular surface and cause staining.

Tear film break-up time

The tear film BUT is abnormal in aqueous tear deficiency and meibomian gland disorders. It is measured as follows:

- Fluorescein 2% or an impregnated fluorescein strip moistened with non-preserved saline is instilled into the lower fornix.
- The patient is asked to blink several times.
- The tear film is examined at the slit lamp with a broad beam using the cobalt blue filter. After an interval, black spots or lines appear in the fluorescein-stained film (Fig. 4.8A), indicating the formation of dry areas.
- The BUT is the interval between the last blink and the appearance of the first randomly distributed dry spot. A BUT of less than 10 seconds is suspicious.

The development of dry spots always in the same location may indicate a local corneal surface abnormality (e.g. epithelial basement membrane disease) rather than an intrinsic instability of the tear film.

Schirmer test

The Schirmer test is a useful assessment of aqueous tear production. The test involves measuring the amount of wetting of a special (no. 41 Whatman) filter paper, 5 mm wide and 35 mm long. The test can be performed with or without topical anaesthesia. In theory, when performed with an anaesthetic (Schirmer 2) basic secretion is measured and without anaesthetic (Schirmer 1) it measures maximum basic plus reflex secretion. In practice, however, topical anaesthesia cannot abolish all sensory and psychological stimuli for reflex secretion. The test is performed as follows:

- Excess tears are delicately dried. If topical anaesthesia is applied the excess should be removed from the inferior fornix with filter paper.
- The filter paper is folded 5 mm from one end and inserted at the junction of the middle and outer third of the lower lid, taking care not to touch the cornea or lashes (Fig. 4.8B).
- The patient is asked to keep the eyes gently closed.
- After 5 minutes the filter paper is removed and the amount of wetting from the fold measured.
- Less than 10 mm of wetting after 5 minutes without anaesthesia or less than 6 mm with anaesthesia is considered abnormal.

Results can be variable and a single Schirmer test should not be used as the sole criterion for diagnosing dry eye, but repeatedly abnormal tests are highly supportive.

Ocular surface staining

- **Fluorescein** stains corneal and conjunctival epithelium (see Figs 4.4 and 4.6) where there is sufficient damage to allow the dye to enter the tissues.
- **Rose Bengal** is a dye that has an affinity for dead or devitalized epithelial cells that have a lost or altered mucous layer (Fig. 4.8C). Corneal filaments and plaques (see Fig. 4.6B) are also shown up more clearly by the dye and the use of a red-free filter may help visualization. A 1% solution of rose Bengal or a moistened impregnated strip can be used. The dye may cause intense stinging that can last for up to a day, particularly in patients with severe KCS; to minimize irritation a very small drop should be used, immediately preceded by a drop of topical anaesthetic, and the excess washed out with saline.
- **Lissamine green** stains in a similar fashion to rose Bengal but causes less irritation and may be preferred.
- **The pattern** of staining may aid diagnosis:
  ○ Interpalpebral staining of the cornea and conjunctiva (see Fig. 4.4B) is common in aqueous tear deficiency.
  ○ Superior conjunctival stain may indicate superior limbic keratoconjunctivitis.
  ○ Inferior corneal and conjunctival stain is often present in patients with blepharitis or exposure.

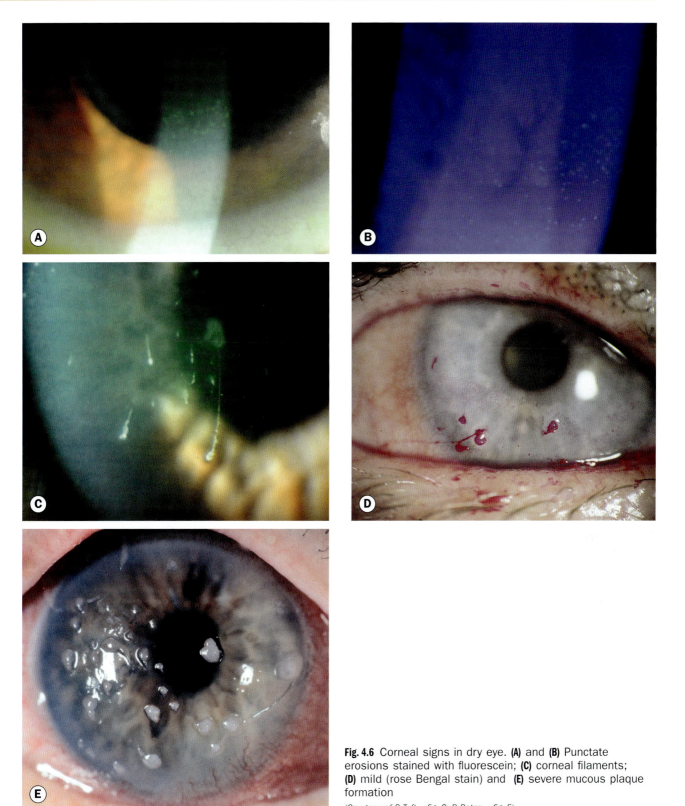

Fig. 4.6 Corneal signs in dry eye. **(A)** and **(B)** Punctate erosions stained with fluorescein; **(C)** corneal filaments; **(D)** mild (rose Bengal stain) and **(E)** severe mucous plaque formation

(Courtesy of S Tuft – fig. C; R Bates – fig. E)

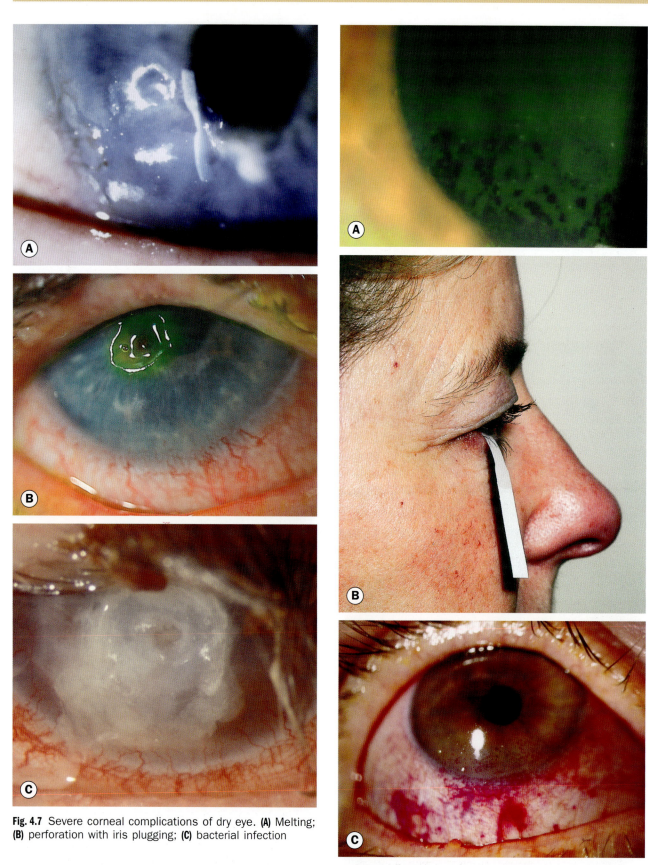

Fig. 4.7 Severe corneal complications of dry eye. **(A)** Melting; **(B)** perforation with iris plugging; **(C)** bacterial infection

Fig. 4.8 Diagnostic tests in dry eye. **(A)** Tear film break-up time – numerous dry spots are present in a fluorescein-stained tear film; **(B)** Schirmer test; **(C)** corneal and conjunctival staining with rose Bengal

Other investigations

The following tests are rarely performed in clinical practice.

- **Fluorescein clearance test** and the tear function index may be assessed by placing 5 μl of fluorescein on the ocular surface and measuring the residual dye in a Schirmer strip placed on the lower lateral lid margin at set intervals. Delayed clearance is observed in all dry eye states.
- **Tear film osmolarity** measurement techniques are available; this may be a particularly accurate means of diagnosis.
- **Tear constituent** measurement. Tear samples can be assayed for the presence of markers known to be elevated (e.g. matrix metalloproteinase-9) or decreased (e.g. lactoferrin) in dry eye.
- **Phenol red thread test** uses a thread impregnated with a pH-sensitive dye. The end of the thread is placed over the lower lid and the length wetted (the dye changes from yellow to red in tears) is measured after 15 seconds. A value of 6 mm is abnormal. It is comparable to the Schirmer test but takes less time to perform.
- **Tear meniscometry** is a technique to quantify the height and thus the volume of the lower lid meniscus.
- **Impression cytology** can determine goblet cell numbers.

TREATMENT

Strategy

The underlying causative processes of dry eye are generally not reversible and management is therefore structured around the control of symptoms and the prevention of surface damage. DEWS have produced guidelines based on earlier International Taskforce Guidelines for Dry Eye, in which suggested treatment options depend on the level of severity of disease graded from 1 to 4. The DEWS guidelines can also be applied in a graded approach, proceeding to the next level if the preceding measures are inadequate.

Level 1

- **Education and environmental/dietary modifications**
  - Establishment of realistic expectations and emphasis on the importance of compliance.
  - Lifestyle review including the importance of blinking whilst reading, watching television or using a computer screen (which should be orientated below eye level to minimize palpebral aperture size), and the management of contact lens wear.
  - Environmental review, e.g. increasing humidity may be possible for some environments.
  - Instillation aids for eye drops (manufacturer-supplied or makeshift, such as nut-crackers to hold plastic bottles) should be advocated for patients with reduced dexterity (e.g. rheumatoid arthritis).
  - Caution the patient that laser refractive surgery can exacerbate dry eye.
- **Systemic medication review** to exclude contributory effects and eliminate offending agents. Discontinuation of toxic/preserved topical medication if possible.
- **Artificial tear substitutes including gels and ointments** – see below; some authorities advocate that use of preserved drops should fall within level 1, and categorize non-preserved drops as a level 2 measure. Mucolytic agents may be specifically indicated for some patients.
- **Eyelid therapy.** Basic measures such as warm compresses and lid hygiene for blepharitis; reparative lid surgery (e.g. entropion, ectropion, excessive lid laxity or scleral show) may be considered as an early measure. Nocturnal lagophthalmos can be addressed by taping the lids closed at bedtime, wearing swimming goggles during sleep, or in extreme cases by lateral tarsorrhaphy.

Level 2

- **Non-preserved tear substitutes** are categorized as level 2 treatment by some authorities.
- **Anti-inflammatory agents** such as topical steroids, oral omega fatty acids and other agents such as topical ciclosporin.
- **Tetracyclines** (for meibomianitis, rosacea).
- **Punctal plugs.**
- **Secretagogues**, e.g. pilocarpine, cevilemine, rebamipide.
- **Moisture chamber spectacles and spectacle side shields.**

Level 3

- **Serum eye drops.** Autologous or umbilical cord serum.
- **Contact lenses.**
- **Permanent punctal occlusion.**

Level 4

- **Systemic anti-inflammatory agents.**
- **Surgery**
  - Eyelid surgery, such as tarsorrhaphy.
  - Salivary gland autotransplantation.
  - Mucous membrane or amniotic membrane transplantation for corneal complications.

Tear substitutes

Tear substitutes have a relatively simple formulation that cannot approximate the complex components and structure of the normal tear film. Their delivery is also periodic rather than continuous. Almost all are based on replacement of the aqueous phase of the tear film. There are no mucus substitutes, and paraffin is only an approximation to the action of tear lipids. The optimal frequency of instillation varies with agent and with severity

- **Drops and gels.** A large range of preparations is available; one agent or category of preparation has not demonstrated superiority, and particular agents are often preferred by individual patients with limited rationale.
  - Cellulose derivatives (e.g. hypromellose, methylcellulose) are appropriate for mild cases.

- Carbomer gels adhere to the ocular surface and so are longer-lasting, but some patients are troubled by slight blurring.
- Other agents include polyvinyl alcohol (PVA), which increases the persistence of the tear film and is useful in mucin deficiency, sodium hyaluronate, povidone, glycerine, propylene glycol, polysorbate and others.
- Diquafosol is a newer agent that works as a topical secretagogue.
- **Ointments** containing petrolatum (paraffin) mineral oil can be used at bedtime to supplement daytime drops or gel instillation; daytime use is precluded by marked blurring. Some practitioners do not prescribe these for long-term use.
- **Eyelid sprays** are applied to the closed eye and typically contain a liposome-based agent that may stabilize the tear film and reduce evaporation.
- **Artificial tear inserts** emplaced once or twice daily offer extended duration treatment and are preferred by some patients.
- **Mucolytic agents.** Acetylcysteine 5% drops may be useful in patients with corneal filaments and mucous plaques, which acetylcysteine dissolves; it may cause stinging on instillation. Acetylcysteine is malodorous and has a limited shelf life. Manual debridement of filaments may also be useful.
- **Preservatives** can be a potent source of toxicity, especially after punctal occlusion. Numerous non-preserved drops are now available, including some multi-dose products, and in general should be used in preference to preservative-containing preparations in any more than mild disease or with instillation more than three or four times daily. If possible, preservative-free formulations should also be used for dry eye patients when other topical medication is required, for example in the treatment of glaucoma. Newer preservatives such as Polyquad and Purite seem to exhibit lower ocular surface toxicity than older agents such as benzalkonium chloride.

Punctal occlusion

Punctal occlusion reduces drainage and thereby preserves natural tears and prolongs the effect of artificial tears. It is of greatest value in patients with moderate to severe KCS who have not responded to frequent instillation of topical agents.

- **Temporary** occlusion can be achieved by inserting collagen plugs into the canaliculi; these dissolve over a number of weeks. The main aim is to ensure that epiphora does not occur following permanent occlusion.
  - Initially the inferior puncta are occluded and the patient is reviewed after 1 or 2 weeks.
  - If the patient is now asymptomatic and without epiphora, the plugs can be removed and the inferior canaliculi permanently occluded (see below).
  - In severe KCS both the inferior and superior canaliculi can be plugged.
- **Reversible** prolonged occlusion can be achieved with silicone (Fig. 4.9) or long-acting (2–6 months) collagen plugs.

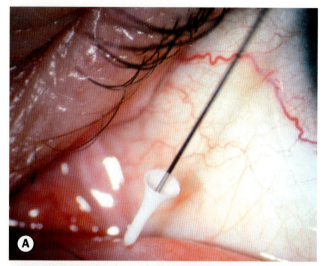
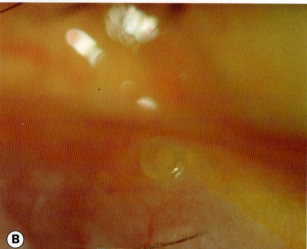

Fig. 4.9 (A) Insertion of a silicone plug; **(B)** plug in place
(Courtesy of S Tuft – fig. A)

- Problems include extrusion, granuloma formation and distal migration.
- Plugs that pass into the horizontal portion of the canaliculus cannot be visualized and although they can usually be flushed out with saline, if they cause epiphora this is not always possible and surgical retrieval may be needed.
- **Permanent** occlusion should be undertaken only in patients with severe dry eye who have had a positive response to temporary plugs without epiphora. It should be avoided in patients, especially if young, who may have reversible pathology. All four puncta should not be occluded at the same time.
  - Permanent occlusion is performed following punctal dilatation by coagulating the proximal canaliculus with cautery; following successful occlusion, it is important to watch for signs of recanalization.
  - Laser cautery seems to be less consistently effective than surgical thermal coagulation.

Anti-inflammatory agents

- **Topical steroids**, generally low-intensity preparations such as fluorometholone, are effective supplementary treatment for acute exacerbations. The risks of longer-term treatment must be balanced against the potential benefits in each case.
- **Omega fatty acid supplements** (e.g. omega-3 fish oil, flax seed oil) can have a dramatic effect on symptoms and may facilitate the reduction of topical medication.
- **Oral tetracyclines** for an extended course, often 3 months at a relatively low dose, may control associated blepharitis, especially meibomianitis, and reduce tear levels of inflammatory mediators. Doxycycline may be preferred to minocycline on the grounds of adverse effect profile.
- **Topical ciclosporin** (usually 0.05%) reduces T-cell mediated inflammation of lacrimal tissue, resulting in an increase in the number of goblet cells and reversal of squamous metaplasia of the conjunctiva.

Contact lenses

Although contact lens wear can exacerbate dry eye, particularly due to inflammatory, sensory and evaporative effects, these can be outweighed by the reservoir effect of fluid trapped behind the lens, and they are effective at relieving symptoms from secondary corneal changes. Patients should be cautioned regarding the possibility of bacterial keratitis.

- **Low water** content HEMA lenses may be successfully fitted to moderately dry eyes.
- **Silicone** rubber lenses that contain no water and readily transmit oxygen are effective in protecting the cornea in extreme tear film deficiency, although deposition of debris on the surface of the lens can blur vision and be problematic. The continued availability of these lenses is in doubt.

- **Occlusive** gas permeable scleral contact lenses provide a reservoir of saline over the cornea. They can be worn on an extremely dry eye with exposure.

Optimization of environmental humidity

- **Reduction of room temperature** to minimize evaporation of tears.
- **Room humidifiers** may be tried but are frequently disappointing because much apparatus is incapable of significantly increasing the relative humidity of an average-sized room. A temporary local increase in humidity can be achieved with moist chamber goggles or side shields to glasses but may be cosmetically unacceptable.

Miscellaneous options

- **Botulinum toxin injection** to the orbicularis muscle may help control the blepharospasm that often occurs in severe dry eye. Injected at the medial canthus it can also reduce tear drainage, presumably by limiting lid movement.
- **Oral cholinergic agonists** such as pilocarpine (5 mg four times daily) and cevilemine may reduce the symptoms of dry eye and dry mouth in patients with Sjögren syndrome. Adverse effects including blurred vision and sweating may be less marked with cevilemine.
- **Submandibular gland transplantation** for extreme dry eye requires extensive surgery and may produce excessive levels of mucus in the tear film.
- **Serum eye drops.** Autologous or umbilical cord serum (20–100%), the blood component remaining after clotting, has produced subjective and objective improvements in studies in patients with dry eye; they may aid the healing of persistent epithelial defects. Their production and storage carries practical challenges.

Conjunctiva

INTRODUCTION

Anatomy

The conjunctiva is a transparent mucous membrane that lines the inner surface of the eyelids and the anterior surface of the globe, terminating at the corneoscleral limbus. It is richly vascular, supplied by the anterior ciliary and palpebral arteries. There is a dense lymphatic network, with drainage to the preauricular and submandibular nodes corresponding to that of the eyelids. It has a key protective role, mediating both passive and active immunity. Anatomically, it is divided into the following:

- **The palpebral conjunctiva** starts at the mucocutaneous junction of the lid margins and is firmly attached to the posterior tarsal plates. The tarsal blood vessels are vertically orientated.
- **The forniceal conjunctiva** is loose and redundant.
- **The bulbar conjunctiva** covers the anterior sclera and is continuous with the corneal epithelium at the limbus. Radial ridges at the limbus form the palisades of Vogt, the likely reservoir of corneal stem cells. The stroma is loosely attached to the underlying Tenon capsule, except at the limbus, where the two layers fuse. The plica semilunaris (semilunar fold) is present nasally, medial to which lies a fleshy nodule (caruncle) consisting of modified cutaneous tissue.

Histology

- **The epithelium** is non-keratinizing and around five cell layers deep (Fig. 5.1). Basal cuboidal cells evolve into flattened polyhedral cells, subsequently being shed from the surface. Mucus-secreting goblet cells are located within the epithelium, being most dense inferonasally and in the fornices.
- **The stroma** (substantia propria) consists of richly vascularized loose connective tissue. The accessory lacrimal glands of Krause and Wolfring are located deep within the stroma. Secretions from the accessory lacrimal glands are essential components of the tear film.

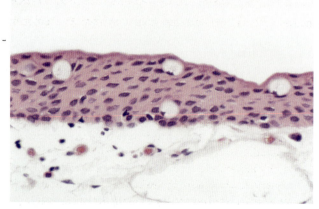

Fig. 5.1 Histology of the conjunctiva
(Courtesy of J Harry)

- **Conjunctiva-associated lymphoid tissue (CALT)** is critical in the initiation and regulation of ocular surface immune responses. It consists of lymphocytes within the epithelial layers, lymphatics and associated blood vessels, with a stromal component of lymphocytes and plasma cells, including follicular aggregates.

Clinical features of conjunctival inflammation

Symptoms

Non-specific symptoms include lacrimation, grittiness, stinging and burning. Itching is the hallmark of allergic disease, although it may also occur to a lesser extent in blepharitis and dry eye. Significant pain, photophobia or a marked foreign body sensation suggest corneal involvement.

Discharge

- **Watery** discharge is composed of a serous exudate and tears, and occurs in acute viral or acute allergic conjunctivitis.
- **Mucoid** discharge is typical of chronic allergic conjunctivitis and dry eye.
- **Mucopurulent** discharge typically occurs in chlamydial or acute bacterial infection.
- **Moderately purulent** discharge occurs in acute bacterial conjunctivitis.
- **Severe purulent** discharge is suggestive of gonococcal infection.

Conjunctival reaction

- **Hyperaemia** that is diffuse, beefy-red and more intense away from the limbus is usual in bacterial infection (Fig. 5.2A). This 'conjunctival injection' should be distinguished from the ciliary injection of iridocyclitis (see Ch. 11).
- **Haemorrhages** may occur in viral conjunctivitis, when they are often multiple, small and discrete ('petechial' – Fig. 5.2B), and severe bacterial conjunctivitis, when they are larger and diffuse.
- **Chemosis** (conjunctival oedema) is seen as a translucent swelling (Fig. 5.2C), which when severe may protrude through the eyelids. Acute chemosis usually indicates a hypersensitivity response (e.g. pollen), but can also occur in severe infective conjunctivitis. Subacute or chronic chemosis has numerous causes:
  - Local, e.g. thyroid eye disease, chronic allergic conjunctivitis, ocular or eyelid surgery, trauma.
  - Increased systemic vascular permeability, e.g. allergic conditions, infections including meningitis, vasculitis.
  - Increased venous pressure, e.g. superior vena cava syndrome, right-sided heart failure.
  - Decreased plasma oncotic pressure, e.g. nephrotic syndrome.

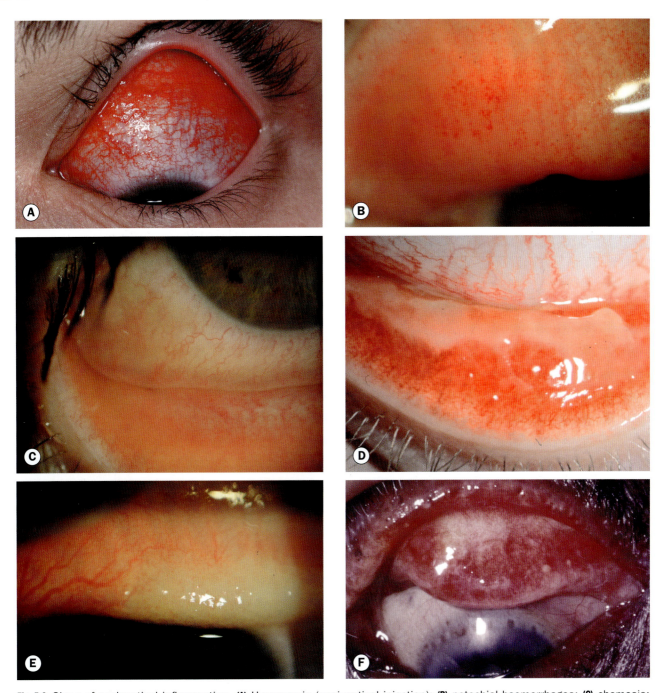

Fig. 5.2 Signs of conjunctival inflammation. **(A)** Hyperaemia (conjunctival injection); **(B)** petechial haemorrhages; **(C)** chemosis; **(D)** pseudomembrane; **(E)** infiltration; **(F)** scarring
(Courtesy of P Saine –fig. A; S Tuft – fig. B; C Barry – fig. F)

- **Membranes**
  - Pseudomembranes (Fig. 5.2D) consist of coagulated exudate adherent to the inflamed conjunctival epithelium. They can be peeled away leaving the underlying epithelium intact.
  - True membranes involve the superficial layers of the conjunctival epithelium so that attempted removal leads to tearing. The distinction between a true membrane and a pseudomembrane is rarely clinically helpful and both can leave scarring following resolution.

  - Causes include severe adenoviral conjunctivitis, gonococcal and some other bacterial conjunctivitides (*Streptococcus* spp., *Corynebacterium diphtheriae*), ligneous conjunctivitis and Stevens–Johnson syndrome.
- **Infiltration** represents cellular recruitment to the site of chronic inflammation and typically accompanies a papillary response. It is recognized by loss of detail of the normal tarsal conjunctival vessels, especially on the upper lid (Fig. 5.2E).
- **Subconjunctival cicatrization** (scarring) may occur in trachoma and other severe conjunctivitides (Fig. 5.2F).

Severe scarring is associated with loss of goblet cells and accessory lacrimal glands, and can lead to cicatricial entropion.

- **Follicles**
  - ○ Signs. Multiple, discrete, slightly elevated lesions resembling translucent grains of rice, most prominent in the fornices (Fig. 5.3A). Blood vessels run around or across rather than within the lesions.
  - ○ Histology shows a subepithelial lymphoid germinal centre with central immature lymphocytes and mature cells peripherally (Fig. 5.3B).
  - ○ Causes include viral and chlamydial conjunctivitis, Parinaud oculoglandular syndrome and hypersensitivity to topical medications. Small follicles are a normal finding in childhood (folliculosis), as are follicles in the fornices and at the margin of the upper tarsal plate in adults.
- **Papillae** can develop only in the palpebral conjunctiva and in the limbal bulbar conjunctiva where it is attached to the deeper fibrous layer.
  - ○ Signs. In contrast to follicles, a vascular core is present. Micropapillae form a mosaic-like pattern of elevated red dots as a result of the central vascular channel,

macropapillae (<1 mm – Fig. 5.3C) and giant papillae (>1 mm) develop with prolonged inflammation. Apical infiltrate or staining with fluorescein or the presence of mucus can be present with marked activity. Limbal papillae have a gelatinous appearance.
  - ○ Histology shows folds of hyperplastic conjunctival epithelium with a fibrovascular core and subepithelial stromal infiltration with inflammatory cells (Fig. 5.3D). Late changes include superficial stromal hyalinization, scarring and the formation of crypts containing goblet cells.
  - ○ Causes include bacterial conjunctivitis, allergic conjunctivitis, chronic blepharitis, contact lens wear, superior limbic keratoconjunctivitis and floppy eyelid syndrome.

Lymphadenopathy

The most common cause of lymphadenopathy associated with conjunctivitis is viral infection. It may also occur in chlamydial and severe bacterial conjunctivitis (especially gonococcal), and Parinaud oculoglandular syndrome. The preauricular site is typically affected.

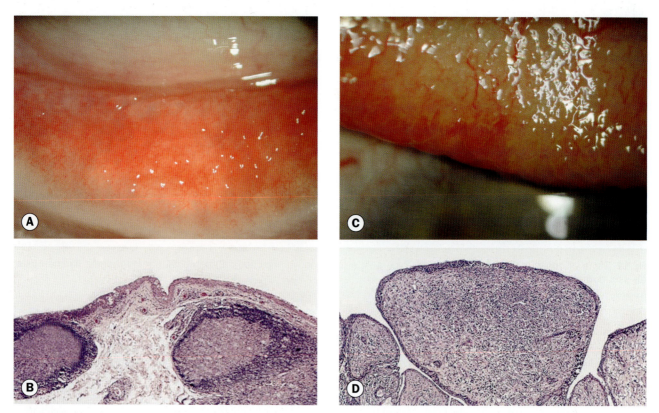

Fig. 5.3 (A) Conjunctival follicles; **(B)** histology of a follicle showing two subepithelial germinal centres with immature lymphocytes centrally and mature cells peripherally; **(C)** conjunctival macropapillae; **(D)** histology of a papilla showing folds of hyperplastic conjunctival epithelium with a fibrovascular core and subepithelial stromal infiltration with inflammatory cells

(Courtesy of J Harry – figs B and D)

BACTERIAL CONJUNCTIVITIS

Acute bacterial conjunctivitis

Acute bacterial conjunctivitis is a common and usually self-limiting condition caused by direct contact with infected secretions. The most common isolates are *Streptococcus pneumoniae*, *Staphylococcus aureus*, *Haemophilus influenzae* and *Moraxella catarrhalis*. A minority of cases, usually severe, are caused by the sexually transmitted organism *Neisseria gonorrhoeae*, which can readily invade the intact corneal epithelium. Meningococcal (*Neisseria meningitidis*) conjunctivitis is rare, and usually affects children.

Diagnosis

- **Symptoms**
  - Acute onset of redness, grittiness, burning and discharge.
  - Involvement is usually bilateral although one eye may become affected 1–2 days before the other.
  - On waking, the eyelids are frequently stuck together and may be difficult to open.
  - Systemic symptoms may occur in patients with severe conjunctivitis associated with gonococcus, meningococcus, *Chlamydia* and *H. influenzae*. In children, the possibility of progression to systemic involvement should always be borne in mind.
- **Signs** are variable and depend on the severity of infection.
  - Eyelid oedema and erythema (Fig. 5.4A) may occur in severe infection, particularly gonococcal.
  - Conjunctival injection as previously described (Fig. 5.4B and see Fig. 5.2A).
  - The discharge can initially be watery, mimicking viral conjunctivitis, but rapidly becomes mucopurulent (Fig. 5.4C).
  - Hyperacute purulent discharge (Fig. 5.4D) may signify gonococcal or meningococcal conjunctivitis.
  - Superficial corneal punctate epithelial erosions are common.
  - Peripheral corneal ulceration may occur in gonococcal and meningococcal infection, and may rapidly progress to perforation.
  - Lymphadenopathy is usually absent except in severe gonococcal and meningococcal infection.

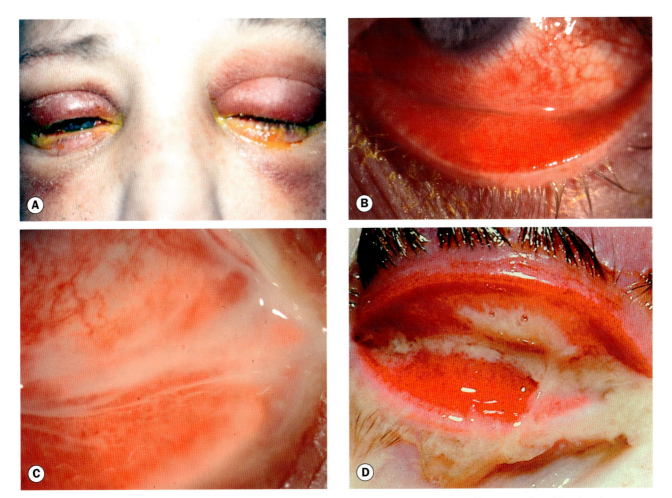

Fig. 5.4 Bacterial conjunctivitis. **(A)** Eyelid oedema and erythema in severe infection; **(B)** diffuse tarsal and forniceal conjunctival hyperaemia (injection); **(C)** mucopurulent discharge; **(D)** profuse purulent discharge

- **Investigations** are not performed routinely but may be indicated in the following situations:
  - In severe cases, binocular conjunctival swabs and scrapings should be taken for urgent Gram staining, particularly to exclude gonococcal and meningococcal infection (Gram-negative kidney-shaped intracellular diplococci).
  - Culture should include enriched media such as chocolate agar or Thayer–Martin for *N. gonorrhoeae*.
  - Polymerase chain reaction (PCR) may be required for less severe cases that fail to respond to treatment, particularly to rule out the possibility of chlamydial and viral infection.

Treatment

About 60% resolve within 5 days without treatment.

- **Topical antibiotics**, usually four times daily for up to a week but sometimes more intensively, are frequently administered to speed recovery and prevent re-infection and transmission. There is no evidence that any particular antibiotic is more effective. Ointments and gels provide a higher concentration for longer periods than drops but daytime use is limited because of blurred vision. The following antibiotics are available:
  - Chloramphenicol, aminoglycosides (gentamicin, neomycin, tobramycin), quinolones (ciprofloxacin, ofloxacin, levofloxacin, lomefloxacin, gatifloxacin, moxifloxacin, besifloxacin), macrolides (erythromycin, azithromycin) polymyxin B, fusidic acid and bacitracin.
  - Some practitioners, particularly in the United States, believe that chloramphenicol should not be used for routine treatment because of a possible link with aplastic anaemia.
  - Gonococcal and meningococcal conjunctivitis should be treated with a quinolone, gentamicin, chloramphenicol or bacitracin 1–2 hourly as well as systemic therapy (see below).
- **Systemic antibiotics** are required in the following circumstances:
  - Gonococcal infection is usually treated with a third-generation cephalosporin such as ceftriaxone; quinolones and some macrolides are alternatives. It is essential to seek advice from a microbiologist and/or genitourinary specialist.
  - *H. influenzae* infection, particularly in children, is treated with oral amoxicillin with clavulanic acid; there is a 25% risk of developing otitis and other systemic problems.
  - Meningococcal conjunctivitis, also particularly in children, in whom early systemic prophylaxis may be life-saving as up to 30% develop invasive systemic disease. The advice of paediatric and infectious disease specialists must be sought but if in doubt treatment with intramuscular benzylpenicillin, ceftriaxone or cefotaxime, or oral ciprofloxacin should not be delayed.
  - Preseptal or orbital cellulitis (see Ch. 3).

- **Topical steroids** may reduce scarring in membranous and pseudomembranous conjunctivitis, although evidence for their use is unclear.
- **Irrigation** to remove excessive discharge may be useful in hyperpurulent cases.
- **Contact lens wear** should be discontinued until at least 48 hours after complete resolution of symptoms. Contact lenses should not be worn whilst topical antibiotic treatment continues.
- **Risk of transmission should be reduced** by hand-washing and the avoidance of towel sharing.
- **Review** is unnecessary for most mild/moderate adult cases, although patients should be cautioned to seek further advice in the event of deterioration.
- **Statutory notification of public health authorities** may be required locally for some causes.

Giant fornix syndrome

Giant fornix syndrome is an uncommon entity causing chronic relapsing pseudomembranous purulent conjunctivitis. It is believed to be due to retained debris in a voluminous upper fornix acting as a focus for persistent bacterial colonization (usually *S. aureus*) in an elderly patient with levator disinsertion. Large protein aggregations may be visualized in the upper fornix, though double eversion with a retractor may be necessary to identify these. Secondary corneal vascularization and lacrimal obstruction are common. It is frequently unilateral. Treatment involves repeated sweeping of the fornix with a cotton-tipped applicator and topical and systemic antibiotics; intensive topical steroid may be helpful. Surgical forniceal reconstruction may be necessary in recalcitrant cases.

Adult chlamydial conjunctivitis

Pathogenesis

Chlamydia trachomatis (Fig. 5.5) is a species of Chlamydiae, a phylum of bacteria that cannot replicate extracellularly and hence depends on host cells. They exist in two principal forms: (a) a robust infective extracellular 'elementary body' and (b) a fragile intracellular replicating 'reticular body'. Adult chlamydial (inclusion) conjunctivitis is an oculogenital infection usually caused by serovars (serological variants) D–K of *C. trachomatis*, and affects 5–20% of sexually active young adults in Western countries. Transmission is by autoinoculation from genital secretions, although eye-to-eye spread probably accounts for about 10%. The incubation period is about a week.

Urogenital infection

- **In males** chlamydial infection is the most common cause of non-gonococcal urethritis (NGU), also termed non-specific urethritis (NSU). It should be noted that the latter term is also sometimes used to mean urethritis in which both gonococcal and chlamydial infection have been ruled out.

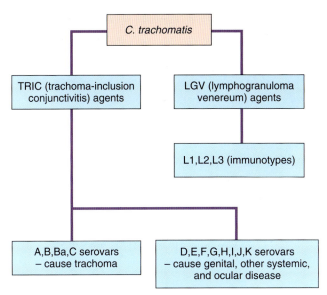

Fig. 5.5 Classification of *Chlamydia trachomatis*

Chlamydial urethritis is frequently asymptomatic in men. *C. trachomatis* may also cause epididymitis, and can act as a trigger for Reiter syndrome.

- **In females** chlamydial urethritis typically causes dysuria and discharge. It may progress to pelvic inflammatory disease (PID), carrying a risk of infertility; 5–10% of women with PID develop perihepatitis (Fitz-Hugh–Curtis syndrome).

Diagnosis

- **Symptoms** consist of the subacute onset of unilateral or bilateral redness, watering and discharge. Untreated, the conjunctivitis becomes chronic, and though self-limiting may persist for several months. It is important to enquire about sexual exposure if chlamydial conjunctivitis is suspected.
- **Signs**
  - Watery or mucopurulent discharge.
  - Tender preauricular lymphadenopathy.
  - Large follicles are often most prominent in the inferior fornix (Fig. 5.6A) and may also involve the upper tarsal conjunctiva (Fig. 5.6B).
  - Superficial punctate keratitis is common.
  - Perilimbal subepithelial corneal infiltrates (Fig. 5.6C) may appear after 2–3 weeks.
  - Chronic cases have less prominent follicles and commonly develop papillae.
  - Mild conjunctival scarring and superior corneal pannus (Fig. 5.6D) are not uncommon.
- **Investigations.** Tarsal conjunctival scrapings are obtained using a spatula or the blunt side of a scalpel blade.
  - Nucleic acid amplification tests such as PCR are likely to be the investigation of choice in time but validation for ocular specimens is limited at present.
  - Giemsa staining for basophilic intracytoplasmic bodies is performed by applying scrapings onto a glass slide.
  - Direct immunofluorescence detects free elementary bodies with about 90% sensitivity and specificity.
  - Enzyme immunoassay for direct antigen detection is also useful.
  - McCoy cell culture is highly specific.
  - Swabs can be taken for bacterial culture, and serology may be helpful in selected cases.

Treatment

Empirical treatment may be given if the clinical picture is convincing pending investigation results, or if investigations are negative.

- **Referral to a genitourinary specialist** is mandatory in confirmed cases, particularly for the exclusion of other sexually transmitted infections, contact tracing and pregnancy testing.
- **Systemic** therapy involves one of the following:
  - Azithromycin 1 g repeated after 1 week is generally the treatment of choice, although a second or a third course is required in up to 30% of cases. Some guidelines advocate only a single 1 g dose.
  - Doxycycline 100 mg twice daily for 10 days (tetracyclines are relatively contraindicated in pregnancy/breastfeeding and in children under 12 years of age).
  - Erythromycin, amoxicillin and ciprofloxacin are alternatives.
- **Topical** antibiotics such as erythromycin or tetracycline ointment are sometimes used to achieve rapid relief of ocular symptoms, but are insufficient alone.
- **Reduction of transmission risk** involves abstinence from sexual contact until completion of treatment (1 week after azithromycin), together with other precautions as for any infectious conjunctivitis.
- **Re-testing** for persistent infection should take place 6–12 weeks after treatment.

It is important to be aware that symptoms commonly take weeks to settle, and that follicles and corneal infiltrates can take months to resolve due to a prolonged hypersensitivity response to chlamydial antigen.

Trachoma

Pathogenesis

Trachoma is the leading cause of preventable irreversible blindness in the world. It is related to poverty, overcrowding and poor hygiene, the morbidity being a consequence of the establishment of re-infection cycles within communities. Whereas an isolated episode of trachomatous conjunctivitis may be relatively innocuous, recurrent infection elicits a chronic immune response consisting of a cell-mediated delayed hypersensitivity (Type IV) reaction to the intermittent presence of chlamydial antigen and can lead to loss of sight. Prior contact with the organism confers short-term partial immunity but also leads to a heightened inflammatory reaction upon reinfection. Vaccination has an effect similar to primary infection in sensitizing the individual, and so

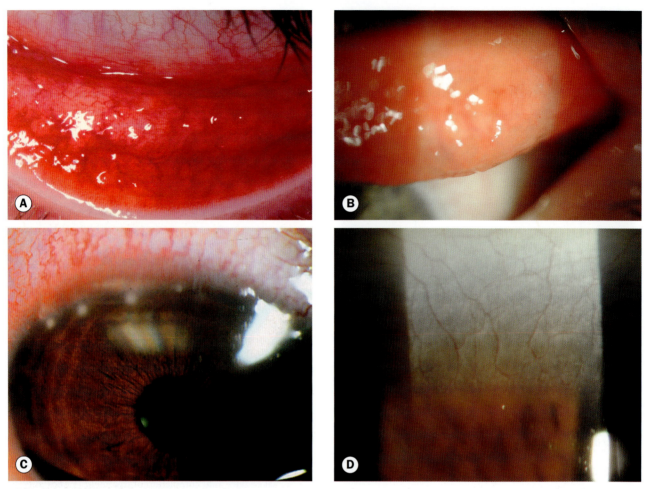

Fig. 5.6 Adult chlamydial conjunctivitis. **(A)** Large forniceal follicles; **(B)** superior tarsal follicles; **(C)** peripheral corneal infiltrates; **(D)** superior pannus

is not helpful. The family childcare group is the most important re-infection reservoir, and consequently young children are particularly vulnerable. The fly is an important vector, but there may be direct transmission from eye or nasal discharge. Trachoma is associated principally with infection by serovars A, B, Ba and C of *Chlamydia trachomatis*, but the serovars D–K conventionally associated with adult inclusion conjunctivitis, and other species of the Chlamydiaceae family such as *Chlamydophila psittaci* and *Chlamydophila pneumoniae* have also been implicated.

Diagnosis

Features of trachoma are divided into an 'active' inflammatory stage and a 'cicatricial' chronic stage, with considerable overlap. A World Health Organization (WHO) grading system is in use (Table 5.1).

- **Active trachoma** is most common in pre-school children and is characterized by the following:
  - Mixed follicular/papillary conjunctivitis (Fig. 5.7A) associated with a mucopurulent discharge. In children under the age of 2 years the papillary component may predominate.

Table 5.1 WHO grading of trachoma
TF = trachomatous inflammation (*follicular*): five or more follicles (>0.5 mm) on the superior tarsal plate
TI = trachomatous inflammation (*intense*): diffuse involvement of the tarsal conjunctiva, obscuring 50% or more of the normal deep tarsal vessels; papillae are present
TS = trachomatous conjunctival scarring: easily visible fibrous white tarsal bands
TT = trachomatous trichiasis: at least one lash touching the globe
CO = corneal opacity sufficient to blur details of at least part of the pupillary margin

- Superior epithelial keratitis and pannus formation (Fig. 5.7B).
- **Cicatricial trachoma** is prevalent in middle age.
  - Linear or stellate (Fig. 5.7C) conjunctival scars in mild cases, or broad confluent scars (Arlt line – Fig. 5.7D) in severe disease.

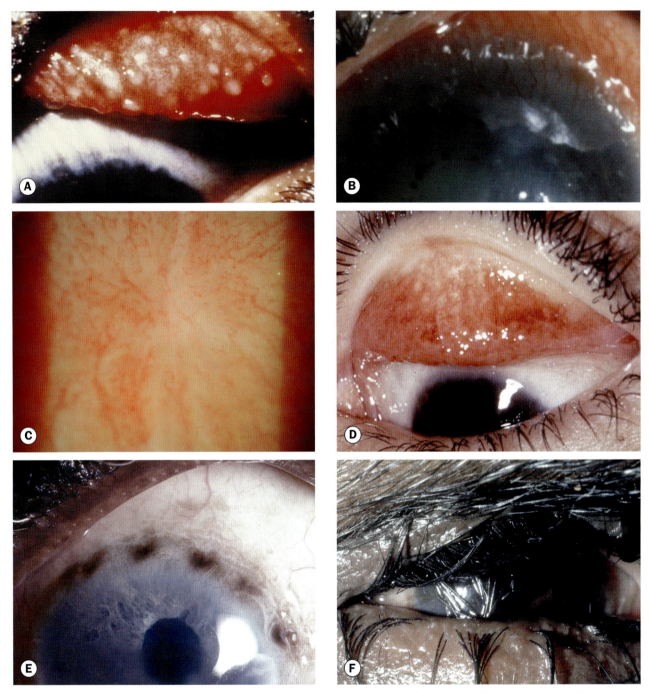

Fig. 5.7 Trachoma. **(A)** Typical white subtarsal follicles; **(B)** marked pannus; **(C)** stellate conjunctival scarring; **(D)** Arlt's line and conjunctival follicles; **(E)** Herbert pits; **(F)** cicatricial entropion

(Courtesy of C Barry – figs A, B, D–F)

- o Although the entire conjunctiva is involved, the effects are most prominent on the upper tarsal plate.
- o Superior limbal follicles may resolve to leave a row of shallow depressions (Herbert pits – Fig. 5.7E).
- o Trichiasis, distichiasis, corneal vascularization and cicatricial entropion (Fig. 5.7F).
- o Severe corneal opacification.

- o Dry eye caused by destruction of goblet cells and the ductules of the lacrimal gland.
- **Investigations** are rarely used in the affected areas, diagnosis being made on clinical features in most cases. Various field techniques (e.g. dipstick enzyme immunoassay) are available and investigations otherwise are similar to those for adult inclusion conjunctivitis.

Management

The SAFE strategy for trachoma management supported by the WHO and other agencies encompasses **S**urgery for trichiasis, **A**ntibiotics for active disease, **F**acial hygiene and **E**nvironmental improvement.

- **Antibiotics** should be administered to those affected and to all family members. A single antibiotic course is not always effective in eliminating infection in an individual, and communities may need to receive annual treatment to suppress infection.
  - A single dose of azithromycin (20 mg/kg up to 1 g) is the treatment of choice.
  - Erythromycin 500 mg twice daily for 14 days or doxycycline 100 mg twice daily for 10 days (tetracyclines are relatively contraindicated in pregnancy/breastfeeding and in children under 12).
  - Topical 1% tetracycline ointment is less effective than oral treatment.
- **Facial cleanliness** is a critical preventative measure.
- **Environmental improvement**, such as access to adequate water and sanitation, as well as control of flies, is important.
- **Surgery** is aimed at relieving entropion and trichiasis and maintaining complete lid closure, principally with bilamellar tarsal rotation.

Neonatal conjunctivitis

Neonatal conjunctivitis (ophthalmia neonatorum) is defined as conjunctival inflammation developing within the first month of life. It is the most common infection of any kind in neonates, occurring in up to 10%. It is identified as a specific entity distinct from conjunctivitis in older infants because of its potentially serious nature (both ocular and systemic complications) and because it is often the result of infection transmitted from mother to infant during delivery.

Causes

- **Organisms acquired during vaginal delivery:**
  C. trachomatis, N. gonorrhoeae (now rare in wealthier countries, but previously responsible for 25% of childhood blindness) and herpes simplex virus (HSV, typically HSV-2). With all of these, conjunctivitis is not uncommonly associated with severe ocular or systemic complications. *C. trachomatis* is the most common cause in cases involving moderate to severe conjunctival inflammation.
- **Staphylococci are usually responsible for mild conjunctivitis**; other bacterial causes include streptococci, *H. influenzae* and various Gram-negative organisms.
- **Topical preparations** used as prophylaxis against infection (see below), may themselves cause conjunctival irritation (chemical conjunctivitis).
- **Congenital nasolacrimal obstruction.** Despite poor neonatal tear production, a persistently mildly watery eye with recurrent mild bacterial conjunctivitis may be secondary to an as yet uncanalized tear duct.

Diagnosis

- **Timing of onset**
  - Chemical irritation: first few days.
  - Gonococcal: first week.
  - Staphylococci and other bacteria: end of the first week.
  - HSV: 1–2 weeks.
  - *Chlamydia*: 1–3 weeks.
- **History**
  - Instillation of a prophylactic chemical preparation.
  - Parental symptoms of sexually transmitted infection (STI).
  - Recent conjunctivitis in close contacts.
  - Features of systemic illness in the child: pneumonitis, rhinitis and otitis in chlamydial infection, skin vesicles and features of encephalitis in HSV; disseminated gonococcal infection is relatively rare.
  - Prior persistent watering without inflammation may indicate an uncanalized nasolacrimal duct.
- **Signs**
  - A mildly sticky eye may occur in staphylococcal infection, or with delayed nasolacrimal duct canalization (mucopurulent reflux on pressure over the lacrimal sac).
  - Discharge is characteristically watery in chemical and HSV infection, mucopurulent in chlamydial infection, purulent (Fig. 5.8) in bacterial infection, and hyperpurulent in gonococcal conjunctivitis.
  - Severe eyelid oedema occurs in gonococcal infection; it may be difficult to distinguish severe conjunctivitis from preseptal or orbital infection. Signs of dacrocystitis should be excluded.
  - Eyelid and periocular vesicles may occur in HSV infection, and can critically aid early diagnosis and treatment.

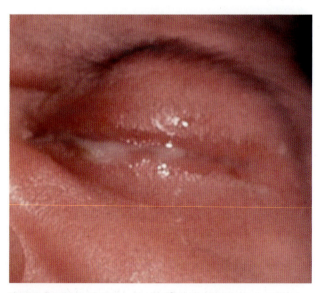

Fig. 5.8 Eyelid oedema and purulent discharge in neonatal conjunctivitis

○ Corneal examination is mandatory, and is particularly important if gonococcal infection is suspected, as ulceration with rapid progression is common. Use of a pen torch, insertion of an eyelid speculum and fluorescein drops may be helpful; the latter may facilitate identification of a dendritic or geographic epithelial lesion that may be present in HSV infection (in contrast to the punctate epitheliopathy seen in older children with primary herpetic conjunctivitis).

○ Pseudomembranes are not uncommon in chlamydial conjunctivitis.

○ Congenital glaucoma may masquerade as neonatal conjunctivitis and should always be considered, particularly in monocular cases.

- **Investigations** are tailored to the clinical picture:
  ○ The results of any parental prenatal testing for STI should be obtained.
  ○ Conjunctival scrapings are taken for nucleic acid amplification (PCR), particularly for *Chlamydia* and HSV.
  ○ Separate conjunctival scrapings are applied to a glass slide for Gram and Giemsa staining. Multinucleated giant cells may be present on Gram stain in HSV infection.
  ○ Conjunctival swabs are taken with a calcium alginate swab or a sterile cotton-tipped applicator, for standard bacterial culture and chocolate agar or Thayer–Martin (for *N. gonorrhoeae*).
  ○ Epithelial cells infected with HSV may show eosinophilic intranuclear inclusions on Papanicolaou smear.
  ○ Conjunctival scrapings or fluid from skin vesicles can be sent for viral culture for HSV.
  ○ Specimens should be taken prior to fluorescein instillation if immunofluorescent testing is planned.

Treatment

- **Prophylaxis** is routinely performed but there is no standard protocol.
  ○ A single instillation of povidone-iodine 2.5% solution is effective against common pathogens.
  ○ Erythromycin 0.5% or tetracycline 1% ointment.
  ○ Silver nitrate 1% solution agglutinates gonococci and is still utilized in areas where gonococcal infection is common. It should be administered in conjunction with a single intramuscular dose of benzylpenicillin when maternal infection is present.
- **Chemical conjunctivitis** does not require treatment apart from artificial tears.
- **Mild conjunctivitis.** A mildly sticky eye is extremely common in neonates. Investigation is often unnecessary and a low-intensity regimen with a broad-spectrum topical antibiotic such as chloramphenicol, erythromycin or fusidic acid ointment is adequate in most cases. Further investigation and treatment can be instituted if the condition fails to settle.

- **Moderate to severe** cases should be investigated as above; microscopy with Gram staining alone is highly sensitive and will often provide a working diagnosis.
  ○ If the diagnosis is uncertain but chlamydial infection is a reasonable possibility, oral erythromycin can be commenced on an empirical basis after samples have been collected.
  ○ If bacteria are evident on Gram stain, a broad-spectrum topical antibiotic (e.g. chloramphenicol, erythromycin or bacitracin for Gram-positive organisms, neomycin, ofloxacin or gentamicin for Gram-negatives) should be used until sensitivities are available; additional systemic treatment should be considered in more severe cases.
- **Severe conjunctivitis**, or when systemic illness is suspected, requires hospital admission. Samples should be taken for a range of investigations, including urgent microscopy, and a broad-spectrum topical antibiotic, such as erythromycin, commenced. The ocular risk is usually most acute from gonococcal infection, so empirical topical treatment should cover this, and in most cases consideration given to systemic treatment such as parenteral ceftriaxone.
- **Chlamydial infection** is treated with oral erythromycin for 2 weeks; a longer or supplementary course may be needed. Erythromycin or tetracycline ointment can be used in addition, but is probably unnecessary.
- **Gonococcal conjunctivitis** is treated systemically with a third-generation cephalosporin and often with supplementary topical treatment. Co-treatment for *Chlamydia* is prudent. Saline irrigation to remove excessive discharge should be considered.
- **Herpes simplex infection** should always be regarded as a systemic condition and is treated with high-dose intravenous aciclovir under paediatric specialist care. Early diagnosis and treatment of encephalitis (PCR of cerebrospinal fluid (CSF) is positive in 95%) may be life-saving or prevent serious neurological disability. Topical aciclovir may be considered in addition.
- **Microbiological** advice should be sought in severe cases, especially regarding local antibiotic sensitivities.
- **Paediatric** specialist involvement is mandatory when systemic disease may be present.
- **Genitourinary** referral for the mother and her sexual contacts is important when an STI is diagnosed. The neonate should be screened for other STIs.
- **Notification** of a case of neonatal conjunctivitis to the local public health authority is a statutory requirement in many countries.

VIRAL CONJUNCTIVITIS

Introduction

Viral conjunctivitis is a common external ocular infection, adenovirus (a non-enveloped double-stranded DNA virus) being the most frequent (90%) causative agent. It may be sporadic, or occur in epidemics in environments such as workplaces (including hospitals), schools and swimming pools. The spread of this highly contagious infection is facilitated by the ability of viral particles to survive on dry surfaces for weeks, and by the fact that viral shedding may occur for many days before clinical features are apparent. Transmission is generally by contact with respiratory or ocular secretions, including via fomites such as contaminated towels.

Presentation

The spectrum of viral conjunctivitis varies from mild subclinical disease to severe inflammation with significant morbidity. There will often be a history of a close contact with acute conjunctivitis.

- **Non-specific acute follicular conjunctivitis** is the most common clinical form of viral conjunctivitis, and is typically due to adenoviral infection by a range of serological variants. Unilateral watering, redness, irritation and/or itching, and mild photophobia occur, the contralateral eye generally being affected 1–2 days later, often less severely. The condition is usually milder than the other clinical forms of adenoviral conjunctivitis; patients may have accompanying (usually mild) systemic symptoms, such as a sore throat or common cold.
- **Pharyngoconjunctival fever (PCF)** is caused mainly by adenovirus serovars 3, 4 and 7. It is spread by droplets within families with upper respiratory tract infection. Keratitis develops in about 30% of cases but is seldom severe. Symptoms are essentially as above, though sore throat is typically prominent.
- **Epidemic keratoconjunctivitis (EKC)** is caused mainly by adenovirus serovars 8, 19 and 37, and is the most severe ocular adenoviral infection. Keratitis, which may be marked, develops in about 80%; photophobia may be correspondingly prominent.
- **Acute haemorrhagic conjunctivitis** usually occurs in tropical areas. It is typically caused by enterovirus and coxsackievirus, though other microorganisms may present similarly. It has a rapid onset, and resolves within 1–2 weeks. Conjunctival haemorrhage is generally marked.
- **Chronic/relapsing adenoviral conjunctivitis** giving a chronic non-specific follicular/papillary clinical picture can persist over years, but is rare and eventually self-limiting.
- **Herpes simplex virus (HSV)** can cause a follicular conjunctivitis, particularly in primary infection; this is usually unilateral and there are often associated skin vesicles.
- **Systemic viral infections** such as those common in childhood, e.g. varicella, measles and mumps, can feature an associated follicular conjunctivitis; varicella-zoster virus secondary infection commonly causes a conjunctivitis as part of ophthalmic shingles. An HIV conjunctivitis is recognized.
- **Molluscum contagiosum** is a skin infection caused by a human specific double-stranded DNA poxvirus that typically affects otherwise healthy children, with a peak incidence between the ages of 2 and 4 years. Transmission is by

contact, with subsequent autoinoculation. A chronic follicular conjunctivitis can be associated, and is due to skin lesion shedding of viral particles. Chronic unilateral ocular irritation and mild discharge is typical. The eyelash line should be examined carefully in patients with chronic conjunctivitis so as not to overlook a molluscum lesion.

Signs

- **Eyelid oedema** ranges from negligible to severe.
- **Lymphadenopathy** is common: tender pre-auricular.
- **Conjunctival** hyperaemia and follicles (Fig. 5.9A) are typically prominent; papillae may also be seen, particularly in the superior tarsal conjunctiva.
- **Severe inflammation** may be associated with conjunctival haemorrhages (usually petechial in adenoviral infection – see Fig. 5.2B), chemosis, membranes (rare) and pseudomembranes (Fig. 5.9B), sometimes with conjunctival scarring after resolution (Fig. 5.9C).
- **Keratitis** (adenoviral):
  - Epithelial microcysts (non-staining) are common at an early stage.
  - Punctate epithelial keratitis (staining) may occur, usually within 7–10 days of the onset of symptoms, typically resolving within 2 weeks.
  - Focal white subepithelial/anterior stromal infiltrates (Fig. 5.9D) often develop beneath the fading epithelial lesions, probably as an immune response to the virus; they may persist or recur over months or years.
  - Small pseudodendritic epithelial formations sometimes occur.
- **Anterior uveitis** is sometimes present, but is mild.
- **Molluscum contagiosum**.
  - A pale, waxy, umbilicated nodule on the lid margin (Fig. 5.10A) associated with follicular conjunctivitis (Fig. 5.10B) and mild watery and mucoid discharge.
  - Bulbar nodules and confluent cutaneous lesions may occur in immunocompromised patients.

Investigation

Investigation is generally unnecessary, but should be considered if the diagnosis is in doubt or there is failure of resolution.

- **Giemsa stain** shows predominantly mononuclear cells in adenoviral conjunctivitis and multinucleated giant cells in herpetic infection.
- **Nucleic acid amplification** techniques such as PCR are sensitive and specific for viral DNA.
- **Viral culture** with isolation is the reference standard but is expensive and fairly slow (days to weeks), and requires specific transport media. Sensitivity is variable but specificity is around 100%.
- A **'point-of-care' immunochromatography** test takes 10 minutes to detect adenoviral antigen in tears; sensitivity and specificity are excellent.
- **Serology** for IgM or rising IgG antibody titres to adenovirus has limitations and is rarely used.

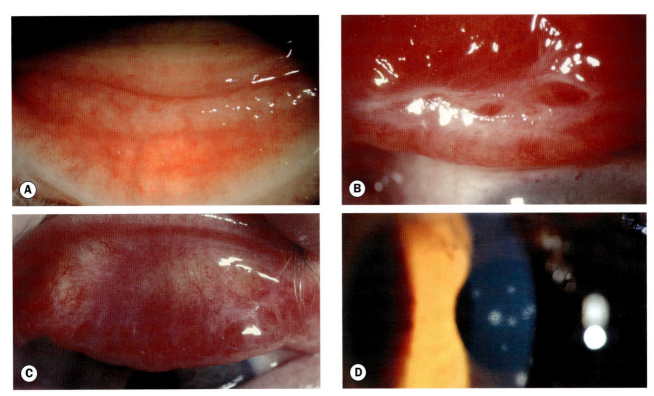

Fig. 5.9 Adenoviral keratoconjunctivitis. **(A)** Follicular conjunctivitis; **(B)** pseudomembrane; **(C)** residual scarring; **(D)** subepithelial infiltrates

(Courtesy of S Tuft – figs B and C)

- **Investigation for other causes** such as chlamydial infection may be indicated in non-resolving cases.

Treatment

The treatment of herpetic ocular surface disease is addressed in Chapter 6.

- **Spontaneous resolution** of adenoviral infection usually occurs within 2–3 weeks, so specific treatment is typically

unnecessary. No antiviral agent with clinically useful activity against adenovirus has yet been produced.

- **Reduction of transmission risk** by meticulous hand hygiene, avoiding eye rubbing and towel sharing. There should be scrupulous disinfection of instruments and clinical surfaces after examination of an infected patient (e.g. sodium hypochlorite, povidone-iodine).

- **Molluscum contagiosum.** Although lesions are self-limiting in immunocompetent patients, removal is often necessary to

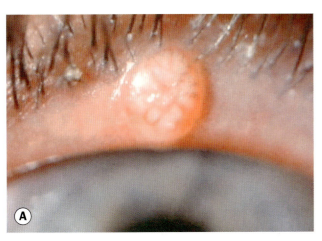

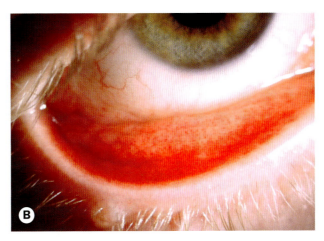

Fig. 5.10 (A) Molluscum eyelid lesion; **(B)** follicular conjunctivitis associated with a molluscum lesion

address secondary conjunctivitis or for cosmetic reasons. Expression is facilitated by making a small nick in the skin at the margin of the lesion with the tip of a needle.

- **Topical steroids** such as prednisolone 0.5% four times daily may be required for severe membranous or pseudomembranous adenoviral conjunctivitis. Symptomatic keratitis may require weak topical steroids but these should be used with caution as they do not speed resolution but only suppress inflammation, and lesions commonly recur after premature discontinuation. Steroids may enhance viral replication and extend the period during which the patient remains infectious. Intraocular pressure should be monitored if treatment is prolonged.
- **Other measures**
  - Discontinuation of contact lens wear until resolution of symptoms.
  - Artificial tears four times daily may be useful for symptomatic relief. Preservative-free preparations may give superior comfort, and if supplied in single-dose units may reduce transmission risk.
  - Cold (or warm) compresses for symptomatic relief.
  - Topical antihistamines and vasoconstrictors may improve symptoms, particularly itching.
  - The place of non-steroidal anti-inflammatory drops is not well established, but may be effective in some circumstances such as steroid weaning. They are not thought to promote viral replication.
  - Removal of symptomatic pseudomembranes or membranes.
  - Topical antibiotics if secondary bacterial infection is suspected.
  - Povidone-iodine is very effective against free (although less so against intracellular) adenovirus, and has been proposed as a means of decreasing infectivity.

ALLERGIC CONJUNCTIVITIS

Atopy is a genetically determined predisposition to hypersensitivity reactions upon exposure to specific environmental antigens. Clinical manifestations include the various forms of allergic conjunctivitis, as well as hay fever (seasonal allergic rhinitis), asthma and eczema. Allergic conjunctivitis is a Type I (immediate) hypersensitivity reaction, mediated by degranulation of mast cells in response to the action of IgE; there is evidence of an element of Type IV hypersensitivity in at least some forms.

Acute allergic conjunctivitis

Acute allergic conjunctivitis is a common condition caused by an acute conjunctival reaction to an environmental allergen, usually pollen. It is typically seen in younger children after playing outside in spring or summer. Acute itching and watering are common, but the hallmark is chemosis (Figs 5.11A and B), which is frequently dramatic and worrying to the child and parents. Treatment is not usually required and the conjunctival swelling

settles within hours as the acute increase in vascular permeability resolves. Cool compresses can be used and a single drop of adrenaline 0.1% may reduce extreme chemosis.

Seasonal and perennial allergic conjunctivitis

These common subacute conditions are distinguished from each other by the timing of exacerbations, thought to relate principally to differing stimulating allergens in each.

- **Seasonal allergic conjunctivitis** ('hay fever eyes'), worse during the spring and summer, is the more common. The most frequent allergens are tree and grass pollens, although the specific allergen varies with geographic location.
- **Perennial allergic conjunctivitis** causes symptoms throughout the year, generally worse in the autumn when exposure to house dust mites, animal dander and fungal

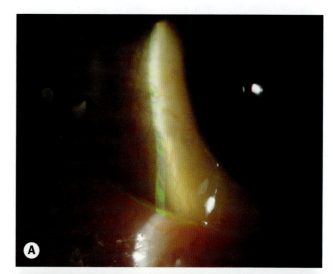

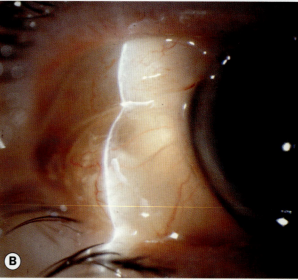

Fig. 5.11 (A) Mild and **(B)** severe chemosis in acute allergic conjunctivitis

allergens is greatest. It is less common and tends to be milder than the seasonal form.

Diagnosis

- **Symptoms.** Transient acute or subacute attacks of redness, watering and itching, associated with sneezing and nasal discharge.
- **Signs.** Conjunctival hyperaemia with a relatively mild papillary reaction, variable chemosis and lid oedema.
- **Investigations** are generally not performed although conjunctival scraping in more active cases may demonstrate the presence of eosinophils. Skin testing for particular allergens is rarely required.

Treatment

- **Artificial tears** for mild symptoms.
- **Mast cell stabilizers** (e.g. sodium cromoglicate, nedocromil sodium, lodoxamide) must be used for a few days before exerting maximal effect, but are suitable (except lodoxamide) for long-term use if required.
- **Antihistamines** (e.g. emedastine, epinastine, levocabastine, bepotastine) can be used for symptomatic exacerbations and are as effective as mast cell stabilizers.
- **Dual action antihistamine and mast cell stabilizers** (e.g. azelastine, ketotifen, olopatadine) act rapidly and are often very effective for exacerbations.
- **Combined preparation** of an antihistamine and a vasoconstrictor (e.g. antazoline with xylometazoline).
- **Non-steroidal anti-inflammatory preparations** (e.g. diclofenac) can provide symptomatic relief but are rarely used.
- **Topical steroids** are effective but rarely necessary.
- **Oral antihistamines** may be indicated for severe symptoms. Some, such as diphenhydramine, cause significant drowsiness and may be useful in aiding sleep; others, such as loratadine, have a far less marked sedative action.

Vernal keratoconjunctivitis

Pathogenesis

Vernal keratoconjunctivitis (VKC) is a recurrent bilateral disorder in which both IgE- and cell-mediated immune mechanisms play important roles. It primarily affects boys and onset is generally from about the age of 5 years onwards. There is remission by the late teens in 95% of cases, although many of the remainder develop atopic keratoconjunctivitis. VKC is rare in temperate regions but relatively common in warm dry climates such as the Mediterranean, sub-Saharan Africa and the Middle East. In temperate regions over 90% of patients have other atopic conditions such as asthma and eczema and two-thirds have a family history of atopy. VKC often occurs on a seasonal basis, with a peak incidence over late spring and summer, although there may be mild perennial symptoms.

Classification

- **Palpebral VKC** primarily involves the upper tarsal conjunctiva. It may be associated with significant corneal disease as a result of the close apposition between the inflamed conjunctiva and the corneal epithelium.
- **Limbal** disease typically affects black and Asian patients.
- **Mixed VKC** has features of both palpebral and limbal disease.

Diagnosis

The diagnosis is clinical; investigations are generally not indicated. Eosinophils may be abundant in conjunctival scrapings.

- **Symptoms** consist of intense itching, which may be associated with lacrimation, photophobia, a foreign body sensation, burning and thick mucoid discharge. Increased blinking is common.
- **Palpebral disease**
  - Early-mild disease is characterized by conjunctival hyperaemia and diffuse velvety papillary hypertrophy on the superior tarsal plate (Fig. 5.12A).
  - Macropapillae (<1 mm) have a flat-topped polygonal appearance reminiscent of cobblestones; focal (Fig. 5.12B) or diffuse (Fig. 5.12C) whitish inflammatory infiltrates may be seen in intense disease.
  - Progression to giant papillae (>1 mm) can occur, as adjacent smaller lesions amalgamate when dividing septa rupture (Fig. 5.12D).
  - Mucus deposition between giant papillae (Fig. 5.12E).
  - Decreased disease activity is characterized by milder conjunctival injection and decreased mucus production (Fig. 5.12F).
- **Limbal disease**
  - Gelatinous limbal conjunctival papillae that may be associated with transient apically located white cellular collections (Horner–Trantas dots – Fig. 5.13A–C).
  - In tropical regions, limbal disease may be severe (Fig. 5.13D).
- **Keratopathy** is more frequent in palpebral disease and may take the following forms:
  - Superior punctate epithelial erosions associated with layers of mucus on the superior cornea (Fig. 5.14A).
  - Epithelial macroerosions caused by a combination of epithelial toxicity from inflammatory mediators and a direct mechanical effect from papillae (Fig. 5.14B–D).
  - Plaques and 'shield' ulcers (Fig. 5.15A and B) may develop in palpebral or mixed disease when the exposed Bowman membrane becomes coated with mucus and calcium phosphate, leading to inadequate wetting and delayed re-epithelialization. This development is serious and warrants urgent attention to prevent secondary bacterial infection.
  - Subepithelial scars that are typically grey and oval (Fig. 5.15C), and may affect vision.

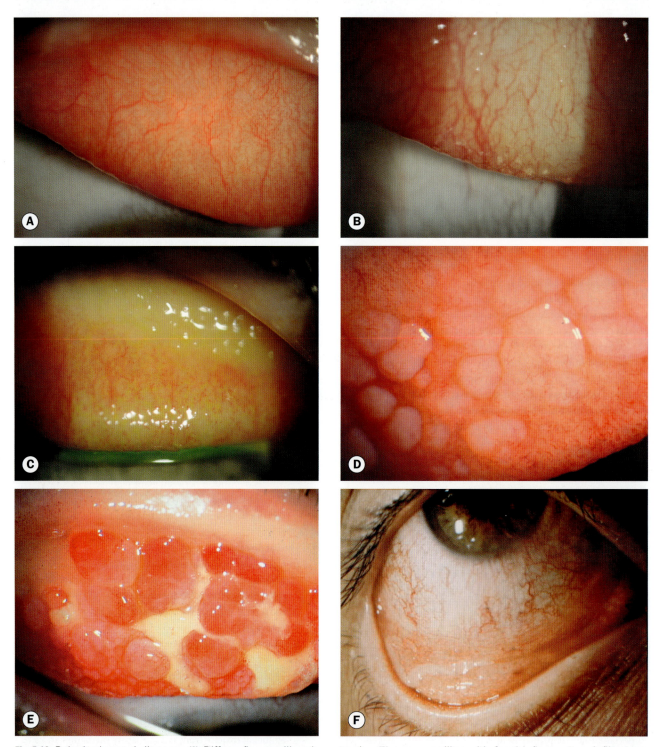

Fig. 5.12 Palpebral vernal disease. **(A)** Diffuse fine papillary hypertrophy; **(B)** macropapillae with focal inflammatory infiltrates; **(C)** macropapillae with diffuse infiltrate; **(D)** giant papillae; **(E)** intense disease with mucus; **(F)** milder disease; note mucous discharge

(Courtesy of S Tuft – fig. D)

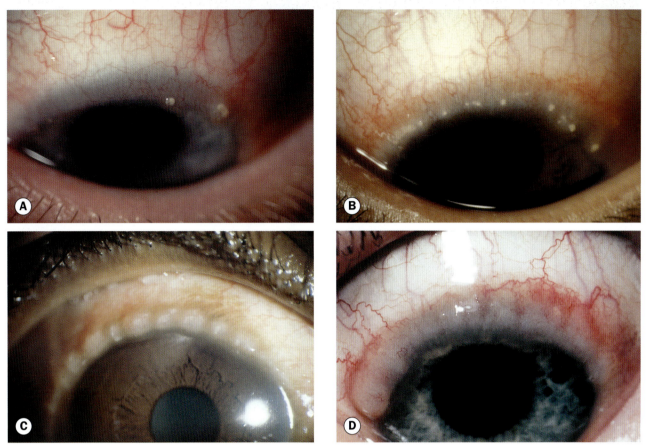

Fig. 5.13 Limbal vernal disease. **(A)** Sparse limbal papillae; **(B)** papillae with Horner–Trantas dots; **(C)** extensive papillae; **(D)** severe features

(Courtesy of S Tuft – fig. B)

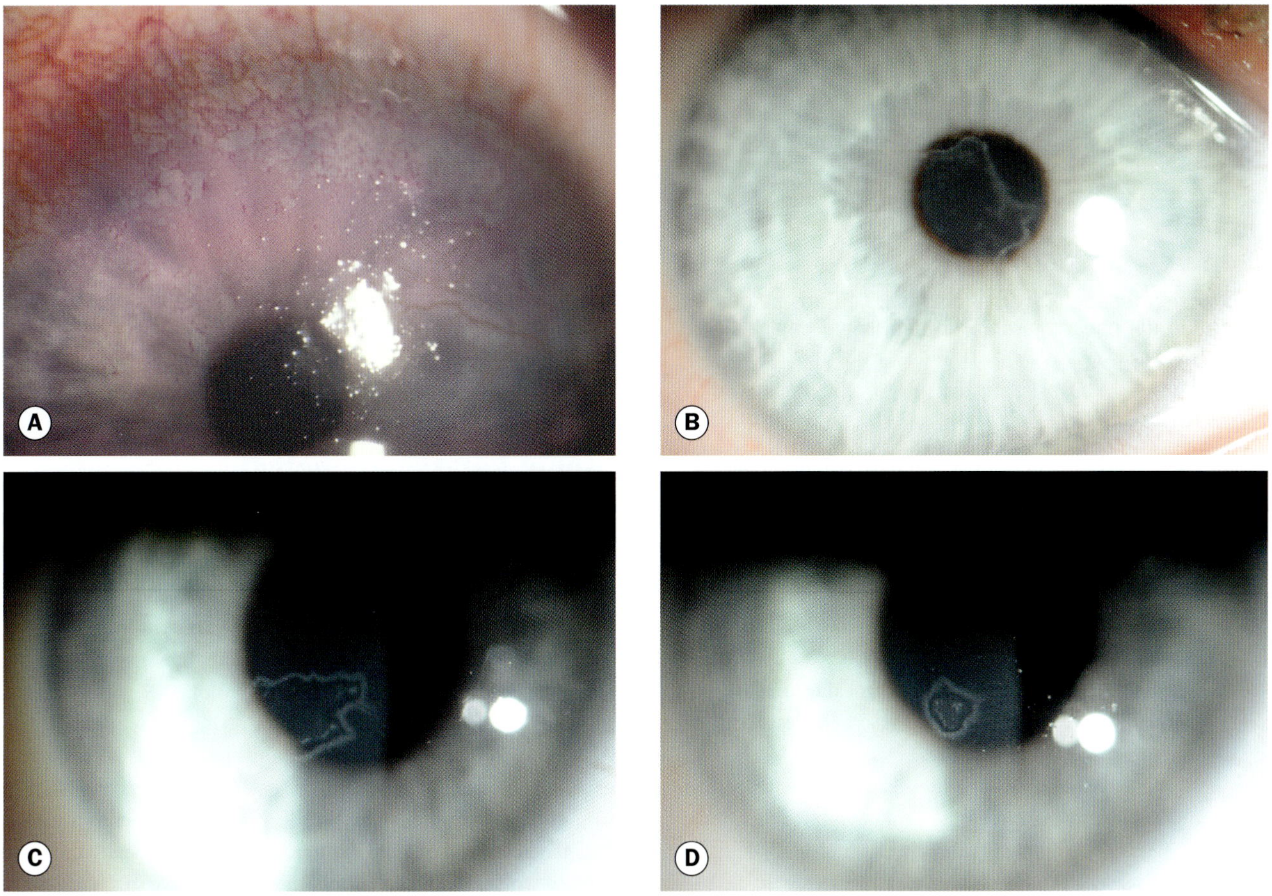

Fig. 5.14 Keratopathy in vernal disease. **(A)** Superior punctate erosions and mucus stained with rose Bengal; **(B-D)** gradual resolution of a macroerosion over months of treatment

(Courtesy of S Tuft – fig. A)

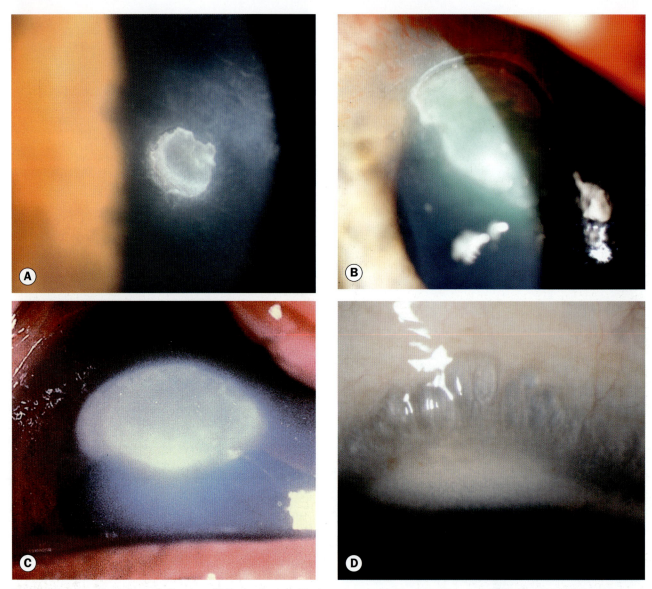

Fig. 5.15 Keratopathy in vernal disease. **(A)** Early plaque; **(B)** plaque and shield ulcer; **(C)** subepithelial scarring following ulceration; **(D)** pseudogerontoxon and limbal papillae
(Courtesy of S Tuft – figs A and D)

○ Pseudogerontoxon can develop in recurrent limbal disease. It is characterized by a paralimbal band of superficial scarring resembling arcus senilis (Fig. 5.15D), adjacent to a previously inflamed segment of the limbus.

○ Vascularization does not tend to be prominent, though some peripheral superficial vessel ingrowth is common, especially superiorly.

○ Keratoconus and other forms of corneal ectasia are more common in VKC and are thought to be at least partly due to persistent eye rubbing.

○ Herpes simplex keratitis is more common than average, though less so than in atopic keratoconjunctivitis. It can be aggressive and is occasionally bilateral.

• **Eyelid disease** is usually mild, in contrast to atopic keratoconjunctivitis.

Atopic keratoconjunctivitis

Pathogenesis

Atopic keratoconjunctivitis (AKC) is a rare bilateral disease that typically develops in adulthood (peak incidence 30–50 years) following a long history of atopic dermatitis (eczema); asthma is also extremely common in these patients. About 5% have suffered from childhood VKC. There is little or no gender preponderance. AKC tends to be chronic and unremitting, with a relatively low expectation of eventual resolution, and is associated with significant visual morbidity. Whereas VKC is more frequently seasonal and generally worse in the spring, AKC tends to be perennial and is often worse in the winter. Patients are sensitive to a wide range of airborne environmental allergens.

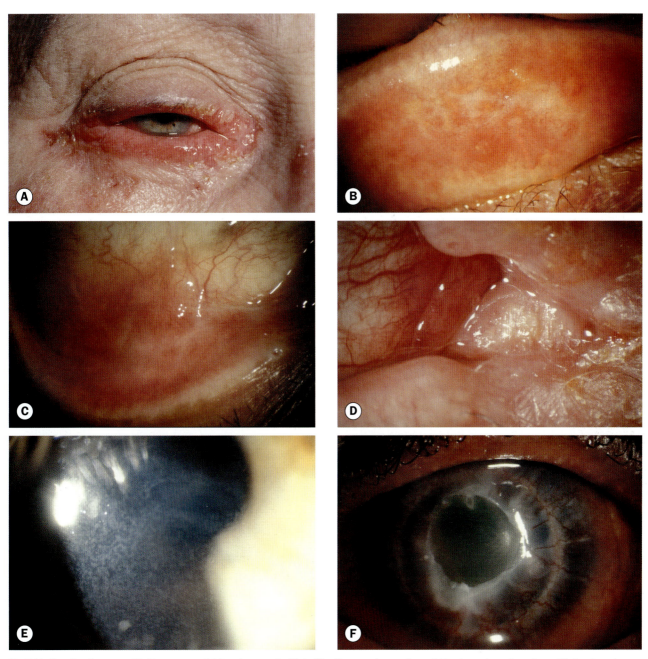

Fig. 5.16 Atopic disease. **(A)** Severe eyelid involvement; **(B)** infiltration and scarring of the tarsal conjunctiva; **(C)** forniceal shortening; **(D)** keratinization of the caruncle; **(E)** dense punctate epithelial erosions; **(F)** persistent epithelial defect and peripheral corneal vascularization; a penetrating keratoplasty interface can be seen

(Courtesy of S Tuft)

Diagnosis

The distinction between AKC and VKC is essentially clinical; eosinophils tend to be less common in conjunctival scrapings than with VKC.

- **Symptoms** are similar to those of VKC, but are frequently more severe and unremitting.
- **Eyelids**
  - Skin changes (Fig. 5.16A) are more prominent than in VKC, and are typically eczematoid: erythema, dryness,
    scaliness and thickening, sometimes with disruption to epidermal integrity such as fissuring and scratches (excoriation), the latter due to intense itching.
  - Associated chronic staphylococcal blepharitis and madarosis are common.
  - There may be keratinization of the lid margin.
  - Hertoghe sign: absence of the lateral portion of the eyebrows.
  - Dennie–Morgan folds: lid skin folds caused by persistent rubbing.

o Tightening of the facial skin may cause lower lid ectropion and epiphora.

o Ptosis is not uncommon.

- **Conjunctival** involvement is preferentially inferior palpebral, whereas in VKC it is worse superiorly.

  o Discharge is generally more watery than the stringy mucoid discharge in VKC.

  o Hyperaemia; chemosis is not uncommon during active inflammation.

  o Papillae are initially smaller than in VKC although larger lesions may develop later.

  o Diffuse conjunctival infiltration and scarring may give a whitish, featureless appearance (Fig. 5.16B).

  o Cicatricial changes can lead to moderate symblepharon formation, forniceal shortening (Fig. 5.16C) and keratinization of the caruncle (Fig. 5.16D).

  o Limbal involvement similar to that of limbal VKC can be seen, including Horner–Trantas dots.

- **Keratopathy**

  o Punctate epithelial erosions over the inferior third of the cornea are common and can be marked (Fig. 5.16E).

  o Persistent epithelial defects (Fig. 5.16F), sometimes with associated focal thinning, can occasionally progress to perforation with descemetocoele (US spelling – descemetocele) formation.

  o Plaque formation may occur (see Figs 5.15A and B).

  o Peripheral vascularization and stromal scarring are more common than in VKC.

  o Predisposition to secondary bacterial and fungal infection, and to aggressive herpes simplex keratitis.

  o Keratoconus is common (about 15%) and as with VKC may be secondary to chronic ocular rubbing.

- **Cataract**

  o Presenile shield-like anterior or posterior subcapsular cataracts are common and may be exacerbated by long-term steroid therapy.

  o Because of the high lid margin carriage of *S. aureus*, cataract surgery carries an increased risk of endophthalmitis.

- **Retinal detachment** is more common than in the general population, and is a particular risk following cataract surgery.

Treatment of VKC and AKC

The management of VKC does not differ substantially from that of AKC, although the latter is generally less responsive and requires more intensive and prolonged treatment.

General measures

- **Allergen avoidance**, if possible. An allergy specialist opinion may be requested; allergen (e.g. patch) testing is sometimes useful, but often gives non-specific results.
- **Cool compresses** may be helpful.
- **Lid hygiene** should be used for associated staphylococcal blepharitis. Moisturizing cream such as E45 can be applied to dry, fissured skin.

- **Bandage contact lens** wear to aid healing of persistent epithelial defects.

Local treatment

- **Mast cell stabilizers** (e.g. sodium cromoglicate, nedocromil sodium, lodoxamide) reduce the frequency of acute exacerbations and the need for steroids and so form the basis of many regimens, but are seldom effective in isolation. Several days to weeks of treatment are needed for a reasonable response and long-term therapy may be needed (lodoxamide is not licensed for long-term use).
- **Topical antihistamines** (e.g. emedastine, epinastine, levocabastine, bepotastine) when used in isolation are about as effective as mast cell stabilizers. They are suitable for acute exacerbations but generally not for continuous long-term use, and courses of several preparations are licensed for use only in courses of limited duration. A trial of several different agents may be worthwhile.
- **Combined antihistamine and vasoconstrictor** (e.g. antazoline with xylometazoline) may offer relief in some cases.
- **Combined action antihistamine/mast cell stabilizers** (e.g. azelastine, ketotifen, olopatadine) are helpful in many patients and have a relatively rapid onset of action.
- **Non-steroidal anti-inflammatory** preparations (e.g. ketorolac, diclofenac) may improve comfort by blocking non-histamine mediators. Combining one of these with a mast cell stabilizer is an effective regimen in some patients.
- **Topical steroids** (e.g. fluorometholone 0.1%, rimexolone 1%, prednisolone 0.5%, loteprednol etabonate 0.2% or 0.5%) are used for (a) severe exacerbations of conjunctivitis and (b) significant keratopathy; reducing conjunctival activity generally leads to corneal improvement. They are usually prescribed in short but intensive (e.g. 2-hourly initially) courses, aiming for very prompt tapering. Although the risk of elevation of intraocular pressure is low, monitoring is advisable if long-term treatment is necessary. Stronger preparations such as prednisolone 1% can be used but carry a higher risk of steroid-induced glaucoma.
- **Steroid ointment** (e.g. hydrocortisone 0.5%) may be used to treat the eyelids in AKC, though as with eye drops, the duration of treatment should be minimized and the intraocular pressure (IOP) monitored.
- **Antibiotics** may be used in conjunction with steroids in severe keratopathy to prevent or treat bacterial infection.
- **Acetylcysteine** is a mucolytic agent that is useful in VKC for dissolving mucus filaments and deposits, and addressing early plaque formation.
- **Immune modulators**

  o Ciclosporin (0.05–2% between two and six times daily) may be indicated if steroids are ineffective, inadequate or poorly tolerated, or as a steroid-sparing agent in patients with severe disease. The effects typically take some weeks to be exerted, and relapses may occur if treatment is stopped suddenly. Irritation and blurred vision are common.

- ○ **Calcineurin inhibitors** show increasing promise as an alternative to steroids in the treatment of allergic eye disease. Tacrolimus 0.03% ointment can be effective in AKC for severe eyelid disease. Instillation into the fornices has been effective in modulating conjunctival inflammation in refractory cases.
- **Supratarsal steroid injection** may be considered in severe palpebral disease or for non-compliant patients. The injection is given into the conjunctival surface of the anaesthetized everted upper eyelid; 0.1 ml of betamethasone sodium phosphate 4 mg/ml, dexamethasone 4 mg/ml or triamcinolone 40 mg/ml is given.

Systemic treatment

- **Oral antihistamines** help itching, promote sleep and reduce nocturnal eye rubbing. Because other inflammatory mediators are involved besides histamines, effectiveness is not assured. Some antihistamines (e.g. loratadine) cause relatively little drowsiness.
- **Antibiotics** (e.g. doxycycline 50–100 mg daily for 6 weeks, azithromycin 500 mg once daily for 3 days) may be given to reduce blepharitis-aggravated inflammation, usually in AKC.
- **Immunosuppressive agents** (e.g. steroids, ciclosporin, tacrolimus, azathioprine) may be effective at relatively low doses in AKC unresponsive to other measures. Short courses of high-dose steroids may be necessary to achieve rapid control in severe disease. Monoclonal antibodies against T cells have shown some promise in refractory cases.
- **Other treatments** that may be effective in some patients include aspirin in VKC (avoided in children and adolescents due to Reye syndrome risk), allergen desensitization, and plasmapheresis in patients with high serum IgE levels.

Surgery

- **Superficial keratectomy** may be required to remove plaques or debride shield ulcers and allow epithelialization. Medical treatment must be maintained until the cornea has re-epithelialized in order to prevent recurrences. Excimer laser phototherapeutic keratectomy is an alternative.
- **Surface maintenance/restoration surgery** such as amniotic membrane overlay grafting or lamellar keratoplasty, or **eyelid procedures** such as botulinum toxin-induced ptosis or lateral tarsorrhaphy, may be required for severe persistent epithelial defects or ulceration. Gluing may be appropriate for focal ('punched-out') corneal perforations.

Non-allergic eosinophilic conjunctivitis

Non-allergic eosinophilic conjunctivitis (NAEC) is a recently proposed chronic non-atopic condition said to occur predominantly in middle-aged women in whom dry eye is also commonly present; it has been suggested that it is relatively common but under-

diagnosed. It is thought to be of similar pathogenesis to non-allergic eosinophilic rhinitis; conjunctival eosinophilia is present without significant IgE levels in the serum or tear film. Symptoms are similar to those of allergic conjunctivitis – itching, redness, foreign body sensation and mild watery discharge. Treatment is with a 1–2 week course of topical steroid for exacerbations followed by maintenance with topical mast cell stabilizers, non-steroidal anti-inflammatory agents or antihistamines.

Contact allergic blepharoconjunctivitis

Analogous to contact dermatitis, this refers to the acute or sub-acute T-cell-mediated delayed hypersensitivity reaction seen most commonly by ophthalmologists as a reaction to eye drop constituents and by optometrists as a reaction to contact lens solutions. Mascara is a less common cause. There may be a conjunctival reaction, but signs predominantly involve the eyelid skin: erythema, thickening, induration and sometimes fissuring occur (Fig. 5.17). Treatment is by removal or discontinuation of the precipitant, sometimes with a mild topical steroid ointment.

Giant (mechanically induced) papillary conjunctivitis

Pathogenesis

Mechanically induced papillary conjunctivitis, the severe form of which is known as giant papillary conjunctivitis (GPC), can occur secondary to a variety of mechanical stimuli of the tarsal conjunctiva. It is most frequently encountered with contact lens (CL) wear, when it is termed contact lens-associated papillary conjunctivitis (CLPC). The risk is increased by the build-up of proteinaceous deposits and cellular debris on the contact lens surface. Ocular prostheses (Fig. 5.18), exposed sutures and scleral buckles, corneal surface irregularity and filtering blebs can all be responsible. A related phenomenon is the so-called 'mucus fishing syndrome', when, in a variety of underlying anterior segment disorders, patients develop or exacerbate a chronic papillary

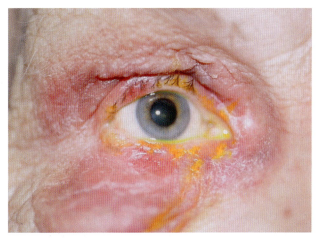

Fig. 5.17 Contact allergic blepharoconjunctivitis

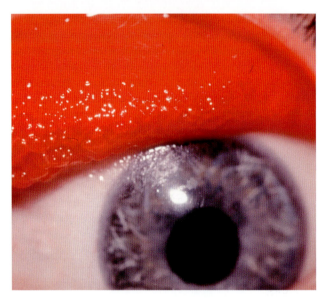

Fig. 5.18 Ocular prosthesis causing giant papillary conjunctivitis

reaction due to repetitive manual removal of mucus. Giant papillae can also be seen in other conditions such as VKC and AKC.

Diagnosis

- **Symptoms** consist of a foreign body sensation, redness, itching, increased mucus production, blurring and loss of CL tolerance. Symptoms may be worse after lens removal. Patients should be questioned about CL cleaning and maintenance.
- **Signs**
  - Variable mucous discharge.
  - Substantial CL protein deposits may be present.
  - Excessive CL mobility due to upper lid capture.
  - Superior tarsal hyperaemia and papillae; by definition, 'giant' papillae are >1.0 mm in diameter, but the clinical syndrome of mechanically induced papillary conjunctivitis commonly features only fine/medium papillae, particularly in early or mild disease.
  - Focal apical ulceration and whitish scarring may develop on larger papillae.
  - Keratopathy is rare because of the relatively subdued secretion of inflammatory cytokines.
  - Ptosis may occur, mainly as a result of irritative spasm and tissue laxity secondary to chronic inflammation.

Treatment

Other causes of conjunctival papillae should be excluded, as well as CL intolerance due to other causes, such as a reaction to lens cleaning solutions and dry eyes.

- **Removal of the stimulus**
  - CL wear should be discontinued for several weeks and the current lenses replaced. For mild–moderate disease, this may be adequate for resolution, sometimes in conjunction with reduced wearing time. In severe CLPC a longer interval without lens wear may be needed.

  - Removal of other underlying causes, such as exposed sutures or a scleral buckle.
  - Assessment of the status and fit of an ocular prosthesis.
  - Filtering bleb: partial excision, revision with non-penetrating drainage surgery or glaucoma drainage device implantation.
- **Ensure effective cleaning of CL or prosthesis**
  - Changing the type of CL solution, particularly discontinuation of preservative-containing preparations.
  - Switching to monthly then daily disposable CL if the condition persists after renewing non-disposable lenses.
  - Rigid lenses carry a lesser risk of CLPC (5%), probably because they are easier to clean effectively.
  - Cessation of contact lens wear, substituting spectacles or refractive surgery, may be necessary for severe or refractory disease.
  - Regular (at least weekly) use of contact lens protein removal tablets.
  - Prosthesis: polishing, cleaning with detergent, coating.
- **Topical**
  - Mast cell stabilizers should be non-preserved in patients wearing soft contact lenses, or can be instilled when the lenses are not in the eye, with a delay of perhaps half an hour after drop instillation prior to lens insertion. Most can be continued long-term if necessary.
  - Antihistamines, non-steroidal anti-inflammatory agents and combined antihistamines/mast cell stabilizers may each be of benefit.
  - Topical steroids can be used for the acute phase of resistant cases, particularly those where effective removal of the stimulus is difficult, as in bleb-related disease.

CONJUNCTIVITIS IN BLISTERING MUCOCUTANEOUS DISEASE

Mucous membrane pemphigoid

Introduction

Mucous membrane pemphigoid (MMP), also known as cicatricial pemphigoid (CP), comprises a group of chronic autoimmune mucocutaneous blistering diseases. An unknown trigger leads to a Type II (cytotoxic) hypersensitivity response resulting in antibodies binding at the basement membrane zone (BMZ), the activation of complement and the recruitment of inflammatory cells, with localized separation of the epidermis from the dermis at the BMZ and subsequent progression to scarring.

A wide range of epithelial tissues can be involved, including the skin and various mucous membranes. Particular clinical forms of MMP tend to involve specific target tissues: bullous pemphigoid (BP) shows a predilection for skin, and ocular mucous membrane pemphigoid (OMMP, also known as ocular cicatricial pemphigoid – OCP) involves the conjunctiva in the majority of cases and causes progressive scarring (cicatrization). The disease typically presents in old age and affects females more commonly than males by a 2:1 ratio. Other causes of cicatrizing conjunctivitis include Stevens–Johnson syndrome, trachoma, drug-induced, trauma and severe or chronic conjunctivitis of many types. MMP should not be confused with pemphigus, a distinct group of disorders.

Ocular features

Diagnosis is principally clinical, but biopsy of involved mucous membrane often shows supportive changes (linear antibody and complement BMZ deposition). Progression has been divided into stages, from stage I (chronic conjunctivitis) to stage IV (immobile globe with a keratinized cornea).

- **Symptoms.** Insidious or relapsing–remitting non-specific bilateral conjunctivitis; misdiagnosis (e.g. dry eye) is common.
- **Conjunctiva**
  - Papillary conjunctivitis, diffuse hyperaemia, oedema and subtle fibrosis (Fig. 5.19A).
  - Fine lines of subconjunctival fibrosis and shortening of the inferior fornices; symblepharon (plural symblephara) formation refers to adhesion between the bulbar and palpebral conjunctiva (Fig. 5.19B).
  - Necrosis in severe cases.
  - Flattening of the plica and keratinization of the caruncle (Fig. 5.19C).
  - Dry eye due to destruction of goblet cells and accessory lacrimal glands, and occlusion of the main lacrimal ductules.
  - Monitoring should include the measurement of forniceal depth and noting the position of adhesions.
- **Eyelids**
  - Aberrant (trichiatic) lashes, chronic blepharitis and keratinization of the lid margin.
  - Ankyloblepharon is an adhesion at the outer canthus between the upper and lower lids (Fig. 5.19D).
- **Cornea**
  - Epithelial defects (Fig. 5.20A) associated with drying and exposure.
  - Infiltration and peripheral vascularization (Fig. 5.20B).

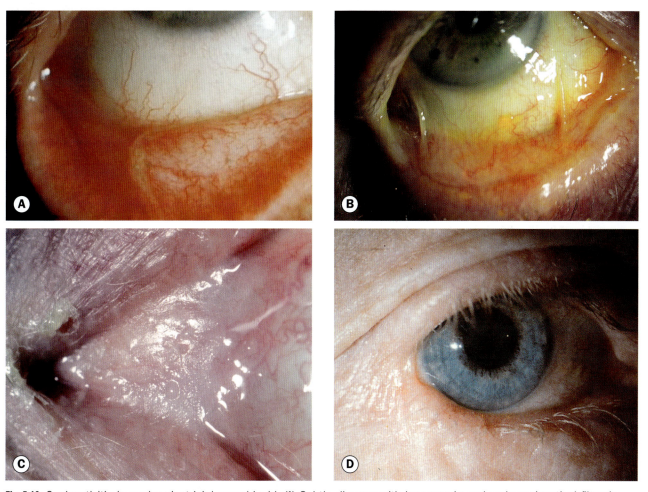

Fig. 5.19 Conjunctivitis in ocular cicatricial pemphigoid. **(A)** Subtle disease with hyperaemia and early conjunctival fibrosis; **(B)** moderate fibrosis with forniceal shortening and symblepharon formation; **(C)** flat plica and keratinized caruncle; **(D)** ankyloblepharon
(Courtesy of S Tuft – fig. C)

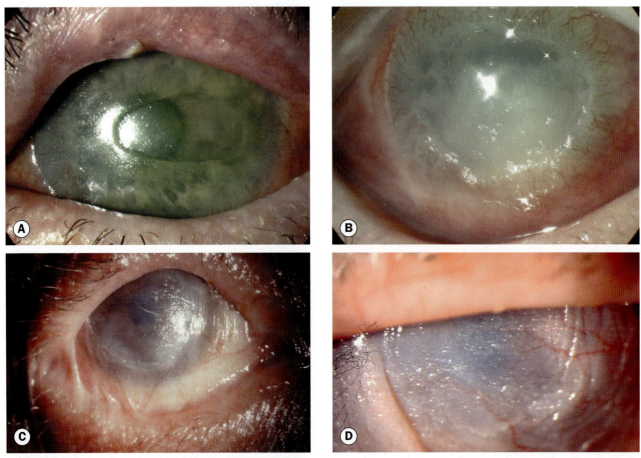

Fig. 5.20 Keratopathy in ocular cicatricial pemphigoid. **(A)** Epithelial defect; **(B)** peripheral vascularization and infiltration; **(C)** keratinization with ankyloblepharon; **(D)** end-stage disease
(Courtesy of S Tuft – figs A–C)

  ○ Keratinization and conjunctivalization of the corneal surface (Fig. 5.20C) due to epithelial stem cell failure.
  ○ End-stage disease is characterized by total symblepharon and corneal opacification (Fig. 5.20D).

Systemic features

- **Mucosal** involvement is very common and is characterized by subepidermal blisters, most frequently oral (Fig. 5.21A). Severe manifestations include oesophageal and laryngeal strictures.
- **Skin** lesions are less common (25%) and present as tense blisters and erosions of the head and neck, groin and extremities (Fig. 5.21B).

Systemic treatment

Systemic treatment is the mainstay of management; any detectable inflammatory activity should be suppressed.

- **Dapsone** (diaminodiphenylsulfone) is a useful first-line treatment in patients with mild–moderate disease; approximately 70% of patients respond. It is contraindicated in glucose-6-phosphate dehydrogenase deficiency. Sulfasalazine is sometimes better tolerated.

- **Antimetabolites** (e.g. azathioprine, methotrexate, mycophenolate mofetil) are alternatives for mild–moderate disease if dapsone is contraindicated, ineffective or poorly tolerated, and are suitable for long-term therapy. Dapsone can be used in conjunction if necessary. Cyclophosphamide may be reserved for severe or refractory disease.
- **Steroids** (prednisolone 1–1.5 mg/kg) are effective for rapid disease control, but adverse effects limit long-term use. IOP should be monitored.
- **Other measures** include intravenous immunoglobulin therapy and rituximab; remission has been reported with a combination regimen.

Local treatment

- **Topical**
  - Artificial tears are an integral part of most regimens.
  - Topical steroids, ciclosporin or tacrolimus may be used as an adjunct to systemic immunosuppressive treatment.
  - Retinoic acid may reduce keratinization.
  - Antibiotics when indicated.
  - Lid hygiene and low-dose oral tetracycline for blepharitis.

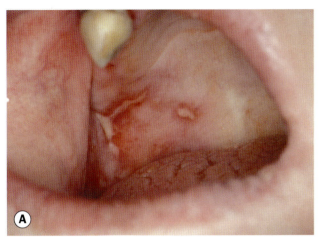 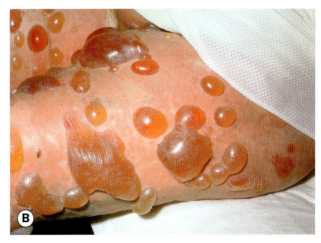

Fig. 5.21 Mucous membrane pemphigoid. **(A)** Oral blisters; **(B)** severe skin blistering
(Courtesy of S Tuft – fig. A)

- **Subconjunctival** mitomycin C and/or steroid injection may be used as a temporizing aid or if systemic immunosuppression is not possible.
- **Contact lenses** may be used with caution to protect the cornea from aberrant lashes and from dehydration.

Reconstructive surgery

Reconstructive surgery, preferably under systemic steroid cover, should be considered when active disease is controlled.

- Aberrant eyelashes (see Ch. 1).
- Punctal occlusion to aid tear retention.
- Lateral tarsorrhaphy or botulinum toxin-induced ptosis may be used to promote healing of corneal epithelial defects.
- Entropion repair: conjunctival incision is avoided if possible.
- Cataract surgery is commonly required.
- Mucous membrane autografting or amniotic membrane transplantation for conjunctival resurfacing and forniceal restoration.
- Limbal stem cell transfer may be attempted for corneal re-epithelialization.
- Keratoplasty carries a high risk of failure; lamellar grafts may be effective for perforation.
- Keratoprosthesis (Fig. 5.22) may be the only option in end-stage disease.

Stevens–Johnson syndrome/ toxic epidermal necrolysis (Lyell syndrome)

Introduction

The terms 'Stevens–Johnson syndrome (SJS)' and 'erythema multiforme major' have historically been used synonymously.

However, it is now believed that erythema multiforme (without the 'major') is a distinct disease, milder and recurrent, with somewhat dissimilar clinical features. Toxic epidermal necrolysis (TEN – Lyell syndrome) is a severe variant of SJS. SJS/TEN patients tend to be young adults, though other groups may be affected. The condition involves a cell-mediated delayed hypersensitivity reaction, usually related to drug exposure. A wide range of medications have been incriminated, including antibiotics (especially sulfonamides and trimethoprim), analgesics including paracetamol (acetaminophen), cold remedies and anticonvulsants. Infections due to microorganisms such as *Mycoplasma pneumoniae* and herpes simplex virus, and some cancers have also been implicated. Because symptoms often take weeks to develop, in many cases the precipitant cannot be identified. Mortality overall is around 5% in SJS (death is commonly due to infection), but is considerably higher in TEN.

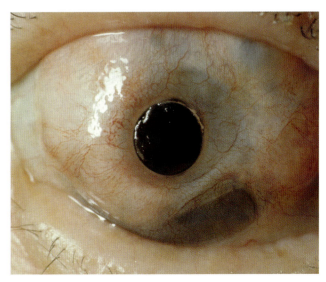

Fig. 5.22 Keratoprosthesis for severe conjunctival scarring

Ocular features

In the acute stage there are often practical obstacles to standard slit lamp examination; the patient may be bedridden and undergoing barrier nursing; a portable slit lamp may be helpful.

- **Symptoms.** Acute ocular symptoms may include redness, mild–severe grittiness, photophobia, watering and blurring.
- **Acute signs**
  - Haemorrhagic crusting of the lid margins (Fig. 5.23A) is characteristic; skin lesions may be confluent and it is often difficult for an examiner to open the eyes without causing marked discomfort.
  - Papillary conjunctivitis, which can range from mild, transient and self-limiting to severe (Fig. 5.23B).
  - Conjunctival membranes and pseudomembranes (Fig. 5.23C), severe hyperaemia, haemorrhages, blisters and patchy infarction.
  - Keratopathy: a spectrum of lesions from punctate erosions to large epithelial defects, secondary bacterial keratitis and occasionally perforation.
  - Iritis is not infrequent, and panophthalmitis has been reported.
- **Late signs**
  - Conjunctival cicatrization (Fig. 5.23D) with forniceal shortening and symblepharon formation.
  - Keratinization of the conjunctiva and lid margin (Fig. 5.23E), sometimes with abrasive plaque formation.
  - Eyelid complications include cicatricial entropion and ectropion, trichiasis, metaplastic lashes and ankyloblepharon.
  - Keratopathy including scarring, vascularization and keratinization (Fig. 5.23F) as a result of the primary inflammation and/or infection, as well as cicatricial entropion and aberrant lashes.
  - Watery eyes due to fibrosis of the lacrimal puncta. Dry eyes may also occur as a result of fibrosis of lacrimal gland ductules and conjunctival metaplasia with loss of goblet cells.

Systemic features

Skin biopsy may help to establish the diagnosis but is rarely necessary.

- **Symptoms.** Flu-like symptoms, which can be severe, may last up to 14 days before the appearance of lesions. In many cases the patient is very ill and hospitalization is required. Symptoms of systemic mucosal involvement include nasal pain and discharge, pain on micturition, diarrhoea, cough, shortness of breath, and pain on eating and drinking.
- **Signs**
  - Mucosal involvement is characterized by blistering and haemorrhagic crusting of the lips (Fig. 5.24A). The blisters may also involve the tongue, oropharynx, nasal mucosa and occasionally the genitalia.
  - Small purpuric, vesicular, haemorrhagic or necrotic skin lesions involving the extremities, face and trunk

(Fig. 5.24B). These are usually transient but may be widespread. Healing usually occurs within 1–4 weeks, leaving a pigmented scar.
  - Widespread sloughing of the epidermis is uncommon.
  - 'Target' lesions showing the classic three zones are now viewed as characteristic of erythema multiforme rather than SJS/TEN.

Systemic treatment

- **Removal of the precipitant** if possible, such as discontinuation of drugs and treatment of suspected infection.
- **General supportive measures** such as maintenance of adequate hydration, electrolyte balance and nutrition (especially protein replacement) are critical. Management in a specialist burns unit should reduce the chance of infection when the extent of skin involvement is substantial.
- **Systemic steroids** remain controversial. There are reports of increased mortality in older papers, but later research has raised the possibility that early short-term high-dose intravenous treatment may improve outcomes.
- **Other immunosuppressants** including ciclosporin, azathioprine, cyclophosphamide and intravenous immunoglobulin may be considered in selected cases, but are controversial and controlled trials are lacking.
- **Systemic antibiotics** may be given as prophylaxis against skin or other systemic infection, avoiding those known to be at higher risk of precipitating SJS/TEN.

Ocular treatment

- **Acute disease.** Daily review is advisable initially in most patients to check the corneas and exclude symblepharon formation.
  - Topical lubricants are used as frequently as necessary, e.g. hypromellose 0.3% preservative-free up to hourly, high-viscosity ointment during sleep.
  - Prevention of corneal exposure, e.g. moisture chambers, gel pads if mechanically ventilated.
  - Topical steroids may be used for iritis and for conjunctival inflammation, though a benefit for the latter has not been demonstrated conclusively.
  - Topical cycloplegia (e.g. atropine 1% once or twice daily) may improve comfort.
  - Lysis of developing symblephara with a sterile glass rod or damp cotton bud.
  - A scleral ring, consisting of a large haptic lens, may help to prevent symblepharon formation (Fig. 5.25).
  - Pseudomembrane/membrane peeling can be considered, although the benefit is unproven.
  - Treatment of acute corneal problems such as bacterial keratitis; the use of prophylactic topical antibiotics is common, but as there may be a propensity to adverse drug reactions a decision should be made on a case basis.
  - Conjunctival swabs should be considered for prophylactic culture.

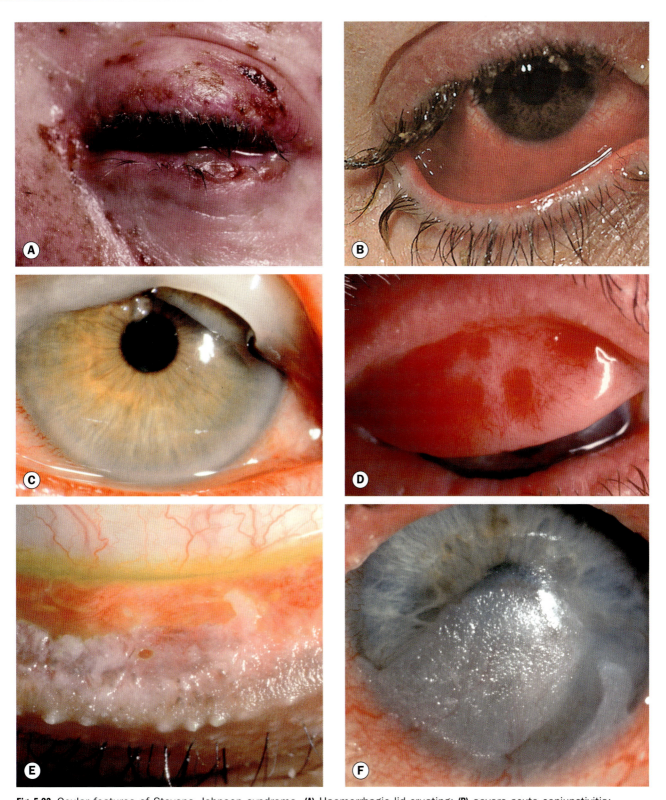

Fig. 5.23 Ocular features of Stevens–Johnson syndrome. **(A)** Haemorrhagic lid crusting; **(B)** severe acute conjunctivitis; **(C)** pseudomembrane; **(D)** conjunctival scarring; **(E)** keratinization with severe lid margin involvement; **(F)** corneal keratinization

(Courtesy of R Bates – fig. A; S Tuft – figs D, E and F)

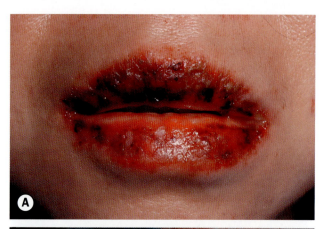

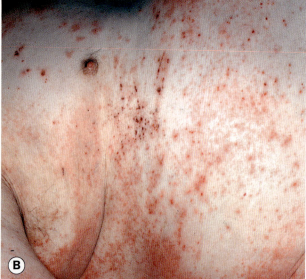

Fig. 5.24 Systemic features in Stevens–Johnson syndrome.
(A) Haemorrhagic lip crusting; **(B)** extensive purpuric lesions

(Courtesy of M Zatouroff, from Physical Signs in General Medicine, *Mosby–Wolfe 1996 – fig. B)*

- IOP monitoring may be prudent, using portable tonometry if necessary.
- **Chronic disease**
  - Adequate lubrication, including punctal occlusion if required.
  - Topical transretinoic acid 0.01% or 0.025% may reverse keratinization.
  - Treatment of aberrant lashes (see Ch. 1).
  - Bandage contact lenses (typically gas permeable scleral lenses) to maintain surface moisture, protect the cornea from aberrant lashes and address irregular astigmatism.
  - Mucous membrane grafting (e.g. buccal mucosa autograft) for forniceal reconstruction.
  - Corneal rehabilitation may involve superficial keratectomy for keratinization, lamellar corneal grafting for superficial scarring (preferred to penetrating keratoplasty), amniotic membrane grafting, limbal stem cell transplantation, and keratoprosthesis implantation in end-stage disease.

Superior limbic keratoconjunctivitis

Introduction

Superior limbic keratoconjunctivitis (SLK) is a relatively uncommon chronic disease of the superior limbus and the superior bulbar and tarsal conjunctiva. It affects one or both eyes of middle-aged women, approximately 50% of whom have abnormal thyroid function (usually hyperthyroidism); approximately 3% of patients with thyroid eye disease have SLK. The condition is probably under-diagnosed because symptoms are typically more severe than signs. The course can be prolonged over years although remission eventually occurs spontaneously. There are similarities to mechanically induced papillary conjunctivitis, and a comparable clinical picture has been described with contact lens wear and following upper lid surgery or trauma. The condition is believed to be the result of blink-related trauma between the upper lid and the superior bulbar conjunctiva, precipitated in many cases by tear film insufficiency and an excess of lax conjunctival tissue. With increased conjunctival movement there is mechanical damage to the tarsal and bulbar conjunctival surfaces, the resultant inflammatory response leading to increasing conjunctival oedema and redundancy, with the creation of a self-perpetuating cycle. It may be analogous to conjunctivochalasis affecting the lower bulbar conjunctiva (see Ch. 2).

Diagnosis

Enquiry should be made about contact lens wear, and previous eyelid surgery or trauma.

- **Symptoms** include a foreign body sensation, burning, mild photophobia, mucoid discharge and frequent blinking, and are often intermittent.

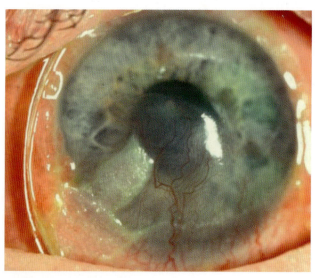

Fig. 5.25 Scleral ring used to prevent symblepharon formation in Stevens–Johnson syndrome

(Courtesy of S Tuft)

- **Conjunctiva**
  - Papillary hypertrophy of the superior tarsal plate, often having a diffuse velvety appearance (Fig. 5.26A).
  - Hyperaemia of a radial band of the superior bulbar conjunctiva (Fig. 5.26B) that stains with rose Bengal and may be best seen macroscopically.
  - Limbal papillary hypertrophy (also Fig. 5.26B); limbal palisades may be lost superiorly.
  - Light downward pressure on the upper lid results in a fold of redundant conjunctiva crossing the upper limbus (Fig. 5.26C).
  - Petechial haemorrhages may be present.
  - Keratinization can be demonstrated on biopsy or impression cytology.
- **Cornea**
  - Superior punctate corneal epithelial erosions are common and are often separated from the limbus by a zone of normal epithelium.
  - Superior filamentary keratitis (Fig. 5.26D) develops in about one-third of cases.
  - Mild superior pannus resembling arcus senilis may be seen in long-standing disease.
  - Keratoconjunctivitis sicca is present in only about 50%.

- **Investigation**
  - Thyroid function testing should be performed if the patient is not known to have thyroid disease.
  - Biopsy or impression cytology may reveal keratinization of the superior bulbar conjunctiva.

Treatment

- **Topical**
  - Lubricants (preservative-free may be preferred) to reduce friction between the tarsal and bulbar conjunctiva should be used regularly and frequently.
  - Acetylcysteine 5% or 10% four times daily to break down filaments and provide lubrication.
  - Mast cell stabilizers and steroids to address any inflammatory component; steroids may be best used in short intensive courses with rapid tapering, and should be reserved for severe cases.
  - Promising results have been reported with topical rebamipide.
  - Ciclosporin 0.05% twice daily as primary or adjunctive therapy, particularly in the presence of coexisting keratoconjunctivitis sicca.

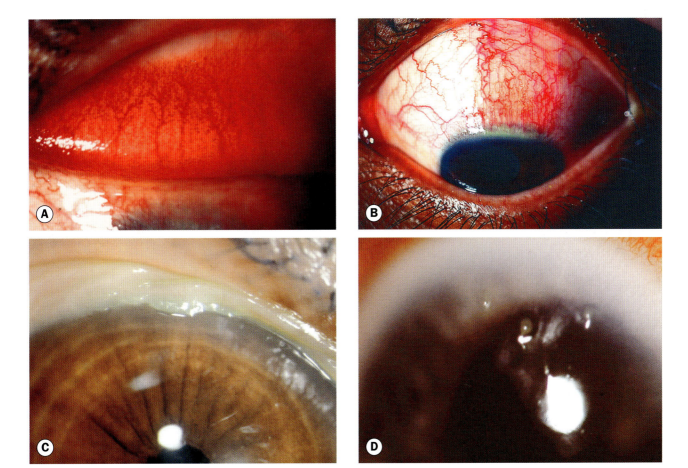

Fig. 5.26 Superior limbic keratoconjunctivitis. **(A)** Diffuse velvety papillary hypertrophy; **(B)** hyperaemic band of superior bulbar conjunctiva with limbal papillae, stained with rose Bengal; **(C)** fold of redundant conjunctiva; **(D)** superior corneal filaments
(Courtesy of S Tuft – fig. C)

- ○ Retinoic acid to retard keratinization.
- ○ Autologous serum 20% drops can be beneficial but may require instillation up to 10 times a day.
- **Soft contact lenses**, which intervene between the lid and the superior conjunctiva, are effective in some cases. Interestingly, a unilateral lens may provide bilateral relief.
- **Supratarsal steroid injection.** 0.1 ml of triamcinolone 40 mg/ml may break the inflammatory cycle.
- **Temporary superior and/or inferior punctal occlusion.**
- **Resection** of the superior limbal conjunctiva, either in a zone extending 2 mm from the superior limbus or of the area staining with rose Bengal, is often effective in resistant disease. Lax conjunctiva is removed, with regrowth tending to be firmly anchored. There is no consensus as to whether underlying Tenon capsule should be excised.
- **Conjunctival ablation** by applying silver nitrate 0.5% (not cautery sticks) or thermocautery to the affected area.
- **Treatment of associated thyroid dysfunction** may improve SLK.

Ligneous conjunctivitis

Introduction

Ligneous conjunctivitis is a very rare potentially sight- and even life-threatening disorder characterized by recurrent, often bilateral fibrin-rich pseudomembranous lesions of wood-like consistency that develop mainly on the tarsal conjunctiva. It is generally a systemic condition and may involve the periodontal tissue, the upper and lower respiratory tract, kidneys, middle ear and female genitalia; death can occasionally occur from pulmonary involvement. It is thought that in susceptible patients patterns of damage repair are abnormal, notably a failure of normal clearance of products of the acute stages of the healing process. This is manifested predominantly in mucosal tissue. A deficiency in plasmin-mediated fibrinolysis may be a key common factor in many patients. Episodes may be triggered by relatively minor trauma, or by systemic events such as fever and antifibrinolytic therapy.

Diagnosis

- **Presentation** is with nonspecific conjunctivitis, usually in childhood (median age 5 years), although onset may be at any age. A conjunctival lesion is commonly noted by parents.
- **Signs**
  - ○ Gradually enlarging red–white lobular conjunctival masses (Fig. 5.27A and B); may be covered by a thick yellow–white mucoid discharge.
  - ○ Corneal scarring, vascularization, infection or melting.
- **Histopathology** shows amorphous subepithelial deposits of eosinophilic material consisting predominantly of fibrin (Fig. 5.27C).

Treatment

Treatment tends to be unsatisfactory and spontaneous resolution is rare. It is important to discontinue any antifibrinolytic drugs.
- **Surgical removal** (Fig. 5.27D) with meticulous diathermy of the base of the lesion. Preoperative topical plasminogen may soften pseudomembranes and facilitate removal.
- **Topical**
  - ○ Following membrane removal, hourly heparin and steroids are commenced immediately and continued until the wound has re-epithelialized, with subsequent tapering over several weeks until all signs of inflammation have disappeared.
  - ○ Recurrence may be retarded by long-term ciclosporin and steroid instillation.
- **Other modalities**
  - ○ Intravenous or topical plasminogen.
  - ○ Amniotic membrane transplantation to the conjunctiva following lesion removal.
  - ○ Prophylactic heparin treatment may be of benefit prior to ocular surgery in at-risk patients.

Parinaud oculoglandular syndrome

Parinaud oculoglandular syndrome is a rare condition consisting of chronic low-grade fever, unilateral granulomatous conjunctivitis (Fig. 5.28) with surrounding follicles, and ipsilateral regional (preauricular) lymphadenopathy. It is virtually synonymous with cat scratch disease (caused by *Bartonella henselae* – see Ch. 11), although several other causes have been implicated, including tularaemia, insect hairs (ophthalmia nodosum), *Treponema pallidum*, sporotrichosis, tuberculosis, and acute *C. trachomatis* infection.

Factitious conjunctivitis

Introduction

Self-injury (factitious keratoconjunctivitis) is most often intentional, but can also occur inadvertently, as in mucus fishing syndrome and removal of contact lenses. Damage may be the result of either mechanical trauma or of the instillation of irritant but readily accessible household substances, such as soap. Occasionally over-instillation of prescribed ocular medication is responsible.

Diagnosis

- **Symptoms.** Reported symptoms may seem disproportionate to signs; the patient may have sought multiple medical opinions over an extended period, often from a range of specialists for different complaints.
- **Signs**
  - ○ Inferior conjunctival injection and staining with rose Bengal (Fig. 5.29), with quiet superior bulbar conjunctiva.
  - ○ Linear corneal abrasions, persistent epithelial defects and occasionally focal corneal perforation.

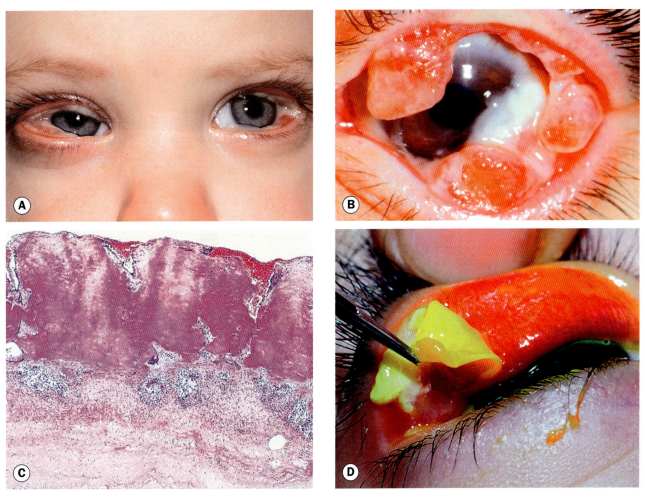

Fig. 5.27 Ligneous conjunctivitis. **(A)** and **(B)** Multiple ligneous lesions; **(C)** histology shows eosinophilic fibrinous coagulum on the conjunctival surface; **(D)** lesion removal

(Courtesy of JH Krachmer, MJ Mannis and EJ Holland, from Cornea, Mosby 2005 *– fig. B; J Harry and G Misson, from* Clinical Ophthalmic Pathology, Butterworth-Heinemann 2001 *– fig. C; J Dart – fig. D)*

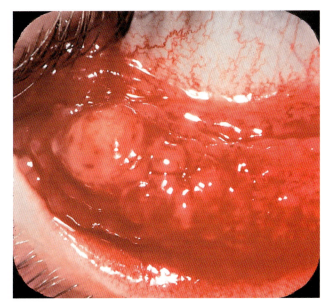

Fig. 5.28 Granulomatous conjunctivitis in Parinaud syndrome

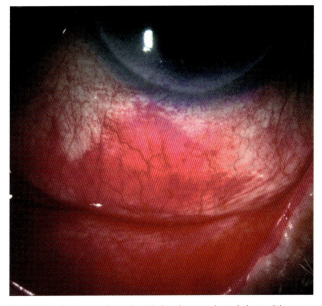

Fig. 5.29 Inferior conjunctival injection and staining with rose Bengal in factitious conjunctivitis

(Courtesy of S Tuft)

○ Secondary infection with *Candida* spp.
○ Sterile ring infiltrate and hypopyon.
○ Corneal scarring.

Management

- Exclude other diagnoses.
- Close observation may be required.
- Confrontation often leads to failure to return for review.
- A psychiatric opinion may be appropriate.

DEGENERATIONS

Pinguecula

Introduction

A pinguecula (plural pingueculae) is an innocuous but extremely common asymptomatic elastotic degeneration of the conjunctival stroma. A yellow–white mound or aggregation of smaller mounds is seen on the bulbar conjunctiva adjacent to the limbus (Fig. 5.30A). It is more frequently located at the nasal than the temporal limbus, but is frequently present at both. Calcification (Fig. 5.30B) is occasionally present. The cause is believed to be actinic damage, similar to the aetiology of pterygium (see below), which pinguecula resembles histologically; the distinction is that the limbal barrier to extension has remained intact with a pinguecula, though transformation can occur. Occasionally a pingueculum may become acutely inflamed (pingueculitis – Fig. 5.30C), often if the lesion is prominent or overlying calcification leads to epithelial breakdown.

Treatment

Treatment is usually unnecessary because growth is absent or very slow.
- Irritation may be treated with topical lubrication.
- Pingueculitis can be treated with lubrication if mild or with a short course of topical steroid.
- Excision may be indicated for cosmetic reasons or for significant irritation; in contrast to pterygium (see next), the recurrence rate is very low and simple excision is usually adequate.
- Thermal laser ablation can be effective; gentian violet marking may be necessary to ensure adequate absorption in lighter-skinned individuals.

Pterygium

Introduction

A pterygium (plural pterygia) is a triangular fibrovascular subepithelial ingrowth of degenerative bulbar conjunctival tissue over the limbus onto the cornea. It typically develops in patients who have been living in hot climates and, as with pinguecula, may represent a response to ultraviolet exposure and to other factors

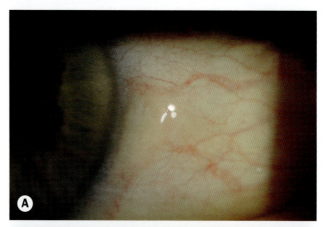

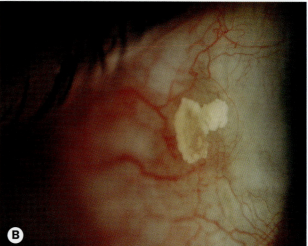

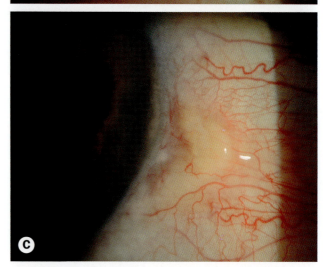

Fig. 5.30 (A) Pinguecula; **(B)** developing calcification; **(C)** pingueculitis

such as chronic surface dryness. A pterygium is histologically similar to a pinguecula and shows elastotic degenerative changes in vascularized subepithelial stromal collagen (Fig. 5.31A). In contrast to pingueculae, pterygia encroach onto the cornea, invading the Bowman layer. Pseudopterygium appears similar clinically but is caused by a band of conjunctiva adhering to an area of compromised cornea at its apex. It forms as a response to an acute

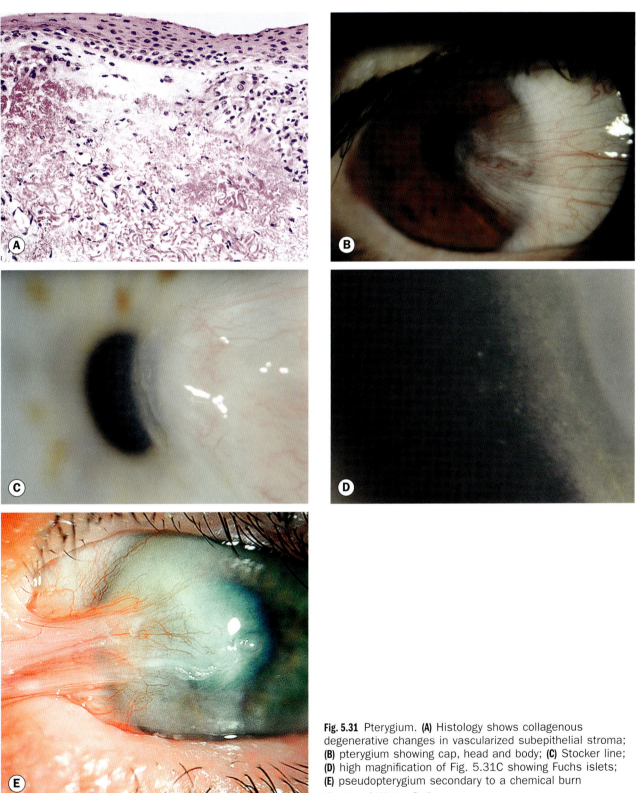

Fig. 5.31 Pterygium. **(A)** Histology shows collagenous degenerative changes in vascularized subepithelial stroma; **(B)** pterygium showing cap, head and body; **(C)** Stocker line; **(D)** high magnification of Fig. 5.31C showing Fuchs islets; **(E)** pseudopterygium secondary to a chemical burn

(Courtesy of J Harry – fig. A)

inflammatory episode such as a chemical burn, corneal ulcer (especially if marginal), trauma and cicatrizing conjunctivitis.

Clinical features

- **Symptoms.** Patients who present with a history of recent enlargement are more likely to require early excision for subsequent aggressive growth. Aggressive growth or an atypical appearance should prompt excision biopsy.
  - Most small lesions are asymptomatic.
  - Irritation and grittiness are caused by a dellen – localized drying – effect at the advancing edge due to interference with the precorneal tear film (more likely if the head of the pterygium is especially elevated).
  - Patients who wear contact lenses may develop symptoms of irritation at an earlier stage due to edge lift.
  - Lesions may interfere with vision by obscuring the visual axis or inducing astigmatism.
  - There may be intermittent inflammation similar to pingueculitis.
  - Cosmesis may be a significant problem.
  - Extensive lesions, particularly if recurrent, may be associated with subconjunctival fibrosis extending to the fornices that may cause restricted ocular excursion.
  - If pseudopterygium is suspected, there may be a history of a causative episode.
- **Signs**
  - A pterygium is made up of three parts: a 'cap' (an avascular halo-like zone at the advancing edge), a head and a body (Fig. 5.31B).
  - Linear epithelial iron deposition (Stocker line) may be seen in the corneal epithelium anterior to the head of the pterygium (Fig. 5.31C).
  - Fuchs islets (Fig. 5.31D) are small discrete whitish flecks consisting of clusters of pterygial epithelial cells often present at the advancing edge.
  - A pseudopterygium (Fig. 5.31E) is classically distinguished by both location away from the horizontal (though this may also be seen with true pterygia) and firm attachment to the cornea only at its apex (head).

Treatment

- **Medical** treatment of symptomatic patients is as for pinguecula. The patient may be advised to wear sunglasses to reduce ultraviolet exposure in order to decrease the growth stimulus.
- **Surgery.** Simple excision ('bare sclera' technique) is associated with a high rate of recurrence (around 80%), often with more aggressive behaviour than the original lesion.
  - Simple conjunctival flap.
  - Conjunctival autografting (Fig. 5.32A). The donor conjunctival patch is usually harvested from the superior or superotemporal paralimbal region (Fig. 5.32B) the site generally heals rapidly, even without suturing. Amniotic membrane patch grafting is an alternative. Both

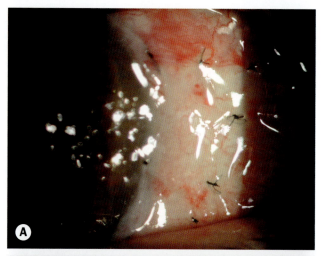

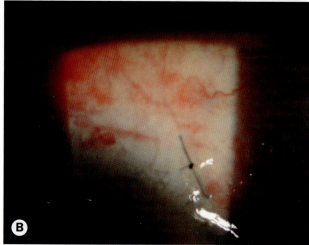

Fig. 5.32 Surgical treatment of pterygium. **(A)** Excision site one week postoperatively showing sutured conjunctival autograft; **(B)** autograft donor site at superior limbus

  conjunctival grafts and amniotic membranes can be secured with tissue glue rather than sutured, shortening operating time and reducing postoperative irritation.
  - Adjunctive treatment with mitomycin C or beta-irradiation are sometimes used in place of patching techniques.
  - Peripheral lamellar keratoplasty may be required for deep lesions.

Concretions

Concretions are extremely common and are usually associated with ageing, although they can also form in patients with chronic conjunctival inflammation such as trachoma. They appear as multiple tiny cysts containing yellowish–white deposits of epithelial debris including keratin, commonly located subepithelially in the inferior tarsal and forniceal conjunctiva (Fig. 5.33A). They can become calcified and, particularly if large, may erode the overlying epithelium (Fig. 5.33B) and cause marked irritation. Treatment if symptomatic involves removal at the slit lamp with a needle under topical anaesthesia.

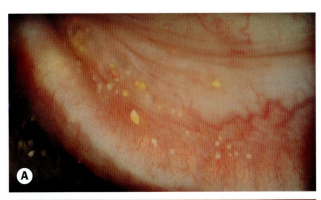

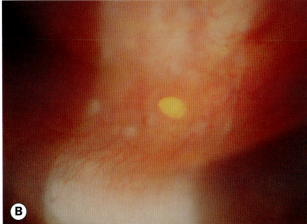

Fig. 5.33 (A) Multiple small concretions; **(B)** large concretion eroding through the conjunctival surface

Conjunctivochalasis

Conjunctivochalasis usually appears as a fold of redundant conjunctiva interposed between the globe and lower eyelid, protruding over the lid margin (Fig. 5.34). It is probably a normal ageing change that may be exacerbated by inflammation and mechanical stress related to dry eye and lid margin disease. Symptoms include watering of the eye due to obstruction of the inferior punctum and interference with the marginal tear meniscus. Treatment consists of topical lubricants and treatment of any blepharitis. A short

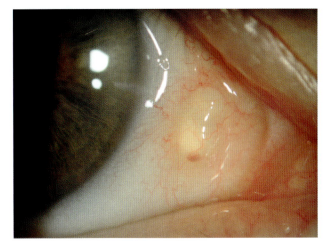

Fig. 5.35 Conjunctival cyst

course of topical steroids or other anti-inflammatory agent may be helpful. Conjunctival resection can be performed in severe cases (see also Ch. 2).

Retention (primary epithelial inclusion) cyst

Conjunctival retention cysts are thin-walled lesions on the bulbar conjunctiva containing clear (Fig. 5.35) or occasionally turbid fluid. They do not usually cause discomfort but may be a mild cosmetic blemish. Histology shows a fluid-filled internal cavity lined by a double epithelial layer. Treatment, if required, is initially by simple puncture with a needle under topical anaesthesia, but recurrence is common. Bleeding should be encouraged within the ruptured cyst as it may promote adhesion of the walls and reduce the chance of recurrence. Cyst wall excision under topical anaesthesia can be carried out for recurrences. The differential diagnosis includes secondary inclusion cysts following conjunctival surgery, and lymphangiectasia. The latter is characterized by strings of cystic or sausage-shaped clear-walled channels, which may become filled with blood (haemorrhagic lymphangiectasia – Fig. 5.36).

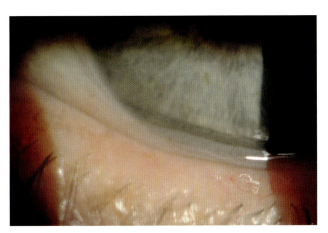

Fig. 5.34 Conjunctivochalasis

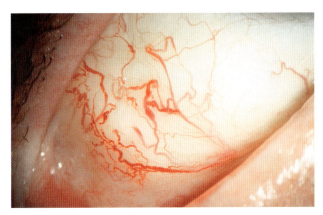

Fig. 5.36 Haemorrhagic lymphangiectasia

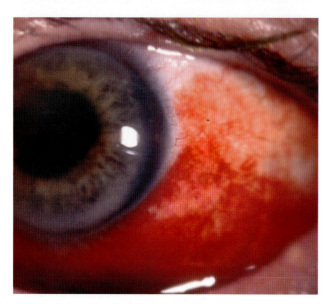

Fig. 5.37 Subconjunctival haemorrhage

SUBCONJUNCTIVAL HAEMORRHAGE

Subconjunctival haemorrhage (Fig. 5.37) is a very common phenomenon that may result from surgery, conjunctivitis and trauma (from minor unnoticed to severe skull base), but is often idiopathic and apparently spontaneous, particularly in older patients. The bleed is usually asymptomatic until noticed by the patient or others; a momentary sharp pain or a snapping or popping sensation is sometimes felt. Coughing, sneezing and vomiting are common precipitants. In younger people contact lens wear is a common association, and in older individuals systemic vascular disease is prevalent, especially hypertension, and blood pressure should be checked. A local ocular cause should be ruled out by slit lamp examination. Bleeding diatheses are a very rare association, but vitamin C deficiency and abusive trauma should always be considered in infants. The vision is usually unaffected unless a substantially elevated haemorrhage leads to a large localized corneal wetting deficit (dellen), which is often uncomfortable. A large bleed can track into the eyelids. Spontaneous resolution over a week or two is typical, but two or three narrowly spaced episodes are not uncommon.

INTRODUCTION

Anatomy and physiology

General

The cornea is a complex structure which, as well as having a protective role, is responsible for about three-quarters of the optical power of the eye. The normal cornea is free of blood vessels; nutrients are supplied and metabolic products removed mainly via the aqueous humour posteriorly and the tears anteriorly. The cornea is the most densely innervated tissue in the body, and conditions such as abrasions and bullous keratopathy are associated with marked pain, photophobia and reflex lacrimation; a subepithelial and a deeper stromal nerve plexus are both supplied by the first division of the trigeminal nerve.

Dimensions

The average corneal diameter is 11.5 mm vertically and 12 mm horizontally. It is 540 μm thick centrally on average, and thicker towards the periphery. Central corneal thickness varies between individuals and is a key determinant of the intraocular pressure (IOP) measured with conventional techniques.

Structure

The cornea consists of the following layers (Fig. 6.1):
- **The epithelium** is stratified squamous and non-keratinized, and is composed of:
  - A single layer of columnar basal cells attached by hemidesmosomes to an underlying basement membrane.
  - Two to three strata of 'wing' cells.
  - Two layers of squamous surface cells.
  - The surface area of the outermost cells is increased by microplicae and microvilli that facilitate the attachment of the tear film and mucin. After a lifespan of a few days superficial cells are shed into the tear film.
  - Corneal stem cells are located at the corneoscleral limbus, possibly in the palisades of Vogt. Deficiency may result in chronic epithelial defects and 'conjunctivalization' (epithelial instability, vascularization and the appearance of goblet cells). They are thought to be critical in the maintenance of a physiological barrier, preventing conjunctival tissue from growing onto the cornea (e.g. pterygium). Deficiency may be addressed by stem cell auto- or allotransplantation.
- **The Bowman layer** is the acellular superficial layer of the stroma, and is formed from collagen fibres.
- **The stroma** makes up 90% of corneal thickness. It is arranged in regularly orientated layers of collagen fibrils whose spacing is maintained by proteoglycan ground substance (chondroitin sulphate and keratan sulphate) with interspersed modified fibroblasts (keratocytes). Maintenance

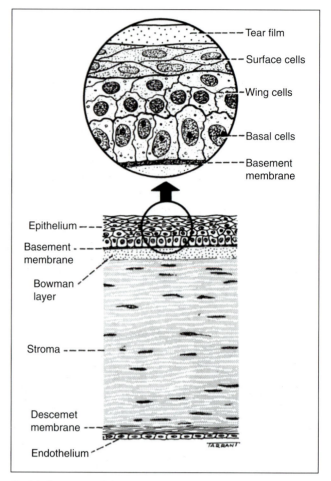

Fig. 6.1 Anatomy of the cornea

of the regular arrangement and spacing of the collagen is critical to optical clarity. The stroma can scar, but cannot regenerate following damage.
- **Descemet membrane** is a discrete sheet composed of a fine latticework of collagen fibrils that are distinct from the collagen of the stroma. The membrane consists of an anterior banded zone that is deposited *in utero* and a posterior non-banded zone laid down throughout life by the endothelium, for which it serves as a modified basement membrane. It has regenerative potential.
- **The endothelium** consists of a monolayer of polygonal cells. Endothelial cells maintain corneal deturgescence throughout life by pumping excess fluid out of the stroma. The young adult cell density is about 3000 cells/mm². The number of cells decreases at about 0.6% per year and neighbouring cells enlarge to fill the space; the cells cannot regenerate. At a density of about 500 cells/mm² corneal oedema develops and transparency is impaired.
- The existence of a sixth corneal layer between the stroma and Descemet membrane has recently been proposed, though some authorities believe this to be a previously described continuation of the posterior stroma.

Signs of corneal disease

Superficial

- **Punctate epithelial erosions (PEE)**, tiny epithelial defects that stain with fluorescein (Figs 6.2A and B) and rose Bengal, are generally an early sign of epithelial compromise. Causes include a variety of stimuli; the location of the lesions may give an indication of aetiology:
  - ○ Superior – vernal disease, chlamydial conjunctivitis, superior limbic keratoconjunctivitis, floppy eyelid syndrome and mechanically induced keratoconjunctivitis.
  - ○ Interpalpebral – dry eye (can also be inferior), reduced corneal sensation and ultraviolet keratopathy.
  - ○ Inferior – chronic blepharitis, lagophthalmos, eye drop toxicity, self-induced, aberrant eyelashes and entropion.
  - ○ Diffuse – some cases of viral and bacterial conjunctivitis, and toxicity to drops.
  - ○ Central – prolonged contact lens wear.

- **Punctate epithelial keratitis (PEK)** appears as granular, opalescent, swollen epithelial cells, with focal intraepithelial infiltrates (Fig. 6.2C). They are visible unstained but stain well with rose Bengal and variably with fluorescein. Causes include:
  - ○ Infections: adenoviral, chlamydial, molluscum contagiosum, early herpes simplex and herpes zoster, microsporidial and systemic viral infections (e.g. measles, varicella, rubella).
  - ○ Miscellaneous: Thygeson superficial punctate keratitis and eye drop toxicity.

- **Subepithelial infiltrates.** Tiny subsurface foci of non-staining inflammatory infiltrates. Causes include severe or prolonged adenoviral keratoconjunctivitis, herpes zoster keratitis, adult inclusion conjunctivitis, marginal keratitis, rosacea and Thygeson superficial punctate keratitis.

- **Superficial punctate keratitis** is a non-specific term describing any corneal epithelial disturbance of dot-like morphology.

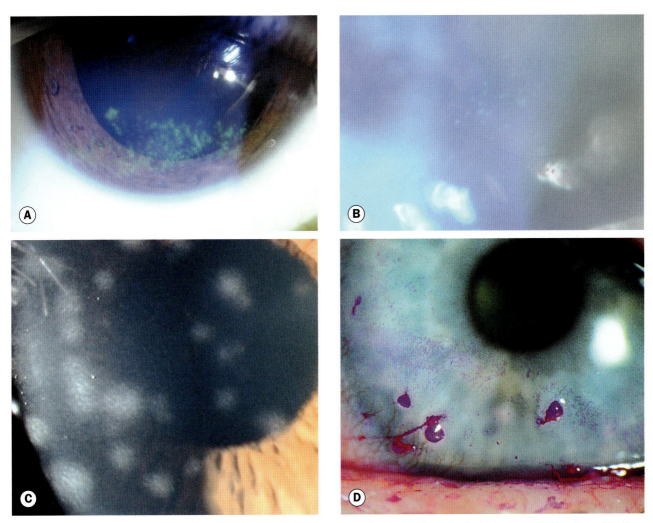

Fig. 6.2 Superficial corneal lesions. **(A)** Punctate epithelial erosions stained with fluorescein in dry eye; **(B)** high-magnification view of punctate epithelial erosions; **(C)** punctate epithelial keratitis; **(D)** filaments stained with rose Bengal;

Continued

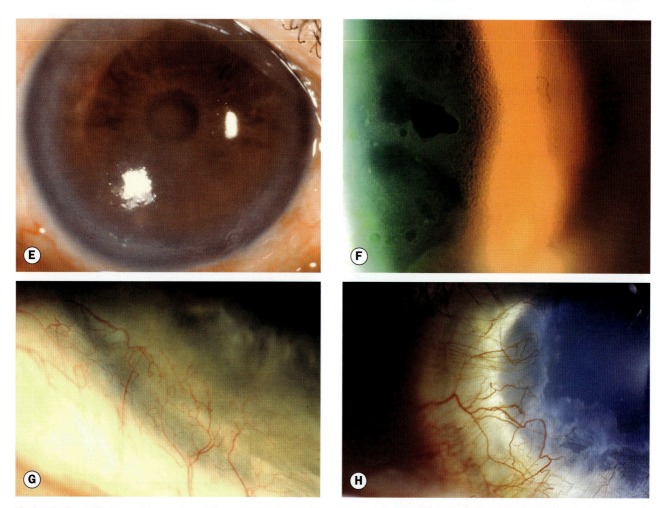

Fig. 6.2, Continued (E) loss of lustre in mild corneal oedema; **(F)** corneal oedema with bullae; **(G)** superficial vascularization; **(H)** pannus

(Courtesy of Chris Barry – figs E and H)

- **Filaments.** Strands of mucus admixed with epithelium, attached at one end to the corneal surface, that stain well with rose Bengal (Fig. 6.2D). The unattached end moves with each blink. Grey subepithelial opacities may be seen at the site of attachment. Dry eye is by far the most common cause; others include superior limbic keratoconjunctivitis, neurotrophic keratopathy, long-term ocular patching and essential blepharospasm.
- **Epithelial oedema.** Subtle oedema may manifest with loss of normal corneal lustre (Fig. 6.2E), but more commonly, abundant tiny epithelial vesicles are seen; bullae form in moderate–severe cases (Fig. 6.2F). The cause is endothelial decompensation, including that due to severe acute elevation of IOP.
- Superficial neovascularization (Fig. 6.2G) is a feature of chronic ocular surface irritation or hypoxia, as in contact lens wear.
- Pannus describes superficial neovascularization accompanied by degenerative subepithelial change (Fig. 6.2H).

Deep

- **Infiltrates** are yellow– or grey–white opacities located initially within the anterior stroma (Fig. 6.3A), usually associated with limbal or conjunctival hyperaemia. They are stromal foci of acute inflammation composed of inflammatory cells, cellular and extracellular debris including necrosis. The key distinction is between sterile and infective lesions (Table 6.1); 'PEDAL' mnemonic: **P**ain, **E**pithelial defects, **D**ischarge, **A**nterior chamber reaction, **L**ocation. Suppurative keratitis is caused by active infection with bacteria, fungi, protozoa and occasionally viruses. Non-infectious 'sterile keratitis' is due to an immune hypersensitivity response to antigen as in marginal keratitis and with contact lens wear.

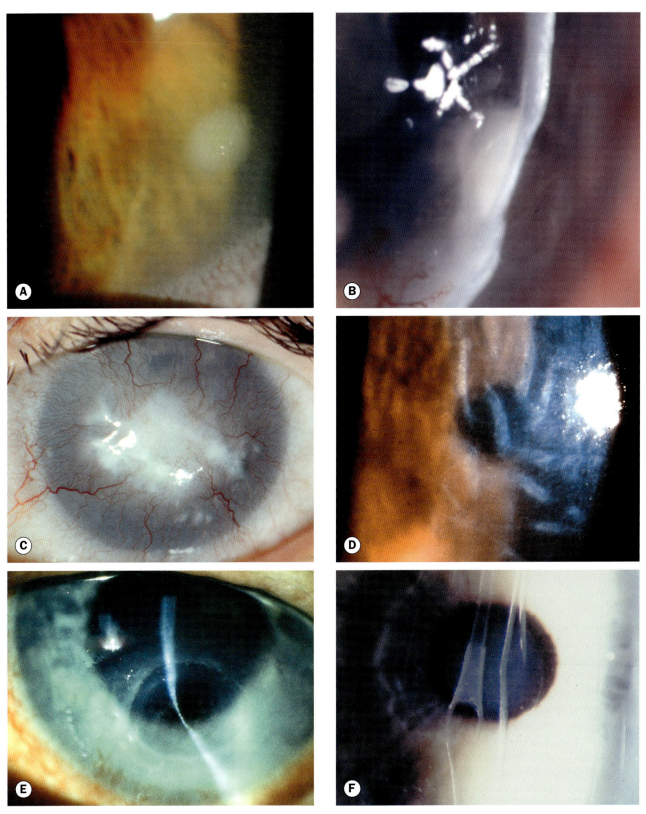

Fig. 6.3 Deeper corneal lesions. **(A)** Infiltration; **(B)** ulceration; **(C)** lipid deposition with vascularization; **(D)** folds in Descemet membrane; **(E)** descemetocoele; **(F)** traumatic breaks in Descemet membrane

(Courtesy of C Barry – figs C–D; R Curtis – fig. F)

Table 6.1 Characteristics of infective versus sterile corneal infiltrates

	Infective	Sterile
Size	Tend to be larger	Tend to be smaller
Progression	Rapid	Slow
Epithelial defect	Very common and larger when present	Much less common and if present tends to be small
Pain	Moderate–severe	Mild
Discharge	Purulent	Mucopurulent
Single or multiple	Typically single	Commonly multiple
Unilateral or bilateral	Unilateral	Often bilateral
Anterior chamber reaction	Severe	Mild
Location	Often central	Typically more peripheral
Adjacent corneal reaction	Extensive	Limited

- **Ulceration** refers to tissue excavation associated with an epithelial defect (Fig. 6.3B), usually with infiltration and necrosis.
- **'Melting'** describes tissue disintegration in response to enzymatic activity, often with mild or no infiltrate, e.g. peripheral ulcerative keratitis.
- **Vascularization** occurs in response to a wide variety of stimuli. Venous channels are easily seen, whereas arterial feeding vessels are smaller and require higher magnification. Non-perfused deep vessels appear as 'ghost vessels', best detected by retroillumination.
- **Lipid** deposition (Fig. 6.3C) may follow chronic inflammation with leakage from corneal new vessels.
- **Folds in Descemet membrane**, also known as striate keratopathy (Fig. 6.3D), may result from corneal oedema exceeding the capacity of the endothelium to maintain normal turgescence. Causes include inflammation, trauma (including surgery) and ocular hypotony.
- **Descemetocoele** (US spelling – descemetocele) is a bubble-like herniation of Descemet membrane into the cornea (Fig. 6.3E), plugging a defect that would otherwise be full-thickness.
- **Breaks in Descemet membrane** (Fig. 6.3F) may be due to corneal enlargement (Haab striae in infantile glaucoma) or deformation such as keratoconus and birth trauma. Acute influx of aqueous into the corneal stroma (acute hydrops) can occur.
- **The Seidel test** demonstrates aqueous leakage. A drop of 1% or 2% fluorescein is applied and the slit lamp with cobalt blue filter is used to detect the change from dark orange to bright yellow–green occurring with localized dilution at a site of leakage.

Documentation of clinical signs

Clinical signs should be illustrated with a colour-coded labelled diagram; including lesion dimensions is particularly useful to facilitate monitoring (Fig. 6.4). Slit lamp photography is an increasingly used supplement or alternative, but must be of high quality.

- **Opacities** such as scars and degenerations are drawn in black.
- **Epithelial oedema** is represented by fine blue circles, stromal oedema as blue shading and folds in Descemet membrane as wavy blue lines.
- **Hypopyon** is shown in yellow.
- **Blood vessels** are added in red. Superficial vessels are wavy lines that begin outside the limbus and deep vessels are straight lines that begin at the limbus.
- **Pigmented lesions** such as iron lines and Krukenberg spindles are shown in brown.

Specular microscopy

Specular microscopy is the study of corneal layers under very high magnification (100 times greater than slit lamp biomicroscopy). It is mainly used to assess the endothelium, which can be analysed for cellular size, shape, density and distribution. The healthy endothelial cell is a regular hexagon (Fig. 6.5A) and the normal cell density in a young adult is about 3000 cells/mm².

- **Physics.** When a light beam of the specular photomicroscope passes through the cornea it encounters a series of interfaces between optically distinct regions. Some light is reflected specularly (i.e. like a mirror) back towards the photomicroscope and forms an image that can be photographed and analysed.
- **Indications**
  - Evaluation of the functional reserve of the corneal endothelium prior to intraocular surgery is the most common indication. A clear cornea with normal thickness on pachymetry is not necessarily associated with normal endothelial morphology or cell density.

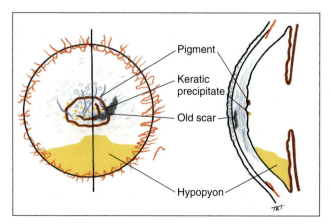

Fig. 6.4 Documentation of corneal lesions

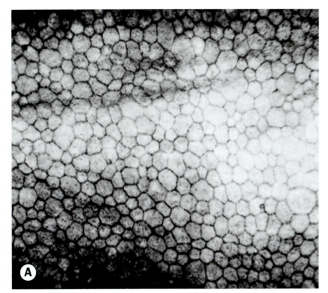

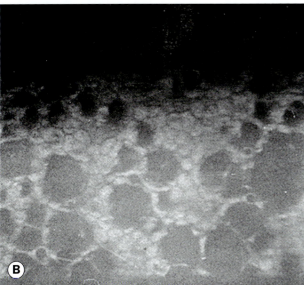

Fig. 6.5 Specular micrograph. **(A)** Normal corneal endothelium; **(B)** cornea guttata with marked loss of endothelial mosaic

(Courtesy of T Casey and K Sharif, from A Colour Atlas of Corneal Dystrophies and Degenerations, Wolfe 1991 – fig. B)

Corneal oedema is considerably more likely to occur with a cell density below 700 cells/mm² but unlikely above 1000 cells/mm².

○ Donor cornea evaluation.
○ To demonstrate pathology, particularly cornea guttata (Fig. 6.5B), Descemet membrane irregularities and posterior polymorphous dystrophy.

Corneal topography

Corneal topography is used to image the cornea by projecting a series of concentric rings of light on the anterior surface, constituting a Placido image. The reflected light is analysed using computer

software to produce a detailed surface map. A major application is the detection and management of corneal ectasia, principally keratoconus; screening for corneal ectasia is especially important prior to refractive surgery. It is used in the management of refractive error, again in relation to refractive surgery as well as sometimes for contact lens fitting, and can be used to measure corneal thickness. Scheimpflug imaging is a newer technology that may offer advantages in topographic imaging. Anterior segment optical coherence tomography (OCT) and ultrasound biomicroscopy can also be used to image the cornea.

Principles of treatment

Control of infection and inflammation

- **Antimicrobial agents** should be started as soon as preliminary investigations have been performed. The choice of agent is determined by the likely aetiology according to clinical findings. Broad-spectrum treatment is generally used initially, with more selective agents introduced if necessary when the results of investigation are available.
- **Topical steroids** should always be used with caution as they may promote replication of some microorganisms, notably herpes simplex virus and fungi, and retard reparative processes such as re-epithelialization. Nevertheless, they are vital in a range of conditions for the suppression of destructive vision-compromising inflammation.
- **Systemic immunosuppressive agents** are useful in some conditions, particularly autoimmune disease.

Promotion of epithelial healing

Re-epithelialization is of great importance in any corneal disease, as thinning seldom progresses if the epithelium is intact.

- **Reduction of exposure** to toxic medications and preservatives wherever possible.
- **Lubrication** with artificial tears (unpreserved if possible) and ointment. Taping the lids closed temporarily (Fig. 6.6A) is often used as a nocturnal adjunct.
- **Antibiotic ointment** prophylaxis should be considered.
- **Bandage soft contact lenses** should be carefully supervised to exclude superinfection, and duration kept to a minimum. Indications include:
  ○ Promotion of healing by mechanically protecting regenerating corneal epithelium from the constant rubbing of the eyelids.
  ○ To improve comfort, particularly in the presence of a large corneal abrasion.
  ○ To seal a small perforation (Fig. 6.6B).
- **Surgical eyelid closure** is particularly useful in exposure and neurotrophic keratopathies as well as in persistent epithelial defects. Lid closure may be used as a conservative method to heal an infective ulcer in selected cases, such as an eye with no visual potential in a patient with severe dementia.
  ○ Botulinum toxin injection into the levator muscle to induce a temporary (2–3 months) ptosis.

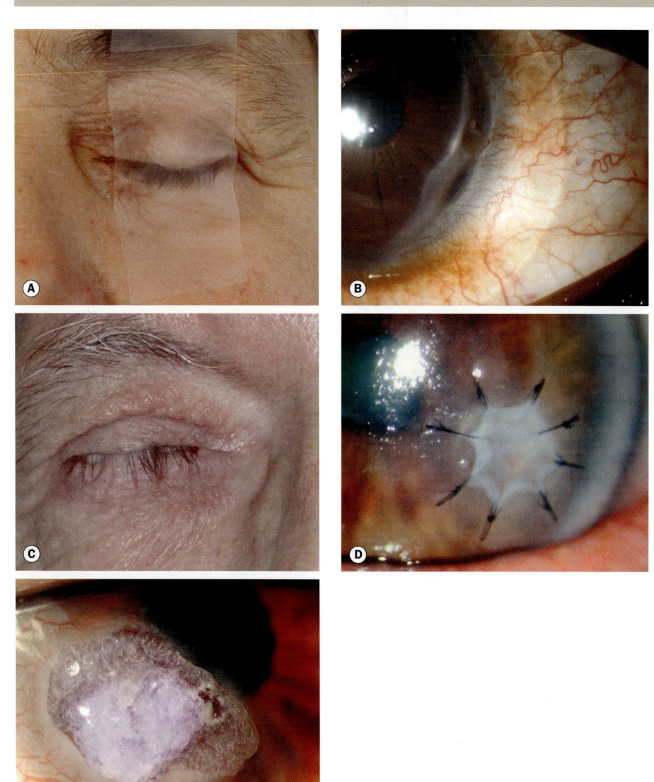

Fig. 6.6 Methods of promoting epithelial healing. **(A)** Taping the lids temporarily; **(B)** bandage contact lens in an eye with a small perforation; **(C)** central tarsorrhaphy; **(D)** amniotic membrane graft over a persistent epithelial defect; **(E)** tissue glue under a bandage contact lens in an eye with severe thinning

(Courtesy of S Tuft – figs A, B, D and E; S Chen – fig. C)

○ Temporary or permanent lateral tarsorrhaphy or medial canthoplasty, and occasionally central tarsorrhaphy (Fig. 6.6C).

- **Conjunctival (Gundersen) flap** will protect and tend to heal a corneal epithelial defect and is particularly suitable for chronic unilateral disease in which the prognosis for restoration of useful vision is poor. Buccal mucous membrane is an alternative.
- **Amniotic membrane patch grafting** (Fig. 6.6D) for persistent unresponsive epithelial defects.
- **Tissue adhesive** (cyanoacrylate glue) to seal small perforations. The glue can be applied to one side of a bespoke trimmed patch of sterile plastic drape, which is pressed over the defect after the edges are dried with a cellulose sponge. The patch remains in place to seal the defect, and a bandage contact lens is inserted for comfort and to aid retention of the patch (Fig. 6.6E).
- **Limbal stem cell transplantation** may be used if there is stem cell deficiency as in chemical burns and cicatrizing conjunctivitis. The source of the donor tissue may be the fellow eye (autograft) in unilateral disease or a living or cadaver donor (allograft) when both eyes are affected. A newer technique involves the *in vitro* replication of the patient's own stem cells with subsequent re-implantation of the enhanced cell population.
- **Smoking** retards epithelialization and should be discontinued.

BACTERIAL KERATITIS

Pathogenesis

Pathogens

Bacterial keratitis usually develops only when ocular defences have been compromised (see below). However, some bacteria, including *Neisseria gonorrhoeae, Neisseria meningitidis, Corynebacterium diphtheriae* and *Haemophilus influenzae* are able to penetrate a healthy corneal epithelium, usually in association with severe conjunctivitis. It is important to remember that infections may be polymicrobial, including bacterial and fungal co-infection. Common pathogens include:

- *Pseudomonas aeruginosa* is a ubiquitous Gram-negative bacillus (rod) commensal of the gastrointestinal tract. The infection is typically aggressive and is responsible for over 60% of contact lens-related keratitis.
- *Staphylococcus aureus* is a common Gram-positive and coagulase-positive commensal of the nares, skin and conjunctiva. Keratitis tends to present with a focal and fairly well-defined white or yellow–white infiltrate.
- Streptococci. *S. pyogenes* is a common Gram-positive commensal of the throat and vagina. *S. pneumoniae* (pneumococcus) is a Gram-positive commensal of the upper respiratory tract. Infections with streptococci are often aggressive.

Risk factors

- **Contact lens wear**, particularly if extended, is the most important risk factor. Corneal epithelial compromise secondary to hypoxia and minor trauma is thought to be important, as is bacterial adherence to the lens surface. Wearers of soft lenses are at higher risk than those of rigid gas permeable and other types. Infection is more likely if there is poor lens hygiene but it can also occur even with apparently meticulous lens care, and with daily disposable lenses.
- **Trauma**, including refractive surgery (particularly LASIK – laser-assisted *in situ* keratomileusis), has been linked to bacterial infection, including with atypical mycobacteria. In developing countries agricultural injury is the major risk factor, when fungal infection should be considered.
- **Ocular surface disease** such as herpetic keratitis, bullous keratopathy, dry eye, chronic blepharitis, trichiasis and entropion, exposure, severe allergic eye disease and corneal anaesthesia.
- **Other factors** include local or systemic immunosuppression, diabetes and vitamin A deficiency.

Clinical features

- **Presentation** is with pain, photophobia, blurred vision and mucopurulent or purulent discharge.
- **Signs**
  ○ An epithelial defect with infiltrate involving a larger area, and significant circumcorneal injection (Fig. 6.7A and B).
  ○ Stromal oedema, folds in Descemet membrane and anterior uveitis, commonly with a hypopyon (Fig. 6.7C) and posterior synechiae in moderate–severe keratitis. Plaque-like keratic precipitates can form on the endothelium contiguous with the affected stroma.
  ○ Chemosis and eyelid swelling in moderate–severe cases.
  ○ Severe ulceration may lead to descemetocoele formation and perforation, particularly in *Pseudomonas* infection (Fig. 6.7D).
  ○ Scleritis can develop, particularly with severe perilimbal infection.
  ○ Endophthalmitis is rare in the absence of perforation.
  ○ Improvement is usually heralded by a reduction in eyelid oedema and chemosis, shrinking of the epithelial defect, decreasing infiltrate density and a reduction in anterior chamber signs.
  ○ Subsequent scarring may be severe, including vascularization; in addition to opacification irregular astigmatism may limit vision.
- **Reduced corneal sensation** may suggest associated neurotrophic keratopathy, particularly where there is no other major risk factor. Sensation may also be reduced in chronic surface disease, herpetic keratitis and long-term contact lens wear.
- **IOP** should be monitored.

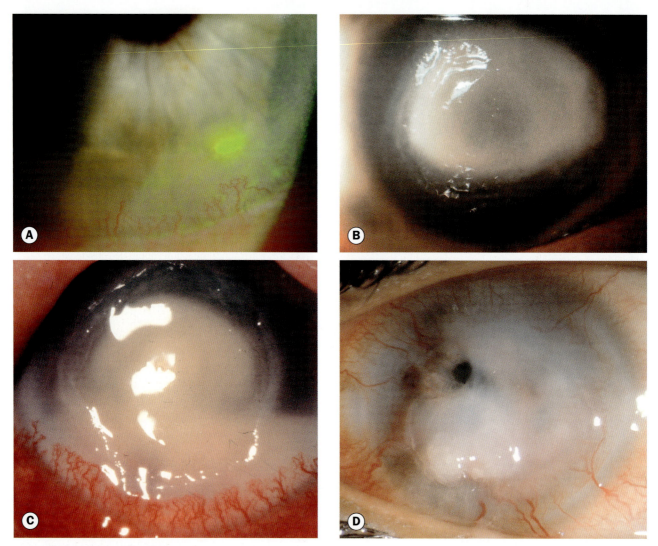

Fig. 6.7 Bacterial keratitis. **(A)** Early ulcer; **(B)** large ulcer; **(C)** advanced disease with hypopyon; **(D)** perforation associated with *Pseudomonas* infection
(Courtesy of C Barry – fig. B; S Tuft – fig. D)

- **Differential diagnosis** includes keratitis due to other microorganisms (fungi, acanthamoeba, stromal herpes simplex keratitis and mycobacteria), marginal keratitis, sterile inflammatory corneal infiltrates associated with contact lens wear, peripheral ulcerative keratitis and toxic keratitis.

Investigations

- **Corneal scraping.** This may not be required for a small infiltrate, particularly one without an epithelial defect and away from the visual axis.
  - A non-preserved topical anaesthetic is instilled (preservatives may lower bacterial viability for culture); one drop of proxymetacaine 0.5% is usually sufficient; tetracaine may have a greater bacteriostatic effect.
  - Scrapings are taken either with a disposable scalpel blade (e.g. No. 11 or Bard Parker), the bent tip of a larger

diameter (e.g. 20- or 21-gauge) hypodermic needle, or a sterile spatula (e.g. Kimura).
  - The easiest way to 'plate' scrapings without breaking the gel surface is with a spatula. If a fresh spatula is not available for each sample a single instrument should be flame-sterilized between scrapes (heat for 5 seconds, cool for 20–30 seconds). Alternatively, a fresh scalpel blade or needle can be used for each pass. Calcium alginate swabs may also be satisfactory.
  - Loose mucus and necrotic tissue should be removed from the surface of the ulcer prior to scraping.
  - The margins and base (except if very thin) of the lesion are scraped (Fig. 6.8A).
  - A thin smear is placed on one or two glass slides for microscopy, including Gram stain (see below). A surface is provided on one side of one end of the slide (conventionally 'up') for pencil labelling. The sample is

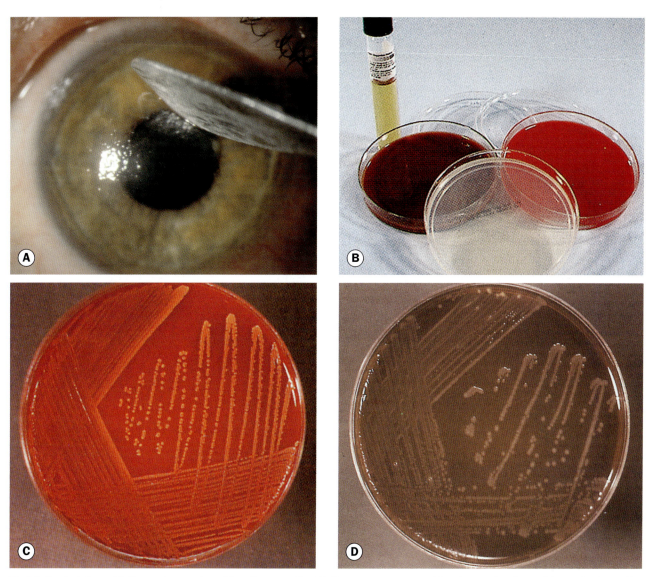

Fig. 6.8 Bacteriology. **(A)** Corneal scraping; **(B)** culture media; **(C)** *S. aureus* grown on blood agar forming golden colonies with a shiny surface; **(D)** *N. gonorrhoeae* grown on chocolate agar

(Courtesy of J Harry – fig. A; R Emond, P Welsby and H Rowland, from Colour Atlas of Infectious Diseases, Mosby 2003 – figs B–D)

allowed to dry in air at room temperature for several minutes then placed in a slide carrier.

○ Re-scraping is performed for each medium and samples are plated onto culture media (Table 6.2), taking care not to break the surface of the gel.

○ Routinely, blood, chocolate and Sabouraud media (Fig. 6.8B–D) are used initially and the samples are placed in an incubator until transported to the laboratory. Refrigerated media should be gently warmed to room temperature prior to sample application.

○ A blade or needle can be placed directly into bottled media such as brain–heart infusion (BHI). There is evidence that a single scrape, sent in BHI to the laboratory where it is homogenized and plated, provides similar results to the traditional multi-scrape method.

○ Scraping may be delayed without treatment for 12 hours if antibiotics have previously been commenced.

- **Conjunctival swabs** may be worthwhile in addition to corneal scraping, particularly in severe cases, as occasionally an organism may be cultured when a corneal scrape is negative. Cotton wool, calcium alginate and synthetic swabs have all been found to have some bacteriostatic effect; calcium alginate may be the best option.
- **Contact lens cases**, as well as bottles of solution and lenses themselves, should be obtained when possible and sent to the laboratory for culture. The case should not be cleaned by the patient first!
- **Gram staining**
  ○ Differentiates bacterial species into 'Gram-positive' and 'Gram-negative' based on the ability of the dye (crystal violet) to penetrate the cell wall.
  ○ Bacteria that take up crystal violet are Gram-positive and those that allow the dye to wash off are Gram-negative.

Table 6.2 Culture media for corneal scrapings

Medium	Notes	Specificity
Blood agar	5–10% sheep or horse blood	Most bacteria and fungi except *Neisseria*, *Haemophilus* and *Moraxella*
Chocolate agar	Blood agar in which the cells have been lysed by heating. Does not contain chocolate!	Fastidious bacteria, particularly *H. influenzae*, *Neisseria* and *Moraxella*
Sabouraud dextrose agar	Low pH and antibiotic (e.g. chloramphenicol) to deter bacterial growth	Fungi
Non-nutrient agar seeded with *Escherichia coli*	*E. coli* is a food source for *Acanthamoeba*	*Acanthamoeba*
Brain–heart infusion	Rich lightly buffered medium providing a wide range of substrates	Difficult-to-culture organisms; particularly suitable for streptococci and meningococci. Supports yeast and fungal growth
Cooked meat broth	Developed during the First World War for the growth of battlefield anaerobes	Anaerobic (e.g. *Propionibacterium acnes*) as well as fastidious bacteria
Löwenstein–Jensen	Contains various nutrients together with bacterial growth inhibitors	Mycobacteria, *Nocardia*

○ Other stains, generally not requested at initial investigation, are listed in Table 6.3.
- **Culture and sensitivity reports** should be obtained as soon as possible. The type of bacteria alone will generally provide an indication of the antibiotic category to be used. An indication of resistance on standard sensitivity testing does not necessarily extrapolate to topical antibiotic instillation, where very high tissue levels can be achieved.

Treatment

General considerations

- **Hospital admission** should be considered for patients who are not likely to comply or are unable to self-administer

Table 6.3 Stains for corneal and conjunctival scrapings

Stain	Organism
Gram	Bacteria, fungi, microsporidia
Giemsa	Bacteria, fungi, *Acanthamoeba*, microsporidia
Calcofluor white (fluorescent microscope)	*Acanthamoeba*, fungi, microsporidia
Acid-fast stain (AFB) e.g. Ziehl–Neelsen, auramine O (fluorescent)	*Mycobacterium*, *Nocardia* spp.
Grocott–Gömöri methenamine-silver	Fungi, *Acanthamoeba*, microsporidia
Periodic acid-Schiff (PAS)	Fungi, *Acanthamoeba*

treatment. It should also be considered for aggressive disease, particularly if involving an only eye.
- **Discontinuation of contact lens wear** is mandatory.
- **A clear plastic eye shield** should be worn between eye drop instillation if significant thinning (or perforation) is present.
- **Decision to treat**
  ○ Intensive treatment may not be required for small infiltrates that are clinically sterile and may be treated by lower-frequency topical antibiotic and/or steroid, and by temporary cessation of contact lens wear.
  ○ It is important to note that the causative organism cannot be defined reliably from the ulcer's appearance.
  ○ Empirical broad-spectrum treatment is usually initiated before microscopy results are available.

Local therapy

Topical therapy (Table 6.4) can achieve high tissue concentration and initially should consist of broad-spectrum antibiotics that cover most common pathogens. Initially instillation is at hourly intervals day and night for 24–48 hours, and then is tapered according to clinical progress.
- **Antibiotic monotherapy** has the major advantage over duotherapy of lower surface toxicity, as well as greater convenience.
  ○ A commercially available fluoroquinolone is the usual choice for empirical monotherapy and appears to be about as effective as duotherapy.
  ○ Ciprofloxacin or ofloxacin are used in countries where widespread resistance to earlier-generation fluoroquinolones has not been identified. Activity against some Gram-positive organisms, particularly some streptococci, may be limited.

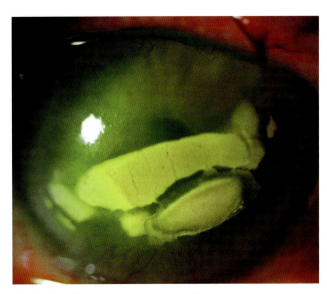

Fig. 6.9 Ciprofloxacin corneal precipitates

○ Resistance to fluoroquinolones has been reported in some areas (e.g. *Staphylococcus* spp. in the USA and *Pseudomonas* in India). Moxifloxacin, gatifloxacin and besifloxacin are new generation fluoroquinolones that largely address this, and also have better activity against Gram-positive pathogens. Moxifloxacin has superior ocular penetration. Novel drug preparations, with higher concentrations or modified vehicles, have been introduced to enhance antibacterial activity.

○ Ciprofloxacin instillation is associated with white corneal precipitates (Fig. 6.9) that may delay epithelial healing.

● **Antibiotic duotherapy** may be preferred as first-line empirical treatment in aggressive disease or if microscopy suggests streptococci or a specific microorganism that may be more effectively treated by a tailored regimen (see Table 6.4).

○ Empirical duotherapy usually involves a combination of two fortified antibiotics, typically a cephalosporin and an aminoglycoside, in order to cover common Gram-positive and Gram-negative pathogens.

○ The antibiotics are not commercially available and must be specially prepared (Table 6.5). A standard parenteral or lyophilized antibiotic preparation is combined with a compatible vehicle such that the antibiotic does not precipitate. Optimally, constitution should take place in the sterile preparation area of a pharmaceutical dispensary.

Table 6.4 Antibiotics for the treatment of keratitis

Isolate	Antibiotic	Concentration
Empirical treatment	Fluoroquinolone monotherapy or cefuroxime + 'fortified' gentamicin duotherapy	Varies with preparation 5% 1.5%
Gram-positive cocci	Cefuroxime vancomycin or teicoplanin	0.3% 5% 1%
Gram-negative rods	'Fortified' gentamicin or fluoroquinolone or ceftazidime	1.5% Varies with preparation 5%
Gram-negative cocci	Fluoroquinolone or ceftriaxone	Varies with preparation 5%
Mycobacteria	Amikacin or clarithromycin	2% 1%
Nocardia	Amikacin or trimethoprim + sulfamethoxazole	2% 1.6% 8%

○ Disadvantages of fortified antibiotics include high cost, limited availability, contamination risk, short shelf-life and the need for refrigeration.

● **Subconjunctival antibiotics** are usually only indicated if there is poor compliance with topical treatment.

● **Mydriatics** (cyclopentolate 1%, homatropine 2% or atropine 1%) are used to prevent the formation of posterior synechiae and to reduce pain.

● **Steroids**

○ Steroids reduce host inflammation, improve comfort, and minimize corneal scarring. However, they promote replication of some microorganisms, particularly fungi, herpes simplex and mycobacteria and are contraindicated if a fungal or mycobacterial agent is suspected (beware prior refractive surgery and trauma involving vegetation). By suppressing inflammation, they also retard the eye's response to bacteria and this can be clinically significant, particularly if an antibiotic is of limited effect or bacteriostatic rather than bactericidal.

○ Evidence that they improve the final visual outcome is mainly empirical, but the recent Steroids for Corneal Ulcers Trial (SCUT) found no eventual benefit in most

Table 6.5 Preparation of fortified antibiotics

Antibiotic	Method	Concentration	Shelf-life
Cephalosporins: cefazolin, cefuroxime, or ceftazidime	500 mg parenteral antibiotic is diluted with 2.5 ml sterile water and added to 7.5 ml of preservative-free artificial tears	50 mg/ml (5%)	24 hours at room temperature; at least 4 days if refrigerated
Gentamicin	2 ml parenteral antibiotic (40 mg/ml) is added to 5 ml commercially available gentamicin ophthalmic solution (0.3%)	15 mg/ml (1.5%)	Up to 14 days if refrigerated

cases, though severe cases (counting fingers vision or large ulcers involving the central 4 mm of the cornea) tended to do better; a positive culture result was an inclusion criterion, and steroids were introduced after 48 hours of moxifloxacin.

- ○ Epithelialization may be retarded by steroids and they should be avoided if there is significant thinning or delayed epithelial healing; corneal melting can occasionally be precipitated or worsened.
- ○ Many authorities do not commence topical steroids until evidence of clinical improvement is seen with antibiotics alone, typically 24–48 hours after starting treatment. Others delay their use at least until the sensitivity of the isolate to antibiotics has been demonstrated, or do not use them at all.
- ○ Regimens vary from minimal strength preparations at low frequency to dexamethasone 0.1% every 2 hours; a reasonable regimen is prednisolone 0.5–1% four times daily.
- ○ Early discontinuation may lead to a rebound recurrence of sterile inflammation.
- ○ The threshold for topical steroid use may be lower in cases of corneal graft infection, as they may reduce the risk of rejection.

Systemic antibiotics

Systemic antibiotics are not usually given, but may be appropriate in the following circumstances:

- **Potential for systemic involvement**, when microbiological/ infectious disease specialist advice should optimally be sought but should not delay treatment:
  - ○ *N. meningitidis*, in which early systemic prophylaxis may be life-saving. Treatment is usually with intramuscular benzylpenicillin, ceftriaxone or cefotaxime, or oral ciprofloxacin.
  - ○ *H. influenzae* infection should be treated with oral amoxicillin with clavulanic acid.
  - ○ *N. gonorrhoeae* requires a third-generation cephalosporin such as ceftriaxone.
- **Severe corneal thinning** with threatened or actual perforation requires:
  - ○ Ciprofloxacin for its antibacterial activity.
  - ○ A tetracycline (e.g. doxycycline 100 mg twice daily) for its anticollagenase effect.
- **Scleral involvement** may respond to oral or intravenous treatment.

Management of apparent treatment failure

It is important not to confuse ongoing failure of re-epithelialization with continued infection. Drug toxicity, particularly following frequent instillation of fortified aminoglycosides, may give increasing discomfort, redness and discharge despite the eradication of infection.

- If no improvement is evident following 24–48 hours of intensive treatment, the antibiotic regimen should be reviewed, including contact with the microbiology laboratory to obtain the latest report.
- There is no need to change the initial therapy if this has induced a favourable response, even if cultures show a resistant organism.
- If there is still no improvement after a further 48 hours, suspension of treatment should be considered for 24 hours then re-scraping performed with inoculation on a broader range of media (see Table 6.2) and additional staining techniques requested (see Table 6.3). Consideration should be given to the possibility of a non-bacterial causative microorganism.
- If cultures remain negative, it may be necessary to perform a corneal biopsy for histology and culture.
- Excisional keratoplasty, penetrating or deep lamellar, may be considered in cases resistant to medical therapy, or for incipient or actual perforation (see below).

Perforation

A small perforation in which infection is controlled may be manageable with a bandage contact lens; tissue glue is often adequate for slightly larger dehiscences. A penetrating keratoplasty or corneal patch graft may be necessary for larger perforations, or in those where infection is extensive or inadequately controlled. Occlusive surface repair techniques may be appropriate in some circumstances, such as an eye with no useful visual potential.

Endophthalmitis

No clear protocol exists for the management of this rare complication, but a similar approach to postoperative endophthalmitis should be considered, whilst continuing specific management of the corneal infection. Secondary sterile intraocular inflammation should not be mistaken for intraocular infection.

Visual rehabilitation

- Keratoplasty (lamellar may be adequate) may be required for residual dense corneal scarring.
- Rigid contact lenses may be required for irregular astigmatism but are generally only introduced at least 3 months after re-epithelialization.
- Cataract surgery may be required because secondary lens opacities are common following severe inflammation. Even in the absence of severe corneal opacification, surgery may be hampered by corneal haze, posterior synechiae and zonular fragility.

FUNGAL KERATITIS

Introduction

Pathogenesis

Fungi are a group of microorganisms that have rigid walls and a distinct nucleus with multiple chromosomes containing both

DNA and RNA. Fungal keratitis is rare in temperate countries but is a major cause of visual loss in tropical and developing countries. Though often evolving insidiously, fungal keratitis can elicit a severe inflammatory response – corneal perforation is common, and the outlook for vision is frequently poor. Two main types of fungi cause keratitis:

- **Yeasts** (e.g. genus *Candida*), ovoid unicellular organisms that reproduce by budding, are responsible for most cases of fungal keratitis in temperate climates.
- **Filamentous fungi** (e.g. genera *Fusarium* and *Aspergillus*), multicellular organisms that produce tubular projections known as hyphae. They are the most common pathogens in tropical climates, but are not uncommon in cooler regions; the keratitis frequently follows an aggressive course.

Predisposing factors

Common predisposing factors include chronic ocular surface disease, the long-term use of topical steroids (often in conjunction with prior corneal transplantation), contact lens wear, systemic immunosuppression and diabetes. Filamentary keratitis may be associated with trauma, often relatively minor, involving plant matter or gardening/agricultural tools.

Candidal and filamentous keratitis

Clinical features

The diagnosis is frequently delayed unless there is a high index of suspicion, and often bacterial infection will initially have been presumed. Clinical signs are not a definitive means of distinguishing bacterial and fungal corneal infection; signs such as satellite infiltrates (see below) can be caused by other microorganisms.

- **Symptoms.** Gradual onset of pain, grittiness, photophobia, blurred vision and watery or mucopurulent discharge.
- **Candidal keratitis**
  ○ Yellow–white densely suppurative infiltrate is typical (Fig. 6.10A).
- **Filamentous keratitis**
  ○ Grey or yellow–white stromal infiltrate with indistinct fluffy margins (Fig. 6.10B).
  ○ Progressive infiltration, often with satellite lesions (Fig. 6.10C and D).
  ○ Feathery branch-like extensions or a ring-shaped infiltrate (Fig. 6.10E) may develop.
  ○ Rapid progression with necrosis and thinning can occur.
  ○ Penetration of an intact Descemet membrane may occur and lead to endophthalmitis without evident perforation.
- **An epithelial defect** is not invariable and is sometimes small when present.
- **Other features** include anterior uveitis, hypopyon, endothelial plaque, raised IOP, scleritis and sterile or infective endophthalmitis.
- **Differential diagnosis** includes bacterial, herpetic and acanthamoebal keratitis. Bacterial infection may sometimes present subacutely, particularly when atypical organisms are

responsible. It is important to beware of co-infection, including with an additional fungal species.

Investigations

Samples for laboratory investigation should be acquired before commencing antifungal therapy.

- **Staining**
  ○ Potassium hydroxide (KOH) preparation with direct microscopic evaluation is a rapid diagnostic tool that can be highly sensitive.
  ○ Gram and Giemsa staining are both about 50% sensitive.
  ○ Other stains include periodic acid–Schiff, calcofluor white and methenamine silver.
- **Culture.** Corneal scrapes should be plated on Sabouraud dextrose agar, although most fungi will also grow on blood agar or in enrichment media. It is important to obtain an effective scrape from the ulcer base. Sensitivity testing for antifungal agents can be performed in reference laboratories but the relevance of these results to clinical effectiveness is uncertain. If applicable, contact lenses and cases should be sent for culture.
- **Polymerase chain reaction (PCR) analysis** of specimens is rapid and highly sensitive (up to 90%) and may be the current investigation of choice. Calcium-containing swabs can inhibit polymerase activity and local collection protocols should be ascertained prior to specimen collection.
- **Corneal biopsy** is indicated in suspected fungal keratitis in the absence of clinical improvement after 3–4 days and if no growth develops from scrapings after a week. A 2–3 mm block should be taken, similar to scleral block excision during trabeculectomy; filamentous fungi tend to proliferate just anterior to Descemet membrane and a deep stromal specimen may be required. The excised block is sent for culture and histopathological analysis.
- **Anterior chamber tap** has been advocated in resistant cases with endothelial exudate, because organisms may penetrate the endothelium.
- **Confocal microscopy** frequently permits identification of organisms *in vivo*, but is not widely available outside tertiary centres.

Treatment

Improvement may be slow in comparison to bacterial infection.

- **General measures** are as for bacterial keratitis although hospital admission is usually required.
- **Removal of the epithelium** over the lesion may enhance penetration of antifungal agents. It may also be helpful to regularly remove mucus and necrotic tissue with a spatula.
- **Topical antifungals** should initially be given hourly for 48 hours and then reduced as signs permit. Because most antifungals are only fungistatic, treatment should be continued for at least 12 weeks.
  ○ *Candida* infection is treated with amphotericin B 0.15% or econazole 1%; alternatives include natamycin 5%, fluconazole 2%, clotrimazole 1% and voriconazole 1 or 2%.

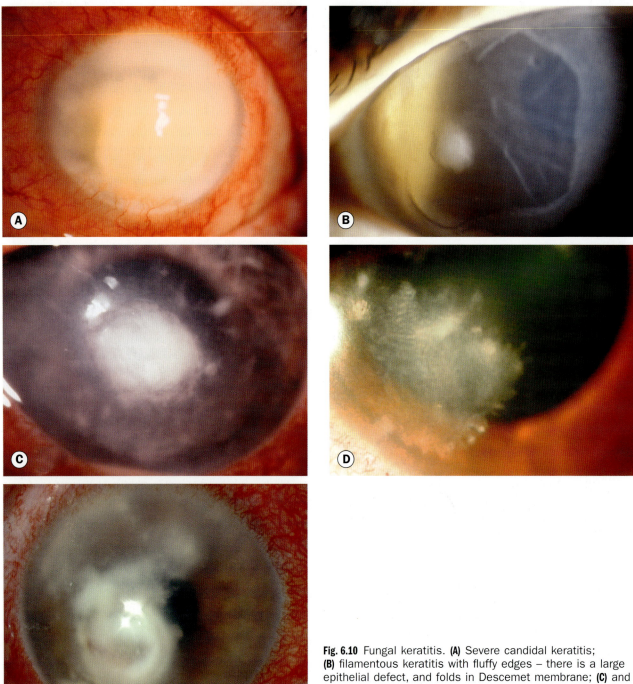

Fig. 6.10 Fungal keratitis. **(A)** Severe candidal keratitis; **(B)** filamentous keratitis with fluffy edges – there is a large epithelial defect, and folds in Descemet membrane; **(C)** and **(D)** satellite lesions; **(E)** ring infiltrate, with satellite lesions and a hypopyon

(Courtesy of S Tuft – figs B and E; R Fogla – fig. D)

- ○ Filamentous infection is treated with natamycin 5% or econazole 1%; alternatives are amphotericin B 0.15%, miconazole 1% and voriconazole 1 or 2%.
- ○ Several others are available.
- **A broad-spectrum antibiotic** might also be considered to address or prevent bacterial co-infection.
- **Cycloplegia** as for bacterial keratitis.
- **Subconjunctival** fluconazole may be used in severe cases.

- **Systemic antifungals** may be given in severe cases, when lesions are near the limbus, and for suspected endophthalmitis. Options include voriconazole 400 mg twice daily for one day then 200 mg twice daily, itraconazole 200 mg once daily, reduced to 100 mg once daily, or fluconazole 200 mg twice daily.
- **Tetracycline** (e.g. doxycycline 100 mg twice daily) may be given for its anticollagenase effect when there is significant thinning.

- **IOP** should be monitored.
- **Perforation** – actual or impending – is managed as for bacterial keratitis.
- **Superficial keratectomy** can be effective to de-bulk a lesion.
- **Therapeutic keratoplasty** (penetrating or deep anterior lamellar) is considered when medical therapy is ineffective or following perforation.
- **Anterior chamber washout** with intracameral antifungal injection may be considered for unresponsive cases in which there is a stable corneal infiltrate but enlarging endothelial exudation.

Microsporidial keratitis

Introduction

Microsporidia (phylum Microspora) are obligate intracellular single-celled parasites previously thought to be protozoa but now reclassified as fungi. They rarely cause disease in the immunocompetent and until the advent of acquired immunodeficiency syndrome (AIDS) were rarely pathogenic for humans. The most common general infection is enteritis and the most common ocular manifestation is keratoconjunctivitis.

Diagnosis

- **Signs**
  - Bilateral chronic diffuse punctate epithelial keratitis (Fig. 6.11A).
  - Unilateral slowly progressive deep stromal keratitis (Fig. 6.11B) may rarely affect immunocompetent patients.
  - Sclerokeratitis and endophthalmitis are rare.
- **Biopsy** shows characteristic spores and intracellular parasites.
- **PCR** of scrapings may have relatively low sensitivity.

Treatment

- **Medical** therapy of epithelial disease is with topical fumagillin. Highly active antiretroviral therapy (HAART) for associated AIDS may also help resolution. Stromal disease is treated with a combination of topical fumagillin and oral albendazole 400 mg once daily for 2 weeks, repeated 2 weeks later with a second course. Patients should be closely monitored for hepatic toxicity. Long-term fumagillin treatment may be required and it is difficult to eradicate the parasites in immunocompromised patients.
- **Keratoplasty** may be indicated although recurrence of disease can occur in the graft periphery; cryotherapy to the residual tissue may reduce this risk.

HERPES SIMPLEX KERATITIS

Introduction

Herpetic eye disease is the most common infectious cause of corneal blindness in developed countries. As many as 60% of

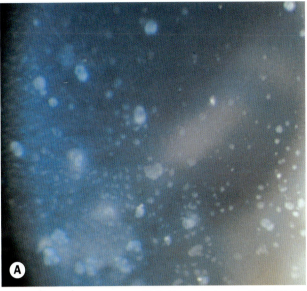

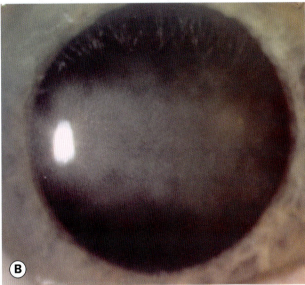

Fig. 6.11 Microsporidial keratitis. **(A)** Diffuse punctate epithelial keratitis; **(B)** deep stromal infiltrates
(Courtesy of S Tuft)

corneal ulcers in developing countries may be the result of herpes simplex virus and 10 million people worldwide may have herpetic eye disease.

Herpes simplex virus (HSV)

HSV is enveloped with a cuboidal capsule and has a linear double-stranded DNA genome. The two subtypes are *HSV-1* and *HSV-2*, and these reside in almost all neuronal ganglia. *HSV-1* causes infection above the waist (principally the face, lips and eyes), whereas *HSV-2* causes venereally acquired infection (genital herpes). Rarely *HSV-2* may be transmitted to the eye through infected secretions, either venereally or at birth (neonatal conjunctivitis). HSV transmission is facilitated in conditions of crowding and poor hygiene.

Primary infection

Primary infection, without previous viral exposure, usually occurs in childhood and is spread by droplet transmission, or less frequently by direct inoculation. Due to protection by maternal antibodies, it is uncommon during the first 6 months of life, though occasionally severe neonatal systemic disease may occur in which early diagnosis and intravenous antiviral treatment are critical to reduce mortality and disability; the presence of maternal antibodies means that dendritic corneal ulcers may be seen. Most primary infections with HSV are subclinical or cause only mild fever, malaise and upper respiratory tract symptoms. Blepharitis and follicular conjunctivitis may develop but are usually mild and self-limited. Treatment, if necessary, involves topical aciclovir ointment for the eye and/or cream for skin lesions, and occasionally oral antivirals. There is unfortunately no evidence that antiviral treatment at this stage reduces the likelihood of recurrent disease.

Recurrent infection

Recurrent disease (reactivation in the presence of cellular and humoral immunity) occurs as follows:

- **After primary infection** the virus is carried to the sensory ganglion for that dermatome (e.g. trigeminal ganglion) where latent infection is established. Latent virus is incorporated in host DNA and cannot be eradicated with presently available treatment.
- **Subclinical reactivation** can periodically occur, during which HSV is shed and patients are contagious.
- **Clinical reactivation.** A variety of stressors such as fever, hormonal change, ultraviolet radiation, trauma, or trigeminal injury may cause clinical reactivation, when the virus replicates and is transported in the sensory axons to the periphery.
- **The pattern of disease** depends on the site of reactivation, which may be remote from the site of primary disease. Hundreds of reactivations can occur during a lifetime.
- **The rate of ocular recurrence** after one episode is about 10% at 1 year and 50% at 10 years. The higher the number of previous attacks the greater the risk of recurrence.
- **Risk factors for severe disease**, which may be frequently recurrent, include atopic eye disease, childhood, immunodeficiency or suppression, malnutrition, measles and malaria. Inappropriate use of topical steroids may enhance the development of geographic ulceration (see below).

Epithelial keratitis

Clinical features

Epithelial (dendritic or geographic) keratitis is associated with active virus replication.

- **Symptoms.** Mild–moderate discomfort, redness, photophobia, watering and blurred vision.

- **Signs** in approximately chronological order:
  - Swollen opaque epithelial cells arranged in a coarse punctate or stellate (Fig. 6.12A) pattern.
  - Central desquamation results in a linear-branching (dendritic) ulcer (Fig. 6.12B), most frequent located centrally; the branches of the ulcer have characteristic terminal buds and its bed stains well with fluorescein.
  - The virus-laden cells at the margin of the ulcer stain with rose Bengal (Fig. 6.12C), and this may help distinction from alternative diagnoses, particularly an atypical recurrent corneal abrasion.
  - Corneal sensation is reduced.
  - Inadvertent topical steroid treatment may promote progressive enlargement of the ulcer to a geographical or 'amoeboid' configuration (Fig. 6.12D).
  - Mild associated subepithelial haze is typical.
  - Anterior chamber activity may be present, but is usually mild.
  - Follicular conjunctivitis may be associated; topical antivirals can also cause this.
  - Vesicular eyelid lesions may coincide with epithelial ulceration.
  - Elevated IOP is not uncommon (tonometry should be performed on the unaffected eye first; a disposable prism should be used, or a re-usable tonometer prism carefully disinfected after use).
  - Following healing, there may be persistent punctate epithelial erosions and irregular epithelium (Fig. 6.12E) which settle spontaneously and should not be mistaken for persistent active infection. A whorled epithelial appearance commonly results from assiduous, especially prolonged, topical antiviral instillation.
  - Mild subepithelial haze (Fig. 6.12F) may persist for weeks after the epithelium heals; in some cases mild scarring may develop, which tends to become more evident after each recurrence and may eventually substantially threaten vision.
- **Investigation** is generally unnecessary as the diagnosis is principally clinical, but pre-treatment scrapings can be sent in viral transport medium for culture. PCR and immunocytochemistry are also available. Giemsa staining shows multinucleated giant cells. HSV serological titres rise only on primary infection, but can be used to confirm previous viral exposure, usually in cases of stromal disease when the diagnosis is in doubt.
- **Differential diagnosis** of dendritic ulceration includes herpes zoster keratitis, healing corneal abrasion (pseudodendrite), acanthamoeba keratitis, epithelial rejection in a corneal graft, tyrosinaemia type 2, the epithelial effects of soft contact lenses, and toxic keratopathy secondary to topical medication.

Treatment

Treatment of HSV disease is predominantly with nucleoside (purine or pyrimidine) analogues that disrupt viral DNA. The

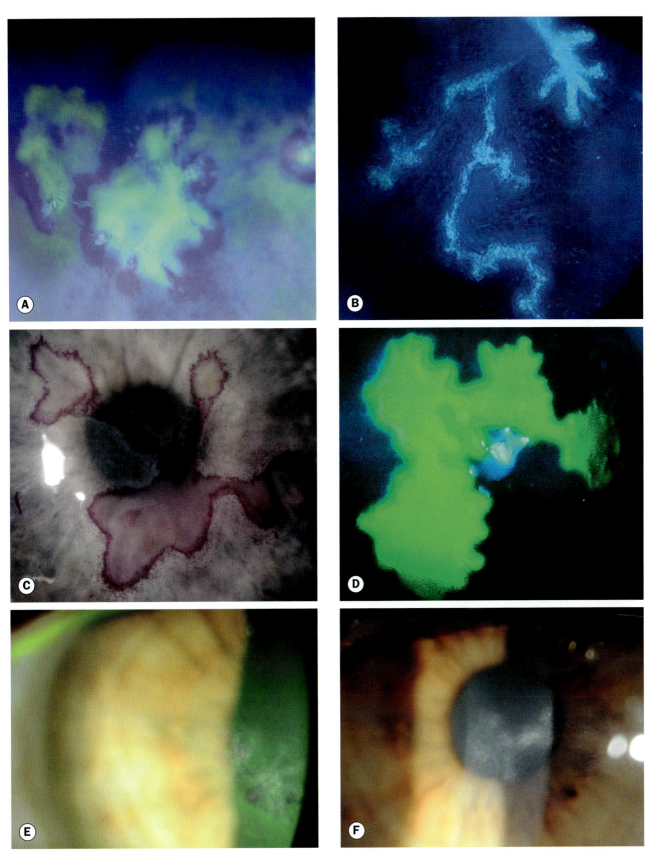

Fig. 6.12 Epithelial herpes simplex keratitis. **(A)** Stellate lesions; **(B)** bed of a dendritic ulcer stained with fluorescein; **(C)** margins of a dendritic ulcer stained with rose Bengal; **(D)** geographic ulcer; **(E)** persistent epithelial changes following resolution of active infection; **(F)** residual subepithelial haze

(Courtesy of C Barry – fig. B; S Tuft – fig. C)

majority of dendritic ulcers will eventually heal spontaneously without treatment, though scarring and vascularization may be more significant.

- **Topical.** The most frequently used drugs are aciclovir 3% ointment and ganciclovir 0.15% gel, each administered five times daily. Trifluridine is an alternative but requires instillation up to nine times a day. The drugs are relatively non-toxic, even when given for up to 60 days. They have approximately equivalent effect, acting preferentially on virus-laden epithelial cells, and penetrating effectively into the stroma; 99% of ulcers heal within two weeks. Idoxuridine and vidarabine are older drugs that are probably less effective and more toxic.
- **Debridement** may be used for resistant cases. The corneal surface is wiped with a sterile cellulose sponge or cotton-tipped applicator (cotton bud). Epithelium should be removed 2 mm beyond the edge of the ulcer, since involvement extends beyond the visible dendrite. The removal of the virus-containing cells protects adjacent healthy epithelium from infection and eliminates the antigenic stimulus to stromal inflammation. A topical antiviral agent should be used in conjunction.
- **Signs of treatment toxicity** include superficial punctate erosions, waves of whorled epithelium, follicular conjunctivitis and, rarely, punctal occlusion. Absence of epithelial whorling with a persistent epithelial lesion raises the possibility of poor or non-compliance.
- **Oral antiviral** therapy (e.g. aciclovir 200–400 mg five times a day for 5–10 days, famciclovir or valaciclovir) is indicated in most immunodeficient patients, in children and patients with marked ocular surface disease. It is an effective alternative to topical treatment when the latter is poorly tolerated, or in resistant cases. The newer oral agents may be better tolerated than aciclovir, and require less frequent dosing, but optimal regimens are not yet defined.
- **Interferon monotherapy** does not seem to be more effective than antivirals, but the combination of a nucleoside antiviral with either interferon or debridement seems to speed healing.
- **Skin lesions** (see Ch. 1) may be treated with aciclovir cream five times daily, as for cold sores, and if extensive an oral antiviral may be given.
- **Cycloplegia,** e.g. homatropine 1% once or twice daily can be given to improve comfort if necessary.
- **Topical antibiotic prophylaxis** is recommended by some practitioners.
- **IOP control.** If glaucoma treatment is necessary, prostaglandin derivatives should probably be avoided as they may promote herpes virus activity and inflammation generally.
- **Topical steroids** are not used unless significant disciform keratitis is also present (see below).
- **Slow healing or frequent recurrence** may indicate the presence of a resistant viral strain, and an alternative topical agent or debridement may be tried. In especially refractory cases, a combination of two topical agents with oral

valaciclovir or famciclovir may be effective. A significant minority of resistant cases are due to varicella-zoster virus.

Disciform keratitis

The aetiopathogenesis of disciform keratitis (endotheliitis) is controversial. It may be the result of active HSV infection of keratocytes or endothelium, or a hypersensitivity reaction to viral antigen in the cornea.

Clinical features

- **Symptoms.** Blurred vision of gradual onset, which may be associated with haloes around lights. Discomfort and redness are common, but tend to be milder than in purely epithelial disease. A clear past history of epithelial ulceration is not always present, and the possibility of a mimicking infection such as acanthamoeba or fungal keratitis should be borne in mind.
- **Signs**
  - A central zone of stromal oedema, often with overlying epithelial oedema (Fig. 6.13A); occasionally the lesion is eccentric.
  - Large (granulomatous) keratic precipitates underlying the oedema (Fig. 6.13B).
  - Folds in Descemet membrane in severe cases.
  - A surrounding (Wessely) immune ring of deep stromal haze (Fig. 6.13C) signifies deposition of viral antigen and host antibody complexes.
  - The IOP may be elevated.
  - Reduced corneal sensation; this may aid in distinguishing other forms of infection.
  - Healed lesions often have a faint ring of stromal or subepithelial opacification and thinning.
  - Consecutive episodes may be associated with gradually worsening subepithelial and/or stromal scarring and superficial or deep vascularization (Fig. 6.13D).
  - Mid-stromal scarring from disciform keratitis is a cause of interstitial keratitis.

Treatment

A broad approach to management is set out below, but in practice regimens should be tailored individually. Careful monitoring and adequate treatment, dependent on severity of inflammation, is critical to minimize progression of scarring. Patients should be cautioned to seek treatment at the first suggestion of recurrence, though some authorities feel that minimal inflammation may not warrant treatment or can be addressed with cycloplegia alone.

- **Initial** treatment is with topical steroids (prednisolone 1% or dexamethasone 0.1%) with antiviral cover, both four times daily. As improvement occurs, the frequency of administration of both is reduced in parallel over not less than 4 weeks. It is prudent to keep steroid intensity and duration to the minimum required for effective control of inflammation. IOP should be monitored. Cycloplegia can be used to improve comfort if necessary, and some practitioners recommend topical antibacterial prophylaxis.

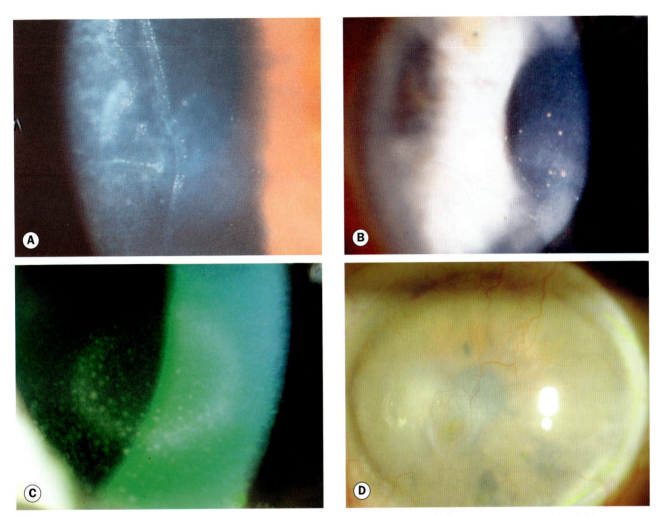

Fig. 6.13 Disciform herpes simplex keratitis. **(A)** Epithelial and stromal oedema, with Descemet membrane folds; **(B)** underlying keratic precipitates; **(C)** Wessely ring; **(D)** scarring from recurrent disease

- Subsequently **prednisolone** 0.5% once daily is usually a safe dose at which to stop topical antiviral cover. Some patients require a weaker steroid such as fluorometholone 0.1% or loteprednol 0.2% on alternate days for many months. Periodic attempts should be made to stop the steroid altogether.
- With active epithelial ulceration it is reasonable to try to keep the steroid intensity as low as possible for adequate effect, with a more frequent antiviral regimen, e.g. initially topical antiviral five times daily, with steroid two or three times daily, titrated according to the signs of activity of both; oral antiviral treatment may be helpful but its efficacy in this situation has not been established.
- Oral steroids are sometimes used in severe stromal inflammation as an adjunct, or to reduce steroid-induced IOP elevation, and/or to avoid viral promotion in infectious viral keratitis.
- Topical ciclosporin 0.05% may be useful, particularly in the presence of epithelial ulceration and to facilitate tapering of topical steroids such as in steroid-related IOP elevation.

- Fine needle diathermy and laser techniques have been reported as successfully addressing established corneal neovascularization and improving vision.

Necrotizing stromal keratitis

This rare condition is thought to result from active viral replication within the stroma, though immune-mediated inflammation is likely to play a significant role. It may be difficult to distinguish from severe disciform keratitis and there may be a spectrum of disease, including overlap with neurotrophic keratopathy. As with disciform keratitis, a similar clinical picture may be caused by other infections.

- **Signs**
  - Stromal necrosis and melting, often with profound interstitial opacification (Fig. 6.14).
  - Anterior uveitis with keratic precipitates underlying the area of active stromal infiltration.
  - An epithelial defect may be present.
  - Progression to scarring, vascularization and lipid deposition is common.

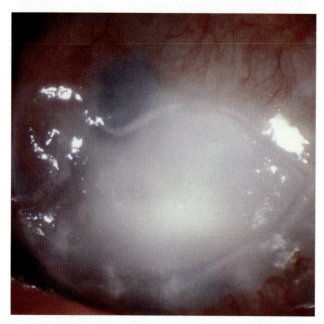

Fig. 6.14 Necrotizing stromal herpes simplex keratitis
(Courtesy of S Tuft)

- **Treatment** is broadly similar to that of aggressive disciform keratitis, but oral antiviral supplementation, initially at the upper end of the dose range, is commonly used. The restoration of epithelial integrity is critical.

Neurotrophic keratopathy

Neurotrophic keratopathy (see also separate topic) is caused by failure of re-epithelialization resulting from corneal anaesthesia, often exacerbated by other factors such as drug toxicity.

- **Signs**
  - A non-healing epithelial defect (Fig. 6.15), sometimes after prolonged topical treatment, is an early sign.
  - The stroma beneath the defect is grey and opaque and may become thin.
  - Secondary bacterial or fungal infection may occur.
- **Treatment** is that of persistent epithelial defects; topical steroids to control any inflammatory component should be kept to a minimum.

Iridocyclitis

Herpetic iridocyclitis can occur without signs of active corneal inflammation, and may be associated with direct viral activity. IOP elevation is common and is often presumed to be due to trabeculitis; steroid-induced IOP elevation may also be relatively common in herpetic iritis. The aetiology may be missed unless there is a history of previous herpes simplex keratitis; patchy iris atrophy (Fig. 6.16A) may provide a clue; transillumination (Fig. 6.16B) may demonstrate subtle lesions. Aqueous sampling for PCR may be diagnostic. Treatment is primarily with topical steroids, but adjunctive oral aciclovir may be given.

Other considerations

Prophylaxis

- **Long-term oral aciclovir** reduces the rate of recurrence of epithelial and stromal keratitis by about 50% and is usually tolerated well. Prophylaxis should be considered in patients with frequent debilitating recurrences, particularly if bilateral or involving an only eye. The standard daily dose of aciclovir is 400 mg twice daily but if necessary a higher dose can be tried, based on practice in the management of systemic herpes simplex infection; continual use for many years has been documented for systemic indications. The prophylactic effect decreases or disappears when the drug is stopped. Excretion is via the kidney, so renal function should be checked periodically during long-term treatment.
- **Oral valaciclovir** (500 mg once daily) or famciclovir are alternatives that are probably as effective as aciclovir, require less frequent dosing and may be better tolerated.
- **Topical.** Oral prophylaxis tends to be preferred to long-term topical administration. Epithelial toxicity may be problematic, with mild blurring and persistent discomfort; allergy and punctal stenosis are also potential problems.
- **Vaccination.** Therapeutic vaccination strategies are under investigation.

Complications

- **Secondary infection.** Herpetic eye disease is a major predisposing factor for microbial keratitis.
- **Glaucoma** secondary to inflammation or chronic steroid use may progress undetected, particularly if there is a poor view of the optic disc. Corneal thinning and distortion may give rise to an inaccurate reading on applanation and alternative forms of tonometry may be superior in these cases.

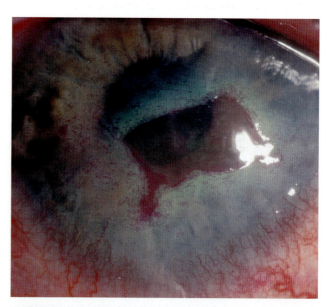

Fig. 6.15 Neurotrophic epithelial defect stained with rose Bengal
(Courtesy of S Tuft)

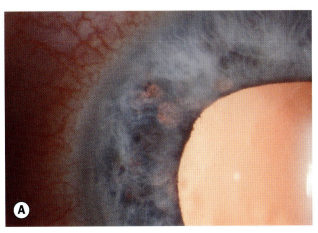 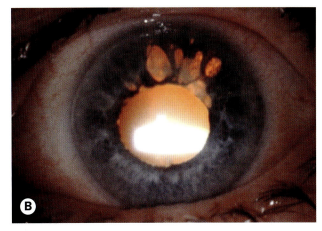

Fig. 6.16 Iris atrophy in herpetic iridocyclitis. **(A)** Characteristic patchy appearance; **(B)** transillumination
(Courtesy of S Tuft – fig. A)

- **Cataract** secondary to inflammation or prolonged steroid use.
- **Iris atrophy** secondary to keratouveitis (see Fig. 6.16).

Keratoplasty

A trial of a rigid contact lens is often worthwhile prior to committing to surgery. Recurrence of herpetic eye disease and rejection are common and threaten the survival of corneal grafts.

- **Topical** antivirals given during a rejection episode may reduce epithelial viral reactivation but toxicity may delay re-epithelialization.
- **Prophylactic oral aciclovir** (400 mg twice daily) improves graft survival and should be given to patients undergoing penetrating keratoplasty for herpetic eye disease; it should also be considered in patients with severe atopic eye disease but no history of ocular HSV involvement. The duration of treatment and the optimum dose has not been established. Immunohistochemistry should be performed on the excised tissue to confirm the presence of herpes antigen.

HERPES ZOSTER OPHTHALMICUS

Introduction

Pathogenesis

Herpes zoster ophthalmicus (HZO) is the term used for shingles involving the dermatome supplied by the ophthalmic division of the fifth cranial (trigeminal) nerve. The globe is commonly affected in HZO; ocular involvement can also occur (though is rarely clinically significant) when the disease affects the maxillary division alone. Varicella-zoster virus (VZV) causes both chickenpox (varicella) and shingles (herpes zoster); VZV belongs to the same subfamily of the herpes virus group as HSV – the viruses are morphologically identical but antigenically distinct. After an episode of chickenpox the virus travels in a retrograde manner to the dorsal root and cranial nerve sensory ganglia, where it may remain dormant for decades, with reactivation thought to occur after VZV-specific cell-mediated immunity has faded. Re-exposure to VZV via contact with chickenpox, or by vaccination, may reinforce immunity and protect against the development of shingles.

Mechanisms of ocular involvement

- **Direct viral invasion** may lead to conjunctivitis and epithelial keratitis.
- **Secondary inflammation** and occlusive vasculitis may cause episcleritis, scleritis, keratitis, uveitis (including segmental iris infarction), optic neuritis and cranial nerve palsies. Inflammation and destruction of the peripheral nerves or central ganglia, or altered signal processing in the central nervous system (CNS) may be responsible for post-herpetic neuralgia. Cicatrizing complications may arise following severe eyelid, periocular skin and conjunctival involvement.
- **Reactivation** causes necrosis and inflammation in the affected sensory ganglia, causing corneal anaesthesia that may result in neurotrophic keratopathy.

Risk of ocular involvement

- **The Hutchinson sign** describes involvement of the skin supplied by the external nasal nerve, a branch of the nasociliary nerve supplying the tip, side and root of the nose (Fig. 6.17A). The sign correlates strongly with ocular involvement, but there is no apparent correlation between the severity of the nasal rash and that of ocular complications.
- **Age.** HZO occurs most frequently in the sixth and seventh decades. In the elderly, signs and symptoms tend to be more severe and of longer duration.
- **AIDS** patients tend to have more severe disease, and shingles can be an early indicator of human immunodeficiency virus (HIV) infection; a lower threshold for HIV testing should be adopted in populations at particular risk. The development of shingles in children or young adults classically has prompted a search for immunodeficiency or malignancy, though the requirement for this has been questioned as an abnormality will be found in only a small minority.

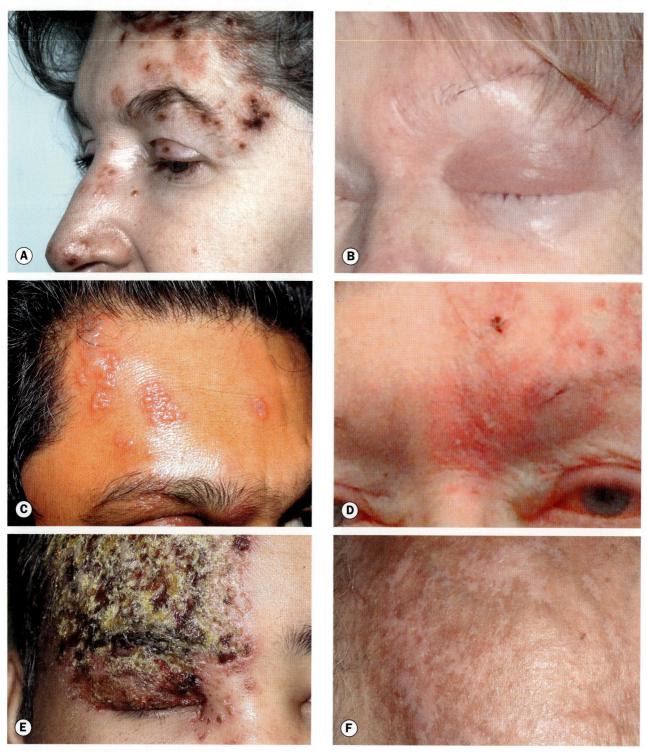

Fig. 6.17 Herpes zoster ophthalmicus. **(A)** Hutchinson sign – rash involving the side of the nose; **(B)** early erythema and oedema; **(C)** vesicular stage; **(D)** mixed vesicular and pustular rash beginning to show crusting – note the boggy oedema affecting the medial part of both upper lids; **(E)** severe rash in a patient with AIDS; **(F)** typical healed appearance with mild to moderate scarring and depigmentation

(Courtesy of S Chen – figs E and F)

Acute shingles

General features

- **A prodromal phase** precedes the appearance of the rash. It lasts 3–5 days and is characterized by tiredness, fever, malaise and headache. Symptoms involving the affected dermatome vary from a superficial itching, tingling or burning sensation to a severe boring or lancing pain that is either constant or intermittent. Older patients with early severe pain and a larger area of involvement are at particular risk of post-herpetic neuralgia.
- **Skin lesions**
  - Painful erythematous areas with a maculopapular rash develop (Fig. 6.17B), and may be confused with cellulitis or contact dermatitis.
  - The rash respects the midline, which may aid in distinguishing shingles from HSV skin infection; pain is also markedly worse in shingles. Bilateral disease is very rare.
  - Within 24 hours, groups of vesicles (Fig. 6.17C) appear and these become confluent over 2–4 days.
  - Although the rash itself does not affect the lower eyelid in HZO, boggy oedema of the upper and lower lids is common (see Fig. 6.17B) and often spreads to the contralateral side of the face.
  - The vesicles often pass through a pustular phase before they crust (Fig. 6.17D) and dry after 2–3 weeks.
  - Large, deep haemorrhagic lesions are more common in immunodeficient patients (Fig. 6.17E).
  - The lesions heal to leave residual skin destruction and depigmented scars (Fig. 6.17F).
  - Zoster sine herpete is shingles without a rash; this may be more common than previously realized.
- **Disseminated zoster** involving multiple dermatomes and organ systems may develop in immunodeficiency or malignancy, and with the advent of PCR testing complications such as meningoencephalitis have increasingly been identified in immunocompetent individuals.
- **Investigation.** In the event that clinical diagnosis is uncertain, typically in immunodeficiency, vesicular fluid can be sent for PCR, immunomicroscopy or (now rarely) culture. A viraemia lasting a few days occurs in acute shingles; PCR of plasma for VZV DNA may be positive (40%), especially in immunosuppressed patients and can be particularly useful if zoster sine herpete is suspected. IgM antibodies to VZV are found in only a minority of early stage and convalescent patients.

Treatment

- **Oral antiviral treatment**, optimally given within 72 hours of rash onset, reduces the severity and duration of the acute episode and the risk of post-herpetic neuralgia. The incidence of late ophthalmic complications is also reduced by about 50%. Patients presenting later than 72 hours but still at the vesicular stage also derive benefit from treatment. Aciclovir (800 mg five times daily for 7–10 days) has been the mainstay of treatment, but newer agents such as valaciclovir 1 g three times daily or famciclovir 250–500 mg three times daily have more convenient regimens, are better tolerated and are at least as effective as aciclovir. Brivudine is available in some countries; fatal interactions with 5-fluoropyrimidines have been reported and it should not be used in combination with even regional 5-fluorouracil.
- **Intravenous aciclovir** 5–10 mg/kg three times daily is generally indicated only for severe disease, particularly encephalitis, and for moderate–severe immunocompromise.
- **Systemic steroids** (e.g. prednisolone 60 mg daily for 4 days, then 40 mg for 4 days, then 20 mg for 4 days) remain somewhat controversial but are commonly used in moderate–severe disease, particularly for neurological complications. They should be given only in conjunction with a systemic antiviral, the course of which will typically require extension. They should probably be avoided in immunodeficiency. A moderate reduction in acute pain and accelerated skin healing is conferred, but steroids have no effect on the incidence or severity of post-herpetic neuralgia.
- **Immunocompromised patients** require the input of an infectious diseases specialist. Antiviral treatment should be extended and intravenous treatment may be optimal. Systemic steroids should probably be avoided.
- **Symptomatic** treatment of skin lesions is by drying, antisepsis and cold compresses. The benefit of topical antibiotic-steroid combinations is uncertain.
- **Patients with shingles can transmit chickenpox** so that contact with people not known to be immune (particularly pregnant women) and immunodeficient individuals should be avoided at least until crusting is complete.
- **VZV uveitis** is considered in depth in Chapter 11.

Eye disease

Acute eye disease

- **Acute epithelial keratitis** develops in over 50% of patients within 2 days of the onset of the rash and usually resolves spontaneously within a few days. It is characterized by dendritic lesions that are smaller and finer than herpes simplex dendrites, and have tapered ends without terminal bulbs (Figs 6.18A and B). The lesions stain better with rose Bengal than with fluorescein. Treatment, if required, is with a topical antiviral.
- **Conjunctivitis** (follicular and/or papillary) is common; it often occurs in conjunction with lid margin vesicles. Treatment is not required in the absence of corneal disease, though some practitioners give topical antibiotic and/or antiviral prophylaxis.
- **Episcleritis** occurs at the onset of the rash and usually resolves spontaneously. A mild non-steroidal anti-inflammatory may be used if necessary.

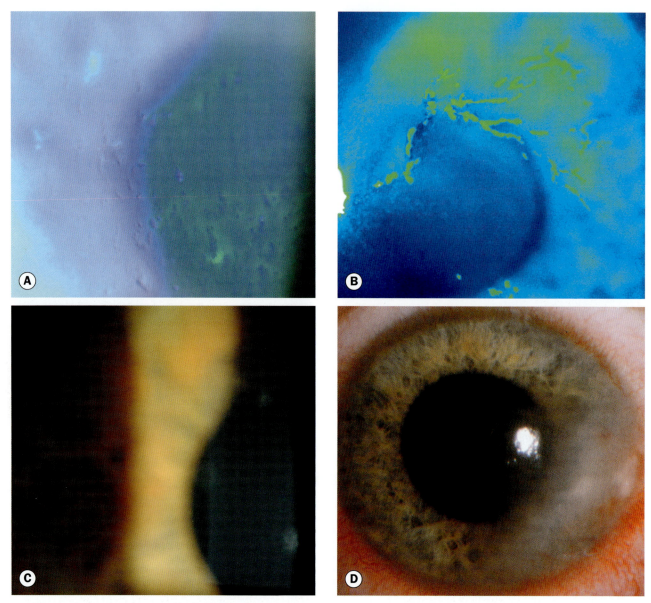

Fig. 6.18 Acute lesions in herpes zoster ophthalmicus. **(A)** and **(B)** Dendritic epithelial lesions with tapered ends; **(C)** nummular keratitis; **(D)** stromal keratitis
(Courtesy of J Krachmer, M Mannis and E Holland, from Cornea, Elsevier 2005 – fig. B; C Barry – fig. D)

- **Scleritis** and sclerokeratitis are uncommon but may develop at the end of the first week. Treatment of indolent lesions is with oral flurbiprofen 100 mg three times daily. Oral steroids with antiviral cover may be required for severe involvement.
- **Nummular keratitis** usually develops at the site of epithelial lesions about 10 days after the onset of the rash. It is characterized by fine granular subepithelial deposits surrounded by a halo of stromal haze (Fig. 6.18C). The lesions fade in response to topical steroids but recur if treatment is discontinued prematurely.
- **Stromal (interstitial) keratitis** (Fig. 6.18D) develops in about 5% 3 weeks after the onset of the rash; significant scarring can occur (Fig. 6.19A). It usually responds to topical

steroids but can become chronic and require slow tapering.
- **Disciform keratitis** (immune-mediated endotheliitis) is less common than with herpes simplex infection but may lead to corneal decompensation. Treatment is with topical steroids.
- **Anterior uveitis** affects at least a third of patients and can be associated with sectoral iris ischaemia and atrophy (Figs 6.19B and C).
- **Posterior uveitis** (see Ch. 11). Progressive retinal necrosis is an aggressive retinitis usually occurring in immunodeficient individuals. Acute retinal necrosis can also be caused by VZV. Posterior segment examination should always be performed in patients with HZO; retinal vasculitis has also been reported.

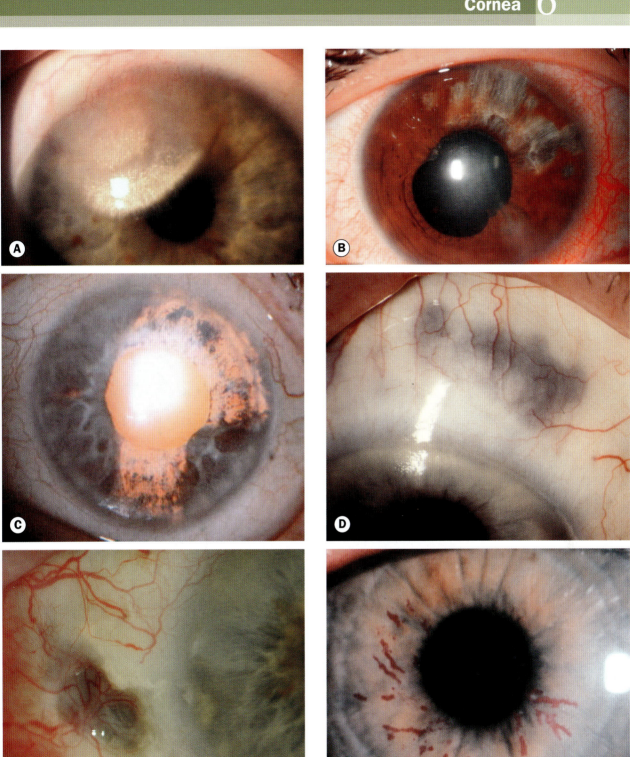

Fig. 6.19 Chronic lesions in herpes zoster ophthalmicus. **(A)** Scarring following stromal keratitis, with crystalline lipid degeneration; **(B)** iris atrophy in a typical sectoral pattern; **(C)** more severe sectoral iris atrophy on transillumination; **(D)** and **(E)** scleral atrophy; **(F)** mucous plaque keratitis

(Courtesy of R Marsh – fig. F)

- **IOP** should be monitored as elevation is common, including steroid-induced. Prostaglandin derivatives should be avoided if treatment is necessary.
- **Neurological complications** may require intravenous antivirals and systemic steroids.
  - Cranial nerve palsies affecting the third (most common), fourth and sixth nerves usually recover within 6 months.
  - Optic neuritis is rare.
  - CNS manifestations are rare but include encephalitis, cranial arteritis, and Guillain–Barré syndrome.

Chronic eye disease

- **Neurotrophic keratopathy** similar to that seen in HSV infection develops in up to about 50%, but is usually relatively mild and settles over several months. Prolonged severe disease occurs in a minority (see also separate topic).
- **Scleritis** may become chronic and lead to patchy scleral atrophy (Figs 6.19D and E).
- **Mucous plaque keratitis** develops in about 5%, most commonly between the third and sixth months. It is characterized by elevated mucous plaques staining with rose Bengal (Fig. 6.19F). Treatment involves a combination of topical steroid and acetylcysteine. Untreated, plaques resolve after a few months, leaving a faint diffuse corneal haze.
- **Lipid degeneration** may develop in eyes with persistent severe nummular or disciform keratitis (see Fig. 6.19A).
- **Lipid-filled granulomata** similar to those resulting from chronic irritation may develop in the tarsal conjunctiva, and may progress to erosive calcified concretions.
- **Subconjunctival scarring** may occur.
- **Eyelid scarring** may result in ptosis, cicatricial entropion and occasionally ectropion, trichiasis, lid notching and madarosis.

Relapsing eye disease

In the relapsing phase lesions may reappear years after an acute episode, which may have been forgotten; eyelid scarring may be the only diagnostic clue. Reactivation of keratitis, episcleritis, scleritis or iritis can occur.

Post-herpetic neuralgia

Post-herpetic neuralgia is defined as pain that persists for more than one month after the rash has healed. It develops in up to 75% of patients over 70 years of age. Pain may be constant or intermittent, worse at night and aggravated by minor stimuli (allodynia), touch and heat. It generally improves slowly over time, with only 2% of patients affected after 5 years. Neuralgia can impair the quality of life, and may lead to depression of sufficient severity to present a danger of suicide. Patients severely affected should be referred to a specialist pain clinic. Treatment may involve the following:

- **Local**
  - Cold compresses.
  - Topical capsaicin 0.075% or lidocaine 5% patches.

- **Systemic treatment** may be used in a staged fashion
  - Simple analgesics such as paracetamol.
  - Stronger analgesics such as codeine.
  - Tricyclic antidepressants, e.g. nortriptyline, amitriptyline, initially 25 mg nightly adjusted up to 75 mg for several weeks if necessary.
  - Carbamazepine 400 mg daily for lancinating pain.
  - Gabapentin (300–600 mg up to three times daily), sustained-release oxycodone (10–30 mg twice daily), or both.

INTERSTITIAL KERATITIS

Introduction

Interstitial keratitis (IK) is an inflammation of the corneal stroma without primary involvement of the epithelium or endothelium. In most cases, the inflammation is thought to be an immune-mediated process triggered by an appropriate antigen. The term is most commonly used to refer to the late appearance of feathery mid-stromal scarring with ghost vessels rather than the acute presentation; the former is typically an incidental finding. Syphilitic IK is the archetype, but the relative frequency of causes varies markedly by geographic region. There is a wide range of aetiology; herpetic keratitis (including chickenpox) and other viral infections, tuberculosis, Lyme disease and numerous other infections (parasitic diseases are an important cause in areas where these are endemic), sarcoidosis, Cogan syndrome and other non-infectious inflammatory conditions. Patients should be thoroughly investigated, in particular to exclude a cause with the potential for severe systemic involvement.

Syphilitic IK

IK of syphilitic origin is usually the result of congenital infection, though acquired syphilis can also be responsible. All patients with acute IK, or with the incidental discovery of its chronic appearance, should be investigated to exclude congenital (and acquired) syphilis, irrespective of the presence of systemic clinical signs; there are numerous reported cases of congenital syphilis being identified for the first time in later life on this basis, averting life-threatening complications such as neurosyphilis.

Congenital syphilis

Infection of the fetus can occur transplacentally, leading to stillbirth, subclinical infection, or a range of clinical features.

- **Early systemic features** include failure to thrive, a maculopapular rash, mucosal ulcers, characteristic fissures around the lips (rhagades) and a range of organ involvement.
- **Late systemic signs** include sensorineural deafness, saddle-shaped nasal deformity (Fig. 6.20A), sabre tibiae (Fig. 6.20B), bulldog jaw (mandibular prominence due to maxillary underdevelopment), Hutchinson teeth (notched, small, widely spaced teeth – Fig. 6.20C), and Clutton joints (painless effusions in large joints, especially the knees).

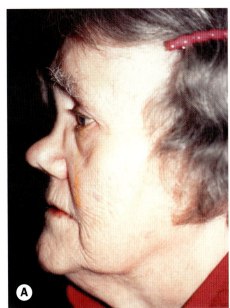

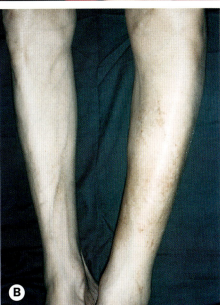

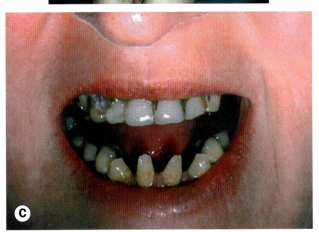

Fig. 6.20 Systemic signs of congenital syphilis. **(A)** Saddle-shaped nasal deformity; **(B)** sabre tibiae; **(C)** Hutchinson teeth

(Courtesy of R Marsh and S Ford – fig. C)

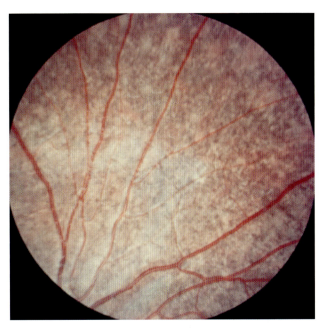

Fig. 6.21 Salt and pepper retinopathy following congenital syphilitic infection

- **Ocular features** include anterior uveitis, IK (see below), dislocated/subluxated lens, cataract, optic atrophy, salt and pepper pigmentary retinopathy (Fig. 6.21) and Argyll Robertson pupils.

Presentation of syphilitic IK

- **Symptoms.** The presentation of IK following congenital syphilitic infection is usually between the ages of 5 and 25 years. The initial symptoms are those of acute anterior uveitis with severe blurring. Involvement is bilateral in 80%, although usually not simultaneous. In acquired disease IK is less common and usually unilateral, typically occurring years after the age at which the disease was contracted, although it can occur as part of the syndrome of primary infection.
- **Signs**
  ○ Profoundly decreased visual acuity is typical in the active stage.
  ○ Limbitis associated with deep stromal vascularization, with cellular infiltration and clouding that may obscure the still-perfused vessels to give the characteristic pinkish 'salmon patch' appearance (Fig. 6.22A).
  ○ Granulomatous anterior uveitis.
  ○ After several months the cornea begins to clear and the vessels become non perfused ('ghost vessels' – Fig. 6.22B).
  ○ If the cornea later becomes inflamed, the vessels may re-fill with blood and, rarely, bleed into the stroma (Fig. 6.22C).
  ○ The healed stage is characterized by ghost vessels, feathery deep stromal scarring (Fig. 6.22D), and sometimes thinning, astigmatism and band keratopathy.

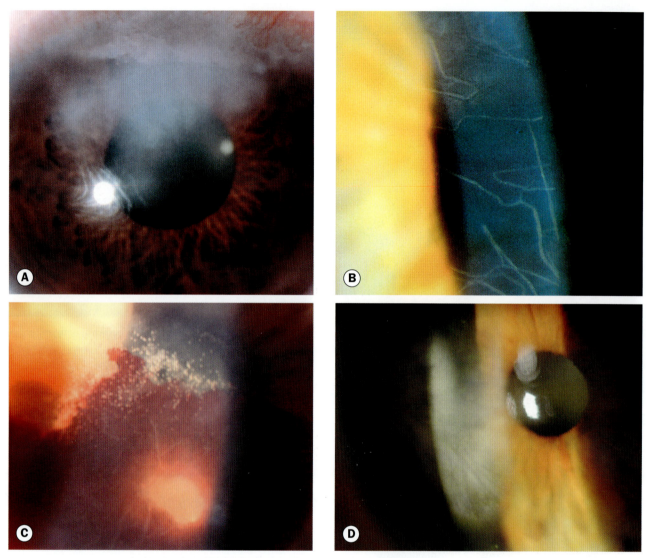

Fig. 6.22 Syphilitic interstitial keratitis. **(A)** Salmon patch; **(B)** ghost vessels; **(C)** intrastromal corneal haemorrhage from re-perfused vessels; **(D)** typical feathery scarring – the tracks of ghost vessels are clearly seen
(Courtesy of J Krachmer, M Mannis and E Holland from Cornea, Mosby 2005 – fig. A)

- **Treatment** of active syphilitic IK is with topical steroids and cycloplegics, as well as immediate systemic therapy under the care of a genitourinary or infectious diseases specialist.

Cogan syndrome

Introduction

Cogan syndrome is a rare systemic autoimmune vasculitis characterized by intraocular inflammation and vestibuloauditory dysfunction (particularly neurosensory) developing within months of each other. The disease primarily occurs in young adults, with both sexes affected equally; children can also be affected. Systemic features occur in 30% and may include multisystem vasculitis that can be life-threatening; multispecialty management is vital.

Diagnosis

Ocular and inner ear symptoms are often separated by a substantial period; the acute phase may last from months to years. Susac syndrome (retinocochleocerebral vasculopathy) should be considered in the differential diagnosis.

- **Vestibuloauditory symptoms.** Deafness, tinnitus and vertigo.
- **Ocular symptoms.** Redness, pain, photophobia and blurred vision.
- **Ocular signs.** Corneal involvement commences with faint bilateral peripheral anterior stromal opacities; deeper opacities and corneal neovascularization (mid-stromal vascular loops) then ensue (Fig. 6.23A), often with central progression (Fig. 6.23B). Uveitis, scleritis and retinal vasculitis may develop.

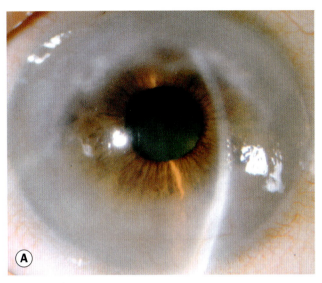

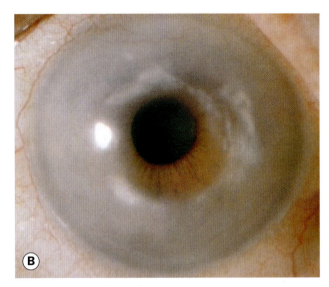

Fig. 6.23 Old interstitial keratitis in Cogan syndrome. **(A)** Peripheral; **(B)** more central scarring
(Courtesy of R Curtis)

- **Investigations**
  - Erythrocyte sedimentation rate (ESR) and C-reactive protein (CRP) may be elevated; elevated white cell count.
  - Antibodies to inner ear antigens may be detectable.
  - MRI may show inner ear and other abnormalities.

Treatment

- **Topical steroids** for keratitis, with additional measures as appropriate.
- **Systemic steroids.** Vestibuloauditory symptoms require immediate treatment with 1–2 g/kg prednisolone to prevent hearing loss; immunosuppressive therapy may also be required. Systemic steroids may also be required for scleritis or retinal vasculitis.

PROTOZOAN KERATITIS

Acanthamoeba

Introduction

Acanthamoeba spp. are ubiquitous free-living protozoa commonly found in soil, fresh or brackish water and the upper respiratory tract. The cystic form (Fig. 6.24A) is highly resilient. Under appropriate environmental conditions, the cysts turn into trophozoites, with tissue penetration and destruction. In developed countries acanthamoeba keratitis is most frequently associated with contact lens wear, especially if tap water is used for rinsing.

Diagnosis

Early misdiagnosis as herpes simplex keratitis is relatively common, and with more advanced signs the possibility of fungal keratitis should be remembered.

- **Symptoms.** Blurred vision and discomfort; pain is often severe and characteristically disproportionate to the clinical signs.
- **Signs**
  - In early disease the epithelial surface is irregular and greyish (Fig. 6.24B).
  - Epithelial pseudodendrites resembling herpetic lesions may form.
  - Limbitis with diffuse or focal anterior stromal infiltrates (Fig. 6.24C).
  - Characteristic perineural infiltrates (radial keratoneuritis) are seen during the first few weeks and are virtually pathognomonic (Fig. 6.24D).
  - Gradual enlargement and coalescence of infiltrates to form a ring abscess (Figs 6.25A and B) is typical.
  - Scleritis may develop and is generally reactive rather than an extension of infection.
  - Slowly progressive stromal opacification and vascularization.
  - Corneal melting may occur at any stage when there is stromal disease. The melt often develops at the periphery of the area of infiltrate (Fig. 6.25C).
- **Investigations**
  - Staining of corneal scrapings using periodic acid–Schiff or calcofluor white (a fluorescent dye with an affinity for amoebic cysts and fungi). Gram and Giemsa stains may also demonstrate cysts.
  - Culture. Non-nutrient agar seeded with dead *E. coli*, which trophozoites consume.
  - Other investigations include immunohistochemistry, PCR and *in vivo* confocal microscopy. Corneal biopsy may be necessary for diagnosis.

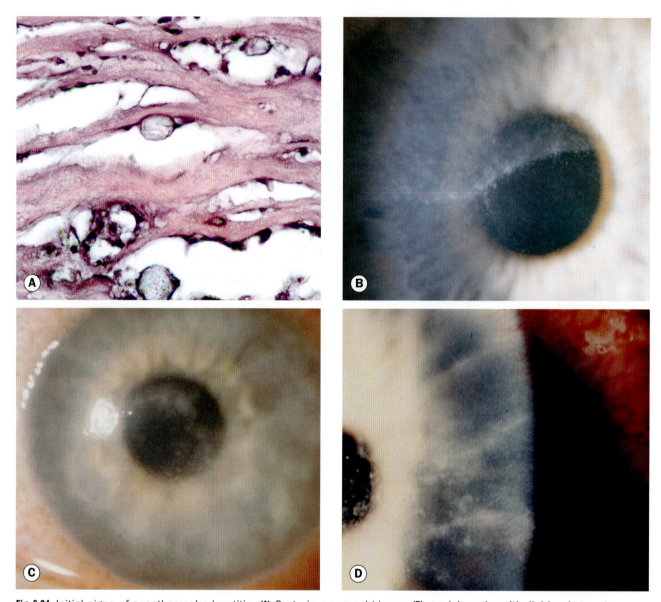

Fig. 6.24 Initial signs of acanthamoeba keratitis. **(A)** Cysts in a corneal biopsy; **(B)** greyish early epithelial involvement; **(C)** focal anterior stromal infiltrates; **(D)** radial perineuritis
(Courtesy of J Harry – fig. A)

Treatment

It is important to maintain a high index of suspicion for *Acanthamoeba* in any patient with a limited response to antibacterial therapy. The outcome is very much better if treatment is started early.

- **Debridement** of involved epithelium is believed to be helpful; it may facilitate eye drop penetration.
- **Topical amoebicides.** *Acanthamoeba* cysts are resistant to most antimicrobial agents, and although successful outcomes have been reported using a variety of topical preparations, it is likely that some of these are active only against the trophozoite stage.
  - Polyhexamethylene biguanide (PHMB) 0.02% and chlorhexidine (0.02%) kill trophozoites and are cysticidal.
  - Hexamidine or propamidine (Brolene); the former probably has greater activity.
  - Voriconazole and other azole antifungals may be effective.
  - An optimal regimen has not been established. Examples include PHMB as duotherapy with chlorhexidine, or either of these in combination with hexamidine or propamidine. Instillation is hourly at first, and gradually reduced; a clear response may take 2 weeks.
  - Simultaneous antibacterial treatment for co-infection may be considered if the clinical picture suggests this.
  - Relapses are common as treatment is tapered, and it may be necessary to continue treatment for many months.

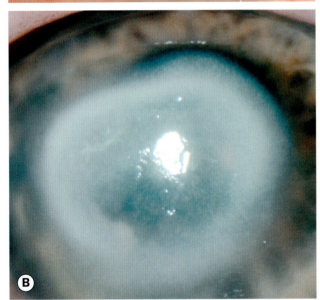

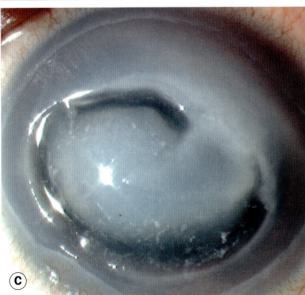

Fig. 6.25 Advanced acanthamoeba keratitis. **(A)** Progression of infiltration, with incipient formation of a ring abscess and early melting; **(B)** ring abscess; **(C)** melting
(Courtesy of S Tuft – figs B and C)

- **Topical steroids** should be avoided if possible although low-dose therapy delayed for at least 2 weeks after starting anti-amoebic treatment may be useful for persistent inflammation. Amoebicidal treatment should be continued in concert with and for several weeks after steroids.
- **Pain control** is with an oral non-steroidal anti-inflammatory agent.
- **Therapeutic keratoplasty** may be necessary for resistant cases, including perforation. Late scarring may also require penetrating keratoplasty.

HELMINTHIC KERATITIS

Onchocerciasis

Onchocerciasis ('river blindness') is discussed in Chapter 11. Keratitis is a common feature.

BACTERIAL HYPERSENSITIVITY-MEDIATED CORNEAL DISEASE

Marginal keratitis

Introduction

Marginal keratitis is believed to be caused by a hypersensitivity reaction against staphylococcal exotoxins and cell wall proteins with deposition of antigen-antibody complexes in the peripheral cornea (antigen diffusing from the tear film, antibody from the blood vessels) with a secondary lymphocytic infiltration. The lesions are culture-negative but *S. aureus* can frequently be isolated from the lid margins.

Diagnosis

- **Symptoms.** Mild discomfort, redness and lacrimation; may be bilateral.
- **Signs**
  - Chronic blepharitis is typical.
  - Inferior punctate epitheliopathy is an early manifestation.
  - Subepithelial marginal infiltrates separated from the limbus by a clear zone, often associated with an adjacent area of conjunctival hyperaemia (Fig. 6.26A).
  - Characteristically, any epithelial defect will be considerably smaller than the area of infiltrate (Fig. 6.26B).
  - Coalescence and circumferential spread (Fig. 6.26C).

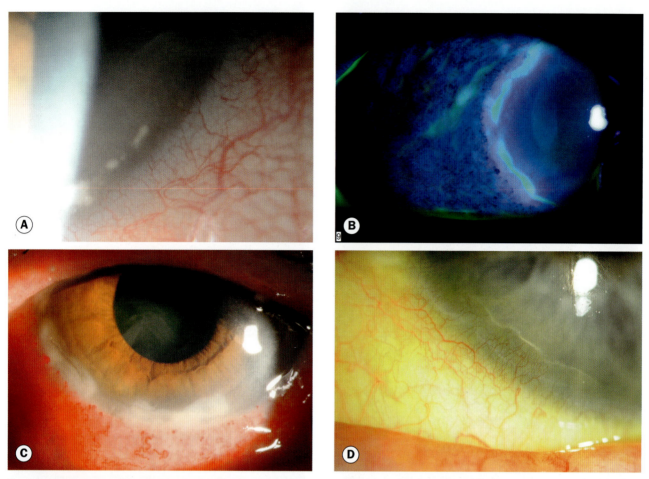

Fig. 6.26 Marginal keratitis. **(A)** Marginal infiltrates; **(B)** fluorescein staining characteristically demonstrates a smaller epithelial defect than infiltrate area; **(C)** substantial marginal infiltrate – note the relatively quiet eye despite the area of involvement; **(D)** mild scarring and pannus

○ Usually little or no anterior chamber reaction, even with large infiltrates.

○ Without treatment, resolution generally occurs in 1–4 weeks, depending on severity. Occasionally there is residual superficial scarring and slight thinning with mild pannus (Fig. 6.26D). Iris new vessels may develop in the presence of persistent large lesions, but resolve when inflammation settles.

Treatment

A weak topical steroid such as fluorometholone or prednisolone 0.5% is instilled four times daily for 1–2 weeks, sometimes combined with a topical antibiotic. An oral tetracycline course (erythromycin in children, breastfeeding and pregnancy) may be required for recurrent disease. Blepharitis is treated as necessary.

Phlyctenulosis

Introduction

Phlyctenulosis is usually a self-limiting disease but may rarely be severe. Most cases in developed countries are the result of a presumed delayed hypersensitivity reaction to staphylococcal antigen, sometimes associated with rosacea. In developing countries the majority are associated with tuberculosis or helminthic infestation, but causation may be uncertain and a range of other agents has been implicated.

Diagnosis

• **Symptoms.** Photophobia, lacrimation and blepharospasm, often in a child or young adult.

• **Signs**

○ A small white limbal (Fig. 6.27A) or conjunctival nodule associated with intense local hyperaemia.

○ A limbal phlycten may extend onto the cornea (Fig. 6.27B).

○ Spontaneous resolution usually occurs within 2–3 weeks; a healed lesion often leaves a triangular limbal-based scar associated with superficial vascularization and thinning (Fig. 6.27C) but occasionally severe thinning and even perforation can ensue.

○ Very large necrotizing or multiple (miliary) lesions may occur.

• **Investigation** for tuberculosis is generally indicated only in endemic areas or in the presence of specific risk factors.

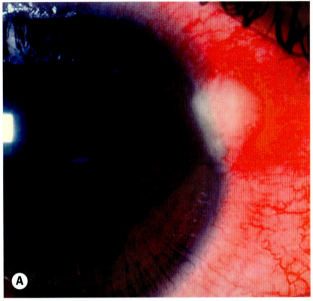

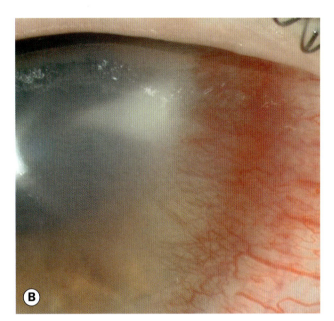

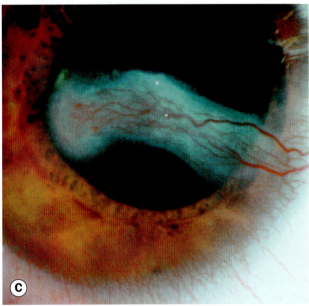

Fig. 6.27 Phlyctenulosis. **(A)** Limbal phlycten; **(B)** corneal phlycten; **(C)** healed phlycten

(Courtesy of J Harry and G Misson, from Clinical Ophthalmic Pathology, Butterworth-Heinemann 2002 – fig. A; S Tuft – fig. B; J Krachmer, M Mannis and E Holland, from Cornea, Mosby 2005 – fig. C)

Treatment

A short course of topical steroid accelerates healing and is often given with a topical antibiotic. Recurrent troublesome disease may require an oral tetracycline, and it is important to treat associated blepharitis.

ROSACEA

Introduction

Rosacea (acne rosacea) is a common chronic idiopathic dermatosis involving the sun-exposed skin of the face and upper neck. Ocular complications develop in 6–18% of patients. Facial telangiectasia, papule and pustule formation, rhinophyma and facial flushing may occur (Fig. 6.28). In contrast to acne vulgaris, comedones (blackheads or whiteheads) are absent.

The aetiology is probably multifactorial and may involve vascular factors, together with an abnormal response to commensal skin bacteria and *Demodex* follicular mites. Exacerbation by *H. pylori* infection has been suspected.

Ocular rosacea

- **Symptoms** include non-specific irritation and lacrimation.
- **Lid** signs include margin telangiectasia (Fig. 6.29A) and posterior blepharitis, often associated with recurrent meibomian cyst formation.
- **Conjunctival** hyperaemia, especially bulbar. Rarely, cicatricial conjunctivitis, conjunctival granulomas and phlyctenulosis may occur.

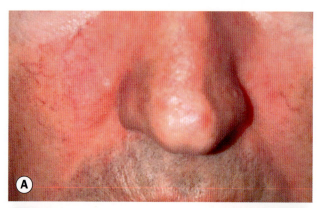

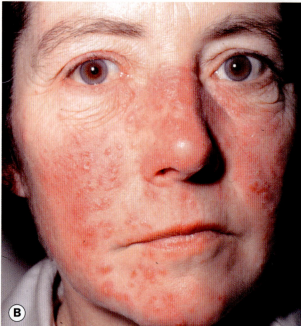

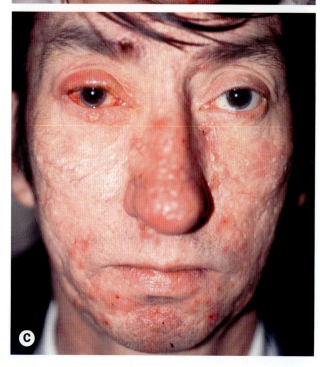

Fig. 6.28 Acne rosacea. **(A)** Nasal and malar telangiectasia; **(B)** papulopustular signs; **(C)** rhinophyma

- **Cornea**
  - Inferior punctate epithelial erosions.
  - Peripheral vascularization (Fig. 6.29B).
  - Marginal keratitis (see Fig. 6.26).
  - Focal or diffuse corneal thinning (Fig. 6.29C), usually inferiorly, in severe cases.
  - Perforation may occur as a result of severe peripheral or central melting, and may be precipitated by secondary bacterial infection.
  - Corneal scarring and vascularization (Fig. 6.29D).
- **Topical treatment**
  - Lubricants (preferably unpreserved) for mild symptoms.
  - Hot compresses and lid hygiene.
  - Topical antibiotics (e.g. fusidic acid, erythromycin, azithromycin) to the lid margins at bedtime for 4 weeks.
  - Steroids are helpful for exacerbations; the lowest potency preparation compatible with improvement should be used in order to minimize the promotion of thinning.
- **Systemic therapy**
  - Tetracyclines may work by altering meibomian gland function to lower free fatty acid production in conjunction with a reduction in lid flora, and probably by a direct anti-inflammatory effect. They also have an anticollagenase action and so may retard thinning. In relatively low dose but extended duration (e.g. doxycycline, which has a longer half-life than tetracycline, 100 mg once daily for 4 weeks then 50 mg daily if required) they may confer an improvement lasting several months but if necessary can be continued long term; tetracyclines should not be used in children and pregnant or breastfeeding women, in whom erythromycin is an alternative. Efficacy has also been reported with other antibiotics.
  - Severe disease may require immunosuppression, e.g. azathioprine.
  - Retinoids can be helpful, but can worsen some features. They are absolutely contraindicated in pregnancy.

PERIPHERAL CORNEAL ULCERATION/THINNING

Introduction

Peripheral corneal ulceration/thinning, known as 'peripheral ulcerative keratitis' (PUK) when inflammatory, refers to a presentation characterized by thinning and/or ulceration preferentially affecting the peripheral rather than central cornea, and spreading around the margin. It should be noted that any cause of corneal ulceration can affect the periphery.

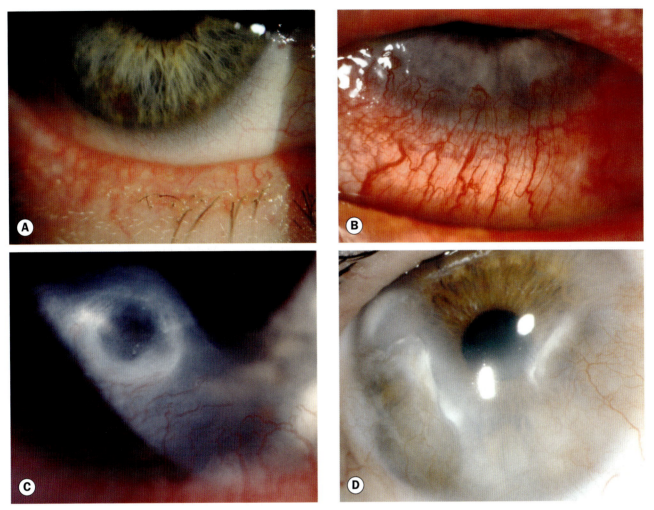

Fig. 6.29 Anterior segment in rosacea. **(A)** Eyelid margin telangiectasia; **(B)** peripheral corneal vascularization; **(C)** focal corneal thinning; **(D)** severe scarring and vascularization

- **Marginal keratitis.** This is discussed above.
- **Mooren ulcer.**
- **Terrien marginal degeneration.**
- **Dellen.** Localized corneal disturbance associated with drying of a focal area, usually associated with an adjacent elevated lesion (e.g. pinguecula or a large subconjunctival haemorrhage – Fig. 6.30A) that impairs physiological lubrication. Generally mild though can occasionally be severe, including descemetocoele formation/corneal perforation.
- Associated with **systemic autoimmune disease**.
- **Others.** Ocular rosacea, furrow degeneration (mild peripheral thinning in the elderly, usually benign – Fig. 6.30B), pellucid marginal degeneration.

Mooren ulcer

Introduction

Mooren ulcer is a rare autoimmune disease characterized by progressive circumferential peripheral stromal ulceration with later central spread. There are two forms: the first affects mainly older patients, often in only one eye, and usually responds well to medical therapy. The second is more aggressive and likely to need systemic immunosuppression, carries a poorer prognosis, may be bilateral and associated with severe pain, and tends to occur in younger patients, including widespread reports in men from the Indian subcontinent. In at least some (usually milder) cases, there is a precipitating corneal insult such as surgery or infection. Associated systemic autoimmune disease and corneal infection should always be ruled out.

Diagnosis

- **Symptoms.** Pain is prominent and may be severe. There is photophobia and blurred vision.
- **Signs**
  - Peripheral ulceration involving the superficial one-third of the stroma (Fig. 6.31A), with variable epithelial loss. Several distinct foci may be present and subsequently coalesce.

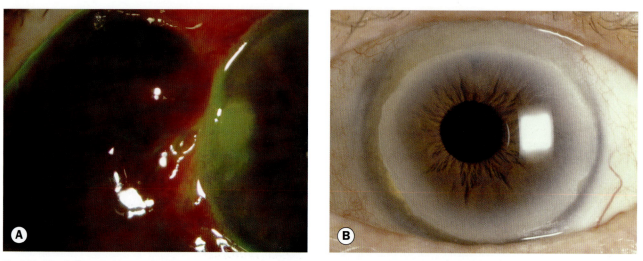

Fig. 6.30 Non-inflammatory peripheral corneal thinning. **(A)** Fluorescein-stained dellen secondary to large subconjunctival haemorrhage following cataract surgery; **(B)** extensive furrow degeneration

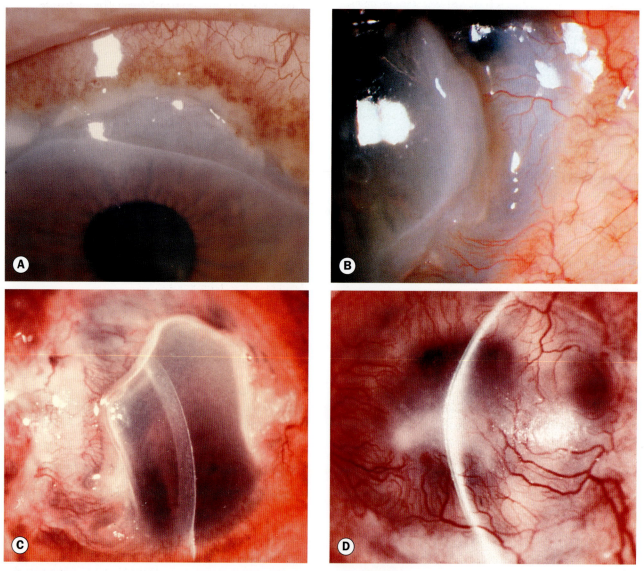

Fig. 6.31 Mooren ulcer. **(A)** Local peripheral ulceration; **(B)** undermined and infiltrated central edge; **(C)** advanced disease; **(D)** healed stage

○ An undermined and infiltrated leading edge is characteristic (Fig. 6.31B).
○ Limbitis may be present, but not scleritis, which aids in distinguishing from systemic disease-associated PUK.
○ Progressive circumferential and central stromal thinning (Fig. 6.31C).
○ Vascularization involving the bed of the ulcer up to its leading edge but not beyond.
○ The healing stage is characterized by thinning, vascularization and scarring (Fig. 6.31D).
○ Iritis is not uncommon.
• **Complications** include severe astigmatism, perforation following minor trauma (spontaneous perforation is rare), secondary bacterial infection, cataract and glaucoma.

Treatment

• **Topical steroids** as frequently as hourly are combined with a low-frequency prophylactic topical antibiotic. If an effective response is seen, treatment is tapered over several months.
• **Topical ciclosporin** (up to 2%) may be effective, but can take weeks to exert a significant effect.
• **Adjunctive** topical therapy includes artificial tears and collagenase inhibitors such as acetylcysteine 10–20%.
• **Conjunctival resection**, which may be combined with excision of necrotic tissue, is performed if there is no response to topical steroids. The excised area should extend 4 mm back from the limbus and 2 mm beyond the circumferential margins. Keratoepithelioplasty (suturing of a donor corneal lenticule onto the scleral bed) may be combined to produce a physical barrier against conjunctival regrowth and further melting. Steroids are continued postoperatively.
• **Systemic immunosuppression** may be needed, including steroids for rapid effect, and should be instituted earlier for bilateral disease, or if involvement is advanced at first examination. Biological blockers show some promise.
• **Systemic collagenase inhibitors** such as doxycycline may be beneficial.
• **Lamellar keratectomy** involving dissection of the residual central island in advanced disease may remove the stimulus for further inflammation.
• **Perforations.** Management is as discussed earlier in this chapter.
• **Visual rehabilitation.** Keratoplasty (with immunosuppressive cover) may be considered once inflammation has settled.

Peripheral ulcerative keratitis associated with systemic autoimmune disease

Introduction

PUK may precede or follow the onset of systemic features. Severe peripheral corneal infiltration, ulceration or thinning unexplained by evident ocular disease should prompt investigation for a (potentially life-threatening) systemic collagen vascular disorder. The mechanism includes immune complex deposition in peripheral cornea, episcleral and conjunctival capillary occlusion with secondary cytokine release and inflammatory cell recruitment, the upregulation of collagenases and reduced activity of their inhibitors. Systemic associations include:

• **Rheumatoid arthritis** (RA – the most common). PUK is bilateral in 30% and tends to occur in advanced RA.
• **Wegener granulomatosis** is the second most common systemic association of PUK. In contrast to RA ocular complications are the initial presentation in 50%.
• **Other conditions** include polyarteritis nodosa, relapsing polychondritis and systemic lupus erythematosus.

Clinical features

• **Crescentic ulceration** with an epithelial defect, thinning and stromal infiltration at the limbus (Fig. 6.32A). Spread is circumferential and occasionally central; in contrast to Mooren ulcer, extension into the sclera may occur.
• **Limbitis, episcleritis or scleritis** are usually present; as with a Mooren ulcer, there is no separation between the ulcerative process and the limbus.
• **Advanced disease** may result in a 'contact lens' cornea (Fig. 6.32B) or perforation.
• **Rheumatoid paracentral ulcerative keratitis (PCUK)** is thought to be a distinct entity, with a punched-out more centrally located lesion with little infiltrate in a quiet eye (Fig. 6.32C). Perforation can occur rapidly, and there is usually a good response to topical ciclosporin, with bandage contact lens and tissue glue application if necessary, rather than systemic treatment.

Treatment

Treatment is principally with systemic immunosuppression in collaboration with a rheumatologist.

• **Systemic steroids**, sometimes via pulsed intravenous administration, are used to control acute disease, with immunosuppressive therapy and biological blockers for longer-term management.
• **Topical lubricants** (preservative-free).
• **Topical antibiotics** as prophylaxis if an epithelial defect is present.
• **Oral tetracycline** (e.g. doxycycline 100 mg once or twice daily) for its anticollagenase effect.
• **Topical steroids** may worsen thinning so are generally avoided; relapsing polychondritis may be an exception.
• **Surgical management** is generally as for Mooren ulcer, including conjunctival excision if medical treatment is ineffective.

Terrien marginal degeneration

Terrien disease is an uncommon idiopathic thinning of the peripheral cornea occurring in young adult to elderly patients. Although

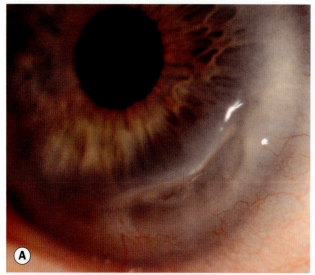

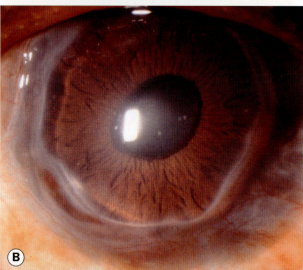

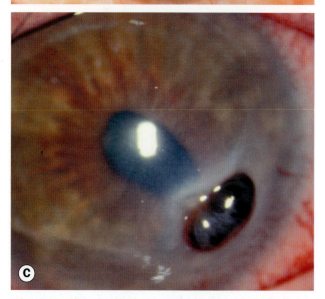

Fig. 6.32 Keratitis in systemic collagen vascular disease. **(A)** Early peripheral ulcerative keratitis; **(B)** contact lens cornea; **(C)** rheumatoid paracentral ulcerative keratitis with iris prolapsing through a perforation

usually categorized as a degeneration, some cases are associated with episodic episcleritis or scleritis. About 75% of affected patients are male and the condition is usually bilateral but may be asymmetrical.

Diagnosis

- **Symptoms.** The condition is commonly asymptomatic, but gradual visual deterioration can occur due to astigmatism. A few patients experience episodic pain and inflammation.
- **Signs**
  - Fine yellow–white refractile stromal opacities, frequently associated with mild superficial vascularization, usually start superiorly, spread circumferentially and are separated from the limbus by a clear zone (Fig. 6.33A). There is no epithelial defect, and on cursory examination the condition may resemble arcus senilis.
  - Slowly progressive circumferential thinning results in a peripheral gutter, the outer slope of which shelves gradually, while the central part rises sharply. A band of lipid is commonly present at the central edge (Fig. 6.33B).
  - Perforation is rare but may be spontaneous or follow blunt trauma.
  - Pseudopterygia sometimes develop (Fig. 6.33C).

Treatment

- **Safety spectacles** (e.g. polycarbonate) if thinning is significant.
- **Contact lenses** for astigmatism. Scleral or soft lenses with rigid gas permeable 'piggybacking'.
- **Surgery** – crescentic or annular excision of the gutter with lamellar (Fig. 6.33D) or full-thickness transplantation – gives reasonable results and may arrest progression.

NEUROTROPHIC KERATOPATHY

Introduction

Neurotrophic keratopathy occurs when there is loss of trigeminal innervation to the cornea resulting in partial or complete anaesthesia. In addition to loss of the protective sensory stimulus, reduced innervation results in intracellular oedema, exfoliation, loss of goblet cells and epithelial breakdown with persistent ulceration. Causes include trigeminal ganglion surgical ablation for neuralgia, stroke, tumour, peripheral neuropathy (e.g. diabetes) and ocular disease such as herpes simplex and herpes zoster keratitis (when sensation loss may be sectoral).

Diagnosis

A full cranial nerve examination is mandatory.
- **Signs**
  - Corneal sensation is reduced.
  - Stage 1: interpalpebral epithelial irregularity and staining, with mild opacification, oedema and tiny focal defects (Fig. 6.34A).

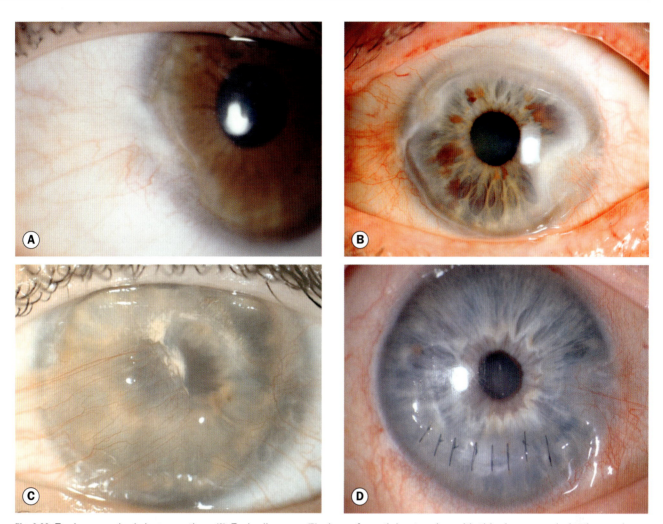

Fig. 6.33 Terrien marginal degeneration. **(A)** Early disease; **(B)** circumferential extension with thinning, vascularization and a lipid band at the central edge; **(C)** pseudopterygia; **(D)** gutter excision with lamellar graft repair
(Courtesy of C Barry – figs C and D)

○ Stage 2: larger persistent epithelial defect with rolled and thickened edges (Fig. 6.34B), subsequently assuming a punched-out configuration with underlying stromal oedema (Fig. 6.34C).
○ Stage 3: stromal melting, often with minimal discomfort.
○ Perforation is uncommon but may occur rapidly, especially with secondary infection (Fig. 6.34D).

Treatment

- **Discontinuation**, if possible, of potentially toxic medications.
- **Topical lubricants** (non-preserved) for associated dry eye or corneal exposure. Topical insulin-like growth factor-1, substance P and neurogenic growth factor have been evaluated but are not commercially available.
- **Anticollagenase agents**: topical (e.g. acetylcysteine, tetracycline ointment) or systemic (e.g. tetracyclines).
- **Protection of the ocular surface**
  ○ Simple taping of the lids, particularly at night, may provide modest protection.

○ Botulinum toxin-induced ptosis.
○ Tarsorrhaphy: temporary or permanent, lateral or central, according to the underlying pathology and visual potential.
○ Therapeutic silicone contact lenses may be fitted, provided the eye is carefully monitored for infection.
○ Amniotic membrane patching with temporary central tarsorrhaphy.
- **Perforation** is dealt with as discussed earlier in the chapter.

EXPOSURE KERATOPATHY

Introduction

Exposure keratopathy is the result of incomplete lid closure (lagophthalmos), with drying of the cornea despite normal tear production. Lagophthalmos may only be present on blinking or gentle lid closure, with full forced lid closure. Causes include neuroparalytic, especially facial nerve palsy, reduced muscle tone as

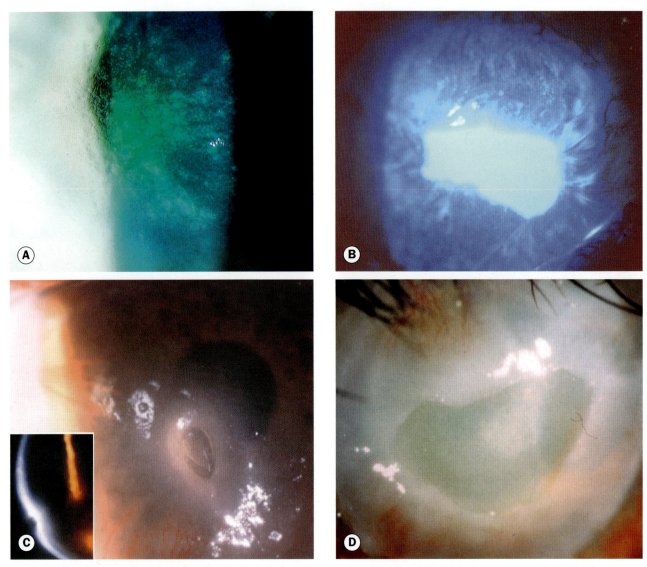

Fig. 6.34 Neurotrophic keratopathy. **(A)** Early central epithelial changes; **(B)** persistent epithelial defect with rolled edges; **(C)** punched-out epithelial defect with underlying stromal oedema and early melting; **(D)** secondary infection with marked thinning
(Courtesy of S Bonini – figs B–D)

in parkinsonism, mechanical such as lid scarring, eczematous skin tightening and post-blepharoplasty, and proptosis.

Diagnosis

- **Symptoms** are those of dry eye.
- **Signs**
  - Mild punctate epithelial changes involving the inferior third of the cornea, particularly with nocturnal lagophthalmos.
  - Epithelial breakdown (Fig. 6.35A).
  - Stromal melting (Fig. 6.35B), occasionally leading to perforation.
  - Inferior fibrovascular change with Salzmann degeneration may develop over time.
  - Secondary infection (Fig. 6.35C).

Treatment

Treatment depends on the severity of exposure and whether recovery is anticipated.

- **Reversible exposure**
  - Artificial tears (unpreserved) during the day and ointment at night.
  - Taping the lid closed at night may be an alternative to ointment.
  - Bandage silicone hydrogel or scleral contact lenses.
  - Management of proptosis by orbital decompression if necessary.
  - Temporary tarsorrhaphy, Frost suture or overlay amniotic membrane grafting.
- **Permanent exposure**
  - Permanent tarsorrhaphy.
  - Gold weight upper lid insertion for facial nerve palsy.

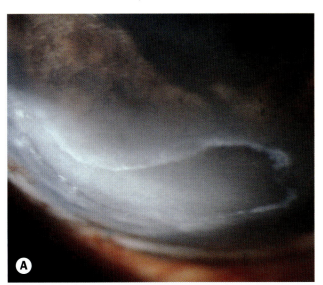

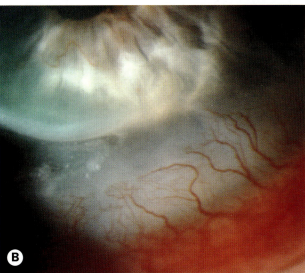

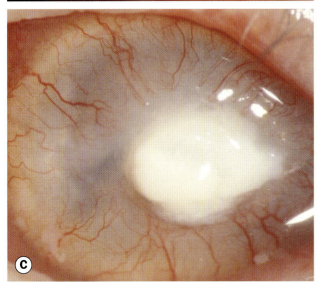

Fig. 6.35 Exposure keratopathy. **(A)** Inferior epithelial defect; **(B)** stromal melting; **(C)** secondary bacterial infection

(Courtesy of S Tuft – fig. C)

○ Permanent central tarsorrhaphy, amniotic membrane grafting or conjunctival flap when vision is poor.

MISCELLANEOUS KERATOPATHIES

Infectious crystalline keratopathy

Infectious crystalline keratopathy is a rare indolent infection usually occurring in a patient on long-term topical steroid therapy with an associated epithelial defect, most frequently following penetrating keratoplasty. *Streptococcus viridans* is most commonly isolated, although numerous other bacteria and fungi have been implicated.

Slowly progressive, grey–white, branching stromal opacities are seen, associated with minimal inflammation and usually intact overlying epithelium (Fig. 6.36). Culture or biopsy is performed

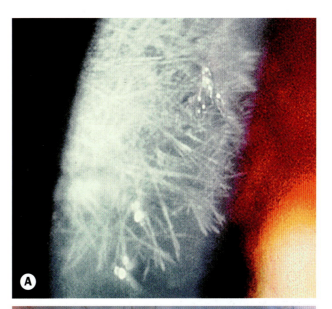

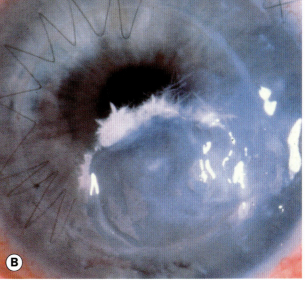

Fig. 6.36 (A) Infectious crystalline keratitis; **(B)** crystalline keratitis in a graft

(Courtesy of M Kerr-Muir – fig. A)

to determine the organism, and topical antibiotics instilled for several weeks.

Thygeson superficial punctate keratitis

Thygeson superficial punctate keratitis is an uncommon idiopathic, usually bilateral, condition characterized by exacerbations and remissions. It is commonly of onset in young adulthood but can affect patients of any age, and may recur over decades.

Diagnosis

- **Symptoms** consist of recurrent attacks of irritation, photophobia, blurred vision and watering.
- **Signs**
  - Granular, coarse, slightly elevated greyish epithelial lesions that stain with fluorescein and mainly involve the central cornea (Fig. 6.37A).
  - A mild subepithelial haze may be present (Fig. 6.37B), especially if topical antivirals have been used.
  - There is little or no conjunctival hyperaemia.
- **Differential diagnosis** includes post-adenoviral keratitis.

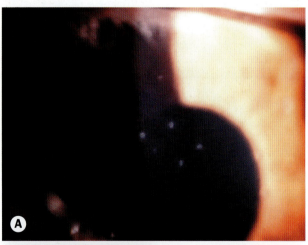

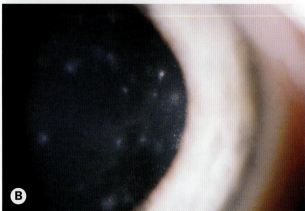

Fig. 6.37 (A) Thygeson superficial punctate keratitis; **(B)** associated subepithelial haze
(Courtesy of R Curtis – fig. B)

Treatment

- **Topical**
  - Lubricants may suffice in mild cases.
  - Steroids. A low-potency preparation is used twice daily initially, with gradual tapering to as little as once-weekly instillation. Higher intensity treatment may sometimes be needed initially.
  - Ciclosporin 0.05% is generally used if the response to steroids is inadequate, or as an alternative in longer-term therapy; some authorities recommend ciclosporin for initial treatment. Tacrolimus may also be effective.
  - Antivirals have not been found to be consistently helpful.
- **Contact lenses** (extended wear or daily disposable soft) may be considered if steroids are ineffective or contraindicated, as an alternative to ciclosporin.
- **Phototherapeutic keratectomy** brings short-term relief but recurrence is likely.

Filamentary keratopathy

Introduction

Filamentary keratopathy is a common condition that can cause considerable discomfort. It is thought that a loose area of epithelium acts as a focus for deposition of mucus and cellular debris. The causes are shown in Table 6.6.

Diagnosis

- **Symptoms** consist of discomfort with foreign body sensation, redness and sometimes photophobia.
- **Signs**
  - Strands of degenerated epithelial cells and mucus that move with blinking and are typically attached to the cornea at one end (Fig. 6.38A).
  - Filaments stain well with rose Bengal (Fig. 6.38B) and to a lesser extent with fluorescein.
  - A small epithelial defect may be present at the base of a filament.
  - Chronic filaments may form plaques.

Treatment

- **Any underlying cause** should be treated.
- **Topical medication** should be changed if a toxic effect is suspected, and unpreserved preparations used where possible.

Table 6.6 Causes of filamentary keratopathy

Aqueous deficiency (keratoconjunctivitis sicca)
Excessive contact lens wear
Corneal epithelial instability (recurrent erosion syndrome, corneal graft, cataract surgery, refractive surgery and drug toxicity)
Superior limbic keratoconjunctivitis
Bullous keratopathy
Neurotrophic keratopathy
Prolonged or frequent eye closure

and their basement membrane. Minor trauma, such as eyelid–cornea interaction during sleep, can be sufficient to precipitate detachment. Erosions may be associated with previous trauma or rarely corneal surgery, and with some corneal dystrophies. Intervals between episodes can be very variable, even in the same patient, but may occur in spates over a short period.

Diagnosis

- **Symptoms.** Severe pain, photophobia, redness, blepharospasm and watering typically waken the patient during the night or are present on awaking in the morning. There is usually (but not invariably) a prior history of corneal abrasion, sometimes years previously, which may have been minor compared to the recurrent symptoms.
- **Signs**
  - An epithelial defect (Fig. 6.39A) may not be present by the time the patient is examined, as healing can often be very rapid (hours), but the extent of loose epithelium may be highlighted by areas of pooling of fluorescein and rapid tear film breakup.

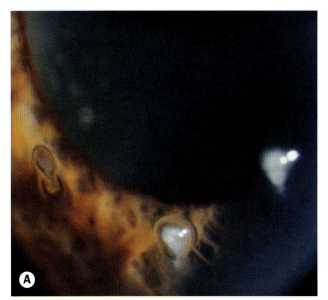

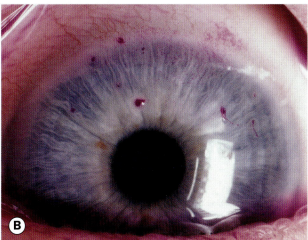

Fig. 6.38 Corneal filaments. **(A)** Comma-shaped lesions attached to the cornea at one end; **(B)** stained with rose Bengal

(Courtesy of S Tuft – fig. A; R Bates – fig. B)

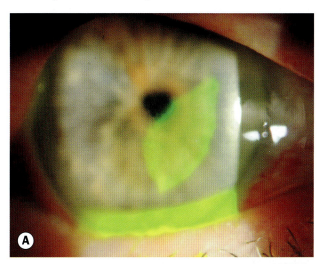

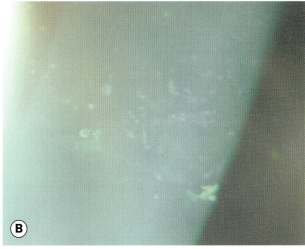

Fig. 6.39 Recurrent corneal erosion syndrome. **(A)** Epithelial defect stained with fluorescein; **(B)** epithelial basement membrane abnormalities, predominantly non-staining, signify the region of abnormal healing

- **Mechanical removal** of filaments gives short-term symptomatic relief.
- **Mucolytics** such as 5% or 10% acetylcysteine drops.
- **Non-steroidal anti-inflammatory drops**, e.g. diclofenac.
- **Hypertonic saline** (5% drops four times daily, ointment at bedtime) may encourage adhesion of loose epithelium.
- **Bandage contact lenses** may protect the cornea from the shearing action of the lids.

Recurrent corneal epithelial erosion

Introduction

Recurrent corneal epithelial erosion is caused by an abnormally weak attachment between the basal cells of the corneal epithelium

○ Infiltrate should not be present, though greyish sloughed and rolled epithelium may sometimes be reminiscent of this.

○ There may be no sign of abnormality once a defect has healed, but signs of epithelial basement membrane disturbance, such as microcysts, punctate or linear/fingerprint opacities are often present (Fig. 6.39B). These will typically be bilateral in a stromal dystrophy and unilateral if injury is the cause.

Treatment

- **Acute symptoms**
  ○ Antibiotic ointment four times daily and cyclopentolate 1% twice daily.
  ○ Pressure patching should not be used as it may impair healing and does not improve comfort.
  ○ In severe cases a bandage contact lens alleviates pain but may not improve healing; antibiotic drops rather than ointment should be used.
  ○ Debridement of heaped/scrolled areas of epithelium with a sterile cellulose sponge or cotton-tipped applicator (cotton bud) may improve comfort and allow healing from the edges of the defect; irregular underlying Bowman layer will often be appreciated in the involved area.
  ○ Topical diclofenac 0.1% reduces pain.
  ○ Topical anaesthetic dramatically relieves pain but should not be dispensed for patient use.
  ○ Hypertonic sodium chloride 5% drops four times daily and ointment at bedtime may improve epithelial adhesion.
  ○ Following resolution, some authorities advise using a prophylactic topical lubricant such as carbomer gel three or four times daily for several months.
- **Recurrent symptoms**
  ○ Topical lubricant gel or ointment, or hypertonic saline ointment, instilled at bedtime used long term may be sufficient.
  ○ Simple debridement of the epithelium in involved areas, which may be followed by smoothing of Bowman layer with a diamond burr or excimer laser.
  ○ Long-term extended-wear bandage contact lenses.
  ○ Anterior stromal puncture for localized areas off the visual axis; it may not be necessary to remove the epithelium to facilitate this.

Xerophthalmia

Introduction

Vitamin A is essential for the maintenance of the body's epithelial surfaces, for immune function and for the synthesis of retinal photoreceptor proteins. Xerophthalmia refers to the spectrum of ocular disease caused by inadequate vitamin A intake, and is a late manifestation of severe deficiency. Lack of vitamin A in the diet may be caused by malnutrition, malabsorption, chronic alcoholism or by highly selective dieting. The risk in infants is increased if their mothers are malnourished and by coexisting diarrhoea or measles.

Diagnosis

A World Health Organization (WHO) grading system is set out in Table 6.7.

Table 6.7 WHO grading of xerophthalmia

XN = night blindness
X1 = conjunctival xerosis (X1A) with Bitot spots (X1B)
X2 = corneal xerosis
X3 = corneal ulceration, less than one-third (X3A); more than one-third (X3B)
XS = corneal scar
XF = xerophthalmic fundus

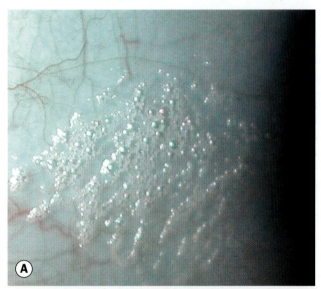

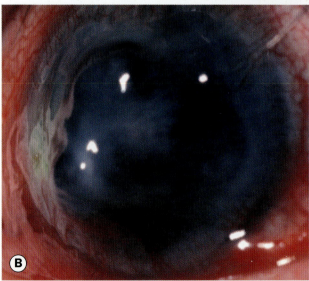

Fig. 6.40 Xerophthalmia. **(A)** Bitot spot; **(B)** keratomalacia and perforation
(Courtesy of N Rogers – fig. A; S Kumar Puri – fig. B)

- **Symptoms** are night blindness (nyctalopia), discomfort and loss of vision.
- **Conjunctiva**
  - Xerosis is characterized by dryness of the conjunctiva in the interpalpebral zone with loss of goblet cells, squamous metaplasia and keratinization.
  - Bitot spots are triangular patches of foamy keratinized epithelium (Fig. 6.40A) in the interpalpebral zone thought to be caused by *Corynebacterium xerosis.*
- **Cornea**
  - Lustreless appearance due to secondary xerosis.
  - Bilateral punctate corneal epithelial erosions in the interpalpebral zone can progress to epithelial defects but are reversible with treatment.
  - Keratinization.
  - Sterile corneal melting by liquefactive necrosis (keratomalacia), which may lead to perforation (Fig. 6.40B).
- **Retinopathy**, characterized by yellowish peripheral dots, may occur in advanced cases and is associated with decreased electroretinogram amplitude.

Treatment

Keratomalacia is an indicator of very severe vitamin A deficiency and should be treated as a medical emergency due to the risk of death, particularly in infants.

- **Systemic** treatment involves oral (oil-based 200 000 IU) or intramuscular (aqueous-based 100 000 IU) vitamin A for keratomalacia. Multivitamin supplements and dietary sources of vitamin A are also administered.
- **Local** treatment consists of intense lubrication, topical retinoic acid and management of perforation.

CORNEAL ECTASIAS

Keratoconus

Introduction

Keratoconus (KC) is a progressive disorder in which central or paracentral corneal stromal thinning occurs, accompanied by apical protrusion and irregular astigmatism. Approximately 50% of normal fellow eyes will progress to KC within 16 years. Both eyes are affected eventually, at least on topographical imaging, in almost all cases. It can be graded by the highest axis of corneal power on keratometry as mild (<48 D), moderate (48–54 D) or severe (>54 D). Most patients do not have a family history, with only about 10% of offspring developing KC; autosomal dominant transmission with incomplete penetrance has been proposed. Presentation is commonly during the teens or twenties, with features initially in only one eye. Systemic associations include Down, Ehlers–Danlos and Marfan syndromes and osteogenesis imperfecta; ocular associations include vernal keratoconjunctivitis, blue

sclera, aniridia, Leber congenital amaurosis, retinitis pigmentosa, as well as persistent eye rubbing from any cause.

Diagnosis

- **Symptoms.** Unilateral impairment of vision due to progressive myopia and astigmatism; occasionally, initial presentation is with acute hydrops (see below).
- **Signs**
  - Direct ophthalmoscopy from a distance of half a metre shows a fairly well delineated 'oil droplet' reflex (Fig. 6.41A).
  - Retinoscopy shows an irregular 'scissoring' reflex.
  - Slit lamp biomicroscopy shows very fine, vertical, deep stromal stress lines (Vogt striae – Fig. 6.41B), which disappear with pressure on the globe.
  - Epithelial iron deposits, best seen with a cobalt blue filter, may surround the base of the cone (Fleischer ring – Fig. 6.41C).
  - Progressive corneal protrusion in a cone configuration (Fig. 6.41D), with thinning maximal at the apex.
  - Bulging of the lower lid in downgaze (Munson sign).
  - Acute hydrops is caused by a rupture in the stretched Descemet membrane that allows a sudden influx of aqueous into the cornea (Figs 6.42A and B), with accompanying pain, photophobia and decreased vision. Although the break usually heals within 6–10 weeks and the oedema clears, a variable amount of stromal scarring (Fig. 6.42C) may develop; this sometimes gives improved vision by flattening the cornea. Acute episodes are initially treated with cycloplegia, hypertonic (5%) saline ointment and patching or a soft bandage contact lens. Accelerated resolution has been reported with intracameral gas injection in the acute stage.
- **Keratometry** readings are steep.
- **Corneal topography** (videokeratography) and various novel corneal profiling techniques are highly sensitive for detection and essential in monitoring. Characteristically, astigmatism progresses from a symmetrical bow-tie pattern, through an asymmetrical appearance to an inferotemporally displaced steep-sided cone (Fig. 6.43). Sometimes a central ('nipple') cone may develop. Contact lens warpage can sometimes appear similar to a cone on topography, but is generally more arcuate-shaped.

Treatment

LASIK is contraindicated; patients should be screened for KC prior to corneal refractive surgery.

- **Eye rubbing** should be avoided.
- **Spectacles** or soft contact lenses are generally sufficient in early cases. If thinning is marked, it may be prudent to consider wearing safety spectacles over contact lenses.
- **Rigid contact lenses,** sometimes scleral, are required for higher degrees of astigmatism to provide a regular refracting surface.

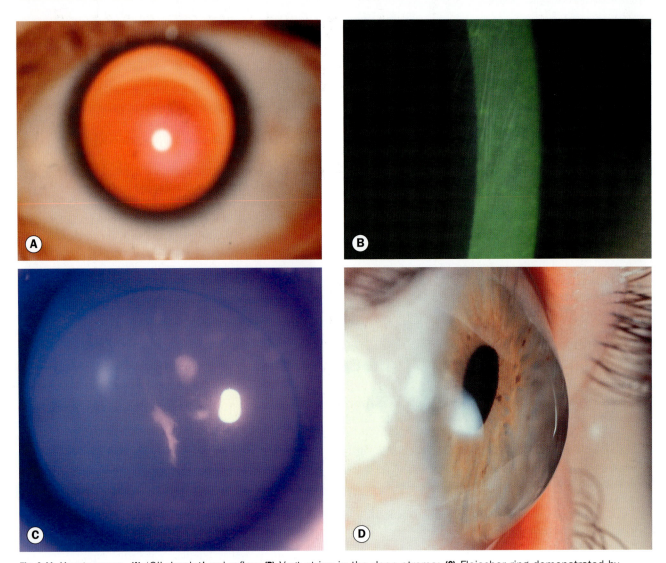

Fig. 6.41 Keratoconus. **(A)** 'Oil droplet' red reflex; **(B)** Vogt striae in the deep stroma; **(C)** Fleischer ring demonstrated by cobalt blue light as a blue circle; **(D)** typical cone
(Courtesy of R Fogla – fig. C; C Barry – fig. D)

- **Corneal collagen cross-linking (CXL)**, using riboflavin drops to photosensitize the eye followed by exposure to ultraviolet-A light, may stabilize or even reverse ectasia, but is not without adverse effects. It can be combined with ring segment insertion. CXL is commonly used only after progression has been documented.
- **Intracorneal ring segment implantation** (Fig. 6.44) using laser or mechanical channel creation is relatively safe, and typically provides at least a moderate visual improvement, facilitating contact lens tolerance in advanced cases.
- **Keratoplasty**, either penetrating or deep anterior lamellar (DALK), may be necessary in patients with severe disease. A history of hydrops is a contraindication to DALK due to the presence of a Descemet membrane discontinuity. Outcomes may be compromised by residual astigmatism and by anisometropia, necessitating contact lens correction for optimal acuity.

Pellucid marginal degeneration

Pellucid marginal degeneration is a rare progressive peripheral corneal thinning disorder, typically involving the inferior cornea in both eyes. Presentation is usually in adulthood.

Diagnosis

- **Symptoms.** Slowly progressive blurring due to astigmatism.
- **Signs**
  - Bilateral, slowly progressive, crescentic 1–2 mm band of inferior corneal thinning extending from 4 to 8 o'clock, 1 mm from the limbus (Fig. 6.45A).
  - The epithelium is intact, and the cornea above the thinned area is ectatic and flattened.
  - In contrast to keratoconus, Fleischer rings and Vogt striae do not occur and acute hydrops is rare.

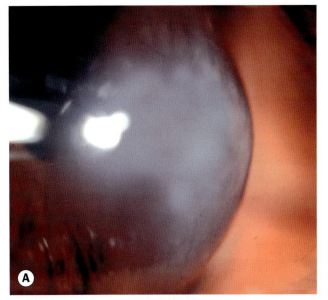

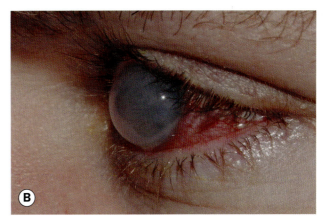

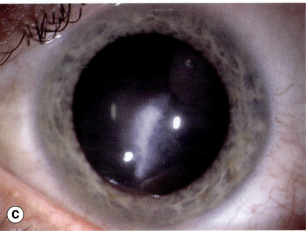

Fig. 6.42 Acute hydrops. **(A)** Localized corneal oedema;
(B) severe diffuse oedema; **(C)** late scarring
(Courtesy of C Barry – figs B and C)

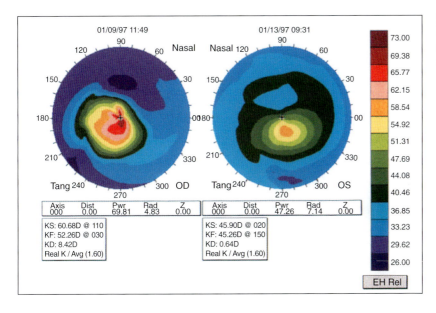

Fig. 6.43 Corneal topography showing
severe keratoconus in the right eye and
an early paracentral cone in the left
(Courtesy of E Morris)

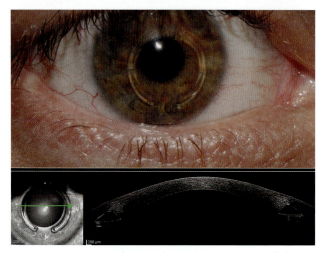

Fig. 6.44 Intracorneal ring segments *in situ*
(Courtesy of C Barry)

- **Corneal topography** shows a 'butterfly' pattern, with severe astigmatism and diffuse steepening of the inferior cornea (Fig. 6.45B).

Treatment

Early cases are managed with spectacles and contact lenses. Surgical options, none of which is ideal, in patients intolerant to contact lenses include large eccentric penetrating keratoplasty, thermocauterization, crescentic lamellar keratoplasty, wedge resection of diseased tissue, epikeratoplasty and intracorneal ring segment implantation. Results of collagen cross-linking are encouraging.

Keratoglobus

Keratoglobus is an extremely rare condition that can be present at birth when differential diagnosis is from congenital glaucoma and megalocornea and associations may be present, or acquired, with onset in adulthood. In contrast to keratoconus, the cornea develops globular rather than conical ectasia; corneal thinning is generalized (Fig. 6.46). Acute hydrops is rare, but the cornea is more prone to rupture on relatively mild trauma. Corneal topography shows generalized steepening. Surgery is difficult and contact lens wear is often unsatisfactory. Intrastromal ring segments and cross-linking may have utility. Special care should be taken to protect the eyes from trauma.

CORNEAL DYSTROPHIES

The corneal dystrophies are a group of progressive, usually bilateral, variable corneal opacifying disorders, many of which are associated with decreased vision and discomfort. Based on biomicroscopical and histopathological features they are classified into epithelial, Bowman layer, stromal, and Descemet membrane and endothelial. One or more underlying genetic abnormalities have been identified for most.

Epithelial dystrophies

Cogan (epithelial basement membrane) dystrophy

Epithelial basement membrane (map-dot-fingerprint) is the most common corneal dystrophy. Despite this, it is often misdiagnosed, principally due to its variable appearance.

- **Inheritance.** The condition is usually sporadic, and these cases may be degenerations rather than true dystrophies, in contrast to the rare familial (autosomal dominant – AD) cases.

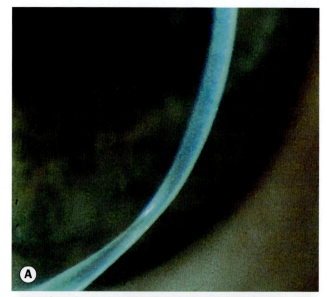

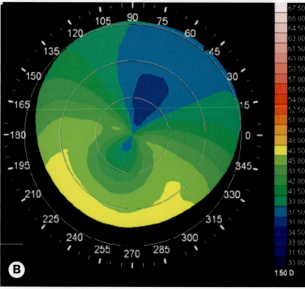

Fig. 6.45 (A) Pellucid marginal degeneration; **(B)** topography shows severe astigmatism and diffuse steepening of the inferior cornea
(Courtesy of R Visser – fig. A; R Fogla – fig. B)

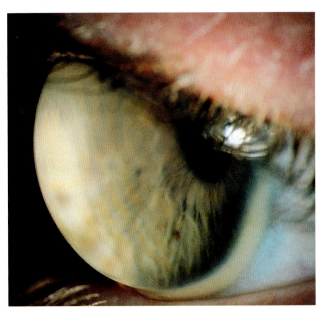

Fig. 6.46 Keratoglobus

- **Histology** shows thickening of the basement membrane with deposition of fibrillary protein between the basement membrane and the Bowman layer. Basal epithelial cell hemidesmosomes are deficient.
- **Onset** is in the second decade. About 10% of patients develop recurrent corneal erosions in the third decade and the remainder are asymptomatic throughout life. The occurrence of bilateral recurrent erosions with no history of trauma suggests basement membrane dystrophy.
- **Signs.** Lesions are often best visualized by retroillumination or scleral scatter. Over time pattern and distribution varies; they may be absent or subtle in a fellow eye. Similar features can be seen with recurrent erosions from any cause.
  ○ Dot-like and microcystic epithelial lesions (Fig. 6.47A).
  ○ Subepithelial map-like patterns surrounded by a faint haze (Fig. 6.47B).
  ○ Whorled fingerprint-like lines.
  ○ Bleb-like subepithelial pebbled glass pattern.
- **Treatment** is that of recurrent corneal erosions.

Meesmann epithelial dystrophy

Meesmann dystrophy is a rare non-progressive abnormality of corneal epithelial metabolism, underlying which mutations in the genes encoding corneal epithelial keratins have been reported.
- **Inheritance.** AD.
- **Histology** shows irregular thickening of the epithelial basement membrane and intraepithelial cysts.
- **Symptoms.** Patients may be asymptomatic, or there may be recurrent erosions and blurring (usually mild).
- **Signs**
  ○ Myriad tiny intraepithelial cysts of uniform size but variable density are maximal centrally and extend towards but do not reach the limbus (Fig. 6.47C).

  ○ The cornea may be slightly thinned and sensation reduced.
- **Treatment** other than lubrication is not normally required.

Others

Other epithelial and subepithelial dystrophies are Lisch epithelial corneal dystrophy (Figs 6.47D and E), subepithelial mucinous corneal dystrophy and gelatinous drop-like corneal dystrophy (Fig. 6.47F).

Bowman layer/anterior stromal dystrophies

Reis–Bücklers corneal dystrophy

This may be categorized as an anterior variant of granular stromal dystrophy (GCD type 3 – see below) and is also known as corneal basement dystrophy type I (CBD1).
- **Inheritance** is AD; the affected gene is *TGFB1*.
- **Histology.** Replacement of the Bowman layer by connective tissue bands.
- **Symptoms.** Severe recurrent corneal erosions in childhood. Visual impairment may occur.
- **Signs**
  ○ Grey–white geographic subepithelial opacities, most dense centrally (Fig. 6.48), increasing in density with age to form a reticular pattern. Histopathology, including electron microscopy, may be required for definitive distinction from Thiel–Behnke dystrophy in some cases.
  ○ Corneal sensation is reduced.
- **Treatment** is directed at the recurrent erosions. Excimer keratectomy achieves satisfactory control in some patients.

Thiel–Behnke corneal dystrophy

Also termed honeycomb-shaped corneal dystrophy and corneal basement dystrophy type II (CBD2); features are generally less severe than Reis–Bücklers.
- **Inheritance.** AD; gene *TGFB1* and at least one other.
- **Histology.** Bowman layer 'curly fibres' on electron microscopy.
- **Symptoms.** Recurrent erosions in childhood.
- **Signs.** Subepithelial opacities are less individually defined than the granular dystrophy-type lesions (see below) seen in Reis–Bücklers dystrophy. They develop in a network of tiny rings or honeycomb-like morphology, predominantly involving the central cornea (Fig. 6.49).
- **Treatment** is not always necessary.

Stromal dystrophies

Lattice corneal dystrophy, TGFB1 type

This is usually regarded as the classic form of lattice dystrophy. Clinical variants (e.g. IIIA – Fig. 6.50) associated with

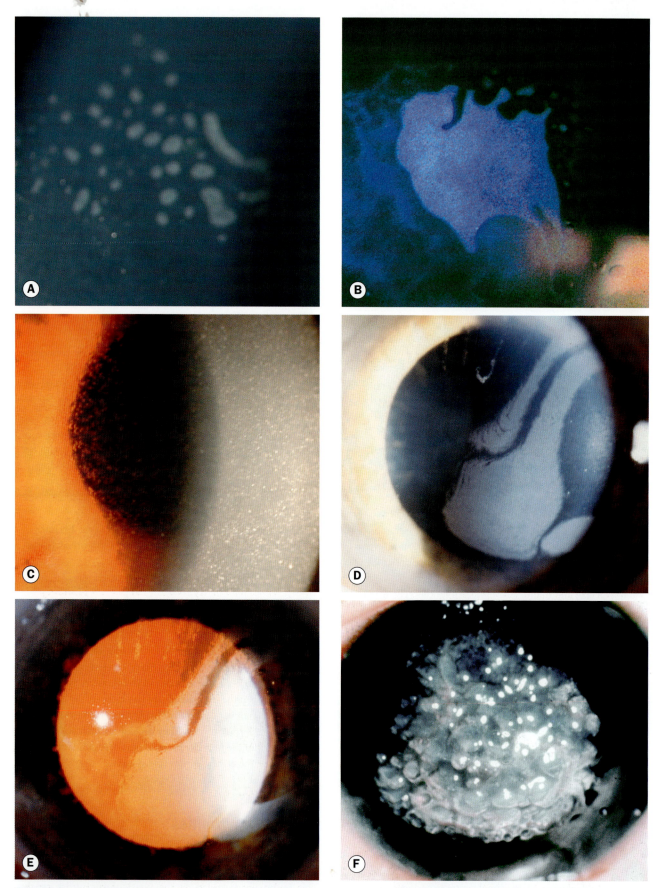

Fig. 6.47 Corneal epithelial and subepithelial dystrophies. **(A)** Cogan – dots and microcysts; **(B)** Cogan – map-like pattern; **(C)** Meesmann – myriad intraepithelial cysts; **(D)** Lisch – grey bands with a whorled configuration; **(E)** Lisch – retroillumination shows densely crowded microcysts; **(F)** gelatinous drop-like dystrophy

(Courtesy of R Fogla – fig. C; W Lisch – figs D and E; D Palay, from J Krachmer, M Mannis and E Holland, Cornea, Mosby 2005 – fig. F)

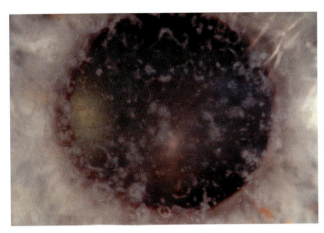

Fig. 6.48 Reis–Bücklers dystrophy – typical moderately discrete geographical opacities
(Courtesy of W Lisch)

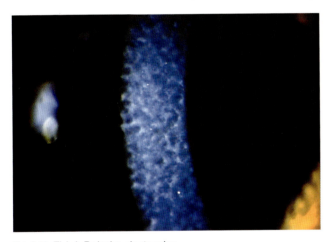

Fig. 6.49 Thiel–Behnke dystrophy

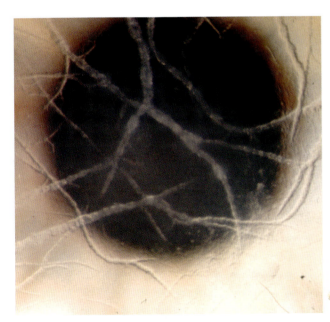

Fig. 6.50 Lattice dystrophy type IIIA

more than 25 heterozygous mutations in *TGFB1* have been described.

- **Inheritance.** AD; gene *TGFB1*.
- **Histology.** Amyloid, staining with Congo red (Fig. 6.51A) and exhibiting green birefringence with a polarizing filter.
- **Symptoms.** Recurrent erosions occur at the end of the first decade in the classic form, when typical stromal signs may not yet be present. Blurring may occur later.
- **Signs**
  ○ Refractile anterior stromal dots (Fig. 6.51B), coalescing into a relatively fine filamentous lattice that spreads gradually but spares the periphery (Fig. 6.51C).
  ○ A generalized stromal haze (Fig. 6.51D) may progressively impair vision.
  ○ Corneal sensation is reduced.
- **Treatment** by penetrating or deep lamellar keratoplasty is frequently required. Recurrence is not uncommon.

Lattice corneal dystrophy, gelsolin type

Also known as LCD2 and Meretoja syndrome, this is a systemic condition rather than a true corneal dystrophy.

- **Inheritance.** AD; gene *GSN*.
- **Histology** shows amyloid deposits in the corneal stroma.
- **Ocular symptoms.** Ocular irritation and late impairment of vision; erosions are rare.
- **Ocular signs**
  ○ Sparse stromal lattice lines spread centrally from the periphery.
  ○ Corneal sensation is impaired.
- **Systemic features.** Progressive cranial and peripheral neuropathy, mask-like facies and autonomic features. Homozygous disease is rare but severe.
- **Treatment.** Keratoplasty may rarely be required in later life.

Granular corneal dystrophy, type 1 (classic)

- **Inheritance.** AD; gene *TGFB1*. Homozygous disease gives more severe features.
- **Histology.** Amorphous hyaline deposits staining bright red with Masson trichrome (Fig. 6.52A).
- **Symptoms.** Glare and photophobia, with blurring as progression occurs. Recurrent erosions are uncommon.
- **Signs**
  ○ Discrete white central anterior stromal deposits resembling sugar granules, breadcrumbs or glass splinters separated by clear stroma (Fig. 6.52B).
  ○ Gradual increase in number and size of the deposits with deeper and outward spread, sparing the limbus (Fig. 6.52C).
  ○ Gradual confluence and diffuse haze leads to visual impairment (Fig. 6.52D).
  ○ Corneal sensation is impaired.
- **Treatment** by penetrating or deep lamellar keratoplasty is usually required by the fifth decade. Superficial recurrences may require repeated excimer laser keratectomy.

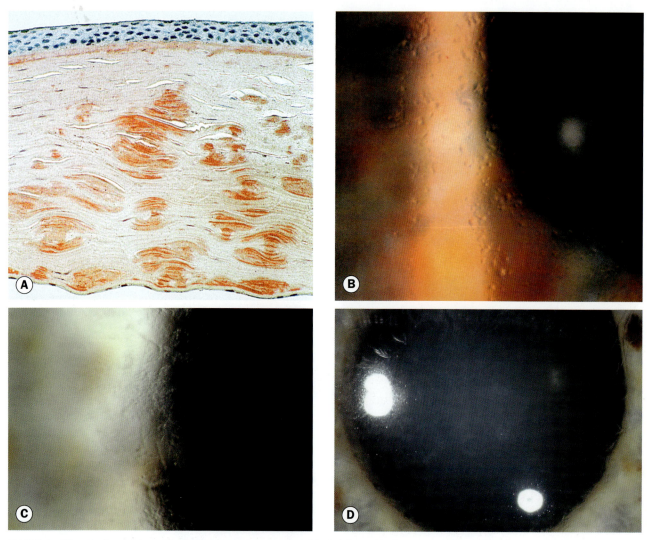

Fig. 6.51 Lattice dystrophy type 1. **(A)** Histology shows amyloid staining with Congo red; **(B)** glassy dots in the anterior stroma; **(C)** fine lattice lines; **(D)** early central stromal haze

(Courtesy of J Harry – fig. A; C Barry – figs C and D)

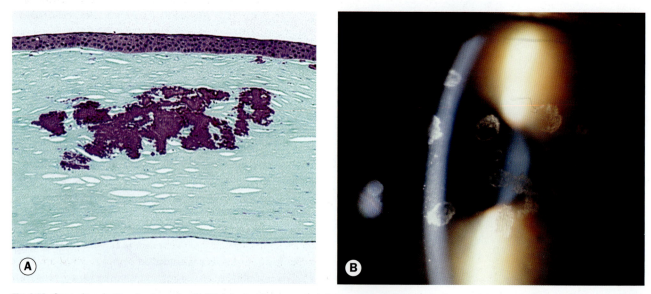

Fig. 6.52 Granular dystrophy type 1. **(A)** Histology shows red-staining material with Masson trichrome; **(B)** sharply demarcated crumb-like opacities;

Continued

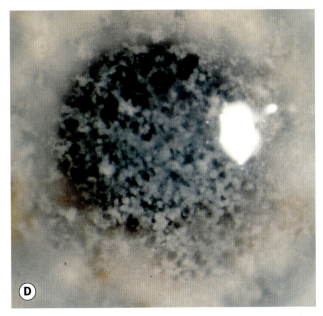

Fig. 6.52, Continued **(C)** increase in number and outward spread; **(D)** confluence
(Courtesy of J Harry – fig. A)

Granular corneal dystrophy, type 2

Also known as Avellino and combined granular-lattice dystrophy.

- **Inheritance.** AD; gene *TGFB1*.
- **Histology** shows both hyaline and amyloid.
- **Symptoms.** Recurrent erosions tend to be mild. Visual impairment is a later feature.
- **Signs** are usually present by the end of the first decade in heterozygotes. Fine superficial opacities progress to form stellate or annular lesions (Fig. 6.53), sometimes associated with deeper linear opacities.

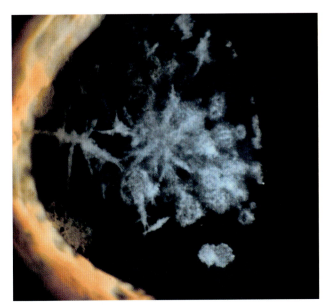

Fig. 6.53 Granular dystrophy type 2 (Avellino)
(Courtesy of W Lisch)

- **Treatment** is usually not required. Corneal trauma accelerates progression; refractive surgery is contraindicated.

Macular corneal dystrophy

- **Inheritance.** Autosomal recessive (AR); gene *CHST6*; the condition is relatively common in Iceland.
- **Histology.** Aggregations of glycosaminoglycans intra- and extracellularly; stain with Alcian blue and colloidal iron (Fig. 6.54A).
- **Symptoms.** Early (end of first decade) visual deterioration; recurrent erosions are very common.
- **Signs**
  ○ Dense but poorly delineated greyish-white spots centrally in the anterior stroma and peripherally in the posterior stroma (Figs 6.54B and C). There is no clear delineation between opacities, which may be elevated.
  ○ Progression of the lesions occurs in conjunction with anterior stromal haze, initially involving the central cornea (Fig. 6.54D).
  ○ There is eventual involvement of full-thickness stroma, extending to the limbus with no clear zone.
  ○ Thinning is a fairly early feature, with late thickening from oedema due to endothelial dysfunction.
  ○ Sensation is reduced.
- **Treatment.** Penetrating keratoplasty. Recurrence is common.

Schnyder (crystalline) corneal dystrophy

This is a disorder of corneal lipid metabolism, associated in some patients with systemic dyslipidaemia. The use of crystalline in the name is no longer recommended as corneal crystals are not a ubiquitous feature.

- **Inheritance.** AD; gene *UBIAD1*.
- **Histology.** Phospholipid and cholesterol deposits.

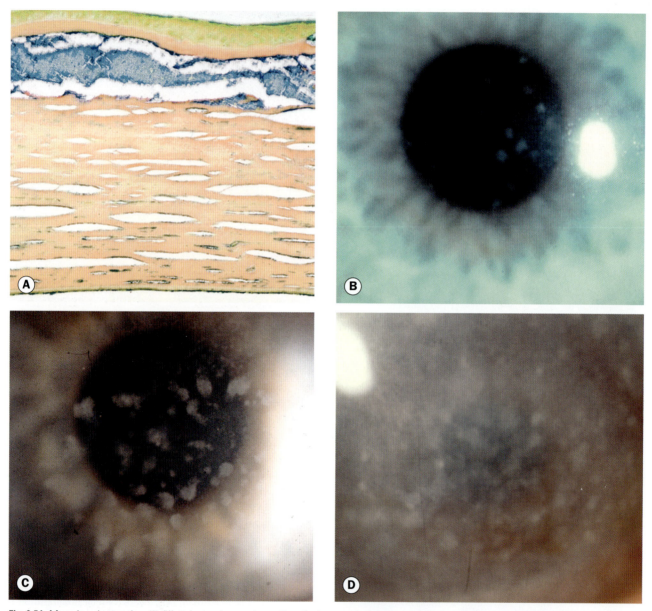

Fig. 6.54 Macular dystrophy. **(A)** Histology shows deposits of abnormal glycosaminoglycans that appear blue with colloidal iron stain; **(B)** and **(C)** poorly delineated deposits increasing in number; **(D)** increase in size and confluence of lesions, with stromal haze

(Courtesy of J Harry and G Misson, from Clinical Ophthalmic Pathology, Butterworth-Heinemann, 2001 – fig. A; A Ridgway – figs B, C and D)

- **Symptoms.** Visual impairment and glare.
- **Signs**
  - Central haze is an early feature (Fig. 6.55A), progressing to more widespread full-thickness involvement over time (Fig. 6.55B).
  - Subepithelial crystalline opacities are present in only around 50%.
  - Prominent corneal arcus is typical, and gradually progresses centrally leading to diffuse haze.
- Treatment is by excimer keratectomy or corneal transplantation.

François central cloudy dystrophy

It is not certain that this entity is a dystrophy; it may be clinically indistinguishable from the degeneration posterior crocodile shagreen.

- **Inheritance.** AD has been reported, but not clearly established.
- **Symptoms.** Almost always none.
- **Signs**
  - Cloudy greyish polygonal or rounded posterior stromal opacities, most prominent centrally (Fig. 6.56).
- Treatment is not required.

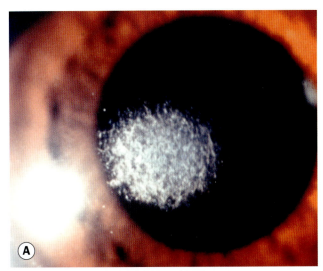

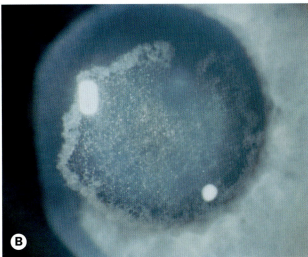

Fig. 6.55 Schnyder dystrophy. **(A)** Early lesion; **(B)** late more diffuse haze – a prominent arcus is present
(Courtesy of K Nischal – fig. A, W Lisch – fig. B)

Others

Congenital stromal corneal dystrophy, fleck corneal dystrophy, posterior amorphous corneal dystrophy and pre-Descemet corneal dystrophy.

Descemet membrane and endothelial dystrophies

Fuchs endothelial corneal dystrophy

This disorder is characterized by bilateral accelerated endothelial cell loss. It is more common in women and is associated with a slightly increased prevalence of open-angle glaucoma.

- **Inheritance.** Most are sporadic, with occasional AD inheritance. Mutation in *COL8A2* has been identified in an early-onset variant.

- **Symptoms.** Gradually worsening blurring, particularly in the morning, due to corneal oedema. Onset is usually in middle age or later.
- **Signs**
  - ○ Cornea guttata: the presence of irregular warts or 'excrescences' on Descemet membrane secreted by abnormal endothelial cells (Fig. 6.57A).
  - ○ Specular reflection shows tiny dark spots caused by disruption of the regular endothelial mosaic (Fig. 6.57B); progression occurs to a 'beaten metal' appearance (Fig. 6.57C).
  - ○ Endothelial decompensation gradually leads to central stromal oedema and blurred vision, worse in the morning.
  - ○ Epithelial oedema develops in more advanced cases, with the formation of microcysts and bullae (bullous keratopathy – Fig. 6.57D) accompanied by discomfort; rupture of bullae is associated with marked acute pain, thought to be due to the exposure of nerve fibres. Subepithelial scarring and peripheral vascularization may be seen in longstanding cases.
- **Treatment**
  - ○ Conservative options include topical sodium chloride 5% drops or ointment, reduction of intraocular pressure and use of a hair dryer for corneal dehydration.
  - ○ Ruptured bullae can be made more comfortable by the use of bandage contact lenses, cycloplegia, antibiotic ointment and lubricants. Anterior stromal puncture may be helpful.
  - ○ Posterior lamellar (e.g. Descemet membrane-stripping endothelial keratoplasty – DSAEK – or Descemet membrane endothelial keratoplasty – DMEK) and penetrating keratoplasty (see Ch. 7) have a high success rate.

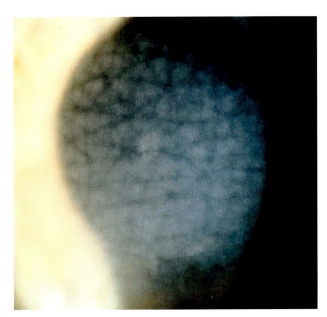

Fig. 6.56 Marked signs in François central cloudy dystrophy
(Courtesy of W Lisch)

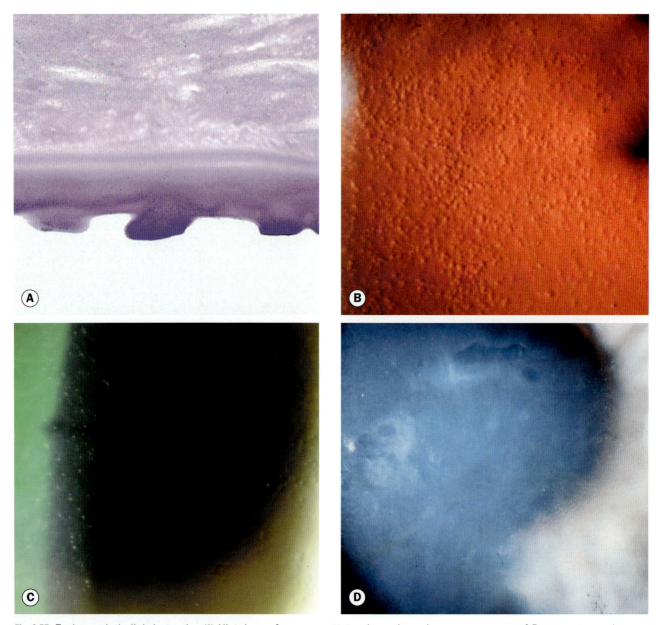

Fig. 6.57 Fuchs endothelial dystrophy. **(A)** Histology of cornea guttata shows irregular excrescences of Descemet membrane – PAS stain; **(B)** cornea guttata seen on specular reflection; **(C)** 'beaten-bronze' endothelium; **(D)** bullous keratopathy
(Courtesy of J Harry – fig. A; W Lisch – fig. D)

○ Options in eyes with poor visual potential include conjunctival flaps and amniotic membrane transplantation.

○ A promising new treatment, topical Rho-kinase inhibitor with prior transcorneal endothelial cryotherapy, seems to stimulate endothelial cell proliferation and improve function.

• **Cataract surgery** may worsen the corneal status via significant endothelial cell loss, and protective steps should be taken. A 'triple procedure' (combined cataract surgery, lens implantation and keratoplasty) may be considered in eyes with corneal oedema.

Posterior polymorphous corneal dystrophy

There are three forms of posterior polymorphous dystrophy, PPCD1–3. Associations include iris abnormalities, glaucoma and Alport syndrome. The pathological basis involves metaplasia of endothelial cells.

• **Inheritance** is usually AD; the gene *VSX1* has been implicated in PPCD1, PPCD2 is caused by mutations in *COL8A2*, and PPCD3 by *ZEB1* mutations.

• **Symptoms.** Typically absent, with incidental diagnosis.

• **Signs.** Subtle vesicular, band-like or diffuse endothelial lesions (Fig. 6.58)

• **Treatment** is not required.

Congenital hereditary endothelial dystrophy

Congenital hereditary endothelial dystrophy (CHED) is a rare dystrophy in which there is focal or diffuse thickening of Descemet membrane and endothelial degeneration. CHED2 is a more common, and more severe, form than CHED1, and is occasionally associated with deafness (Harboyan syndrome).

- **Inheritance**
  - CHED1 is AD with the gene locus on chromosome 20. CHED1 may not be distinct from PPCD.
  - CHED2 is AR; gene *SLC4A11*.
- **Symptoms.** Photophobia and watering are common in CHED1, but not in CHED2.
- **Signs**
  - Corneal clouding and thickening (Fig. 6.59) is neonatal in CHED2, and develops during the first year or two in CHED1.
  - Visual impairment is variable and visual acuity may surpass that expected from the corneal appearance.
  - Nystagmus is more common in CHED2.
- **Treatment.** Lamellar or penetrating keratoplasty.

CORNEAL DEGENERATIONS

Age-related degenerations

Arcus senilis

Arcus senilis (gerontoxon, arcus lipoides) is the most common peripheral corneal opacity; it frequently occurs without any predisposing systemic condition in elderly individuals, but may be associated with dyslipidaemia in younger patients (arcus juvenilis).

- **Signs**
  - Stromal lipid deposition, initially in the superior and inferior perilimbal cornea, progressing circumferentially to form a band about 1 mm wide (Fig. 6.60A).
  - The band is usually wider in the vertical than horizontal meridian.
  - The central border is diffuse and the peripheral edge is sharp and separated from the limbus by a clear zone that may undergo mild thinning.

Vogt limbal girdle

Vogt limbal girdle is an innocuous condition that is present in up to 60% of individuals over 40 years of age, more commonly in women. It consists of whitish crescentic limbal bands composed of chalk-like flecks centred at 9 and/or 3 o'clock, more often nasally. There may be irregular central extension. **Type I** may be a variant of band keratopathy, featuring a 'Swiss cheese' hole pattern and a clear area separating the lesion from the scleral margin (Fig. 6.60B). **Type II** is more prevalent, and is distinguished by the absence of holes and typically also of a juxtalimbal clear zone (Fig. 6.60C); histologically the changes in both are similar to pinguecula and pterygium.

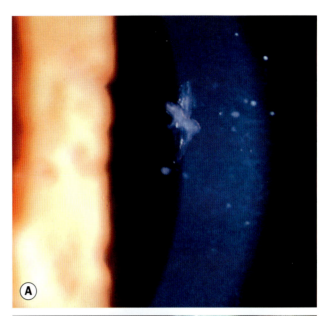
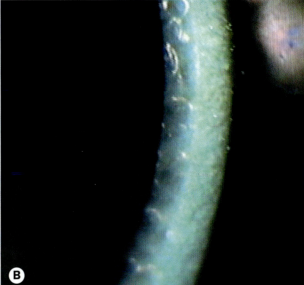
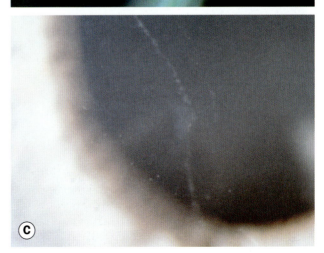

Fig. 6.58 Posterior polymorphous dystrophy. **(A)** Vesicles; **(B)** confluent vesicles; **(C)** band-like lesions
(Courtesy of W Lisch – fig. B)

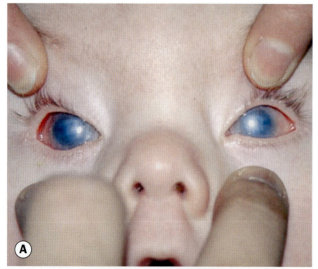

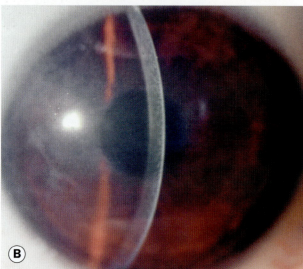

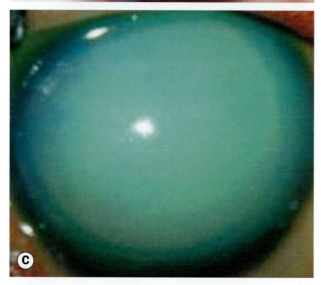

Fig. 6.59 Congenital hereditary endothelial dystrophy.
(A) Bilateral perinatal corneal opacification; **(B)** mild; **(C)** very severe
(Courtesy of K Nischal – figs A and C; J Krachmer, M Mannis and E Holland, from Cornea, Mosby 2005 – fig. B)

Cornea farinata

Cornea farinata is a visually insignificant condition characterized by bilateral, minute, flour-like deposits in the deep stroma, most prominent centrally (Fig. 6.60D).

Crocodile shagreen

Crocodile shagreen is characterized by asymptomatic, greyish–white, polygonal stromal opacities separated by relatively clear spaces (Fig. 6.60E). The opacities most frequently involve the anterior two-thirds of the stroma (anterior crocodile shagreen), although on occasion they may be found more posteriorly (posterior crocodile shagreen). It may be indistinguishable from François central cloudy dystrophy; conventionally the distinction is on the basis of François dystrophy being inherited, but this has been questioned.

Lipid keratopathy

- **Primary** lipid keratopathy is rare and occurs apparently spontaneously. It is characterized by white or yellowish, often with a crystalline element, stromal deposits consisting of cholesterol, fats and phospholipids and is not associated with vascularization (Fig. 6.61).
- **Secondary** lipid keratopathy is much more common and is associated with previous ocular injury or disease that has resulted in corneal vascularization. The most common causes are herpes simplex and herpes zoster keratitis (see Fig. 6.19A).
- **Treatment** is primarily aimed at medical control of the underlying inflammatory disease. Other options include:
  - Photocoagulation or needle cautery (suture needle grasped with cautery forceps) of feeder vessels.
  - Penetrating keratoplasty may be required in advanced but quiescent disease, though vascularization, thinning and hypoaesthesia may prejudice the outcome.

Band keratopathy

Band keratopathy consists of the age-related deposition of calcium salts in the Bowman layer, epithelial basement membrane and anterior stroma.

- **Causes**
  - Ocular. Chronic anterior uveitis (particularly in children), phthisis bulbi, silicone oil in the anterior chamber, chronic corneal oedema and severe chronic keratitis.
  - Age-related; affects otherwise healthy individuals.
  - Metabolic (metastatic calcification). This is rare and includes increased serum calcium and phosphorus, hyperuricaemia and chronic renal failure.
  - Hereditary causes include familial cases and ichthyosis.
- **Signs**
  - Peripheral interpalpebral calcification with clear cornea separating the sharp peripheral margins of the band from the limbus (Fig. 6.62A).

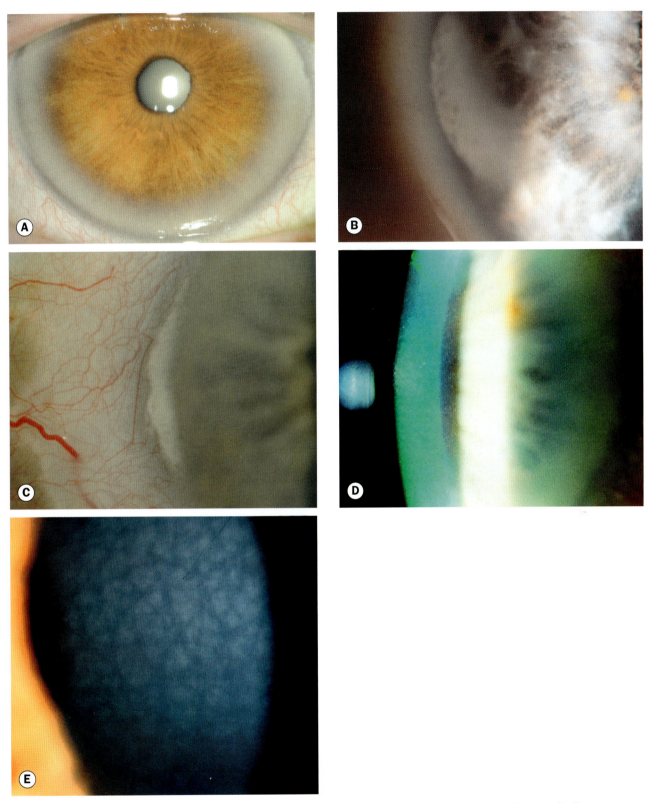

Fig. 6.60 Age-related degenerations. **(A)** Arcus senilis; **(B)** Vogt limbal girdle type I; **(C)** Vogt limbal girdle type II; **(D)** cornea farinata; **(E)** crocodile shagreen

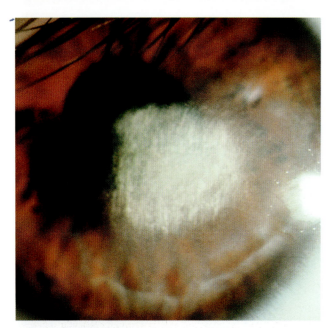

Fig. 6.61 Primary lipid keratopathy

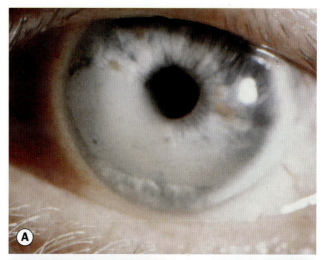

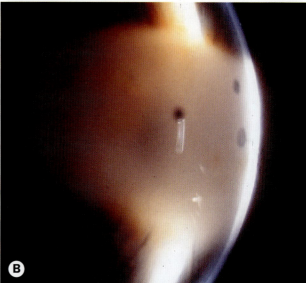

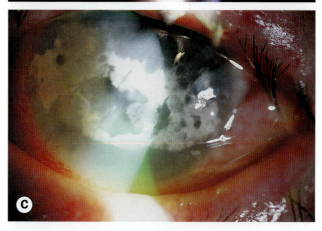

Fig. 6.62 Band keratopathy. **(A)** Moderate; **(B)** typical appearance with small holes; **(C)** advanced disease with overlying epithelial breakdown

○ Gradual central spread to form a band-like chalky plaque containing transparent small holes (Fig. 6.62B) and occasionally clefts.
○ Advanced lesions may become nodular and elevated with considerable discomfort due to epithelial breakdown (Fig. 6.62C).
- **Treatment** is indicated if vision is threatened or if the eye is uncomfortable. It is important to recognize and treat any underlying condition.
○ Chelation is simple and effective for relatively mild cases and is performed using a microscope. The corneal epithelium overlying the opacity and a solid layer of calcification are first scraped off with forceps and a scalpel blade (e.g. No. 15). The cornea is then rubbed with a cotton-tipped applicator dipped in a solution of ethylenediaminetetraacetic acid (EDTA) 1.5–3.0% until all calcium has been removed; adequate time (15–20 minutes) must be allowed for chelation to occur, and more than one session may be necessary. Re-epithelialization can take many days.
○ Other modalities: diamond burr, excimer laser keratectomy and lamellar keratoplasty.

Spheroidal degeneration

Spheroidal degeneration (Labrador keratopathy, climatic droplet keratopathy) typically occurs in men whose working lives are spent outdoors. Ultraviolet exposure is likely to be an aetiological factor. The condition is relatively innocuous but visual impairment may rarely occur. A secondary form can follow inflammation or injury.

- **Histology.** Irregular proteinaceous deposits in the anterior stroma that replace the Bowman layer.

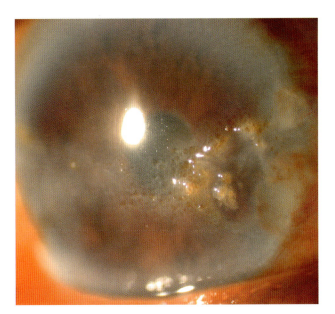

Fig. 6.63 Spheroidal degeneration
(Courtesy of R Fogla)

- **Signs**
  - Amber-coloured granules in the superficial stroma of the peripheral interpalpebral cornea.
  - Increasing opacification, coalescence and central spread.
  - Advanced lesions commonly protrude above the corneal surface (Fig. 6.63) and the surrounding stroma is often hazy; the conjunctiva can be involved.
- **Treatment.** Protection against ultraviolet damage with sunglasses, and superficial keratectomy or lamellar keratoplasty in a minority.

Salzmann nodular degeneration

Salzmann nodular degeneration consists of nodules of hyaline tissue, usually located anterior to the Bowman layer. It can occur in any form of chronic corneal irritation or inflammation such as trachoma, dry eye, chronic blepharitis and chronic allergic keratoconjunctivitis.

- **Signs**
  - Superficial stromal opacities progressing to elevated whitish or blue–grey nodular lesions that may be round or elongated (Fig. 6.64).
  - The base of a nodule may be associated with pannus and epithelial iron deposition.
- **Treatment** consists mainly of lubrication together with control of the cause. Removal is via manual superficial keratectomy – the lesions can often be 'peeled' away and the surface flattened with a diamond burr. Adjunctive mitomycin C applied for 10 seconds with a sponge may reduce the recurrence rate, though some authorities restrict its use to reoperations. Excimer laser phototherapeutic keratectomy or lamellar keratoplasty are occasionally required.

Advancing wave-like epitheliopathy

Advancing wave-like epitheliopathy (AWE) is characterized by an irregular advancing epithelial plaque encroaching gradually on the cornea, typically originating at the superior limbus (Fig. 6.65) and sometimes extending circumferentially from a pterygium. Topical fluorescein generally demonstrates the lesion well. Irritation and redness are common; the vision may be affected with central involvement. Reported risk factors include contact lens wear, certain contact lens solutions, topical glaucoma medication, prior ocular surgery and some skin conditions such as rosacea. Treatment of the cause may be curative, but otherwise is with 1% silver nitrate solution to the adjacent limbus or cryotherapy (1–2 seconds twice) to the limbus and abnormal tissue. Distinction from neoplasia may occasionally warrant impression cytology or excision biopsy.

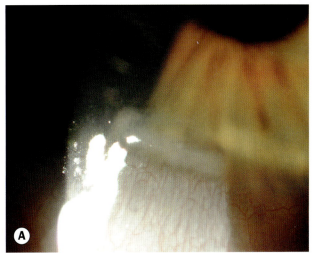

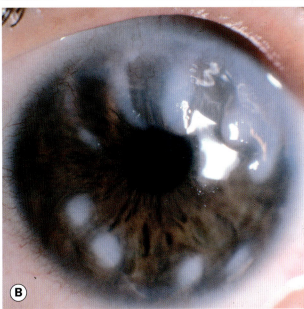

Fig. 6.64 Salzmann nodular degeneration. **(A)** Solitary early elongated lesion; **(B)** multiple lesions
(Courtesy of R Bates – fig. B)

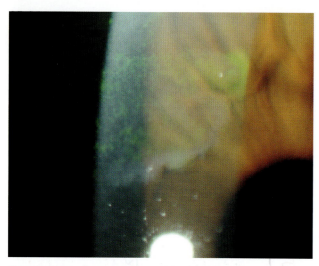

Fig. 6.65 Advancing wave-like epitheliopathy

METABOLIC KERATOPATHIES

Cystinosis

Cystinosis is a rare AR (gene: *CTNS*) lysosomal storage disorder characterized by widespread tissue deposition of cystine crystals, leading to paediatric renal failure and a range of other severe systemic problems. Non-nephropathic (ocular), nephropathic and intermediate forms can occur. Keratopathy may develop in the first year, with progressive deposition of crystals in the cornea (Fig. 6.66A) and conjunctiva associated with photophobia, epithelial erosions and visual impairment. Systemic treatment is with cysteamine, which can be given in eye drop form to reverse corneal crystal formation.

Mucopolysaccharidoses

The mucopolysaccharidoses (MPS) are a group of lysosomal storage disorders involving enzyme dysfunction along the pathways for breakdown of glycosaminoglycans, long chain carbohydrates formerly known as mucopolysaccharides. Altered metabolites accumulate intracellularly in various tissues. Inheritance is mainly AR. Systemic features vary with the type of MPS, but can include facial coarseness, skeletal anomalies, heart disease and learning difficulties. Keratopathy comprises punctate corneal opacification and diffuse stromal haze (Fig. 6.66B), and occurs in all MPS except Hunter and Sanfilippo. Other ocular features may include pigmentary retinopathy and optic atrophy.

Wilson disease

Wilson disease (hepatolenticular degeneration) is a rare condition involving the widespread abnormal deposition of copper in tissues. It is caused by a deficiency of caeruloplasmin, the major copper-carrying blood protein. Presentation is with liver disease, basal ganglia dysfunction or psychiatric disturbances. A Kayser–Fleischer ring is present in 95% of patients with neurological signs, and consists of a brownish-yellow zone of fine copper dusting in

peripheral Descemet membrane (Fig. 6.66C); this is best detected on gonioscopy when subtle. The deposits are preferentially distributed in the vertical meridian and may disappear with penicillamine therapy. Anterior capsular 'sunflower' cataract is seen in some patients.

Lecithin-cholesterol-acyltransferase deficiency

Lecithin-cholesterol-acyltransferase (LCAT) deficiency is a disorder of lipoprotein metabolism that has complete (Norum disease, with systemic manifestations including renal failure) and partial (fish eye disease, causing only corneal opacification) forms that are both AR (gene: *LCAT*). Keratopathy is characterized by numerous minute greyish dots throughout the stroma, often concentrated in the periphery in an arcus-like configuration (Fig. 6.66D).

Immunoprotein deposition

Diffuse or focal immunoprotein deposition is a relatively uncommon manifestation of several systemic diseases, including multiple myeloma, Waldenström macroglobulinaemia, monoclonal gammopathy of unknown cause, some lymphoproliferative disorders and leukaemia. Corneal involvement may be the earliest manifestation. Bands of punctate flake-like opacities are seen, mostly at the level of the posterior stroma (Fig. 6.66E). Treatment is that of the underlying disease; severe corneal involvement may require corneal transplantation.

Tyrosinaemia type 2

Tyrosinaemia type 2 (oculocutaneous tyrosinaemia, Richner–Hanhart syndrome) is a very rare AR disease (gene: *TAT*) in which an enzyme deficiency leads to elevated plasma tyrosine levels. Ocular involvement may occasionally be the presenting feature. Painful palmar and plantar hyperkeratotic lesions and variable central nervous system involvement are seen. A bilateral pseudo-dendritic keratitis with crystalline edges often begins in childhood and causes photophobia, watering and redness.

Fabry disease

Fabry disease is an X-linked lysosomal storage disorder caused by a deficiency of the enzyme alpha-galactosidase A that leads to abnormal tissue accumulation of a glycolipid. All males with the gene develop the disease, and some heterozygous females. Systemic features include periodic burning pain in the extremities (acroparaesthesia) and GI tract, angiokeratomas (Fig. 6.67A), cardiomyopathy and renal disease. Ocular manifestations include white to golden-brown corneal opacities in a vortex pattern (75%) that may be the first feature of the disease (Fig. 6.67B), facilitating early intervention; wedge- or spoke-shaped posterior cataract (Fabry cataract); conjunctival vascular tortuosity (corkscrew vessels) and aneurysm formation (Fig. 6.67C); and retinal vascular tortuosity.

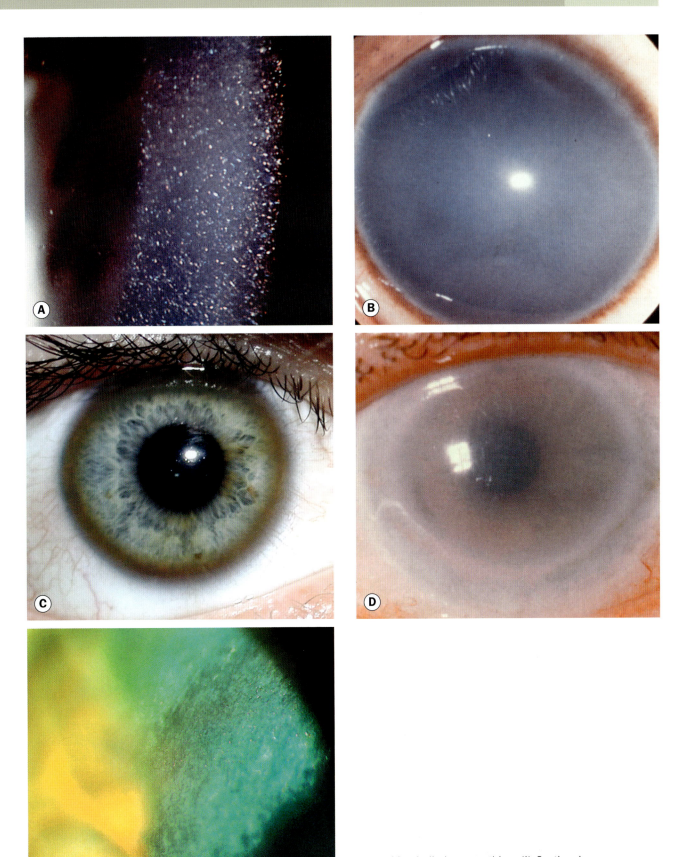

Fig. 6.66 Metabolic keratopathies. **(A)** Cystinosis;
(B) typical appearance in a mucopolysaccharidosis;
(C) Wilson disease; **(D)** LCAT (see text) deficiency;
(E) immunoprotein deposits

(Courtesy of L Merin – fig. A; S Chen – fig. C; W Lisch – fig. D)

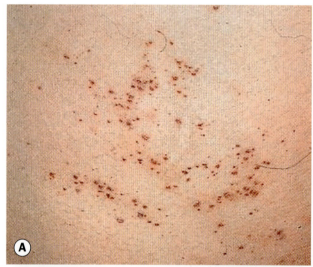

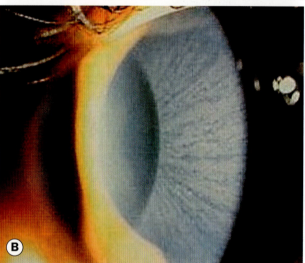

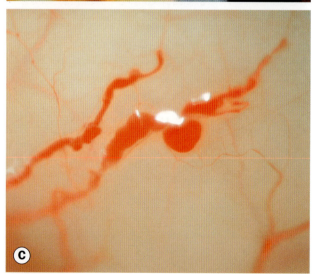

Fig. 6.67 Fabry disease. **(A)** Angiokeratomas; **(B)** vortex keratopathy; **(C)** conjunctival vessel tortuosity and aneurysms

CONTACT LENSES

Therapeutic uses

The risks of fitting a contact lens to an already compromised eye are greater than with lens wear for cosmetic reasons. The benefit–risk balance should be considered in each case individually, with education and regular review to ensure early diagnosis and treatment of complications. The choice of lens type is dictated by the nature of the ocular pathology.

Optical

Optical indications are aimed at improving visual acuity when this cannot be achieved by spectacles in the following situations:

- **Irregular astigmatism** associated with keratoconus can be corrected with rigid contact lenses after spectacles have failed and before corneal grafting becomes necessary. Patients with astigmatism following corneal grafting may also benefit.
- **Superficial corneal irregularities** can be neutralized by rigid contact lenses, which provide a smoother and optically more regular surface. Visual acuity can only be substantially improved if irregularities are not too severe.
- **Anisometropia** in which binocular vision cannot be achieved by spectacles due to aniseikonia, such as may occur following monocular cataract surgery with high refractive error correction.

Promotion of epithelial healing

- **Persistent epithelial defects** often heal if the regenerating corneal epithelium is protected from the constant rubbing of the lids, allowing the development of hemidesmosomal attachments to the basement membrane.
- **Recurrent corneal erosions** associated with basement membrane dystrophy may require long-term contact lens wear to reduce the recurrence rate. In post-traumatic cases, lens wear can usually be discontinued after a few weeks. Lens wear also improves comfort.

Pain relief

- **Bullous keratopathy** can be managed with soft bandage lenses that relieve pain by protecting the exposed corneal nerve endings from the shearing forces of the lids during blinking. The lens may also flatten bullae into diffuse fine epithelial cysts.
- **Filamentary keratopathy** resistant to topical treatment will usually achieve some relief from soft contact lens wear.
- **Other indications** include Thygeson superficial punctate keratitis and protection of the corneal epithelium from aberrant lashes in trichiasis; they can also be used as a temporizing measure in entropion prior to definitive surgery.

Preservation of corneal integrity

- **A descemetocoele** can be temporarily capped with a tight-fitting, large-diameter soft or scleral lens to prevent perforation and encourage healing.
- **Splinting** and apposition of the edges of a small corneal wound can be achieved by means of a contact lens. Slightly larger perforations may be sealed with glue followed by insertion of a bandage contact lens to both protect the glue and prevent irritation of the lids from the glue's irregular surface.

Miscellaneous indications

- **Ptosis props** to support the upper lids in patients with ocular myopathies.
- **Maintenance of the fornices** to prevent symblepharon formation in cicatrizing conjunctivitis.
- **Drug delivery** enhancement by a hydrogel lens imbued with topical medication is an occasional indication.

Complications

Mechanical and hypoxic keratitis

- **Pathogenesis.** Insufficient oxygen transmission through the lens. A tightly fitting contact lens that does not move with blinking will impair tear circulation under the lens. This is exacerbated by lid closure if the lens is worn during sleep. Hypoxia leads to anaerobic metabolism and lactic acidosis that inhibits the normal barrier and pump mechanisms of the cornea.
- **Superficial punctate keratitis** is the most common complication. The pattern may give a clue as to the aetiology. For example, staining at 3 and 9 o'clock is associated with incomplete blinking and drying in rigid lens wearers.
- **The tight lens syndrome** is characterized by indentation and staining of the conjunctival epithelium in a ring around the cornea.
- **Acute hypoxia** is characterized by epithelial microcysts (Fig. 6.68A) and necrosis, and endothelial blebs. Very painful macroerosions may develop several hours after lenses are removed following a period of overwear.
- **Chronic hypoxia** may result in vascularization and lipid deposition (Fig. 6.68B); superficial peripheral neovascularization of <1.5 mm is common in myopic contact lens wearers and can be monitored.
- **Treatment** depends on the cause but may involve:
  - Increasing oxygen permeability by refitting with a thinner lens, a gas permeable rigid lens or a silicone hydrogel soft lens.
  - Modifying lens fit to increase movement.
  - Reducing lens wearing time.

Immune response (hypersensitivity) keratitis

A hypersensitivity response to bacterial antigen or the chemicals used in lens care can lead to the development of sterile marginal corneal infiltrates; the mechanism is thought to be similar to that of marginal keratitis.

- **Signs.** Mildly red eye associated with infiltrates, often marginally located, with no or minimal epithelial defects (Fig. 6.68C).
- **Treatment** involves cessation of lens wear until resolution occurs. Topical antibiotics and steroids may be used in some cases, but if the diagnosis is uncertain, treatment should be that of bacterial keratitis.

Toxic keratitis

- **Pathogenesis.** Acute chemical injury may be caused by inadvertently placing a contact lens on the eye without first neutralizing toxic cleaning agents such as hydrogen peroxide. Chronic toxicity can result from long-term exposure to disinfecting preservatives such as thiomersal or benzalkonium chloride.
- **Signs**
  - Acute pain, redness, and chemosis on lens insertion, which may take 48 hours to resolve completely.
  - Vascularization and scarring of the cornea (Fig. 6.68D) and limbal conjunctiva in chronic cases.
- **Treatment** may involve switching to daily disposable lenses or using a non-preserved disinfectant such as hydrogen peroxide.

Suppurative keratitis

Contact lens wear is the greatest risk factor for the development of bacterial keratitis; the risk is probably least for rigid contact lenses. Bacteria in the tear film are normally unable to bind to the corneal epithelium, but following an abrasion and in association with hypoxia, they can attach and invade the epithelium. Micro-organisms may also be introduced onto the corneal surface by poor lens hygiene or the use of tap water for rinsing.

Contact lens-associated giant papillary conjunctivitis

See Chapter 5.

CONGENITAL ANOMALIES OF THE CORNEA AND GLOBE

Microcornea

The normal neonatal corneal diameter is 10 mm, and the adult diameter of 12 mm is usually reached by the age of 2 years. Micro-cornea is a rare autosomal dominant (sometimes sporadic) uni-lateral or bilateral condition in which the horizontal corneal diameter is 10 mm or less over 2 years of age (Fig. 6.69A), or less than 9 mm in the newborn; there may be hypermetropia and a shallow anterior chamber but other dimensions are normal. Ocular associations include glaucoma (angle-closure and open-angle), congenital cataract, leukoma (Fig. 6.69B), persistent fetal vasculature, coloboma, optic nerve hypoplasia, aniridia and

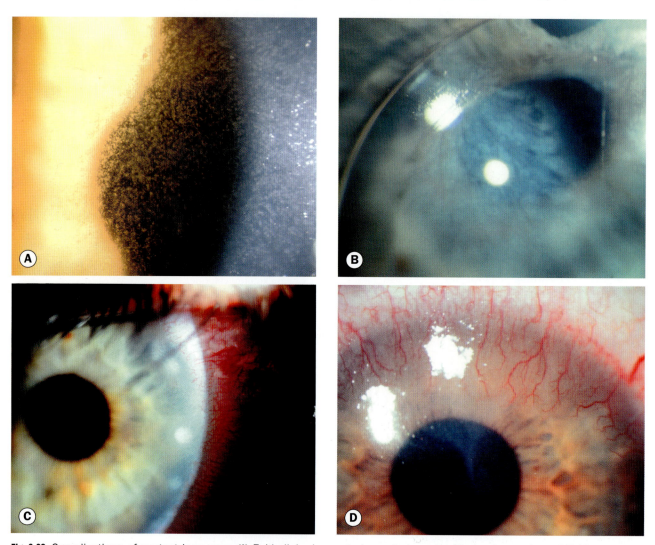

Fig. 6.68 Complications of contact lens wear. **(A)** Epithelial microcysts in acute hypoxia; **(B)** ghost vessels and lipid deposition from chronic hypoxia; **(C)** marginal infiltrates in immune response keratitis; **(D)** vascularization and scarring in chronic toxic keratitis

(Courtesy of S Tuft – figs A and B; J Dart – fig. D)

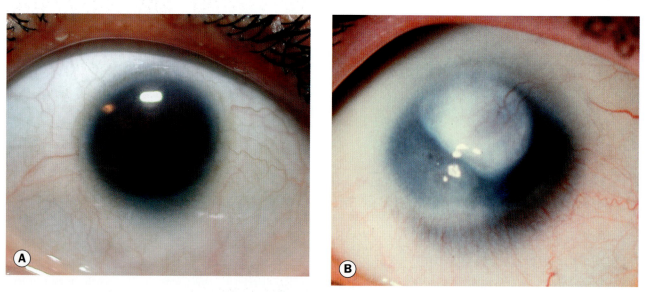

Fig. 6.69 (A) Severe microcornea; **(B)** microcornea and corneal opacity – leukoma

(Courtesy of R Fogla – fig. A)

nanophthalmos. Systemic associations have been reported. Refractive error and amblyopia should be managed appropriately.

Microphthalmos

Microphthalmos (microphthalmia – Fig. 6.70A) is a condition in which the entire eye is small, with an axial length at least two standard deviations below the mean for age. Simple or pure microphthalmos (nanophthalmos – see below) refers to an eye that is structurally normal apart from a short length, and complex microphthalmos to eyes with other features of dysgenesis; a coloboma (Fig. 6.70B) or orbital cyst (Fig. 6.70C) and a range of other ocular abnormalities. It may be unilateral or bilateral; when unilateral, abnormalities may be present in the fellow eye. Vision is variably affected, in conjunction with severity. It is typically sporadic; mutations in numerous genes have been implicated. Around 50% of cases may be associated with systemic abnormalities, including of the central nervous system. Potential environmental causes include fetal alcohol syndrome and intrauterine infections.

Nanophthalmos

In nanophthalmos (simple microphthalmos) the entire eye is small but is structurally normal; both eyes are usually affected. Ocular associations include uveal effusions associated with thickened sclera, glaucoma (especially angle-closure as the lens is large relative to the size of the eye), hypermetropia, ametropia, often bilateral, amblyopia and strabismus. In childhood, management of refractive error and amblyopia are critical. Cataract surgery poses particular technical problems; a custom high-power lens implant may be considered to avoid polypseudophakia with its attendant risk of precipitating angle-closure.

Anophthalmos

Anophthalmos (anophthalmia) refers to the complete absence of any visible globe structure (Fig. 6.71A), though a microphthalmic remnant or cyst may be present (Fig. 6.71B). It is associated with other abnormalities such as absence of extraocular muscles, a short conjunctival sac and microblepharon. Causative factors are probably broadly similar to those of microphthalmos.

Megalocornea

Megalocornea is a rare bilateral non-progressive condition that is usually X-linked recessive; 90% of affected individuals are male. The adult horizontal corneal diameter is 13 mm or more, with a very deep anterior chamber (Fig. 6.72A). There is typically high myopia and astigmatism but normal corrected visual acuity. Lens subluxation may occur due to zonular stretching, and pigment dispersion syndrome (see Ch. 10) is very common (Fig. 6.72B). Numerous systemic associations have been reported.

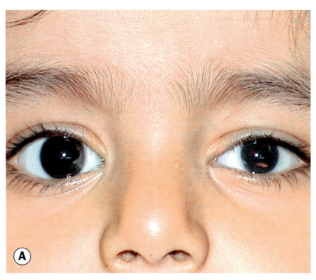

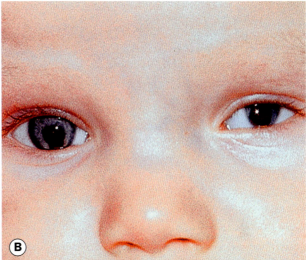

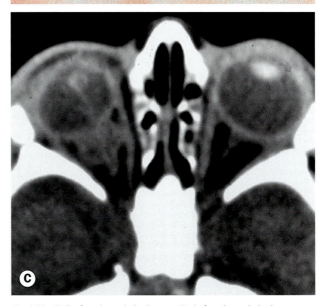

Fig. 6.70 (A) Left microphthalmos; **(B)** left microphthalmos and bilateral iris colobomas; **(C)** axial CT shows right microphthalmos with cyst
(Courtesy of L MacKeen – fig. C)

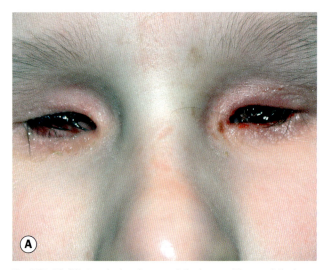

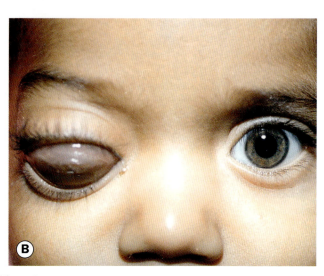

Fig. 6.71 (A) Bilateral simple anophthalmos; **(B)** anophthalmos with cyst
(Courtesy of U Raina – fig. B)

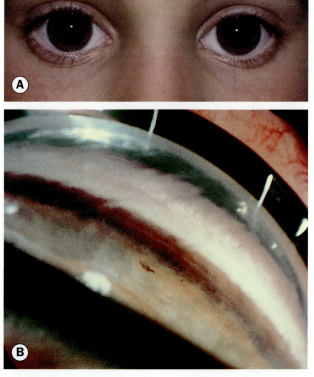

Fig. 6.72 Megalocornea. **(A)** Clinical appearance; **(B)** trabecular hyperpigmentation due to pigment dispersion
(Courtesy of C Barry – fig. A)

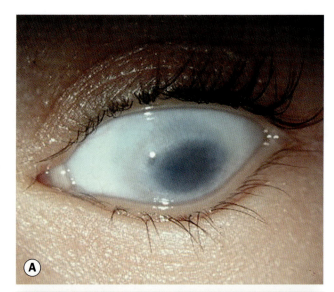

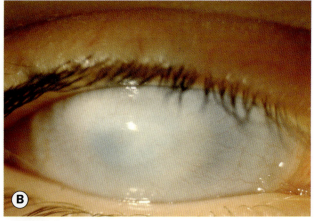

Fig. 6.73 Sclerocornea. **(A)** Moderate; **(B)** severe
(Courtesy of K Nischal – fig. A)

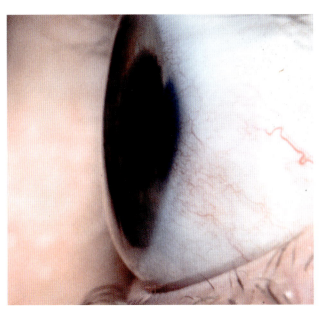

Fig. 6.74 Cornea plana
(Courtesy of R Visser)

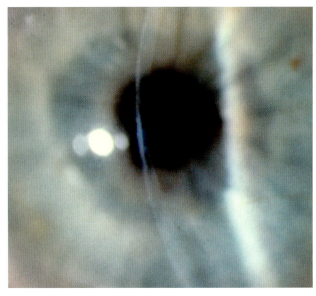

Fig. 6.76 Posterior keratoconus
(Courtesy of S Johns)

Sclerocornea

Sclerocornea is a very rare, usually bilateral, condition that may be associated with cornea plana (see below). Sporadic cases are common, but a milder form can be inherited as AD and a more severe form as AR. Peripheral corneal opacification, with no visible border between the sclera and cornea, confers the

appearance of apparently reduced corneal diameter in mild–moderate disease (Fig. 6.73A); occasionally the entire cornea is involved (Fig. 6.73B).

Cornea plana

This is an extremely rare bilateral condition in which the cornea is flatter than normal (Fig. 6.74) – the radius of curvature is larger. There is a corresponding reduction in refractive power resulting in high hypermetropia. Two forms are described, cornea plana 1 (CNA1) being milder than cornea plana 2. Associated ocular abnormalities are common.

Keratectasia

Keratectasia is a very rare, usually unilateral, condition thought to be the result of intrauterine keratitis and perforation. It is characterized by protuberance between the eyelids of a severely opacified and sometimes vascularized cornea (Fig. 6.75). It is often associated with raised intraocular pressure.

Posterior keratoconus

Posterior keratoconus is a sporadic condition in which there is unilateral non-progressive increase in curvature of the posterior corneal surface. The anterior surface is normal and visual acuity relatively unimpaired because of the similar refractive indices of the cornea and aqueous humour. Generalized (involvement of the entire posterior corneal surface) and localized (paracentral or central posterior indentation – Fig. 6.76) types are described.

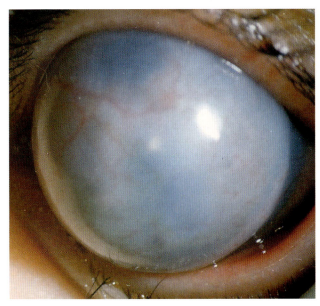

Fig. 6.75 Keratectasia

Chapter 7

Corneal and refractive surgery

KERATOPLASTY

Introduction

Corneal transplantation (grafting) refers to the replacement of diseased host corneal tissue by healthy donor cornea. A corneal graft (keratoplasty) may be partial-thickness (anterior or posterior lamellar) or full-thickness (penetrating).

General indications

- **Optical** keratoplasty is performed to improve vision. Important indications include keratoconus, scarring, corneal dystrophies (Fig. 7.1A), pseudophakic bullous keratopathy and corneal degenerations.
- **Tectonic** grafting may be carried out to restore or preserve corneal integrity in eyes with severe structural changes such as thinning with descemetocoele (US spelling – descemetocele; Fig. 7.1B).
- **Therapeutic** corneal transplantation facilitates removal of infected corneal tissue in eyes unresponsive to antimicrobial therapy (Fig. 7.1C).
- **Cosmetic** grafting may be performed to improve the appearance of the eye, but is a rare indication.

Donor tissue

Donor tissue should be removed within 12–24 hours of death. There is an attempt to age-match donors and recipients; corneas from infants (3 years and under) are used only very occasionally, even for paediatric transplants, as they are associated with surgical, refractive and rejection problems. Most corneas are stored in coordinating 'eye banks' prior to transplantation, where pre-release evaluation includes medical history review and donor blood screening to exclude contraindications, and microscopic examination of the cornea including endothelial cell count determination. Corneas are preserved in hypothermic storage (up to 7–10 days) or organ culture medium (4 weeks) until needed; culture allows extended testing for infective contamination. Contraindications to ocular tissue donation are set out below, though there is international variation and the list is not exhaustive:

- Death from unknown cause.
- Certain systemic infections such as human immunodeficiency virus (HIV), viral hepatitis, syphilis, congenital rubella, tuberculosis, septicaemia and active malaria.
- Prior high-risk behaviour for HIV and hepatitis such as sex with someone HIV-positive, men who have sex with men, intravenous drug abuse and prostitution.
- Within the last 12 months: sex with someone who has engaged in high-risk behaviour, or who lives in parts of Africa, or who has received blood clotting factor concentrates; tattooing, acupuncture or ear/body piercing; imprisonment.
- Infectious and possibly infectious diseases of the central nervous system, such as Creutzfeldt–Jakob disease, systemic

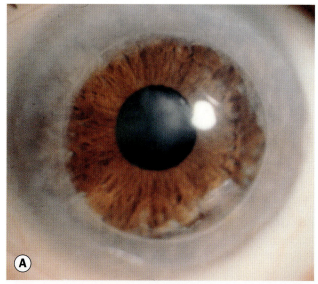

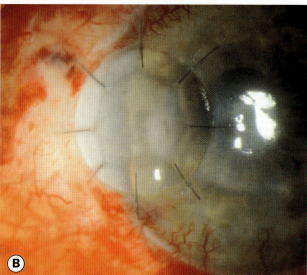

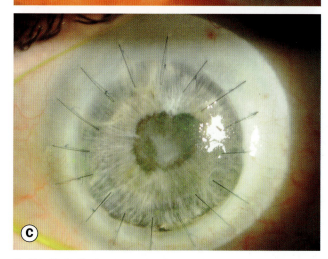

Fig. 7.1 (A) Optical penetrating keratoplasty for macular corneal dystrophy; **(B)** tectonic lamellar patch graft for descemetocoele; **(C)** penetrating keratoplasty for pseudomonas keratitis – a dense cataract and posterior synechiae are visible
(Courtesy of S Tuft – fig. B)

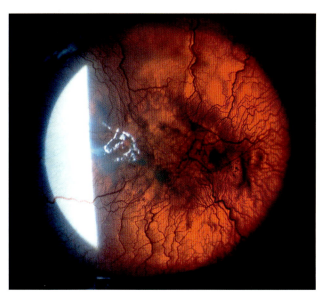

Fig. 7.2 Retroillumination of heavily vascularized cornea resulting from recurrent herpes simplex keratitis
(Courtesy of C Barry)

sclerosing panencephalitis, progressive multifocal leukoencephalopathy, encephalitis, Alzheimer disease and other dementias, Parkinson disease, multiple sclerosis and motor neurone disease.
- Receipt of a transplanted organ.
- Receipt of human pituitary-derived growth hormone.
- Brain or spinal surgery before 1992.
- Most haematological malignancies.
- Ocular disease such as inflammation and disease likely to compromise graft outcome, some malignant ocular tumours (e.g. retinoblastoma) and corneal refractive surgery.

Recipient prognostic factors

The following host factors may adversely affect the prognosis of a corneal graft and if possible should be optimized prior to surgery. In general, the most favourable cases are keratoconus, localized scars and dystrophies.
- Severe stromal vascularization (Fig. 7.2), absence of corneal sensation, extreme thinning at the proposed host–graft junction and active corneal inflammation.
- Abnormalities of the eyelids, such as blepharitis, ectropion, entropion and trichiasis; these should be addressed before surgery.
- Recurrent or progressive forms of conjunctival inflammation, such as atopic conjunctivitis and ocular cicatricial pemphigoid.
- Tear film dysfunction.
- Anterior synechiae.
- Uncontrolled glaucoma.
- Uveitis.

Penetrating keratoplasty

Component layer grafting of the cornea is increasingly utilized, but full-thickness keratoplasty remains commonly performed and

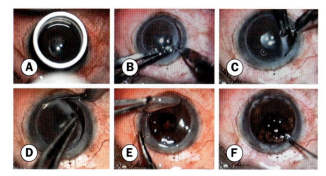

Fig. 7.3 Excision of host tissue. **(A)** Partial-thickness trephination; **(B)** incision into the anterior chamber; **(C)**, **(D)** and **(E)** completion of excision; **(F)** injection of viscoelastic bed
(Courtesy of R Fogla)

is the appropriate procedure for disease involving all layers of the cornea. Key surgical points include:
- A common graft size is 7.5 mm; smaller grafts may give high astigmatism, and larger diameters are associated with an increasing tendency to peripheral anterior synechiae formation and raised intraocular pressure (IOP).
- The donor button is usually about 0.25 mm larger in diameter than the host site.
- Preparation of donor cornea should always precede excision of host tissue (Fig. 7.3), in case a problem with the former means that the surgery cannot be completed.
- Either mechanically guided manual or automated (including laser) trephination is commonly used.
- The graft may be secured with either interrupted (see Fig. 7.1C) or continuous (Fig. 7.4) suture techniques, or a combination of both.

Postoperative management

- **Topical steroids** (e.g. prednisolone acetate 1%, dexamethasone phosphate 0.1%) are used to decrease the risk of immunological graft rejection. Initial administration

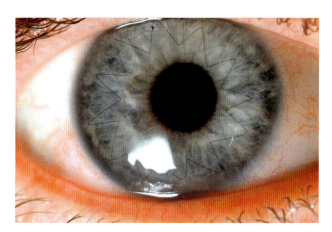

Fig. 7.4 Penetrating keratoplasty secured by continuous sutures
(Courtesy of C Barry)

is typically every 2 hours with gradual tapering depending on the likelihood of rejection and clinical progress. Long-term instillation at low intensity, such as once daily for a year or more, is usual.

- **Other immunosuppressants** such as oral azathioprine and topical and systemic ciclosporin are usually reserved for high-risk patients.
- **Cycloplegia** (e.g. homatropine 2% twice daily) is typically used for 1–2 weeks.
- **Oral aciclovir** may be used in the context of pre-existing herpes simplex keratitis to minimize the risk of recurrence.
- **Monitoring of IOP.** Applanation tonometry is relatively unreliable so measurement is commonly performed during the early postoperative period with a non-applanation method.
- **Removal of sutures** is performed when the graft–host junction has healed. This is often after 12–18 months, although in elderly patients it may take much longer.

Removal of broken or loose individual sutures is performed as soon as identified, to avoid promoting rejection.

Postoperative complications

- **Early** complications include persistent epithelial defects, loose or protruding sutures (risk of infection – Fig. 7.5A, marked sterile reaction, papillary hypertrophy), wound leak (sometimes with flat anterior chamber or iris prolapse), uveitis, elevation of intraocular pressure, traumatic graft rupture (Fig. 7.5B), cystoid macular oedema, microbial keratitis (Fig. 7.5C), endophthalmitis (Fig. 7.5D) and rejection (see below). A rare complication is a fixed dilated pupil (Urrets–Zavalia syndrome).
- **Late** complications include astigmatism, recurrence of underlying disease, late wound dehiscence, retrocorneal membrane formation, glaucoma, rejection (see below) and failure without rejection.

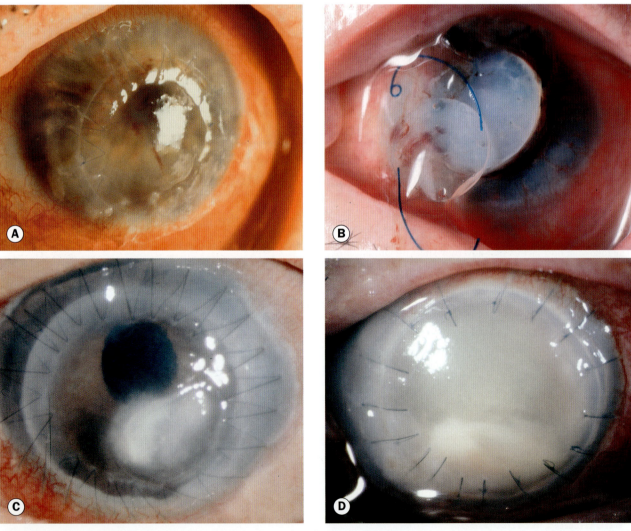

Fig. 7.5 Early postoperative complications. **(A)** Loose continuous suture with probable infection and rejection; **(B)** traumatic graft rupture and extrusion of intraocular lens implant; **(C)** microbial keratitis; **(D)** endophthalmitis
(Courtesy of C Barry – fig. A; R Bates – fig. B; S Tuft – fig. D)

Corneal graft rejection

Immunological rejection of any layer of the cornea can occur. Rejection of separate layers (endothelial, stromal and epithelial) can occur in isolation, but typically a combination is present. Simple graft failure can occur in the absence of rejection, although rejection is a common contributory factor.

- **Pathogenesis.** The corneal graft is immunologically privileged, with an absence of blood vessels and lymphatics and the presence of relatively few antigen-presenting cells; inflammation and neovascularization contribute to loss of this privilege. Important predisposing factors for rejection include eccentric or larger grafts (over 8 mm in diameter), infection (particularly herpetic), glaucoma and previous keratoplasty. If the host becomes sensitized to histocompatibility antigens present in the donor cornea, rejection may result. Human leukocyte antigen (HLA) matching has a small beneficial effect on graft survival.

- **Symptoms.** Blurred vision, redness, photophobia and pain are typical, but many cases are asymptomatic until rejection is established. The timing of onset is very variable, occurring from days to years after keratoplasty.

- **Signs** vary depending on the type of graft.
  - Ciliary injection associated with anterior uveitis is an early manifestation (Fig. 7.6A).
  - Epithelial rejection may be accompanied by an elevated line of abnormal epithelium (Fig. 7.6B) in a quiet or mildly inflamed eye, occurring at an average of 3 months; increased treatment may not be required.
  - Subepithelial rejection is characterized by subepithelial infiltrates, reminiscent of adenoviral infection (Krachmer spots – Fig. 7.6C) on the donor cornea, with deeper oedema and infiltrative opacification.
  - Stromal rejection features deeper haze. It can be chronic or hyperacute, the latter in association with endothelial rejection.

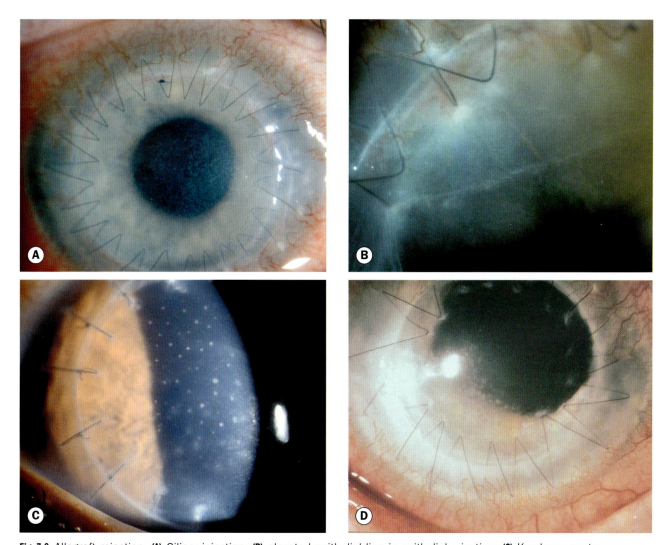

Fig. 7.6 Allograft rejection. **(A)** Ciliary injection; **(B)** elevated epithelial line in epithelial rejection; **(C)** Krachmer spots; **(D)** endothelial rejection with Khodadoust line
(Courtesy of S Tuft – figs A, B and C)

○ Endothelial rejection is characterized by a linear pattern of keratic precipitates (Khodadoust line – Fig. 7.6D) associated with an area of inflammation at the graft margin.

○ Stromal oedema is indicative of endothelial failure.

• **Management.** Early intensive treatment greatly improves the likelihood of reversing the rejection. The most aggressive regimen is generally required for endothelial rejection, followed in order of severity by stromal, subepithelial and epithelial. Intraocular pressure monitoring is critical.

○ Preservative-free topical steroids hourly for 24 hours are the mainstay of therapy. The frequency is reduced gradually over several weeks. Steroid ointment can be used at bedtime as the regimen is tapered. High-risk patients can be maintained on the highest tolerated topical dose (e.g. prednisolone acetate 1% four times daily) for an extended period.

○ Topical cycloplegia (e.g. homatropine 2% or atropine 1% once or twice daily).

○ Topical ciclosporin 0.05% to 2% may be of benefit, but the onset of action is delayed.

○ Systemic steroids. Oral prednisolone 1 mg/kg/day for 1–2 weeks with subsequent tapering; if given within 8 days of onset intravenous methylprednisolone 500 mg daily for up to 3 days may be particularly effective, suppressing rejection and reducing the risk of further episodes.

○ Subconjunctival steroid injection (e.g. 0.5 ml of 4 mg/ml dexamethasone) is sometimes used.

○ Other systemic immunosuppressants such as ciclosporin, tacrolimus or azathioprine.

• **Differential diagnosis** includes graft failure (no inflammation), infective keratitis including fungal and herpetic, uveitis, sterile suture reaction, raised IOP and epithelial ingrowth.

Superficial lamellar keratoplasty

This involves partial-thickness excision of the corneal epithelium and stroma so that the endothelium and part of the deep stroma are left behind as a bed for appropriately partial-thickness donor cornea. The area grafted depends on the extent of the disease process to be addressed.

• **Indications**
○ Opacification of the superficial one-third of the corneal stroma not caused by potentially recurrent disease.

○ Marginal corneal thinning or infiltration as in recurrent pterygium, Terrien marginal degeneration, and limbal dermoids or other tumours.

○ Localized thinning or descemetocoele formation (see Fig. 7.1B).

Deep anterior lamellar keratoplasty

Deep anterior lamellar keratoplasty (DALK) is a technique in which corneal tissue is removed almost to the level of Descemet membrane. A theoretical advantage is the decreased risk of rejection because the endothelium, a major target for rejection, is not

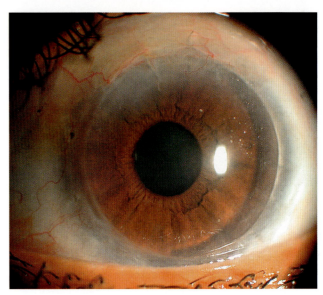

Fig. 7.7 Deep anterior lamellar keratoplasty for chemical injury. A superior conjunctival limbal autograft has also been performed

transplanted. The major technical difficulty lies in judging the depth of the corneal dissection as close as possible to Descemet membrane without perforation, and if this is not achieved the visual outcome may be compromised.

• **Indications**
○ Disease involving the anterior 95% of corneal thickness with normal endothelium and the absence of breaks or scars in Descemet membrane (e.g. keratoconus without a history of acute hydrops, superficial trauma – Fig. 7.7).

○ Chronic inflammatory disease such as atopic keratoconjunctivitis that carries an increased risk of graft rejection.

• **Advantages**
○ No risk of endothelial rejection, although epithelial/subepithelial/stromal rejection may occur.

○ Less astigmatism and a structurally stronger globe compared with penetrating keratoplasty.

○ Increased availability of graft material since endothelial quality is irrelevant.

• **Disadvantages**
○ Difficult and time-consuming with a high risk of perforation.

○ Interface haze may limit the best final visual acuity.

• **Postoperative management** is similar to penetrating keratoplasty except that lower intensity topical steroids are needed and sutures can usually be removed after 6 months.

Endothelial keratoplasty

Endothelial keratoplasty involves removal only of diseased endothelium along with Descemet membrane (DM) through a corneoscleral or corneal incision. Folded donor tissue is introduced through the same small (2.8–5.0 mm) incision. Descemet

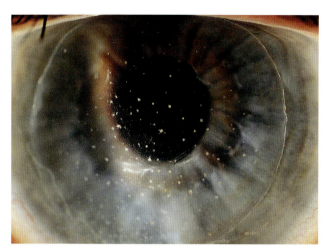

Fig. 7.8 Endothelial graft undergoing rejection
(Courtesy of C Barry)

stripping (automated) endothelial keratoplasty (DSAEK), uses an automated microkeratome to prepare donor tissue and is currently the most commonly performed technique; a small amount of posterior stromal thickness is transplanted along with DM and endothelium. Descemet membrane endothelial keratoplasty (DMEK) is a more recently introduced procedure in which only the DM and endothelium are transplanted; better visual outcomes and lower rejection rates seem to be achieved, but intraoperative complication rates are higher.

- **Indications** include endothelial disease such as Fuchs endothelial corneal dystrophy.
- **Advantages**
  - Relatively little refractive change and a structurally more intact globe.
  - Faster visual rehabilitation than penetrating keratoplasty.
  - Suturing is minimized.
- **Disadvantages**
  - Significant learning curve.
  - Specialized equipment is required.
  - Endothelial rejection can still occur (Fig. 7.8).

Limbal stem cell grafting

Various techniques have been described to attempt to replenish the limbal stem cell population in patients with severe ocular surface disease and associated stem cell deficiency. These include transplantation of a limbal area of limited size from a healthy fellow eye (see Fig. 7.7), complete limbal transplantation of a donor annulus and *ex vivo* expansion by culture of either host or donor stem cells with subsequent transplantation. A consistently successful technique has not yet been established, and research is ongoing.

KERATOPROSTHESES

Keratoprostheses (Fig. 7.9A) are artificial corneal implants used in patients unsuitable for keratoplasty. The modern osteo-odontokeratoprosthesis consists of the patient's own tooth root

and alveolar bone supporting a central optical cylinder, and is usually covered with a buccal mucous membrane graft. Surgery is difficult and time-consuming and is performed in two stages, 2–4 months apart.

- **Indications**
  - Bilateral blindness from severe but inactive anterior segment disease with no realistic chance of success from conventional keratoplasty, e.g. Stevens–Johnson syndrome, ocular cicatricial pemphigoid, chemical burns and trachoma.
  - Visual acuity of counting finger or less in the better eye.
  - Intact optic nerve and retinal function, without marked glaucomatous optic neuropathy.
  - High patient motivation.
- **Complications** include glaucoma (up to 75%), retroprosthesis membrane formation (Fig. 7.9B), tilting or extrusion, retinal detachment and endophthalmitis. Glaucoma management is inevitably extremely challenging.

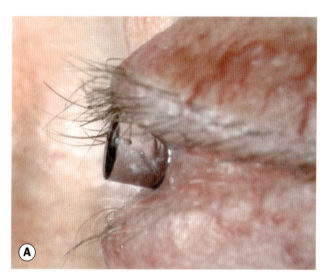

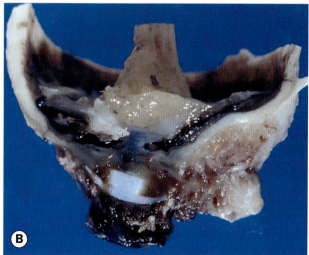

Fig. 7.9 (A) Keratoprosthesis; **(B)** retroprosthesis membrane formation with associated funnel-shaped retinal detachment
(Courtesy of C Barry)

- **Results.** Approximately 80% of patients achieve visual acuity between counting fingers and 6/12, and occasionally even better. A poor outcome is often associated with pre-existing optic nerve or retinal dysfunction.

REFRACTIVE PROCEDURES

Introduction

Refractive surgery encompasses a range of procedures aimed at changing the refraction of the eye by altering the cornea or lens, the principal refracting components. Myopia, hypermetropia (hyperopia) and astigmatism can all be addressed, though correction of presbyopia is yet to be achieved on a consistently satisfactory basis.

Correction of myopia

- **Surface ablation procedures** (see below) can correct low–moderate degrees of myopia.
- **Laser *in situ* keratomileusis** (LASIK – see below) can correct moderate to high myopia depending on initial corneal thickness, but for very high refractive errors one of the intraocular procedures below is necessary.
- **Refractive lenticule extraction** (see below) is a newer technique for the correction of myopia and myopic astigmatism.
- **Clear lens exchange** gives very good visual results but carries a small risk of the complications of cataract surgery (see Ch. 9), particularly retinal detachment in high myopes.
- **Iris clip** ('lobster claw') implant is attached to the iris (Fig. 7.10A). Complications include subluxation or dislocation due to dislodgement of one or both attachments (Fig. 7.10B), an oval pupil, endothelial cell loss, cataract, pupillary-block glaucoma and retinal detachment.
- **Phakic posterior chamber implant** (implantable contact lens, ICL) is inserted behind the iris and in front of the lens (Fig. 7.10C), and supported in the ciliary sulcus. The lens is composed of material derived from collagen (Collamer) with a power of −3 D to −20.50 D. Visual results are usually very good but complications include uveitis, pupillary block, endothelial cell loss, cataract formation and retinal detachment.
- **Radial keratotomy** (Fig. 7.11) is now predominantly of historical interest.

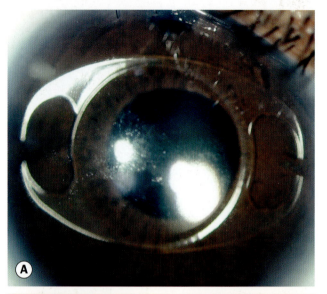

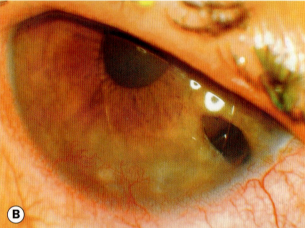

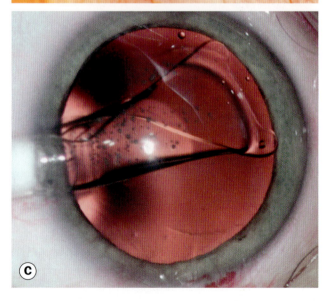

Fig. 7.10 Phakic intraocular implants for correction of myopia. **(A)** Anterior chamber iris claw implant with anterior iris attachment at 3 and 9 o'clock; **(B)** inferior subluxation with resultant inferior endothelial decompensation – note also an iridectomy to prevent pupillary block; **(C)** emplacement of a posterior chamber phakic implant between the iris and anterior lens surface

(Courtesy of Y Kerdraon – fig. B; J Krachmer, M Mannis and E Holland, from Cornea, Mosby 2005 – fig. C)

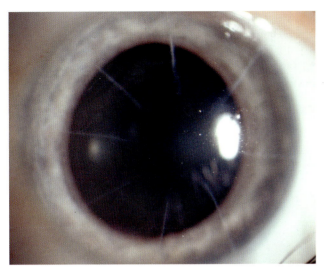

Fig. 7.11 Radial keratotomy
(Courtesy of C Barry)

Correction of hypermetropia (hyperopia)

- **Surface ablation procedures** can correct low degrees of hypermetropia.
- **LASIK** can correct up to 4 D.
- **Conductive keratoplasty (CK)** involves the application of radiofrequency energy to the corneal stroma and can correct low–moderate hypermetropia and hypermetropic astigmatism. Burns are placed in one or two rings in the corneal periphery using a probe. The resultant thermally induced stromal shrinkage is accompanied by an increase in central corneal curvature. Significant regression may occur but the procedure can be repeated. CK may also be helpful for presbyopia (see below). Complications are infrequent.
- **Laser thermal keratoplasty** with a holmium laser can correct low hypermetropia. Laser burns are placed in one or two rings in the corneal mid-periphery (Fig. 7.12). As with

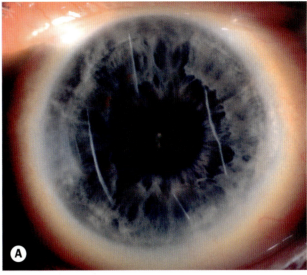

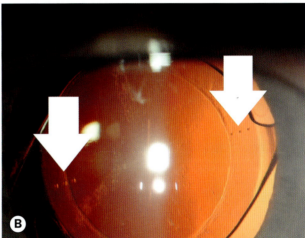

Fig. 7.13 Correction of astigmatism. **(A)** Arcuate keratotomies; **(B)** toric intraocular implant in site – markings incorporated in the lens (arrows) facilitate correct orientation
(Courtesy of C Barry – fig. A)

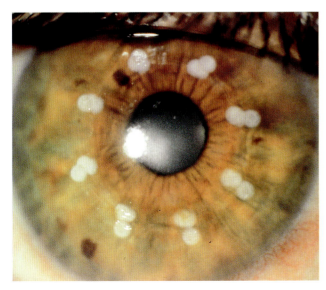

Fig. 7.12 Thermal keratoplasty
(Courtesy of H Nano Jr)

CK, thermally induced stromal shrinkage is accompanied by increased corneal curvature. Correction decays over time but treatment can be repeated.
- **Other modalities** include clear lens extraction and phakic lens implants as described above for myopia; intraocular surgical procedures are the only options for high degrees of refractive error.

Correction of astigmatism

- **Limbal relaxing incisions/arcuate keratotomy** involves making paired arcuate incisions on opposite sides of the cornea (Fig. 7.13A) in the axis of the correcting 'plus' cylinder (the steep meridian). The resultant flattening of the steep meridian coupled with a smaller steepening of the flat meridian at 90° to the incisions reduces astigmatism. The desired result can be controlled by varying the length and depth of the incisions and their distance from the optical centre of the cornea. Arcuate keratotomy may be combined with compression sutures placed in the perpendicular meridian, when treating large degrees of astigmatism such as can occur following penetrating keratoplasty.

- **PRK** and **LASEK** can correct up to 3 D.
- **LASIK** can correct up to 5 D.
- **Lens surgery** involves using a 'toric' intraocular implant incorporating an astigmatic correction (Fig. 7.13B). Postoperative rotation of the implant away from the desired axis occurs in a small minority of cases.
- **Conductive keratoplasty** (see 'Correction of hypermetropia' above).

Correction of presbyopia

- **Lens extraction**, either to treat cataract or for purely refractive purposes. Acronyms used include clear lens exchange (CLE), refractive lens exchange (RLE) and presbyopic lens exchange (PreLEx). Much research effort is being applied to the development of effective accommodating prosthetic lenses.
  - Implantation of a multifocal, bifocal or 'accommodating'/ pseudoaccommodative intraocular lens implant (IOL) can optically restore some reading vision; reading glasses commonly still have to be used for some tasks. Although many recipients of multifocal IOLs are very happy with the visual outcome, dissatisfaction occurs in a significant minority, mainly due to nocturnal glare and reduced contrast sensitivity. Around 10% of patients receiving multifocal IOLs subsequently undergo higher-risk IOL exchange surgery. In some jurisdictions, implantation of a multifocal IOL is a contraindication to the holding of a private or commercial pilot's licence, or to military service.
  - 'Monovision' consists of the targeting of IOL-induced refractive outcomes so that one eye (usually the dominant) is optimized for clear uncorrected distance vision and the other for near or intermediate vision, in order to facilitate both good distance and near vision when the eyes are used together.
  - Some studies show similar levels of functional near vision using bilateral distance-optimized monofocal IOLs compared to multifocal IOLs.
- **Conductive keratoplasty** (see 'Correction of hypermetropia' above); there is some evidence that CK can impart a degree of multifocal functionality to the cornea.
- **Laser-induced monovision** refers to the use of laser refractive surgery to optimize one eye for distance and the fellow for near or intermediate vision (see above under 'Lens extraction').
- **Corneal multifocality.** Several different approaches are under development utilizing a laser procedure to alter the shape of the cornea such that a bifocal or transitional effect is induced.

- **Scleral expansion surgery.** Results have been inconsistent and unpredictable and this technique has not achieved sustained popularity.
- **Intracorneal inlays** (Fig. 7.14A–D) commonly provide substantial benefit in presbyopia, though in the past the biocompatibility of some materials has been relatively poor, and complications such as extrusion (Fig. 7.14E) can mandate explantation.
- **Laser modification of the natural lens.** Research is ongoing into the use of a femtosecond laser to modulate crystalline lens elasticity.

Laser refractive procedures

To settle any contact lens-induced corneal distortion prior to definitive keratometry, soft contact lenses should probably be discontinued for 2 weeks and hard/rigid gas permeable lenses for at least 3 weeks (some surgeons suggest 1 week for each year of wear to date).

Laser in situ keratomileusis

Laser (or laser-assisted) *in situ* keratomileusis (LASIK) is a very common refractive procedure. The excimer laser, which can ablate tissue to a precise depth with negligible disruption of surrounding areas, is used to reshape corneal stroma exposed by the creation of a superficial flap; the flap remains attached by a hinge to facilitate accurate and secure repositioning. Myopia is corrected by central ablative flattening, and hypermetropia by ablation of the periphery so that the centre becomes steeper. LASIK can generally be used to treat higher refractive errors than surface ablation techniques (see below): hypermetropia up to 4 D, astigmatism up to 5 D and myopia up to 12 D depending on initial corneal thickness. To decrease the risk of subsequent ectasia, a residual corneal base at least 250 μm thick must remain after ablation. The amount of tissue removed, and so the amount of refractive error correctable, is therefore limited by the original corneal thickness; very high refractive errors can be addressed only by an intraocular procedure. In addition to treatment of a wider range of refractive errors, advantages over surface ablation include greater postoperative comfort, faster visual rehabilitation, more rapid stabilization of refraction and milder stromal haze. The major disadvantage is the potential for serious flap-related complications.

- **Technique**
  - A suction ring centred on the cornea is applied to the globe; this raises the intraocular pressure substantially.
  - The ring stabilizes the eye and provides the guide track for a mechanical microkeratome, which is advanced across the cornea to create a thin flap. The flap can also be created using a femtosecond (and recently a picosecond) laser microkeratome.
  - The flap is reflected (Fig. 7.15A) and the bed reshaped, followed by flap repositioning.
- **Intraoperative complications** include 'buttonholing' (penetration) of the flap, flap amputation, incomplete or irregular flap creation and rarely penetration into the anterior chamber.

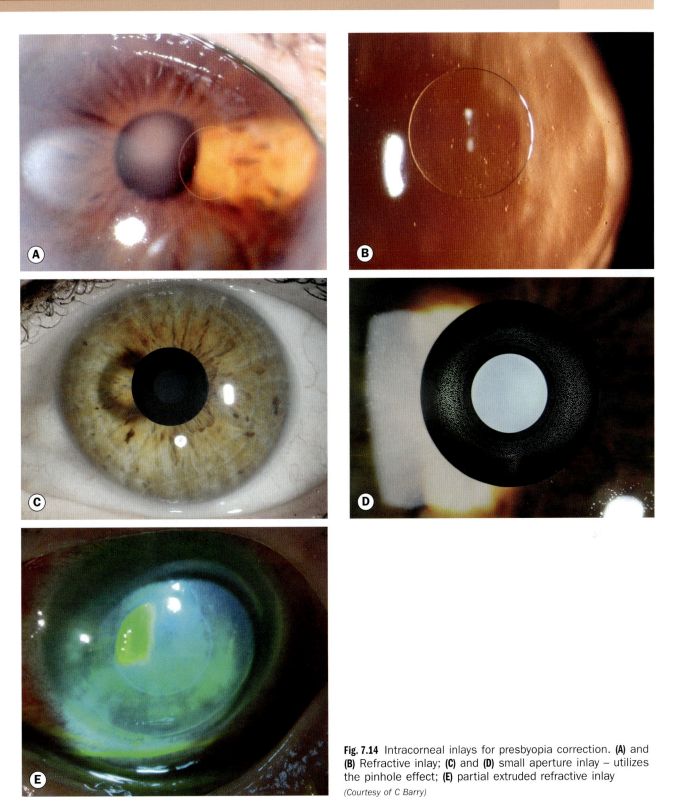

Fig. 7.14 Intracorneal inlays for presbyopia correction. **(A)** and **(B)** Refractive inlay; **(C)** and **(D)** small aperture inlay – utilizes the pinhole effect; **(E)** partial extruded refractive inlay
(Courtesy of C Barry)

- **Postoperative complications**
  - ○ Tear instability is almost universal and may require treatment.
  - ○ Wrinkling (Fig. 7.15B), distortion or dislocation of the flap.
  - ○ Subepithelial haze (Fig. 7.15C) with resultant glare, especially at night.
  - ○ Persistent epithelial defects.
  - ○ Epithelial ingrowth under the flap (Fig. 7.15D).
  - ○ Diffuse lamellar keratitis ('sands of the Sahara' – Fig. 7.15E) may develop 1–7 days following LASIK. It is characterized by granular deposits at the flap interface. Treatment is with intensive topical antibiotic and steroid.

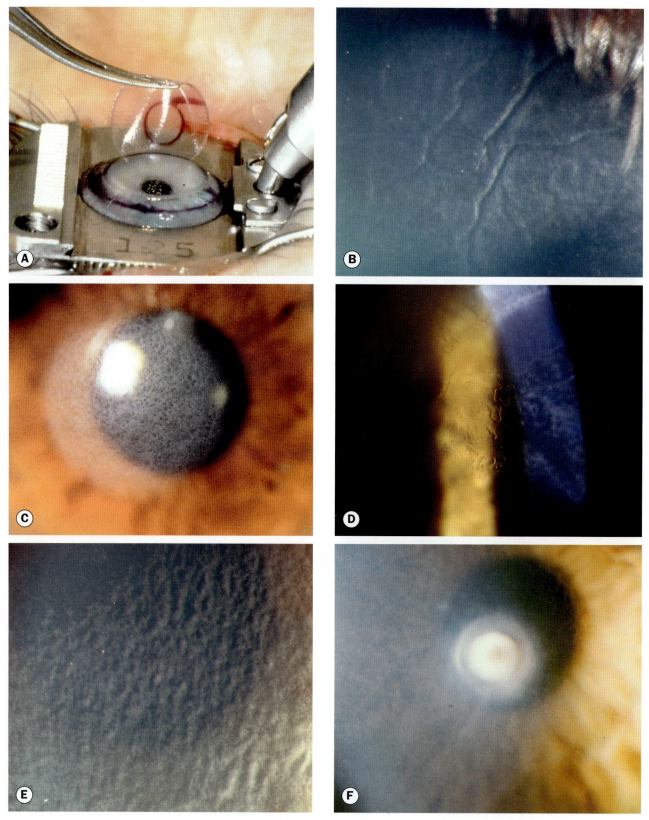

Fig. 7.15 Laser *in situ* keratomileusis (LASIK). **(A)** Elevating the flap; **(B)** wrinkling of the flap; **(C)** subepithelial haze; **(D)** epithelial ingrowth; **(E)** diffuse lamellar keratitis ('sands of the Sahara'); **(F)** bacterial keratitis

(Courtesy of Eye Academy – fig. A; S Tuft – figs B and E; H Nano Jr – fig. C; C Barry – fig. D; R Bates – fig. F)

○ Bacterial keratitis (Fig. 7.15F) is rare.

○ Corneal ectasia (see Ch. 6). 'Forme fruste' (occult/mild) keratoconus and a low post-ablation corneal thickness are the major risk factors, and careful pre-procedure screening should be performed to detect any predisposition.

Surface ablation procedures

Like LASIK, photorefractive keratectomy (PRK) employs excimer laser ablation to reshape the cornea. PRK is able to correct myopia up to 6 D (sometimes higher), astigmatism up to around 3 D and low–moderate hypermetropia. The main disadvantages compared with LASIK are the somewhat lower degrees of refractive error correctable, and variably slower epithelial healing with unpredictable postoperative discomfort. However, as a flap is not created there is a lower risk of serious complications than with LASIK, including corneal ectasia and late flap dislocation, and it may be the procedure of choice for patients at higher than average occupational or leisure-related risk of eye injury. It is also suitable for patients rendered ineligible for LASIK due to low corneal thickness; other indications for surface ablation rather than LASIK include epithelial basement membrane disease, prior corneal transplantation or radial keratotomy, and large pupil size.

- **Technique**
  ○ The corneal epithelium is removed prior to ablation; methods used may include a sponge, an automated brush (Amoils epithelial scrubber) and alcohol.
  ○ Ablation of the Bowman layer and anterior stroma (Fig. 7.16) is performed, generally taking 30–60 seconds. In

modern systems, sophisticated tracking mechanisms adjust laser targeting with eye movement, and will pause the procedure if the eye is significantly decentred.

  ○ The epithelium usually heals within 48–72 hours. A bandage contact lens is generally used to minimize discomfort. Subepithelial haze invariably develops within 2 weeks and commonly persists for several weeks to months. Diminished final visual acuity is rare but there may be decreased contrast and nocturnal glare. Intraoperative application of mitomycin C (mitomycin-LASEK or M-LASEK) may reduce haze.

- **Complications** include slowly healing epithelial defects, corneal haze with blurring and haloes, poor night vision and regression of refractive correction. Uncommon problems include decentred ablation, scarring, abnormal epithelial healing, irregular astigmatism, hypoaesthesia, sterile infiltrates, infection and acute corneal necrosis.

- **Variations of PRK.** A range of procedural variations with correspondingly varying terminology have been described. LASEK (laser epithelial keratomileusis or laser-assisted subepithelial keratectomy), Epi-LASIK (epipolis or epithelial LASIK; epipolis is a Greek word meaning superficial), modified PRK, advanced surface (laser) ablation (ASA or ASLA) and Trans-PRK (trans-epithelial PRK) are variations of PRK that utilize a variety of techniques to try to reduce discomfort and post-laser haze, and to speed visual recovery; ASA and modified PRK are sometimes used generally to refer to all surface ablative procedures. In LASEK the epithelium is detached and peeled back after pre-treatment with dilute alcohol; laser is then applied and the epithelium repositioned. Epi-LASIK employs a mechanical device, an epikeratome, to elevate a hinged sheet of epithelium with an oscillating blunt plastic blade, and alcohol application is not usually required. Some recent reports suggest that healing occurs more rapidly if the epithelium is simply detached entirely without replacement (flap-off Epi-LASIK). In Trans-PRK, epithelial ablation is performed with the laser prior to the refractive ablation, reducing operative time and possibly conferring other benefits.

Refractive lenticule extraction

Refractive lenticule extraction (ReLEx) is a relatively new technique that uses a femtosecond laser to cut a lens-shaped piece of corneal tissue (a lenticule) within the intact cornea. This is then removed via either a LASIK-style flap or more recently using a minimally invasive 4 mm incision (small incision lenticule extraction – SMILE). Potential advantages include less marked biomechanical and neurological corneal disturbance than LASIK and a likely lower risk of infection and other flap complications. Surface disturbance is minimal in comparison to surface ablation procedures.

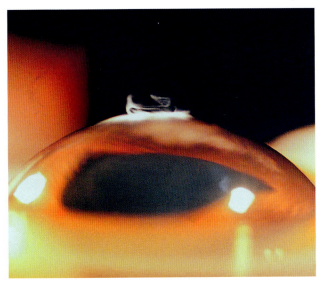

Fig. 7.16 Corneal ablation during photorefractive keratectomy (PRK or advanced surface (laser) ablation – ASA/ASLA)
(Courtesy of C Barry)

Episclera and sclera

ANATOMY

The scleral stroma is composed of collagen bundles of varying size and shape that are not uniformly orientated as in the cornea, and so are not transparent. The inner layer of the sclera (lamina fusca) blends with the uveal tract. Anteriorly the episclera consists of a connective tissue layer between the superficial scleral stroma and Tenon capsule. There are three pre-equatorial vascular layers:

- **Conjunctival vessels** are the most superficial; arteries are tortuous and veins straight.
- **Superficial episcleral plexus** vessels are straight with a radial configuration. In episcleritis, maximal congestion occurs at this level (Fig. 8.1A). Topical phenylephrine 2.5% will also constrict the conjunctival and 10% also the superficial episcleral vessels.
- **Deep vascular plexus** lies in the superficial part of the sclera and shows maximal congestion in scleritis (Fig. 8.1B); a purplish hue, best seen in daylight, is characteristic.

EPISCLERITIS

Episcleritis is a common, usually idiopathic and benign, recurrent and frequently bilateral condition. Females may be affected more commonly than males, except possibly in children, in whom

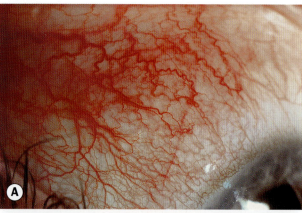

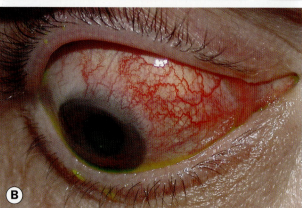

Fig. 8.1 (A) Diffuse episcleritis with maximal vascular congestion in the superficial episcleral plexus; **(B)** scleritis with congestion of the deep vascular plexus
(Courtesy of P Watson – fig. A; S Chen – fig. B)

episcleritis is rare; the average patient is middle-aged. It is typically self-limiting and tends to last from a few days up to 3 weeks, but rarely longer. Associated disease, either ocular (e.g. dry eye, rosacea, contact lens wear) or systemic (e.g. collagen vascular disorders such as rheumatoid arthritis, herpes zoster ophthalmicus, gout and others) has been identified in up to a third of patients seen at tertiary centres, with ocular disease the most common. Infectious causes are very rare but a wide range has been reported. Investigation of recurrent cases is as for scleritis (see later).

Simple episcleritis

Simple episcleritis accounts for 75% of cases. It has a tendency to recur (60%), decreasing in frequency with time. Features often peak within 24 hours, gradually fading over the next few days.

- **Symptoms.** Redness; discomfort ranges from absent (up to 50%) to moderate and occasionally severe, when scleritis should be excluded. Grittiness is common, and photophobia may occur.
- **Signs.** More than half of cases are simultaneously bilateral.
  - Visual acuity is almost always normal.
  - Redness may be sectoral (two-thirds – Fig. 8.2A) or diffuse (Fig. 8.2B). Often it has an interpalpebral distribution, in a triangular configuration with the base at the limbus.
  - Chemosis, ocular hypertension, anterior uveitis and keratitis are all rare.
- **Treatment**
  - If mild, no treatment is required; cool compresses or refrigerated artificial tears may be helpful.
  - A weak topical steroid four times daily for 1–2 weeks is usually sufficient, though occasionally more intensive instillation is needed initially or a more potent preparation can be used with rapid tapering. A topical non-steroidal anti-inflammatory (NSAID) is an alternative, though may be less effective.
  - An oral NSAID is occasionally required (e.g. ibuprofen 200 mg three times daily, or occasionally a more potent agent such as indometacin). It is very rare for more aggressive systemic treatment to be required, and this is typically in patients with a known systemic association.

Nodular episcleritis

Nodular episcleritis also tends to affect females but has a less acute onset and a more prolonged course than the simple variant.

- **Symptoms.** A red eye is typically first noted on waking. Over the next 2–3 days the area of redness enlarges and becomes more uncomfortable.
- **Signs.** Attacks usually clear without treatment, but tend to last longer than simple episcleritis.
  - A tender red vascular nodule, almost always within the interpalpebral fissure (Fig. 8.3A). Occasionally more than one focus is present.
  - A slit lamp section shows an underlying flat anterior scleral surface, indicating the absence of scleritis (Fig. 8.3B).

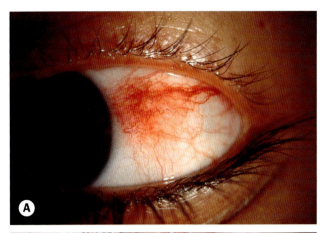

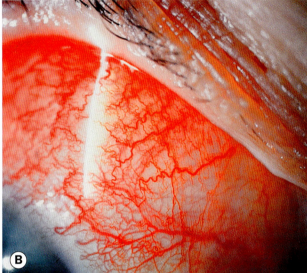

Fig. 8.2 Simple episcleritis. **(A)** Sectoral; **(B)** diffuse
(Courtesy of JH Krachmer, MJ Mannis and EJ Holland, from Cornea, *Mosby 2005 – fig. B)*

- Intraocular pressure (IOP) is very occasionally elevated.
- An anterior chamber reaction may be present, but is uncommon (10%).
- After several episodes inflamed vessels may become permanently dilated.
- It is important to exclude other causes of a nodule such as phlyctenulosis (a phlycten is within rather than beneath the conjunctiva) or a conjunctival granuloma.
- **Treatment** is similar to that of simple episcleritis but is more commonly indicated.

IMMUNE-MEDIATED SCLERITIS

Scleritis is an uncommon condition characterized by oedema and cellular infiltration of the entire thickness of the sclera. Immune-mediated (non-infectious) scleritis is the most common type, and is frequently associated with an underlying systemic inflammatory condition, of which it may be the first manifestation. Scleritis is much less common than episcleritis and comprises a spectrum from trivial and self-limiting disease to a necrotizing process that

can involve adjacent tissues and threaten vision. A classification of non-infectious scleritis is shown in Table 8.1; recurrences tend to be of the same type, though 10% progress to more aggressive disease.

Anterior non-necrotizing scleritis

Diffuse

Diffuse disease is slightly more common in females and usually presents in the fifth decade.

- **Symptoms.** Ocular redness progressing a few days later to pain that may radiate to the face and temple. The discomfort typically wakes the patient in the early hours of the morning and improves later in the day; it responds poorly to common analgesics.

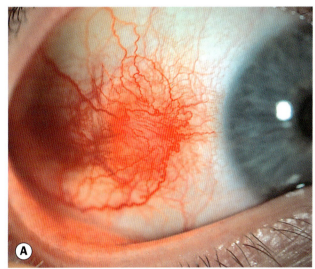

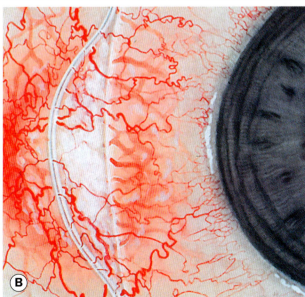

Fig. 8.3 (A) Nodular episcleritis; **(B)** slit illumination shows that the deep beam is not displaced above the scleral surface

Table 8.1 Classification of immune-mediated (non-infectious) scleritis

Anterior
• Non-necrotizing
• Diffuse
• Nodular
• Necrotizing with inflammation
• Vaso-occlusive
• Granulomatous
• Surgically induced (can also be infective)
• Scleromalacia perforans (necrotizing without inflammation)
Posterior

- **Signs**
  - Vascular congestion and dilatation associated with oedema. If treatment is started early, which rarely happens, the disease can be completely inhibited.
  - The redness may be generalized (Fig. 8.4A) or localized to one quadrant. If confined to the area under the upper eyelid the diagnosis may be missed.
  - Secondary features can include chemosis, eyelid swelling, anterior uveitis and raised IOP.
  - As the oedema resolves, the affected area often takes on a slight grey/blue appearance because of increased scleral translucency (Fig. 8.4B); this is due to rearrangement of scleral fibres rather than a decrease in scleral thickness.
  - Recurrences at the same location are common unless an underlying cause is treated.
- **Prognosis.** The average duration of disease is around 6 years, with the frequency of recurrences decreasing after the first 18 months. The long-term visual prognosis is very good.

Nodular

The incidence of nodular and diffuse anterior scleritis is the same but a disproportionately large number of those with nodular disease have had a previous attack of herpes zoster ophthalmicus. The age of onset is similar to that of diffuse scleritis.

- **Symptoms.** The insidious onset of pain followed by increasing redness, tenderness of the globe and the appearance of a scleral nodule.
- **Signs**
  - Scleral nodules may be single or multiple and most frequently develop in the interpalpebral region close to the limbus (Fig. 8.5A). They have a deeper blue–red colour than episcleral nodules and are immobile.
  - In contrast to episcleritis, a slit lamp beam shows an elevated anterior scleral surface (Fig. 8.5B).
  - Multiple nodules may expand and coalesce if treatment is delayed.
  - Instillation of 10% phenylephrine drops will constrict the conjunctival and superficial episcleral vasculature but not the deep plexus overlying the nodule.
  - As the inflammation in the nodule subsides, increased translucency of the sclera becomes apparent.

- The duration of the disease is similar to diffuse scleritis.
- More than 10% of patients with nodular scleritis develop necrotizing disease, but if treatment is instituted early superficial necrosis does not occur and the nodule heals from the centre leaving a small atrophic scar.

Anterior necrotizing scleritis with inflammation

Necrotizing disease is the aggressive form of scleritis. The age at onset is later than that of non-necrotizing scleritis, averaging 60 years. The condition is bilateral in 60% of patients and unless

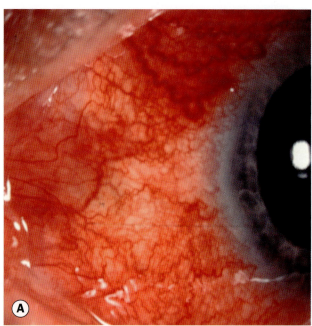

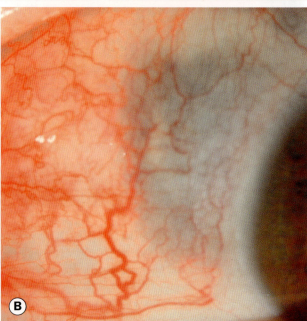

Fig. 8.4 (A) Diffuse non-necrotizing anterior scleritis; **(B)** scleral translucency following recurrent disease
(Courtesy of M Jager – fig. B)

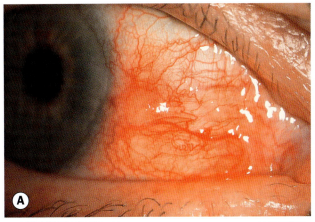

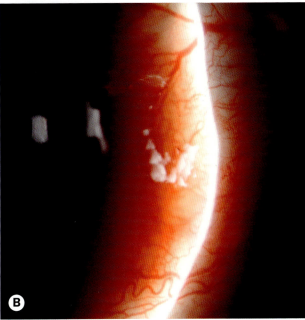

Fig. 8.5 (A) Nodular non-necrotizing anterior scleritis; **(B)** slit illumination shows superficial displacement of the entire beam
(Courtesy of P Watson – fig. A)

appropriately treated, especially in its early stages, may result in severe visual morbidity and even loss of the eye.

Clinical features

- **Symptoms.** Gradual onset of pain that becomes severe and persistent and radiates to the temple, brow or jaw; it frequently interferes with sleep and responds poorly to analgesia.
- **Signs** vary according to the following three types of necrotizing disease.
  - Vaso-occlusive is commonly associated with rheumatoid arthritis. Isolated patches of scleral oedema with overlying non-perfused episclera and conjunctiva are seen (Fig 8.6A). The patches coalesce, and if unchecked rapidly proceed to scleral necrosis (Fig. 8.6B).
  - Granulomatous may occur in conjunction with conditions such as granulomatosis or polyarteritis

nodosa. The disease typically starts with injection adjacent to the limbus and then extends posteriorly. Within 24 hours, the sclera, episclera, conjunctiva and adjacent cornea become irregularly raised and oedematous (Fig. 8.7).
  - Surgically induced scleritis typically starts within 3 weeks of a procedure, though much longer intervals have been reported. It may be induced by any type of surgery including strabismus repair, trabeculectomy (Fig. 8.8) and scleral buckling, and excision of pterygium with adjunctive mitomycin C. The necrotizing process starts at the site of surgery and extends outwards, but tends to remain localized to one sector.

Investigations

- **Laboratory.** These should be employed as adjuncts to clinical assessment, and evaluation by a general physician or rheumatologist should be considered. Specific tests may

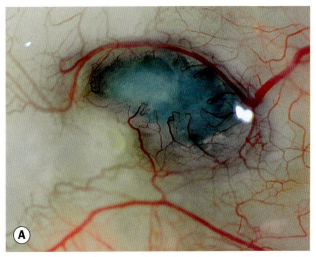

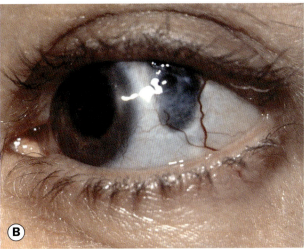

Fig. 8.6 Vaso-occlusive necrotizing scleritis with inflammation. **(A)** Early stage; **(B)** moderate disease – inflammatory signs are commonly more marked than in these cases
(Courtesy of C Barry – fig. B)

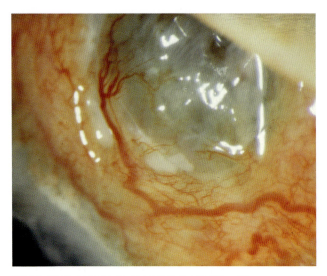

Fig. 8.7 Granulomatous necrotizing scleritis with inflammation
(Courtesy of P Watson)

include erythrocyte sedimentation rate (ESR), C-reactive protein (CRP), full blood count (e.g. anaemia related to inflammatory connective tissue disease, eosinophilia for polyarteritis nodosa, atopy or Churg–Strauss syndrome), rheumatoid factor, antinuclear antibodies (ANA), antineutrophil cytoplasmic antibodies (ANCA) and anti-cyclic citrullinated peptide (CCP) antibodies, serum uric acid, syphilis serology, Lyme serology, hepatitis B surface antigen (polyarteritis nodosa) and antiphospholipid antibodies. Investigation for tuberculosis, sarcoidosis or ankylosing spondylitis may be appropriate (see Ch. 11).

- **Radiological imaging.** Chest, sinus, joint and other imaging may be indicated in the investigation of a range of conditions such as tuberculosis, sarcoidosis, Churg–Strauss syndrome, Wegener granulomatosis, ankylosing spondylitis and other conditions.

- **Angiography.** Fluorescein angiography of the anterior segment helps to distinguish necrotizing disease by the presence of non-perfusion, and can be used for monitoring; occlusion is predominantly venular in inflammatory disease, and mainly arteriolar in scleromalacia perforans (see below). Indocyanine green is a more accurate indicator of disease activity.
- **Ultrasonography** can help to detect associated posterior scleritis (see below).
- **Biopsy.** This may be considered in resistant cases, especially if infection is suspected.

Complications of anterior scleritis

- **Acute infiltrative stromal keratitis** may be localized or diffuse.
- **Sclerosing keratitis**, characterized by chronic thinning and opacification in which the peripheral cornea adjacent to the site of scleritis resembles sclera.
- **Peripheral ulcerative keratitis** is characterized by progressive melting and ulceration (Fig. 8.9), and may constitute a severe risk to the integrity of the eye. In granulomatous scleritis the destruction extends directly from the sclera into the limbus and cornea; this characteristic pattern is seen in Wegener granulomatosis, polyarteritis nodosa and relapsing polychondritis. Peripheral corneal ulceration can occur at any stage of a necrotizing scleritis and, in rare cases, precede its onset. (See also Ch. 6.)
- **Uveitis**, if severe, may denote aggressive scleritis.
- **Glaucoma** is the most common cause of eventual loss of vision. The intraocular pressure can be very difficult to control in the presence of active scleritis.
- **Hypotony** (rarely phthisis) may be the result of ciliary body detachment, inflammatory damage or ischaemia.
- **Perforation** of the sclera as a result of the inflammatory process alone is extremely rare.

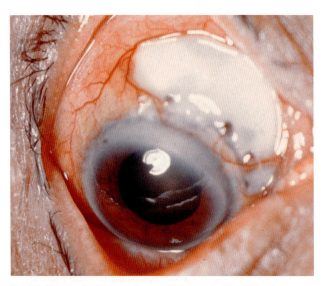

Fig. 8.8 Surgically induced necrotizing scleritis following trabeculectomy

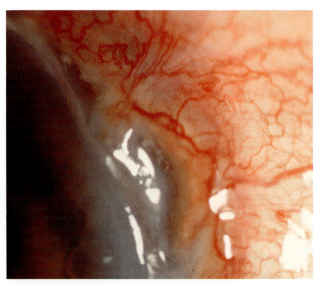

Fig. 8.9 Peripheral ulcerative keratitis secondary to necrotizing scleritis

Scleromalacia perforans

- Scleromalacia perforans (5% of scleritis) is a specific type of progressive scleral thinning without inflammation that typically affects elderly women with longstanding rheumatoid arthritis, but has also been described in association with other systemic disorders. Despite the nomenclature, perforation of the globe is extremely rare as integrity is maintained by a thin layer of fibrous tissue. Differential diagnosis is from the innocuous scleral hyaline plaque and senile scleromalacia (see below).
- **Symptoms.** Mild non-specific irritation; pain is absent and vision unaffected, and keratoconjunctivitis sicca may be suspected.
- **Signs**
  - ○ Necrotic scleral plaques near the limbus without vascular congestion (Fig. 8.10A).
  - ○ Coalescence and enlargement of necrotic areas.
  - ○ Slow progression of scleral thinning with exposure of underlying uvea (Figs 8.10B and C).
- **Treatment** may be effective in patients with early disease but by the time of typical presentation, either no treatment is needed or progression has been marked.
  - ○ Consistent benefit from any agent has not been demonstrated, though frequent lubricant instillation, local (including topical sodium versenate) or systemic anticollagenase agents, immunosuppressives (including topical and oral, but not periocular injection of, steroids, and topical ciclosporin) and biological blockers have been used.
  - ○ Underlying systemic disease should be treated aggressively.
  - ○ Protection from trauma is important.
  - ○ Surgical repair of scleral perforation (e.g. patch grafting) is mandatory to prevent phthisis bulbi.

Posterior scleritis

Posterior scleritis is a potentially blinding condition in which diagnosis is commonly delayed, with an adverse prognostic effect. The inflammatory changes in posterior and anterior scleral disease are identical and can arise in both segments simultaneously or separately. The age at onset is often less than 40 years; young patients are usually otherwise healthy but about a third over the age of 55 have associated systemic disease.

Diagnosis

- **Symptoms.** Pain does not correlate well with the severity of inflammation but tends to be more severe in those with accompanying orbital myositis; photophobia is not a dominant feature.
- **Signs.** The disease is bilateral in 35%.
  - ○ Choroidal folds (see Ch. 14) are usually confined to the posterior pole and orientated horizontally (Fig. 8.11A).
  - ○ Exudative retinal detachment occurs in around 25%; yellowish-brown subretinal exudative material can be mistaken for a choroidal tumour.

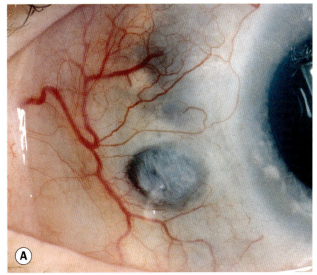
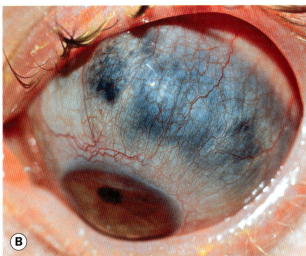
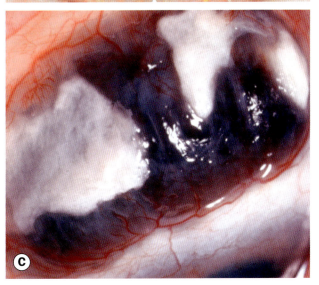

Fig. 8.10 Progression of scleromalacia perforans. **(A)** Asymptomatic necrotic patch; **(B)** moderate and **(C)** severe thinning and exposure of underlying uvea *(Courtesy of R Bates – fig. A; C Barry – figs B and C)*

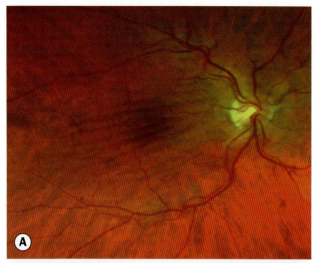

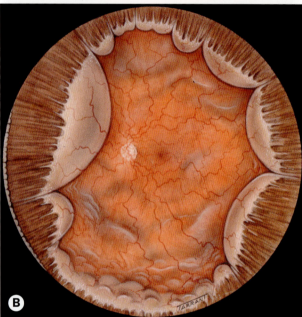

Fig. 8.11 Signs of posterior scleritis. **(A)** Choroidal folds; **(B)** uveal effusion

(Courtesy of S Chen – fig. A)

○ Uveal effusion with choroidal detachment may be present (Fig. 8.11B).
○ Disc oedema with accompanying reduction of vision is common, and is caused by spread of inflammation into the orbital tissue and optic nerve; treatment must not be delayed in these patients as permanent visual loss can ensue rapidly.
○ Myositis is common and gives rise to diplopia, pain on eye movement, tenderness to touch and redness around a muscle insertion.
○ Proptosis is usually mild and is frequently associated with ptosis.
○ Occasional features include raised IOP, periorbital oedema and chemosis. Associated anterior scleritis is a useful diagnostic aid but occurs only in a minority.

• **Ultrasonography** may show increased scleral thickness, scleral nodules, separation of Tenon capsule from sclera, disc oedema, choroidal folds and retinal detachment. Fluid in the Tenon space may give a characteristic 'T' sign, the stem of the T being formed by the optic nerve and the cross bar by the fluid-containing gap (Fig. 8.12).
• **MR** and **CT** may show scleral thickening and proptosis.

Differential diagnosis

• **Subretinal mass.** Alternative lesions include miscellaneous granulomatous conditions and choroidal neoplasia.
• **Choroidal folds**, retinal striae and disc oedema may also occur in orbital tumours, orbital inflammatory disease, thyroid eye disease, papilloedema and hypotony.
• **Exudative retinal detachment.** Vogt–Koyanagi–Harada (VKH) syndrome and central serous retinopathy.
• **Orbital cellulitis** may cause proptosis and periocular oedema but is associated with marked pyrexia.

Important systemic associations of scleritis

Rheumatoid arthritis

The autoimmune disease rheumatoid arthritis (RA) is the most common systemic association of scleritis, and is characterized by a symmetrical deforming inflammatory polyarthropathy, with a spectrum of possible extra-articular manifestations. Presentation is commonly in the third decade with joint swelling, usually of the hands (Fig. 8.13A). It is much more common in females than males. Rheumatoid factor autoantibodies are present in 80–90%. All forms of immune-mediated scleritis have been described in RA, and the clinical course is often more aggressive than when

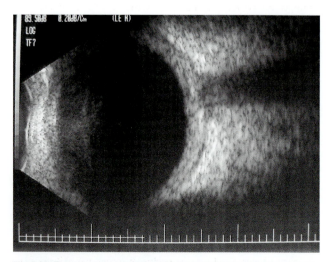

Fig. 8.12 B-scan ultrasonography in posterior scleritis shows scleral thickening and fluid in the sub-Tenon space, with the characteristic 'T sign' (see text)

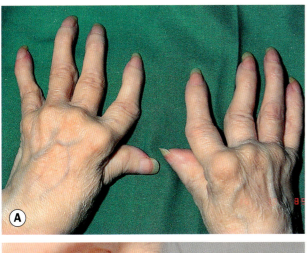
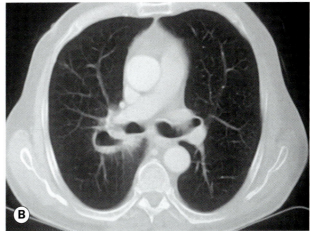
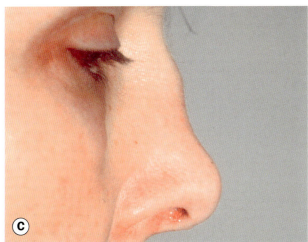
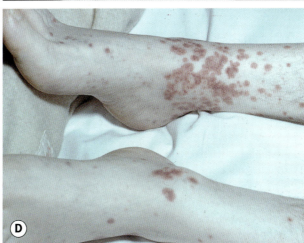

Fig. 8.13 Important systemic associations of scleritis. **(A)** Severe deformities of the hands in rheumatoid arthritis; **(B)** CT showing lung cavitation in Wegener granulomatosis; **(C)** saddle-shaped nasal deformity in relapsing polychondritis; **(D)** purpura in polyarteritis nodosa

(Courtesy of M Zatouroff, from Physical Signs in General Medicine, *Mosby 1996 – fig. A; J Nerad, K Carter and M Alford, from 'Oculoplastic and Reconstructive Surgery', in* Rapid Diagnosis in Ophthalmology, *Mosby 2008 – fig. B; C Pavesio – fig. C)*

there is no systemic association. Other ocular manifestations of RA include keratoconjunctivitis sicca (secondary Sjögren syndrome), ulcerative keratitis and acquired superior oblique tendon sheath syndrome (very rare).

Wegener granulomatosis

Wegener granulomatosis (granulomatosis with polyangiitis) is an idiopathic multisystem granulomatous disorder characterized by small vessel vasculitis typically affecting primarily the paranasal sinuses, lower respiratory tract (Fig. 8.13B) and the kidneys. There is a male predominance. Presentation is in the fifth decade on average, often with pulmonary symptoms. Antineutrophil cytoplasmic antibodies (cANCA) are found in over 90% of patients with active disease. Scleritis is often rapidly progressive, necrotizing and granulomatous. Other ocular manifestations include peripheral ulcerative keratitis, occlusive retinal vasculitis, orbital inflammatory disease, nasolacrimal obstruction, dacryocystitis and, rarely, tarsal–conjunctival disease.

Relapsing polychondritis

Relapsing polychondritis is a rare idiopathic condition characterized by small vessel vasculitis involving cartilage resulting in recurrent, often progressive, inflammatory episodes involving multiple organ systems such as the ears, respiratory system (Fig. 8.13C), heart and joints. Presentation is frequently in middle age. Scleritis is often intractable and may be necrotizing or non-necrotizing. Isolated anterior uveitis may also occur.

Polyarteritis nodosa

Polyarteritis nodosa (PAN) is an idiopathic aneurysmal vasculitis affecting medium-sized and small arteries, with a wide range of manifestations across multiple organ systems (Fig. 8.13D). Presentation is in the third to sixth decades, often with constitutional symptoms. The male : female ratio is about 3 : 1. Ocular involvement may precede the systemic manifestations by several years. About a third of patients have hepatitis B infection. Scleritis is often aggressive and necrotizing. Peripheral ulcerative keratitis, orbital pseudotumour and occlusive retinal periarteritis are other reported ocular features.

Treatment of immune-mediated scleritis

- **Topical steroids** do not affect the natural history of the scleral inflammation, but may relieve symptoms and oedema in non-necrotizing disease.
- **Systemic NSAIDs** should be used alone only in non-necrotizing disease; it is often necessary to try a number of different drugs before finding one that provides adequate relief of symptoms. A cyclooxygenase (COX)-2 inhibitor may be optimal for elderly patients or if there is a history of peptic ulceration, noting concerns regarding cardiovascular adverse effects for these and some other NSAIDs such as diclofenac.
- **Periocular steroid injections** may be used in non-necrotizing disease but their effects are usually transient; some authorities view them as contraindicated in necrotizing scleritis.
- **Systemic steroids** (e.g. prednisolone is 1–1.5 mg/kg/day) are used when NSAIDs are inappropriate or inadequate (necrotizing disease). Intravenous methylprednisolone may be used for emergent cases.
- **Immunosuppressives** and/or **biological blockers** should be considered if control is incomplete with steroids alone, as a steroid-sparing measure in long-term treatment or for underlying systemic disease. A wide range of drugs may be utilized, including cytostatics (e.g. cyclophosphamide, azathioprine, methotrexate), drugs acting on immunophilins (e.g. ciclosporin, tacrolimus) and others; in necrotizing disease, rituximab may be particularly effective.

INFECTIOUS SCLERITIS

Infectious scleritis is rare but may present diagnostic difficulty as the initial clinical features are similar to those of immune-mediated disease. In some cases infection may follow surgical or accidental trauma, endophthalmitis, or may occur as an extension of corneal infection.

Causes

- **Herpes zoster** is the most common infective cause. Necrotizing scleritis is extremely resistant to treatment and may result in a thinned or punched-out area (Fig. 8.14A).
- **Tuberculous** scleritis is rare and difficult to diagnose. The sclera may be infected by direct spread from a local conjunctival or choroidal lesion, or more commonly by haematogenous spread. Involvement may be nodular (Fig. 8.14B) or necrotizing.
- **Leprosy.** Recurrent necrotizing scleritis can occur, even after apparent systemic cure. Nodular disease may be seen in lepromatous leprosy.
- **Syphilis.** Diffuse anterior scleritis may occur in secondary syphilis, and occasionally scleral nodules may be a feature of tertiary syphilis.

- **Lyme disease.** Scleritis (Fig. 8.14C) is common but typically occurs long after initial infection.
- **Other causes** include fungi (Fig. 8.14D), *Pseudomonas aeruginosa* and *Nocardia*.

Treatment

Once the infective agent has been identified, specific antimicrobial therapy should be initiated. Topical and systemic steroids may also be used to reduce the inflammatory reaction. If appropriate, surgical debridement can be used to debulk a focus of infection and facilitates the penetration of antibiotics.

SCLERAL DISCOLORATION

Alkaptonuria

In this autosomal recessive condition a defect in homogentisic acid oxidase results in the accumulation of homogentisic acid in collagenous tissues such as cartilage and tendon (ochronosis). Systemic features include dark urine and arthropathy. Ocular manifestations include bluish-grey or black generalized pigmentation of the sclera and the tendons of horizontal recti associated with discrete pigmented globules (Fig. 8.15).

Haemochromatosis

The systemic features of haemochromatosis are caused by increased iron deposition in various tissues. Features may be more subtle than the classic triad of a bronze complexion, hepatomegaly and diabetes. Inheritance is autosomal recessive. Dry eye and rusty-brown perilimbal conjunctival and scleral discoloration may develop.

BLUE SCLERA

Blue scleral discoloration is caused by thinning or transparency with resultant visualization of the underlying uvea (Fig. 8.16). Major associations are discussed below; rare associations include Marshall–Smith syndrome (accelerated prenatal skeletal maturation and growth), Russell–Silver syndrome (short stature and other features) and Hallermann–Streiff–François syndrome.

Osteogenesis imperfecta

Osteogenesis imperfecta is an inherited disease of connective tissue, usually caused by defects in the synthesis and structure of type 1 collagen. There are multiple types, at least two of which have ocular features.

- **Type I** is autosomal dominant. Patients suffer few fractures with little or no deformity, hyperextensible joints, dental hypoplasia, deafness and easy bruising. Possible ocular features include blue sclera, megalocornea and corneal arcus.
- **Type IIA** is either sporadic or inherited in an autosomal dominant manner. Systemic features include deafness, dental anomalies, multiple fractures (Fig. 8.17A) and short limbs, with death in infancy from respiratory infection. Ocular manifestations include blue sclera and shallow orbits.

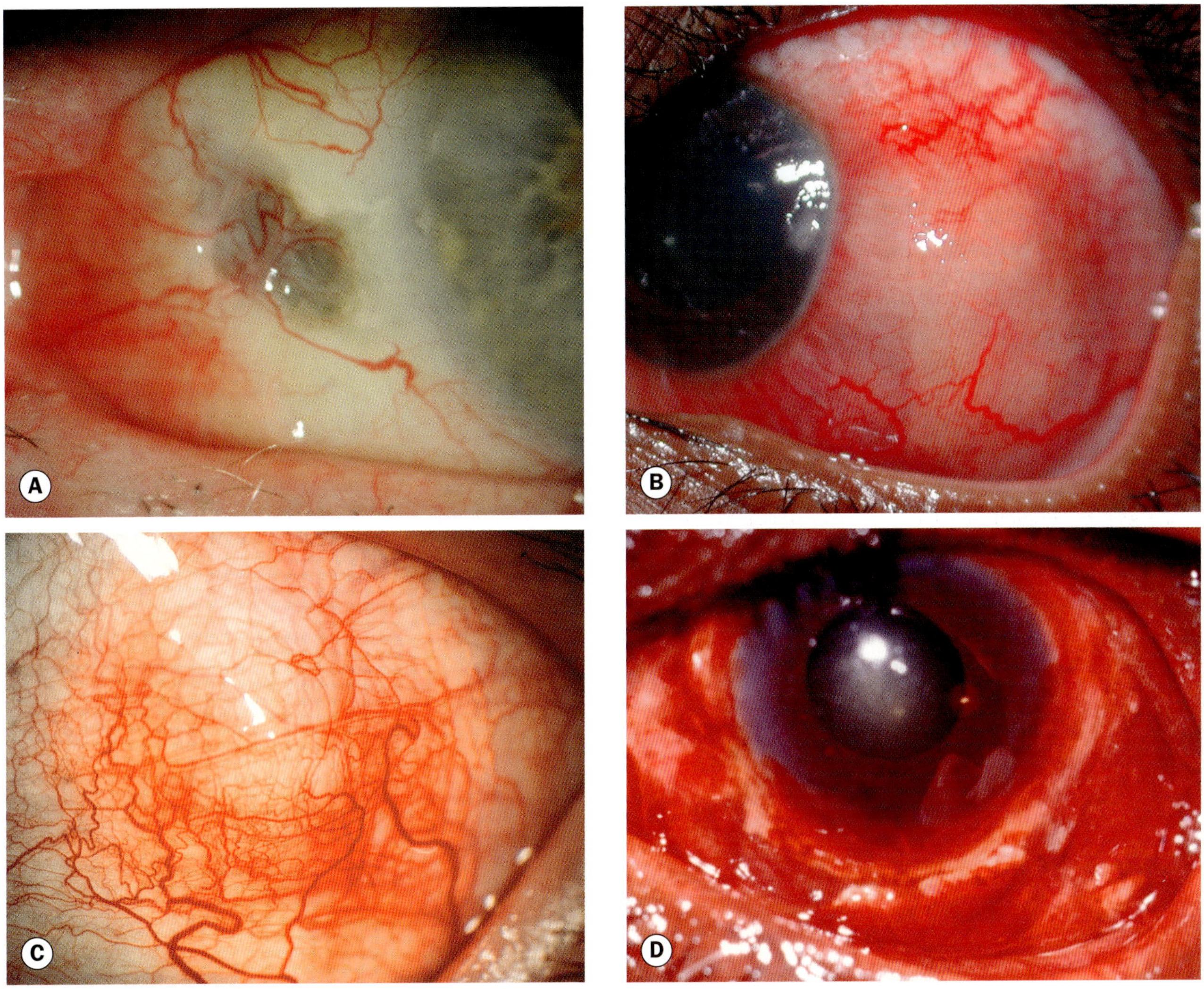

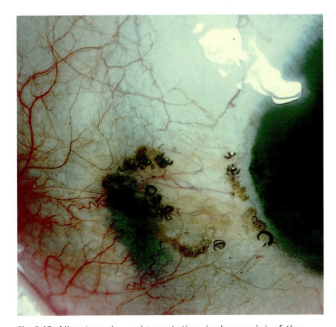

Fig. 8.14 Infectious scleritis. **(A)** Focal necrosis due to herpes zoster; **(B)** nodular tuberculous disease; **(C)** nodular scleritis in Lyme disease; **(D)** fungal infection
(Courtesy of R Fogla – fig. B, P Watson – fig. C; C Barry – fig. D)

Fig. 8.15 Alkaptonuria – pigmentation (ochronosis) of the sclera and horizontal rectus tendons

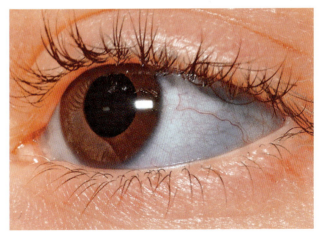

Fig. 8.16 Blue sclera
(Courtesy of P Watson)

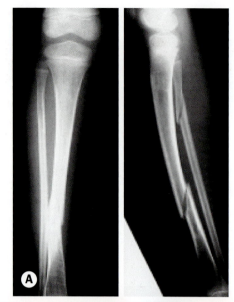

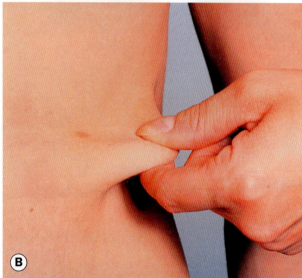

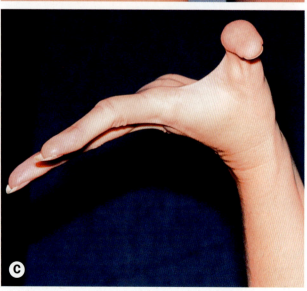

Fig. 8.17 Systemic associations of blue sclera. **(A)** multiple fractures in osteogenesis imperfecta type IIA; **(B)** cutaneous hyperelasticity and **(C)** joint hypermobility in Ehlers–Danlos syndrome type VI

(Courtesy of BJ Zitelli and HW Davis, from Atlas of Pediatric Physical Diagnosis, *Mosby 2002 – fig. A; MA Mir, from* Atlas of Clinical Diagnosis, *Saunders, 2003 – fig. B; JH Krachmer, MJ Mannis and EJ Holland, from* Cornea, *Elsevier 2005 – fig. C)*

Ehlers–Danlos syndrome type VI

Ehlers–Danlos syndrome VI (ocular sclerotic) is an inherited disorder of collagen formation. Patients have thin and hyperelastic skin (Fig. 8.17B) that bruises easily and heals slowly; joints are hypermobile (Fig. 8.17C), which may lead to recurrent dislocation and falls. Cardiovascular disease can be severe, including a bleeding diathesis, dissecting aneurysms, spontaneous rupture of large blood vessels and mitral valve prolapse. There are six major types but type VI and, rarely, type IV, are associated with ocular features. As well as blue sclera, these may include scleral fragility (globe rupture may be caused by mild trauma), epicanthic folds, microcornea, keratoconus, keratoglobus, ectopia lentis, myopia and retinal detachment.

MISCELLANEOUS CONDITIONS

Congenital ocular melanocytosis

Congenital ocular melanocytosis is an uncommon condition characterized by an increase in number, size and pigmentation of melanocytes in the sclera and uvea. The periocular skin, orbit, meninges and soft palate may also be involved.

- **Ocular** melanocytosis, the least common, involves only the eye. Multifocal slate-grey pigmentation is seen within the sclera and episclera (Fig. 8.18A) – the process does not involve the overlying conjunctival layers, unless there is incidental conjunctival pigmentation. The overlying conjunctiva is mobile over the episcleral pigmentation but the pigmentation itself is intrinsic and cannot be moved over the globe. The peripheral cornea is occasionally involved.
- **Dermal** melanocytosis (one-third) involves only the skin.
- **Oculodermal** melanocytosis (naevus of Ota) is the most common type and involves both skin and eye. Naevus of Ota is bilateral in 5%; it occurs frequently in darker-complexioned races but is rare in Caucasians. There is deep bluish hyperpigmentation of the facial skin, most frequently in the distribution of the first and second trigeminal divisions (Fig. 8.18B). It may be subtle in pale-skinned individuals, when it is best detected under good lighting.
- **Ipsilateral associations**
  - Iris hyperchromia is common (Fig. 8.19A).
  - Iris mammillations are uncommon, tiny, regularly spaced villiform lesions (Fig. 8.19B). They may also be found in

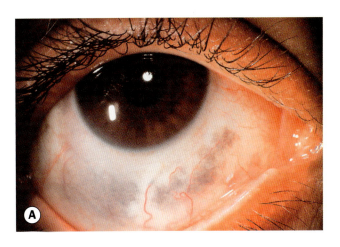
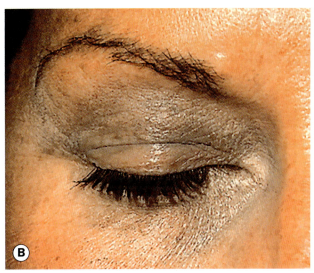

Fig. 8.18 Congenital melanocytosis. **(A)** Episcleral melanocytosis; **(B)** cutaneous melanocytosis in naevus of Ota

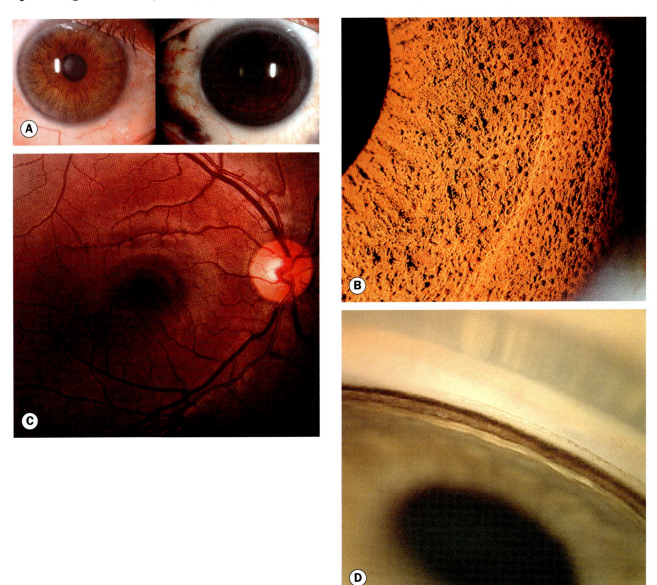

Fig. 8.19 Ipsilateral associations of naevus of Ota. **(A)** Iris heterochromia (hyperchromia); **(B)** iris mammillations; **(C)** fundus hyperpigmentation; **(D)** trabecular hyperpigmentation

(Courtesy of B Gilli – fig. A; L MacKeen – fig. D)

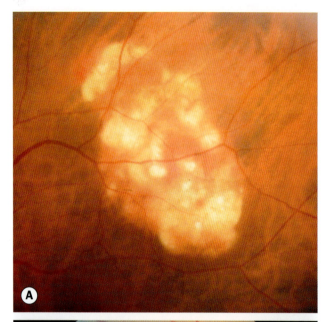

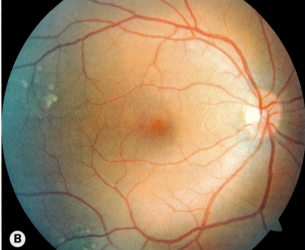

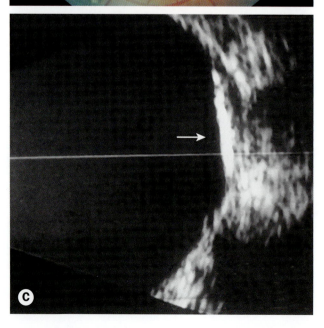

Fig. 8.20 Idiopathic sclerochoroidal calcification. **(A)** Single large lesion; **(B)** early lesions in typical locations associated with the temporal vascular arcades; **(C)** ultrasonogram showing a highly reflective calcific lesion with orbital shadowing

(Courtesy of A Agarwal, from Gass' Atlas of Macular Diseases, Elsevier Saunders 2012 – fig. C)

neurofibromatosis type 1, Axenfeld–Rieger anomaly and Peters anomaly.
○ Fundus hyperpigmentation (Fig. 8.19C).
○ Trabecular hyperpigmentation (Fig. 8.19D); this is associated with glaucoma in about 10% of cases.
○ Uveal melanoma develops in a small minority of patients, and long-term anterior and posterior segment review is required.

Idiopathic sclerochoroidal calcification

Idiopathic sclerochoroidal calcification is an innocuous, age-related condition that usually involves both eyes of an affected older adult.
- **Signs.** Geographical yellow–white fundus lesions with ill-defined margins (Fig. 8.20A), often multiple and located in the superotemporal or inferotemporal mid-periphery associated with the vascular arcades (Fig. 8.20B).
- **Ultrasonography** shows highly reflective choroidal plaque-like lesions with orbital shadowing (Fig. 8.20C).
- **Differential diagnosis** is mainly from osseous metaplasia associated with a choroidal haemangioma, and from

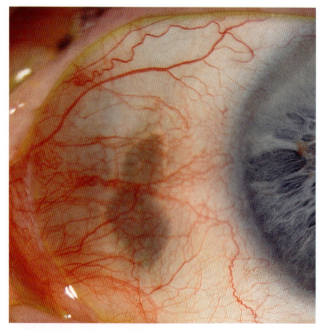

Fig. 8.21 Scleral hyaline plaque

choroidal osteoma, which is usually a single – though often large – lesion that usually (80–90%) involves only one eye.

Scleral hyaline plaque and senile scleromalacia

Scleral hyaline plaques are oval dark-greyish, generally sharply demarcated, areas located close to the insertion of the horizontal rectus muscles (Fig. 8.21). Senile scleromalacia refers to a spontaneously occurring irregular, oval or kidney-shaped partial-thickness scleral defect found at the same location, typically with one or more scleral hyaline plaques at the opposite location in the same eye or in the fellow eye; separation of a scleral hyaline plaque to leave an area of scleromalacia has been described. Both these entities typically affect elderly patients, are innocuous, and should not be confused with scleromalacia perforans (see above), which occurs in somewhat younger patients, may be located anywhere in the anterior sclera, is unassociated with hyaline plaques elsewhere and can progress to a full-thickness scleral defect with uveal exposure.

ACQUIRED CATARACT

Age-related cataract

Subcapsular cataract

Anterior subcapsular cataract lies directly under the lens capsule and is associated with fibrous metaplasia of the lens epithelium. Posterior subcapsular opacity lies just in front of the posterior capsule and has a granular or plaque-like appearance on oblique slit lamp biomicroscopy (Fig. 9.1A), but typically appears black and vacuolated (Fig. 9.1B) on retroillumination; the vacuoles are swollen migratory lens epithelial cells (bladder or Wedl), similar to those commonly seen postoperatively in posterior capsular opacification (see Fig. 9.21A). Due to its location at the nodal point of the eye, a posterior subcapsular opacity often has a particularly profound effect on vision. Patients are characteristically troubled by glare, for instance from the headlights of oncoming cars, and symptoms are increased by miosis, such as occurs during near visual activity and in bright sunlight.

Nuclear sclerotic cataract

Nuclear cataract is an exaggeration of normal ageing change. It is often associated with myopia due to an increase in the refractive index of the nucleus, resulting in some elderly patients being able to read without spectacles again ('second sight of the aged'); in contrast, in the healthy ageing eye (and in occasional cases of cortical and subcapsular cataract) there is mild hypermetropic shift. Nuclear sclerotic cataract is characterized by a yellowish hue due to the deposition of urochrome pigment, and is best assessed with an oblique slit lamp beam (Fig. 9.1C). When advanced, the nucleus appears brown (Fig. 9.1D) or even black, the latter being typical of marked post-vitrectomy opacity.

Cortical cataract

Cortical cataract may involve the anterior, posterior or equatorial cortex. The opacities start as clefts and vacuoles between lens fibres due to cortical hydration. Subsequent opacification results in typical cuneiform (wedge-shaped) or radial spoke-like opacities (Figs 9.2A and B), often initially in the inferonasal quadrant. As with posterior subcapsular opacity, glare is a common symptom.

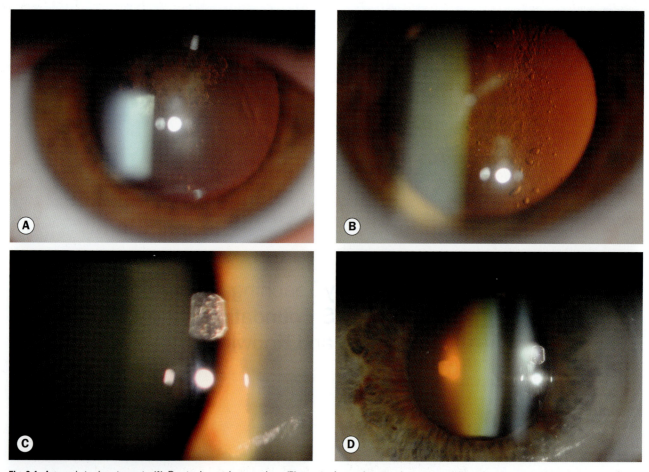

Fig. 9.1 Age-related cataract. **(A)** Posterior subcapsular; **(B)** posterior subcapsular on retroillumination, showing Wedl cells; **(C)** minimal and **(D)** moderate nuclear sclerosis

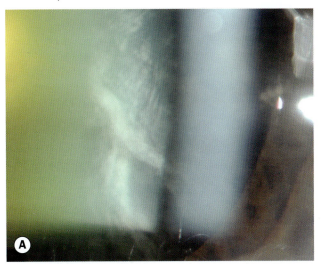

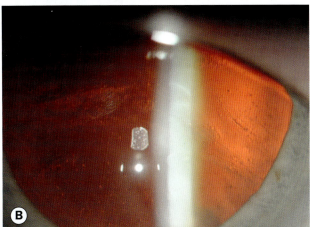

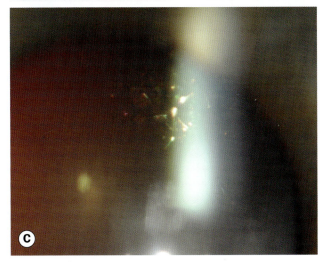

Fig. 9.2 Age-related cataract. **(A)** Cortical; **(B)** cortical on retroillumination; **(C)** Christmas tree

Christmas tree cataract

Christmas tree cataract, which is uncommon, is characterized by polychromatic needle-like formations in the deep cortex and nucleus (Fig. 9.2C).

Cataract maturity

- **Immature** cataract is one in which the lens is partially opaque.
- **Mature** cataract is one in which the lens is completely opaque (Fig. 9.3A).
- **Hypermature** cataract has a shrunken and wrinkled anterior capsule (Fig. 9.3B) due to leakage of water out of the lens.
- **Morgagnian** cataract is a hypermature cataract in which liquefaction of the cortex has allowed the nucleus to sink inferiorly (Fig. 9.3C).

Cataract in systemic disease

Diabetes mellitus

Hyperglycaemia is reflected in a high level of glucose in the aqueous humour, which diffuses into the lens. Here glucose is metabolized into sorbitol, which accumulates within the lens, resulting in secondary osmotic overhydration. In mild degree, this may affect the refractive index of the lens with consequent fluctuation of refraction in line with the plasma glucose level, hyperglycaemia resulting in myopia and vice versa. Cortical fluid vacuoles develop and later evolve into frank opacities. Classic diabetic cataract, which is actually rare, consists of snowflake cortical opacities (Fig. 9.4A) occurring in the young diabetic; it may mature within a few days or resolve spontaneously. Age-related cataract occurs earlier in diabetes mellitus. Nuclear opacities are common and tend to progress rapidly.

Myotonic dystrophy

About 90% of patients with myotonic dystrophy (see Ch. 19) develop fine iridescent cortical opacities in the third decade, sometimes resembling Christmas tree cataract; these evolve into visually disabling wedge-shaped cortical and subcapsular opacities, often star-like in conformation (Fig. 9.4B) by the fifth decade. Later, the opacities may become indistinguishable from typical cortical cataract.

Atopic dermatitis

About 10% of patients with severe atopic dermatitis develop cataracts in the second to fourth decades; these are often bilateral and may mature quickly. Shield-like dense anterior subcapsular plaque that wrinkles the anterior capsule (Fig. 9.4C) is characteristic. Posterior subcapsular opacities may also occur.

Neurofibromatosis type 2

Neurofibromatosis type 2 (NF2; see Ch. 19) is associated with early cataract in more than 60% of patients. Opacities are posterior subcapsular or capsular, cortical or mixed, and tend to develop in early adulthood.

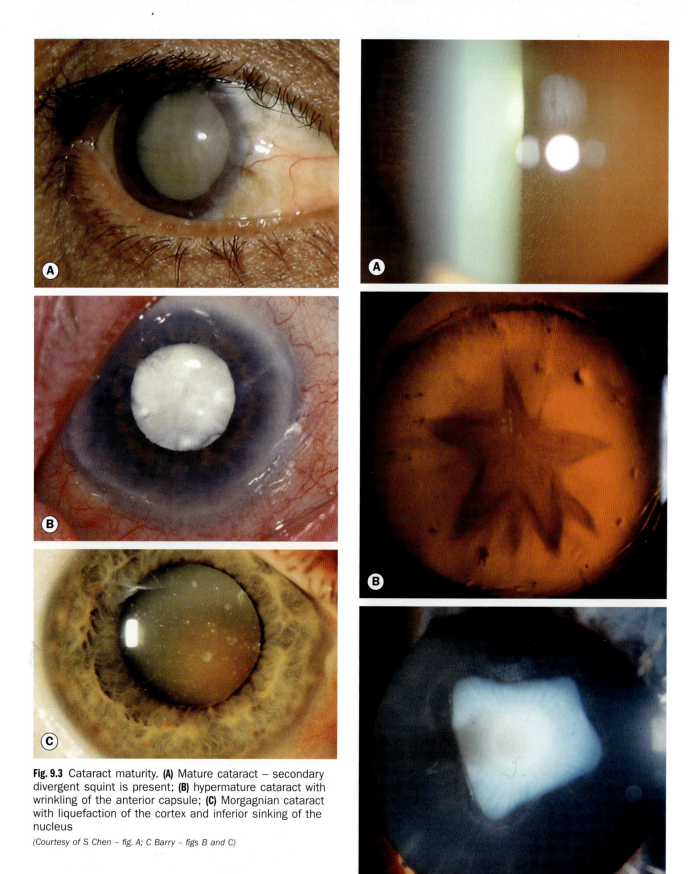

Fig. 9.3 Cataract maturity. **(A)** Mature cataract – secondary divergent squint is present; **(B)** hypermature cataract with wrinkling of the anterior capsule; **(C)** Morgagnian cataract with liquefaction of the cortex and inferior sinking of the nucleus

(Courtesy of S Chen – fig. A; C Barry – figs B and C)

Fig. 9.4 Cataract in systemic disease. **(A)** Diabetic snowflake cataract; **(B)** posterior subcapsular cataract spokes assuming a stellate morphology in myotonic dystrophy; **(C)** shield-like anterior subcapsular cataract in atopic dermatitis

Secondary cataract

A secondary (complicated) cataract develops as a result of other primary ocular disease.

Chronic anterior uveitis

Chronic anterior uveitis is the most common cause of secondary cataract, the incidence being related to the duration and intensity of inflammation. Topical and systemic steroids used in treatment are also causative. The earliest finding is often a polychromatic lustre at the posterior pole of the lens (Fig. 9.5A). If inflammation persists, posterior and anterior opacities (Fig. 9.5B) develop. Cataract appears to progress more rapidly in the presence of posterior synechiae (Fig. 9.5C).

Acute congestive angle closure

Acute congestive angle closure may cause small anterior grey-white subcapsular or capsular opacities, glaukomflecken (Fig. 9.5D), to form within the pupillary area. These represent focal infarcts of the lens epithelium and are almost pathognomonic of prior acute angle-closure glaucoma.

High myopia

High (pathological) myopia can be associated with posterior subcapsular lens opacities and early-onset nuclear sclerosis, which ironically may increase the myopic refractive error.

Hereditary fundus dystrophies

Hereditary fundus dystrophies (see Ch. 15) such as retinitis pigmentosa, Leber congenital amaurosis, gyrate atrophy and Stickler syndrome, may be associated with posterior and, less commonly, anterior subcapsular lens opacities (Fig. 9.5E). Cataract surgery may improve visual function even in the presence of severe retinal changes.

Traumatic cataract

Trauma is the most common cause of unilateral cataract in young individuals.

- **Penetrating trauma** (Fig. 9.6A).
- **Blunt trauma** may cause a characteristic flower-shaped opacity (Fig. 9.6B).
- **Electric shock** is a rare cause of cataract, patterns including diffuse milky-white opacification and multiple snowflake-like opacities, sometimes in a stellate subcapsular distribution (Fig. 9.6C).
- **Infrared radiation**, if intense as in glassblowers, may rarely cause true exfoliation of the anterior lens capsule (Fig. 9.6D).
- **Ionizing radiation** exposure such as for ocular tumour treatment may cause posterior subcapsular opacities (Fig. 9.6E); these may not manifest for months or years.

MANAGEMENT OF AGE-RELATED CATARACT

Preoperative considerations

Indications for surgery

- **Visual improvement** is by far the most common indication for cataract surgery. Operation is indicated when the opacity develops to a degree sufficient to cause difficulty in performing essential daily activities. Clear lens exchange (replacement of the healthy lens with an artificial implant) is an option for the management of refractive error.
- **Medical** indications are those in which a cataract is adversely affecting the health of the eye, for example phacolytic or phacomorphic glaucoma; clear lens exchange usually definitively addresses primary angle closure, but less invasive options are generally preferred (see Ch. 10). Cataract surgery to improve the clarity of the ocular media may also be required in the context of monitoring or treatment of fundus pathology.

Systemic preoperative assessment

For elective surgery, a general medical history is taken and any problems managed accordingly. Table 9.1 sets out suggested further enquiry and action in relation to a range of systemic diseases. Routine preoperative general medical examination, blood tests and electrocardiogram (ECG) are not usually required for local anaesthesia. If general anaesthesia is planned, assessment is according to local protocol, e.g. general examination, urea and electrolytes, random blood glucose, full blood count and ECG; an anaesthetic opinion may be considered for chronically unwell or medically complex patients.

- **Current medication** should be recorded. This will often guide general medical assessment. Medications relevant to eye surgery include:
  - Systemic alpha-blockers (e.g. tamsulosin) are commonly associated with intraoperative floppy iris syndrome (IFIS).
  - Management of anticoagulant therapy or an antiplatelet agent should follow local protocol. Most surgeons do not stop antiplatelet drugs for cataract surgery, though this may be preferred for larger oculoplastic procedures. Anticoagulation status, usually expressed as the international normalized ratio (INR) level, should be within the therapeutic range appropriate for the individual indication (e.g. usually higher for heart valve thrombosis prophylaxis than following deep vein thrombosis); a common approach is to check the INR within the 24 hours prior to surgery in stable patients.
- **Allergy.** True allergy rather than intolerance should be confirmed.
  - Medication, including sulfonamides and antibiotics commonly used following cataract surgery.
  - Iodine or shellfish – the latter may indicate an iodine allergy. If allergy to iodine is present an alternative skin

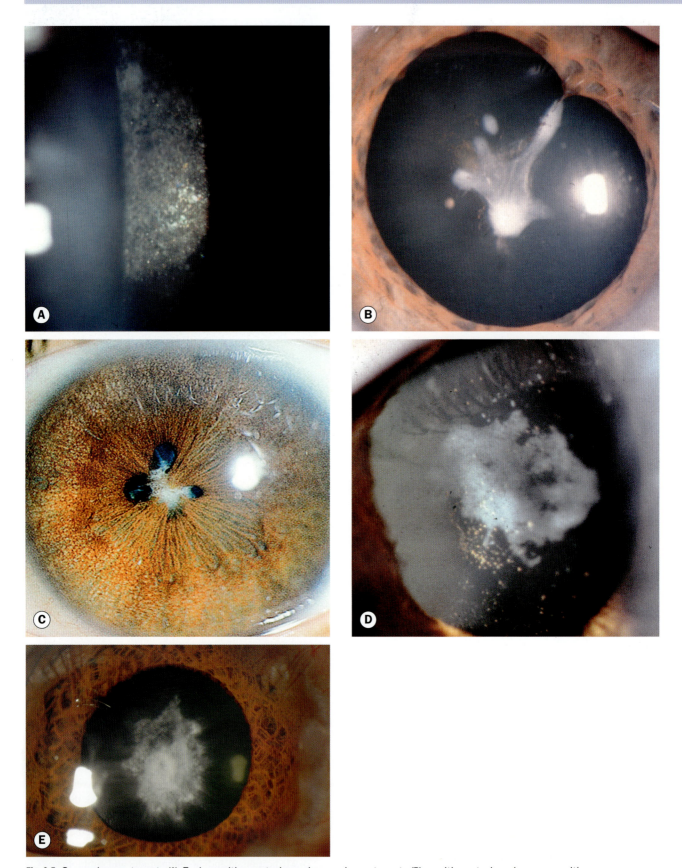

Fig. 9.5 Secondary cataract. **(A)** Early uveitic posterior subcapsular cataract; **(B)** uveitic anterior plaque opacities; **(C)** extensive posterior synechiae and anterior lens opacity; **(D)** glaukomflecken; **(E)** anterior subcapsular cataract in retinitis pigmentosa

(Courtesy of S Chen – fig. E)

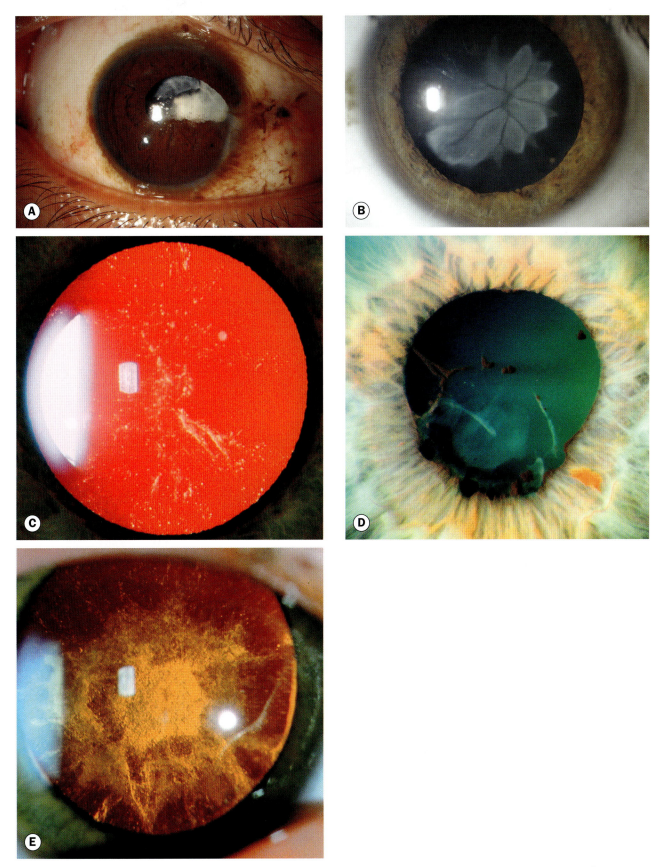

Fig. 9.6 Causes of traumatic cataract. **(A)** Penetrating trauma; **(B)** blunt trauma; **(C)** electric shock and lightning strike;
(D) infrared radiation (glassblower's cataract); **(E)** ionizing radiation

(Courtesy of S Chen – fig. A; C Barry – fig. B; J Schuman, V Christopoulos, D Dhaliwal, M Kahook and R Noecker, from 'Lens and Glaucoma', in Rapid Diagnosis in Ophthalmology, Mosby 2008 – figs C–E)

Table 9.1 Management of general medical conditions prior to elective surgery

Condition	Further questions/examination	Action
Diabetes mellitus	Well-controlled? Will need blood test (finger-prick may be sufficient, consider additional tests if necessary)	If control poor, may need to defer surgery and contact patient's physician Medication and food and drink intake as usual on the day of surgery for local anaesthesia
Systemic hypertension	If systolic >170 mmHg or diastolic >100 mmHg may need physician opinion	Consider contacting physician for optimization; defer surgery if necessary as risk of suprachoroidal haemorrhage may be elevated
Actual or suspected myocardial infarction (MI) in the past	Date of MI?	Defer surgery for 3–6 months from date of MI. Contact physician/anaesthetist if concerns about current cardiovascular status
Angina	Stable/well controlled?	Bring glyceryl trinitrate (GTN) spray on day of surgery. If unstable, contact physician or anaesthetist
Respiratory disease	Is chest function currently optimal? Can the patient lie flat?	If the patient cannot lie flat, may need to discuss with operating surgeon. Trial of lying flat (at least half an hour) Chest function should be optimized as far as possible prior to surgery Remind patient to bring any inhalers to hospital
Leg ulcer or other skin wound	Acute or chronic? Evidence of active infection?	Surgery should be deferred until active infection has resolved. If healing is not possible (e.g. chronic leg ulcer) the lesion should be covered with a sterile dressing during the perioperative period. A preoperative wound swab for culture, and prophylactic oral antibiotics may be considered
Rheumatic fever, transplanted or prosthetic heart valve, previous endocarditis	Does the patient usually require prophylactic antibiotic cover for operations?	Antibiotic prophylaxis only exceptionally required for ophthalmic surgery, e.g. removal of an infected eye
Stroke in the past	Date of stroke? Particular residual difficulties?	Defer surgery for at least 6 months from date of stroke Many have positional/other practical consequences
Rheumatoid arthritis	Does the patient have any problems lying flat or with neck position?	If in doubt about patient's ability to position appropriately, may need to discuss with operating surgeon; intubation for general anaesthesia may be more difficult in some patients
Jaundice or known viral hepatitis in the past	What was the underlying diagnosis?	If viral hepatitis suspected, note prominently as special precautions to avoid needlestick injury may be necessary
Human immunodeficiency virus (HIV) infection	If there are any high-risk factors, has the patient undergone an HIV test in the past?	Special precautions to avoid needlestick injury may be necessary
Sickle status	For patients of southern Asian and Afro-Caribbean ethnic origin, enquire about sickle status	Blood test if unknown and general anaesthesia planned
Parkinson disease or other cause of substantial tremor	Is the patient able to maintain head stability sufficiently to cooperate with local anaesthesia and surgery?	If not, may require general anaesthesia
Epilepsy	Is the condition well controlled?	General anaesthesia may be preferred
Myotonic dystrophy	Has the patient undergone surgery and anaesthesia in the past?	If general anaesthesia is planned, an anaesthetic opinion should be obtained well in advance of surgery

and conjunctival antiseptic such as chlorhexidine should be used.

- ○ Others: latex (latex-free gloves may be necessary), sticking plaster, local anaesthetics, insect bites (cross-reaction with hyaluronidase that is often used with local anaesthesia).
- **Methicillin-resistant *Staphylococcus aureus* (MRSA) carriage.** Relevant national and local protocols for the identification and management of patients at high risk for MRSA carriage should be followed.
- **Transport** (to hospital and to the operating theatre within hospital): special arrangements may be needed for patients with poor mobility or exceptionally high body mass.

For urgent or emergency surgery, medical risks should be assessed individually and according to the circumstances.

Ophthalmic preoperative assessment

A detailed and pertinent ophthalmic evaluation is required. Following the taking of a past ophthalmic history, the following should be considered:

- **Visual acuity** is usually tested using a Snellen chart, despite its limitations (see Ch. 14).
- **Cover test.** A heterotropia may indicate amblyopia, which carries a guarded visual prognosis, or the possibility of diplopia if the vision is improved. A squint, usually a divergence, may develop in an eye with poor vision due to cataract, and lens surgery alone may straighten the eye.
- **Pupillary responses.** Because cataract never produces an afferent pupillary defect, its presence implies substantial additional pathology.
- **Ocular adnexa.** Dacryocystitis, blepharitis, chronic conjunctivitis, lagophthalmos, ectropion, entropion and tear film abnormalities may predispose to endophthalmitis and in most cases optimization should be achieved prior to intraocular surgery.
- **Cornea.** Eyes with decreased endothelial cell counts (e.g. substantial cornea guttata) have increased vulnerability to postoperative decompensation secondary to operative trauma. Specular microscopy and pachymetry may be helpful in assessing risk, and precautions should be taken to protect the endothelium (see below). A prominent arcus senilis is often associated with a surgical view of decreased clarity, as are stromal opacities.
- **Anterior chamber.** A shallow anterior chamber can render cataract surgery difficult. Recognition of a poorly dilating pupil allows intensive preoperative mydriatic drops, planned mechanical dilatation prior to capsulorhexis and/or intracameral injection of mydriatic. A poor red reflex compromises the creation of a capsulorhexis, but can be largely overcome by staining the capsule with trypan blue.
- **Lens.** Nuclear cataracts tend to be harder and may require more power for phacoemulsification, while cortical and subcapsular opacities tend to be softer. Black nuclear opacities are extremely dense and extracapsular cataract extraction rather than phacoemulsification may be the superior option. Pseudoexfoliation indicates a likelihood of weak zonules (phakodonesis – lens wobble – may be present), a fragile capsule and poor mydriasis.
- **Fundus examination.** Pathology such as age-related macular degeneration may affect the visual outcome. Ultrasonography may be required, principally to exclude retinal detachment and staphyloma, in eyes with very dense opacity that precludes fundus examination.
- **Sclera.** If a prominent explant/encircling band has been placed during prior retinal detachment surgery, the eye is particularly large or the sclera thin (e.g. high myopia), peri- and retrobulbar local anaesthesia may be avoided and special care taken with sub-Tenon local anaesthetic infiltration.
- **Current refractive status.** It is critical to obtain details of the patient's preoperative refractive error in order to guide intraocular lens (IOL) implant selection. The keratometry readings (obtained during biometry – see below) should be noted in relation to the refraction, particularly if it is planned to address astigmatism by means of targeted wound placement, a toric IOL or a specific adjunctive procedure. It is particularly important to obtain a postoperative refractive result from an eye previously operated upon so that any 'refractive surprise', even if minor, can be taken into account.

Informed consent

It is essential that the patient has arrived at a fully informed decision to proceed with cataract surgery. As well as discussing the benefits, risks should be conveyed at a level appropriate to each patient's level of understanding, with an explanation of the more common and severe potential problems. Points for discussion with the patient may include:

- Most cataract operations are straightforward, with the patient achieving good vision.
- Most complications can be dealt with effectively and cause no long-term difficulties, but some rare problems can be very serious.
- In about 1 in 1000 cataract operations the eye will be left with little or no sight; in about 1 in 10 000 the patient will lose the eye.
- Some complications mean that a second operation will be necessary.
- Relatively mild and usually easily treatable but common complications include: periocular ecchymosis, allergy to eye drops, intraocular pressure (IOP) spike, iridocyclitis, posterior capsular opacification (currently in decline) and wound leak.
- Moderate to severe but less common complications: posterior capsular rupture/vitreous loss (1% or less for experienced surgeons, higher for trainees dependent on experience), zonular dehiscence, cystoid macular oedema (CMO), dropped nucleus (about 0.2%), corneal decompensation sufficient to need corneal graft, intolerable refractive outcome (may need contact lens wear, lens implant exchange or corneal surgery), retinal detachment (<1%), IOL dislocation, persistent ptosis and diplopia.

- Rare but invariably very serious complications: endophthalmitis (0.1%) and suprachoroidal haemorrhage (0.04%).
- The risks of anaesthesia should be conveyed by the person administering it. Local anaesthesia carries only a low risk of problems, though some rare complications have the potential to be very serious including loss of the eye and even death: allergy to the anaesthetic agent, retrobulbar haemorrhage (see Ch. 21), perforation of the globe, and inadvertent infusion of anaesthetic agent into the cerebrospinal fluid via the optic nerve sheath causing brainstem anaesthesia.
- There is virtually no risk to the other eye; sympathetic ophthalmitis is vanishingly rare following modern cataract surgery.

Biometry

Biometry facilitates calculation of the lens power likely to result in the desired postoperative refractive outcome; in its basic form this involves the measurement of two ocular parameters, keratometry and axial (anteroposterior) length.

- **Keratometry** involves determination of the curvature of the anterior corneal surface (steepest and flattest meridians), expressed in dioptres or in millimetres of radius of curvature. This is commonly carried out with the interferometry apparatus used to determine axial length (see below), but if this is unavailable or unsuitable manual keratometry (e.g. Javal–Schiøtz keratometer) or corneal topography can be performed.
- **Optical coherence biometry** (Figs 9.7A and B) is a non-contact method of axial length measurement that utilizes two coaxial partially coherent low-energy laser beams to produce an interference pattern (partial coherence interferometry). Modern biometry devices also perform keratometry, anterior chamber depth and corneal white-to-white measurement, and are able to calculate IOL power using a range of formulae. Measurements have high reproducibility and generally require less skill than ultrasonic biometry (see below).
- **A-scan ultrasonography** is a generally slightly less accurate method of determining the axial dimension and can be acquired either by direct contact (Fig. 9.7C) or more accurately but with greater technical difficulty by using a water bath over the eye (immersion ultrasonography). The sound beam must be aligned with the visual axis for maximal precision; each reflecting surface is represented by a spike on an oscilloscope display monitor (Fig. 9.7D).
- **IOL power calculation formulae.** Numerous formulae have been developed that utilize keratometry and axial length to calculate the IOL power required to achieve a given refractive outcome. Some formulae incorporate additional parameters such as anterior chamber depth and lens thickness to try to optimize accuracy. The SRK-T, Haigis, Hoffer Q and Holladay 1 and 2 are commonly used. Specific formulae may be superior for very short (possibly the Hoffer

Q) or long eyes, but opinions vary and it is always wise to plan individually for an unusual eye, consulting the latest research and recommendations. Short eyes in particular are prone to unexpected mean spherical and astigmatic errors following surgery.
- **Previous refractive surgery.** Any form of corneal refractive surgery is likely to make a significant difference to the IOL power required, and standard IOL calculations are unsuitable. Several different methods have been described to address this situation. Most involve the calculation of the post-refractive procedure 'true' corneal power using a special process (refractive history method, contact lens method) and insertion of this into a standard (e.g. Hoffer Q) or specific (e.g. Masket) formula, but the Haigis-L regression formula uses statistical data to facilitate calculation on post-refractive surgery eyes using only standard inputs. It may prudent to utilize more than one method of IOL calculation.
- **Contact lenses.** If the patient wears soft contact lenses, these should not be worn for up to a week prior to biometry to allow corneal stabilization; hard/gas permeable lenses may need to be left out for 3 weeks.
- **Personalized A-constant.** If a consistent postoperative refractive deviation is found in most of an individual surgeon's cases, it is assumed that some aspects of personal surgical (or possibly biometric) technique consistently and similarly influence outcome, and a personalized A-constant can be programmed into biometry apparatus to take this into account.

Postoperative refraction

- **Emmetropia** is typically the desired postoperative refraction, though usually spectacles will be needed for near vision since a conventional IOL cannot accommodate. Many surgeons aim for a small degree of myopia (about −0.25 D) to offset possible errors in biometry; postoperative hypermetropia, which necessitates correction for clear vision at all distances, is typically less well tolerated than myopia.
- **Contralateral eye.** Postoperative refractive planning must take account of the contralateral eye. If this has a significant refractive error but is unlikely to require cataract surgery within a few years, the postoperative target for the operated eye might be set for within less than 2.0 D of its fellow, to avoid problems with binocular fusion. In some cases, such as when there is an early lens opacity in the fellow eye or when ametropia is extreme, the patient can be offered lens surgery to the other eye to facilitate targeting both at emmetropia.
- **'Monovision'** is a concept in which the (usually) non-dominant eye is left with between 1 and 2 dioptres of myopia to allow reading, whilst emmetropia is targeted in the dominant eye. This is attractive to some patients, generally those who have previously been using contact lenses or spectacles to achieve monovision.
- **Multifocal** lens options use a variety of optical means to attempt to achieve satisfactory near, distance and intermediate vision. Many patients are very satisfied with the

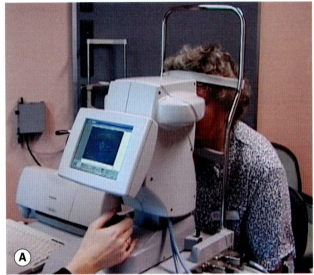

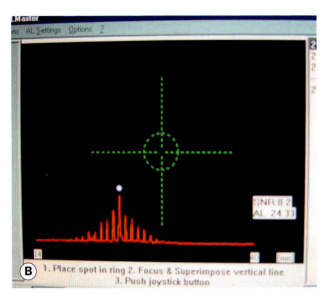

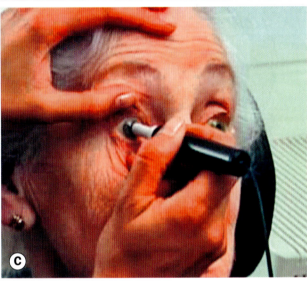

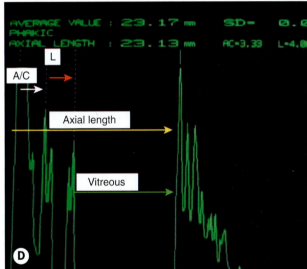

Fig. 9.7 Biometry. **(A)** Optical coherence biometry; **(B)** optical biometry monitor display; **(C)** contact ultrasonic biometry; **(D)** ultrasonographic monitor display (A/C, anterior chamber depth; L, lens thickness)

(Courtesy of D Michalik and J Bolger)

results but a significant minority are unhappy, complaining of phenomena such as glare. Highly accurate refractive outcomes, including very limited astigmatism, are necessary for optimal function and a greater likelihood of tolerance.

- **Younger patients.** With a conventional monofocal IOL, patients younger than about 50 need to be aware that they will experience the sudden loss of active focusing and that it will often take some time to adjust.

Intraocular lenses

Positioning

An IOL (Fig. 9.8A) consists of an optic and haptics. The optic is the central refracting element, and the haptics the arms or loops that sit in contact with peripheral ocular structures to centralize

the optic. Modern cataract surgery, with preservation of the lens capsule, affords positioning of the IOL in the ideal location – 'in the bag' (Fig. 9.8B). Complicated surgery, with rupture of the posterior capsule, may necessitate alternative positioning in the posterior chamber with the haptics in the ciliary sulcus (a three-piece IOL only, not one-piece including those with plate haptics, as these may not be stable), or in the anterior chamber (AC) with the haptics supported in the angle – AC positioning requires a specific lens type. In some circumstances a supplementary IOL may be placed in the sulcus in addition to an IOL in the capsular bag, for instance to address a residual refractive error following primary surgery (secondary pseudopolyphakia), and thin-profile IOLs are available for this purpose. It is preferable to avoid a secondary sulcus IOL (primary pseudopolyphakia) in very short (e.g. nanophthalmic) eyes due to the risk of angle closure; off-the-shelf IOLs of power up to 40 D are available, and custom IOLs can be produced in even higher powers.

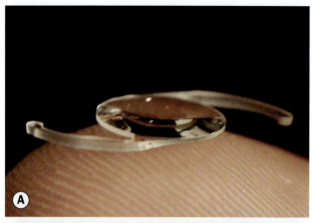

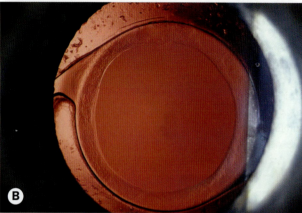

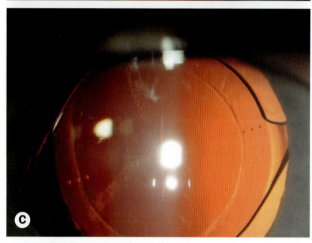

Fig. 9.8 Intraocular lens (IOL). **(A)** One-piece flexible IOL – note the square-edged optic; **(B)** IOL *in situ* in the capsular bag; **(C)** implanted toric IOL showing diametrically opposite sets of three dots marking the lens axis
(Courtesy of C Barry – fig. A)

Design

- **Flexible IOLs** introduced into the eye via an injector and subsequently unrolled inside the eye are now in general use. Injector-based delivery utilizes a very small incision and also allows avoidance of lens contact with the ocular surface, so reducing the risk of bacterial contamination; simple folding of the IOL is an alternative, but requires a larger incision.

Flexible materials available are discussed below; there seems to be no distinct superiority of one material over another.

- ○ Acrylic IOLs. Hydrophobic (water content <1%) acrylic materials have a greater refractive index than hydrophilic lenses and are consequently thinner, though this can result in dysphotopsia (troublesome glare and reflections). They have been reported to produce a greater reaction in uveitic eyes, but outcomes do not seem to be materially affected. Hydrophilic acrylic (hydrogel) in theory offers superior biocompatibility, but the image of hydrogel IOLs has been marred by the occurrence of severe calcification requiring IOL removal in some types, and inflammation in others; these problems have now been resolved by lens manufacturers. Posterior capsular opacification (PCO) rates may be higher with hydrogel IOLs than with other materials.
- ○ Silicone IOLs are available in both loop haptic (one- or three-piece) and plate haptic (one-piece) conformations, the latter consisting of a roughly rectangular leaf with the optic sited centrally. Silicone IOLs may exhibit greater biocompatibility than hydrophobic acrylic IOLs, but may be prone to significant silicone deposition in silicone oil-filled eyes. First-generation silicone materials were associated with a higher rate of PCO than acrylic, but there is no clear difference in rates with later IOLs.
- ○ Collamer is composed of collagen, a poly-HEMA-based copolymer and an ultraviolet-absorbing chromophore. It is marketed principally on the basis of high biocompatibility and a favourable track record.
- **Rigid IOLs** are made entirely from polymethylmethacrylate (PMMA). They cannot be injected or folded so require an incision larger than the diameter of the optic, typically 5 or 6 mm, for insertion. For economic reasons, they continue to be widely used in developing countries. PCO rates are higher with PMMA lenses than silicone and acrylic. Some surgeons favour heparin-coated IOLs (see below) in uveitic eyes, particularly in children.
- **Sharp/square-edged optics** (see Fig. 9.8A) are associated with a significantly lower rate of PCO compared with round-edged optics, and the former is now the predominant design. However, square edges may be associated with a higher rate of dysphotopsia (see below).
- **Blue light filters.** Although essentially all IOLs contain ultraviolet light filters, a number also include filters for blue wavelengths, in order to reduce the possibility of damage to the retina by this higher-energy visible light. The blue filters impart a slight yellow tint to the IOL, though similar only to that of the physiological young adult lens. Some evidence suggests slightly poorer visual function in scotopic conditions of illumination.
- **Aspheric optics** to counteract corneal spherical aberration are widely available, and have been shown to improve contrast, particularly in mesopic conditions. A potential drawback is that the aspheric element of the manufactured IOLs is set at a single standardized level (this differs between manufacturers), but the extent of spherical aberration varies

between individuals; some will be over- and some under-compensated.

- **Heparin coating** reduces the attraction and adhesion of inflammatory cells, and this may have particular application in eyes with uveitis. However, there is no clear evidence about whether heparin surface modification is clinically beneficial, and indeed about which IOL material is superior for use in cataract surgery on eyes with uveitis.
- **Multifocal IOLs** (see also Ch. 7) utilizing refractive or diffractive mechanisms aim to provide clear vision over a range of focal distances. So-called accommodative IOLs attempt to flex and thereby alter focal length but in practice the amplitude of accommodation is slight.
- **Toric IOLs** (Fig. 9.8C) have an integral cylindrical refractive component to compensate for pre-existing corneal astigmatism. The main potential problem is rotation within the capsular bag, which occurs in only a small percentage, and may be corrected by early surgical repositioning.
- **Adjustable IOLs** allow the alteration of refractive power following implantation. One version uses low-level ultraviolet irradiation at the slit lamp about a week after surgery to induce polymerization of its constituent molecules in specific patterns with precise spherical and cylindrical (astigmatism) correction.

Anaesthesia

The majority of cataract surgery is performed under local anaesthesia (LA), sometimes in conjunction with intravenous or oral sedation. General anaesthesia is required in some circumstances, such as children and many young adults, very anxious patients, some patients with learning difficulties, epilepsy, dementia and those with a head tremor.

- **Sub-Tenon block** involves insertion of a blunt-tipped cannula through an incision in the conjunctiva and Tenon capsule 5 mm from the limbus inferonasally (Fig. 9.9A), and passing it around the curve of the globe through the sub-Tenon space. The anaesthetic is injected beyond the equator of the globe (Fig. 9.9B). Although anaesthesia is good and complications minimal, akinesia is variable. Chemosis and subconjunctival haemorrhage are common but penetration of the globe is extremely rare.
- **Peribulbar block** is given through the skin (Figs 9.9C and D) or conjunctiva with a 1-inch (25-mm) needle. It generally provides effective anaesthesia and akinesia. Penetration of the globe is a rare but severe complication, and for this reason peribulbar is avoided, or approached with great caution, in longer eyes (which also tend to have a larger equatorial diameter).
- **Topical anaesthesia** involves drops or gel (proxymetacaine 0.5%, tetracaine 1% drops, lidocaine 2% gel), which can be augmented with intracameral preservative-free lidocaine 0.2%–1%, often infused during hydrodissection; combined viscoelastic/lidocaine preparations are also commercially available. Although analgesia is generally adequate, it tends to be less effective than peribulbar or sub-Tenon blocks.

Despite the absence of akinesia, most patients can cooperate adequately. The intraoperative complication rate is probably higher than with regional blocks, but anaesthesia-related complications are lower. The possibility of a higher rate of endophthalmitis compared to other anaesthetic techniques has been raised, though this may be compensated for by the use of intracameral antibiotic at the end of surgery.

Manual cataract surgery

When posterior chamber IOLs began to be widely used in the 1980s most surgeons adopted extracapsular cataract extraction (ECCE), abandoning the older intracapsular technique (ICCE). In ICCE, a cryoprobe is used to remove the lens complete with its capsule (Fig. 9.10A). In ECCE, after a large anterior capsulotomy is created, an extensive limbal incision (8–10 mm) is completed and the lens nucleus is expressed following hydrodissection to free its cortical attachments (Fig. 9.10B). Cortical matter is then aspirated, leaving behind a sufficiently intact capsular bag to support an IOL. Suturing of the incision is required, sometimes inducing considerable corneal astigmatism. Manual small-incision cataract surgery (MSICS) is a variant of ECCE used to address the requirement for high-volume surgical throughput of dense cataracts in less affluent geographical regions; it involves the creation of a small self-sealing sclerocorneal tunnel (Fig. 9.10C), manual one-piece expression of the nucleus (Fig. 9.10D), manual aspiration of the cortex and IOL implantation. Visual rehabilitation is comparable to phacoemulsification but MSICS is faster and avoids the need for expensive technology.

Phacoemulsification

Introduction

Phacoemulsification ('phaco') is the standard method of cataract extraction in developed countries, and in regional centres in most developing countries.

Phacodynamics

Choosing appropriate settings makes surgery safer and easier.

- **Level of irrigating bottle** above the patient's eye is set to maintain anterior chamber stability with a reasonable IOP. Infusion flow is proportional to the height of the bottle.
- **Aspiration flow rate** (AFR) refers to the volume of fluid removed from the eye in millilitres per minute. For a higher AFR the irrigating bottle must be elevated to compensate for increased fluid loss. High AFR results in attraction of lens material towards the phaco tip, with faster vacuum build-up and swifter removal of lens matter but with less effective power. A high AFR should usually be avoided by trainee surgeons.
- **Vacuum**, measured in mmHg, is generated during occlusion when the pump is attempting to aspirate fluid. Vacuum level determines how tightly material is held by the phaco tip when occluded, providing the ability to manipulate lens

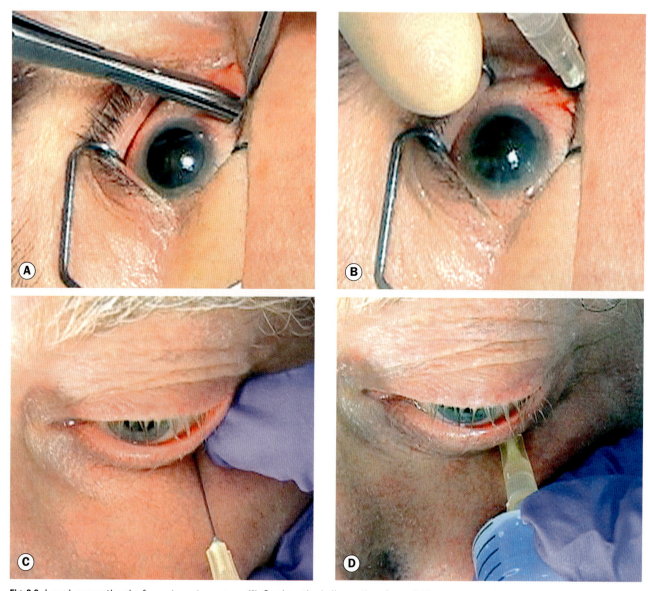

Fig. 9.9 Local anaesthesia for cataract surgery. **(A)** Conjunctival dissection for sub-Tenon anaesthesia; **(B)** sub-Tenon infiltration with a blunt cannula; **(C)** insertion of needle for peribulbar anaesthesia. **(D)** peribulbar infiltration of anaesthetic agent

fragments. High vacuum can decrease the total power required to remove the lens. As with AFR, a lower-vacuum setting slows down the speed of intraocular events, reduces the intensity of surge (see below) and makes inadvertent aspiration of iris or lens capsule less likely.

- **Post-occlusion surge.** When occlusion of the phaco tip by lens material is broken, pent-up energy results in a sudden temporary increase in outflow – 'surge'. This may result in complications such as capsular rupture, and as far as possible is suppressed by modern phaco machines.

Pump type

The main implication of the type of pump employed by a particular phaco machine is the effect on vacuum behaviour.

- **Peristaltic (flow) pumps** pull fluid and lens material into the phaco tip by compressing tubing over variable speed rollers.

Vacuum is generated only when occlusion of the tip occurs, following which the pump slows and stops as a set maximum is achieved.

- **Venturi (vacuum) pumps** create a negative pressure in a vessel by passing compressed gas across its entrance. This has the practical effect of synchronizing vacuum and AFR so there is generally no independent means of adjusting AFR. Depression of the foot pedal increases vacuum towards the preset maximum independent of occlusion, and tip vacuum is therefore always available.
- **Hybrid pumps** are offered by some modern machines.

Handpiece

The phaco handpiece (Fig. 9.11A) features a tip consisting of a hollow titanium needle with an enclosing fluid-cooling sleeve (Fig. 9.11B) to protect the cornea from thermal and mechanical damage.

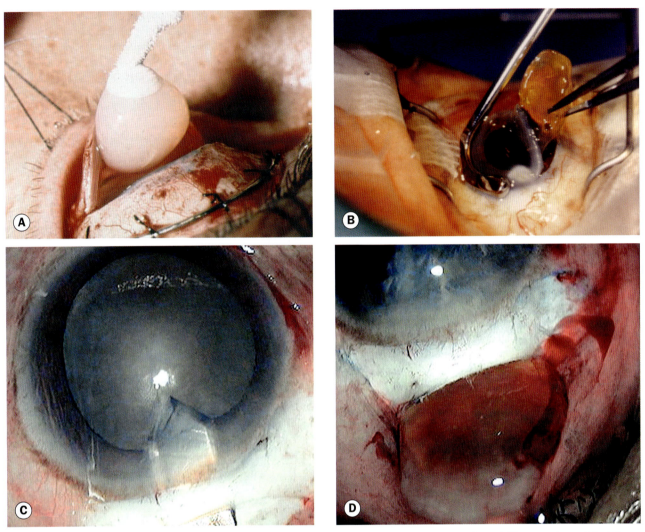

Fig. 9.10 Manual cataract surgery. **(A)** Intracapsular extraction; **(B)** extracapsular extraction; **(C)** and **(D)** manual small-incision cataract surgery
(Courtesy of C Barry – figs A and B; A Hennig – figs C and D)

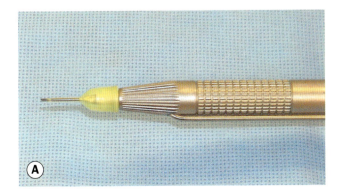

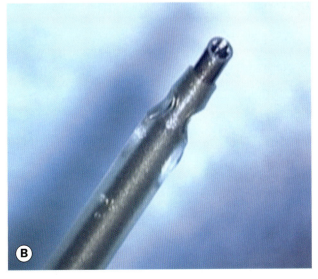

Fig. 9.11 (A) Phaco handpiece with tip; **(B)** phaco tip with sleeve

Its emulsifying action is mediated by very high-frequency (ultrasonic) vibration leading to jackhammer, cavitation and other effects; some machines offer variants such as a torsional phaco action or water jet-mediated phacoemulsification. Phaco tips of differing shapes and sizes are available, each having particular cutting and holding characteristics.

Ophthalmic viscosurgical devices

Ophthalmic viscosurgical devices (OVDs or viscoelastics) are biopolymers playing a critical role in modern cataract surgery.

- **Cohesive** OVDs are used to create and maintain intraocular spaces, for example to maintain the anterior chamber during capsulorhexis and inflation of the capsular bag to facilitate introduction of an IOL. Higher molecular weight variants maintain intraocular space more effectively but tend to promote iris prolapse in shallow anterior chambers and confer a more sustained postoperative IOP rise.
- **Dispersive** OVDs are more adherent to surfaces than cohesive OVDs, and are typically used to protect the endothelium. They are more difficult to remove from the eye than cohesive viscoelastics, but tend to cause a less marked IOP spike. The major practical disadvantage of dispersive OVDs is their tendency to retain air bubbles and lens fragments, compromising the surgical view.
- **Adaptive** OVDs display mixed characteristics.
- **'Soft shell'** technique involves the injection prior to the capsulotomy stage of an outer dispersive layer followed by an inner cohesive nucleus. Some surgeons use this routinely, others only for eyes at higher risk of corneal decompensation (e.g. cornea guttata).
- **Pupillary manipulation.** In eyes with small pupils a high molecular weight cohesive viscoelastic (e.g. Healon GV™) will push the iris away from the lens and help to induce mydriasis. Adaptive OVDs' cohesive effect can be used to dilate a pupil intraoperatively, and their dispersive effect to maintain the dilatation. OVDs can be used to break posterior synechiae with minimal trauma.
- **Cortical manipulation.** OVDs can be useful to dissect cortex away from the lens capsule to minimize traction on fragile zonular ligaments.
- **Capsulorhexis rescue.** If a capsulorhexis shows signs of running out to the periphery, injecting a cohesive viscoelastic will flatten the anterior capsule, aiding the exertion of a centrally directed vector and helping to expand the pupil.
- **Capsular rupture.** In small posterior capsular tears a dispersive viscoelastic (an entire vial may be necessary) will push the vitreous back into the posterior chamber and maintain plugging of the capsular defect, facilitating completion of lens removal. Subsequent creation of a posterior capsulorhexis is possible in some cases.

Technique

- **Preparation**
  - Topical anaesthetic is followed by povidone-iodine 5% (Fig. 9.12A) or chlorhexidine instillation into the conjunctival sac and cleaning of the eyelids (Fig. 9.12B), ensuring thorough eyelash application; the antiseptic should be left to work for a minimum of 3 minutes.
  - Careful draping (Fig. 9.12C) is performed, excluding the lashes and lid margins from the surgical field, and a speculum is inserted.

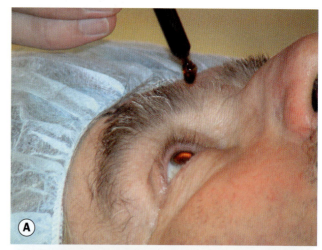

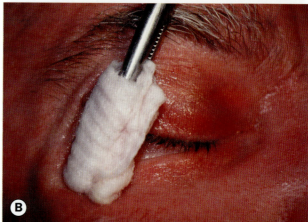

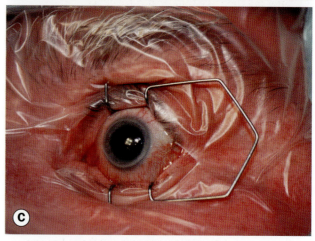

Fig. 9.12 Preparation. **(A)** Povidone-iodine 5% conjunctival fornix instillation; **(B)** cleaning the skin with povidone-iodine; **(C)** plastic drape and speculum isolating the operating field from the eyelids

- **Incisions**
  - A side port incision is made around 60° to the left (in right-handed surgeons) of the main incision; some surgeons prefer two side ports approximately 180° apart.
  - Viscoelastic is injected into the anterior chamber.
  - Many surgeons locate the main corneal incision (Fig. 9.13A) on the steepest corneal axis, others prefer consistent siting. Temporal incisions can provide better access and less induced astigmatism but may be associated with a slightly higher risk of endophthalmitis.
- **Continuous curvilinear capsulorhexis** is performed with a cystotome, a bent hypodermic needle and/or capsule forceps (Fig. 9.13B).
- **Hydrodissection** is performed to separate the nucleus and cortex from the capsule so that the nucleus can be manipulated. A blunt cannula is inserted just beneath the edge of the capsulorhexis and fluid injected gently under the capsule (Fig. 9.13C). A hydrodissection wave should be seen, provided there is an adequate red reflex.
- **'Divide and conquer'** is a widely used, safe technique for removal of the nucleus in which two perpendicular grooves are created (sculpting), the phaco tip and a second instrument engaged in opposite walls of the grooves and the nucleus cracked into quadrants by applying force in opposite directions (Fig. 9.13D). Each of the quadrants is then emulsified and aspirated in turn (Fig. 9.13E).
- **'Phaco chop'** has the advantage of generally greater speed and a lower total phaco energy requirement, but commonly takes longer to learn. In horizontal chopping a blunt-tipped chopper is placed horizontally underneath the capsule and rotated vertically as the equator is reached. Vertical chopping is performed with a pointed-tip chopper that does not need to pass beyond the capsulorhexis. The nucleus is separated into several pieces for emulsification.
- **'Stop and chop'** is a combination technique.
- **Removal of lens cortex.** Cortical lens matter segments are carefully engaged by means of vacuum, peeled away centrally from the lens capsule and aspirated. Automated coaxial, bimanual automated (Fig. 9.13F) and manual aspiration (e.g. Simcoe cannula) methods are available.
- **IOL insertion.** The capsular bag is filled with cohesive viscoelastic. A loaded injector cartridge is introduced through the main section and the IOL slowly injected and unrolled inside the capsular bag; a toric IOL (see Fig. 9.8C) should be rotated to the correct alignment. Viscoelastic may be aspirated prior to or following toric IOL rotation.
- **Completion.** Side port incisions and the main wound may be sealed with corneal stromal saline injection (hydrosealing). Prophylactic measures at the end of surgery may include intracameral (anterior chamber) antibiotic injection, subconjunctival injection of antibiotic and steroid and/or topical antibiotic.

Femtosecond lasers in cataract surgery

Femtosecond lasers, used in refractive surgery for several years, have recently been adopted by many surgeons, replacing several of the manual steps of phacoemulsification with an automated process. The corneal incisions, the capsulorhexis and initial fragmentation of the crystalline lens, as well as astigmatism-relieving incisions (Fig. 9.14), can all be performed with the laser. Potential advantages include greater precision and integrity of incisions, reduced phacoemulsification energy, and possibly improved refractive outcomes due to more precise capsulorhexis placement. Disadvantages include substantially higher cost, longer total operating time and difficulties with technically challenging cases (e.g. small pupils). There is a substantial learning curve.

Operative complications

Rupture of the posterior lens capsule

Capsular rupture may be accompanied by vitreous loss, posterior migration of lens material and, rarely, expulsive haemorrhage. Sequelae to vitreous loss, particularly if inappropriately managed, include CMO, retinal detachment, endophthalmitis, updrawn pupil, uveitis, vitreous touch, vitreous wick syndrome, glaucoma and posterior dislocation of the IOL.

- **Signs**
  - Sudden deepening or shallowing of the anterior chamber and momentary pupillary dilatation.
  - The nucleus falls away and cannot be approached by the phaco tip.
  - Vitreous aspirated into the phaco tip often manifests with a marked slowing of aspiration.
  - The torn capsule or vitreous gel may be directly visible.
- **Management** depends on the magnitude of the tear, the size and type of any residual lens material, and the presence or absence of vitreous prolapse.
  - Dispersive viscoelastic such as Viscoat may be injected (see above). If a complete or nearly complete nucleus remains, conversion to extracapsular extraction may be considered. A vitrector can be employed at this point (see below) to remove vitreous entangled with nuclear fragments.
  - The incision may be enlarged, if necessary, and a lens glide (Sheets) may be passed behind lens fragments to cover the capsular defect (Fig. 9.15), although it is important to confirm that vitreous has first been displaced or removed and will not be put under traction.
  - Residual nuclear fragments are carefully removed by phaco using a low bottle height and low AFR, or, if large, by viscoexpression after extending the main wound.
  - Once nuclear remnants have been removed, a common approach is to re-plug the tear with dispersive OVD, gently filling the anterior chamber with a cohesive viscoelastic and using a manual aspiration cannula with the irrigation off to carefully aspirate residual cortex, topping up the AC with viscoelastic as necessary.

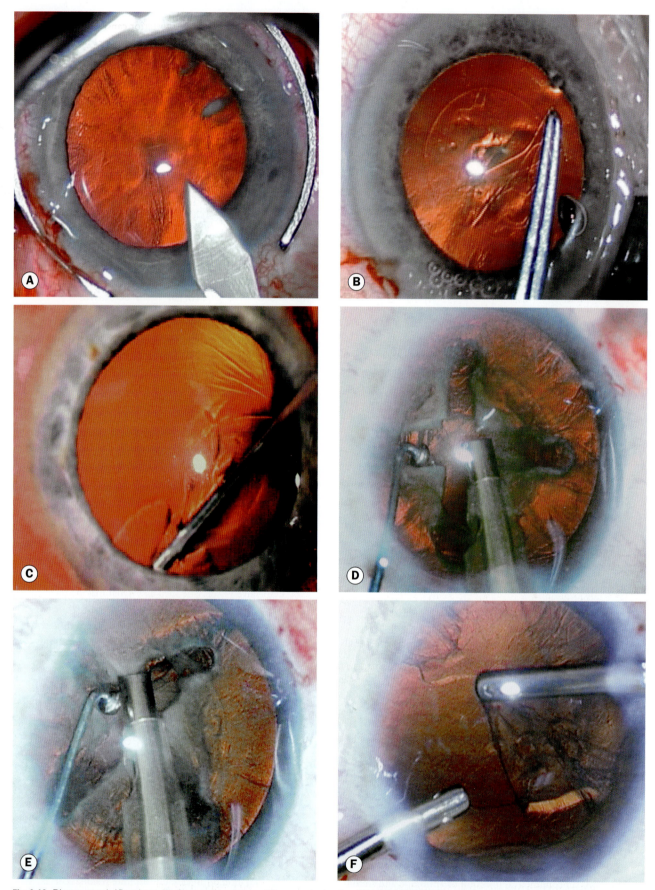

Fig. 9.13 Phacoemulsification. **(A)** Corneal incision; **(B)** capsulorhexis; **(C)** hydrodissection; **(D)** cracking of the nucleus; **(E)** phacoemulsification and aspiration of nuclear quadrants – 'divide and conquer' method; **(F)** cortical aspiration using a bimanual automated technique

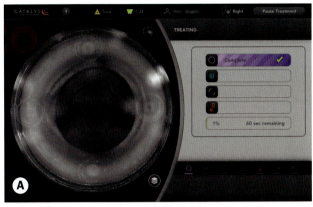

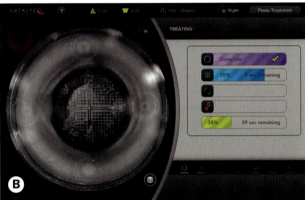

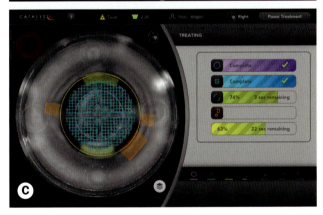

Fig. 9.14 Femtosecond laser for cataract surgery – graphical user interface. **(A)** Capsulotomy completed; **(B)** nuclear fragmentation; **(C)** limbal relaxing incisions for astigmatism
(Courtesy of Abbott Medical Optics)

○ All vitreous is then removed from the AC and the wound with a vitrector, including deep to the capsular tear. A bimanual technique, with separate cutting and infusion instruments, is viewed as superior by many, as vitreous is not pushed away from the cutter; the position of the infusion cannula is kept high and that of the cutter low. The main practical difficulty is visualization of the vitreous gel, and this can be enhanced by the instillation of trypan blue or 0.1 ml of 40 mg/ml triamcinolone (shaken well before use). The infusion bottle height should be sufficient to keep the anterior chamber maintained without intermittent shallowing.

○ A small posterior capsular tear may allow careful in-the-bag implantation of a posterior chamber (PC) IOL; it may be possible to convert a small tear into a posterior capsulorhexis, preventing inadvertent enlargement of the dehiscence.

○ Even a large tear will usually allow ciliary sulcus placement of a three-piece (but not a one-piece) PC IOL. The centre of the haptic loops should be placed at 90° to a peripheral tear. If possible, after placing the IOL in the sulcus the optic should be captured within an intact capsulorhexis of slightly smaller diameter by depressing each side of the optic beneath the capsulorhexis in turn. With capsulorhexis capture, the originally planned IOL power, or possibly 0.5 D less, can be used; without capture, the power is reduced by 0.5–1.0 D.

○ Acetylcholine solution is used to constrict the pupil following implantation of a PC IOL or prior to inserting an AC IOL.

○ Insufficient capsular support may necessitate implantation of an AC IOL (Fig. 9.16); a prior iridectomy is needed to prevent pupillary block. AC IOLs are associated with a higher risk than PC IOLs of complications including bullous keratopathy, hyphaema, iris tuck and pupillary irregularities. An iris-attached anterior (see Fig. 7.10A) or posterior chamber (see Fig. 9.17D) IOL or a sclerally secured posterior chamber IOL are alternatives.

○ A suture should be used to secure the wound following capsular rupture, even if this seems adequately self-sealed.

Posterior loss of lens fragments

Dislocation of fragments of lens material into the vitreous cavity (Fig. 9.17A) after zonular dehiscence or posterior capsule rupture is rare but potentially serious as it may result in glaucoma, chronic

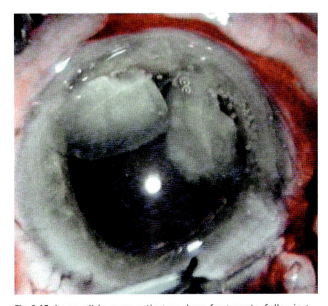

Fig. 9.15 Lens glide supporting nuclear fragments following rupture of the posterior capsule
(Courtesy of R Packard)

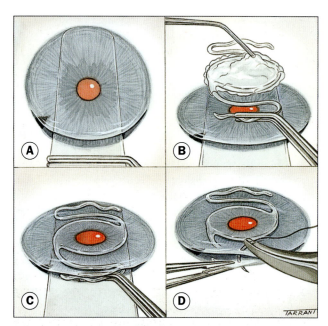

Fig. 9.16 Insertion of an anterior chamber IOL; note that an iridectomy has been created. **(A)** Insertion of a lens glide; **(B)** OVD (see text) coating the anterior surface of the IOL; **(C)** insertion of the IOL; **(D)** suturing of the incision

uveitis, retinal detachment or chronic CMO. Initially, any uveitis or raised IOP must be treated. It may be reasonable to adopt a conservative approach for small (less than a quadrant) fragments, but pars plana vitrectomy will virtually always be required for larger pieces.

Posterior dislocation of IOL

Dislocation of an IOL into the vitreous cavity (Fig. 9.17B) is rare; loss can occur via a posterior capsular dehiscence, or in an eye with fragile zonular attachments (e.g. pseudoexfoliation) the entire capsular bag may dislocate (Fig. 9.17C). Complications include vitreous haemorrhage, retinal detachment, uveitis and chronic CMO. Treatment involves pars plana vitrectomy with IOL removal, repositioning or exchange (Fig. 9.17D) depending on the extent of capsular support.

Suprachoroidal haemorrhage

A suprachoroidal haemorrhage involves a bleed into the suprachoroidal space from a ruptured posterior ciliary artery. If sufficiently severe it may result in extrusion of intraocular contents (expulsive haemorrhage). It is a dreaded complication, but extremely rare (0.04%) with phacoemulsification. Contributing factors include advanced age, glaucoma, increased axial length, systemic cardiovascular disease, vitreous loss and conversion from phacoemulsification to ECCE. A high intraoperative index of suspicion is critical, and if there is any suggestion of a suprachoroidal haemorrhage the operation should be terminated and the incision sutured immediately.

- **Signs**
  - ○ Progressive shallowing of the AC, increased IOP and prolapse of the iris.

  - ○ Vitreous extrusion, loss or partial obscuration of the red reflex and the appearance of a dark mound behind the pupil.
  - ○ In severe cases, posterior segment contents may be extruded into the AC and through the incision.
- **Immediate treatment** involves filling of the AC with a cohesive viscoelastic and sutured closure of the incision. Unless significant glaucomatous damage is present, leaving a substantial quantity of viscoelastic in the eye has been advocated, in order to raise the IOP and tamponade the bleeding vessel; balloon (e.g. Honan) compression to a pressure of 50 mmHg has also been suggested, perhaps for up to 30 minutes. It may be helpful to keep the patient in a sitting rather than lying position. The diagnosis should be confirmed at the slit lamp as soon as possible. IOP-lowering medication such as oral acetazolamide is given to address the pressure spike. Intraoperative posterior sclerotomy is not recommended. Postoperatively, topical and systemic steroids should be used aggressively to reduce intraocular inflammation, with standard postoperative antibiotic treatment and IOP management as indicated. Non-steroidal anti-inflammatory drugs (NSAIDs) should be avoided for analgesia, and any antiplatelet or anticoagulant discontinued short-term, provided this is safe.
- **Subsequent treatment**, if spontaneous absorption fails to occur, consists of drainage of large haemorrhages. This can be performed 7–14 days later, by which time liquefaction of blood clot has taken place. The visual prognosis for large haemorrhages is highly variable; prolonged chorioretinal apposition (>14 days) has a worse prognosis. Pars plana vitrectomy may be considered when the retina appears adherent or detached, though even apposed 'kissing' haemorrhages may resolve spontaneously without apparent retinal problems. If appropriate, completion of cataract surgery may be considered after a further 1–2 weeks.

Acute postoperative endophthalmitis

Pathogenesis

The contemporary reported incidence of acute endophthalmitis following cataract surgery varies substantially between studies, but is probably at least 0.1%. Acute intraocular infection is invariably a severe event. Toxins produced by infecting bacteria and the host inflammatory responses cause rapid and irreversible photoreceptor damage, and ongoing effects can continue long after the ocular contents have been rendered sterile.

- **Risk factors** are difficult to establish but may include operative complications such as posterior capsule rupture, prolonged procedure time, combined procedure (e.g. with vitrectomy), clear corneal sutureless incision, temporal incision, wound leak on the first day, delaying postoperative topical antibiotics until the day after surgery, topical anaesthesia, adnexal disease and diabetes.

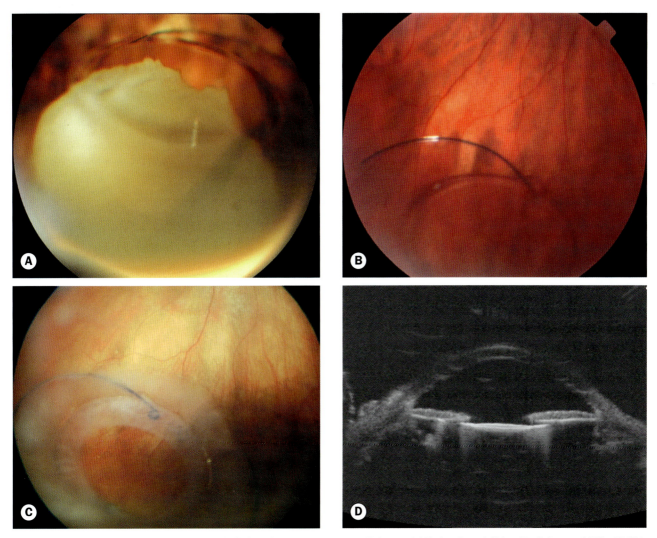

Fig. 9.17 (A) Large nuclear fragment in the inferior vitreous cavity – a dislocated IOL is also visible; **(B)** dislocated IOL; **(C)** IOL within a dislocated capsular bag in a patient with pseudoexfoliation; **(D)** ultrasonogram of iris clip ('lobster claw') IOL attached to the posterior iris surface in the eye shown in (C)

(Courtesy of S Milewski – figs A and B; S Chen – figs C and D)

- **Pathogens.** About 90% of isolates are Gram-positive and 10% Gram-negative. *Staphylococcus epidermidis* is the most common, and with early treatment carries a reasonable prognosis.
- **The source of infection** usually cannot be identified with certainty. It is thought that the flora of the eyelids and conjunctiva are the most frequent source, including contamination via incisions in the early postoperative stages. Other potential sources include contaminated solutions and instruments, environmental air, and the surgeon and other operating room personnel.

Prophylaxis

Because of the low rate of endophthalmitis it is very difficult to establish the effectiveness of any preventative measure.

- **Instillation of 5% povidone-iodine** into the conjunctival fornices and leaving this undisturbed for at least 3 minutes prior to surgery.

- **Scrupulous preparation** of the surgical site, with re-draping if eyelash coverage is inadequate.
- **Treatment of pre-existing infections** such as blepharitis, conjunctivitis, chronic dacryocystitis and infection in the contralateral eye or socket.
- **Antibiotic prophylaxis**
  - Intracameral cefuroxime (1 mg in 0.1 ml) injected into the AC at the end of surgery.
  - Postoperative subconjunctival injection can achieve bactericidal levels in the AC for at least 1–2 hours.
  - Preoperative topical fluoroquinolone antibiotics are frequently given in regimens from 1 hour to 3 days before surgery, but evidence for their efficacy is lacking.
  - Newer-generation quinolones such as moxifloxacin penetrate the eye effectively to give inhibitory concentrations, but their routine prophylactic use might promote the development of resistant organisms.

- **Early resuturing** of leaking wounds rather than observation is likely to be prudent.
- **Reviewing personal surgical practice** to eliminate potentially risk-prone elements, particularly if a significant rate of endophthalmitis is encountered.

Clinical features

- **Symptoms.** Pain, redness and visual loss.
- **Signs** vary according to severity.
  - Eyelid swelling, chemosis, conjunctival injection and discharge.
  - A relative afferent pupillary defect is common.
  - Corneal haze.
  - Fibrinous exudate and hypopyon (Fig. 9.18A).
  - Vitritis with an impaired view of the fundus.
  - Severe vitreous inflammation and debris (Fig. 9.18B) with loss of the red reflex.

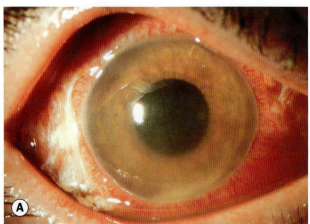

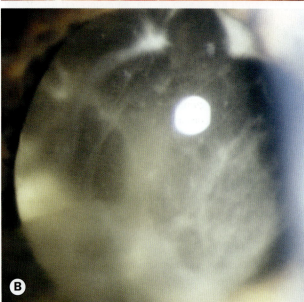

Fig. 9.18 Acute postoperative bacterial endophthalmitis.
(A) Ciliary injection, fibrinous exudate and hypopyon;
(B) severe vitreous involvement
(Courtesy of C Barry – fig. A; S Tuft – fig. B)

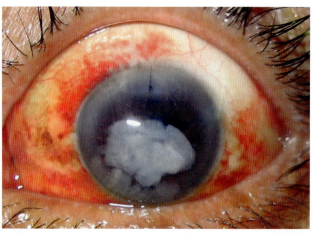

Fig. 9.19 Retained lens fragment in the anterior chamber following cataract surgery
(Courtesy of S Chen)

Differential diagnosis

If there is any doubt about the diagnosis, treatment should be that of infectious endophthalmitis, as early recognition leads to a better outcome.

- **Retained lens material** in the AC (Fig. 9.19) or vitreous may precipitate a severe uveitis, corneal oedema and raised IOP.
- **Vitreous haemorrhage**, especially if blood in the vitreous is depigmented.
- **Postoperative uveitis.** A confident diagnosis of infection is not always straightforward. If signs of inflammation are mild a trial of topical steroid therapy and early review (6–24 hours) is appropriate. If there is no substantial improvement, management should be that of endophthalmitis.
- **Toxic reaction** to the use of inappropriate or contaminated irrigating fluid or viscoelastic. An intense fibrinous reaction with corneal oedema may develop although other signs of infectious endophthalmitis are absent. Treatment is with intensive topical steroids and a cycloplegic.
- **Complicated or prolonged surgery** may result in corneal oedema and uveitis.

Identification of pathogens

Samples for culture should be obtained from aqueous and vitreous to confirm the diagnosis; negative culture does not necessarily rule out infection and treatment should be continued. An operating theatre with experienced staff is the best setting, but samples can be taken in a minor procedures room if necessary to avoid delay.

- **B-scan ultrasound** should be performed prior to vitreous sampling if there is no clinical view, to exclude retinal detachment.
- **Preparation**
  - Povidone-iodine 5% is instilled.
  - Topical and subconjunctival, sub-Tenon or peribulbar anaesthesia is administered; the inflamed eye is often resistant to local anaesthesia and sedation or general anaesthesia may be necessary.

- ○ The eye is draped as for cataract surgery, with insertion of a speculum.
- **Aqueous sampling** – 0.1–0.2 ml of aqueous is aspirated via a limbal paracentesis using a 25-gauge needle on a tuberculin syringe; the syringe is capped and labelled.
- **Vitreous sampling** is more likely to yield a positive culture than aqueous. A 1 or 2 ml syringe and 23-gauge needle may be used, or optimally a disposable vitrector. The vitreous cavity is entered 3.5 mm from the limbus (pseudophakic eye), measured with a calliper. 0.2–0.4 ml is aspirated from the mid-vitreous cavity. If using a disposable vitrector, the tubing is capped and both the vitrector and tubing sent for analysis.
- **Conjunctival swabs** may be taken in addition, as significant culture may be helpful in the absence of a positive result from intraocular samples.
- **Microbiology.** Specimens should be sent to the microbiology laboratory immediately; most laboratories prefer to receive a sample in the acquiring apparatus and will divide the specimen for microscopy and culture. PCR can be helpful in identifying unusual organisms, the cause of culture-negative disease, and organisms after antibiotic treatment has been started. However, its high sensitivity means that contamination can lead to false-positive results.

Treatment

- **Intravitreal antibiotics** are the key to management because levels above the minimum inhibitory concentration of most pathogens are achieved, and are maintained for days. They should be administered immediately after culture specimens have been obtained. Antibiotics commonly used in combination are ceftazidime, which will kill most Gram-negative organisms (including *Pseudomonas aeruginosa*) and vancomycin to address Gram-positive cocci (including methicillin-resistant *Staphylococcus aureus*).
  - ○ The concentrations are ceftazidime 2 mg in 0.1 ml and vancomycin 2 mg in 0.1 ml; amikacin 0.4 mg in 0.1 ml is an alternative to ceftazidime in patients with a definite penicillin allergy, but is more toxic to the retina. Table 9.2 provides details of preparation.
  - ○ The antibiotics are injected slowly into the mid-vitreous cavity using a 25-gauge needle.
  - ○ After the first injection has been given, the syringe may be disconnected but the needle left inside the vitreous cavity so that the second injection can be given through the same needle; alternatively a second needle can be used.
- **Subconjunctival antibiotic injections** are often given but are of doubtful additional benefit if intravitreal antibiotics have been used. Suggested doses are vancomycin 50 mg and ceftazidime 125 mg (or amikacin 50 mg if penicillin-allergic).
- **Topical antibiotics** are of limited benefit and are often used only 4–6 times daily in order to protect the fresh wounds from contamination. Vancomycin 5% (50 mg/ml) or ceftazidime 5% (50 mg/ml) applied intensively may

Table 9.2 Preparation of antibiotics for intravitreal injection

Ceftazidime (broad spectrum, including *Pseudomonas*)
A. Begin with a 500 mg ampoule
B. Add 10 ml water for injection (WFI) or saline and dissolve thoroughly (for a 250 mg vial add 5 ml WFI or saline, for a 1 g vial add 20 ml WFI or saline)
C. Draw up 1 ml of the solution, containing 50 mg of antibiotic
D. Add 1.5 ml WFI or saline giving 50 mg in 2.5 ml
E. Draw up about 0.2 ml (excess to facilitate priming) into a 1 ml syringe. When ready to inject, fit the Rycroft cannula or the needle to be used, and discard all but 0.1 ml (contains 2 mg of antibiotic) for injection

Vancomycin (action primarily against Gram-positive organisms)
Only saline, not WFI, should be used with vancomycin
As A–E above, again preferably starting with a 500 mg ampoule

Amikacin
Alternative to ceftazidime; as it carries a higher risk of retinal infarction, use only if well-defined penicillin or cephalosporin allergy is present; note the lower intravitreal dose than ceftazidime and vancomycin
Note different dilution procedure to ceftazidime and vancomycin
A. Presentation: vial contains 500 mg of amikacin in 2 ml of solution
B. Use a 2.5 ml syringe to draw up 1 ml of amikacin solution then 1.5 ml of WFI
C. Inject 0.4 ml of the solution, containing 40 mg of antibiotic, into a 10 ml syringe and dilute to 10 ml (giving 4 mg per ml)
D. Draw up about 0.2 ml (excess to facilitate priming) into a 1 ml syringe. When ready to inject, fit the needle to be used, and discard all but 0.1 ml (contains 0.4 mg of antibiotic) for injection

penetrate the cornea in therapeutic levels. Third or fourth generation fluoroquinolones achieve effective levels in the aqueous and vitreous, even in uninflamed eyes, and may be considered.
- **Oral antibiotics.** Fluoroquinolones penetrate the eye well and moxifloxacin 400 mg daily for 10 days is recommended; clarithromycin 500 mg twice daily may be helpful for culture-negative infections. Evidence suggests these may attack bacterial biofilm.
- **Oral steroids.** The rationale for the use of steroids is to limit destructive complications of the inflammatory process. Prednisolone 1 mg/kg daily may be considered in severe cases after 12–24 hours provided fungal infection has been excluded from examination of smears. Contraindications must be excluded and gastric protection (e.g. lansoprazole 30 mg once daily) prescribed with appropriate monitoring including baseline blood tests; if necessary, general medical advice should be requested prior to commencement.

- **Periocular steroids.** Dexamethasone or triamcinolone should be considered if systemic therapy is contraindicated.
- **Topical dexamethasone** 0.1% 2-hourly initially for anterior uveitis.
- **Topical mydriatic** such as atropine 1% twice daily.
- **Intravitreal steroids** may reduce inflammation in the short term but do not influence the final visual outcome; some studies even suggest a detrimental effect. Conversely, improvement in outcome in some bacterial sub-groups has been reported.
- **Pars plana vitrectomy.** The Endophthalmitis Vitrectomy Study (EVS) showed a benefit for immediate pars plana vitrectomy in eyes with a visual acuity (VA) of perception of light (*not* hand movements vision or better) at presentation, with a 50% reduction in severe visual loss. If vitrectomy is not immediately available, it is prudent to take samples as above and give intravitreal antibiotics as a temporizing measure. The conclusions of the EVS in post-cataract surgery eyes cannot necessarily be extrapolated to other forms of endophthalmitis.

Subsequent management

Subsequent management should proceed according to culture results and clinical response.

- **Signs of improvement** include contraction of fibrinous exudate and reduction of AC cellular activity and hypopyon. In this situation treatment is not modified irrespective of culture results. Ultrasonography may be useful in vitreous assessment.
- **If the clinical signs are worsening** after 48 hours antibiotic sensitivities should be reviewed and therapy modified accordingly. Pars plana vitrectomy should be considered if not previously performed. Intravitreal antibiotics can be repeated after 2 days; if amikacin has previously been used, repeated administration should probably be avoided to reduce the risk of retinal toxicity.
- **Outcome** is related to the duration of the infection prior to treatment and the virulence of organisms.
  - If VA at presentation is light perception, 30% of eyes achieve 6/12 following treatment. If VA is better than light perception, this figure increases to 60%.
  - Infection with *Bacillus cereus* or streptococci often has a poor visual outcome despite aggressive and appropriate therapy, with 70% and 55% respectively achieving a final VA of 6/60 or less. This poor visual outcome may be related to early retinopathy from exotoxins.
- **Late problems**
  - Persistent vitreous opacification. Aggressive and extended topical, periocular, and if necessary oral steroid treatment will often lead to resolution. Vitrectomy can be considered if unresolving and severe.
  - Maculopathy in the form of epiretinal membrane, cystoid oedema and ischaemia.
  - Hypotony. Wound leak should be excluded and persistent inflammation addressed. Choroidal effusions should be identified and drained if necessary. Retinal detachment and anterior vitreous membranes may require vitrectomy.
  - Other problems include chronic uveitis, secondary glaucoma, retinal detachment and phthisis.

Delayed-onset postoperative endophthalmitis

Pathogenesis

Delayed-onset endophthalmitis following cataract surgery develops when an organism of low virulence such as *P. acnes*, becomes trapped within the capsular bag (saccular endophthalmitis). Organisms can become sequestered within macrophages, protected from eradication but with continued expression of bacterial antigen. Onset ranges from 4 weeks to years (mean 9 months) postoperatively and typically follows uneventful cataract surgery. It may rarely be precipitated by laser capsulotomy release of the organism.

Diagnosis

- **Symptoms.** Painless mild progressive visual deterioration is typical; floaters may be present.
- **Signs**
  - Low-grade anterior uveitis, sometimes with medium-large keratic precipitates (Fig. 9.20A); a degree of vitritis is common.
  - The inflammation initially responds well to topical steroids, but recurs when treatment is stopped and may eventually become steroid-resistant.
  - An enlarging capsular plaque composed of organisms sequestrated in residual cortex within the peripheral capsular bag is common (Fig. 9.20B); gonioscopy under mydriasis may identify an equatorial plaque.
- **Differential diagnosis** is principally from other causes of anterior uveitis, particularly idiopathic, sterile post-surgical and chronic/recurrent viral infection (see Ch. 11).
- **Initial management.** Later-generation fluoroquinolones, such as moxifloxacin, penetrate the eye well, and are concentrated within macrophages. An empirical 10–14-day course of moxifloxacin (alternatives include clarithromycin) may be worthwhile prior to more invasive options.
- **Investigation.** Sampling of aqueous and vitreous should be considered if oral antibiotics are ineffective. Anaerobic culture should be requested if *P. acnes* infection is suspected, and isolates may take 10–14 days to grow. The detection rate can be greatly improved with the use of PCR, which should also screen for the common causes of viral anterior uveitis.
- **Treatment if persistent**
  - Intravitreal antibiotics alone are usually unsuccessful in resolving the infection.
  - Removal of the capsular bag, residual cortex and IOL, requiring pars plana vitrectomy. Secondary IOL

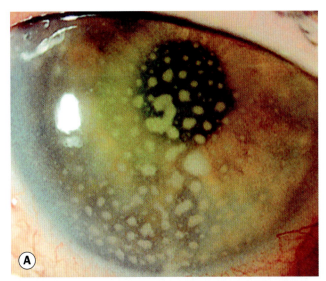

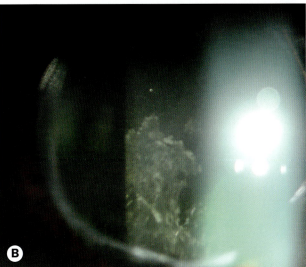

Fig. 9.20 Delayed-onset postoperative endophthalmitis.
(A) Mild anterior uveitis with large keratic precipitates;
(B) capsular plaque

implantation may be considered at a later date. Intravitreal antibiotics are combined: vancomycin (1–2 mg in 0.1 ml) is the antibiotic of choice and can also be irrigated into any capsular remnant. *P. acnes* is also sensitive to methicillin, cefazolin and clindamycin.

Posterior capsular opacification

Visually significant posterior lens capsular opacification (PCO), also known as 'after cataract', is the most common late complication of uncomplicated cataract surgery, historically occurring eventually in up to 50% of patients. It is caused by the proliferation of lens epithelial cells that have remained within the capsular bag following cataract extraction. The incidence of PCO is reduced when the capsulorhexis opening is in complete contact with the anterior surface of the IOL. PMMA (and probably to a lesser extent hydrogel) IOLs are particularly prone to PCO, but otherwise implant design is more important than material; a square

optic edge appears to inhibit PCO (though may have a higher rate of dysphotopsia – see below).

Diagnosis

- **Symptoms** include persistent slowly worsening blurring, glare and sometimes monocular diplopia.
- **VA** is variably reduced, though dysfunction may be more marked on contrast sensitivity testing.
- **Signs** typically include more than one pattern of opacification.
  ○ Vacuolated (pearl-type) PCO (Fig. 9.21A) consists of proliferating swollen lens epithelial cells, similar to the bladder (Wedl) cells seen in posterior subcapsular cataract (see Fig. 9.1B). They are commonly termed 'Elschnig pearls', particularly when grouped into clusters at the edge of a capsulotomy (Fig. 9.21B), though strictly Hirschberg–Elschnig pearls refers to globular or grape-like collections of swollen cells seen following traumatic or surgical anterior capsular rupture.
  ○ Fibrosis-type PCO (Fig. 9.21C) is thought to be due to fibroblastic metaplasia of epithelial cells, which develop contractile qualities.
  ○ A Soemmering ring is a whitish annular or doughnut-shaped proliferation of residual cells that classically formed almost in the periphery of the capsular bag following older methods of cataract surgery, but is clinically uncommon now. It may form at the edge of a capsulorhexis or capsulotomy.

Treatment

Treatment involves the creation of an opening in the posterior capsule, termed a capsulotomy (see Figs 9.21B and D), with the Nd:YAG laser.

- **Indications.** The presence of significant visual symptoms is the main indication; less commonly, capsulotomy is performed to improve an inadequate fundus view impairing assessment and treatment of posterior segment pathology.
- **Technique.** Safe and successful laser capsulotomy involves accurate focusing and use of the minimum energy required. Laser power is initially set at 1 mJ/pulse, and may be increased if necessary. A series of punctures is applied in a cruciate pattern using single-pulse shots, the first puncture aimed at the visual axis. The opening should equate approximately to the size of the physiologically dilated pupil under scotopic conditions – this averages around 4–5 mm in the pseudophakic eye. A larger capsulotomy may be necessary if glare persists, or for retinal examination or treatment, but the capsulotomy should not extend beyond the edge of the optic in case vitreous prolapses around its edge. It may be prudent to adopt a higher threshold for treatment, and minimizing its extent, in eyes at risk of retinal detachment (e.g. high myopia), CMO (e.g. history of uveitis) or lens displacement (e.g. pseudoexfoliation). Some research suggests that the total energy applied should be less than 80 mJ in order to reduce the risk of a significant IOP spike or increase in macular thickness.

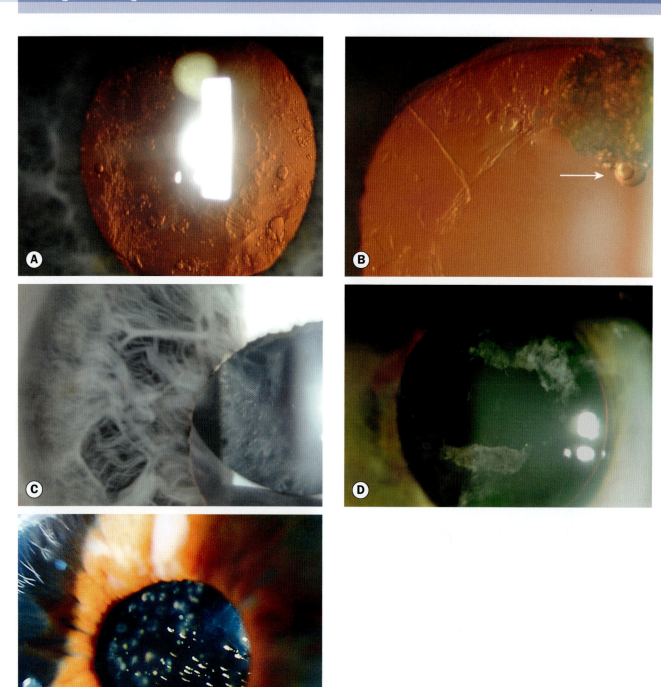

Fig. 9.21 Posterior capsular opacification. **(A)** Vacuolated or pearl-type; **(B)** Elschnig pearl formation (arrow) following laser capsulotomy; **(C)** capsular fibrosis; **(D)** Soemmering ring surrounding a slightly contracted capsulotomy; **(E)** laser pitting of an IOL
(Courtesy of R Curtis – fig. E)

- **Complications** include pitting of the IOL (Fig. 9.21E) that is virtually always visually inconsequential, intraocular pressure elevation (usually mild and transient) and extremely rarely CMO (less common when capsulotomy is delayed for 6 months or more after cataract surgery), retinal detachment and IOL subluxation or dislocation.

Anterior capsular fibrosis and contraction

Since the advent of continuous curvilinear capsulorhexis, contraction of the anterior capsular opening (capsulophimosis – Fig. 9.22) has become a more common complication. It typically progresses

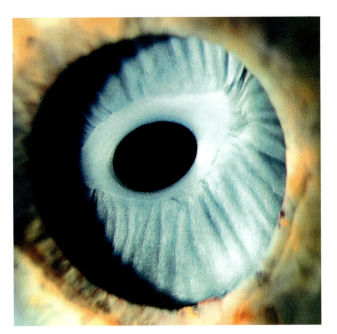

Fig. 9.22 Anterior capsular contraction and fibrosis

over months, and if severe, YAG laser anterior capsulotomy may be required. Risk factors include pseudoexfoliation, retinitis pigmentosa and a small capsulorhexis; it may be highest with plate-haptic silicone IOLs.

Miscellaneous postoperative complications

Cystoid macular oedema

Symptomatic CMO (see Ch. 14) is relatively uncommon following uncomplicated phacoemulsification and in most cases is mild and transient. It occurs more often after complicated surgery and has a peak incidence at 6–10 weeks, although the interval to onset may be much longer.

- **Risk factors** include epiretinal membrane, a history of CMO in the other eye, operative complications such as posterior capsular rupture, particularly with vitreous incarceration into the incision site (Fig. 9.23A), anterior chamber IOL (Fig. 9.23B), secondary IOL implantation, prior topical prostaglandin treatment, diabetes and uveitis.
- **Symptoms.** Blurring, especially for near tasks, and sometimes distortion. Subtle CMO may not be readily visible clinically, but is demonstrated well on OCT.
- **Treatment.** One or a combination of the following modalities may be used.
  - Anterior vitrectomy or YAG laser vitrotomy to vitreous incarceration in the anterior segment if present.
  - Topical NSAIDs (e.g. ketorolac four times daily, bromfenac twice daily, nepafenac) may be beneficial even in long-standing cases; treatment for several months may be necessary.

- Steroids. Topically, by periocular or intravitreal (triamcinolone acetate 0.05–0.1 ml of 40 mg/ml) injection.
- Carbonic anhydrase inhibitors given systemically or topically.
- Intravitreal anti-VEGF agents.
- Pars plana vitrectomy may be useful for CMO refractory to medical therapy, even in eyes without apparent vitreous disturbance.

Dysphotopsia

Up to 1 in 10 patients complain of annoying visual phenomena following uncomplicated cataract surgery with monofocal IOL implantation; multifocal IOLs have particular issues that are discussed separately above. Improvement in and adaptation to the symptoms typically occurs over several months, and the number

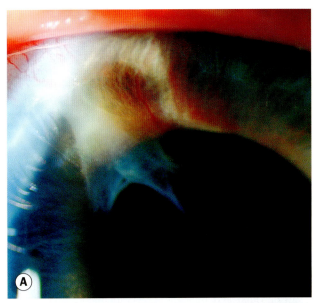

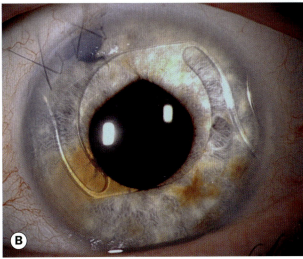

Fig. 9.23 Factors predisposing to cystoid macular oedema. **(A)** Vitreous incarceration in the incision; **(B)** anterior chamber IOL

(Courtesy of S Chen – fig. B)

of monofocal IOL patients actually requiring further surgery for the symptoms is very small. Rounded-edged IOLs may be less prone to negative photopsia, and silicone IOLs may be less liable in general to dysphotopsia than acrylic. Optic and capsulorhexis size may also be important.

- **Symptoms.** A dark shadow in the temporal periphery (negative dysphotopsia – often the most troublesome), scintillations, haloes, peripheral or central flaring or flashes (positive dysphotopsia) and possibly monocular diplopia.
- **Treatment**
  ○ Encouraging the patient that the symptoms usually improve over time, both because of anatomical changes (e.g. capsulorhexis edge thickening) and because the brain is able to ignore unwanted images; patients may be able to accelerate this by trying to avoid paying specific attention to the phenomena.
  ○ Positive nocturnal symptoms can be helped with gentle pupillary constriction (e.g. brimonidine), but dilatation may help negative dysphotopsia.
  ○ Successful alleviation of symptoms has been reported with a variety of techniques, including reverse optic capture (vaulting the optic forward out of the capsular bag, leaving the haptics in place), ciliary sulcus IOL re-implantation, and piggyback IOL implantation in the sulcus; these can also be considered for second-eye surgery.
  ○ IOL exchange (round-edged) may be considered.
  ○ Laser capsulotomy is best avoided as it markedly complicates IOL exchange; in some eyes, YAG laser removal of a sector of capsulorhexis edge has reduced symptoms.

Corneal decompensation

Corneal oedema (see Ch. 6) is very common postoperatively but is usually mild and transient. Eyes with pre-existing corneal endothelial pathology, particularly low cell counts, are at increased risk. Causes of more marked oedema include dense nuclei requiring high phacoemulsification energy, complicated or prolonged surgery, pseudoexfoliation, intraoperative endothelial trauma and elevated postoperative IOP. Use of a dispersive viscoelastic, and possibly a scleral tunnel incision, may help to protect the corneal endothelium during surgery in higher-risk eyes.

Ptosis

Mild ptosis, probably secondary to a variety of mechanisms, is not uncommon after cataract surgery, but usually improves; observation for at least a year postoperatively is recommended in most cases.

Malposition of the IOL

Although uncommon, malposition (Fig. 9.24) may be associated with both optical and structural problems. Significant malposition

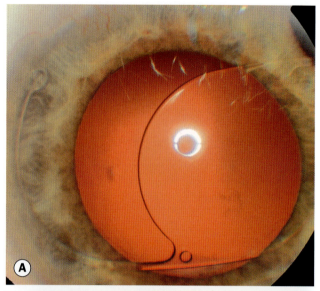

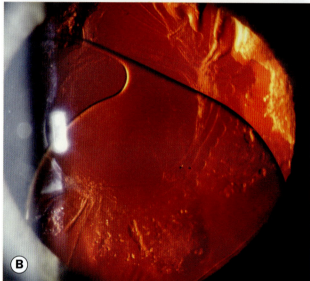

Fig. 9.24 (A) Decentred optic with one haptic in the angle and the other in the bag; **(B)** inferior subluxation of an IOL
(Courtesy of P Gili – fig. B)

may require repositioning or replacement, occasionally with an iris or sclerally fixated lens.

Retinal detachment

Rhegmatogenous retinal detachment (RRD) is uncommon. Preoperative risk factors include lattice degeneration and retinal breaks – both are generally treated prophylactically prior to cataract surgery (and probably laser capsulotomy) – and high myopia. The key intraoperative risk is vitreous loss. Pars plana vitrectomy is usually the surgical modality employed for pseudophakic RRD.

CONGENITAL CATARACT

Aetiology

Congenital cataract occurs in about 3 in 10 000 live births. Two-thirds are bilateral and a cause can be identified in about half of these. Autosomal dominant (AD) inheritance is the most common aetiological factor; others include chromosomal abnormalities, metabolic disorders and intrauterine infections. Isolated inherited congenital cataracts carry a better visual prognosis than those with coexisting ocular and systemic abnormality. Unilateral cataracts are usually sporadic, without a family history or systemic disease, and affected infants are usually otherwise healthy.

Associated metabolic disorders

Galactosaemia

Galactosaemia is an autosomal recessive (AR) condition characterized by impairment of galactose utilization caused by absence of the enzyme galactose-1-phosphate uridyl transferase (GPUT). Unless galactose (milk and milk products) is withheld from the diet, severe systemic complications culminate in early death. 'Oil droplet' lens opacity (see Fig. 9.25D) develops within the first few days or weeks of life in a large percentage of patients. Exclusion of galactose may reverse early lens changes.

Lowe syndrome

Lowe (oculocerebrorenal) syndrome is an X-linked recessive (gene: *OCRL1*) inborn error of amino acid metabolism with neuromuscular, renal and other manifestations. Cataract is universal, and microphakia may also be present. Congenital glaucoma is present in about half of patients. Female carriers may have visually insignificant cortical lens opacities.

Fabry disease

See Chapter 6.

Mannosidosis

Mannosidosis is an AR disorder with deficiency of α-mannosidase. Infantile and juvenile-adult forms are seen, both of which feature progressive mental deterioration, musculoskeletal and other abnormalities. Punctate lens opacities arranged in a spoke-like pattern in the posterior lens cortex are frequent; corneal clouding can also occur but is less common.

Other metabolic disorders

Potential causes include hypo- and pseudohypoparathyroidism, and hypo- and hyperglycaemia.

Associated intrauterine infections

Rubella

Congenital rubella results from transplacental transmission of virus from an infected mother, and may lead to severe fetal malformations. Pearly nuclear or more diffuse unilateral or bilateral cataract occurs in around 15%. (See also Ch. 11.)

Toxoplasmosis

Ophthalmic features of congenital toxoplasmosis include cataract, chorioretinitis, microphthalmos and optic atrophy. (See also Ch. 11.)

Cytomegalovirus infection

Systemic features of congenital cytomegalovirus (CMV) infection include jaundice, hepatosplenomegaly, microcephaly and intracranial calcification. Ocular features apart from cataract include chorioretinitis, microphthalmos, keratitis and optic atrophy.

Varicella

Systemic features include mental handicap, cortical cerebral atrophy, cutaneous scarring and limb deformities; death in early infancy is common. Ocular features may include cataract, microphthalmos, chorioretinitis, optic disc hypoplasia and optic atrophy.

Others

Measles, syphilis, herpes simplex and human immunodeficiency virus (HIV). (See also Ch. 11.)

Other systemic associations

Down syndrome (trisomy 21)

- **Systemic features** include learning difficulties, stunted growth, distinctive facial and peripheral features, thyroid dysfunction, cardiorespiratory disease and reduced life span.
- **Ocular features.** Cataract of varied morphology (75%); the opacities are usually symmetrical and often develop in late childhood. Other features include iris Brushfield spots (see Fig. 12.14B) and hypoplasia, chronic blepharitis, myopia, strabismus and keratoconus.

Edwards syndrome (trisomy 18)

- **Systemic features.** Characteristic facial and peripheral features, deafness, cardiac anomalies, mental handicap and early death.
- **Ocular features** apart from cataract include ptosis, microphthalmos, corneal opacity, uveal and disc coloboma and vitreoretinal dysplasia.

Miscellaneous

Hallermann–Streiff syndrome features impaired growth and other features, with cataract in 90%; Nance–Horan syndrome is an

X-linked condition comprising distinctive dental and facial anomalies together with congenital cataract and microcornea. Female carriers may show Y suture opacities (see Fig. 9.25F).

Management

Ocular assessment

Determination in the neonate of the visual significance of lens opacity is based principally on the appearance of the red reflex and the quality of the fundus view.

- **A very dense cataract** occluding the pupil; the decision to operate is straightforward.
- **A less dense** but still visually significant cataract (e.g. central or posterior opacities over 3 mm in diameter) will permit visualization of the retinal vasculature with the indirect but not with the direct ophthalmoscope.
- **A visually insignificant opacity** will allow clear visualization of the retinal vasculature with both the indirect and direct ophthalmoscope.
- **Other indicators of severe visual impairment** include absence of central fixation, nystagmus and strabismus.
- **Morphology**
  - Blue dot opacities (Fig. 9.25A) are common and innocuous.
  - Nuclear opacities (Fig. 9.25B) are confined to the embryonic or fetal nucleus.
  - Lamellar opacities affect a particular lamella of the lens both anteriorly and posteriorly and may be associated with radial extensions ('riders' – Fig. 9.25C). Lamellar opacities may be autosomal dominant or occur in isolation as well as in association with metabolic disorders and intrauterine infections.
  - Coronary (supranuclear) cataract lies in the deep cortex, surrounding the nucleus like a crown. It is usually sporadic but occasionally hereditary.
  - Central 'oil droplet' opacities (Fig. 9.25D) are characteristic of galactosaemia.
  - Posterior polar cataract (Fig. 9.25E) may be associated with posterior lenticonus or fetal vascular remnants including a Mittendorf dot. This form of opacity is often closely integrated with the lens capsule and/or a pre-existing defect, with a very high risk of dehiscence during surgery.
  - Sutural, in which the opacity follows the anterior or posterior Y suture (Fig. 9.25F); may be seen in female Nance–Horan carriers.
  - Anterior polar cataract may be flat or project into the AC. Occasional associations include persistent pupillary membrane, aniridia, Peters anomaly and anterior lenticonus.
- **Associated ocular pathology** may involve the anterior (e.g. corneal clouding, microphthalmos, glaucoma, persistent fetal vasculature) or posterior segments (e.g. chorioretinitis, Leber amaurosis, rubella retinopathy, foveal or optic nerve

hypoplasia). Its presence may give an additional indication of visual prognosis. The differential diagnosis of leukocoria may apply (see Ch. 12).

- **Assessment of family members** for subclinical familial cataract is prudent.
- **Ultrasonography** should be performed if the fundus is not visible, and may reveal a definitive cause such as persistent fetal vasculature.
- **Special tests** such as forced-choice preferential looking and visual evoked potentials may provide useful supporting information.

Systemic investigations

Investigation of familial cataract is unnecessary, but otherwise the following should be considered. Assessment beyond a search for infection and possibly urinary reducing substance is probably unnecessary in unilateral cases.

- **Screening** for intrauterine infections should usually be performed in all unilateral and bilateral cases.
- **Urine.** Urinalysis for reducing substance after drinking milk (galactosaemia) and chromatography for amino acids (Lowe syndrome).
- **Other investigations** may include fasting blood glucose, serum calcium and phosphorus, red blood cell GPUT and galactokinase levels. Children who have calcium and phosphorus anomalies severe enough to cause cataract are likely to be unwell.
- **Referral to a paediatrician** may be warranted for dysmorphic features or suspicion of other systemic diseases. Chromosome analysis may be useful in this context.

Treatment

The requirement for urgent surgery is balanced by the fact that the earlier this takes place, particularly before 4 weeks of age, the higher the chance of glaucoma developing during the juvenile years.

- **Bilateral dense** cataracts require surgery between 4–10 weeks of age to prevent the development of stimulus deprivation amblyopia. If severity is asymmetrical, the eye with the more dense opacity should be addressed first.
- **Bilateral partial** cataracts may not require surgery until later, or indeed at any stage. In cases of doubt it may be prudent to defer surgery in favour of careful monitoring.
- **Unilateral dense** cataract merits more urgent surgery; there is no consensus regarding timing except that 6 weeks is the latest point at which elective surgery should be performed. Many authorities would advocate surgery between 4 and 6 weeks, followed by aggressive anti-amblyopia therapy, despite which results are often disappointing. If the cataract is detected after 16 weeks of age then the visual prognosis is particularly poor.
- **Partial unilateral** cataract can usually be observed or treated non-surgically with pupillary dilatation and possibly part-time contralateral occlusion.
- **Surgery** involves anterior capsulorhexis, aspiration of lens matter, capsulorhexis of the posterior capsule, limited

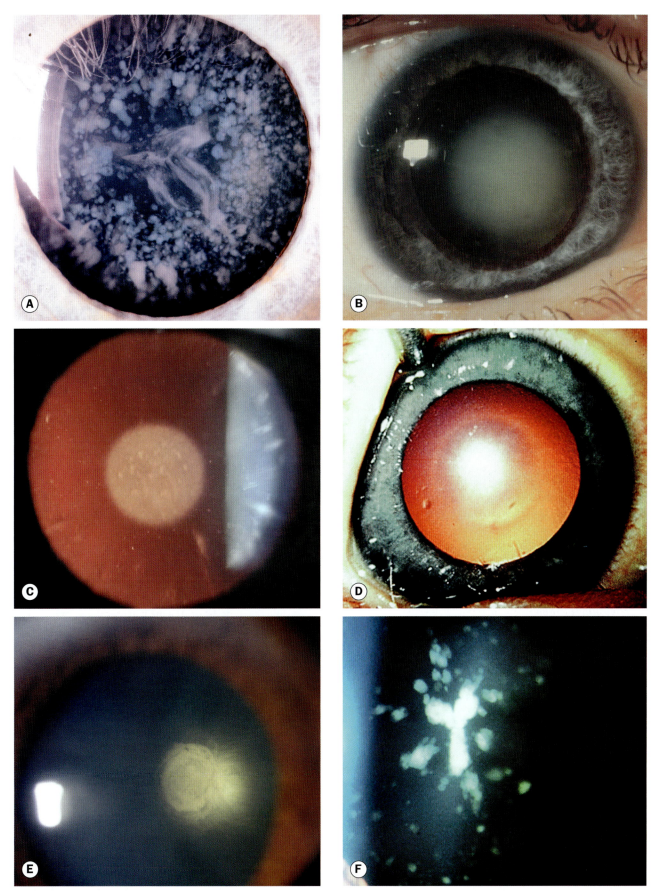

Fig. 9.25 Congenital cataracts. **(A)** Extensive blue dot; **(B)** nuclear; **(C)** lamellar with riders; **(D)** 'oil droplet'; **(E)** posterior polar; **(F)** sutural with blue dots

(Courtesy of R Bates – fig. A; C Barry – figs B, C and E; K Nischal – fig. D)

anterior vitrectomy and IOL implantation, if appropriate. It is important to correct associated refractive errors.

Postoperative complications

Surgery carries a higher incidence of complications than in adults.

- **Posterior capsular opacification** is nearly universal if the posterior capsule is retained, and can have a substantial amblyogenic effect. Posterior capsulorhexis with vitrectomy is generally performed during the primary lens extraction.
- **Secondary membranes** may form across the pupil, particularly if postoperative uveitis is not treated aggressively.
- **Proliferation of lens epithelium** is universal, often forming a Soemmering ring; it is usually visually inconsequential.
- **Glaucoma**
  - Secondary open-angle glaucoma may develop in up to two-thirds of eyes by 10 years after surgery.
  - Angle-closure may occur in the immediate postoperative period secondary to pupillary block, especially in microphthalmic eyes.
- **Retinal detachment** is an uncommon and usually late complication.

Visual rehabilitation

The visual results of cataract surgery in infants are hampered by amblyopia, which should be treated aggressively (see Ch. 18).

- **Spectacles** are useful for older children with bilateral aphakia.
- **Contact lenses** provide a superior optical solution for unilateral or bilateral aphakia. After the age of about 2 years compliance may worsen as the child becomes more independent.
- **IOL implantation** is increasingly being performed in younger children and appears to be effective and safe in selected cases. Hypermetropia (correctable with spectacles) is initially targeted, and as the child ages decay towards emmetropia should occur; however, the final refractive outcome is variable.

ECTOPIA LENTIS

Introduction

Ectopia lentis refers to a hereditary or acquired displacement of the lens from its normal position. The lens may be completely dislocated, rendering the eye functionally aphakic (luxated), or partially displaced, remaining partly within the pupillary area (subluxated). The early stages of subluxation may manifest with a tremulous lens (phacodonesis), demonstrated on the slit lamp by lens wobble on rapid return of the eye to the primary position.

Causes

- **Acquired**
  - Trauma.
  - Pseudoexfoliation.
  - Inflammation, e.g. chronic cyclitis, syphilis.
  - Hypermature cataract.
  - Large eye, e.g. high myopia, buphthalmos.
  - Anterior uveal tumours.
- **Familial ectopia lentis.** This is an AD condition characterized by bilateral symmetrical superotemporal displacement; it may manifest congenitally or later in life.
- **Ectopia lentis et pupillae** is a rare congenital bilateral disorder with AR inheritance characterized by displacement of the pupil and the lens in opposite directions (Fig. 9.26A). The pupils are small and dilate poorly. Microspherophakia may be present.
- **Aniridia** is occasionally associated with ectopia lentis (Fig. 9.26B).
- **Marfan syndrome**
  - AD inheritance (gene: *FBN1*) with variable expressivity.
  - Musculoskeletal features include a tall, thin stature with disproportionately long limbs (arm span > height), long fingers and toes (arachnodactyly), a narrow high-arched ('gothic') palate.
  - Kyphoscoliosis, sternal abnormalities, mild joint laxity, muscular underdevelopment and predisposition to hernias.
  - Cardiovascular lesions include dilatation of the aortic root, mitral valve prolapse and aortic aneurysm formation.
  - Bilateral ectopia lentis (80%); subluxation is most frequently superotemporal. The zonule is frequently intact so that accommodation is retained (Fig. 9.26C), although rarely the lens may dislocate into the AC or vitreous (Fig. 9.26D).
  - Other ocular features: angle anomaly may lead to glaucoma, and lattice retinal degeneration to retinal detachment; there may be hypoplasia of the dilator pupillae, microspherophakia, and strabismus.
- **Weill–Marchesani syndrome** is a rare systemic connective tissue disease, conceptually the converse of Marfan syndrome.
  - Inheritance is AR or AD, the latter resulting from polymorphisms in *FBN1*, the same gene as Marfan syndrome.
  - Systemic features include short stature, short fingers and toes (brachydactyly) and learning difficulties.
  - Ectopia lentis (50%). Subluxation is in an inferior direction and occurs in late childhood or early adulthood. Microspherophakia (Fig. 9.26E) is common, so that pupillary block with angle closure may ensue.
- **Homocystinuria** is an AR disorder in which decreased enzymatic metabolism of the amino acid methionine results in systemic accumulation of methionine and homocysteine.
  - Systemic features include coarse blond hair, blue irides, malar flush, Marfanoid habitus, neurodevelopmental delay, marked thrombotic predisposition and early atherosclerosis.
  - Treatment involves oral pyridoxine, folic acid and vitamin B_{12} to reduce plasma homocysteine and methionine levels.

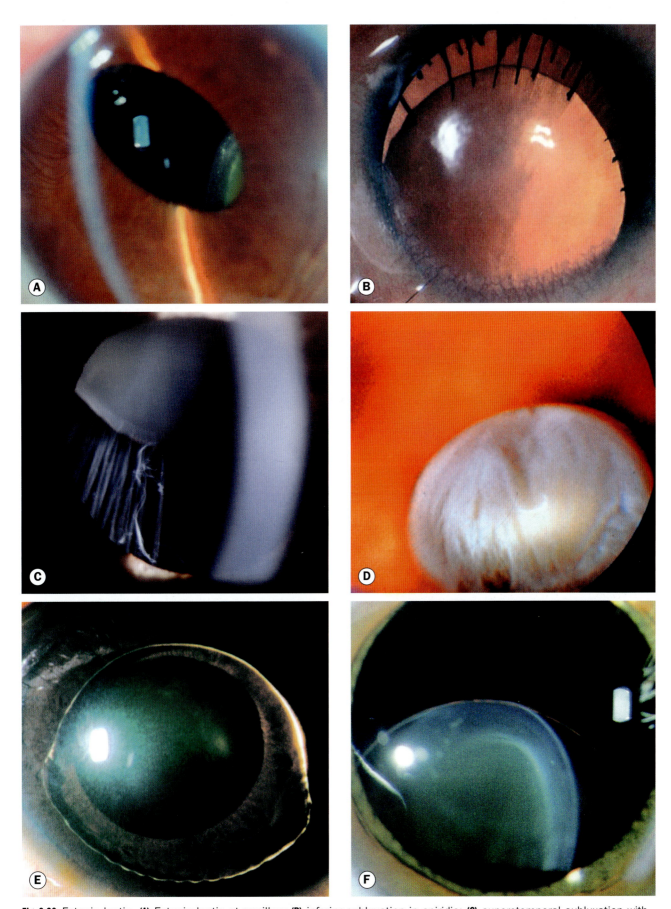

Fig. 9.26 Ectopia lentis. **(A)** Ectopia lentis et pupillae; **(B)** inferior subluxation in aniridia; **(C)** superotemporal subluxation with intact zonule in Marfan syndrome; **(D)** dislocation into the vitreous in Marfan syndrome; **(E)** dislocation of microspheric lens into the anterior chamber in Weill–Marchesani syndrome; **(F)** inferior subluxation with zonular disintegration

(Courtesy of J Schuman, V Christopoulos, D Dhaliwal, M Kahook and R Noecker, from 'Lens and Glaucoma', in Rapid Diagnosis in Ophthalmology, Mosby 2008 *– figs A and F; U Raina – fig. B; R Curtis – fig. E)*

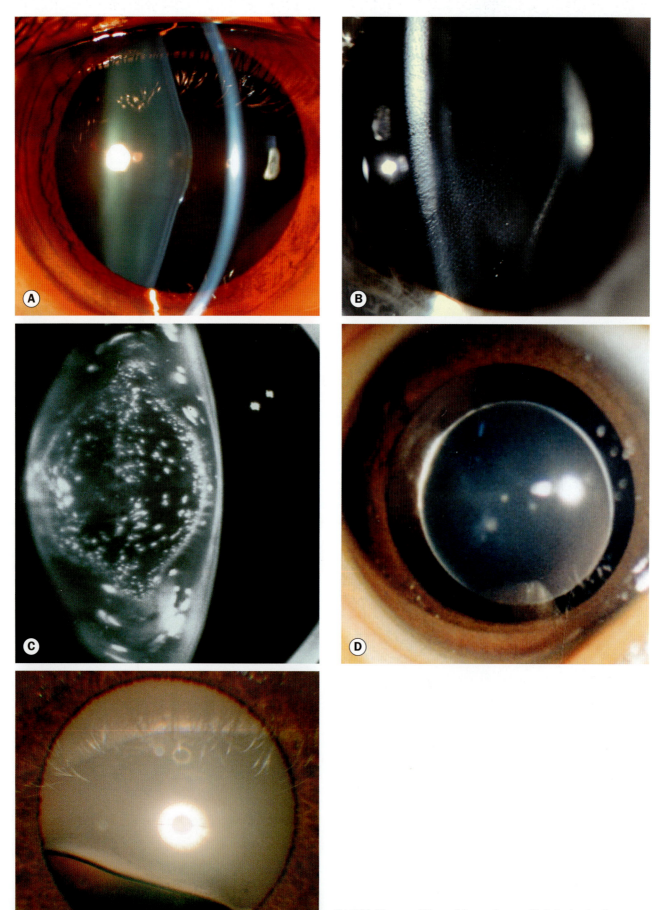

Fig. 9.27 Abnormalities of lens shape. **(A)** Anterior lenticonus; **(B)** posterior lenticonus; **(C)** microspherophakia; **(D)** microphakia; **(E)** lens coloboma

(Courtesy of R Bates – fig. C)

- ○ Ectopia lentis, typically inferonasal, is almost universal by the age of 25 years in untreated cases. The zonule, which normally contains high levels of cysteine (deficient in homocystinuria), disintegrates (Fig. 9.26F) so that accommodation is often lost. Pupillary block may occur.
  - ○ Other ocular features include iris atrophy, optic atrophy, cataract, myopia and retinal detachment.
- **Other systemic conditions** associated with ectopia lentis include sulfite oxidase deficiency (ectopia lentis is universal), and occasionally Stickler syndrome (retinal detachment is the most common ocular manifestation – see Ch. 16), Ehlers–Danlos syndrome and hyperlysinaemia.

Management

The main complications of ectopia lentis are refractive error of any type depending on lens position, optical distortion due to astigmatism and/or lens edge effect, glaucoma (see Ch. 10) and, rarely, lens-induced uveitis.

- **Spectacle correction** may correct astigmatism induced by lens tilt or edge effect in eyes with mild subluxation. Aphakic correction may also afford good visual results if a significant portion of the visual axis is aphakic in the undilated state.
- **Surgical removal** of the lens is indicated for intractable ametropia, meridional amblyopia, cataract, lens-induced glaucoma or uveitis, or endothelial touch.

ABNORMALITIES OF LENS SHAPE

Anterior lenticonus

Anterior lenticonus consists of a bilateral axial projection of the anterior surface of the lens into the anterior chamber (Fig. 9.27A). Almost all patients have Alport syndrome, a hereditary condition characterized by progressive sensorineural deafness and renal disease associated with abnormal glomerular basement membrane; retinal flecks and posterior polymorphous corneal dystrophy may also occur.

Posterior lenticonus

Bulging of the posterior axial lens (Fig. 9.27B) is associated with local thinning or absence of the capsule in posterior lenticonus. Most cases are unilateral, sporadic and not associated with systemic disease. With age, bulging progressively increases and the lens cortex may opacify. Progression of cataract is variable, but an acutely opacified lens is sometimes seen in early childhood.

Lentiglobus

Lentiglobus is a very rare, usually unilateral, generalized hemispherical deformity of the lens; it may be associated with posterior polar opacity.

Microspherophakia and microphakia

The lens is small and spherical in microspherophakia (Fig. 9.27C), which may be seen as an isolated familial (dominant) abnormality, or in association with a number of systemic conditions including Marfan and Weill–Marchesani syndromes, hyperlysinaemia and congenital rubella. Ocular associations include Peters anomaly and familial ectopia lentis et pupillae. Complications can include lenticular myopia, subluxation and dislocation. Microphakia (Fig. 9.27D) is the term used for a lens with a smaller than normal diameter. It may be found in isolation; a systemic association is Lowe syndrome.

Coloboma

This is characterized by congenital indentation of the lens periphery (Fig. 9.27E) and occurs as a result of localized zonular deficiency. It is not a true coloboma, as there is no focal absence of a tissue layer due to failure of closure of the optic fissure, though occasionally a lens coloboma is associated with a coloboma of the iris or fundus.

INTRODUCTION

Aqueous production

Aqueous humour is produced from plasma by the ciliary epithelium of the ciliary body pars plicata, using a combination of active and passive secretion. A high-protein filtrate passes out of fenestrated capillaries (ultrafiltration) into the stroma of the ciliary processes, from which active transport of solutes occurs across the dual-layered ciliary epithelium. The osmotic gradient thereby established facilitates the passive flow of water into the posterior chamber. Secretion is subject to the influence of the sympathetic nervous system, with opposing actions mediated by beta-2 receptors (increased secretion) and alpha-2 receptors (decreased secretion). Enzymatic action is also critical – carbonic anhydrase is among those playing a key role.

Aqueous outflow

Anatomy

- **The trabecular meshwork** (trabeculum) is a sieve-like structure (Fig. 10.1) at the angle of the anterior chamber (AC) through which 90% of aqueous humour leaves the eye. It has three components (Fig. 10.2).
    - The uveal meshwork is the innermost portion, consisting of cord-like endothelial cell-covered strands arising from the iris and ciliary body stroma. The intertrabecular spaces are relatively large and offer little resistance to the passage of aqueous.
    - The corneoscleral meshwork lies external to the uveal meshwork to form the thickest portion of the trabeculum. It is composed of layers of connective tissue strands with overlying endothelial-like cells. The intertrabecular spaces are smaller than those of the uveal meshwork, conferring greater resistance to flow.

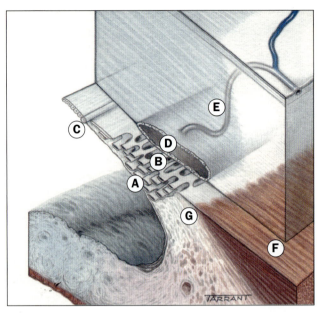

Fig. 10.2 Anatomy of outflow channels: A, Uveal meshwork; B, corneoscleral meshwork; C, Schwalbe line; D, Schlemm canal; E, connector channels; F, longitudinal muscle of the ciliary body; G, scleral spur

- The juxtacanalicular (cribriform) meshwork is the outer part of the trabeculum, and links the corneoscleral meshwork with the endothelium of the inner wall of the canal of Schlemm. It consists of cells embedded in a dense extracellular matrix with narrow intercellular spaces, and offers the major proportion of normal resistance to aqueous outflow.
- The **Schlemm canal** is a circumferential channel within the perilimbal sclera. The inner wall is lined by irregular spindle-shaped endothelial cells containing infoldings (giant vacuoles) that are thought to convey aqueous via the formation of transcellular pores. The outer wall is lined by smooth flat cells and contains the openings of collector channels, which leave the canal at oblique angles and connect directly or indirectly with episcleral veins. Septa commonly divide the lumen into 2–4 channels.

Physiology

Aqueous flows from the posterior chamber via the pupil into the AC, from where it exits the eye via three routes (Fig. 10.3).
- **Trabecular** outflow (90%): aqueous flows through the trabeculum into the Schlemm canal and then the episcleral veins. This is a bulk flow pressure-sensitive route so that increasing IOP will increase outflow.
- **Uveoscleral** drainage (10%): aqueous passes across the face of the ciliary body into the suprachoroidal space, and is drained by the venous circulation in the ciliary body, choroid and sclera.
- **Iris**: some aqueous also drains via the iris.

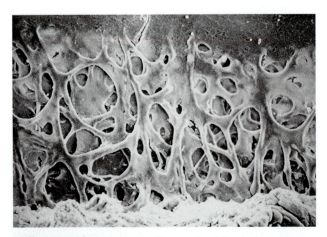

Fig. 10.1 Scanning electron micrograph of the trabecular meshwork

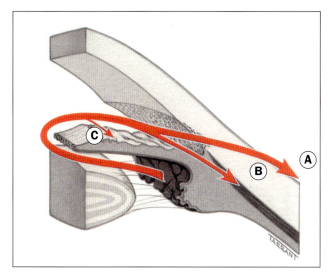

Fig. 10.3 Routes of aqueous outflow: A, trabecular; B, uveoscleral; C, iris

Intraocular pressure

Intraocular pressure (IOP) is determined by the balance between the rate of aqueous production and its outflow, the latter in turn related to factors that include the resistance encountered in the trabeculum and the level of episcleral venous pressure.

Concept of normal intraocular pressure

The average IOP in the general population is around 16 mmHg on applanation tonometry, and a range of about 11–21 mmHg – two standard deviations either side of the average – has conventionally been accepted as normal, at least for a Caucasian population. However, some patients develop glaucomatous damage with IOP less than 21 mm Hg whilst others remain unscathed with IOP well above this level. Whilst reduction of IOP is a key modifiable element in essentially all types of glaucoma, additional incompletely understood factors are critical in determining whether a particular individual or eye develops glaucomatous damage. These include features influencing the IOP reading, such as corneal rigidity, and probably factors affecting the susceptibility of the optic nerve to damage, such as the integrity of its blood supply and structural vulnerability to mechanical stress at the optic nerve head.

Fluctuation

Normal IOP varies with time of day (diurnal variation), heartbeat, blood pressure and respiration. The diurnal pattern varies, with a tendency to be higher in the morning and lower in the afternoon and evening. This is at least partially due to a diurnal pattern in aqueous production, which is lower at night. Glaucomatous eyes exhibit greater than normal fluctuation, the extent of which is directly proportional to the likelihood of progressive visual field damage, and a single reading may therefore be misleading. It is good practice always to note the time of day in conjunction with a recorded IOP.

Overview of glaucoma

Definition

It is difficult to define glaucoma precisely, partly because the term encompasses a diverse group of disorders. All forms of the disease have in common a characteristic potentially progressive optic neuropathy that is associated with visual field loss as damage progresses, and in which IOP is a key modifiable factor.

Classification

Glaucoma may be congenital (developmental) or acquired. Open-angle and angle-closure types are distinguished based on the mechanism by which aqueous outflow is impaired with respect to the AC angle configuration. Distinction is also made between primary and secondary glaucoma; in the latter a recognizable ocular or non-ocular disorder contributes to elevation of IOP.

Epidemiology

Glaucoma affects 2–3% of people over the age of 40 years; 50% may be undiagnosed. Primary open-angle glaucoma (POAG) is the most common form in white, Hispanic/Latino and black individuals; the prevalence is especially high in the latter. On a worldwide basis, primary angle closure (PAC) constitutes up to half of cases, and has a particularly high prevalence in individuals of Asian descent, although with improved assessment such as the routine performance of gonioscopy in a darkened rather than a bright environment, PAC is known to be more prevalent in Caucasian individuals than previously realized.

TONOMETRY

Goldmann tonometry

Principles

Goldmann applanation tonometry (GAT) is based on the Imbert–Fick principle, which states that for a dry thin-walled sphere, the pressure (P) inside the sphere equals the force (F) necessary to flatten its surface divided by the area (A) of flattening (i.e. $P = F/A$). Theoretically, average corneal rigidity (taken as 520 µm for GAT) and the capillary attraction of the tear meniscus cancel each other out when the flattened area has the 3.06 mm diameter contact surface of the Goldmann prism, which is applied to the cornea using the Goldmann tonometer with a measurable amount of force from which the IOP is deduced (Fig. 10.4). The tonometer prism should be disinfected between patients and replaced regularly in accordance with the manufacturer's instructions. Disposable tonometer prisms and caps have been introduced to address concerns of infection from reusable prisms.

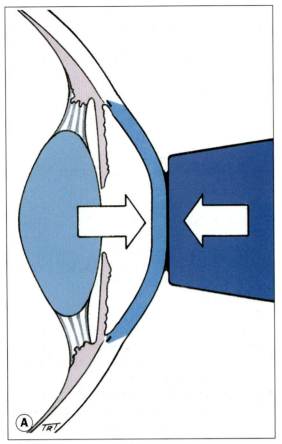

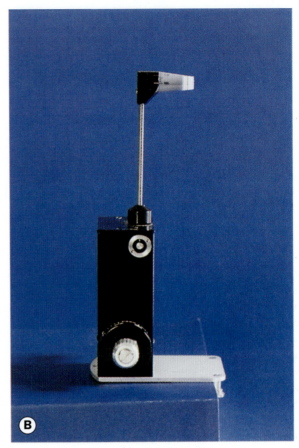

Fig. 10.4 Goldmann tonometry. **(A)** Physical principles; **(B)** tonometer
(Courtesy of J Salmon – fig. B)

Technique

- Topical anaesthetic (commonly proxymetacaine 0.5%) and a small amount of fluorescein are instilled into the conjunctival sac.
- The patient is positioned at the slit lamp with his or her forehead firmly against the headrest and instructed to look straight ahead (often at the examiner's opposite ear) and to breathe normally.
- With the cobalt blue filter in place and illumination of maximal intensity directed obliquely (approximately 60°) at the prism, the prism is centred in front of the apex of the cornea.
- The dial is preset at 1 (i.e. 10 mmHg).
- The prism is advanced until it just touches the apex of the cornea (Fig. 10.5A).
- Viewing is switched to the ocular of the slit lamp.
- A pattern of two green semicircular mires will be seen, one above and one below the horizontal midline, which represent the fluorescein-stained tear film touching the upper and lower outer halves of the prism. Mire thickness should be around 10% of the diameter of its total arc (Fig. 10.5B). Care should be taken to horizontally and vertically centre the mires so that as far as practically possible two centralized semicircles are observed.

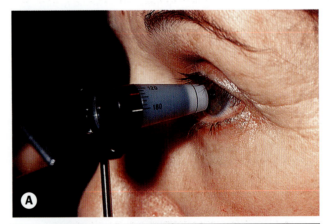

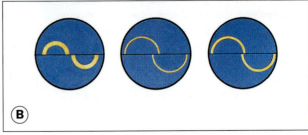

Fig. 10.5 Applanation tonometry. **(A)** Contact between the tonometer prism and the cornea; **(B)** fluorescein-stained semicircular mires – the diagram at right shows the correct end-point using mires of appropriate thickness

- The dial on the tonometer is rotated to vary the applied force; the inner margins of the semicircles align when a circular area of diameter precisely 3.06 mm is flattened.
- The reading on the dial, multiplied by 10, gives the IOP; a version is available that shows IOP on a digital display.

Sources of error

- **Inappropriate fluorescein pattern.** Excessive fluorescein will result in the mires being too thick, with consequent overestimation of IOP; insufficient will make the semicircles too thin, with consequent underestimation (see Fig. 10.5B, left and centre).
- **Pressure on the globe** from the examiner's fingers, eyelid squeezing or restricted extraocular muscles (e.g. thyroid myopathy) may give an anomalously high reading.
- **Central corneal thickness (CCT).** Calculations of IOP by GAT assume that central corneal thickness is 520 μm, with minimal normal variation. If the cornea is thinner, an underestimation of IOP is likely to result, and if thicker, an overestimation. Corneas tend to be thicker than average in individuals with ocular hypertension, and thinner in normal-tension glaucoma (NTG); following refractive surgery procedures the cornea is both thinner and structurally altered such that IOP is likely to be underestimated. Some methods of IOP measurement (e.g. DCT – see below) may reduce the effect of structural confounding variables. Other corneal mechanical factors may also be important but are less well defined.
- **Corneal oedema** may result in artificial lowering of IOP, hypothesized to be due to a boggy softening; the associated increased CCT seems to be more than offset.
- **Astigmatism**, if significant, may give distorted mires as well as leading to mechanically induced errors. If over 3 dioptres, the average reading of two can be taken with the prism rotated 90° for the second, or optimally the prism is rotated so that the red line on the tonometer housing is aligned with the prescription of the minus axis.
- **Incorrect calibration** of the tonometer can result in a false reading, and calibration should optimally be checked before each clinical session using the manufacturer's calibration arm.
- **Wide pulse pressure.** It is normal for there to be a small oscillation of IOP in concert with the rhythm of ocular perfusion. If this 'pulse pressure' is substantial, either the midpoint or the highest level observed may be taken.
- **Repeated readings over a short period** will often be associated with a slight fall in IOP due to a massaging effect on the eye.
- **Other factors** include a tight collar and breath-holding, both of which obstruct venous return and can raise IOP.

Other forms of tonometry

- **Pneumotonometry** (Fig. 10.6A) is based on the principle of applanation, but the central part of the cornea is flattened by a jet of air rather than a prism. The time required to sufficiently flatten the cornea relates directly to the level of IOP. Contact is not made with the eye and topical anaesthesia is not required, so it is particularly useful for screening in the community. The sudden jet of air can startle the patient. Accuracy is improved if an average of at least three readings is taken.
- **Portable applanation tonometry** (Perkins) uses a Goldmann prism in conjunction with a portable light source (Fig. 10.6B). It is hand-held, and can therefore be used in bed-bound or anaesthetized patients.
- **Dynamic contour tonometry (DCT)** (e.g. PASCAL®) uses a solid state sensor and a corneal contour-matching surface, with the aim of measuring IOP relatively independently of corneal mechanical factors such as rigidity. It is mounted on a slit lamp in similar fashion to the Goldmann tonometer, and IOP is shown on a digital display. Studies comparing DCT and GAT IOP readings with manometric intracameral IOP seem to confirm DCT as providing a more physiological measurement.
- **Ocular response analyser** (e.g. Reichert®) is a form of pneumotonometer that measures IOP whilst attempting to compensate for corneal biomechanical properties by using two sequential measurements to assess corneal hysteresis, a function of viscous damping.
- **Electronic indentation/applanation tonometry** (e.g. Tono-Pen® – Fig. 10.6C) is a hand-held electronic contact tonometer (a modified version of the older Mackay–Marg tonometer). The probe tip contains a transducer that measures applied force. Besides portability, its main advantage is the facility to measure IOP reasonably accurately in eyes with distorted or oedematous corneas, and through a soft contact lens.
- **Rebound tonometry** (e.g. iCare® – Fig. 10.6D) involves a 1.8 mm plastic ball attached to a wire; deceleration of the probe upon contact with the cornea is proportional to IOP. Anaesthesia is not required. The instrument can be used for self-monitoring – a tailored personal version is available – and for screening in the community.
- **Indentation (impression) tonometry** (e.g. Schiotz) is a portable device that measures the extent of corneal indentation by a plunger of known weight; it is now seldom used.
- **Implantable tonometers** are under development and if a clinically workable device is realized should facilitate accurate lifelong 24-hour IOP measurement.

GONIOSCOPY

Introduction

Overview

- **Gonioscopy** is a method of evaluating the AC angle, and can be used therapeutically for procedures such as laser trabeculoplasty and goniotomy.

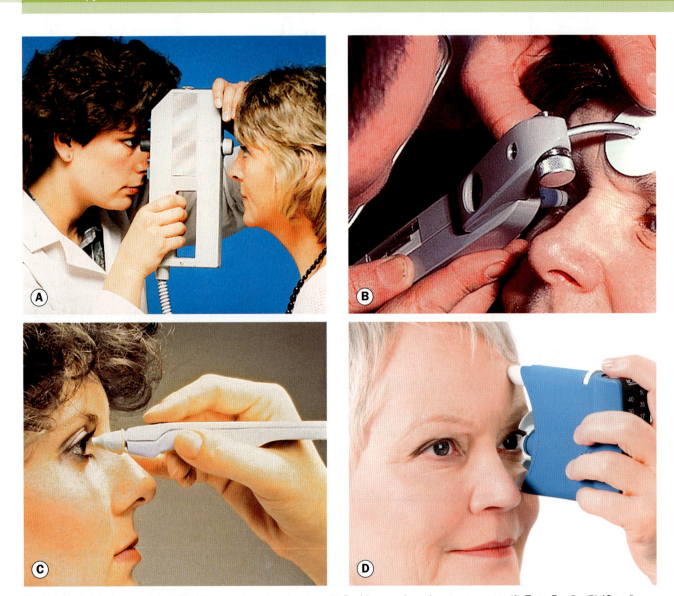

Fig. 10.6 Portable tonometers. **(A)** Keeler pneumotonometer; **(B)** Perkins applanation tonometer; **(C)** Tono-Pen® ; **(D)** iCare®
(Courtesy of Mainline Instruments Ltd – fig. D)

- **Other means** of angle assessment such as anterior segment optical coherence tomography (OCT) and high-frequency ultrasound biomicroscopy (UBM) offer advantages in some aspects of angle analysis, but current clinical opinion suggests they should supplement rather than replace visual gonioscopic analysis.

Optical principles

The angle of the AC cannot be visualized directly through the intact cornea because light from angle structures undergoes 'total internal reflection' at the anterior surface of the precorneal tear film (Fig. 10.7, top). When light travels from a medium of higher to one of lower refractive index (such as cornea to air) it will be reflected at the interface between the two unless the angle of incidence is less than a certain 'critical angle' dependent on their refractive index difference (46° for the tear film–air interface). The phenomenon is utilized in optical fibre signal transmission, where

it ensures that light is retained within the core of a cable. Because the refractive index of a goniolens is similar to that of the cornea, it eliminates total internal reflection by replacing the tear film–air interface with a tear film–goniolens interface (Fig. 10.7, bottom). Light rays can then be viewed as they exit the contact lens, directly or indirectly (see below).

Disinfection

Lenses must be cleaned between patients to remove any particulate matter and then sterilized; a suggested regimen is soaking in 2% hypochlorite solution (this has activity against transmissible spongiform encephalopathies) for at least 5 minutes followed by thorough rinsing in sterile saline, then air-drying.

Indirect gonioscopy

Indirect goniolenses use a mirror to reflect rays from the angle such that they exit the goniolens at much less than the critical

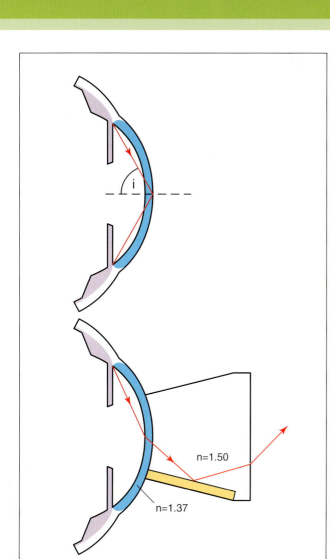

Fig. 10.7 Optical principles of gonioscopy; *n* = refractive index; *i* = angle of incidence

- The size and intensity of the slit beam should be reduced to the absolute minimum compatible with an adequate view, in particular avoiding any of the beam being directed through the pupil.
- The patient is seated at the slit lamp and advised that the lens will touch the eye but will not usually cause discomfort; the forehead must be kept against the headband and both eyes should remain open.
- A drop of local anaesthetic is instilled.
- A drop or two of coupling fluid (e.g. hypromellose 0.3%) is placed on the contact surface of the lens.

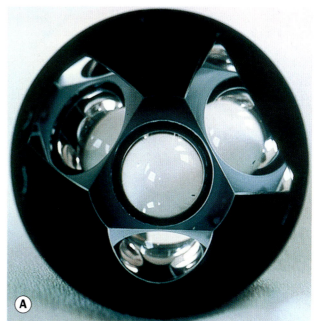

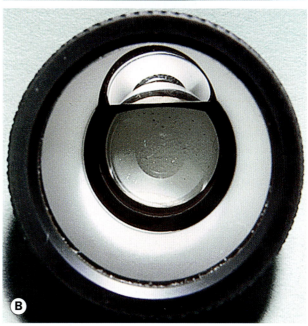

Fig. 10.8 Goldmann goniolens. **(A)** Three mirrors; **(B)** single mirror

angle. They provide a mirror image of the opposite angle and can be used only in conjunction with a slit lamp.

Non-indentation gonioscopy

- **Goniolenses**
  - The classic Goldmann lens consists of three mirrors (Fig. 10.8A), one of which is specifically for gonioscopy; some goniolenses have one (Fig. 10.8B), two or four mirrors.
  - Lenses of similar basic structure but with modifications include the Magna View, Ritch trabeculoplasty and the Khaw direct view.
  - Because the curvature of the contact surface of the lens is steeper than that of the cornea, a viscous coupling substance of refractive index similar to the cornea is required to bridge the gap between cornea and lens.
- **Technique**
  - It is essential that the examination takes place in a room in which the ambient illumination is very low – completely dark if possible.

○ The patient is asked to look upwards and the lens is inserted rapidly so as to avoid loss of the coupling fluid. The patient then looks straight ahead.

○ Indirect gonioscopy gives an inverted view of the portion of the angle opposite the mirror.

○ Once the initial examination has been performed and the findings noted, increasing the level of illumination may help in defining the angle structures.

○ When the view of the angle is obscured by a convex iris, it is possible to see 'over the hill' by asking the patient to look in the direction of the mirror. Only slight movement is permissible, otherwise the structures will be distorted and a closed angle may appear open.

○ Excessive pressure with a non-indentation lens narrows the angle appearance (in contrast to the effect of pressure during indentation gonioscopy – see below). Excessive pressure also causes folds in the cornea that compromise the clarity of the view.

○ In some eyes, suction on the cornea from the lens may artificially open the angle; awareness of the need to avoid retrograde, as well as anterograde, pressure on the lens will tend to prevent inadvertent distortion.

Indentation (dynamic, compression) gonioscopy

- **Goniolenses** include the Zeiss (Fig. 10.9), Posner and Sussman (no handle), all of which are four-mirror gonioprisms.
  - ○ The contact surface of the lenses has a curvature flatter than that of the cornea, negating the need for a coupling substance.
  - ○ The lenses do not stabilize the globe and are relatively unsuitable for laser trabeculoplasty.
  - ○ A common criticism is that it is easy to inadvertently open the angle, giving a misleadingly reassuring impression, especially if inexperienced.
- **Technique**
  - ○ The first stages are as set out above for non-indentation gonioscopy.
  - ○ Indentation is performed by gently pressing the lens posteriorly against the cornea; this forces aqueous into the angle, pushing the peripheral iris posteriorly.
  - ○ If the angle is closed only by apposition between the iris and cornea it will be forced open, allowing visualization of the angle recess (Fig. 10.10).
  - ○ If the angle is closed by adhesions between the peripheral iris and cornea – peripheral anterior synechiae (PAS) – it will remain closed.
  - ○ Dynamic gonioscopy can be invaluable in helping to define the structures in angles that are difficult to assess, such as in distinguishing an extensive or double highly pigmented Schwalbe line from the pigmented meshwork.

Direct gonioscopy

Direct goniolenses work by constructing the viewing surface of the lens in a domed or slanted configuration such that exiting light

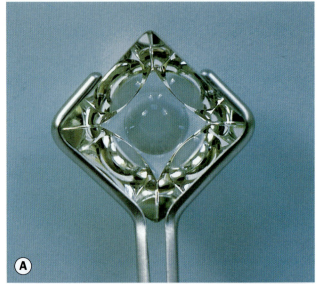

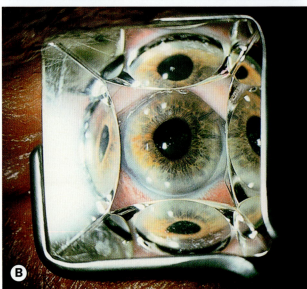

Fig. 10.9 (A) Zeiss goniolens; **(B)** slit lamp view with lens in place on the cornea

rays strike the contact lens/air interface at a steeper than critical angle so that they will pass through to the observer. This approach is called 'direct' because light rays from the angle are viewed directly, without reflection inside the lens. They do not require a slit lamp and are used with the patient in the supine position, typically under general anaesthesia in the evaluation and surgical treatment of infantile glaucoma.

- **Direct goniolenses** include the Koeppe (Fig. 10.11A), Medical Workshop, Barkan and Swan–Jacob (Fig. 10.11B).
- **Technique**
  - ○ Gonioscopy is performed with the patient in the supine position (note that this may deepen the angle) in conjunction with an operating or hand-held microscope or magnifying loupes.

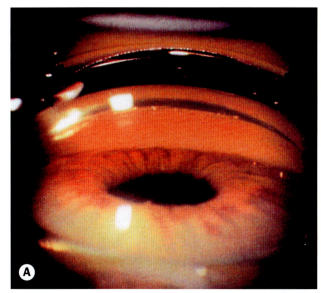

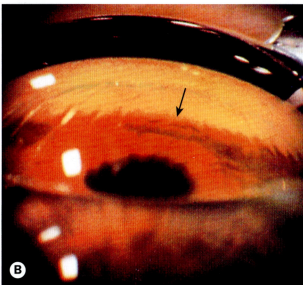

Fig. 10.10 Indentation gonioscopy in appositional angle closure. **(A)** Total angle closure prior to indentation; **(B)** during indentation the entire angle becomes visible (arrow) – the corneal folds seen are typical
(Courtesy of W Alward, from Color Atlas of Gonioscopy, Wolfe 1994)

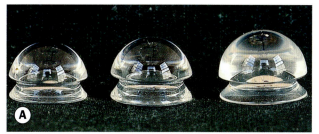

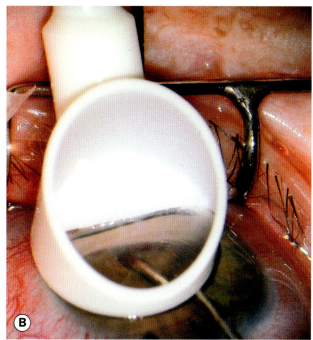

Fig. 10.11 Goniolenses. **(A)** Koeppe; **(B)** Swan–Jacob

○ The technique cannot be used with a desktop slit lamp so clarity, illumination and variable magnification are not comparable with indirect lenses.

Identification of angle structures

Accurate identification of angle structures (Fig. 10.12) is not always straightforward, even for highly experienced gonioscopists.

- **Schwalbe line.** This is the most anterior structure, appearing whitish to variably pigmented. Anatomically it demarcates the peripheral termination of Descemet membrane and the anterior limit of the trabeculum. It may be barely discernible in younger patients. In contrast, there may be pigment deposits on or anterior to the Schwalbe

line – a Sampaolesi line – especially in heavily pigmented angles (e.g. pseudoexfoliation syndrome). It may have a double-line configuration, when the posterior component may be mistaken for the pigmented meshwork.
- **The corneal wedge** is useful in locating an inconspicuous Schwalbe line. Using a narrow slit beam, two distinct linear corneal reflections can be identified, one on the inner and one on the outer corneal surface; the outer reflection will arc round across the corneoscleral interface – due to the sclera being opaque – to meet the inner reflection at the apex of the corneal wedge that coincides with the Schwalbe line.
- **The trabeculum** extends from the Schwalbe line to the scleral spur, with an average width of 600 μm. In younger people it has a ground-glass translucent appearance. The anterior non-functional part lies adjacent to the Schwalbe line and has a whitish colour. The posterior, pigmented functional part lies adjacent to the scleral spur and has a greyish-blue translucent appearance in the young. Trabecular pigmentation is rare prior to puberty, but in older eyes involves the posterior trabeculum to a variable extent, most marked inferiorly. Patchy trabecular pigmentation in a suspiciously narrow angle raises the possibility of intermittent iris contact.

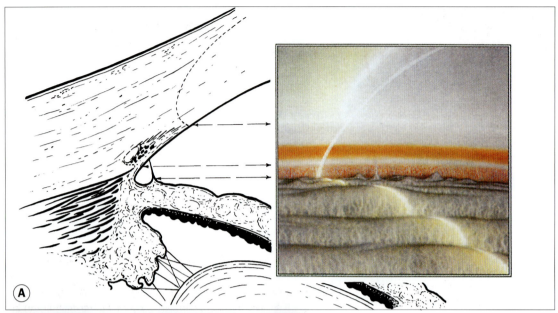

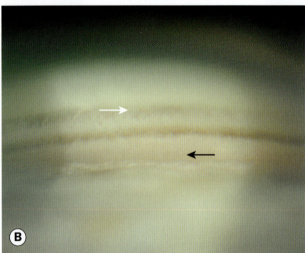

Fig. 10.12 Normal angle structures. **(A)** Schematic representation – inset painting demonstrates corneal wedge; **(B)** goniophotograph – a broad Schwalbe line is indicated by the white arrow, below which are the non-pigmented meshwork, the pigmented meshwork, the scleral spur and the ciliary body (black arrow) – the ciliary body is relatively lightly pigmented

(Courtesy of W Alward, from Color Atlas of Gonioscopy, *Wolfe 1994 – fig. A)*

- **The Schlemm canal** may be identified in the angle, especially if non-pigmented, as a slightly darker line deep to the posterior trabeculum. Blood can sometimes be seen in the canal (Fig. 10.13), either physiologically (sometimes due to excessive pressure on the episcleral veins with a goniolens), or in the presence of low intraocular or raised episcleral venous pressure.
- **The scleral spur** is the most anterior projection of the sclera and the site of attachment of the longitudinal muscle of the ciliary body. Gonioscopically it is situated immediately posterior to the trabeculum and appears as a narrow whitish band that yellows with age.
- **The ciliary body** stands out just behind the scleral spur as a pink, dull brown or slate grey band. Its width depends on the position of iris insertion and it tends to be narrower in hypermetropic eyes and wider in myopic eyes. The angle recess represents the posterior dipping of the iris as it inserts into the ciliary body. It may not be visible in some eyes due

to a physiological anterior iris insertion, though fixed pathological angle narrowing due to peripheral anterior synechiae (PAS) – adhesions between the iris and angle structures – should be excluded.
- **Iris processes** are small, usually tenuous extensions of the anterior surface of the iris that insert at the level of the scleral spur and cover the ciliary body to a varying extent (see Fig. 10.13). They are present in about one-third of normal eyes and are most prominent during childhood and in brown eyes. The processes should not be confused with PAS, which typically extend more anteriorly and are more substantial.
- **Blood vessels.** Radial vessels at the base of the angle recess are often seen in normal eyes. Pathological blood vessels run randomly in various directions. As a general principle, any blood vessel that crosses the scleral spur onto the trabecular meshwork is abnormal. Larger circumferential vessels may also be seen.

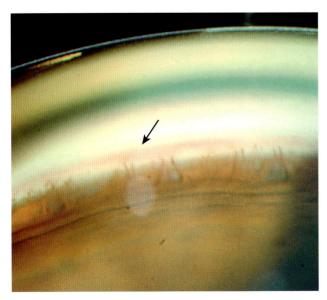

Fig. 10.13 Blood in the Schlemm canal (arrow), and iris processes

(Courtesy of J Schuman, V Christopoulos, D Dhaliwal, M Kahook and R Noecker, from 'Lens and Glaucoma', in Rapid Diagnosis in Ophthalmology, *Mosby 2008)*

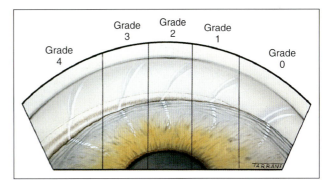

Fig. 10.14 Grading of angle width according to number of visible structures

Grading of angle width

In practice, the angle is graded by many practitioners simply according to the number of structures visible (Fig. 10.14), together with qualifying comments relating to the width of the iris approach; many angles are narrowest superiorly, though this difference may be reduced by decreasing the ambient illumination.

Shaffer system

The Shaffer system records the angle in degrees between two imaginary lines tangential to the inner surface of the trabeculum and the anterior surface of the iris about one-third of the distance from its periphery. The system assigns a numerical grade to each quadrant of the angle.

- **Grade 4** (35–45°) is the widest angle, characteristic of myopia and pseudophakia; the ciliary body can be visualized without tilting the lens.
- **Grade 3** (25–35°) is an open angle in which the scleral spur is visible.

- **Grade 2** (20°) is an angle in which the trabeculum but not the scleral spur can be seen.
- **Grade 1** (10°) is a very narrow angle in which only the Schwalbe line and perhaps the top of the trabeculum can be identified.
- **Slit angle** is one in which there is no obvious iridocorneal contact but no angle structures can be identified.
- **Grade 0** (0°) is closed due to iridocorneal contact.
- Indentation will distinguish appositional from synechial angle closure.

Other systems

- The **Spaeth** system is detailed but underused. It allows formal description of the position of iris insertion, the angular approach and peripheral iris curvature.
- The **Scheie** classification refers to the angle structures visible and allocates a Roman numeral accordingly. In contrast to common clinical use, in the original system a higher numeral (e.g. IV) actually signifies a narrower angle.
- **The van Herick** method (Table 10.1) uses the slit lamp alone to estimate the AC angle width:
  - A thin but bright slit beam is set approximately perpendicularly to the corneal surface (offset from the optics by about 60°) to the patient's temporal side for each eye.
  - The beam is used to estimate the ratio of the corneal thickness to the most peripheral part of the AC.

Table 10.1 Van Herick method for anterior chamber angle assessment

Anterior chamber depth as a proportion of corneal thickness	Description	Grade	Comment
≥1	Peripheral AC space equal to full corneal thickness or larger	4	Wide open
¼–½	Space between one-fourth and one-half corneal thickness	3	Incapable of closure
¼	Space equal to one-fourth corneal thickness	2	Should be gonioscoped
<¼	Space less than one-fourth corneal thickness	1	Gonioscopy will usually demonstrate a dangerously narrowed angle

○ It is useful as a screening tool, but overestimates angle width in a proportion of patients, particularly those with a plateau iris conformation.

Pathological findings

- **Peripheral anterior synechiae**
  ○ Primary angle-closure glaucoma.
  ○ Anterior uveitis.
  ○ Iridocorneal endothelial (ICE) syndrome.
- **Neovascularization**
  ○ Neovascular glaucoma.
  ○ Fuchs heterochromic cyclitis.
  ○ Chronic anterior uveitis.
- **Hyperpigmentation**
  ○ Physiological variant.
  ○ Pigment dispersion syndrome.
  ○ Pseudophakic pigment dispersion.
  ○ Pseudoexfoliation syndrome.
  ○ Blunt ocular trauma.
  ○ Anterior uveitis.
  ○ Following acute angle-closure glaucoma.
  ○ Following YAG laser iridotomy.
  ○ Iris or angle melanoma or naevus.
  ○ Iris pigment epithelial cysts.
  ○ Naevus of Ota.
- **Trauma**
  ○ Angle recession.
  ○ Trabecular dialysis.
  ○ Cyclodialysis.
  ○ Foreign bodies.
- **Blood in the Schlemm canal**
  ○ Physiological variant.
  ○ Carotid–cavernous fistula and dural shunt.
  ○ Sturge–Weber syndrome.
  ○ Obstruction of the superior vena cava.

EVALUATION OF THE OPTIC NERVE HEAD

Normal optic nerve head

Neuroretinal rim

The neuroretinal rim (NRR) is the orange-pink tissue between the outer edge of the cup and the optic disc margin. The inferior rim is the broadest followed by the superior, nasal and temporal (the 'ISNT' rule – Fig. 10.15); this has high sensitivity for glaucoma but is not very specific, i.e. eyes without glaucoma often do not respect the rule.

Cup/disc (C/D) ratio

The C/D ratio indicates the diameter of the cup expressed as a fraction of the diameter of the disc; the vertical rather than the

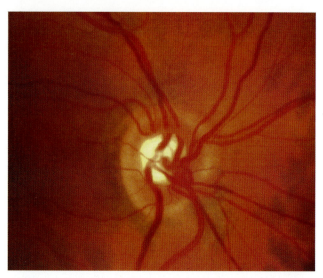

Fig. 10.15 Normal disc that obeys the 'ISNT' rule (see text)

horizontal ratio is generally taken. Small diameter optic discs have small cups (Fig. 10.16A) and vice versa (Fig. 10.16B); only 2% of the population have a C/D ratio greater than 0.7. In any individual, asymmetry of 0.2 or more between the eyes should also be regarded with suspicion, though it is critical to exclude a corresponding difference in overall disc diameter (see next).

Optic disc size

Optic disc size is important in deciding if a cup/disc (C/D) ratio is normal (see above), and is also a prognostic indicator. Large discs are believed to be more likely to sustain damage, particularly in NTG. This may be the result of the larger diameter conferring relative mechanical weakness and hence greater vulnerability to IOP-induced displacement of the lamina cribrosa; the lamina cribrosa has been found to be thinner in eyes with NTG. Disc size varies on average between racial groups, and is largest in black individuals. Imaging can objectively measure disc area, but vertical diameter is the parameter most frequently used clinically; normal median vertical diameter (for non-glaucomatous discs) is 1.5–1.7 mm in a white population.

○ A narrow slit beam is focused on the disc using a fundus lens.
○ The height of the beam is adjusted until it matches the distance between the superior and inferior limits of the NRR (not the scleral rim surrounding the neural tissue), and the diameter in millimetres is read from the slit lamp graticule.
○ A correction factor may be necessary, depending on the lens used (Table 10.2). Refractive error affects measurement only minimally, although myopia above −8 dioptres may distort the result.

Changes in glaucoma

In many cases it is not possible to be certain whether an individual optic disc is glaucomatous. The clinical findings and results of

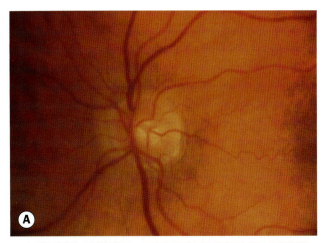

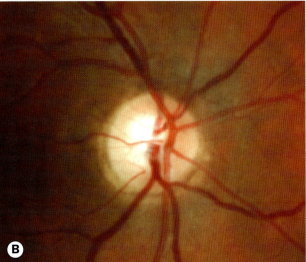

Fig. 10.16 Normal discs. **(A)** Small disc with a low cup/disc ratio; **(B)** larger disc with a proportionally larger cup

investigation should be considered together to guide management. Glaucomatous damage results in characteristic signs involving (a) the optic nerve head, (b) the peripapillary area and (c) the retinal nerve fibre layer.

Optic nerve head

Pathological cupping is caused by an irreversible decrease in the number of nerve fibres, glial cells and blood vessels. A documented

Table 10.2 Correction factors for estimating optic disc diameter

Lens	Correction factor
Volk 60 D	×0.88–1.0
Nikon 60 D	Around 1.0
Volk 90 D	×1.3
Volk 78 D	×1.1
Goldmann 3-mirror	×1.27

increase in cup size is always significant. If an eye with a small optic disc and correspondingly small cup develops glaucoma, the cup will increase in size, but even in the presence of substantial damage may still be smaller than that of a large physiological cup.

Subtypes of glaucomatous damage

Four 'pure' glaucomatous disc appearances have been described, and although the majority of discs are unclassifiable the descriptions encompass a useful overview of patterns of glaucomatous damage, and may provide clues to underlying pathological processes.

- **Focal ischaemic discs** (Fig. 10.17A) are characterized by localized superior and/or inferior notching and may be associated with localized field defects with early threat to fixation.
- **Myopic disc with glaucoma** (Fig. 10.17B) refers to a tilted (obliquely inserted), shallow disc with a temporal crescent of parapapillary atrophy, together with features of glaucomatous damage. Dense superior or inferior scotomas threatening fixation are common. This morphology is most common in younger male patients.
- **Sclerotic discs** (Fig. 10.17C) are characterized by a shallow, saucerized cup and a gently sloping NRR, variable peripapillary atrophy and peripheral visual field loss. The peripapillary choroid is thinner than in other disc types. Patients are older, of either gender, and there is an association with systemic vascular disease.
- **Concentrically enlarging discs** (verified by serial monitoring) are characterized by fairly uniform NRR thinning (Fig. 10.17D) and are frequently associated with diffuse visual field loss. IOP is often significantly elevated at presentation.

Non-specific signs of glaucomatous damage

Other disc signs of glaucomatous damage include:
- **Disc haemorrhages** (Figs 10.18A and B, and see Fig. 10.17A) often extend from the NRR onto the retina, most commonly inferotemporally. Their presence is a risk factor for the development and progression of glaucoma. They are more common in NTG, but can also occur in healthy individuals as well as patients with systemic vascular disease.
- **Baring of circumlinear blood vessels** is a sign of early thinning of the NRR. It is characterized by a space between the neuroretinal rim and a superficial blood vessel (Fig. 10.18C).
- **Bayoneting** is characterized by double angulation of a blood vessel. With NRR loss, a vessel entering the disk from the retina may angle sharply backwards into the disk and then turn towards its original direction to run across the lamina cribrosa (Fig. 10.18D).
- **Collaterals** between two veins at the disc (Fig. 10.18E), similar to those following central retinal vein occlusion (CRVO), are relatively uncommon. They are probably caused by chronic low-grade circulatory obstruction. Retinal vascular tortuosity may also occur.

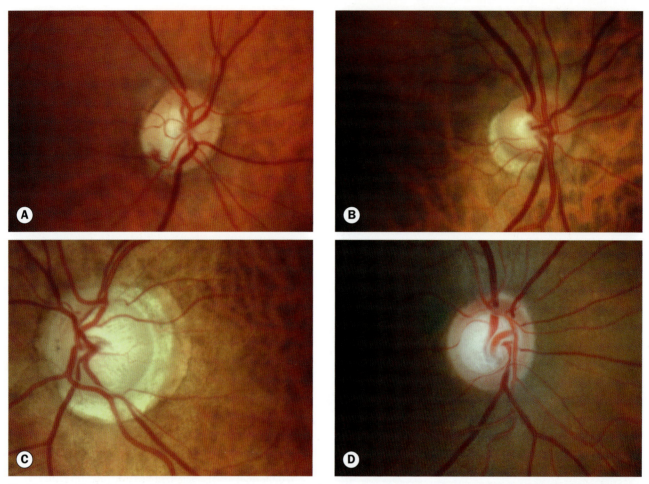

Fig. 10.17 Classic subtypes of glaucomatous damage. **(A)** Focal ischaemic – inferior notch and disc haemorrhage; **(B)** myopic; **(C)** sclerotic; **(D)** concentrically enlarging

- **Loss of nasal NRR** (Fig. 10.18F) is a sign of moderately advanced damage; a space may develop between the NRR and the central retinal vasculature.
- The **laminar dot sign** occurs in advancing glaucoma. Grey dot-like fenestrations in the lamina cribrosa (see Fig. 10.18F) become exposed as the NRR recedes. The fenestrations sometimes appear linear, and this itself may be a sign of advanced damage, indicating distortion of the lamina. The dots may be seen in normal eyes.
- **'Sharpened edge' or 'sharpened rim'** is a sign of advancing damage. As NRR is lost adjacent to the edge of the disc, the disc margin contour assumes a sharper angle backwards. Bayoneting of vessels is often seen at a sharpened edge. This should not be confused with a 'sharpened nasal polar edge', which refers to the sharp angulation of the NRR at the nasal margin of a focal vertical polar notch.

Peripapillary changes

Peripapillary atrophy (PPA) surrounding the optic nerve head may be of significance in glaucoma (Fig. 10.19), and may be a sign of early damage in patients with ocular hypertension.

- **Alpha (outer) zone** is characterized by superficial retinal pigment epithelial changes. It tends to be larger and possibly more common in glaucomatous eyes.
- **Beta (inner) zone** is characterized by chorioretinal atrophy; it is distinct from the scleral rim, the white band of exposed sclera central to the beta zone. The beta zone is larger and more common in glaucoma, and is a risk factor for progression; the location of beta-zone PPA seems to indicate the orientation of likely visual field loss.

Retinal nerve fibre layer

In glaucoma subtle retinal nerve fibre layer (RNFL) defects precede the development of detectable optic disc and visual field changes; their onset often follows disc haemorrhages. Two patterns occur: (a) localized wedge-shaped defects and (b) diffuse defects that are larger and have indistinct borders. Defects are sometimes evident following disc haemorrhages (Fig. 10.20A). Red-free (green) light increases the contrast between normal retina and defects on slit lamp biomicroscopy or fundus photography (Fig. 10.20B) and typically makes identification easier. OCT and scanning laser polarimetry are highly effective means of quantifying the RNFL.

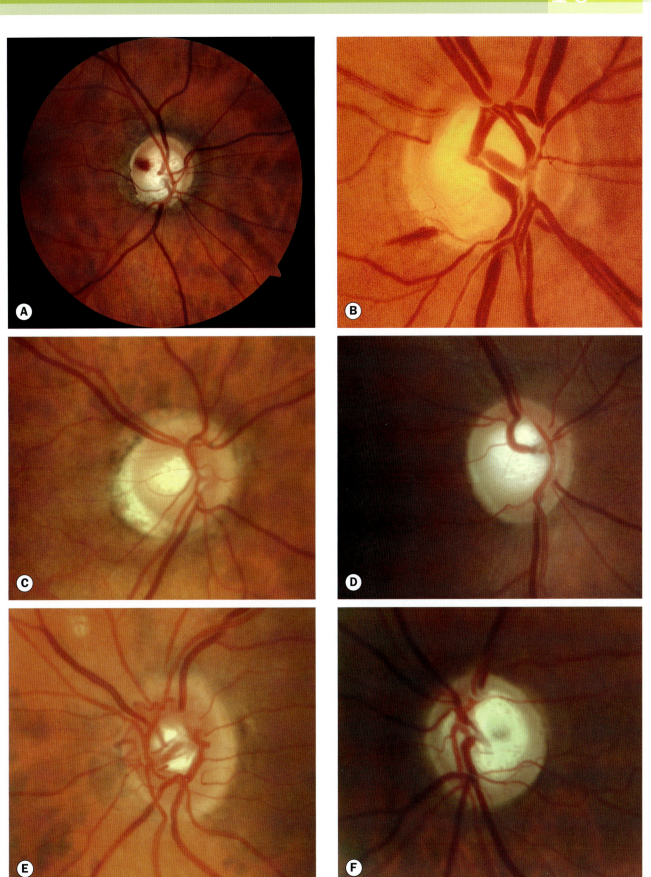

Fig. 10.18 Non-specific signs of glaucomatous damage. **(A)** and **(B)** Disc haemorrhages; **(C)** baring of inferior circumlinear blood vessel; **(D)** bayoneting of blood vessels; **(E)** collateral vessels; **(F)** loss of nasal neuroretinal rim and laminar dot sign

(Courtesy of S Chen – fig. A)

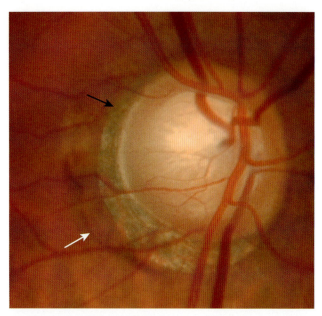

Fig. 10.19 Parapapillary changes. Alpha zone (white arrow) and beta zone (black arrow)

- **Optic nerve head.** Radial cross-sectional scans permit an objective and repeatable assessment of disc morphology, with reasonable discriminatory value. This function has tended to be less commonly used than RNFL analysis in practice.
- **Ganglion cell complex (GCC) analysis** involves measurement of retinal thickness at the macula in an attempt to detect early stage glaucomatous damage. Using older time domain OCT, it was found to be regarded as inferior to assessment of other parameters such as peripapillary RNFL assessment; with newer OCT technology interest in GCC analysis has been renewed and it is regarded as comparable and supplementary.
- **Progression analysis software** has been introduced on several machines, providing a computed assessment of the extent of damage over time presented in graphical form.

It should be noted that RNFL defects are not specific to glaucoma, and can be seen in a range of neurological disease, as well as apparently normal individuals.

IMAGING IN GLAUCOMA

Pachymetry

Pachymetry, the measurement of corneal thickness, in recent years has become an essential part of the assessment of glaucoma patients. Ultrasonic (e.g. Pachmate) and optical methods are available.

Stereo disc photography

Stereo photography has historically been regarded as the reference standard in optic disc imaging, and remains a valuable option. The images are taken by repositioning slightly between shots, either manually or using a stereo separator built into the camera.

Optical coherence tomography

OCT has become a routine part of the management of macular and other retinal disease; the same machine can be used for the assessment of glaucoma (Fig. 10.21) and has been widely adopted for this purpose. Sensitivity and specificity utilizing comparison with a normative database are as high as 90%. The principles are discussed in detail in Chapter 14.

- **Peripapillary retinal nerve fibre layer (RNFL).** This involves the acquisition of a circular scan of the retina around the optic nerve head. Retinal thickness is compared with normals.

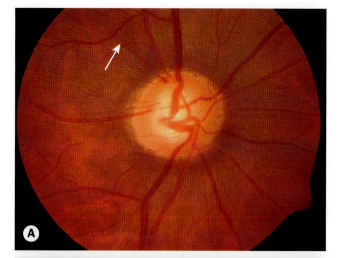

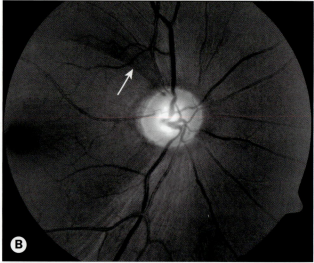

Fig. 10.20 Retinal nerve fibre layer defects. **(A)** Superotemporal wedge-shaped defect associated with a disc margin haemorrhage; **(B)** red-free photograph of the same eye

(Courtesy of P Gili)

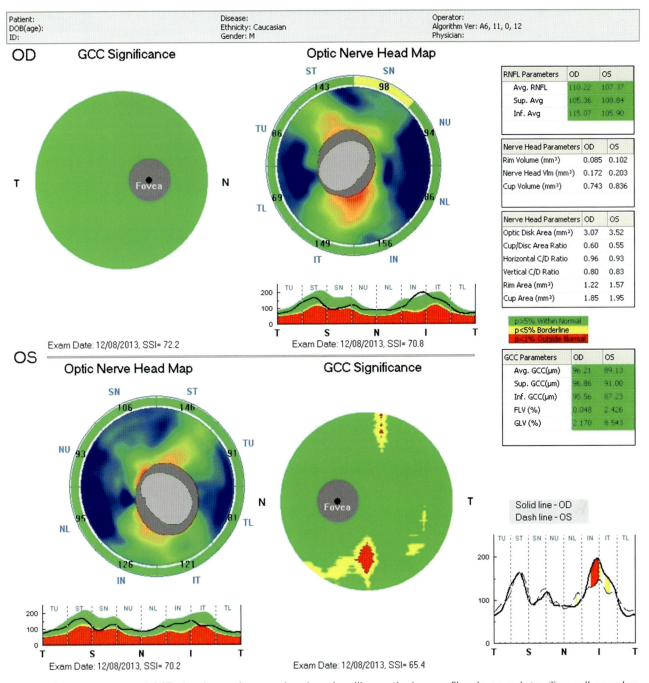

Fig. 10.21 Glaucoma-protocol OCT showing optic nerve head, peripapillary retinal nerve fibre layer and ganglion cell complex analysis

Confocal scanning laser ophthalmoscopy

This employs a scanning laser ophthalmoscope (SLO) to build a three-dimensional image of the optic nerve head and retina.

- The Heidelberg Retinal Tomograph (HRT) is in widespread clinical practice As with the OCT, it is used to distinguish normal from glaucomatous eyes by comparison against a normative database (Moorfields regression analysis), and to monitor disease progression.

- Keratometry values must be entered and significant (>1.0 dioptre) astigmatism corrected by means of a cylindrical lens. High-quality images can usually be acquired without pupillary dilatation and through mild–moderate lens opacity. After image capture, for greatest accuracy the operator must manually mark the contour line defining the edge of the neuroretinal rim.

- Images, data and analysis can be examined on a computer screen or printed (Fig. 10.22).

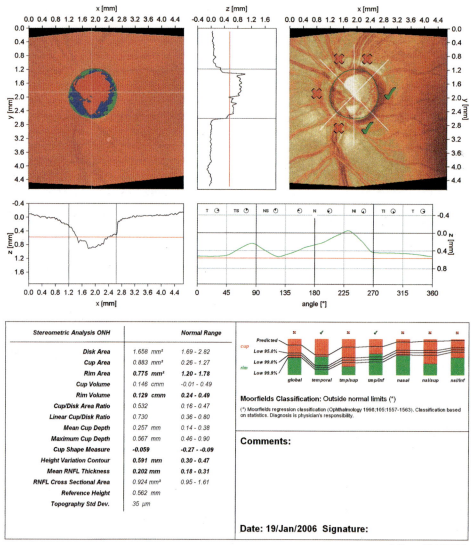

Fig. 10.22 Heidelberg Retinal Tomograph of a glaucomatous eye

- Detailed stereometric data are presented, with abnormal readings identified.

Scanning laser polarimetry

The GDx (Glaucoma Diagnosis) RNFL analyser assesses the nerve fibre layer thickness by using its 'birefringent' (resolving or splitting a light wave into two unequally reflected or transmitted waves) nature to change the polarization of incident polarized diode laser light; the amount of alteration is directly related to the thickness of the layer.

- A display provides colour images of the optic nerve head, together with RNFL maps in four quadrants; deviation maps show the location and magnitude of RNFL defects as tiny colour-coded squares, and parameters for each eye are displayed in a table (Fig. 10.23).

- A global value based on the entire thickness map is the optimal parameter for discriminating normal from glaucoma.

Anterior chamber depth measurement

Objective measurement of the depth of the AC is often clinically useful in glaucoma management. Indications include assessment of PAC risk, and monitoring of progression in conditions where the AC is shallowed, such as post-trabeculectomy hypotony and cilio-lenticular block. Older methods used a slit lamp with or without a special attachment, but an accurate and repeatable measurement can be obtained using ultrasonographic or optical interferometric methods (e.g. Zeiss IOLMaster).

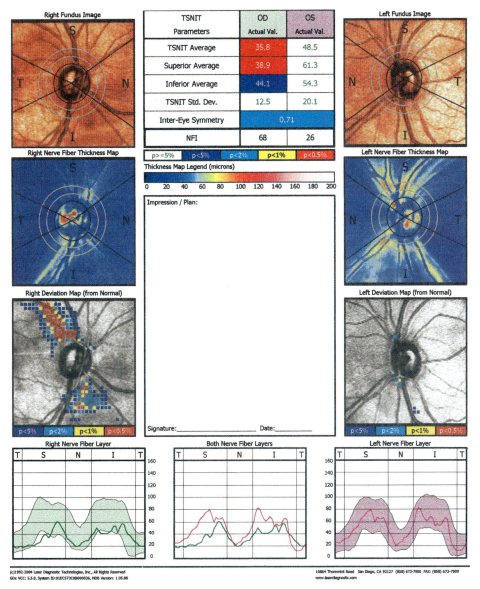

Fig. 10.23 GDx VCC (variable corneal compensation) shows reduction in retinal nerve fibre density in the right eye and abnormal parameters

(Courtesy of J Salmon)

PERIMETRY

Definitions

- **The visual field** can be represented as a three-dimensional structure akin to a hill of increasing sensitivity (Fig. 10.24A). The outer aspect extends approximately 50° superiorly, 60° nasally, 70° inferiorly and 90° temporally. Visual acuity is sharpest at the very top of the hill (i.e. the fovea) and then declines progressively towards the periphery, the nasal slope being steeper than the temporal. The 'bottomless pit' of the blind spot is located temporally between 10° and 20°, slightly below the horizontal.

- **An isopter** is a line connecting points of the same sensitivity, and on a two-dimensional isopter plot encloses an area within which a stimulus of a given strength is visible. When the field is represented as a hill, isopters resemble the contour lines on a map (Fig. 10.24B).

- **A scotoma** is an area of reduced ('relative') or total ('absolute') loss of vision surrounded by a seeing area.

- **Luminance** is the intensity or 'brightness' of a light stimulus, measured in apostilbs (asb). A higher intensity stimulus has a higher asb value; this is related inversely to sensitivity.

- A **logarithmic** rather than a linear scale is used for stimulus intensity and sensitivity, so that for each log unit intensity changes by a factor of 10. With a log scale, greater

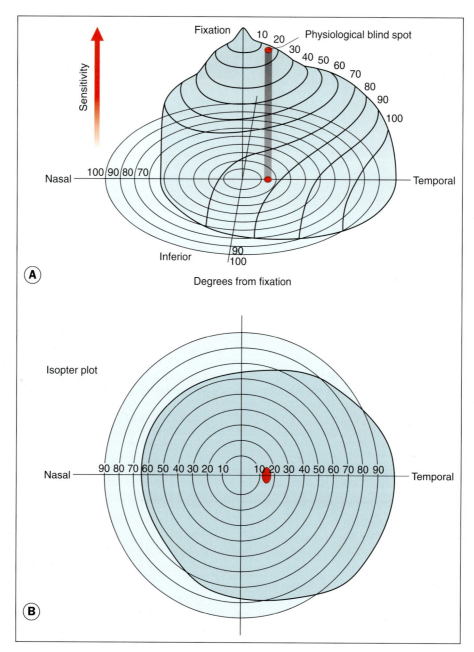

Fig. 10.24 (A) Hill of vision; **(B)** isopter plot

significance is given to the lower end of the intensity range. The normal eye has a very large sensitivity range, and assessment of the lower end of the scale is of critical significance so that early damage can be detected. With a linear scale, the lower end would be reduced to a very small portion of a graphical chart axis. The visual system itself operates on close to a logarithmic scale, so using this method more closely matches the physiological situation.

- **Decibels.** Simple log units are not used in clinical perimetry, but rather 'decibels' (dB), where 10 dB = 1 log unit. Decibels are not true units of luminance but a representation, and vary between visual field machines. Perimetry usually concentrates on the eye's sensitivity rather than the stimulus intensity. Therefore, the decibel reading goes up as retinal sensitivity increases, which obviously corresponds to reducing intensity of the perceived stimulus. This makes the assessment of visual fields more intuitive, as a higher number corresponds with higher retinal sensitivity. If the sensitivity of a test location is 20 dB (= 2 log units), a point with a sensitivity of 30 dB would be the more sensitive. The blind spot has a sensitivity of 0 dB. If, on a given machine, seeing a stimulus of 1000 asb gives a value of 10 dB, a stimulus of 100 asb will give 20 dB.

- **Differential light sensitivity** represents the degree by which the luminance of a target must exceed background luminance in order to be perceived. The visual field is therefore a three-dimensional representation of differential light sensitivity at different points.

- **Threshold** at a given location in the visual field is the brightness of a stimulus at which it can be detected by the subject. It is defined as 'the luminance of a given fixed-location stimulus at which it is seen on 50% of the occasions it is presented'. In practice we usually talk about an eye's *sensitivity* at a given point in the field rather than the stimulus intensity. The threshold sensitivity is highest at the fovea and decreases progressively towards the periphery. After the age of 20 years the sensitivity decreases by about 1 dB per 10 years.

- **Background luminance.** The retinal sensitivity at any location varies depending on background luminance. Rod photoreceptors are more sensitive in dim light than cones, and so owing to their preponderance in the peripheral retina, at lower (scotopic) light levels the peripheral retina becomes more sensitive in proportion to the central retina; the hill of vision flattens, with a central crater rather than a peak at the fovea due to the high concentration of cones, which have low sensitivity in scotopic conditions. Some diseases give markedly different field results at different background luminance levels e.g. in retinitis pigmentosa the field is usually much worse with low background luminance. It should be noted that it takes about 5 minutes to adapt from darkness to bright sunlight and 20–30 minutes from bright sunlight to darkness. The HFA (see below) uses a photopic (preferentially cone) level of background luminance at 31.5 asb.

- **Static perimetry.** A method of assessing fields, usually automated, in which the location of a stimulus remains fixed, with intensity increased until it is seen by the subject (threshold is reached – Fig. 10.25A) or decreased until it is no longer detected.

- **Kinetic (dynamic) perimetry** is now much less commonly performed than static perimetry. A stimulus of constant intensity is moved from a non-seeing area to a seeing area (Fig. 10.25B) at a standardized speed until it is perceived, and the point of perception is recorded on a chart; points from different meridia are joined to plot an isopter for that stimulus intensity. Stimuli of different intensities are used to produce a contour map of the visual field. Kinetic perimetry can be performed by means of a manual (Goldmann) or an automated perimeter if the latter is equipped with an appropriate software program.

- **Manual perimetry** involves presentation of a stimulus by the perimetrist, with manual recording of the response. It was formerly the standard method of field testing but has now largely been superseded by automated methods. It is still used occasionally, particularly in cognitively limited patients unable to interact adequately with an automated system, and for dynamic testing of peripheral fields.

- **Standard automated perimetry (SAP)** is the method used routinely in most clinical situations. Automated perimeters in common use include the Humphrey Field Analyser (HFA), the Octopus, Medmont, Henson and Dicon. These predominantly utilize static testing, though software is available on some machines to perform dynamic assessment.

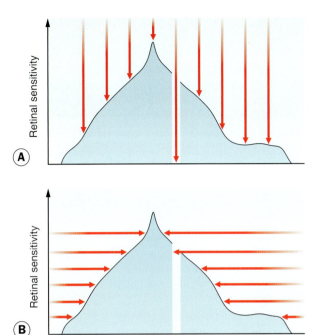

Fig. 10.25 Principles of perimetry. **(A)** Static – stimulus intensity (red arrow) at a single location is increased until perceived – areas of lower sensitivity perceive only stimuli of greater intensity (longer red arrows); **(B)** kinetic – stimulus of constant intensity is moved from a non-seeing area until perceived

Testing algorithms

Threshold

Threshold perimetry is used for detailed assessment of the hill of vision by plotting the threshold luminance value at various locations in the visual field and comparing the results with age-matched 'normal' values. A typical automated strategy is to present a stimulus of higher than expected intensity; if seen, the intensity is decreased in steps (e.g. 4 dB) until it is no longer seen ('staircasing'). The stimulus is then increased again (e.g. 2 dB steps) until seen once more (Fig. 10.26). If the stimulus is not seen initially, its intensity is increased in steps until seen. Essentially, the threshold is crossed in one direction with large increments, then crossed again to 'fine-tune' the result with smaller increments. Threshold testing is commonly used for monitoring glaucoma.

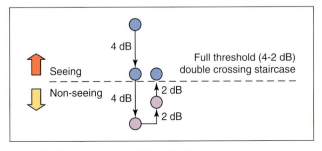

Fig. 10.26 Determination of threshold

Suprathreshold

Suprathreshold perimetry involves testing with stimuli of luminance above the expected normal threshold levels for an age-matched population to assess whether these are detected; in other words, testing to check that a subject can see stimuli that would be seen by a normal person of the same age. It enables testing to be carried out rapidly to indicate whether function is grossly normal or not and is usually reserved for screening.

Fast algorithms

In recent years strategies have been introduced with shorter testing times, providing efficiency benefits with little or no detriment to testing accuracy. The HFA offers the SITA (Swedish Interactive Thresholding Algorithm), which uses a database of normal and glaucomatous fields to estimate threshold values, and takes responses during the test into account to arrive at adjusted estimates throughout the test. Full threshold values are obtained at the start of the test for four points. SITA-Standard and SITA-Fast (Fig. 10.27) versions are available; their relative superiority is subject to debate. The Octopus Perimeter uses G-TOP (Glaucoma Tendency Oriented Perimetry), which again estimates thresholds based on information gathered from more detailed assessment of adjacent points. TOP presents each stimulus once at each location, instead of 4–6 times per location with a standard technique.

Testing patterns

- **Glaucoma**
  - Importance of central area. Most important defects in glaucoma occur centrally – within a 30° radius from the fixation point – so this is the area most commonly tested.
  - 24-2 is a glaucoma-orientated pattern used routinely. '24' denotes the extent in degrees to which the field is tested on the temporal side (to 30° on the nasal side). The number after the hyphen (2) describes the pattern of the points tested. 30-2 is an alternative.
  - 10-2 is used to assess a central area of radius 10°. Glaucomatous defects here may threaten central vision; the 10-2 pattern facilitates more detailed monitoring of the extent of damage, especially in advanced glaucoma.
- **Peripheral field.** Patterns that include central and peripheral points (e.g. FF-120) are typically limited to the assessment of neurological defects.
- **Binocular field testing** (e.g. Esterman strategy) is used to assess statutory driving entitlement in many jurisdictions.

Analysis

SAP provides the clinician with an array of clinically relevant information via monitor display or printout. The patient's name and age are confirmed and a check made that any appropriate refractive error compensation was used. General information should be reviewed, such as the type of algorithm performed, the time taken for the test and the order in which the eyes were tested;

in some cases these must be interpreted to discern likely learning or fatigue-induced effects.

Reliability indices

Reliability indices (see Fig. 10.27, top left corner) reflect the extent to which the patient's results are reliable, but it is important to note that there is relatively little research-based evidence in this area, with limited absolutes in branding a field as clearly reliable or unreliable. With SITA strategies, false negatives or false positives over about 15% should probably be regarded as highly significant, and with full-threshold strategies, fixation losses over 20% and false positives or negatives over 33%. In patients who consistently fail to achieve good reliability it may be useful to switch to a suprathreshold strategy or kinetic perimetry.

- **Fixation losses** indicate steadiness of gaze during the test. Methods of assessment include presentation of stimuli to the blind spot to ensure no response is recorded, and the use of a 'gaze monitor'.
- **False positives** are usually assessed by decoupling a stimulus from its accompanying sound. If the sound alone is presented and the patient still responds, a false positive is recorded. With a high false-positive score the grey scale printout appears abnormally pale (Fig. 10.28). In SITA testing, false positives are estimated based on the response time.
- **False negatives** are registered by presenting a stimulus much brighter than threshold at a location where the threshold has already been determined. If the patient fails to respond, a false negative is recorded. A high false-negative score indicates inattention, tiredness or malingering, but is occasionally an indication of disease severity rather than unreliability. The grey scale printout in individuals with high false-negative responses tends to have a clover leaf shape (Fig. 10.29).

Sensitivity values

- **A numerical display** (see Fig. 10.27, upper left display) gives the measured or estimated (depending on strategy) threshold in dB at each point. In a full-threshold strategy, where the threshold is rechecked either as routine or because of an unexpected (>5 dB) result, the second result is shown in brackets next to the first.
- **A grey scale** represents the numerical display in graphical form (see Fig. 10.27, upper right display) and is the simplest display modality to interpret: decreasing sensitivity is represented by darker tones – the physiological blind spot is a darker area in the temporal field typically just below the horizontal axis. Each change in grey scale tone is equivalent to a 5 dB change in sensitivity at that location.
- **Total deviation** (see Fig. 10.27, middle left display) shows the difference between a test-derived threshold at a given point and the normal sensitivity at that point for the general population, correcting for age. Negative values indicate lower than normal sensitivity, positive values higher than normal.

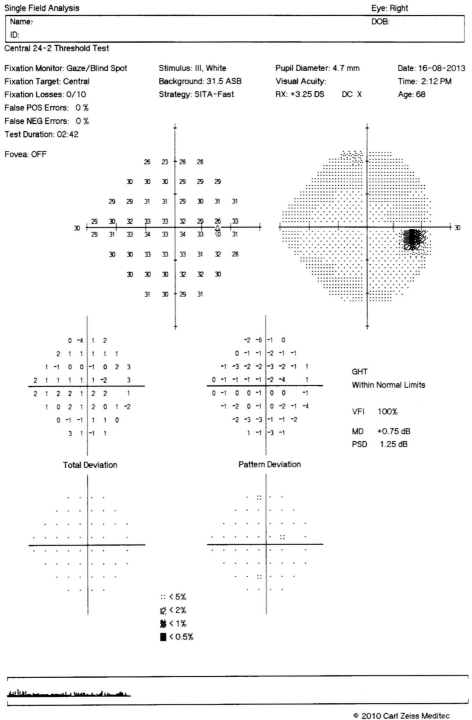

Fig. 10.27 Humphrey perimetry – SITA-Fast printout (see text)

- **Pattern deviation** (see Fig. 10.27, middle right display) is derived from total deviation values adjusted for any generalized decrease in sensitivity in the overall field (e.g. lens opacity), and demonstrates localized defects.
- **Probability value plots** of the total and pattern deviation (see Fig. 10.27, left and right lower displays) are a representation of the percentage (<5% to <0.5%) of the normal population in whom the measured defect at each point would be expected. Darker symbols represent a greater likelihood that a defect is significant.

Summary values

Summary values ('global indices' on the HFA – see Fig. 10.27, right of middle row) represent distilled statistical information,

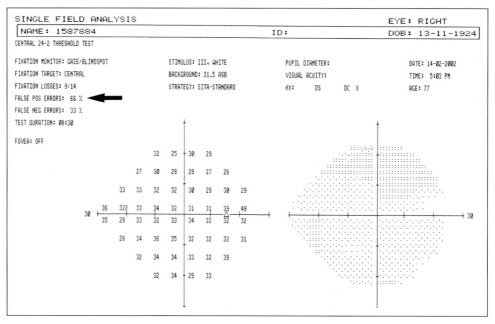

Fig. 10.28 High false-positive score (arrow) with an abnormally pale grey scale display

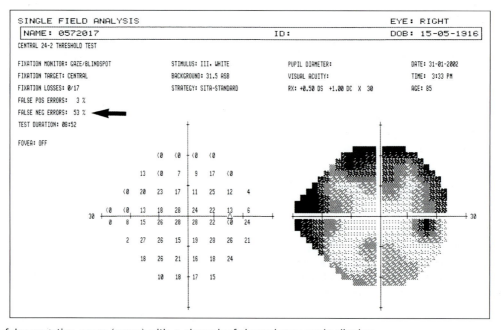

Fig. 10.29 High false-negative score (arrow) with a clover leaf-shaped grey scale display

taking into account age-matched normal data, and are principally used to monitor progression of glaucomatous damage rather than for initial diagnosis.

- **Visual field index (VFI)** in the HFA is a measure of the patient's overall visual field function expressed as a percentage, the normal age-adjusted value being 100%.
- **Mean deviation (MD)** on the HFA (**mean defect** on the Octopus) gives an indication of the overall sensitivity of the field. It is derived from averaging the total deviation values.

- **Pattern standard deviation (PSD)** is a measure of focal loss or variability within the field taking into account any generalized depression in the hill of vision. An increased PSD is therefore a more specific indicator of glaucomatous damage than MD.
- **Loss variance (LV)** is a summary measure on the Octopus perimeter similar to PSD.
- **Probability values.** Abnormal summary values are followed by a probability value, representing the percentage likelihood that an abnormal value of this level will occur in a normal

subject; the lower the *P* value, the more likely the result is abnormal.

- The **glaucoma hemifield test (GHT)** used with some HFA testing patterns assesses the visual field for damage conforming to a pattern commonly seen in glaucoma.

Computer analysis of serial fields

Computed analysis of serial visual fields for progression is now becoming more widespread. A disadvantage is the requirement for several reliable fields to be carried out before analysis is effective. The quality of available software has been improving steadily, with integrated programs such as GPA (Guided Progression Analysis) on the HFA and several trend analysis options on the Octopus.

High-sensitivity field modalities

SAP tends to detect field damage only after substantial ganglion cell loss is established. Attempts at detecting change at an earlier stage include the adoption of stimuli intended to target specific ganglion cell types.

- **Short-wave automated perimetry (SWAP)** uses a blue stimulus on a yellow background. Sensitivity to blue light (mediated by blue cone photoreceptors) is adversely affected relatively early in glaucoma. SWAP is more sensitive to early glaucomatous defects but has not been widely adopted because cataract decreases sensitivity to blue light (the brunescing lens acts as a yellow filter) and patients frequently dislike the lengthy test. It is available on newer HFA models.
- **Frequency-doubling test (FDT).** Large diameter axon (magnocellular) ganglion cells appear to be preferentially lost in early glaucoma. The frequency-doubling illusion is produced when a low spatial frequency sinusoidal grating undergoes high temporal frequency counter phase flicker (>15 Hz). The rapid alternation in which the light bars become dark and vice versa produces the illusion of the grating having doubled its frequency; magnocellular ganglion cells are believed to mediate the pathways used. Screening (Fig. 10.30) and extended testing (Humphrey Matrix) perimeter versions are available, the latter being suitable for detailed assessment and monitoring of glaucoma.

Sources of error

- **Inexperienced or unskilled perimetrist.** Though less important with SAP than manual perimetry, correctly setting up the test, explaining the procedure to and reassuring the patient, and monitoring performance are fundamental to obtaining an accurate field.
- **Incorrect patient details.** The patient's date of birth must be entered correctly to facilitate appropriate normative database matching.
- **Poor patient performance.**
- **Uncorrected refractive error** can cause a significant decrease in central sensitivity. If a hypermetropic patient who usually

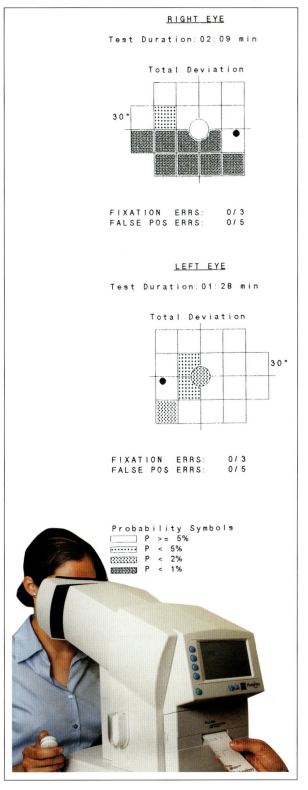

Fig. 10.30 Screening frequency-doubling perimeter with display

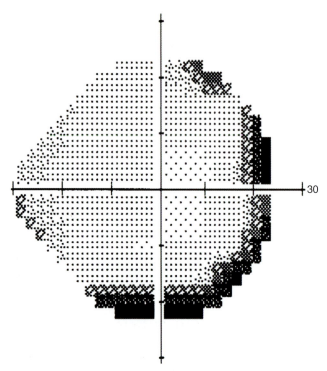

Fig. 10.31 Grey scale display of spectacle rim artefact

wears contact lenses is tested wearing spectacles, this will have the effect of magnifying and enlarging any scotomas as compared with contact lenses. Most perimetry is performed with a stimulus at approximately reading distance, so a near correction should be used for presbyopic patients.

- **Spectacle rim artefact.** Spectacles can cause rim scotomas if small aperture lenses are used or if incorrectly dispensed (Fig. 10.31). Narrow-aperture trial frame lenses are unsuitable for perimetry.
- **Miosis decreases sensitivity** in the peripheral field and increases variability in the central field in both normal and glaucomatous eyes. Pupils less than 3 mm in diameter should therefore be dilated prior to perimetry; a consistent mydriatic should be used for serial tests.
- **Media opacities** (usually cataract) can have a profound effect, exaggerated by miosis.
- **Ptosis,** even if mild, can suppress the superior visual field. Similar effects result from dermatochalasis, prominent eyelashes and deeply set eyes.
- **Inadequate retinal adaptation** may lead to error if perimetry is performed soon after ophthalmoscopy.

MEDICAL TREATMENT OF GLAUCOMA

Introduction

It is important to attempt to maximize compliance by providing an explanation of the disease and the rationale for treatment. A discussion of the medication being prescribed including technique and timing of administration, and its potential adverse effects, is also essential. The provision of written information may be helpful. Most glaucoma medications are administered topically, but significant systemic absorption can still occur, with resultant systemic adverse effects. Systemic absorption may be minimized by lacrimal occlusion following instillation: simply closing the eyes for 3 minutes will reduce systemic absorption by about 50%, and this can be enhanced by applying digital pressure over the lacrimal sac – these measures also prolong eye–drug contact. Effects on the periocular skin may be reduced by blotting overflow from the eyelids with a clean dry tissue immediately after instillation. Glaucoma medications should be avoided in pregnancy if possible, with systemic carbonic anhydrase inhibitors perhaps carrying the greatest risk due to teratogenicity concerns. A promising new route of administration is subconjunctival injection of a liposomal depot preparation of medication that would conventionally be administered topically, which may exert a useful IOP-lowering effect over several months.

Prostaglandin derivatives

Introduction

The major mode of prostaglandin (PG) action is the enhancement of uveoscleral aqueous outflow, although increased trabecular outflow facility and other mechanisms have been identified. Their IOP-lowering effect is typically greater than alternatives, though beta-blockers (see below) are sometimes equivalent. A prostaglandin derivative is now typically preferred to a beta-blocker as first-line treatment for glaucoma due to the latter's potential for systemic side effects. Duration of action may extend for several days, though administration once every day (at bedtime) is generally recommended. Systemic side effects are few; the most commonly troublesome ocular side effect is conjunctival hyperaemia. Periorbital fat loss is common, especially with bimatoprost, manifestations including deepening of the upper lid sulcus. If one prostaglandin fails to show adequate efficacy, inter-individual receptor variation means that an alternative preparation may be superior in a given patient. Although some research has suggested that using more than one PG at a time may have an additive effect, consensus currently is that PG overdosing – twice a day or more – raises the IOP in many patients.

Agents

- **Latanoprost** may cause fewer ocular adverse events than other PG agents and so is often used first line, although as a proportion of patients show no response many practitioners prefer initial use of an alternative.
- **Travoprost** is similar to latanoprost, though it may lower IOP to a slightly greater extent, particularly in black patients. Polyquad® is a novel proprietary preservative introduced by a major pharmaceutical manufacturer in its travoprost formulation that may reduce ocular surface-related adverse effects.

- **Bimatoprost** has been shown to have a greater IOP-lowering effect than the other PG agents in several studies, but may cause more conjunctival hyperaemia but fewer headaches and perhaps also less iris hyperpigmentation. A newer 0.01% (versus the older 0.03%) preparation may have a comparable IOP-lowering effect but with less hyperaemia. Preservative-free bimatoprost is now available.
- **Tafluprost** is a newer prostaglandin derivative, and was the first available in preservative-free form. Its IOP-lowering efficacy may be slightly less than that of other PG agents, but it is well tolerated and seems to cause less disruption of the ocular surface.

Side effects

- **Ocular**
  - Conjunctival hyperaemia is very common.
  - Eyelash lengthening, thickening, hyperpigmentation (Fig. 10.32A) and occasionally increase in number.
  - Irreversible iris hyperpigmentation (Fig. 10.32B) occurs in up to a quarter of patients after 6 months. The highest incidence is in green–brown irides, less in yellow-brown irides and least in blue-grey/brown irides. It is caused by an increase in the number of pigmented granules within the superficial stroma rather than an increase in the number of melanocytes. Iris naevi and freckles are not affected.
  - Hyperpigmentation of periocular skin (see Fig. 10.32B) is common but reversible.
  - Preoperative use of PG agents may increase the likelihood of cystoid macular oedema following cataract surgery.
  - Anterior uveitis is rare, but prostaglandins should be used with caution in inflamed eyes.
  - Promotion of herpetic keratitis can occur, so prostaglandins should be used with caution in patients with a history of the condition.
- **Systemic** side effects include occasional headache, precipitation of migraine in susceptible individuals, malaise, myalgia, skin rash and mild upper respiratory tract symptoms.

Beta-blockers

Introduction

Beta-blockers reduce IOP by decreasing aqueous production, mediated by an effect on the ciliary epithelium. In approximately 10% of cases the response decreases with time (tachyphylaxis), sometimes within only a few days. There may be limited supplementary effect if a topical beta-blocker is added when a patient already takes a systemic beta-blocker; the combination may also involve a relatively high risk of systemic side effects. Beta-blockers should not be instilled at bedtime as they may cause a profound drop in blood pressure while the individual is asleep, thus reducing optic disc perfusion and potentially causing visual field deterioration; the IOP-lowering effect is also believed to be less marked during sleep, as nocturnal aqueous production is normally less than half the daytime rate. However, a beta-blocker may be preferred under some circumstances such as monocular treatment to avoid the cosmetic disadvantage of the asymmetrical periocular

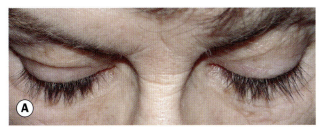
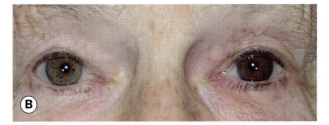
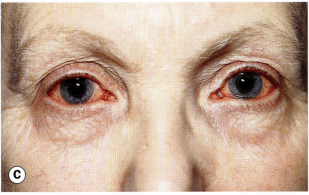
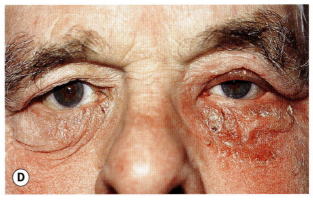

Fig. 10.32 Side effects of topical medication. **(A)** Lengthening and hyperpigmentation of lashes with prostaglandin analogue treatment; **(B)** monocular prostaglandin analogue treatment – darkening of left iris and eyelid skin; **(C)** allergic conjunctivitis due to brimonidine; **(D)** blepharoconjunctivitis due to topical carbonic anhydrase inhibitors

(Courtesy of S Chen – figs A and B; J Salmon – fig. C)

skin darkening and/or conjunctival hyperaemia with prostaglandins. Beta-blockers are also preferred in conditions such as ocular inflammation and cystoid macular oedema, or where there is a history of herpes simplex keratitis.

Side effects

- **Ocular.** Ocular side effects are few but include allergy and punctate keratitis. Granulomatous uveitis has been reported with metipranolol.
- **Systemic.** Though severe problems are extremely rare, numerous deaths have been associated with topical beta-blocker use.
  - Bronchospasm. This may be fatal in asthma or other reversible airways disease, and it is critical to exclude a history of asthma before prescribing a beta-blocker. About 1 in 50 patients without asthma will develop reversible airways disease requiring treatment within 12 months of commencing a topical beta-blocker.
  - Cardiovascular. There is a strong suggestion that cardiovascular mortality is higher in patients taking a topical beta-blocker. Effects include heart block, bradycardia, worsening of heart failure and hypotension, induction of the latter by topical beta-blocker having been reported as a common cause of falls in elderly patients. The pulse should be assessed before prescription. A peripheral vasoconstrictive effect means that they should be avoided or used with caution in patients with peripheral vascular disease, including Raynaud phenomenon.
  - Unpleasant but less severe side effects include sleep disorders, reduced exercise tolerance, hallucinations, confusion, depression, fatigue, headache, nausea, dizziness, decreased libido and dyslipidaemia.

Agents

- **Timolol** is available in various forms, including 0.25% and 0.5% solutions used twice daily; there is no evidence of a clinically significant difference in efficacy between the two solution concentrations. Gel-forming preparations of 0.1%, 0.25% and 0.5% are used once daily.
- **Betaxolol** twice daily has a lower hypotensive effect than timolol. However, optic nerve blood flow may be increased due to a calcium-channel blocking effect, so that visual field preservation may be superior. Betaxolol is relatively cardioselective (beta-1 receptors), so causes less bronchoconstriction.
- **Levobunolol** once or twice daily has a broadly similar profile to timolol.
- **Carteolol** twice daily is similar to timolol and also exhibits intrinsic sympathomimetic activity. It has a more selective action on the eye than on the cardiopulmonary system and so may have a lower systemic side effect incidence.
- **Metipranolol** twice daily is similar to timolol but has been linked with granulomatous anterior uveitis.

Alpha-2 agonists

Introduction

Ocular alpha-2 receptor stimulation decreases aqueous synthesis via an effect on the ciliary epithelium, and increases uveoscleral outflow. There is probably a neuroprotective effect. They cross the blood–brain barrier and should be used with great caution in young children, in whom severe central nervous system (CNS) depression and hypotension been reported, and are contraindicated under the age of 2 years. They may potentiate vascular insufficiency. They should not be given with oral monoamine oxidase inhibitor antidepressants due to the risk of hypertensive crisis.

Agents

- **Brimonidine** 0.2% twice daily in isolation generally has a slightly less marked IOP-lowering effect than timolol. Allergic conjunctivitis (Fig. 10.32C) is relatively common; its onset may be delayed for up to 18 months after commencement of therapy. Granulomatous anterior uveitis can occur, but is rare. Systemic side effects include xerostomia and fatigue, the latter sometimes being severe. A brimonidine preparation, Alphagan-P®, containing a proprietary preservative, Purite®, has been introduced as an alternative to the more common benzalkonium-containing forms and may have greater ocular surface tolerability.
- **Apraclonidine** 1% (or 0.5%) is used principally to prevent or treat an acute rise in IOP following laser surgery on the anterior segment. The 0.5% concentration is typically used as a temporizing measure over the course of several weeks, such as whilst a patient is awaiting glaucoma surgery. It is generally not suitable for long-term use because of a loss of therapeutic effect over weeks to months and a high incidence of local side effects.

Topical carbonic anhydrase inhibitors

Introduction

The carbonic anhydrase inhibitors (CAI) are chemically related to sulfonamide antibiotics. They lower IOP by inhibiting aqueous secretion, and via the topical route are used three times daily as monotherapy or twice daily as adjunctive treatment. In general, they are slightly less effective than beta-blockers but are hypothesized to have a supplementary neuroprotective effect. They may precipitate corneal decompensation in patients with corneal endothelial dysfunction, but some benefit has been reported in the treatment of cystoid macular oedema. Idiosyncratic bone marrow suppression can occur. Though cross-reaction is uncommon, topical (and systemic) CAI are relatively contraindicated in patients allergic to sulfonamide antibiotics. Research suggests that concomitant treatment with a topical and systemic CAI does not usually give an additive effect.

Agents

- **Dorzolamide**. The main adverse effects are stinging and a transient bitter taste following administration; allergic blepharoconjunctivitis (Fig. 10.32D) is not uncommon.
- **Brinzolamide** is similar to dorzolamide, but with a lower incidence of stinging and local allergy. It is a suspension, and a white residue may be left on the eyelids after instillation if excess is not wiped away.

Miotics

Introduction

Miotics are cholinergic agonists that are now predominantly used in the treatment of angle closure, though were formerly a mainstay of the treatment of open-angle glaucoma. In angle-closure glaucoma, miotic-induced contraction of the sphincter pupillae pulls the peripheral iris away from the trabeculum, opening the angle. Miotics also reduce IOP by contraction of the ciliary muscle, which increases the facility of aqueous outflow through the trabecular meshwork. Local side effects include miosis, brow ache, myopic shift and exacerbation of the symptoms of cataract. Visual field defects appear denser and larger. Systemic side effects are rare but include confusion, bradycardia, bronchospasm, gastrointestinal symptoms and urinary frequency.

Agents

- **Pilocarpine** 0.5%, 1%, 2%, or 4% solution as four times daily monotherapy is equal in efficacy to beta-blockers. Pilocarpine gel (Pilogel®) 4% is instilled once daily at bedtime so that induced myopia and miosis are predominantly confined to sleep. Gel, or drops twice daily, may be used to prevent angle closure following laser iridotomy in the presence of a substantial non-pupillary block element.
- **Carbachol** is an alternative to pilocarpine.

Combined preparations

Combined preparations with similar ocular hypotensive effects to the sum of the individual components improve convenience and patient compliance. They are also more cost effective. Proprietary examples include:

- **Cosopt®**: timolol and dorzolamide, administered twice daily.
- **Xalacom®**: timolol and latanoprost once daily.
- **TimPilo®**: timolol and pilocarpine twice daily.
- **Combigan®**: timolol and brimonidine twice daily.
- **DuoTrav®**: timolol and travoprost once daily.
- **Ganfort®**: timolol and bimatoprost once daily.
- **Azarga®**: timolol and brinzolamide twice daily.
- **Simbrinza®**: brimonidine and brinzolamide; a new combination – the only one that does not contain the beta-blocker timolol; administered twice daily.

Systemic carbonic anhydrase inhibitors

Introduction

Systemically administered CAI are generally used for short-term treatment, particularly in patients with acute glaucoma. Because of their systemic side effects, long-term use is reserved for patients at high risk of visual loss. Sulfonamide ('sulfa') allergy is a relative contraindication.

Agents

- **Acetazolamide** is available as 250 mg tablets (250–1000 mg daily in divided doses), sustained-release 250 mg capsules (250–500 mg daily) and 500 mg powder vials for injection (single dose, typically used in acute angle-closure glaucoma).
- **Dichlorphenamide** 50 mg tablets (50–100 mg two or three times daily).
- **Methazolamide** 50 mg tablets (50–100 mg two or three times daily); this has a longer duration of action than acetazolamide but is less widely available.

Side effects

- **Ocular.** Choroidal effusion, particularly after cataract surgery. Angle closure may result.
- **Systemic.** Paraesthesia ('pins and needles' sensation in the extremities), hypokalaemia (reduced blood potassium level – common), malaise and lowered mood, gastrointestinal symptoms, renal stones, Stevens–Johnson syndrome (very rare), dose-related bone marrow suppression, idiosyncratic aplastic anaemia (exceptionally rare but with 50% mortality).

Osmotic agents

Introduction

Osmotic agents lower IOP by creating an osmotic gradient so that water is 'drawn out' from the vitreous into the blood. They are employed when a short-term reduction in IOP is required that cannot be achieved by other means, such as in resistant acute angle-closure glaucoma or when the IOP is very high prior to intraocular surgery. They are of limited value in inflammatory glaucoma, in which the integrity of the blood–aqueous barrier is compromised. Side effects include cardiovascular overload as a result of increased extracellular volume (caution in patients with cardiac or renal disease), urinary retention (especially elderly men), headache, backache, nausea and confusion.

Agents

- **Mannitol** is given intravenously (1 g/kg body weight or 5 ml/kg body weight of a 20% solution in water) over 30–60 minutes; peak action occurs within 30 minutes.

- **Glycerol** is an oral agent (1 g/kg body weight or 2 ml/kg body weight of a 50% solution) with a sweet and sickly taste, and can be given with lemon (not orange) juice to avoid nausea. Peak action occurs within 1 hour. Glycerol is metabolized to glucose, and careful monitoring with insulin cover may be required if administered to a (well-controlled only) diabetic patient.
- **Isosorbide** is a metabolically inert oral agent with a minty taste; the dose is the same as for glycerol. It may be safer for diabetic patients.

LASER TREATMENT OF GLAUCOMA

Laser trabeculoplasty

Introduction

Laser trabeculoplasty (LTP) involves the delivery of laser to the trabecular meshwork with the aim of enhancing aqueous outflow and thereby lowering IOP.

- **Selective laser trabeculoplasty (SLT)** has increased in popularity over recent years and is now widely performed. A 532 nm frequency-doubled, Q-switched Nd:YAG laser is used to selectively target melanin pigment in trabecular meshwork (TM) cells, leaving non-pigmented structures unscathed. It is probably similar in efficacy to medical monotherapy and argon laser trabeculoplasty (see below). The mechanism is incompletely understood, but potentially includes stimulation of TM cell division, macrophage recruitment and extracellular matrix recruitment. Laser application is made easier by a broad targeted and treated area (Fig. 10.33, left), which may lead to more consistent results. Reported protocols (e.g. 180° or 360° TM treatment) and results vary markedly, but IOP reductions of 10–40% can be expected after 6 months in responsive patients, with

25% being common. Probably around two-thirds of patients will achieve a reasonable IOP fall within 6 months of 180° TM treatment. The contralateral untreated eye also tends to sustain a small IOP fall. The effects generally wane over time, but as there is no thermal tissue damage, treatment can be repeated with a successful outcome, even if initial treatment has been unsuccessful. The prior use of topical glaucoma medication does not seem to affect results. Energy delivered to the TM is much lower than with argon laser, and complications are relatively mild but include transient mild inflammation with mild discomfort, PAS formation and IOP elevation; the latter is usually mild but substantial rises have been reported, especially in heavily pigmented angles, for which overtreatment should be avoided. The concern has been raised that the extensive treated area causes damage to corneal endothelial cells, with rare reports of endothelial decompensation. Herpes simplex keratitis reactivation has been reported, as has macular oedema.

- **Argon laser trabeculoplasty (ALT)** is a long-established procedure that uses laser burns to achieve IOP reduction comparable to SLT; there is an extensive body of published research reporting good outcomes. Mechanisms are likely to overlap with those of SLT, and there may also be a mechanical opening of the trabecular spaces. As the TM sustains thermal damage, repeat treatment is of limited benefit and is infrequently performed. Complications include peripheral anterior synechiae, acute elevation of IOP (should be monitored carefully over subsequent weeks in patients with severe glaucomatous damage), cystoid macular oedema and anterior uveitis (usually mild); there is concern that there may be an adverse effect on the outcome of subsequent filtration surgery.
- **Micropulse laser trabeculoplasty (MLT)** is a relatively new modality that uses extremely short duration pulses of laser to deliver thermal energy to the TM to stimulate cells without damage. Unlike SLT and ALT, there is no visible tissue reaction. A smaller area is targeted than in SLT (Fig. 10.33, right), limiting potential collateral effects on adjacent tissue. Initial results suggest a benign safety profile with results comparable to other LTP forms.

Indications

- **Type of glaucoma.** LTP can be used in a range of open-angle glaucomas including primary, pseudoexfoliative and pigmentary, and can also be used in ocular hypertension. Success has been reported in less common circumstances, e.g. steroid-induced glaucoma has been treated with SLT.
- **Primary therapy.** As SLT has increasingly demonstrated a favourable safety profile, its use as a primary alternative to topical medication has increasingly been considered.
- **Failure of compliance** with medical therapy.
- **Adjunctive treatment** to avoid polypharmacy.
- **Intolerance** of topical medication including allergy.
- **Failure of medical therapy**, as a less aggressive treatment measure than surgery.

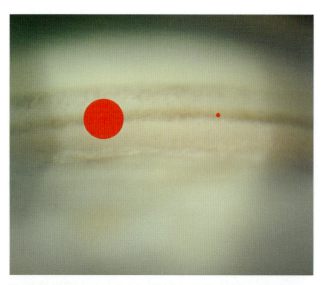

Fig. 10.33 Targeted area in selective (left) and conventional argon (right) and micropulse laser trabeculoplasty

Technique

- LTP is performed under topical anaesthesia.
- A drop of apraclonidine or brimonidine is instilled 30–60 minutes pre-procedure with the aim of preventing or minimizing an early post-laser IOP rise. A similar drop is instilled post-procedure.
- Some practitioners instil a drop of pilocarpine prior to the procedure, particularly if the angle is not wide. There is likely to be greater potential for PAS formation in narrower angles, particularly with ALT, and this should be borne in mind when considering a particular patient's suitability for LTP.
- A goniolens is inserted; with the mirror at the 12 o'clock position, the inferior angle is visualized.
- ALT: initial settings are commonly 50 μm spot size, 0.1 s duration, and 700 mW power (range of 400–1200 mW, largely dependent on angle pigmentation). The aiming beam is focused at the junction of the pigmented and non-pigmented TM ensuring that the spot is round and has a clear edge. The optimal reaction is a very light blanching or the appearance of a minute gas bubble. If the reaction is inadequate, the power is increased by 50–200 mW. Fifty burns are applied at regularly spaced intervals over 180° of the angle. Many practitioners apply initial treatment of 180° of the angle, treating the other 180° if the initial response is unsatisfactory; primary treatment of the entire circumference is associated with a higher risk of IOP spikes. Topical fluorometholone or prednisolone 0.5% four times daily for one week is prescribed post-laser.
- SLT: a common initial power setting is 0.8 mJ; as with ALT, this should be varied depending on angle pigmentation (range 0.3–1.0 mJ); the spot size and duration are fixed at 400 μm and 0.3 ns respectively. The TM is brought into focus rather than the aiming beam; the beam is centred on the pigmented TM and then fired, an optimal reaction consisting of a few tiny ('champagne') bubbles with adjustment of the power higher or lower as required to achieve this. The number of burns applied is as for ALT. The total energy used for SLT is considerably less than for ALT, and it is common not to prescribe any post-laser anti-inflammatory drops, though non-steroidal or weak steroid drops can be used if significant inflammation occurs.
- With practice it is possible to perform LTP by continually rotating the goniolens and applying each burn through the centre of the mirror; using this technique, treatment of the entire inferior half of the angle is accomplished by first rotating the lens to one side (e.g. anticlockwise) by 90° whilst applying 25 shots, then returning to the 12 o'clock position before applying an additional 25 shots whilst rotating the lens to the opposite side (clockwise in this example).
- An IOP check should be performed 30–60 minutes after the laser to exclude a substantial early spike, with further IOP measurement, treatment and review as appropriate if this occurs, depending on each patient's risk profile.

- Medical glaucoma therapy is generally continued.
- Follow-up is dependent on the perceived level of risk; 1–2 weeks is typical in the absence of pertinent considerations.

Laser iridotomy

Introduction

Laser iridotomy is used principally in the treatment of primary angle closure, but may also be indicated in secondary angle closure with pupillary block. It is also sometimes performed in pigment dispersion syndrome, though its effectiveness in this scenario remains under investigation.

Technique

- A topical anaesthetic agent is instilled.
- Apraclonidine or brimonidine is given prophylactically as for LTP.
- The pupil is miosed with topical pilocarpine (e.g. one drop of 2%).
- A special iridotomy contact lens (e.g. Abraham – Fig. 10.34A, Volk MagPlus) is inserted.
- Many practitioners target a site under the upper eyelid between 11 and 1 o'clock, though some prefer 3 or 9 o'clock. The highest risk of monocular diplopia or glare (see below) occurs when an iridotomy is half-covered by the lid margin. Radially, the iridotomy should be located within the outer third in order to reduce the risk of damage to the crystalline lens (see Fig. 10.34D). Targeting an iris crypt, if present, is usually associated with much easier achievement of an adequate opening.
- It is critical to note that effective power settings vary somewhat between machines. The spot size and duration are fixed. Most iridotomies are made with power settings of 4–5 mJ; the risk of crystalline lens damage may be higher at 5 mJ or above. For a thin blue iris the typical required energy level is 2–4 mJ. Some practitioners prefer single pulse shots, others shots of up to three pulses.
- Pre-treatment with thermal (argon or diode) laser is often required in thick dark irides. Suitable parameters include power of 600–900 mW using a small spot size of 50 μm and relatively short duration of 0.03–0.05 s, though larger, lower power, longer duration settings can be equally effective.
- The beam is focused precisely and the laser fired. Successful penetration is characterized by a gush of pigment debris. The number of shots required to produce an adequate iridotomy is very variable. The optimal size is uncertain, recommendations ranging from 150 to 500 μm (Figs 10.34B–D).
- Over-treatment should be avoided due to the risk of substantial postoperative inflammation and pressure spikes; further treatment can be applied after a few days; in urgent circumstances re-treating the same site after allowing a few minutes for pigment and debris to clear, or moving to a different site, may be adequate.

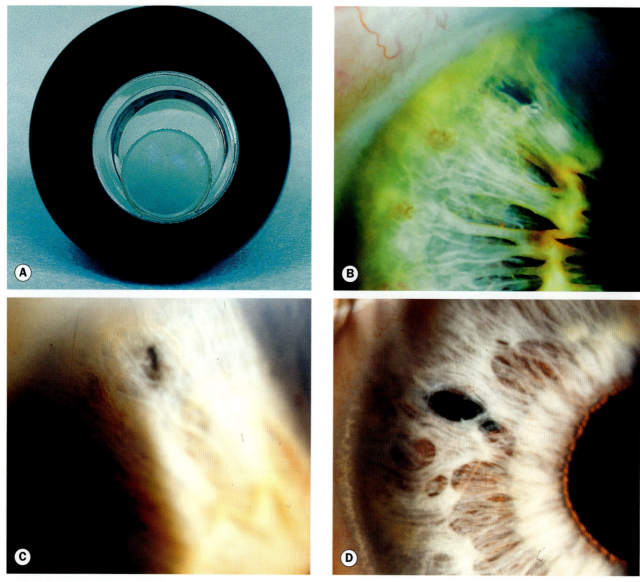

Fig. 10.34 Nd:YAG iridotomy. **(A)** Abraham lens; **(B)** approximately appropriate iridotomy size; **(C)** probably too small; **(D)** probably too large – may also be insufficiently peripheral

- A second drop of apraclonidine is instilled following the procedure; oral acetazolamide may also be given in patients at high risk such as those with advanced glaucomatous damage or high IOP pre-treatment.
- A potent topical steroid (e.g. dexamethasone 0.1%) is prescribed post-procedure. Varying regimens have been described, with a limited evidence base for the optimal approach; four times daily for 1 week is typical, though instillation every hour for several hours immediately post-laser is common.
- The IOP should be checked 1–2 hours after the procedure to exclude an early spike. Routine review is usually at 1 or 2 weeks, with subsequent monitoring according to individual circumstances. Patients with marked glaucomatous damage may require extended ocular hypotensive cover and earlier review.

Complications

- **Bleeding** occurs in around 50% but is usually mild and stops after only a few seconds; persistent bleeding can be terminated by increasing contact lens pressure.
- **IOP elevation**. Usually early and transient but occasionally persistent.
- **Iritis**. Especially if excessive laser is applied or post-laser steroid therapy is inadequate, or in darker irides (including those due to prostaglandin derivative treatment).
- **Corneal burns** may occur if a contact lens is not used or if the AC is shallow; these usually heal very rapidly without sequelae.
- **Cataract.** Localized lens opacities occasionally develop at the treatment site; age-related cataract formation may be accelerated by iridotomy.

- **Glare and/or diplopia** due to a 'second pupil' effect are rare (see above).

Diode laser cycloablation

Diode laser ablation (cyclodiode) lowers IOP by destroying part of the secretory ciliary epithelium, thereby reducing aqueous secretion. In the past it was used mainly in uncontrolled end-stage secondary glaucoma with minimal visual potential, mainly to control pain. However, its use in eyes with good vision, especially those with a poor prognosis for penetrating drainage surgery, has been well described over recent years. More than one treatment session is commonly required for adequate pressure control. Moderate post-procedure pain and anterior segment inflammation are common. A temporary IOP rise is not uncommon during the first few weeks. Serious complications are rare but include chronic hypotony, phthisis bulbi, suprachoroidal haemorrhage, corneal decompensation and retinal detachment.

Technique

- A sub-Tenon or peribulbar anaesthetic is administered.
- Laser settings are 1.5–2 s and 1500–2000 mW; the spot size is fixed.
- The power is adjusted over sequential shots until a 'popping' sound is heard and then reduced to just below that level.
- Approximately 12–24 burns are placed posteriorly to the limbus over 360°, avoiding the neurovascular bundles at 3 and 9 o'clock (Fig. 10.35). Fewer shots (e.g. treatment of only one or two quadrants) can be used for eyes with good vision, in order to reduce the risk of complications; more treatment sessions are likely to be required using this approach.
- A strong topical steroid is prescribed hourly on the day of treatment and then 2-hourly for 2 days and four times daily for at least 2 weeks. A topical antibiotic and a cycloplegic (e.g. cyclopentolate 1% twice daily) are used for 3 days.
- Pre-laser glaucoma treatment may be continued, or reduced slightly.
- Oral non-steroidal anti-inflammatory agents may be prescribed for 2 days.
- Review is generally after 1–4 days, depending on risk, to exclude significant reactive inflammation and/or an IOP spike.

Laser iridoplasty

Laser iridoplasty is performed to widen the anterior chamber angle by contraction of the peripheral iris away from the angle recess (Fig. 10.36). It can be used to attempt to break an episode of acute angle closure, but is more commonly applied on an elective basis, for example in plateau iris syndrome. Complications tend to be mild, but heavy treatment can be associated with a substantial and persistent IOP spike that may be potentiated by heavy iris pigmentation. Altered accommodation is fairly common but almost always transient.

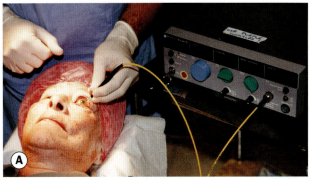

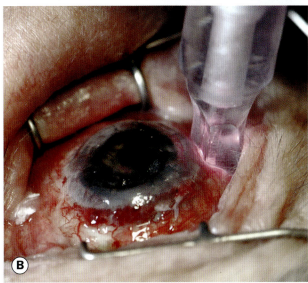

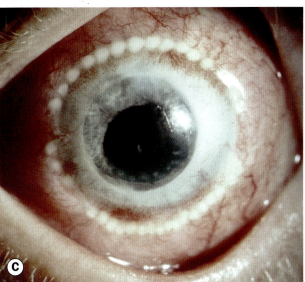

Fig. 10.35 (A) Diode laser cycloablation; **(B)** cyclodiode probe during laser application; **(C)** early postoperative appearance in a patient with prior penetrating keratoplasty

(Courtesy of J Salmon – fig. A; Krachmer, Mannis and Holland, from Cornea, Mosby 2005 – fig. B)

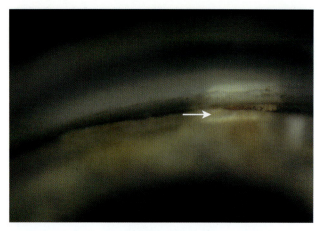

Fig. 10.36 Gonioscopic appearance following treatment of part of the angle circumference with laser iridoplasty – the white arrow indicates a laser burn. The narrower region on the left has not yet been treated

Technique

Numerous modifications are in use; the following description relates predominantly to the classical procedure.

- The pupil is miosed preoperatively (e.g. pilocarpine 2%).
- A bridle suture is inserted (commonly superior cornea or superior rectus muscle).
- A limbal or fornix-based flap of conjunctiva and Tenon capsule is fashioned superiorly.
- Episcleral tissue is cleared, and major vessels cauterized.
- Incisions are made through about 50% of scleral thickness, to create a 'trapdoor' lamellar scleral flap (Fig. 10.38A). This flap may be rectangular (3 × 3–4 mm), trapezoidal or triangular, according to preference.
- The superficial flap is dissected forwards until clear cornea is reached (Fig. 10.38B).
- A paracentesis is made in temporal peripheral clear cornea.

Technique

- A topical anaesthetic is instilled.
- One drop each of 1% pilocarpine and 1% apraclonidine is instilled.
- Via an iridotomy lens, 1–2 burns per clock hour are applied to the periphery, 500 μm size, 100–400 mW, 0.2–0.5 s duration, aiming for slight visible iris contraction.
- Post-procedure 1% apraclonidine is given (oral prophylaxis – e.g. acetazolamide – may be given if significant glaucomatous optic neuropathy is present).
- Topical ketorolac, prednisolone 1% or dexamethasone 0.1% four times daily for a week is a common regimen.
- Review is typically 1–2 hours post-laser, then after 1 week and subsequently depending on progress and glaucomatous damage – patients with significant glaucomatous neuropathy may need frequent review for the first few weeks to exclude an IOP spike.

TRABECULECTOMY

Trabeculectomy is glaucoma filtration surgery that lowers IOP by creating a fistula, protected by a superficial scleral flap, to allow aqueous outflow from the anterior chamber to the sub-Tenon space (Fig. 10.37). Indications include:

- **Failure of conservative therapy** to achieve adequate IOP control.
- **Avoidance of excessive polypharmacy.**
- **Progressive deterioration despite seemingly adequate IOP control** (including poor compliance with medical treatment).
- **Primary therapy.** Advanced disease requiring a very low target pressure may achieve a superior long-term outcome from early surgery, particularly in younger patients.
- **Patient preference.** Occasionally patients express a strong desire to be free of the commitment to chronic medical treatment.

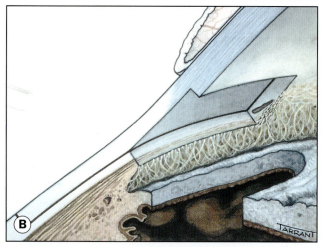

Fig. 10.37 Trabeculectomy principles. **(A)** Pathway of aqueous egress following trabeculectomy; **(B)** schematic representation of appearance from inside the eye following completion

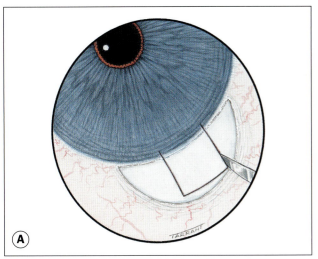 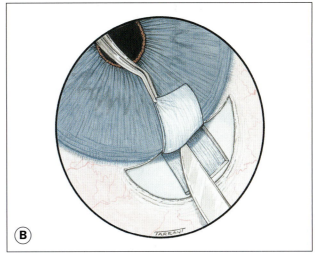

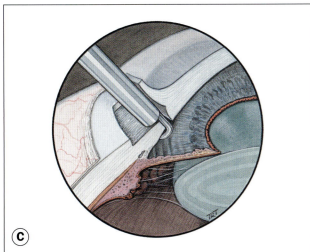 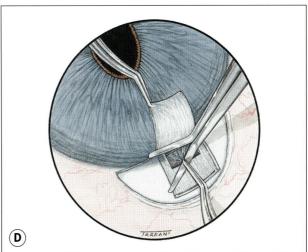

Fig. 10.38 Trabeculectomy technique. **(A)** Outline of superficial scleral flap; **(B)** dissection of superficial scleral flap; **(C)** excision of deep scleral tissue with a punch; **(D)** peripheral iridectomy

- The AC is entered along most of the width of the trapdoor base.
- A block of deep sclera is excised, usually a punch (e.g. Kelly – Fig. 10.38C).
- A peripheral iridectomy is created in order to prevent blockage of the internal opening (Fig. 10.38D); some surgeons omit this step in pseudophakic eyes or those with a deep anterior chamber.
- The superficial scleral flap is sutured at its posterior corners, either so that it is lightly apposed to the underlying bed or tightly with releasable or lysable sutures to reduce the risk of postoperative leakage Some surgeons insert a suture into each of the radial edges to reduce the risk of a substantial lateral leak.
- Balanced salt solution is injected through the paracentesis to deepen the anterior chamber and test the patency of the fistula.

- Conjunctiva/Tenon capsule flap is sutured. Irrigation through the paracentesis is repeated to produce a bleb, which is checked for leakage.
- A drop of atropine 1% is instilled; when no iridectomy has been performed, pilocarpine 2% may be used instead.
- Steroid and antibiotic are injected under the inferior conjunctiva.
- Steroid and antibiotic drops are used four times daily for 2 weeks and then changed to steroid alone for a further 8–12 weeks.

Antimetabolites in filtration surgery

Indications

Adjunctive antimetabolites inhibit the natural healing response that may preclude successful filtration surgery. They should be used with caution because of potential complications, and are usually considered in the presence of risk factors for surgical failure. In uncomplicated glaucoma the use of low-dose antimetabolites may improve long-term control of IOP.

- **High-risk factors** include neovascular glaucoma, previous failed trabeculectomy or filtering device, and certain secondary glaucomas (e.g. inflammatory, post-traumatic angle recession and iridocorneal endothelial syndrome). A glaucoma drainage device would be advocated by many authorities in some or all of these circumstances; a mitomycin C-enhanced trabeculectomy with the Ex-Press™ mini-shunt is an alternative.
- **Intermediate- and lower-risk factors** include patients on topical medication (particularly sympathomimetics) for over 3 years, previous conjunctival or cataract surgery, black ethnicity, and age under 40.

5-fluorouracil

5-fluorouracil (5-FU) inhibits fibroblast proliferation by retarding DNA synthesis. It is a less aggressive antimetabolite than mitomycin C (see below), but substantial complications can still occur, notably persistent corneal epithelial defects and bleb leakage.

- **Intraoperative** use involves the application of one or more small cellulose sponges soaked in a 50 mg/ml solution, placed under the dissected flap of Tenon's capsule at the site of filtration for 5 minutes prior to creation of the scleral trapdoor.
- **Post-operative** subconjunctival injection of 0.1 ml of 25 mg/ml or 50 mg/ml solution can be used; placement may be away from the fistula, even at the opposite limbus. Various regimens are described, including daily injections for several postoperative days, and ad hoc use if a drainage bleb appears to be unduly vascularized or fibrotic; it is also often used as an adjunct to a limited 'needling' revision of a trabeculectomy (see below).

Mitomycin C

Mitomycin C (MMC) is an alkylating agent that inhibits proliferation of fibroblasts and suppresses vascular ingrowth; it is much more potent than 5-FU. It is generally used intraoperatively in the manner described above for 5-FU, a typical exposure protocol being 0.2 mg/ml for 2 minutes, though a higher concentration (e.g. 0.4 mg/ml) may be used for particularly high-risk patients; higher concentrations and extended exposure times are associated with an increased risk of complications; a cystic thin-walled bleb is common following the use of mitomycin C and may predispose to chronic hypotony, late-onset bleb leak and endophthalmitis.

Shallow anterior chamber

A shallow anterior chamber (Figs 10.39A and B) following trabeculectomy may be due to pupillary block, overfiltration or malignant glaucoma. Severe and sustained shallowing is uncommon, the chamber re-forming spontaneously in most cases. However, those that do not may develop severe complications such as peripheral anterior synechiae, corneal endothelial damage (Fig. 10.39C) and cataract (Fig. 10.39D).

Pupillary block

Pupillary block may occur with a non-patent peripheral iridectomy.

- **Signs**
  - High IOP and flat bleb.
  - Negative Seidel test.
  - Iris bombé with a non-patent iridectomy.
- **Treatment** involves YAG laser to the pigment epithelium at the iridectomy site if the anterior iris stroma appears to have been largely removed (common), or the creation of a new laser iridotomy.

Overfiltration

Overfiltration may be caused by insufficient resistance to outflow at the lamellar scleral flap, but bleb leakage through an inadvertent buttonhole or due to inadequate closure of the conjunctiva and Tenon capsule is more common.

- **Signs**
  - Low IOP with a well-formed bleb in a scleral flap leak and flat in a bleb leak.
  - The Seidel test is negative in a scleral flap leak but positive (Fig. 10.40A) in a bleb leak.
  - The cornea may show signs of hypotony such as folds in Descemet membrane.
  - Choroidal detachments (Fig. 10.40B) may be present.
- **Treatment** depends on the cause and degree of shallowing.
  - Initial management in eyes with mild overfiltration such as may be caused by a very small bleb leak, may consist simply of observation, with atropine to prevent PAS formation and reduce the risk of malignant glaucoma.
  - Subsequent treatment if the above measures are ineffective involves temporary tamponade of the conjunctiva to enhance spontaneous healing by simple pressure patching, a large diameter soft bandage contact lens, a collagen shield or a Simmons shell designed for the purpose.
  - Definitive treatment often consists of the insertion of additional conjunctival sutures, and if necessary placement of a transconjunctival scleral flap suture. If potentially serious shallowing is present, the anterior chamber can be reformed with a viscoelastic. Choroidal detachments rarely require drainage.

Malignant glaucoma

Malignant glaucoma is rare but serious. It is caused by anterior rotation of the ciliary processes and iris root, commonly with aqueous misdirection (ciliolenticular block) in which blockage of aqueous flow occurs in the vicinity of the pars plicata of the ciliary body, so that aqueous is forced backwards into the vitreous.

- **Signs**
  - High IOP and absent bleb.
  - Negative Seidel test.

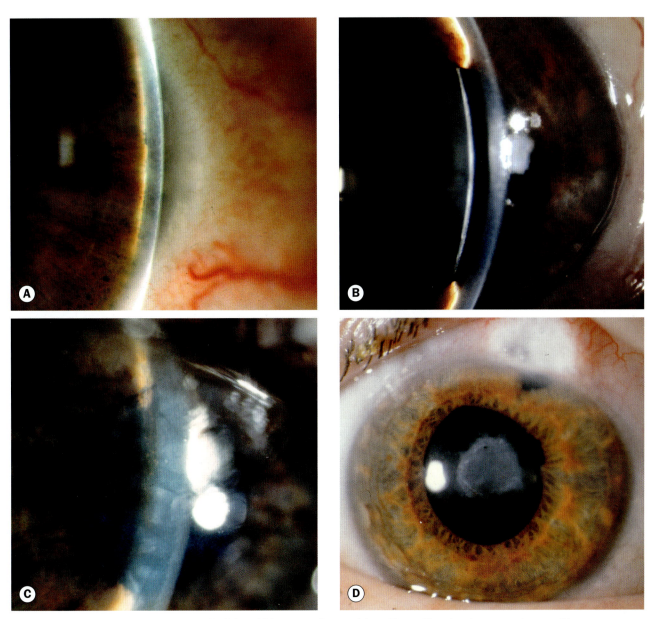

Fig. 10.39 Shallow anterior chamber. **(A)** Peripheral iris–corneal apposition; **(B)** pupillary border–corneal apposition; **(C)** lenticulo-corneal apposition with associated corneal oedema; **(D)** cataract following shallow anterior chamber

(Courtesy of J Schuman, V Christopoulos, D Dhaliwal, M Kahook and R Noecker, from 'Lens and Glaucoma', in Rapid Diagnosis in Ophthalmology, *Mosby 2008 – fig. A)*

- **Treatment**
  - Initial treatment is with mydriatics (atropine 1% and phenylephrine 10%) to dilate the ciliary ring and increase the distance between the ciliary processes and the equator of the lens, thereby tightening the zonule and pulling the lens posteriorly into its normal position. Intravenous mannitol may be used if mydriatics are ineffective, in order to shrink the vitreous gel and allow the lens to move posteriorly.
  - Subsequent treatment if medical therapy fails is with Nd:YAG laser fired through the iridectomy in order to disrupt the anterior hyaloid face, reduce the vitreous volume and break any ciliary block. In pseudophakic

eyes, laser posterior capsulotomy and disruption of the anterior hyaloid face should be performed. Cyclodiode may be effective. Pars plana vitrectomy is performed if laser therapy fails: sufficient vitreous gel is excised to allow free flow of aqueous to the anterior chamber.

Failure of filtration

Diagnosis

A normally functioning bleb should be slightly elevated, relatively avascular (Fig. 10.41A) and show superficial microcysts – tiny

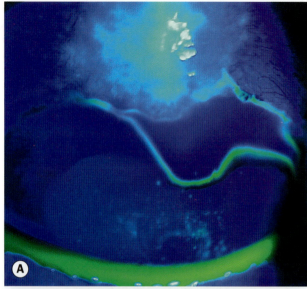

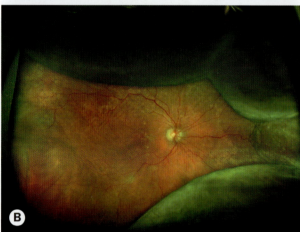

Fig. 10.40 (A) Positive Seidel test – a wave of egressing fluid is delineated by a fluorescein band; **(B)** wide-field image of choroidal detachments
(Courtesy of S Chen – fig. B)

- **Scleral** causes include over-tight suturing of the scleral flap and gradual scarring in the scleral bed.
- **Intraocular** causes are uncommon and include blockage of the sclerostomy by vitreous, blood or uveal tissue or by a variety of thin membranes derived from surrounding cornea or sclera.

Management

Management of filtration failure depends on the cause and may involve one or more of the following:

- **Ocular 'digital massage'** in an effort to force outflow through the surgical fistula may be performed by digital compression through the upper lid whilst looking downwards; this can be carried out by the patient 4–8 times a day for up to several weeks until the bleb is deemed stable.
- **Suture manipulation** may be considered 7–14 days postoperatively if the eye has high IOP, a flat bleb and a deep anterior chamber. Releasable sutures can be cut or released according to the technique of initial placement. Argon or diode laser suture lysis is useful if releasable sutures have not been used. It may be performed through a suture lysis lens or a Zeiss four-mirror goniolens.
- **Needling** of an encysted bleb may be performed at the slit lamp or using an operating microscope under topical anaesthesia. It can be augmented with 5-fluorouracil to enhance the success rate.
- **Subconjunctival injection of 5-fluorouracil** may be used in the first 7–14 days to suppress episcleral fibrosis; 2.5–5 mg (0.1 ml of 25–50 mg/ml solution) is injected (see above) using a 30-gauge needle directed away from the fistula, and can be repeated as necessary.

spherical clear intraepithelial formations thought to indicate the current passage of aqueous across the conjunctival barrier. Poor filtration is indicated by increasing IOP and a bleb with one of the following appearances:

- **Flat** without vascularization (Fig. 10.41B).
- **Vascularized** bleb (Fig. 10.41C) due to episcleral fibrosis.
- **Encapsulated** bleb (Tenon cyst – Fig. 10.41D), characterized by a localized, highly elevated, dome-shaped, fluid-filled cavity of hypertrophied Tenon capsule, often with engorged surface blood vessels.

Causes

Causes of failure can be classified according to the site of obstruction:

- **Extrascleral** causes include subconjunctival and episcleral fibrosis, sometimes with bleb encapsulation.

Late bleb leakage

This occurs due to disintegration of conjunctiva overlying a sclerostomy, typically following peroperative application of antimetabolites, particularly mitomycin C. Necrosis of the surface epithelium results in transconjunctival drainage of aqueous. Complications of untreated leaks include infection and hypotony maculopathy (see Ch. 14).

- **Signs**
  - Low IOP and an avascular cystic bleb (Fig. 10.42).
  - Seidel testing may initially be negative with only multiple punctate staining areas ('sweating'), though this alone may well be sufficient to cause hypotony. The formation of a hole may result in gross leakage with a positive test, and a very low IOP.
  - A shallow anterior chamber and choroidal detachments may be present in severe cases.
- **Treatment** can be difficult. The following are options:
  - Initial treatment is as for early postoperative overfiltration, but is seldom successful.
  - Subsequent treatment depends on whether the leakage involves merely 'sweating' or is due to a hole: sweating

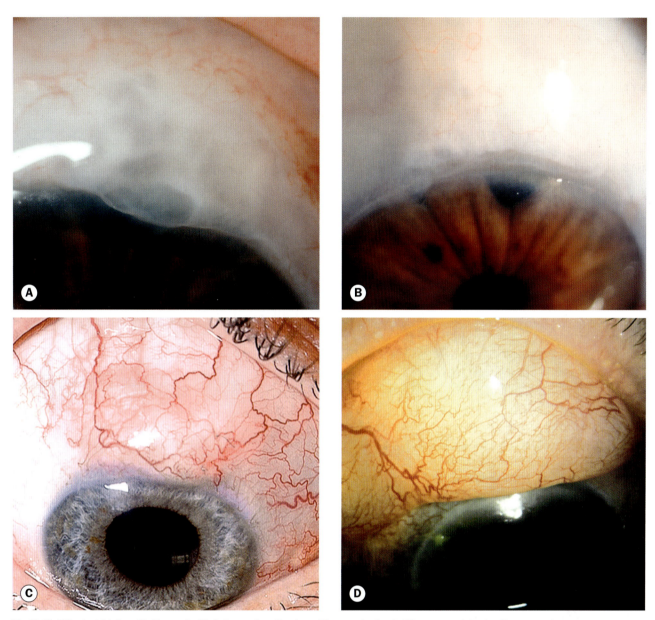

Fig. 10.41 Filtering blebs. **(A)** Normal; **(B)** flat non-functioning; **(C)** vascularized; **(D)** encapsulated – Tenon cyst

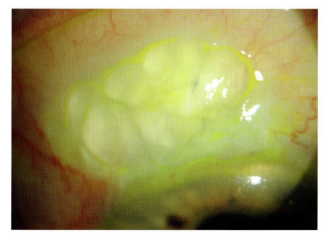

Fig. 10.42 Cystic thin-walled bleb after a mitomycin trabeculectomy

blebs may be treated by injection of autologous blood into the bleb, 'compression' sutures or a transconjunctival scleral flap suture, or sometimes surgery.
○ Full-thickness holes usually require surgical revision, such as conjunctival advancement to hood the existing bleb, a free conjunctival patch autograft or amniotic membrane graft removal of the existing bleb, or a scleral graft to limit flow through the sclerostomy.

Bleb-associated bacterial infection and endophthalmitis

Glaucoma filtration-associated infection is classified as limited to the bleb (blebitis) or endophthalmitis, although there is some overlap. The incidence of blebitis following trabeculectomy with mitomycin has been estimated to be up to 5% per year, though many studies show a far lower rate. Patients who have undergone trabeculectomy should be warned of the possibility of late infection and strongly advised to report immediately should they develop a red and sticky eye, or blurred vision.

- **Risk factors** include blepharitis, antimetabolite use, long-term topical antibiotics, an inferior or nasally placed bleb, and bleb leak. Late bleb leaks should be treated aggressively to reduce the risk of infection.
- **Pathogens**. The most frequent are *Haemophilus influenzae*, *Streptococcus* spp., and *Staphylococcus* spp. The often poor visual prognosis is related to the virulence of these organisms.

Blebitis

Blebitis describes infection without vitreous involvement.
- **Symptoms** consist of a sore, red, photophobic and typically sticky eye.
- **Signs**
  - A white bleb that appears to contain inflammatory material (Fig. 10.43A).
  - Anterior uveitis may be absent or mild, but may be moderate and a hypopyon may be present.
  - The red reflex is normal.

Treatment

  - A conjunctival swab should be taken; a sample should not be aspirated from within the bleb.
  - Broad-spectrum topical antibiotics instilled every hour, e.g. ofloxacin and a cephalosporin; the latter may be prepared from an intravenous ampoule.
  - Oral co-amoxiclav 500/125 mg three times daily, and ciprofloxacin 750 mg twice daily for at least 5 days; azithromycin 500 mg daily is an alternative.
  - The role of topical steroids is undefined; their introduction may be considered after a definite response to antibiotics.

Endophthalmitis

Fistula-related endophthalmitis, even with early treatment, can be associated with a very poor outcome, including blindness or even loss of the eye (Fig. 10.43B).
- **Symptoms** are generally much more severe than those of blebitis.
- **Signs**
  - White milky bleb, as in blebitis but of greater severity.
  - Severe injection.
  - Severe anterior uveitis; a substantial hypopyon is typical (Fig. 10.43C).
  - Vitritis and impairment of the red reflex.
- **Treatment**
  - Vitreous and aqueous samples should be obtained immediately on presentation, though antibiotic treatment should not be delayed if samples cannot be taken straight away.

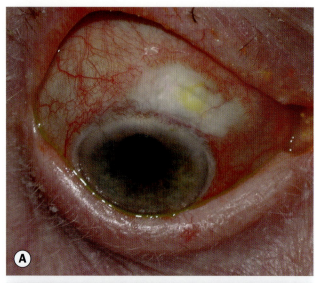

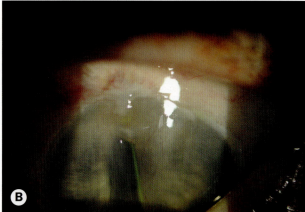

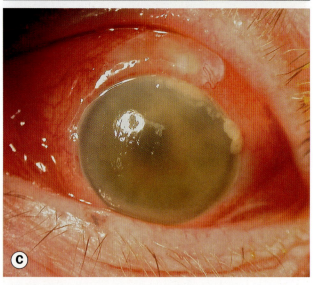

Fig. 10.43 Bacterial infection of a trabeculectomy site. **(A)** Blebitis; **(B)** phthisis following bleb-related endophthalmitis; **(C)** endophthalmitis showing marked anterior chamber involvement including a large hypopyon
(Courtesy of S Chen – figs A and C)

○ Intravitreal antibiotics as for acute postoperative endophthalmitis following cataract extraction (see Ch. 9).

○ Topical and systemic therapy as for blebitis.

NON-PENETRATING GLAUCOMA SURGERY

Overview

In non-penetrating filtration surgery the anterior chamber is not entered and the internal trabecular meshwork is preserved, thus reducing the incidence of postoperative overfiltration with hypotony and its potential sequelae. Two concentric lamellar scleral flaps are fashioned and the deep flap excised leaving behind a thin membrane consisting of trabeculum/Descemet membrane through which aqueous diffuses from the AC to the subconjunctival space. The surgery is technically challenging and requires meticulous dissection of a deep scleral flap to avoid entering the anterior chamber through the delicate Descemet membrane.

Indications

The main indication for non-penetrating surgery is POAG, although other open-angle glaucomas may also be amenable. In general the IOP reduction is less than that achieved by trabeculectomy, so that topical medication often needs to be recommended. Conventional filtration is therefore still the procedure of choice when the target IOP is in the low teens though non-penetrating surgery is probably associated with a lower risk of 'snuffing out' central vision when advanced damage is present.

Technique

- **Deep sclerectomy** (Fig. 10.44). A Descemet window is created to allow aqueous migration from the AC. Subsequent egress is subconjunctival, resulting in a shallow filtration bleb, as well as along deeper suprachoroidal routes. The long-term results can be enhanced by using a collagen implant at the time of surgery and postoperative application of Nd:YAG laser to the meshwork at the surgical site using a gonioscopy lens (goniopuncture).

- **Viscocanalostomy** involves the creation of a filtering window, with identification and dilatation of the Schlemm canal with high density viscoelastic. The superficial scleral flap is sutured tightly so that subconjunctival fluid outflow and bleb formation are minimized. The procedure probably causes inadvertent microscopic ruptures in the juxtacanalicular tissue and meshwork.

- **Canaloplasty** is a variant of viscocanalostomy involving cannulation of the entire circumference of the Schlemm canal with a microcatheter.

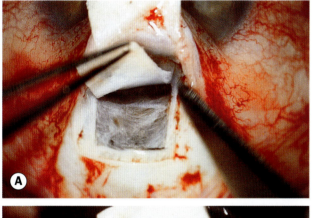
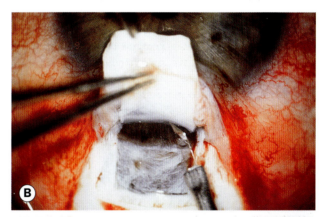
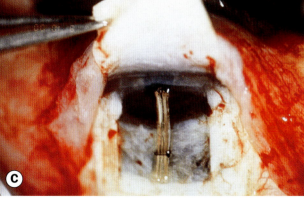
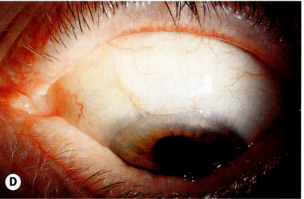

Fig. 10.44 Non-penetrating filtration surgery: deep sclerectomy. **(A)** Dissection of deep scleral flap; **(B)** dissection into clear cornea exposing the Schlemm canal; **(C)** collagen implant; **(D)** shallow diffuse avascular bleb

(Courtesy of A Mermoud)

- **Trabectome.** The Trabectome is a novel microelectrosurgical device that approaches the angle *ab interno* under direct vision using a gonioscopy lens, to remove a strip of trabecular meshwork and inner wall of the Schlemm canal ('trabeculotomy'). Whilst it does not seem to lower the IOP as effectively as trabeculectomy, the safety profile is better.

DRAINAGE SHUNTS

Shunts using episcleral explants

Introduction

Glaucoma drainage devices (GDD) create a communication between the anterior chamber and the sub-Tenon space via a tube attached to a posteriorly explanted episcleral reservoir. Some contain pressure-sensitive valves for the regulation of aqueous flow. Reduction of IOP is due to passive, pressure-dependent flow of aqueous, limited by the wall of a tissue capsule that forms around the explant over the course of several weeks postoperatively. Over recent years the use of GDD has increased, with a large trial, the Tube Versus Trabeculectomy Study, providing good-quality evidence of their safety and comparability to mitomycin C-enhanced trabeculectomy. In practice the threshold for GDD implantation has been lowered, though the number of trabeculectomies being performed remains significantly higher than the rate of GDD implantation. Examples of GDD implants include:

- **Molteno.** This consists of a silicone tube connected to one or two polypropylene plates 13 mm in diameter (Fig. 10.45).
- **Baerveldt.** This implant consists of a silicone tube connected to a silicone plate of large area; silicone may elicit little tissue reaction in comparison with polypropylene.
- **Ahmed.** This is a valved implant consisting of a silicone tube connected to a silicone sheet valve held in a polypropylene body. The valve mechanism consists of two thin silicone elastomer membranes, with the aim of reducing early postoperative hypotony and its complications.

Indications

The circumstances under which GDD may be superior to trabeculectomy are incompletely defined, and many factors must be taken into account, including an individual surgeon's experience and expertise. The introduction of the Ex-Press™ mini-shunt implant modification may have extended the repertoire of trabeculectomy to include some of the previously clearly defined indications for GDD implantation such as ICE syndrome. GDD may be considered in the following cases, though the list is not exhaustive:

- Eyes with severe conjunctival scarring precluding accurate dissection of the conjunctiva.
- Uncontrolled glaucoma despite previous trabeculectomy with adjunctive antimetabolite therapy.
- Secondary glaucoma where routine trabeculectomy, with or without adjunctive antimetabolites, is less likely to be

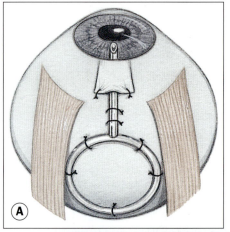

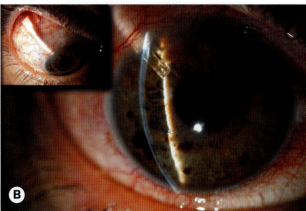

Fig. 10.45 (A) Single-plate Molteno drainage device; **(B)** postoperative appearance
(Courtesy of P Gili – fig. B)

successful. Examples include neovascular glaucoma and glaucoma following traumatic anterior segment disruption.
- Certain congenital glaucomas where conventional procedures have failed.

Complications

The rate of serious complications is similar to that of mitomycin trabeculectomy.

- **Excessive drainage**, resulting in hypotony and a shallow anterior chamber.
- **Malposition** (Fig. 10.46A) may result in endothelial or lenticular touch with corneal decompensation and cataract respectively. Ciliary sulcus or pars plana tube placement can be used in some eyes to negate the possibility of corneal touch.
- **Tube erosion** through the sclera and conjunctiva (Fig. 10.46B).
- **Corneal decompensation** due to endothelial cell loss.
- **Double vision** due to extraocular muscle interference; this may be a higher risk with some implants than others.
- **Early drainage failure** may occur as a result of blockage of the end of the tube by vitreous, blood or iris (Fig. 10.46C).
- **Late drainage failure** occurs in about 10% of cases per year and is comparable to, or perhaps slightly better than, that following trabeculectomy.

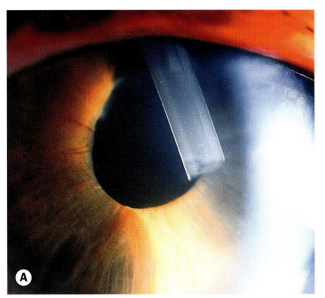

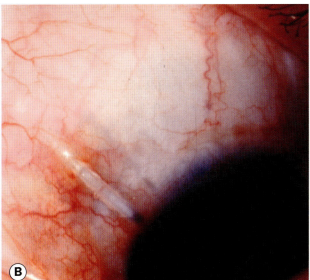

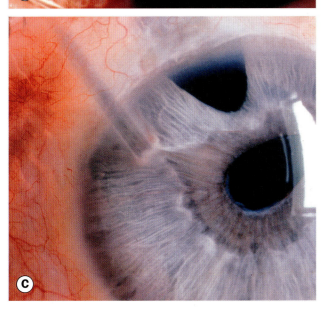

Fig. 10.46 Complications of drainage implants.
(A) Malposition; **(B)** tube erosion; **(C)** blockage by iris
(Courtesy of J Salmon – fig. B; R Bates – fig. C)

Results

The results depend on the type of glaucoma. In general, an IOP in the mid-teens is achieved, though as with trabeculectomy topical medication is frequently required in the medium and longer term. The success rate in some conditions such as neovascular glaucoma is often disappointing. Adjunctive mitomycin C may enhance the success rate of drainage shunt surgery but is associated with a higher complication rate.

Mini-shunts

Ex-Press™ Mini-Shunt

This is a valveless titanium MRI-compatible stent inserted under a scleral flap during a modified trabeculectomy, with a principal aim of increased standardization of drainage (Fig. 10.47). Following creation of the scleral flap as for a standard trabeculectomy, a needle is used to enter the anterior chamber instead of creating a punch sclerostomy. A peripheral iridectomy is not performed. The rate of complications such as hypotony appears to be lower than with standard trabeculectomy, with fewer postoperative interventions, but IOP control is equivalent. It is not generally viewed as suitable in angle-closure glaucoma without prior or contemporaneous cataract surgery.

iStent®

This consists of a tiny hooked titanium tube inserted *ab interno* into the Schlemm canal via the trabecular meshwork (Fig. 10.48), and shows promise for adequate IOP reduction in mild-to-moderate glaucoma. Implantation is considerably more straightforward than conventional glaucoma surgery, and can be performed during phacoemulsification. More than one iStent can be implanted to give more profound IOP reduction.

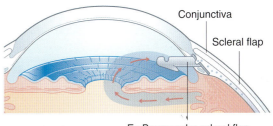

Conjunctiva

Scleral flap

Ex-Press under scleral flap

Fig. 10.47 Ex-Press™ mini-shunt in place under a scleral flap
(Courtesy of E Dahan and A Mermoud, from 'The Ex-Press™ Miniature Glaucoma Implant', in T Shaarawy et al., Glaucoma, Elsevier 2009)

Table 10.3 Risk of developing glaucoma according to IOP (intraocular pressure) and CCT (central corneal thickness)

Mean IOP> 25.75 mmHg	36%	13%	6%
Mean IOP>23.75 to ≤25.75 mmHg	12%	10%	7%
Mean IOP<23.75 mmHg	17%	9%	2%
	CCT ≤ 555 µm	CCT >555 to ≤588 µm	CCT >588 µm

OCULAR HYPERTENSION

Definition

In the general population the mean IOP is 16 mmHg; two standard deviations either side of this gives a 'normal' IOP range of 11–21 mmHg. The distribution is Gaussian with the curve skewed to the right (Fig. 10.49). It is estimated that 4–10% of the population over the age of 40 years have IOP >21 mmHg without detectable glaucomatous damage: 'ocular hypertension' (OHT). An absence of angle closure is implicit, and there should be no detectable cause of secondary glaucoma, though sometimes the term OHT is used to describe raised IOP in these contexts.

Risk factors for developing glaucoma in OHT

The Ocular Hypertension Treatment Study (OHTS) was a multicentre longitudinal trial. In addition to looking at the effect of treatment in ocular hypertensives (IOP <32 mmHg), invaluable information was gained about the effect of a range of putative risks for conversion from OHT to glaucoma; the percentage of OHT patients likely to develop glaucoma taking key factors into account is set out in Tables 10.3 and 10.4; median follow-up was 72 months. Additional considerations are discussed below. Limitations included the possibility that early glaucomatous damage was already present in some of the patients classified as having OHT.

Table 10.4 Risk of developing glaucoma according to vertical C/D ratio and CCT

C/D ratio ≥0.50	22%	16%	8%
C/D ratio >0.30 to <0.50	26%	16%	4%
C/D ratio ≤0.30	15%	1%	4%
	CCT ≤555 µm	CCT >555 to ≤588 µm	CCT >588 µm

The following factors were significant on multivariate analysis:

- **Intraocular pressure.** The risk of developing glaucoma increases with increasing IOP.
- **Age.** Older age is associated with greater risk.
- **Central corneal thickness (CCT).** The risk is greater in eyes with low CCT and lower in eyes with higher CCT. This is probably due to resultant under- and over-estimation of IOP although it has been proposed that associated structural factors, perhaps at the lamina cribrosa, might also be important.
- **Cup/disc (C/D) ratio.** The greater the C/D ratio the higher the risk. This may be because an optic nerve head with a large cup is structurally more vulnerable, or it may be that early damage is already present.

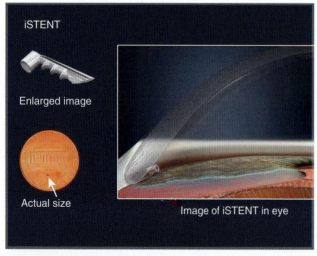

Fig. 10.48 iStent™ trabecular bypass device
(Courtesy of Glaukos Corporation)

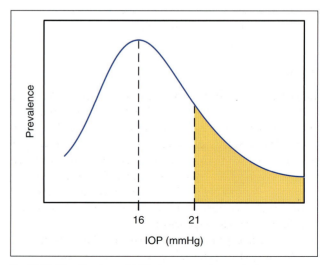

Fig. 10.49 Distribution of IOP the general population

- **Pattern standard deviation (PSD).** A greater PSD result represented a significant risk. It is possible that this signified early glaucomatous field change.

The following factors were significant on univariate analysis only; they were not significant in isolation but were over-ridden when the factors considered above were taken into account.

- **African-American race** was associated with a higher glaucoma risk.
- **Gender.** Males were more likely to convert.
- **Heart disease** was found to be significant.

Factors examined in the OHTS but not found to be significant are listed below.

- **Myopia**, although it is suspected that myopic discs are more susceptible to glaucomatous damage at a lower IOP than emmetropic discs.
- **Diabetes.** An apparent protective effect of diabetes was initially found, but later analysis with refreshed data did not confirm this.
- **Family history of glaucoma** was not found to be a risk factor for conversion.

Other factors that were not examined in the OHTS but may be important include retinal nerve fibre defects (though the presence of these may be taken to indicate pre-perimetric glaucoma – see below) and specific peripapillary atrophic changes.

Clinical evaluation

History and examination should be carried out as for glaucoma (see below). Of particular note, consideration should be given to whether any systemic medication is being taken that might be influencing IOP, either upwards (e.g. steroids) or downwards (e.g. beta-blockers).

Pre-perimetric glaucoma

This concept refers to glaucomatous damage, usually manifested by a suspicious optic disc and/or the presence of retinal nerve fibre layer defects, in which no visual field abnormality has developed. The field testing modality for this purpose is usually taken as standard achromatic automated perimetry.

Management

In the OHTS, untreated patients with ocular hypertension had a 9.5% cumulative risk of developing POAG after 5 years; treatment (which aimed to reduce IOP by 20% or more and to reach 24 mmHg or less) reduced this to 4.4%. Hence, when deciding on whether to start treatment it is important to take into account that it will be necessary to treat a large number of patients in order to prevent the development of glaucoma in a single individual. Various guidelines exist, but there is a high level of disagreement even between glaucoma specialists.

- In general, only those at **higher risk** should be treated, although patient preference may be a decisive factor.
- **Age**, and so life expectancy, is a key point to consider.

- Most practitioners would treat every patient with an **IOP of 30 mmHg or more** (>40% 5-year risk of glaucoma). The decision to treat in patients with varying risk profiles is commonly less than straightforward, and has to be made on an individual basis.
- OHT almost certainly increases the risk of **retinal venous occlusion**, an additional point to take into account when considering whether to start treatment.
- **Treatment options** are the same as for POAG, although a less aggressive pressure-lowering approach is frequently taken, e.g. alternate day prostaglandin dosing and low-intensity selective laser trabeculoplasty have been proposed; filtration surgery is only occasionally indicated. Cataract surgery commonly results in a significant IOP reduction.
- Careful **monitoring** is a reasonable alternative in many circumstances: baseline visual fields and RNFL/disc imaging should be performed.

PRIMARY OPEN-ANGLE GLAUCOMA

Introduction

Definition

Primary open-angle glaucoma (POAG) is a commonly bilateral disease of adult onset. It is characterized by:

- IOP >21 mmHg at some stage.
- Glaucomatous optic nerve damage.
- An open anterior chamber angle.
- Characteristic visual field loss as damage progresses.
- Absence of signs of secondary glaucoma or a non-glaucomatous cause for the optic neuropathy.

POAG is the most prevalent type of glaucoma in individuals of European and African ethnic origin, in a meta-analysis of those older than 70 years of age having a prevalence of 6% in white populations, 16% in black populations and around 3% in Asian populations. It affects both genders equally.

Risk factors

- **IOP.** The higher the IOP, the greater the likelihood of glaucoma. Asymmetry of IOP of 4 mmHg or more is also significant.
- **Age.** POAG is more common in older individuals.
- **Race.** It is significantly (perhaps four times) more common, develops at an earlier age and may be more difficult to control in black individuals than in whites.
- **Family history of POAG.** First-degree relatives of patients with POAG are at increased risk. An approximate risk to siblings is four times and to offspring twice the normal population risk, though surveyed figures vary.
- **Diabetes mellitus.** Many studies suggest a correlation between diabetes and POAG.
- **Myopia** is associated with an increased incidence of POAG and myopic eyes may be more susceptible to glaucomatous

damage. It is speculated that this may be due to mechanical factors, particularly the region of the optic disc.

- **Contraceptive pill.** Recent research suggests that long-term use of the oral contraceptive pill may substantially increase the risk of glaucoma, perhaps by blocking a protective oestrogen effect.
- **Vascular disease.** A range of systemic conditions linked to vascular compromise may be associated, though clear-cut relationships have proved difficult to demonstrate consistently. Systemic hypertension, cardiovascular disease, diabetes and vasospastic conditions such as migraine have all been implicated. Poor ocular perfusion may be a risk factor for glaucoma progression.
- **Translaminar pressure gradient.** Studies suggest that a difference in the levels of IOP and orbital CSF pressure may increase the likelihood of the development and progression of glaucomatous damage, perhaps due to associated deformation of the lamina cribrosa.
- **Optic disc area.** Large discs may be more vulnerable to damage, again with some commentators speculating that causation may be linked to mechanical factors associated with laminar deformation.
- **Ocular perfusion pressure** is the difference between the arterial BP and the intraocular pressure (IOP), and has been shown in population studies to be linked to increased risk for the development and progression of glaucoma.

Genetics

POAG has been associated with at least 20 loci in the human genome, but mutations in only the *MYOC* gene, coding for the protein myocilin that is found in the trabecular meshwork, and the *OPTN* gene, which codes for optineurin, are broadly accepted as causing glaucoma. A number of different mutations have been described in the *MYOC* gene, though the normal function of myocilin and its role in glaucoma is as yet undetermined. If a single family member develops glaucoma prior to age 35 years, the chances of a mutation in the myocilin gene may be as high as 33%. Genetic investigation of a patient and family may be considered if three or more first-degree relatives from two generations are affected, or for research purposes.

Steroid responsiveness

Around one in three individuals develop some degree of elevation of IOP in response to a course of potent topical steroid, dividing the population into steroid 'responders' and 'non-responders'. Responders are more likely than non-responders to develop POAG, and a majority of patients with POAG are responders. Close relatives of patients with POAG are also more likely to exhibit a steroid response. Steroids of greater potency have a greater propensity to elevate IOP, as does higher frequency of instillation, and this tendency is more marked in patients with POAG and their close relatives. Intra- and periocular steroid administration, including periocular application of steroid skin cream and nasal administration, are also prone to elevate IOP.

Systemic steroids are much less prone to cause elevation of IOP, but substantial, probably dose-dependent, rises can occur and some authorities have advocated screening for all patients taking systemic steroids, perhaps dexamethasone in particular. The precise mechanism of the 'steroid response' is uncertain, but it is thought to be mediated by an alteration in the composition and function of the trabeculum, including altered expression of myocilin production.

Pathogenesis of glaucomatous optic neuropathy

Retinal ganglion cell death in glaucoma occurs predominantly through apoptosis (programmed cell death) rather than necrosis. The preterminal event is calcium ion influx into the cell body and an increase in intracellular nitric oxide; glutamine metabolism is intrinsically involved. After initial injury, a cascade of events results in astrocyte and glial cell proliferation, and alterations in the extracellular matrix of the lamina cribrosa, with subsequent optic nerve head remodelling. Multiple factors are likely to be involved, but the mechanisms remain relatively speculative: the process of glaucomatous damage and the relationship with IOP and other potential influences is still poorly understood. One or both of the following mechanisms may be involved:

- **Direct mechanical** damage to retinal nerve fibres at the optic nerve head, perhaps as they pass through the lamina cribrosa; accumulating evidence of the influence of mechanical deformability in the region of the lamina cribrosa supports this.
- **Ischaemic damage**, possibly due to compression of blood vessels supplying the optic nerve head; this may relate to ocular perfusion pressure as a possible risk factor for glaucoma.
- **Common pathways of damage.** Both mechanisms might lead to a reduction in axoplasmic flow, interference with the delivery of nutrients or removal of metabolic products, deprivation of neuronal growth factors, oxidative injury and the initiation of immune-mediated damage.

Screening

Universal population screening for glaucoma has not been demonstrated to be cost-effective, and current practice restricts screening to high-risk groups, such as older individuals, those over the age of 40 with a history of POAG in a close family member, and people of black ethnicity. In these groups, screening tends to be performed sporadically via routes such as commercial optometric eye examinations, which may lead to the relative exclusion of underprivileged economic groups. Population screening with tonometry alone is unsatisfactory, since it will label as normal a significant number of cases with other features of POAG such as cupping and visual field loss, and routine screening eye examinations should include visual field assessment as well as tonometry and ophthalmoscopy.

Diagnosis

History

- **Visual symptoms** will usually be absent, unless damage is advanced. Sometimes symptomatic central field defects may occur at an early stage, in the presence of a relatively normal peripheral field.
- **Previous ophthalmic history.** Specific enquiry should be made about:
  - Refractive status as myopia carries an increased risk of POAG, and hypermetropia of primary angle-closure glaucoma (PACG).
  - Causes of secondary glaucoma such as ocular trauma or inflammation; previous eye surgery, including refractive surgery, may affect IOP readings.
- **Family history**
  - POAG or related conditions such as OHT.
  - Other ocular disease in family members.
- **Past medical history.** Asking specifically about the following may be indicated.
  - Asthma, heart failure or block, peripheral vascular disease: contraindications to the use of beta-blockers.
  - Head injury, intracranial pathology including stroke: may cause optic atrophy or visual field defects.
  - Vasospasm: migraine and Raynaud phenomenon.
  - Diabetes, systemic hypertension and cardiovascular disease may increase the risk of POAG.
  - Oral contraceptive pill for several years may be associated with an increased risk of glaucoma.
- **Current medication**
  - Steroids including skin cream and inhalants.
  - Oral beta-blockers may lower IOP.
- **Social history** including smoking and alcohol intake, especially if toxic/nutritional optic neuropathy is suspected.
- **Allergies,** particularly to any drugs likely to be used in glaucoma treatment, e.g. sulfonamides.

Examination

- **Visual acuity** is likely to be normal except in advanced glaucoma.
- **Pupils.** Exclude a relative afferent pupillary defect (RAPD); if initially absent but develops later, this constitutes an indicator of substantial progression.
- **Colour vision assessment** such as Ishihara chart testing if there is any suggestion of an optic neuropathy other than glaucoma.
- **Slit lamp examination.** Exclude features of secondary glaucomas such as pigmentary and pseudoexfoliative.
- **Tonometry** prior to pachymetry, noting the time of day.
- **Gonioscopy.**
- **Optic disc examination** for glaucomatous changes (see earlier in chapter) should always be performed with the pupils dilated, provided gonioscopy does not show critically narrow angles. Red-free light can be used to detect RNFL defects.

Investigation

- **Pachymetry** for CCT.
- **Perimetry** should usually be performed prior to clinical examination.
- **Imaging** of the optic disc, peripapillary RNFL and/or ganglion cell complex, e.g. red-free photography, stereo disc photography, OCT, confocal scanning laser ophthalmoscopy and/or scanning laser polarimetry.

Visual field defects

Nerve damage in glaucoma is believed to be inflicted at the optic nerve head, and the resultant visual field defect corresponds to the pattern of fibres in the retinal area served.

- **Early changes** include increased variability of responses in areas that subsequently develop defects, and slight asymmetry between the two eyes. Special modalities such as FDT and SWAP may demonstrate defects at an earlier stage.
- **Small paracentral depressions** (Fig. 10.50) can form at a relatively early stage, often superonasally; they are probably more common in NTG.
- **Nasal step** represents a difference in sensitivity above and below the horizontal midline in the nasal field; the defect is bounded by the horizontal midline, corresponding to the retinal nerve fibre layer horizontal raphe. Inferior optic disc and OCT changes with a corresponding superior nasal step are shown in Fig. 10.51.
- **Temporal wedge** is less common than a nasal step but has similar implications.
- **Arcuate defects** (see Fig. 10.51C) develop as a result of coalescence of paracentral scotomas. They typically develop between 10° and 20° of fixation as downward or upward extensions from the blind spot ('baring of the blind spot' – Fig. 10.52) around fixation. With time, they tend to elongate circumferentially along the distribution of arcuate nerve fibres.
- **A ring scotoma** develops when superior and inferior arcuate defects become continuous, usually in advanced glaucoma (Fig. 10.53).
- **End-stage** changes are characterized by a small island of central vision, typically accompanied by a temporal island. The 10-2 perimetry pattern facilitates monitoring of the residual central field.
- **Summary measures** should always be taken into account; on average an annual deterioration in mean total deviation of just over 1.0 dB can be expected in treated patients (Fig. 10.54).

Management

The primary aim of treatment is to prevent functional impairment of vision within the patient's lifetime by slowing the rate of ganglion cell loss closer to that of the normal population. Currently the only proven method of achieving this is the lowering of IOP. Both higher mean IOP and substantial variation in IOP are

Text continued on p. 356

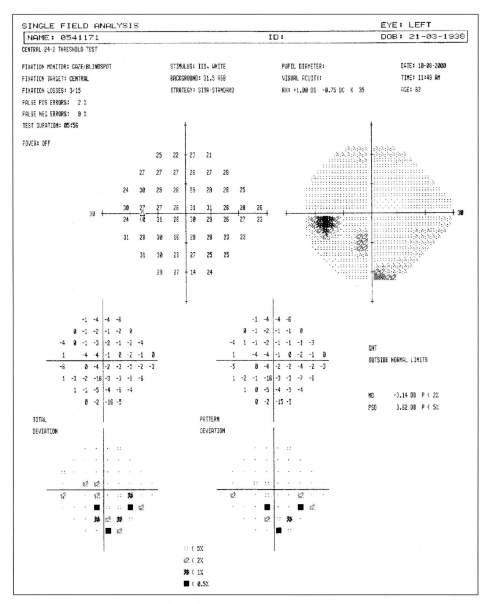

Fig. 10.50 Small paracentral scotoma in mild to moderate glaucoma

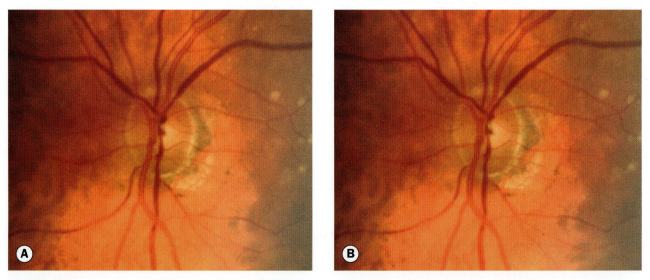

Fig. 10.51 Moderate to marked glaucoma. **(A)** and **(B)** Stereo disc photographs showing inferior neuroretinal rim shelving;

Continued

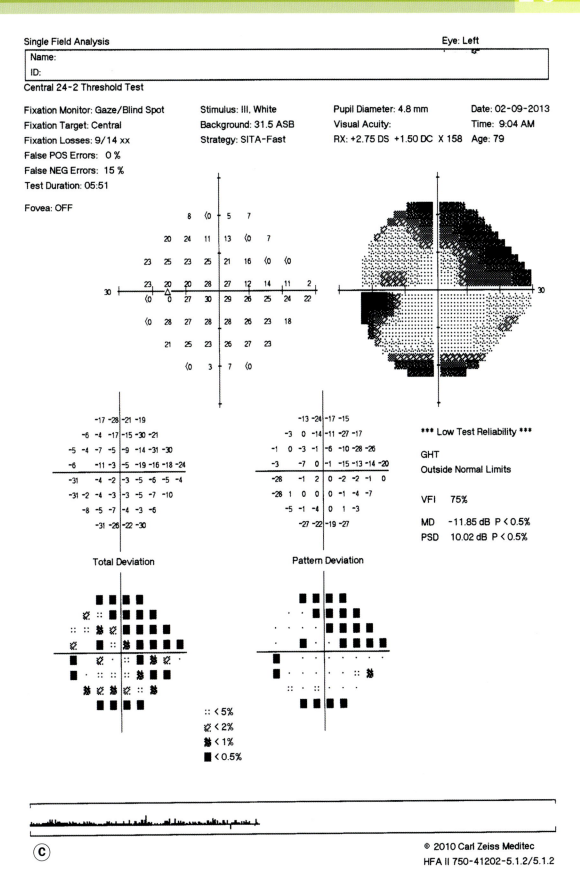

Single Field Analysis   Eye: Left

Name:

ID:

Central 24-2 Threshold Test

Fixation Monitor: Gaze/Blind Spot   Stimulus: III, White   Pupil Diameter: 4.8 mm   Date: 02-09-2013
Fixation Target: Central   Background: 31.5 ASB   Visual Acuity: Time: 9:04 AM
Fixation Losses: 9/14 xx   Strategy: SITA-Fast   RX: +2.75 DS +1.50 DC X 158   Age: 79
False POS Errors: 0 %
False NEG Errors: 15 %
Test Duration: 05:51

Fovea: OFF

```
              8  ⟨0   5   7
          20  24  11  13  ⟨0   7
      23  25  23  25 │ 21  16  ⟨0  ⟨0
   23  20  20  28  27 │ 12  14  11   2
30 ⟨0   0  27  30 │ 29  26  25  24  22          30
   ⟨0  28  27  28 │ 28  26  23  18
      21  25  23 │ 26  27  23
          ⟨0   3   7  ⟨0
```

Total Deviation
```
       -17 -28 -21 -19
     -6  -4 -17 -15 -30 -21
  -5  -4  -7  -5 -9 -14 -31 -30
  -6     -11 -3 -5 -19 -16 -18 -24
 -31    -4  -2 -3 -5  -6  -5  -4
 -31 -2 -4  -3 -3 -5  -7 -10
     -8  -5  -7 -4 -3  -6
       -31 -26 -22 -30
```

Pattern Deviation
```
       -13 -24 -17 -15
     -3   0 -14 -11 -27 -17
  -1   0  -3  -1 -6 -10 -28 -26
  -3     -7   0 -1 -15 -13 -14 -20
 -28    -1   2  0 -2  -2  -1   0
 -28  1  0   0  0 -1  -4  -7
     -5  -1  -4  0  1  -3
       -27 -22 -19 -27
```

*** Low Test Reliability ***

GHT

Outside Normal Limits

VFI   75%

MD   -11.85 dB P < 0.5%
PSD   10.02 dB P < 0.5%

Total Deviation   Pattern Deviation

```
::  < 5%
⟨⟩  < 2%
▨  < 1%
■  < 0.5%
```

Fig. 10.51, Continued (C) visual field from the same eye showing superior arcuate scotoma and nasal step (but note suboptimal reliability);

Continued

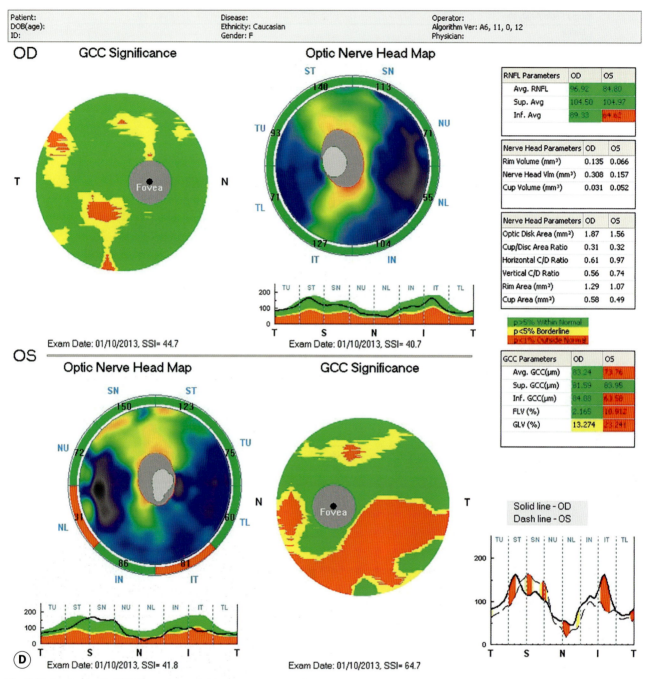

Fig. 10.51, Continued (D) OCT from the same patient – note inferior abnormality on ganglion cell complex analysis of the left eye corresponding to the superior nasal step

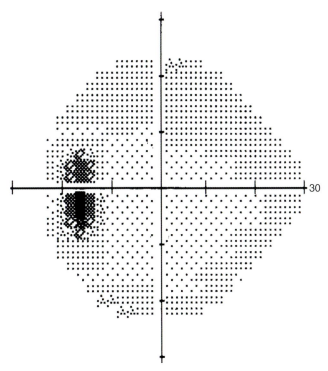

Fig. 10.52 Grey scale display of early upwards arcuate extension from the blind spot – 'baring of the blind spot'

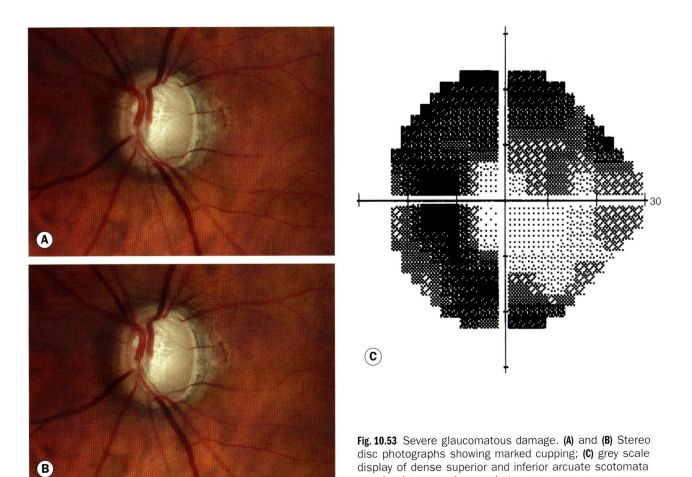

Fig. 10.53 Severe glaucomatous damage. **(A)** and **(B)** Stereo disc photographs showing marked cupping; **(C)** grey scale display of dense superior and inferior arcuate scotomata merging into superior nasal step

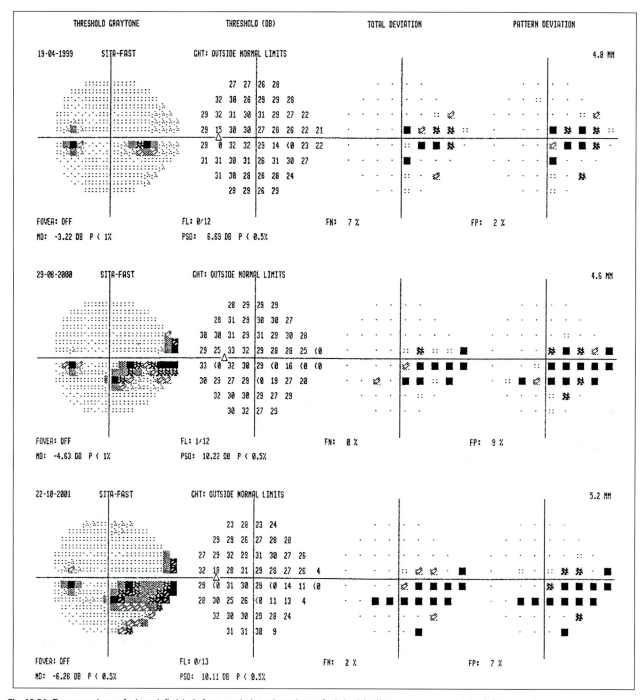

Fig. 10.54 Progression of visual field defect and deterioration of global indices over a period of 30 months

predictive of progressive visual field loss in patients with glaucoma, whether newly diagnosed or advanced, and aggressive treatment should be considered in these circumstances.

Patient instruction

An explanation should be offered concerning the nature of the disease, and relevant literature provided. The timing of medication use should be specified, and the patient educated in the technique of eye drop instillation. At follow-up visits the patient's proficiency at instilling drops should be checked. In order to maximize drug contact time with the anterior segment and to minimize systemic absorption the patient should be instructed either to perform lacrimal sac occlusion by applying fingertip pressure at the medial canthus or to close the eyes for about 3 minutes after instillation. Common or severe potential adverse effects should be explained at the commencement of treatment and their occurrence enquired about at review visits.

Treatment goals

- **Target pressure.** It is assumed that the pre-treatment level of IOP has damaged the optic nerve and will continue to do so. An IOP level is identified below which further damage is considered unlikely: the target pressure. This is identified taking into account the severity of existing damage (particularly a greater vertical C/D ratio and a greater mean deviation on visual fields), the level of IOP, CCT, the rapidity with which damage occurred if known, and the age and general health of the patient; greater age is associated with a higher likelihood of rapid progression, but a shorter life expectancy may also be taken into account. Therapy should maintain the IOP at or below the target level. If not achievable by more conservative measures, a decision is made regarding whether to proceed with surgery or to continue monitoring with an above-target IOP.
- **Proportional reduction.** An alternative strategy is to aim for a reduction in IOP by a certain percentage – often 30% – and then monitor, aiming for a further reduction if progression occurs. There may be a smaller margin for error with this approach if advanced damage is present, and it may not be as well supported by research-based evidence.
- **Response to progression.** As damage progresses the loss of each remaining ganglion cell has a greater proportional impact on visual function, and there is less reserve capacity. If damage progresses despite a target pressure having been reached consistently, the target IOP is set to a lower level; there is evidence that each 1 mmHg reduction in IOP leads to a 10% reduction in the rate of nerve fibre loss. If further damage is sustained despite apparently good IOP control, surgery may be appropriate.

Medical therapy

- **Commencing medical therapy**
  - Any drug chosen should be prescribed in the lowest concentration consistent with the desired therapeutic effect, and administered as infrequently as possible.
  - Ideally the drug with the fewest potential side effects should be used.
  - Initial treatment is usually with one type of medication, typically a prostaglandin analogue or beta-blocker.
- **Review**
  - The interval to review after starting medication is set according to the individual patient, but is usually 4–8 weeks.
  - Response to the drug is assessed against the target IOP.
  - If the response is satisfactory, subsequent assessment is generally set for a further 3–6 months.
  - If there has been little or no response the initial drug is withdrawn and another substituted.
  - If there has been an apparently incomplete response another drug may be added or a fixed combination substituted.
  - When two separate drugs are used the patient should be instructed to wait 5 minutes before instilling the second drug to prevent washout of the first.
  - Sometimes it may be worthwhile to allow a further month or two of treatment before altering a regimen, as response may improve over time.
  - Inadequate drop instillation technique should be considered as a cause of unsatisfactory IOP response.
  - Poor compliance should always be borne in mind, e.g. if progression occurs despite excellent IOP readings at review assessments.
  - When drops are administered in the morning, it is good practice always to enquire about whether that day's dose has been used prior to attendance.
- **Perimetry.** If IOP control is good and glaucomatous damage mild or moderate with no substantial threat to central vision, perimetry every 6–12 months is generally sufficient.
- **Gonioscopy** should be performed annually in most patients because the anterior chamber angle tends to narrow with age.
- **Optic disc examination** should be performed at each visit, as a disc haemorrhage may indicate ongoing damage; a new haemorrhage should be recorded pictorially, optimally by photography.
- **Serial imaging** is increasingly viewed as standard care.
- **Causes of treatment failure**
  - Inappropriate target pressure. If the IOP is maintained in the upper part of the statistically normal range, progressive field loss is relatively common.
  - Poor compliance with therapy occurs in at least 25% of patients.
  - Wide fluctuations in IOP are not uncommon in patients treated medically, and are associated with a tendency to progression.
  - Patients may deteriorate despite apparently good IOP control. Causes include occult compliance failure, undetected diurnal variation, and possibly other mechanisms not readily detectable clinically such as impaired optic nerve perfusion. The possibility of an alternative pathology, particularly a compressive lesion, should always be considered in these circumstances.

Laser trabeculoplasty

SLT is often as effective as medical monotherapy, and has been gaining in popularity as a first-line treatment.

Surgery

Trabeculectomy is the surgical procedure most commonly performed for POAG. Over recent years, the threshold for glaucoma drainage device implantation has been lowered by many surgeons, the procedure having previously been performed only in a small minority of complex cases at very high risk of failure. Non-penetrating surgery (e.g. deep sclerectomy, viscocanalostomy) is utilized extensively in POAG by some authorities. Phacoemulsification alone is frequently associated with a significant fall in IOP, but is generally only offered to patients in whom significant lens opacity is present; it can be combined with a filtration procedure (phacotrabeculectomy). Progressive damage is thought to be less likely after surgery than with medical therapy, probably because the resultant IOP is often significantly lower and less likely to fluctuate, and because compliance is no longer a factor.

Prognosis

The great majority of patients with POAG will not become blind in their lifetime, but the incidence of blindness varies considerably depending on multiple factors such as the presence of advanced damage at diagnosis, non-compliance with treatment and ethnic origin (e.g. the prognosis is better for white than black patients). Data are incomplete, but in a white population with POAG the lifetime chance of blindness in both eyes has historically been 5–10%; given the long-term nature of progression in glaucoma, the prognosis may have been significantly improved with newer treatment strategies. The average period from diagnosis to death has been estimated at around 15 years.

NORMAL-TENSION GLAUCOMA

Introduction

Normal-tension glaucoma (NTG), also referred to as low-tension or normal-pressure glaucoma, is usually regarded as a variant of POAG. It is characterized by:

- IOP consistently equal to or less than 21 mmHg.
- Signs of optic nerve damage in a characteristic glaucomatous pattern.
- An open anterior chamber angle.
- Visual field loss as damage progresses, consistent in pattern with the nerve appearance.
- No features of secondary glaucoma or a non-glaucomatous cause for the neuropathy.

The distinction between NTG and POAG is based on an epidemiologically derived range of normal IOP. It is essentially an arbitrary division that may not have significant clinical value, though it is possible that a spectrum exists in which, towards the NTG end, IOP-independent factors are of increasing relative importance. Up to two-thirds of Japanese patients and 30% of Caucasians with OAG may have normal IOP at initial assessments.

Pathogenesis

Any aetiological factors distinct from those in POAG have not been conclusively determined, although various mechanisms have been postulated including anomalies of local and systemic vascular function, structural optic nerve anomalies and autoimmune disease. With the introduction of widespread central corneal thickness (CCT) assessment, NTG in some patients has been explained by very low CCT, and overall CCT in patients with NTG is lower than in POAG. A small proportion of NTG patients have been found to have marked nocturnal IOP spikes, sometimes only detected on testing in the supine position.

Risk factors

- **Age**. Patients tend to be older than those with POAG, though this may be due to delayed diagnosis.
- **Gender**. Some studies have found a higher prevalence in females.
- **Race**. NTG occurs more frequently in people of Japanese origin than in European or North American Caucasians.
- **Family history**. The prevalence of POAG is greater in families of patients with NTG than in the normal population. Mutations in the *OPTN* gene coding for optineurin have been identified in some patients with NTG, though also in patients with POAG.
- **CCT** is lower in patients with NTG than POAG.
- **Abnormal vasoregulation**, particularly migraine and Raynaud phenomenon, has been found more commonly in NTG than POAG by some investigators; others have found abnormalities just as commonly in POAG. Other systemic diseases associated with vascular risk, such as diabetes, carotid insufficiency, hypertension and hypercoagulability, may also be important.
- **Systemic hypotension** including nocturnal blood pressure dips of >20%, particularly in those on oral hypotensive medication.
- **Obstructive sleep apnoea syndrome** may be associated, perhaps via an effect on ocular perfusion.
- **Autoantibody levels** have been found to be higher in some groups of NTG patients by some investigators.
- **Translaminar pressure gradient.** This may on average be larger than in POAG.
- **Ocular perfusion pressure** may be relatively lower than in POAG.
- **Myopia** is associated with a greater likelihood of glaucoma and of its progression.
- **Thyroid disease** may be more common.

Differential diagnosis

- **Angle closure** should always be ruled out by meticulous dark-room gonioscopy.
- **Low CCT** leading to underestimation of IOP; suspicion has also been raised that a thin posterior ocular wall may increase mechanical stress in the region of the lamina cribrosa. Prior refractive surgery and corneal ectasia also lead to falsely low IOP readings, sometimes dramatically so.
- **POAG** presenting with apparently normal IOP because of wide diurnal fluctuation. Plotting a diurnal IOP curve over an 8-hour period (phasing) during office hours may detect daytime elevation, but detection of nocturnal IOP spikes requires substantial resource commitment.
- **Previous episodes of raised IOP** may have occurred as a result of ocular trauma, uveitis or local or systemic steroid therapy.

- **Masking by systemic treatment** such as an oral beta-blocker, commenced after glaucomatous damage has already been sustained.
- **Spontaneously resolved pigmentary glaucoma.** The typical examination features of pigmentary glaucoma tend to become less evident with increasing age. The IOP in some cases of POAG may also spontaneously normalize over time.
- **Progressive retinal nerve fibre defects not due to glaucoma** such as may occur in myopic degeneration and optic disc drusen.
- **Congenital disc anomalies** simulating glaucomatous cupping, such as disc pits and colobomas.
- **Neurological** lesions causing optic nerve or chiasmal compression can produce visual field defects that may be misinterpreted as glaucomatous, and neuroimaging should be performed if there is any suspicion; some practitioners routinely perform a cranial MRI in all cases of NTG.
- **Previous anterior ischaemic optic neuropathy (AION)** may give rise to a disc appearance and visual field defect consistent with glaucoma. Non-arteritic AION often occurs in a 'crowded' disc, and the fellow eye should be examined for this; prior retinal vascular occlusion should also be considered.
- **Previous acute optic nerve insult** such as hypovolaemic or septicaemic shock, or head injury.
- **Miscellaneous optic neuropathies** including inflammatory, infiltrative and drug-induced pathology will often be clinically obvious, but can occasionally masquerade as NTG.

Clinical features

History and examination are essentially the same as for POAG but specific points warrant attention.

- **History**
  - Migraine and Raynaud phenomenon.
  - Episodes of shock.
  - Head or eye injury.
  - Headache and other neurological symptoms (intracranial lesion).
  - Medication, e.g. systemic steroids, beta-blockers.
- **IOP** is usually in the high teens, but may rarely be in the low teens. In asymmetrical disease the more damaged disc typically corresponds to the eye with the higher IOP.
- **Optic nerve head**
  - The optic nerve head may be larger on average in NTG than in POAG.
  - The pattern of cupping is similar, but acquired optic disc pits and focal nerve fibre layer defects may be more common.
  - Peripapillary atrophic changes may be more prevalent.
  - Disc (splinter, Drance – see Figs 10.18A and B) haemorrhages may be more frequent than in POAG, and are associated with a greater likelihood of progression.
  - Pallor disproportionate to cupping should prompt a suspicion of an alternative diagnosis.
- **Visual field defects** are essentially the same as in POAG although there is some evidence that they tend to be closer to fixation, deeper, steeper and more localized. In probably more than half of patients, field changes are non-progressive over a period of 5 years or more without treatment. However, perhaps because of delayed diagnosis, patients tend to present with more advanced damage than in POAG. A high level of suspicion for a deficit pattern suggesting a lesion posterior to the optic nerve is important.
- **Other investigations** are as for POAG although in selected patients the following can be considered.
  - Assessment of systemic vascular risk factors.
  - Blood pressure measurement can be used to calculate ocular perfusion pressure; 24-hour ambulatory monitoring will exclude nocturnal systemic hypotension in selected patients.
  - Blood tests for other causes of non-glaucomatous optic neuropathy such as vitamin B_{12}, red cell folate, full blood count, erythrocyte sedimentation rate/C-reactive protein, treponemal serology including Lyme disease, serum angiotensin-converting enzyme level, plasma protein electrophoresis and autoantibody screen.
  - Cranial MRI.
  - Carotid Duplex imaging.
  - Ocular blood flow assessment (e.g. laser flowmetry) may have useful clinical potential.

Treatment

Further lowering of IOP is effective in reducing progression in many or most patients. However, as a large proportion of untreated patients will not deteriorate (approximately 50% at 5 years), in many cases progression should be demonstrated before commencing treatment. Exceptions include advanced glaucomatous damage, particularly if threatening central vision, and young age. Regular assessment including perimetry should be performed at 4–6 monthly intervals initially.

- **Medical treatment.** The alpha-2 agonist brimonidine may have a neuroprotective effect on the retina and optic nerve in addition to its IOP-lowering effect and may be superior to beta-blockers. Carbonic anhydrase inhibitors, particularly dorzolamide, may improve ocular perfusion. Prostaglandin derivatives tend to have a greater ocular hypotensive effect, which may be an over-riding consideration. Topical beta-blockers can have a dramatic effect on BP in a minority, and may contribute to nocturnal dips, though selective blockade (e.g. betaxolol) may actually have a beneficial effect on optic nerve perfusion.
- **Laser trabeculoplasty**, particularly SLT, is a reasonable option to achieve IOP targets.
- **Surgery** may be considered if progression occurs despite IOP in the low teens; antimetabolite enhancement of trabeculectomy is likely to be indicated in order to achieve a satisfactorily low pressure.
- **Control of systemic vascular disease** such as diabetes, hypertension and hyperlipidaemia may be important, in order theoretically to optimize optic nerve perfusion.
- **Systemic calcium-channel blockers** to address vasospasm have been advocated by some authorities.

- **Antihypotensive measures.** If significant nocturnal dips in BP are detected, it may be necessary to reduce antihypertensive medication, especially if taken at bedtime. Non-selective topical beta-blockers in particular may cause a profound drop in systemic blood pressure in some individuals. Selected patients might be encouraged to increase their salted food intake, in consultation with the patient's cardiovascular physician.
- **Neuroprotective agents** of proven benefit are not yet available; memantine is used to retard neuronal death in some CNS disorders, and its use has been adopted in glaucoma by some practitioners. Ginkgo biloba (40 mg three times daily) or an antiplatelet agent may confer some benefit in selected cases.

PRIMARY ANGLE-CLOSURE GLAUCOMA

Introduction

Overview

The term 'angle closure' refers to occlusion of the trabecular meshwork by the peripheral iris (iridotrabecular contact – ITC), obstructing aqueous outflow. Angle closure can be primary, when it occurs in an anatomically predisposed eye, or secondary to another ocular or systemic factor. PACG may be responsible for up to half of all cases of glaucoma globally, with a particularly high prevalence in individuals of Far Eastern descent. It is typically associated with greater rapidity of progression and visual morbidity than POAG.

Classification

As knowledge about the epidemiology and mechanisms of angle closure has increased, classification has moved away from a symptom-based approach (acute, subacute and chronic) to reflect the stages in the natural history of the disease. This takes into account the fact that the majority of patients are asymptomatic, and can be linked to prognosis and management. The scheme below has been suggested by a consensus group of the Association of International Glaucoma Societies.

- **Primary angle closure suspect (PACS)**
  - Gonioscopy shows posterior meshwork ITC (Fig. 10.55A) in three or more quadrants but no PAS.
  - Many patients with less ITC have evidence of intermittent angle closure, and a lower threshold for diagnosis such as two quadrants of ITC, pigment smudging (Figs 10.55B and C) or even a very narrow angle approach (perhaps 20° or less – Fig. 10.55D) may be justified.
  - Normal IOP, optic disc and visual field.
  - No peripheral anterior synechiae (PAS).
  - The risk of PACG at 5 years may be around 30%.
- **Primary angle closure (PAC)**
  - Gonioscopy shows three or more quadrants of ITC (Fig. 10.56A) with raised IOP and/or PAS (Fig. 10.56B), or excessive pigment smudging on the TM.

  - Normal optic disc and field.
  - Some authorities further classify PAC into non-ischaemic and ischaemic, the latter showing anterior segment evidence of prior substantial IOP elevation such as iris changes or glaukomflecken (see Fig. 10.61).
- **Primary angle-closure glaucoma (PACG)**
  - ITC in three or more quadrants, with glaucomatous optic neuropathy.
  - Optic nerve damage from an episode of severe IOP elevation, such as acute angle closure, may not appear as typical glaucomatous cupping.

Mechanism

The mechanisms involved in angle closure can be categorized according to the anatomical level (anterior to posterior) at which causative forces act. In many patients more than one level is contributory.

- **Relative pupillary block**
  - Failure of physiological aqueous flow through the pupil leads to a pressure differential between the anterior and posterior chambers, with resultant anterior bowing of the iris (Fig. 10.57).
  - Usually anatomically relieved by iridotomy, which equalizes anterior and posterior chamber pressure. Control of IOP if elevated will be achieved provided the angle has opened adequately; this may not occur if there are substantial PAS or an additional mechanism of angle closure is in effect. TM damage can prevent normalization of IOP even with an anatomically open angle.
  - The lens vault quantifies the portion of the lens located anterior to the anterior chamber angle; a common definition is the distance between the anterior pole of the lens and a horizontal line joining the scleral spur at diametrically opposite locations. A large lens vault is independently associated with angle closure, though it is not clear whether this is entirely via a pupillary block or non-pupillary block (see next) mechanism, or both.
- **Non-pupillary block**
  - Thought to be important in many Far Eastern patients.
  - Associated with a deeper anterior chamber (AC) than pure pupillary block.
  - Patients with non-pupillary block, particularly those with plateau iris, tend to be younger than those with pure pupillary block.
  - An element of pupillary block is invariably present, but angle closure is not fully relieved by iridotomy. The term 'mixed mechanism' has been suggested to describe glaucoma in which both significant pupillary block and non-pupillary block iris-induced mechanisms coexist.
  - Specific anatomical causative factors include plateau iris (anteriorly positioned/rotated ciliary processes – Fig. 10.58), and a thicker or more anteriorly positioned iris; a 'thick peripheral iris roll' concept has been introduced by some authorities. A thicker peripheral iris may be relatively important in patients of Far Eastern ethnic origin.

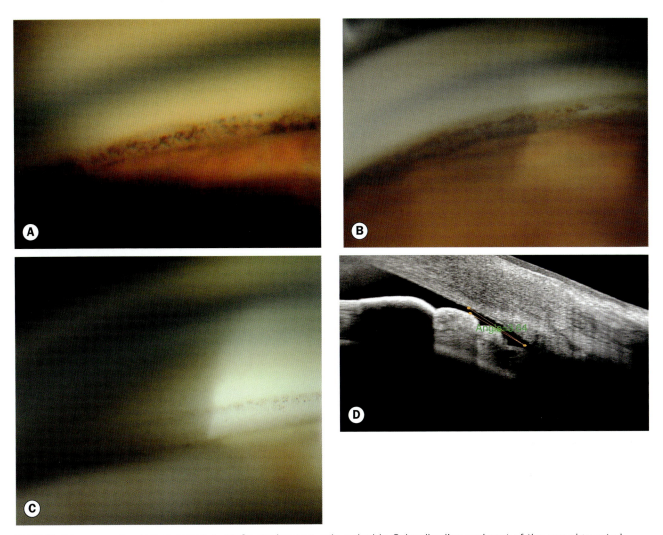

Fig. 10.55 Primary angle closure suspect. **(A)** On gonioscopy only a double Schwalbe line and part of the non-pigmented trabecular meshwork are visible – the iris is apposed to the pigmented meshwork; **(B)** pigment smudging of the non-pigmented meshwork seen on indentation gonioscopy; **(C)** moderately but not critically narrow angle for comparison – sparsely pigmented Schwalbe line, non-pigmented and pigmented meshwork; **(D)** very narrow angle on dark-room anterior segment OCT

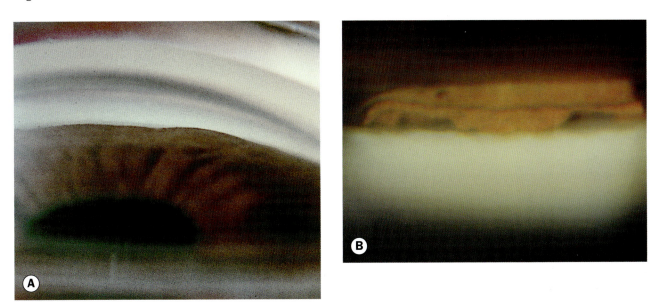

Fig. 10.56 Primary angle closure. **(A)** Closed inferior angle on gonioscopy; **(B)** PAS on indentation gonioscopy – superior angle
(Courtesy of L MacKeen – fig. A)

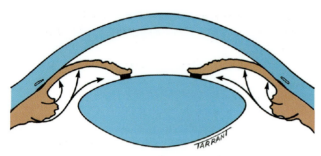

Fig. 10.57 Angle closure due to pupillary block, with anterior iris bowing and iridocorneal contact

○ Plateau iris *configuration* is characterized by a flat or only slightly convex central iris plane, often in association with normal or only slightly shallow central anterior chamber depth. The angle recess is typically very narrow, with a sharp backward iris angulation over anteriorly positioned and/or orientated ciliary processes. A characteristic 'double hump' sign is seen on indentation gonioscopy, the central hump being due to the underlying central lens supporting the iris and the peripheral hump resulting from the underlying ciliary processes.

○ Plateau iris *syndrome* describes the persistence of gonioscopic angle closure despite a patent iridotomy in a patient with morphological plateau iris; factors such as a dark environment or pharmacological pupillary dilatation may be necessary to demonstrate the angle closure. It is divided into a complete form in which occlusion of the functional TM is present and the IOP is elevated, and an incomplete form with occlusion to a lesser extent and normal IOP.

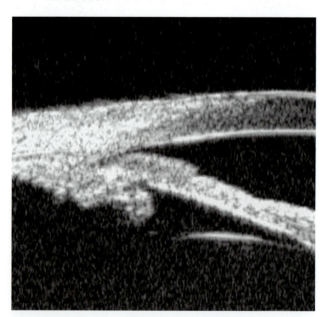

Fig. 10.58 Ultrasound biomicroscopy in plateau iris configuration shows loss of the ciliary sulcus due to anteriorly located ciliary processes

(Courtesy of J Schuman, V Christopoulos, D Dhaliwal, M Kahook and R Noecker, from 'Lens and Glaucoma', in Rapid Diagnosis in Ophthalmology, Mosby 2008)

- **Lens-induced angle-closure.** Angle closure that is predominantly lens-induced or due to a retrolenticular cause is often categorized as secondary (see below).
  ○ Includes only those cases in which a sudden change in lens volume and/or position leads to an acute or subacute IOP rise.
  ○ Usually rapid progression of lens intumescence (phacomorphic glaucoma) or anterior lens subluxation.
  ○ Virtually all pupillary block can be said to have a phacomorphic element that increases with age as the lens enlarges.
- **Retrolenticular**
  ○ Malignant glaucoma ('ciliolenticular block' – see previous).
  ○ Posterior segment causes of secondary angle closure (see below).
- **'Combined mechanism'** has been proposed as a formal label for the combination of angle-closure and open-angle elements.
- **Reduced aqueous outflow** in angle closure has been postulated to be caused by the following mechanisms in varying degree:
  ○ Appositional obstruction by the iris.
  ○ Degeneration of the TM itself due to chronic or intermittent contact with the iris or damage sustained due to elevated IOP.
  ○ Permanent occlusion of the TM by PAS; the prognosis for IOP control correlates well with the extent of PAS.

Risk factors

- **Age.** The average age of relative pupillary block is about 60 years at presentation. Non-pupillary block forms of primary angle closure tend to occur at a younger age.
- **Gender.** Females are more commonly affected than males.
- **Race.** Particularly prevalent in Far Eastern and Indian Asians; in the former non-pupillary block is relatively more significant.
- **Family history.** Genetic factors are important but poorly defined, with an increased prevalence of angle closure in family members.
- **Refraction.** Eyes with 'pure' pupillary block are typically hypermetropic, although this is not as clear-cut with non-pupillary block, which can occur in myopic eyes. Up to one in six patients with hypermetropia of one dioptre or more are primary angle closure suspects, so routine gonioscopy should be considered in all hypermetropes.
- **Axial length.** Short eyes tend to have a shallow AC (Fig. 10.59); eyes with nanophthalmos have a very short eye with a proportionally large lens and are at particular risk.

Diagnosis

Symptoms

- Most patients with angle closure are asymptomatic, including a majority of those with intermittently or chronically elevated IOP.

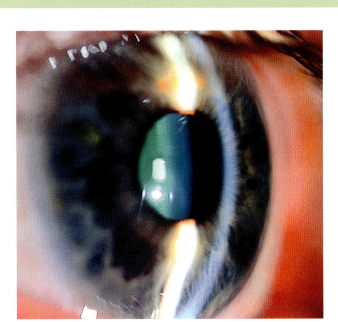

Fig. 10.59 Shallow anterior chamber

- Presentation can be with intermittent mild symptoms of blurring ('smoke-filled room') and haloes ('rainbow around lights') due to corneal epithelial oedema, or acutely with markedly decreased vision, redness and ocular/periocular pain and headache; abdominal pain and other gastrointestinal symptoms may occur.
- Precipitating factors include watching television in a darkened room, pharmacological mydriasis or rarely miosis, adoption of a semiprone position (e.g. reading), acute emotional stress and occasionally systemic medication: parasympathetic antagonists or sympathetic agonists including inhalers, motion sickness patches and cold/flu remedies (mydriatic effect), topiramate and other sulfa derivatives (ciliary body effusion).

Signs

- **Chronic presentation**
  - VA is normal unless damage is advanced.
  - The AC is usually shallower in relative pupillary block than non-pupillary block.
  - IOP elevation may be only intermittent.
  - 'Creeping' angle closure is characterized by a gradual band-like anterior advance of the apparent insertion of the iris. It starts in the deepest part of the angle and spreads circumferentially.
  - Intermittent ITC may be associated with the formation of discrete PAS, individual lesions having a pyramidal ('saw-tooth') appearance.
  - Optic nerve signs depend on the severity of damage.
- **Acute primary angle closure (APAC)**
- VA is usually 6/60 to HM.
- The IOP is usually very high (50–100 mmHg).
- Conjunctival hyperaemia with violaceous circumcorneal injection.
- Corneal epithelial oedema (Fig. 10.60A; see also Ch. 6).

- The AC is shallow, and aqueous flare is usually present.
- An unreactive mid-dilated vertically oval pupil is classic (Fig. 10.60B).
- The fellow eye typically shows an occludable angle; if not present, secondary causes should be considered.
- **Resolved APAC**
  - Early: low IOP (ciliary body shutdown and effect of intensive treatment), folds in Descemet membrane if IOP has reduced rapidly (Fig. 10.61A), optic nerve head congestion, choroidal folds.
  - Late: iris atrophy with a spiral-like configuration, glaukomflecken (white foci of necrosis in the superficial lens) and other forms of cataract, and irregular pupil due to iris sphincter/dilator damage and posterior synechiae (Fig. 10.61B); the optic nerve may be normal or exhibit varying signs of damage, including pallor and/or cupping (Fig. 10.61C).

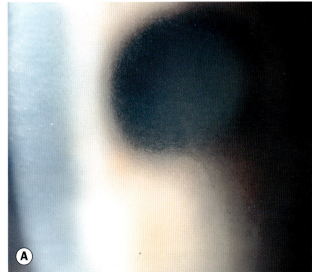

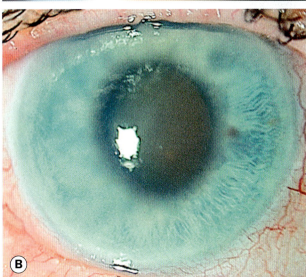

Fig. 10.60 Acute (congestive) primary angle closure. **(A)** Corneal epithelial oedema, with very numerous tiny epithelial cysts; **(B)** mid-dilated vertically oval pupil

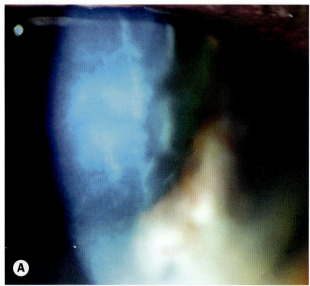

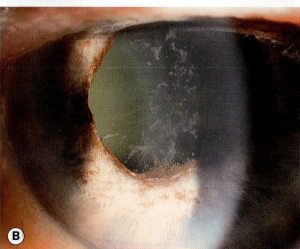

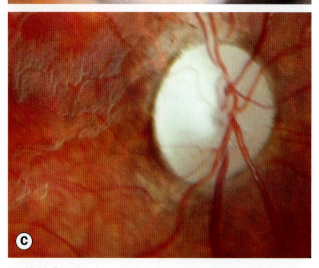

Fig. 10.61 Resolved acute primary angle closure. **(A)** Stromal corneal oedema and folds in Descemet membrane; **(B)** glaukomflecken, spiral-shaped atrophic iris, dilated pupil and posterior synechiae; **(C)** optic atrophy – combined pallor and cupping

○ The greater (i) the duration of an attack of APAC and (ii) the extent of post-APAC PAS, the lower the likelihood of IOP control with medical treatment alone.

- **Subacute angle closure** is sometimes used to describe the clinical scenario of intermittent episodes of spontaneously resolving mild/moderate APAC, usually in patients with predominant pupillary block. The clinical course may be chronic, or may culminate in a more severe/unresolving episode of APAC.

Investigation

- **Anterior segment OCT** (AS-OCT – see Fig. 10.55D), ultrasound biomicroscopy or Scheimpflug photography may be useful to supplement gonioscopic findings and for patient education.
- **Anterior chamber depth measurement** is helpful in some cases.
- **Biometry** if lens extraction is considered.
- **Posterior segment ultrasonography** in atypical cases to exclude causes of secondary angle closure.
- **Provocative testing.** This may aid decision-making in some circumstances, such as to assess the propensity to develop a steep increase in IOP with only partially opened angles post-iridotomy, and hence determine whether further intervention (e.g. iridoplasty) might be appropriate.
  ○ Pharmacological mydriasis probably discriminates poorly. It carries a small risk of precipitating APAC in susceptible patients without a patent iridotomy.
  ○ Dark room/prone provocative test (DRPPT): the patient sits in a dark room, face down for one hour without sleeping (sleep induces miosis). The IOP is checked (immediately after the test, as IOP can normalize very rapidly), and an IOP rise of 8 mmHg or more is frequently taken as being of significance; a positive result is not uncommon in normal eyes, so AS-OCT or gonioscopy without indentation should be used to confirm a compatible angle appearance. A positive response is virtually always abolished following lens extraction.

Differential diagnosis of acute IOP elevation

- **Lens-induced angle closure** due to a swollen or subluxated lens.
- **Malignant glaucoma**, especially if recent intraocular surgery.
- **Other causes of secondary angle closure**, with or without pupillary block; see below.
- **Neovascular glaucoma** may occasionally cause the sudden onset of pain and congestion.
- **Hypertensive uveitis**, e.g. iridocyclitis with trabeculitis (particularly herpetic including cytomegalovirus), glaucomatocyclitic crisis (Posner–Schlossman syndrome).
- **Scleritis** (rarely episcleritis) with or without angle closure.
- **Pigment dispersion**.
- **Pseudoexfoliation.**

- **Orbital/retro-orbital lesions** including orbital inflammation, retrobulbar haemorrhage and carotid-cavernous fistula.

Treatment

PACS

- Laser iridotomy (Fig. 10.62).
- If significant ITC persists after iridotomy, options include observation (most), laser iridoplasty, and long-term pilocarpine prophylaxis, e.g. 1% twice daily; provocative testing may be helpful in some patients. If symptomatic cataract is present, lens extraction usually definitively opens the angle. If IOP is elevated, then by definition PAC is present.

PAC and PACG

- Management is as for PACS, but with a lower threshold for further intervention if angle widening is inadequate after iridotomy, particularly if IOP remains elevated.
- Urgency and intensity of treatment, and frequency of review is tailored to the individual patient, taking into account IOP, extent of angle closure and glaucomatous damage, if present.
- Medical treatment as for POAG may be required for eyes with substantial synechial closure or with persistently elevated IOP despite an opened angle.

APAC

- **Initial treatment**
  - The patient should assume a supine position to encourage the lens to shift posteriorly under the influence of gravity.
  - Acetazolamide 500 mg is given intravenously if IOP >50 mmHg, and orally (not slow-release) if IOP is <50 mmHg.
  - If treatment is intravenous an additional oral dose of acetazolamide 500 mg may be given provided the patient is not of low body weight. Contraindications include sulfonamide allergy and angle closure secondary to topiramate/other sulfa derivatives).
  - A single dose of each of apraclonidine 0.5% or 1%, timolol 0.5%, and prednisolone 1% or dexamethasone 0.1% to the affected eye, leaving 5 minutes between each.
  - Pilocarpine 2–4% one drop to the affected eye, repeated after half an hour; one drop of 1% into the fellow eye. Some practitioners omit pilocarpine until a significant IOP fall, as when IOP is high ischaemia may compromise its action, and excessive dosing carries a toxicity risk and may exert a forward vector.
  - Analgesia and an antiemetic may be required.
- **Resistant cases**
  - Central corneal indentation with a squint hook or indentation goniolens to force aqueous into the angle; epithelial oedema can be cleared first with topical 50% glycerol to improve visualization and avoid abrasion.
  - Further pilocarpine 2–4%, timolol 0.5%, apraclonidine 1% and topical steroid.
  - Mannitol 20% 1–2 g/kg intravenously over 1 hour, oral glycerol 50% 1 g/kg, or oral isosorbide 1–1.5 g/kg, having checked for contraindications.
  - Early laser iridotomy or iridoplasty after clearing corneal oedema with glycerol.
  - Paracentesis can be performed, but carries significant risks.
  - Surgical options: peripheral iridectomy, lens extraction, goniosynechialysis, trabeculectomy and cyclodiode.
- **Subsequent medical treatment**
  - Pilocarpine 2% four times daily to the affected eye and 1% four times daily to the fellow eye.
  - Topical steroid (prednisolone 1% or dexamethasone 0.1%) four times daily if the eye is acutely inflamed.
  - Any or all of the following should be continued as necessary according to response: timolol 0.5% twice daily, apraclonidine 1% three times daily and oral acetazolamide 250 mg four times daily.

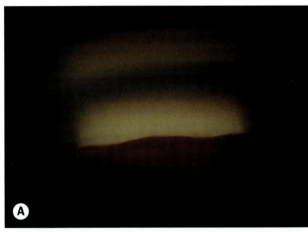

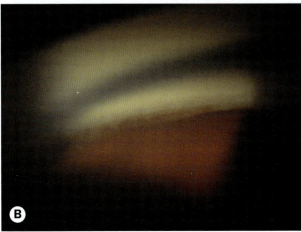

Fig. 10.62 Effect of peripheral iridotomy. **(A)** Very narrow angle before treatment; **(B)** substantially wider angle following laser – pigment smudging is present

- **Bilateral laser iridotomy** is performed once an attack has been broken, signified by a clear cornea and preferably normalized IOP. Topical steroids and any necessary hypotensives are continued for at least a week.
- **Subsequent management** is as for post-iridotomy chronic PAC/PACG. A low threshold may be adopted for cataract surgery, particularly if a significant phacomorphic element is suspected. Trabeculectomy is occasionally necessary for persistent IOP elevation despite a successfully opened angle.

CLASSIFICATION OF SECONDARY GLAUCOMA

Open-angle

Secondary open-angle glaucoma can be subdivided on the basis of the site of aqueous outflow obstruction.

- **Pre-trabecular**, in which aqueous outflow is obstructed by a membrane covering the trabeculum (Fig. 10.63A), which may consist of:
  - Fibrovascular tissue (neovascular glaucoma).
  - Endothelial cellular membranous proliferation (iridocorneal endothelial syndrome).
  - Epithelial cellular membranous proliferation (epithelial ingrowth).
- **Trabecular**, in which the obstruction occurs as a result of 'clogging up' of the meshwork (Fig. 10.63B) and secondary degenerative changes.
  - Pigment particles (pigmentary glaucoma).
  - Red blood cells (red cell glaucoma).
  - Degenerate red cells (ghost cell glaucoma).
  - Macrophages and lens proteins (phacolytic glaucoma).
  - Proteins (probably an element in hypertensive uveitis).
  - Pseudoexfoliative material (pseudoexfoliation glaucoma).
  - Trabecular glaucomas may also be caused by alteration of the trabecular fibres themselves by oedema (e.g. trabeculitis in hypertensive uveitis) or scarring (e.g. post-traumatic angle recession).
- **Post-trabecular** in which the trabeculum itself is normal but aqueous outflow is impaired as a result of elevated episcleral venous pressure.
  - Carotid-cavernous fistula.
  - Sturge–Weber syndrome.
  - Obstruction of the superior vena cava.

Angle-closure

- **With pupillary block** (Fig. 10.63C)
  - Seclusio pupillae (360° posterior synechiae), usually secondary to recurrent iridocyclitis.
  - Subluxated lens.
  - Phacomorphic glaucoma.
  - Capsular block syndrome with 360° iris–capsule adhesion in a pseudophakic eye.
  - Aphakic pupillary block.

- Anterior chamber lens implant without a patent iridotomy.
- **Without pupillary block** (Fig. 10.63D)
  - Secondary causes of PAS such as advanced neovascular glaucoma and chronic anterior uveitis.
  - Cilio-choroidal effusion.
  - Capsular block syndrome without iris–capsule adhesion.
  - Ciliary body/iris cyst or other ciliary body or posterior segment tumour.
  - Contraction of retrolenticular fibrovascular tissue such as in proliferative vitreoretinopathy and retinopathy of prematurity.
  - Malignant glaucoma (cilio-lenticular block).

PSEUDOEXFOLIATION

Introduction

Pseudoexfoliative material (PXF), the presence of which in the eye is termed pseudoexfoliation syndrome (PXS), is a common cause of secondary open-angle glaucoma, but is easily overlooked if signs are mild. It is rare before the age of 50, though after this age its prevalence increases rapidly. It is more common in women than men. The prevalence is up to 5% in many older populations but is particularly common in Scandinavia and several other areas, including parts of Africa; rates of 25% or more have been reported in members of some ethnic groups with symptomatic cataract. The incidence of glaucoma (PXG) at diagnosis of PXS is 15–30%, and the cumulative risk of eyes with PXS requiring glaucoma treatment may be as high as 60% at 5 years. It should be distinguished from true capsular exfoliation, which occurs due to chronic infrared exposure ('glassblower's cataract' – see Fig. 9.6D).

Pathogenesis

PXF is a grey-white fibrillary amyloid-like material; it may derive from abnormal extracellular matrix metabolism in ocular and other tissues. The material is deposited on various ocular structures including the lens capsule (Fig. 10.64), zonular fibres, iris, trabeculum and conjunctiva. PXF has been found in skin and visceral organs, leading to the concept of PXS as the ocular manifestation of a systemic disorder; PXS is associated with an increased prevalence of vascular disorders, hearing loss and Alzheimer disease. Plasma homocysteine tends to be higher than controls, and inadequate dietary folate intake (folate reduces homocysteine) may be a risk factor. The aetiopathogenesis is multifactorial, but in at least some populations almost all patients with PXS have certain single nucleotide polymorphisms (SNPs) in the *LOXL1* gene, which is involved in elastin fibre production. However, the SNPs are very common in the general population and most individuals with them do not develop PXS. Open-angle glaucoma associated with PXF (sometimes termed capsular glaucoma) is conventionally due to elevated IOP, likely mechanisms including trabecular obstruction by PXF and liberated iris pigment, with secondary degenerative outflow dysfunction. However, a high prevalence of glaucomatous optic neuropathy has been reported

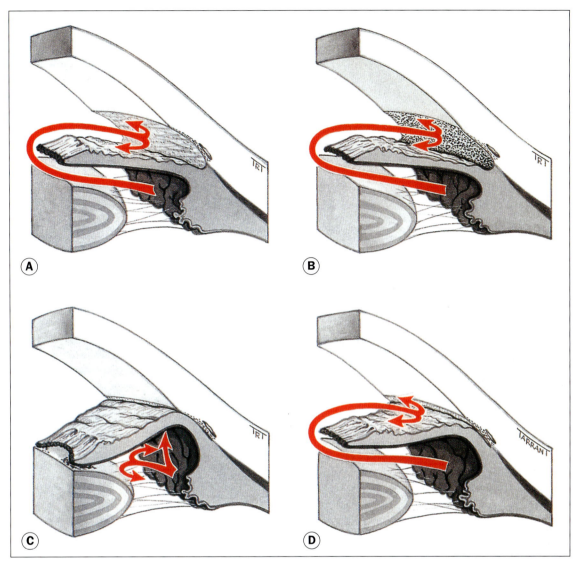

Fig. 10.63 Pathogenesis of secondary glaucoma. **(A)** Pre-trabecular obstruction; **(B)** trabecular obstruction; **(C)** angle closure with pupillary block; **(D)** angle closure without pupillary block

in eyes with visible PXF but normal IOP, and in fellow eyes of PXS with no visible PXF and apparently normal IOP. Aggressive investigation such as conjunctival biopsy will usually reveal subclinical PXF in fellow eyes.

Clinical features

- **Diagnosis** is usually incidental, though follows vision loss from advanced glaucoma more commonly than POAG.
- **Cornea.** PXF may be deposited on the endothelium, and scattered pigment deposits are common; a vertical (Krukenberg) spindle may rarely form, similar to that seen in pigment dispersion syndrome. Endothelial cell abnormalities such as low density are more common than average.
- **Anterior chamber.** PXF particles are sometimes seen; mild aqueous flare from an impaired blood–aqueous barrier is common.

- **Iris.** Granular PXF deposits (Fig. 10.65A), pupillary ruff loss and patchy transillumination defects (Figs 10.65B and C) at the pupillary margin.
- **Lens.** The anterior lens capsule typically shows a central disc and a radially indented peripheral layer of PXF material, separated by a clear zone maintained by pupillary abrasion (Fig. 10.65D). Peripheral capsular deposition is often visible only with pupillary dilatation (Fig. 10.65E). Deposits may be flaky, with scrolled edges. Cataract is more common than average. Phacodonesis (lens instability) due to zonular weakness may be present, but spontaneous subluxation is rare.
- **Anterior chamber angle.** Regular gonioscopy – at least annually in most cases – is important.
  - Patchy trabecular and Schwalbe line hyperpigmentation is common, especially inferiorly.
  - A Sampaolesi line is seen in PXF and other causes of a heavily pigmented angle: an irregular band of

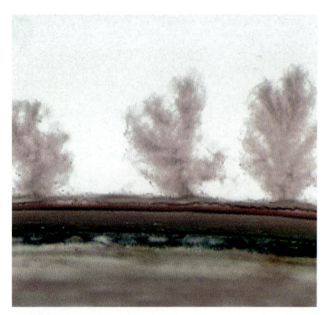

Fig. 10.64 Christmas-tree like deposits of pseudoexfoliative material on the lens capsule

(Courtesy of J Harry and G Misson, from Clinical Ophthalmic Pathology, *Butterworth-Heinemann 2001)*

pigment running on or anterior to the Schwalbe line (Fig. 10.65F).

○ Dandruff-like PXF angle deposits may be seen.

○ There is an increased risk of angle closure and of post-surgical malignant glaucoma (cilio-lenticular block), probably due to zonular laxity.

- **IOP.** In most eyes the presence of glaucomatous damage is associated with elevated IOP. The majority of patients have a chronic open-angle glaucoma that is usually unilateral at first. Occasionally the IOP may rise acutely despite a wide angle, mimicking acute angle closure.

- **Investigation** is similar to that of POAG.

- **Prognosis.** This is worse than POAG; the IOP is often higher and may exhibit marked fluctuation. Severe damage may be present at diagnosis, or can develop rapidly. It is therefore important to monitor patients closely, and it may be prudent for review in patients with PXS to take place at intervals of no more than 6 months.

Treatment

- **Medical** treatment is similar to that of POAG, but failure is more common.

- **Laser trabeculoplasty** is probably more effective than in POAG, with mean IOP reduction around 30% following SLT. Care should be taken not to apply excessive energy, as trabecular pigmentation may confer higher absorption; transient IOP spikes are not uncommon.

- **Phacoemulsification** alone may significantly lower IOP, though it may give better control combined with trabeculectomy. There is a higher risk of complications, due to poor mydriasis, increased fragility of the zonule and lens capsule, and endothelial deficiency; there is also an increased risk of a postoperative IOP spike, postoperative corneal oedema, capsular opacification, capsulorhexis contraction (capsular phimosis) and late IOL decentration or dislocation.

- **Filtration surgery** in PXG has a similar success rate to POAG.

- **Trabecular aspiration** alone seems to confer at least a short-term benefit, and can be performed at the same time as other intraocular procedures.

PIGMENT DISPERSION

Introduction

Pigment dispersion syndrome (PDS) is characterized by the liberation of pigment granules from iris pigment epithelium (IPE), and their deposition throughout the anterior segment. Secondary pigmentary glaucoma (PG) is common. PDS and PG are more common in males, particularly young myopic white men; there is also a cluster of disease in older hypermetropic black women. About a third of patients with PDS will have developed elevated IOP or glaucoma after 15 years. Although PDS is rare in black individuals, PG tends to be more severe than in whites. AD inheritance with incomplete penetrance seems to be present in at least some families; a range of genetic loci have been linked, with any genetic basis likely to be multifactorial. Myopia is a risk factor for clinical manifestation, higher degrees of myopia being associated with earlier and more severe glaucoma. Secondary pigment dispersion can occur, causes including trauma, intraocular tumour and rubbing of a malpositioned IOL on the IPE.

Pathogenesis

In primary PDS/PG, pigment shedding is precipitated by rubbing of the posterior pigment layer of the iris against the zonule as a result of excessive posterior bowing of the mid-peripheral portion of the iris (Fig. 10.66A). It is believed that an increase in anterior chamber pressure relative to the posterior chamber occurs due to reverse pupillary block, supported by the observation that peripheral iridotomy flattens the iris and decreases iridozonular contact (Fig. 10.66B). The pigment epithelium itself may be abnormally susceptible to shedding in affected individuals. Pigment shedding decreases from middle age onwards due to physiological changes resulting in decreased iridozonular contact. Acute IOP elevation can occur due to direct trabecular obstruction by shed melanin granules; chronic elevation appears to be caused by pigmentary obstruction of the intertrabecular spaces and damage to the trabeculum secondary to denudation, collapse and sclerosis. Patients with pigmentary glaucoma have an increased incidence of steroid responsiveness.

Diagnosis

- **Presentation.** PDS and PG are typically detected at a routine eye examination; the myopic patients who tend to develop the conditions are likely to be under regular optometric

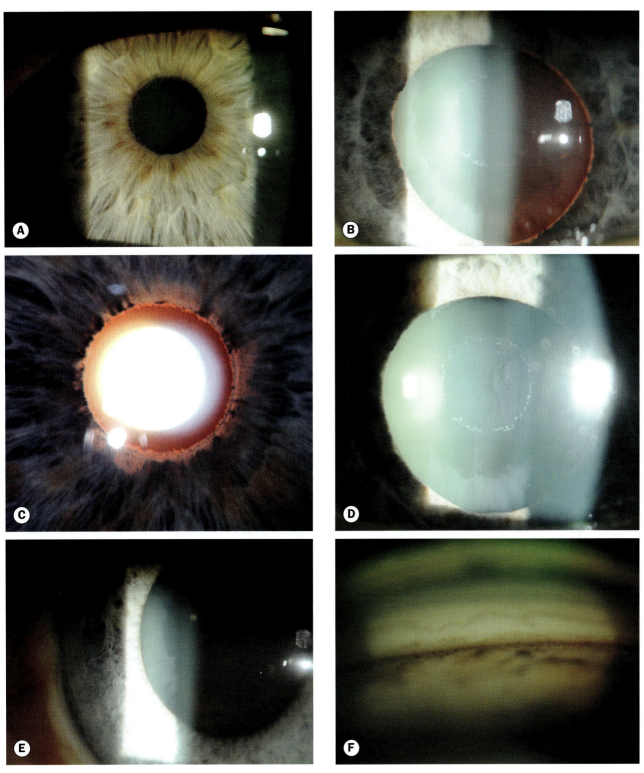

Fig. 10.65 Anterior segment signs in pseudoexfoliation syndrome. **(A)** PXF on the pupillary margin; **(B)** and **(C)** loss of the pupillary ruff and marginal transillumination defects corresponding to iris sphincter atrophy; **(D)** and **(E)** PXF on the lens; **(F)** gonioscopy shows patchy trabecular hyperpigmentation and a markedly irregular Sampaolesi line

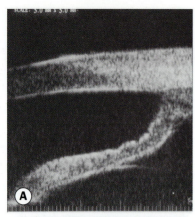
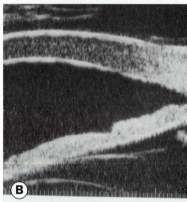

Fig. 10.66 Ultrasound biomicroscopy in pigment dispersion syndrome. **(A)** Very deep anterior chamber and posterior bowing of the peripheral iris; **(B)** flattening of the peripheral iris following laser iridotomy

(Courtesy of J Salmon)

review. Occasionally symptoms from glaucomatous visual loss lead to attendance, or from corneal oedema due to an acute IOP rise following the release of pigment granules (particularly after physical exercise). Signs of PDS are usually bilateral; they may be subtle and go undetected.

- **Cornea.** Pigment is deposited on the endothelium in a vertical spindle shape (Krukenberg spindle – Fig. 10.67A) in many patients, and its presence may mean that progression to PG is more likely. The spindle tends to shrink in long-standing cases.
- **Anterior chamber (AC).** The AC is typically deep. Melanin granules may be seen in the aqueous.
- **Iris.** Characteristic radial spoke-like transillumination defects (Fig. 10.67B) are seen in lighter, but often not in dark, irides. To best demonstrate these, the room should be minimally illuminated and a short, narrow but intense slit beam directed through the pupil; visualization may be aided by asking the patient to look up. Melanin granules may be present on the surface of the iris, usually inferiorly (Fig. 10.67C), but in extreme cases conferring a general increase in pigmentation. There may be partial loss of the pupillary ruff. The iris (and other) signs tend to lessen with age.

- **Gonioscopy.** The angle is wide in the myopic patients who constitute the majority, and there is often a characteristic mid-peripheral iris concavity where the iris bows backwards. The trabecular meshwork is heavily pigmented, with a dense homogeneous circumferential posterior meshwork band (Fig. 10.67D). Pigment may also be seen on or anterior to the Schwalbe line, forming a Sampaolesi line (see Fig. 10.65F). Pigmentation of the angle typically reduces with increasing age.
- **Lens.** Pigment granules may be deposited on the anterior surface. There may be a line (Scheie stripe) or a (Zentmayer) ring of pigment on the peripheral/equatorial surface around the zonular insertions.
- **IOP.** This may be volatile, some patients exhibiting higher levels and wider fluctuations of IOP than in POAG. Over time the control of IOP may become easier as pigment liberation decreases and occasionally the IOP may revert to normal. NTG can be erroneously diagnosed if the IOP has normalized spontaneously and the PDS signs resolved.
- **Posterior segment.** Peripheral retinal pigmentation may be seen, and lattice degeneration may be more common than in myopic patients without PDS or PG; the incidence of retinal detachment may also be higher. Glaucomatous optic neuropathy is dependent on disease stage and extent and may be markedly asymmetrical; it is common to find advanced disease in one eye and relatively mild damage in the other.

Treatment

It is important to review patients with PDS regularly – at least annually in low-risk cases – to exclude the development of raised IOP and/or glaucomatous damage.

- **Lifestyle measures.** Forms of exercise involving jolting have been associated with acute iris pigment liberation, and it may be better to avoid activities such as jogging and running up and down stairs. Pilocarpine may have a prophylactic effect in exercise.
- **Medical** treatment is similar to that of POAG. Miotics are theoretically of particular benefit because they decrease iridozonular contact in addition to facilitating aqueous outflow. However, they have the disadvantage of exacerbating myopia, and also carry a risk of precipitating retinal detachment in short-sighted eyes. They are often not tolerated well by younger patients. Topical thymoxamine, a selective alpha-adrenergic antagonist, induces miosis without causing spasm of accommodation, but is also poorly tolerated as it causes irritation.
- **Laser trabeculoplasty** is often effective. It is important not to over-treat eyes with heavily pigmented angles.
- **Laser iridotomy** has been proposed to retard pigment liberation by reversing iris concavity and eliminating iridozonular contact. It may have utility especially in patients under the age of 40 years but benefit has not been conclusively demonstrated.

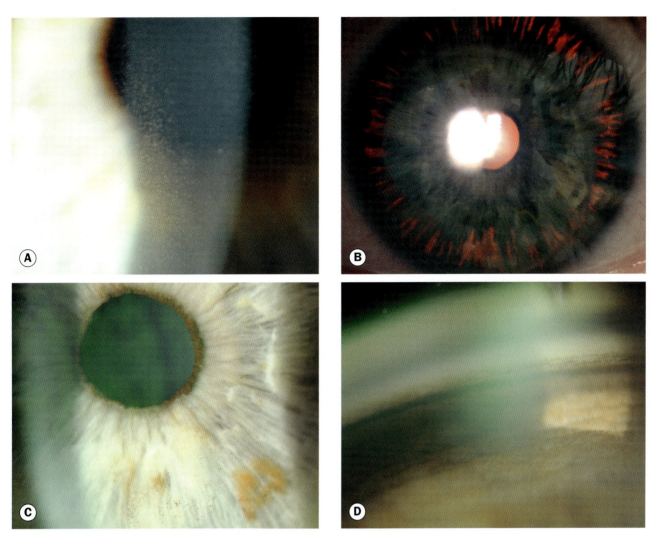

Fig. 10.67 Pigment dispersion syndrome. **(A)** Krukenberg spindle; **(B)** radial spoke-like iris transillumination defects; **(C)** pigment granules on the inferior iris surface; **(D)** homogeneous band of trabecular hyperpigmentation

- **Filtration surgery** is indicated more commonly than in POAG. The use of adjunctive antimetabolites may improve surgical outcome, particularly in younger patients in whom the risk of failure is higher. Post-surgical hypotony may be more common in young myopic eyes.

Acute bilateral iris pigment loss with raised IOP

Bilateral acute depigmentation of the iris (BADI) and bilateral acute iris transillumination (BAIT) have recently been proposed as distinct idiopathic clinical syndromes involving pigment dispersal from the iris into the anterior chamber. They are said to be more common in young to middle-aged women, occurring spontaneously or following a flu-like illness and possibly after oral antibiotic treatment, especially moxifloxacin. It is possible that the primary process is uveitic, but there is evidence that the mechanism is phototoxicity following sensitization in predisposed individuals. Presentation is usually with acute bilateral ocular redness and photophobia. Both may be associated with an IOP rise, but

this has been reported to be more severe and resistant in BAIT. Findings described in the two differ in that pigment is lost from the iris stroma in BADI and the iris pigment epithelium in BAIT, with marked iris transillumination defects and irregular mydriasis in the latter. It is possible that BADI and BAIT represent different points on a common disease spectrum. Differential diagnosis is principally from viral anterior uveitis and pigment dispersion syndrome.

NEOVASCULAR GLAUCOMA

Pathogenesis

Neovascular glaucoma (NVG) occurs as a result of aggressive iris neovascularization (rubeosis iridis). The common aetiological factor is severe, diffuse and chronic retinal ischaemia. It is postulated that hypoxic retinal tissue produces angiogenic factors in an attempt to revascularize hypoxic areas; the most important of these is probably vascular endothelial growth factor (VEGF). The mediators induce both retinal and anterior segment neovascularization, the latter initially impairing aqueous outflow in the presence of an open angle, with subsequent progression to typically severe and relentless secondary synechial angle-closure glaucoma (Fig. 10.68A).

Causes

- **Ischaemic central retinal vein occlusion** accounts for over a third of cases. Up to 50% of eyes develop NVG following ischaemic CRVO. Extensive peripheral retinal capillary non-perfusion on fluorescein angiography is a useful predictor of the risk of subsequent NVG. Glaucoma typically occurs 3 months after the occlusive event ('100-day glaucoma') but intervals from 4 weeks to 2 years have been documented.
- **Diabetes mellitus** accounts for a slightly smaller proportion. The risk of glaucoma is decreased by appropriate panretinal photocoagulation, but may be increased by cataract extraction. Pars plana vitrectomy in diabetics may precipitate NVG (7% overall in a large study), especially if angle neovascularization is present preoperatively.
- **Arterial retinal vascular disease** such as central retinal artery occlusion and ocular ischaemic syndrome are less common causes.
- **Miscellaneous** causes include intraocular tumours, long-standing retinal detachment (RD) and chronic intraocular inflammation.

Clinical features

- **Symptoms** vary from none to severe pain, decreased vision, redness and photophobia.
- **Cornea.** Elevated IOP, particularly when substantial and acute, leads to corneal oedema.
- **IOP** may be normal early in the disease process, but is frequently extremely high later on. The anterior segment will often be congested once progression to elevated IOP has occurred. In advanced disease hypotony may supervene.
- **Anterior chamber.** Flare, cells and posterior synechiae may be present, depending on severity and stage. Presentation is sometimes with anterior chamber haemorrhage (Fig. 10.68B).
- **Pupillary margin.** Subtle vessels at the pupillary margin are often an early sign (Fig. 10.68C), but may be missed unless the iris is examined carefully under high magnification. Diagnosis at this stage is likely to substantially improve the prognosis.
- **Iris surface.** New vessels grow radially over the surface of the iris towards the angle (Fig. 10.68D), sometimes joining dilated blood vessels at the collarette. At this stage the IOP may still be normal, but elevation can occur fairly acutely.
- **Gonioscopy.** Angle neovascularization may commonly occur without other signs, particularly after CRVO, and it is important to perform careful non-mydriatic gonioscopy in eyes at risk; early signs may be very subtle, even in the presence of moderate IOP elevation. Neovascular tissue

proliferates across the face of the angle, forming an obstructing fibrovascular membrane that subsequently contracts to close the angle. The angle closes circumferentially (Fig. 10.68E) leading to very high IOP, severe visual impairment, congestion of the globe and pain; the visual prognosis is generally poor by this stage, but aggressive management can achieve comfort and retain useful sight in some cases.

- **Cataract** is common once ischaemia is established (Fig. 10.68F).
- **Posterior segment.** Signs correspond to aetiology. Glaucomatous optic neuropathy may be present.
- **Investigations.** FA may be helpful in confirming aetiology and delineating ischaemia. B-scan ultrasonography will help to exclude potential causes such as RD when the posterior segment view is impaired. Anterior segment OCT has been proposed as a useful tool for angle assessment.

Treatment

It is critical to address the cause of the neovascularization as well as the elevated IOP; appropriate management of systemic disease is also key.

- **Review.** Frequent review during high-risk periods is critical: the first few months following an ischaemic CRVO, and the first few weeks following diabetic vitrectomy.
- **Medical treatment of elevated IOP** is as for POAG but miotics should be avoided, and prostaglandin derivatives used with relative caution due to their inflammation-promoting potential. Topical atropine 1% once or twice daily will resist posterior synechiae and PAS formation, and topical steroids should be given if significant inflammation is present, watching for secondary raised IOP. Steroids and atropine alone may be adequate if there is no visual potential. Topical apraclonidine and oral acetazolamide may be useful temporizing measures; acetazolamide can be associated with renal dysfunction in diabetes, especially type 1, and should be used with caution in these patients.
- **Panretinal photocoagulation (PRP)** is usually effective in inducing regression of neovascularization and, if performed early, preventing progression to glaucoma. It will not reverse an established fibrovascular membrane. The timing of PRP in CRVO is discussed in Chapter 13. If the retinal view is poor, indirect ophthalmoscopic application may provide better access, if necessary performed in the operating room with iris hooks to open a small pupil caused by posterior synechiae. Trans-scleral cryotherapy may be used in eyes with opaque media or as an adjunct for increasing peripheral retinal coverage.
- **Goniophotocoagulation.** Laser application directly to angle new vessels has been described, but has largely been supplanted by intravitreal anti-VEGF injection (see below). Photodynamic therapy to the iris and angle has also been described.
- **Intraocular VEGF inhibitors**, e.g. bevacizumab (Avastin®) at a dose of 1.25 mg in 0.05 ml, can be an effective adjunctive

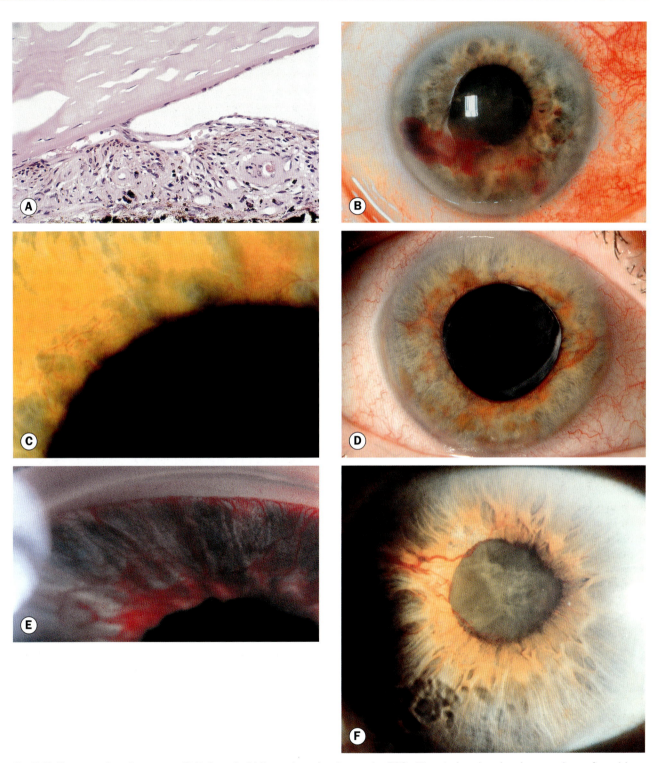

Fig. 10.68 Neovascular glaucoma. **(A)** Rubeosis iridis and angle closure by PAS; **(B)** anterior chamber haemorrhage from iris new vessels; **(C)** early pupillary margin neovascularization; **(D)** extension of new vessels across the iris surface; **(E)** progressive synechial angle closure; **(F)** cataract associated with established rubeosis iridis

(Courtesy of J Harry and G Misson, from Clinical Ophthalmic Pathology, *Butterworth-Heinemann 2001 – fig. A; C Barry – figs B and F; S Chen – figs C and D)*

measure whilst waiting for PRP to take effect, particularly if fibrovascular angle closure has not yet supervened. Intracameral (AC) injection is an alternative to the intravitreal route. The duration of control from a single injection is limited. There may be a substantial risk of CRAO in ocular ischaemic syndrome.

- **Retinal detachment repair** should be performed where this is a factor, including reattachment of a diabetic tractional detachment.
- **Ciliary body ablative procedures.** Cyclodiode or – now rarely – cyclocryotherapy should be considered if medical IOP control is not possible. These have conventionally been used only in eyes with poor visual potential, but can be employed if there is reasonable vision in order to prevent severe glaucomatous damage occurring whilst neovascularization is brought under control. Lowering a substantially raised IOP generally improves comfort, and clearing corneal oedema may facilitate an adequate retinal view for PRP. Care should be taken not to use excessive treatment, which can lead to hypotony. Endoscopic cyclophotocoagulation is an alternative to trans-scleral treatment.
- **Filtration surgery** may be considered if VA is HM or better. Options include an artificial filtering shunt (glaucoma drainage device) and trabeculectomy with mini-shunt implantation, adjunctive mitomycin C and postoperative subconjunctival 5-fluorouracil. Active neovascularization and inflammation should be controlled preoperatively (perhaps including preoperative anti-VEGF treatment) to improve the chances of surgical success; there is a relatively high risk of hypotony. Postoperative anti-inflammatory treatment should be aggressive and may include systemic steroids.
- **Pars plana vitrectomy** with peroperative endolaser at an early stage may improve the prognosis in eyes with vitreous haemorrhage, especially in CRVO. Preoperative intravitreal anti-VEGF may be of benefit.
- **Retrobulbar alcohol injection** is useful in relieving pain but may cause permanent ptosis and does not relieve congestion.
- **Enucleation** may be considered if all else fails.

INFLAMMATORY GLAUCOMA

Introduction

Overview

Elevation of IOP secondary to intraocular inflammation frequently presents a diagnostic and therapeutic challenge. The elevation of IOP may be transient and innocuous, or persistent and severely damaging. The prevalence of secondary glaucoma increases with chronicity and severity of disease. Secondary glaucoma is particularly common in Fuchs uveitis syndrome and chronic anterior uveitis associated with juvenile idiopathic

arthritis. Posterior uveitis is less likely to affect the aqueous outflow pathway and consequently less likely to lead to IOP elevation.

Diagnostic dilemmas

- **IOP fluctuation** may be dramatic in uveitic glaucoma and phasing may be helpful in patients with borderline IOP.
- **Ciliary body shutdown** caused by acute exacerbation of chronic anterior uveitis is frequently associated with lowering of IOP that may mask the underlying tendency to glaucoma. Even eyes with considerably elevated IOP (30–35 mmHg) may become hypotonous during acute exacerbations of uveitis. Return of ciliary body function with subsidence of uveitis may be associated with a rise in IOP in the presence of permanently compromised outflow facility.
- **Pathogenesis** of elevation of IOP may be uncertain; multiple mechanisms may be involved. Steroid-responders often represent a therapeutic challenge.
- **Assessment of glaucomatous damage** may be hampered by a small pupil or opacities in the media. Poor visual acuity may also compromise accurate perimetry.
- **Iris vessels** may give rise to diagnostic confusion with neovascular glaucoma.

Angle-closure glaucoma with pupillary block

Pathogenesis

Secondary angle closure is caused by posterior synechiae extending for 360° (seclusio pupillae), which obstruct aqueous flow from the posterior to the anterior chamber (Fig. 10.69A). The resultant increased pressure in the posterior chamber produces anterior bowing of the peripheral iris (iris bombé – Fig. 10.69B) resulting in shallowing of the anterior chamber and apposition of the iris to the trabeculum and peripheral cornea (Fig. 10.69C). Such an inflamed iris easily sticks to the trabeculum and the iridocorneal contact may become permanent, with the development of peripheral anterior synechiae (PAS).

Diagnosis

- **Slit lamp biomicroscopy** shows seclusio pupillae, iris bombé and a shallow anterior chamber.
- **Gonioscopy** shows angle closure from iridotrabecular contact. Indentation may be used to assess the extent of appositional as opposed to synechial angle closure.

Angle-closure glaucoma without pupillary block

- **Pathogenesis.** Chronic anterior uveitis causes the deposition of inflammatory cells and debris in the angle (Figs 10.70A and B). Subsequent organization and contraction pulls the peripheral iris over the trabeculum, causing gradual and progressive synechial angle closure (Fig. 10.70C) and

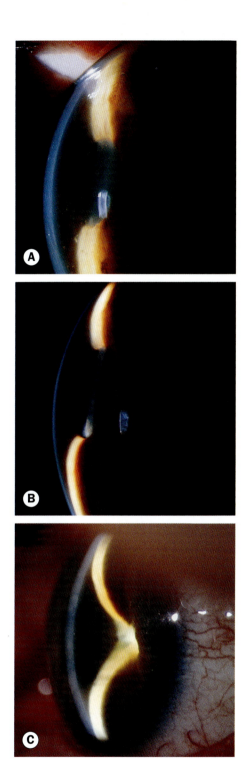

Fig. 10.69 Secondary angle closure with pupillary block.
(A) Seclusio pupillae; **(B)** iris bombé; **(C)** iridocorneal contact

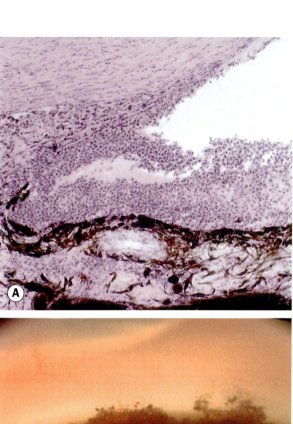

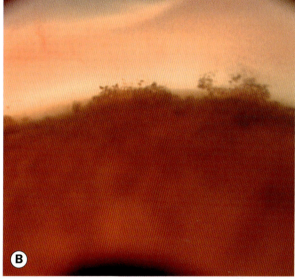

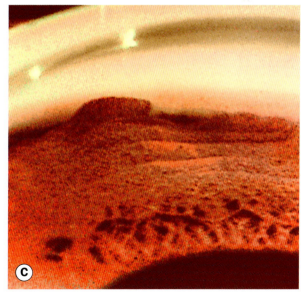

Fig. 10.70 Secondary angle closure without pupillary block.
(A) Deposition of inflammatory cells in the angle;
(B) gonioscopy showing inflammatory debris; **(C)** synechial
angle closure

*(Courtesy of J Harry and G Misson, from Clinical Ophthalmic Pathology,
Butterworth-Heinemann 2001 – fig. A)*

eventual elevation of IOP. The eye with a pre-existing narrow angle may be at higher risk.

- **Diagnosis.** The anterior chamber is deep but gonioscopy shows extensive angle closure by PAS.

Open-angle glaucoma

In acute anterior uveitis

In acute anterior uveitis the IOP is usually normal or subnormal due to concomitant ciliary shutdown. Occasionally, however, secondary open-angle glaucoma develops due to obstruction of aqueous outflow, most commonly as acute inflammation is subsiding and ciliary body function returning. This effect, which is often transient and innocuous, may be steroid-induced or caused by a combination of the following mechanisms:

- **Trabecular obstruction** by inflammatory cells and debris, which may be associated with increased aqueous viscosity due to leakage of protein from inflamed iris blood vessels.
- **Acute trabeculitis** involving inflammation and oedema of the trabecular meshwork with secondary diminution of intertrabecular porosity may result in a reduction in outflow facility. It is thought that this is especially relevant in anterior uveitis associated with herpes zoster, herpes simplex, other viral anterior uveitides and toxoplasma retinitis.

In chronic anterior uveitis

In chronic anterior uveitis the main mechanism for reduced outflow facility is thought to be trabecular scarring and/or sclerosis secondary to chronic trabeculitis. The importance of this mechanism is, however, difficult to determine as most eyes also have some degree of synechial angle closure. Because of the variable appearance of the angle on gonioscopy, definitive diagnosis of trabecular damage is difficult. In some eyes, a gelatinous exudate is seen on the trabeculum.

Treatment

Medical

- Medical control of IOP is more likely to be achieved if the angle is completely open.
- The target IOP is lower in eyes with advanced glaucomatous optic neuropathy.
- Long-acting depot steroid preparations should be used with caution, and minimized in known or suspected steroid-responders.
- The effect of ocular hypotensive drugs is less predictable in uveitis, e.g. some cases may be unexpectedly sensitive to topical carbonic anhydrase inhibitors (CAI).
- A beta-blocker is usually the drug of first choice.
- Prostaglandin derivatives should be avoided if possible as they may promote inflammation and macular oedema.

- The choice of additional agents often depends on the IOP level. If this is very high, oral acetazolamide may be required. For moderate elevation (e.g. less than 35 mmHg on a beta-blocker) in the absence of significant glaucomatous damage, an alpha-adrenergic agonist or topical CAI might be adequate.
- Miotics are contraindicated as they increase vascular permeability, and as miosis promotes the formation of posterior synechiae.

Laser iridotomy

- Laser iridotomy is performed to re-establish communication between the posterior and anterior chambers in eyes with pupillary-block angle-closure glaucoma.
- An iridotomy is likely to become occluded in the presence of active uveitis, and intensive topical steroid should be used following the laser.
- Correction of pupillary block alone may not control the IOP if there is insufficient exposed functional angle, though a patent iridotomy may retard progressive PAS formation.
- Surgical iridectomy is the definitive method of preventing further pupil block, and may be required if laser fails to maintain a viable iridotomy.

Surgery

- **Preoperative preparation**
  - Control of chronic uveitis for a minimum of 3 months before surgery is ideal but often impractical.
  - Preoperative topical steroids should be used, not only as prophylaxis against recurrent inflammation but also to reduce the conjunctival inflammatory cell population.
  - In patients with particularly labile inflammatory disease oral prednisolone should be considered (0.5 mg/kg/day).
- **Trabeculectomy with mitomycin C enhancement or glaucoma drainage device implantation** are the major options; modification of the former with an Ex-Press™ mini-shunt may improve outcomes.
  - Combined cataract and glaucoma surgery is relatively contraindicated, but may sometimes be performed in conjunction with goniosynechialysis; occasionally cataract surgery alone can be appropriate. In most cases cataract surgery should be deferred for at least 6 months after trabeculectomy.
  - Postoperative hypotony is a particular risk as a delicate balance may exist between reduced aqueous production and restricted outflow.
  - Following surgery, steroids are tapered more slowly than in non-inflammatory glaucomas.
- **Cyclodestructive** procedures should be used with caution as they may exacerbate inflammation. Possible underlying ciliary body insufficiency also carries the risk of profound hypotony that may progress to phthisis bulbi.

Posner–Schlossman syndrome (PSS)

Introduction

PSS (glaucomatocyclitic crisis) is a rare condition characterized by recurrent attacks of unilateral acute raised IOP associated with mild anterior uveitis. The mechanism is speculated to be acute trabeculitis, and there is evidence that infection, possibly cytomegalovirus (CMV) or *H. pylori*, may play a role; anterior chamber sampling for viral PCR is sometimes employed. PSS typically affects young to middle-aged adults. Males are affected more frequently than females. Episodes are unilateral, although 50% of patients have involvement of the other eye at different times. The intervals between attacks vary, but usually become longer with time. Patients should be followed even after the attacks have completely subsided, because a significant proportion will develop chronic IOP elevation, with the fellow eye also at risk.

Diagnosis

An acute IOP rise in PDS and demonstrable CMV or other viral anterior uveitis can present in an almost identical manner; the signs of the former may be atypical in older patients and those with dark irides. Simple IOP volatility in POAG, especially the juvenile variant, must also be distinguished.

- **Presentation** is with mild discomfort, haloes around lights and slight blurring of vision in one eye, and sometimes redness.
- **Slit lamp biomicroscopy** typically shows a few anterior chamber cells and one to several fine white central keratic precipitates. Injection is likely to be absent or minimal. Mild corneal epithelial oedema is frequent.
- **Mydriasis** is common; posterior synechiae are not a feature.
- **IOP** is typically raised to over 40 mmHg, out of proportion to iritis severity, and untreated persists for hours to weeks; elevation precedes the inflammatory signs.
- **Gonioscopy** shows an open angle; PAS do not form.
- **Glaucomatous optic neuropathy** is relatively uncommon in most cases. Reversible cupping has been described.

Treatment

Topical steroids are used to control inflammation, with aqueous suppressants to lower the IOP. Topical or oral non-steroidal anti-inflammatory agents may also be beneficial. The benefit of antiviral treatment is unclear.

LENS-RELATED GLAUCOMA

Phacolytic glaucoma

Introduction

Phacolytic glaucoma is a secondary open-angle glaucoma occurring in association with a hypermature cataract. Trabecular obstruction is caused by high molecular-weight lens proteins that leak through the intact capsule into the aqueous humour leading to trabecular obstruction; macrophages containing lens proteins may also contribute (Fig. 10.71A). Phacolytic glaucoma should not be confused with phacogenic (previously phacoanaphylactic) uveitis, an autoimmune granulomatous reaction to exposed lens proteins occurring with a compromised lens capsule (see Ch. 11).

Diagnosis

- **Presentation** is with pain; vision is poor due to cataract.
- **Slit lamp biomicroscopy** shows corneal oedema, a hypermature cataract and a deep anterior chamber. There may be large floating white particles in the AC, consisting of lens protein and protein-containing macrophages (Fig. 10.71B), which may impart a milky appearance to the aqueous if very dense (Fig. 10.71C), and can form a pseudohypopyon (Figs 10.71B–D).
- **Gonioscopy**, if a reasonable view can be obtained, shows an open angle with lens-derived material and inflammatory cells that are most substantial inferiorly.

Treatment

After IOP is controlled medically, proteinaceous material is washed out from the anterior chamber and the cataract is removed. Care should be taken not to rupture the zonule, which is likely to be more fragile than usual.

Phacomorphic glaucoma

Pathogenesis

Phacomorphic glaucoma is an acute secondary angle-closure glaucoma precipitated by an intumescent cataractous lens. Equatorial age-related growth of the lens slackens the suspensory ligament and allows the lens to move anteriorly. Associated anteroposterior growth leads to increased iridolenticular contact and potentiates pupillary block and iris bombé.

Diagnosis

- **Presentation** is similar to acute PACG with a shallow anterior chamber (AC) and mid-dilated pupil; cataract is evident (Fig. 10.72).
- **The fellow eye.** Phacomorphic glaucoma is more likely in eyes with a shorter axial length and shallower AC, but the fellow eye may demonstrate a deep AC and an open angle.
- **Anterior segment OCT** or US biomicroscopy may be useful.

Treatment

- **Medical** treatment is initially similar to that of acute PACG.
- **Miotics** are omitted as they tend to increase iris–lens apposition and shift the lens anteriorly; dilatation is sometimes helpful but should be implemented with caution.
- **Systemic hyperosmotic agents** may be required more commonly than in PACG.

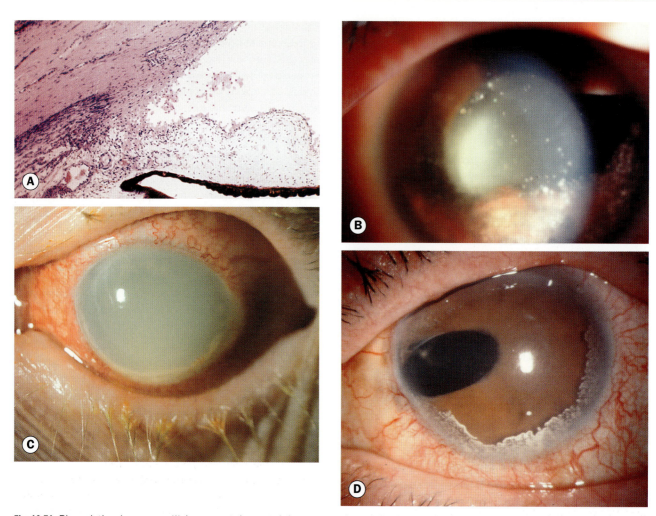

Fig. 10.71 Phacolytic glaucoma. **(A)** Lens protein-containing macrophages in the angle; **(B)** hypermature cataract, lens protein-containing macrophages floating in the aqueous, and a pseudohypopyon; **(C)** dense milky aqueous with pseudohypopyon; **(D)** mature pseudohypopyon

(Courtesy of J Harry – fig. A)

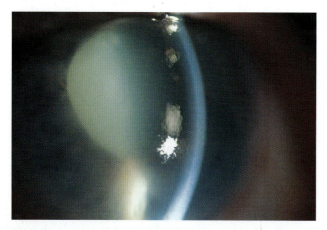

Fig. 10.72 Intumescent cataract, shallow anterior chamber, dilated pupil and corneal oedema in phacomorphic glaucoma

- **Laser iridotomy** may be worthwhile but is often not possible (due to corneal oedema or lens–cornea proximity) or ineffective. A similar procedure should be considered for the fellow eye.
- **Laser iridoplasty** may be a useful temporizing measure.
- **Cataract extraction** constitutes the definitive treatment, ideally once the IOP has been normalized and the eye is quiet; the surgery can be difficult and carries a higher risk of complications.

Pupillary block from disruption of lens position

Causes

- **Blunt ocular trauma**, even if relatively trivial, may result in lens dislocation in eyes with a weak zonule as in pseudoexfoliation and homocystinuria.

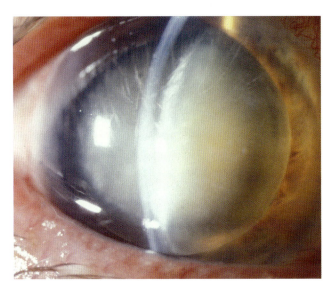

Fig. 10.73 Lens-induced pupillary block glaucoma – dislocated lens incarcerated in the pupil
(Courtesy of C Barry)

- **Congenitally small lens** (microspherophakia), e.g. Weill–Marchesani syndrome.

Dislocation may be into the AC, the zonules may be stretched or only part of the attachments may be disrupted so that the intact part acts as a hinge, and the lens may remain fully or partially in the posterior chamber. Vitreous herniation may be contributory.

Diagnosis

A lens fully or partially dislocated into the anterior chamber will usually be evident (Fig. 10.73). Acute pupillary block will cause a sudden severe elevation of IOP with associated visual impairment. Imaging such as ultrasound biomicroscopy may be diagnostic.

Treatment

The IOP is initially reduced with osmotic agents, which reduce vitreous volume. Treatment should be urgent; prolonged lenticulocorneal contact, particularly in the presence of high IOP, may cause permanent endothelial damage.

- **Initial treatment.** The patient should adopt a supine posture with the pupil dilated, to attempt to reposition the lens in the posterior chamber, following which a miotic can be used with caution. Bilateral laser iridotomy may provide extended control in some cases, but lens extraction may be necessary.
- **Definitive treatment** consists of surgical lens extraction; the approach will be dictated by the clinical situation. An anterior chamber-, iris- or sclerally fixated IOL will be necessary.

TRAUMATIC GLAUCOMA

Hyphaema

Introduction

Although most traumatic hyphaemas (see Ch. 21) are relatively small (Fig. 10.74), innocuous and transient, IOP elevation may result from trabecular obstruction by red blood cells or occasionally from angle closure due to pupillary occlusion by a blood clot. Severe and prolonged elevation of IOP may cause corneal blood staining and damage the optic nerve. The size of a hyphaema is a useful indicator of visual prognosis and risk of complications: if the entire anterior chamber is occupied by blood, eventual good vision is achieved in only about one in three eyes, though impairment is commonly due to injury sustained during the initial insult. Secondary haemorrhage, often more severe than the primary bleed, may develop within 3–5 days of the initial injury and is associated with a poorer visual outcome. Patients with sickle-cell haemoglobinopathy are at increased risk of complications, especially IOP elevation due to trabecular meshwork obstruction by deformed red cells, and vascular occlusion due to elevated IOP.

Treatment

- **General**
  - A coagulation abnormality, particularly a haemoglobinopathy, should be excluded.
  - Any current anticoagulant medication should be discontinued after liaison with a general physician to assess the risk; NSAIDs should not be used for analgesia. Likewise, specialist advice should be sought regarding the management of a patient with a haemoglobinopathy, particularly before administering high-risk medication (see below).

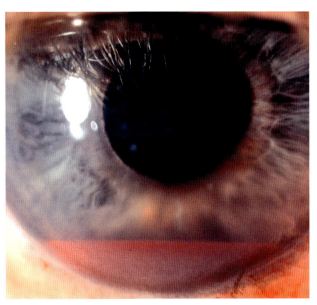

Fig. 10.74 Small hyphaema with a low risk of glaucoma

○ Hospital admission may be required for a large hyphaema.

○ Strict bed rest is probably unnecessary, but substantially limiting activity is prudent, and the patient should remain in a sitting or semi-upright posture, including during sleep.

○ A protective eye shield should be worn.

- **Medical**

○ A beta-blocker and/or a topical or systemic CAI is administered, depending on the IOP; CAI are avoided in sickle haemoglobinopathies if possible. Miotics should also be avoided as they may increase pupillary block and disrupt the blood–aqueous barrier, and prostaglandins as they may promote inflammation. Alpha-agonists can be useful, but are avoided in small children and sickling disorders.

○ Occasionally a hyperosmotic agent is needed, though as with CAI and alpha-agonists a high threshold is adopted in sickle patients.

○ Topical steroids should be used since they reduce inflammation and possibly the risk of secondary haemorrhage.

○ Atropine is recommended by some authorities to achieve constant mydriasis and reduce the chance of secondary haemorrhage, but clear evidence is lacking.

○ Antifibrinolysis with systemic aminocaproic acid (ACA) or tranexamic acid or with topical ACA may be considered under higher-risk circumstances such as recurrent bleeding.

- **Laser photocoagulation** of angle bleeding points via a gonioprism has been described, though gonioscopy should probably be deferred for 5–6 days post-injury.

- **Surgical evacuation** of blood is required in around 5%. If a total hyphaema or persistently intolerable IOP lasts for more than 5 days surgery should be considered to reduce the risk of permanent corneal staining (rare) and optic atrophy, and to prevent the occult development of peripheral anterior synechiae and chronic secondary glaucoma; a lower threshold is required in haemoglobinopathy patients (even moderate pressure elevation can lead to optic atrophy), patients with prior glaucomatous optic neuropathy and in young children with a risk of amblyopia. A glaucoma filtration procedure may be necessary in some cases. A bleeding point should be cauterized if possible.

- **On discharge** the patient should be advised to avoid any activity with a risk of even minor eye trauma for several weeks; symptoms of a rebleed should prompt immediate review.

Angle recession glaucoma

Introduction

Angle recession involves rupture of the face of the ciliary body, the portion between the iris root and the scleral spur, due to blunt trauma. Although a large percentage of eyes with traumatic hyphaema exhibit some degree of angle recession, glaucoma only develops in fewer than 10% after 10 years. The rise in IOP is secondary to associated trabecular damage rather than from angle recession itself; but the risk of glaucoma is directly related to the extent of angle recession.

Diagnosis

- **Presentation** is with unilateral chronic glaucoma.

- **Slit lamp examination** may show signs of previous blunt trauma; these may be mild, such as a small sphincter rupture.

- **Gonioscopy** may initially reveal irregular widening of the ciliary body face (Fig. 10.75A). In long-standing cases, the

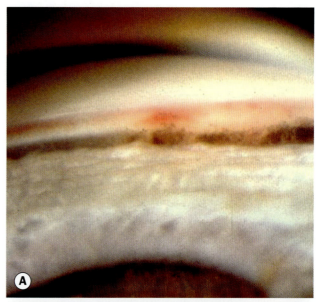

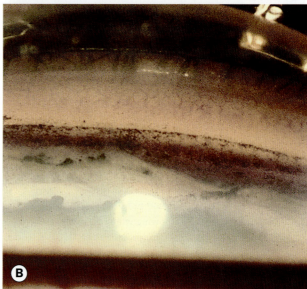

Fig. 10.75 **(A)** Angle recession; **(B)** old angle recession with hyperpigmentation
(Courtesy of R Curtis – fig. A)

cleft may become obscured by fibrosis and the angle may show hyperpigmentation (Fig. 10.75B).

Treatment

- **Long-term regular review** of patients at risk is required.
- **Medical** treatment is as for other types of secondary open-angle glaucoma but is frequently unsatisfactory; laser trabeculoplasty is likely to be of little benefit.
- **Trabeculectomy** with adjunctive antimetabolite is generally effective.
- **An artificial filtering shunt or cyclodiode** should be considered if trabeculectomy fails.

IRIDOCORNEAL ENDOTHELIAL SYNDROME

Introduction

Iridocorneal endothelial (ICE) syndrome typically affects one eye of a middle-aged woman. It consists of the following three clinical presentations: Chandler syndrome, progressive (also termed essential) iris atrophy and iris naevus (Cogan–Reese) syndrome. The pathological basis in all three is an abnormal corneal endothelial cell layer with a predilection for proliferation and migration across the anterior chamber angle and onto the surface of the iris, with subsequent progression to glaucoma (50%) and corneal decompensation in a substantial proportion of involved eyes. Glaucoma is due to trabecular obstruction by proliferating tissue followed by angle closure secondary to contraction. PCR shows the presence of herpes simplex virus DNA in a substantial percentage of ICE syndrome corneal specimens, suggesting a possible viral aetiology.

Diagnosis

Clear differentiation between the three presentations may be difficult; apparent transition from one to another has been reported. Differentiation depends primarily on iris appearance, but there is often substantial overlap. Gonioscopically visible changes in some patients may be subtle despite elevated IOP, particularly in early disease. The specular microscopic appearance is characteristic.

- **Chandler syndrome** is the most common clinical presentation and is characterized by an abnormal corneal endothelial appearance said to resemble hammered silver (Fig. 10.76A). It frequently presents with blurred vision and haloes due to corneal oedema (Fig. 10.76B). Iris atrophy is absent in about 60% and in the remainder is variable in severity; corectopia is mild to moderate when present. When glaucoma occurs it is usually less severe than in the other two presentations.
- **Progressive (essential) iris atrophy** is characterized by severe iris changes including corectopia (pupil malposition – Fig. 10.77A), pseudopolycoria (supernumerary false pupil – Fig. 10.77B), ectropion uveae, iris atrophy of varying severity

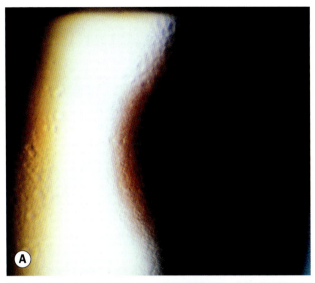

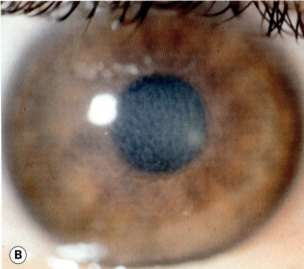

Fig. 10.76 Chandler syndrome. **(A)** 'Hammered silver' endothelial changes; **(B)** corneal oedema due to endothelial decompensation
(Courtesy of J McAllister – fig. B)

(Figs 10.77C–E) and broad-based PAS that often extend anterior to the Schwalbe line (Fig. 10.77F).
- **Iris naevus (Cogan–Reese) syndrome** is characterized by either a diffuse naevus that covers the anterior iris, or by iris nodules (Fig. 10.78). Iris atrophy is absent in 50% of cases and in the remainder it is usually mild to moderate, although corectopia may be severe. The appearance may be mimicked by a diffuse iris melanoma.

Treatment

- **Medical** treatment of glaucoma is often ineffective in the longer term.

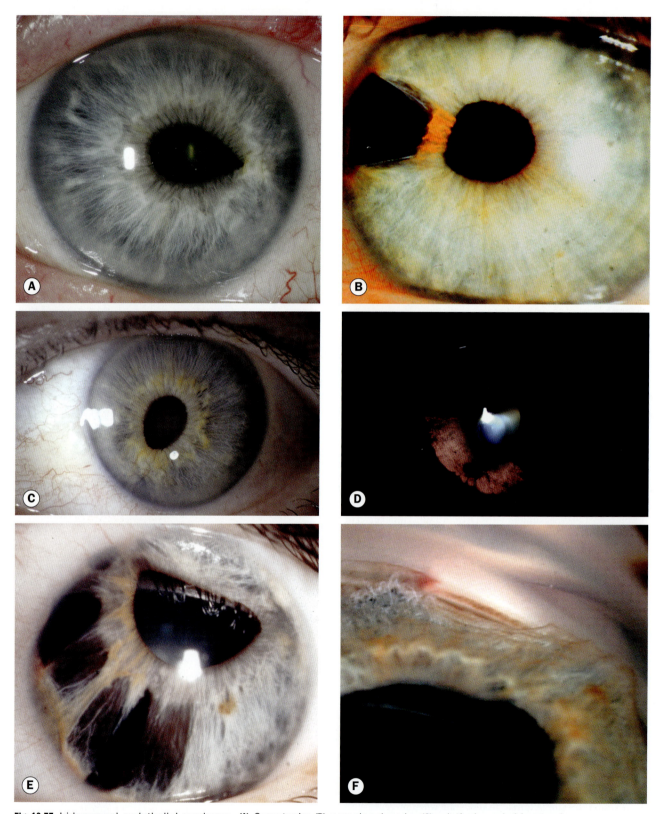

Fig. 10.77 Iridocorneal endothelial syndrome. **(A)** Corectopia; **(B)** pseudopolycoria; **(C)** relatively early iris atrophy; **(D)** transillumination of the eye in (C); **(E)** marked iris atrophy; **(F)** broad peripheral anterior synechiae

(Courtesy of C Barry – figs A, C and D; L MacKeen – fig. F)

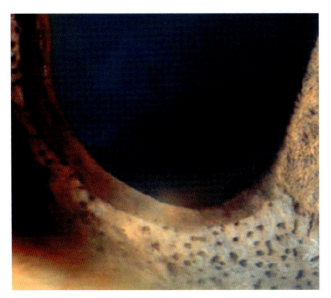

Fig. 10.78 Iris nodules in Cogan–Reese syndrome
(Courtesy of R Martincova)

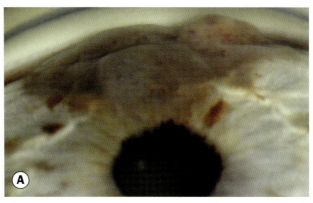

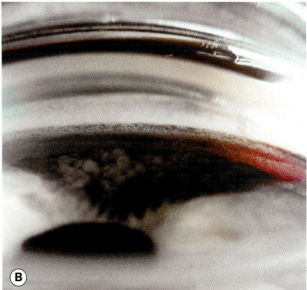

- **Trabeculectomy** with mitomycin C is frequently unsuccessful; the Ex-Press™ mini-shunt may afford a better prognosis.
- **Glaucoma drainage device or cyclodiode** is eventually required in many cases.
- **Corneal treatment.** Oedema can be treated with topical hypertonic saline in early disease and transplantation later on.

GLAUCOMA ASSOCIATED WITH INTRAOCULAR TUMOURS

Approximately 5% of eyes with intraocular tumours develop a secondary elevation of IOP. Potential mechanisms are set out below:

- **Trabecular block.** Distinction between different mechanisms may not be possible clinically.
  - ○ Angle invasion by a solid iris melanoma (Fig. 10.79A).
  - ○ Trabecular infiltration by neoplastic cells originating from an iris melanoma (Fig. 10.79B). Rarely, tumour seeding from a retinoblastoma may also invade the trabeculum.
  - ○ Melanomalytic glaucoma may occur in some eyes with iris melanoma; it is due to trabecular blockage by macrophages that have ingested pigment and tumour cells, similar to phacolytic glaucoma (Fig. 10.79C).
- **Secondary angle closure**
  - ○ Neovascular glaucoma is the most common mechanism in eyes with choroidal melanoma or retinoblastoma.
  - ○ Anterior displacement of iris–lens diaphragm may occur in an eye with a ciliary body melanoma or a large tumour of the posterior segment.

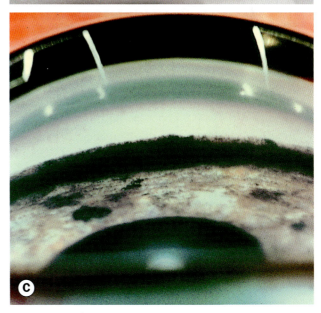

Fig. 10.79 Glaucoma secondary to intraocular melanoma. **(A)** Angle invasion by a solid iris melanoma; **(B)** melanoma cells infiltrating the trabeculum; **(C)** melanomalytic glaucoma
(Courtesy of J Harry – fig. B; R Curtis – fig. C)

GLAUCOMA SECONDARY TO EPITHELIAL INGROWTH

Introduction

Epithelial ingrowth (downgrowth) is a rare but potentially blinding complication of anterior segment surgery or trauma, occurring when conjunctival or corneal epithelial cells migrate through a wound and proliferate in the anterior segment (Fig. 10.80A). Elevation of IOP is due to trabecular obstruction by one or more of an epithelial membrane, secondary synechial angle closure, and desquamated epithelial and inflammatory cells. The associated glaucoma can be particularly intractable and the prognosis poor.

Diagnosis

- Persistent postoperative anterior uveitis.
- Diffuse epithelialization characterized by a greyish translucent membrane with a scalloped border that involves the posterior corneal surface in the area of a surgical or traumatic wound (Fig. 10.80B).
- Cystic and fibrous proliferative patterns sometimes occur, and tend to have a better prognosis.
- Pupillary distortion.

Treatment

The aim of treatment is the eradication of all invading epithelium to avoid recurrence.

- **Block excision** involves the simultaneous excision of adjacent iris and pars plicata of the ciliary body, together with all layers of the sclera and cornea in contact with the lesion. The resultant defect is covered with a tectonic corneoscleral graft. The area of iris involvement may be delineated by applying argon laser burns, which will cause whitening of the affected area.
- **Cryotherapy** may be applied trans-sclerally to devitalize the epithelium remaining on the posterior surface of the cornea, in the angle and on the ciliary body. Intraocular air is used to insulate other tissues from the effects of the cryotherapy.
- **5-fluorouracil.** Favourable results have been reported with a novel technique using intracameral 5-fluorouracil.
- **Glaucoma drainage devices** are of value for medically uncontrolled glaucoma associated with extensive epithelial ingrowth unsuitable for surgical excision. Antimetabolite-enhanced trabeculectomy with mini-shunt implantation is an alternative.

IRIDOSCHISIS

Iridoschisis is a rare condition typically affecting both eyes of an older patient; glaucoma, particularly angle-closure, is associated in up to 90%. The mechanism is incompletely understood, but it has been proposed that in many cases intermittent substantial elevation of IOP results in iris atrophy, with severity ranging from stromal atrophy to fibrillar disintegration of the anterior layer; changes are more marked inferiorly (Fig. 10.81). The anterior

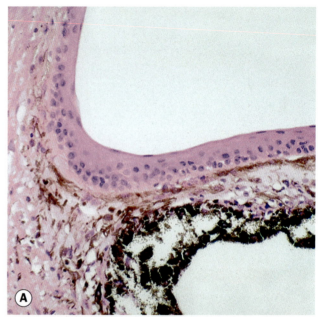

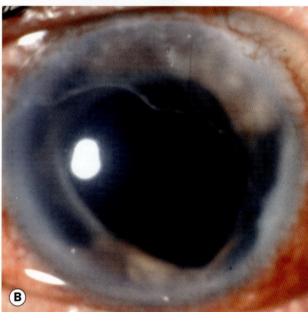

Fig. 10.80 Diffuse epithelial ingrowth. **(A)** Stratified squamous epithelium lining the anterior iris surface and filtration angle; **(B)** translucent membrane with a scalloped border involving the posterior corneal surface
(Courtesy of J Harry and G Misson, from Clinical Ophthalmic Pathology, Butterworth-Heinemann 2001 – fig. A)

chamber is typically shallow. Gonioscopy commonly shows an occludable angle, often with PAS. Angle closure is treated if present, with a laser iridotomy initially.

PRIMARY CONGENITAL GLAUCOMA

Introduction

Primary congenital glaucoma (PCG) is rare, with an incidence of 1:10 000 in many populations; boys are more commonly affected

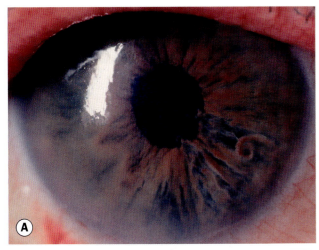

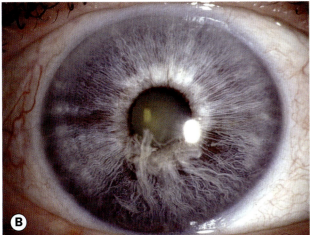

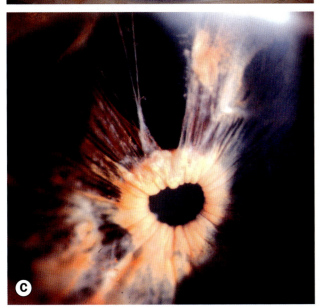

Fig. 10.81 Iridoschisis. **(A)** Mild; **(B)** moderate; **(C)** severe
(Courtesy of R Bates – fig. A; S Chen – fig. B)

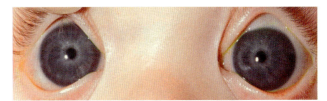

Fig. 10.82 Bilateral buphthalmos
(Courtesy of C Barry)

in most surveys. Involvement is more often bilateral, but frequently asymmetrical. It can be classified as follows:

- **True congenital glaucoma** (40%) in which IOP is elevated during intrauterine life.
- **Infantile glaucoma** (55%) which manifests prior to age 3.
- **Juvenile glaucoma**, the least common, in which IOP rises between 3 and 16 years of age.

PCG, by definition unassociated with other major ocular abnormalities, is thought to be caused by impaired aqueous outflow due to maldevelopment of the anterior chamber angle (trabeculodysgenesis). It is usually sporadic, but approximately 10% are AR with variable penetrance. Several genes have been implicated, prominently *CYP1B1*. The prognosis is dependent on severity and age at onset/diagnosis; in true congenital glaucoma, legal blindness is the outcome in at least 50% of eyes. Secondary infantile glaucoma can be caused by a range of conditions including tumours such as retinoblastoma, persistent fetal vasculature (persistent hyperplastic primary vitreous) and uveitis.

Diagnosis

- **Presentation** usually occurs when an abnormality such as corneal haze, large (buphthalmos – see below) or asymmetrical eyes (Fig. 10.82), watering, photophobia or blepharospasm (Fig. 10.83) is noticed by parents or a health professional.

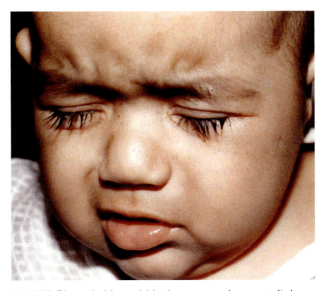

Fig. 10.83 Photophobia and blepharospasm in congenital glaucoma
(Courtesy of U Raina)

- **Corneal haze** (Fig. 10.84A) is due to diffuse oedema secondary to raised IOP, or localized oedema due to breaks in Descemet membrane.
- **Buphthalmos** (Fig. 10.84B) is a large eye as a result of stretching due to elevated IOP prior to the age of 3 years. The thinned sclera often appears blue due to increased visualization of the underlying uvea. Complications include myopia and lens subluxation.
- **Haab striae** (Fig. 10.84C) are curvilinear healed breaks in Descemet membrane.
- **Corneal scarring and vascularization** (Fig. 10.84D).
- **Optic disc cupping** in infants may regress once IOP is normalized. Most normal infants exhibit no apparent cup.
- **Evaluation under general anaesthesia** is generally required; intravenous ketamine lowers IOP less than other agents.
  - ○ IOP measurement should be performed first, optimally with more than one method (e.g. Perkins, Tono-Pen, iCare). It is preferable where possible for this to be measured in a conscious or sedated child; 10–12 mmHg is normal.
  - ○ Anterior chamber examination with an operating microscope and/or portable slit lamp.
  - ○ Optic disc examination; asymmetry or a cup/disc ratio of >0.3 is suspicious.
  - ○ Corneal diameter measurement; >12 mm prior to the age of one year is highly suspicious.
  - ○ Gonioscopy using a direct goniolens may be normal or reveal trabeculodysgenesis, vaguely characterized by an anteriorly located iris insertion and a hypoplastic-appearing peripheral iris (Fig. 10.85). An older concept of a discrete (Barkan) membrane has not been definitively confirmed.
  - ○ Refraction.

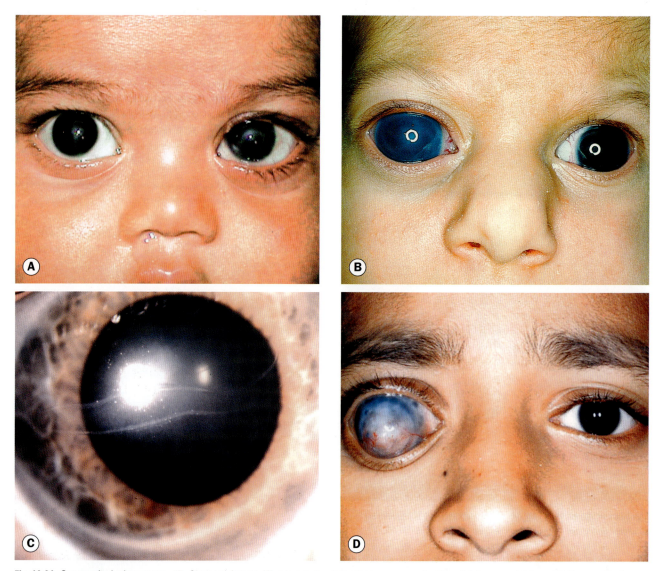

Fig. 10.84 Congenital glaucoma. **(A)** Corneal haze; **(B)** severe buphthalmos, worse in the right eye, which exhibits marked diffuse corneal oedema; **(C)** Haab striae; **(D)** corneal scarring and vascularization

(Courtesy of M Parulekar – fig. A; U Raina – fig. D)

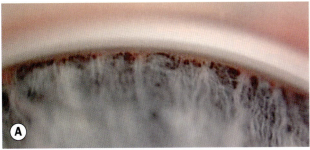

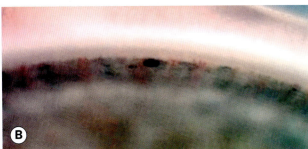

Fig. 10.85 (A) Normal infant angle shows the iris root, prominent ciliary body band but no discernible scleral spur and trabeculum; **(B)** one angle variant in congenital glaucoma shows the iris root but not the ciliary body band due to translucent amorphous tissue that obscures the trabeculum

(Courtesy of K Nischal)

Treatment

Management is essentially surgical; angle surgery alone is successful in 80–90%. Medication may be used as temporary or supplementary therapy; caution is required with selection of medication in young children, as most are relatively contraindicated.

- **Goniotomy.** Under direct gonioscopic visualization, an incision is made at the midpoint of the trabecular meshwork (Fig. 10.86).

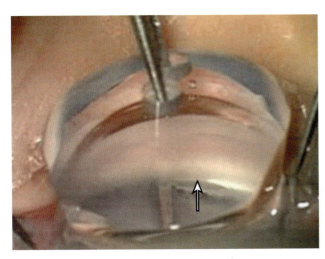

Fig. 10.86 Goniotomy – arrow shows the cleft
(Courtesy of K Nischal)

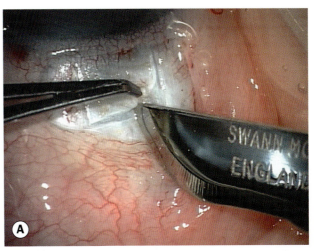

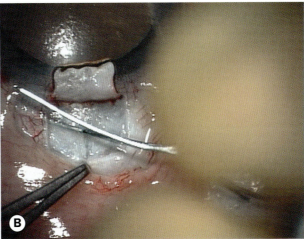

Fig. 10.87 Trabeculotomy (see text)
(Courtesy of K Nischal)

- **Trabeculotomy** may be necessary if corneal clouding prevents an adequate view of the angle, and is also an option when repeated goniotomy has failed. A partial-thickness scleral flap is created (Fig. 10.87A), and a trabeculotome (Fig. 10.87B) inserted into the Schlemm canal and rotated into the anterior chamber.
- **Other procedures** when angle surgery fails include trabeculectomy, tube shunt implantation and ciliary body ablative procedures.
- **Monitoring** of IOP, corneal diameter and other parameters is required long term.
- **Amblyopia and refractive error** should be managed aggressively.

Differential diagnosis

- **Cloudy cornea**
  - Birth trauma.
  - Rubella keratitis; congenital rubella is also associated with congenital glaucoma.
  - Metabolic disorders such as mucopolysaccharidoses and mucolipidoses.

- ○ Congenital hereditary endothelial dystrophy.
- ○ Sclerocornea.
- **Large cornea**
  - ○ Megalocornea.
  - ○ High myopia.
- **Epiphora**
  - ○ Delayed/failed canalization of the nasolacrimal duct.
  - ○ Lacrimation secondary to ocular irritation, e.g. conjunctivitis, aberrant eyelashes, entropion.

IRIDOCORNEAL DYSGENESIS

Posterior embryotoxon

Posterior embryotoxon refers to a prominent and anteriorly displaced Schwalbe line, seen as a thin grey-white arcuate ridge adjacent to the limbus on the inner surface of the cornea (Fig. 10.88A). It is an innocuous isolated finding in up to 15% of the general population, but is one of the features of Axenfeld–Rieger anomaly; it is seen as well in the multisystem genetic disorder Alagille syndrome, in which optic disc drusen are also common.

Axenfeld–Rieger syndrome

Introduction

Axenfeld–Rieger syndrome is the umbrella term for a spectrum of disorders featuring bilateral developmental ocular anomalies: Axenfeld anomaly, Rieger anomaly and Rieger syndrome. It is caused by defective neural crest cell-related processes during fetal development; an abnormal endothelial cell membrane has been identified on anterior segment structures in some patients. The key implication of the syndrome is a 50% risk of glaucoma. Associated variants in several different genes have been found, including *PITX2, PAX6, FOXC1* and *RIEG2*; that is, different genetic abnormalities can give a similar clinical picture. Cases may be sporadic, but a family history is common, when inheritance is autosomal dominant with variable expressivity but very high penetrance. There is no gender predilection.

Clinical features

- **Axenfeld anomaly** is characterized by posterior embryotoxon (see Fig. 10.88A) with attached strands of peripheral iris, the latter best viewed with gonioscopy (Figs 10.88B and C).
- **Rieger anomaly** often manifests with an anterior segment appearance similar to that of iridocorneal endothelial (ICE) syndrome.
  - ○ Posterior embryotoxon.
  - ○ Iris stromal hypoplasia (Figs 10.89A and B).
  - ○ Ectropion uveae (Fig. 10.89C).
  - ○ Corectopia and full-thickness iris defects (Fig. 10.89D).

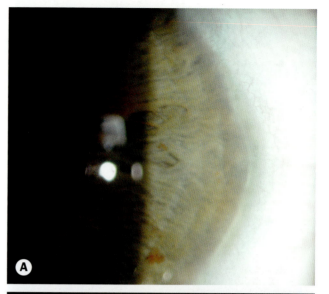

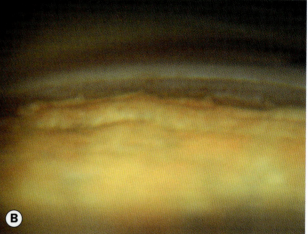

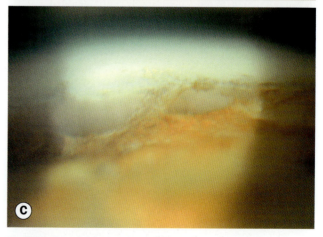

Fig. 10.88 Axenfeld anomaly. **(A)** Posterior embryotoxon; **(B)** and **(C)** gonioscopy showing strands of peripheral iris tissue extending to the cornea
(Courtesy of Y Kerdraon)

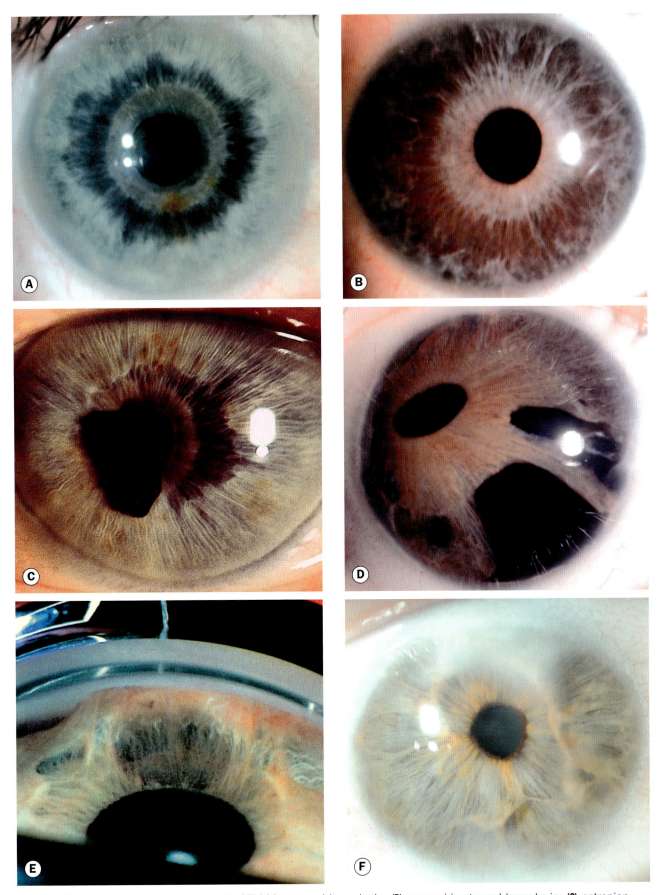

Fig. 10.89 Rieger anomaly and syndrome. **(A)** Mild iris stromal hypoplasia; **(B)** severe iris stromal hypoplasia; **(C)** ectropion uveae; **(D)** corectopia and full-thickness iris defects – pseudopolycoria; **(E)** peripheral anterior synechiae; **(F)** iris adhesion to anterior cornea

(Courtesy of Y Kerdraon – fig. F)

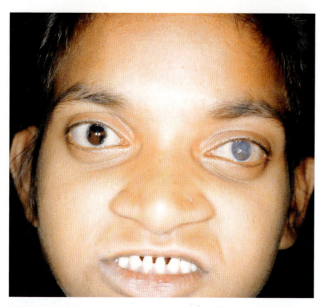

Fig. 10.90 Facial and dental anomalies in Rieger syndrome
(Courtesy of U Raina)

- **Gonioscopy** in mild cases shows the Axenfeld anomaly. In severe cases, broad leaves of iris adhere to the cornea anterior to the Schwalbe line (Figs 10.89E and F).
- **Glaucoma** develops in about 50%, usually during childhood or early adulthood. Surgical management is often necessary.
- **Rieger syndrome** is characterized by the Rieger anomaly together with extraocular malformations that, as with the ocular features, are caused by defective neural crest cell-related tissue development (Fig. 10.90):
  ○ Dental anomalies: hypodontia (few teeth) and microdontia (small teeth).
  ○ Facial anomalies: maxillary hypoplasia, broad nasal bridge, telecanthus and hypertelorism.
  ○ Other anomalies include redundant paraumbilical skin and hypospadias. Hearing loss, hydrocephalus, cardiac and renal anomalies and congenital hip dislocation are rare.

Peters anomaly

Introduction

Peters anomaly is a rare but often severe condition that is bilateral in more than half of cases. It is the result of defective neural crest cell migration during fetal development. Manifestations range from mild to severe. Most cases are sporadic, although autosomal recessive inheritance has been described.

Clinical features

Peters type I affects the cornea alone, type II shows both corneal and lens abnormalities.

- **Central corneal opacity** of variable density (Fig. 10.91A).

- **Posterior corneal defect** involving the posterior stroma, Descemet membrane and endothelium with or without iridocorneal (Fig. 10.91B) or lenticulocorneal (Fig. 10.91C) adhesions.
- **Glaucoma** occurs in about 50% due to associated angle anomaly. Onset is usually in infancy but occasionally in childhood or later. The prognosis tends to be worse than in primary congenital glaucoma.
- **Systemic associations** including craniofacial and central nervous system anomalies have been reported. 'Peters plus' syndrome includes a particular constellation of systemic abnormalities.

Aniridia

Genetics

Aniridia (AN) is a rare bilateral condition that may have life-threatening associations. It occurs as a result of abnormal neuro-ectodermal development secondary to a mutation in the *PAX6* gene. *PAX6* is adjacent to gene *WT1*, mutation of which predisposes to Wilms tumour.

- **Autosomal dominant** aniridia accounts for about two-thirds of cases and has no systemic implications. Penetrance is complete (all patients with the genotype will have the phenotype) but expressivity (severity) is variable.
- **Sporadic**, including WARG, previously known as Miller, syndrome (Wilms tumour, Aniridia, mental Retardation, Genitourinary abnormalities), includes about a third of patients. Children with sporadic aniridia have about a 30% chance of developing Wilms tumour.
- **Gillespie syndrome** accounts for only about 1% of cases. Inheritance is AR but is not caused by *PAX6* mutations. Cerebellar ataxia and mental handicap are features.

Diagnosis

All patients with sporadic aniridia should have abdominal ultrasonography every 3 months until 5 years of age, every 6 months until 10 years of age and annually until 16 years of age to detect the development of Wilms tumour or until molecular genetic analysis confirms the absence of a *WT1* mutation.

- **Presentation** is typically at birth with nystagmus and photophobia. The parents may have noticed the absence of irides or apparently large pupils.
- **Aniridia** is variable in severity, ranging from minimal, detectable only by retroillumination, to total absence (Figs 10.92A and B).
- **Lids** often show meibomian gland dysfunction.
- **Cornea**
  ○ Tear film instability, dry eye and epithelial defects are common.
  ○ Limbal stem cell deficiency may result in 'conjunctivalization' of the peripheral cornea.

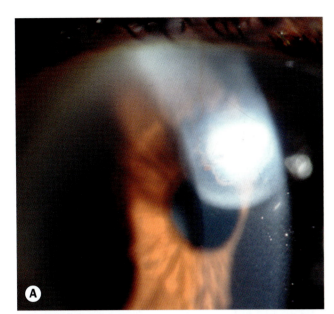

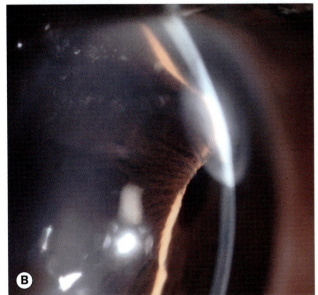

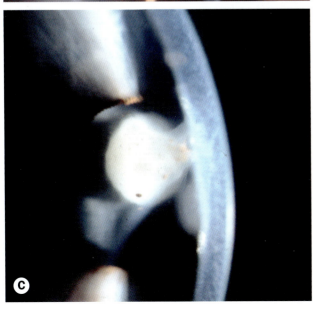

Fig. 10.91 Peters anomaly. **(A)** Corneal opacity; **(B)** iridocorneal adhesion; **(C)** lenticulocorneal adhesion

○ Total corneal central stromal scarring and vascularization may occur in end-stage disease.
- **Lens** changes can include cataract (Fig. 10.92C) and subluxation (usually superiorly – Fig. 10.92D).
- **Fundus.** Possible abnormalities include foveal (Fig. 10.92E) and/or optic nerve hypoplasia and choroidal coloboma.
- **Gonioscopy** even in eyes with apparently total aniridia usually shows a hypoplastic or rudimentary frill of iris tissue (Fig. 10.93A).
- **Glaucoma** (75%) usually presents in late childhood or adolescence. It is caused by synechial angle closure secondary to the contraction of rudimentary iris tissue (Fig. 10.93B). Treatment is difficult and the prognosis guarded.

Treatment

- **Glaucoma**
  ○ Medical treatment is usually inadequate in the longer term.
  ○ Goniotomy may be helpful if performed before the development of irreversible angle closure.
  ○ Trabeculectomy or combined trabeculectomy–trabeculotomy may be successful; an antimetabolite and a mini-shunt may be utilized.
  ○ Glaucoma drainage devices may be effective.
  ○ Diode laser cycloablation may be necessary if other modalities fail.
- **Painted contact lenses** may be used to create an artificial pupil and improve both vision and cosmesis; simple tinted lenses are an alternative; both may improve nystagmus.
- **Lubricants** are frequently required for associated keratopathy.
- **Cataract surgery** is often required; a tinted artificial lens implant may be used to try to improve photophobia. Trauma to the corneal limbus should be minimized in order to preserve stem cell function.
- **Prosthetic iris implantation** has been described in pseudophakic aniridic eyes, but may be complicated by, or worsen, glaucoma.
- **Limbal stem cell transplantation** with or without keratoplasty may be required.
- **Refractive errors, amblyopia and squint** should be managed aggressively.

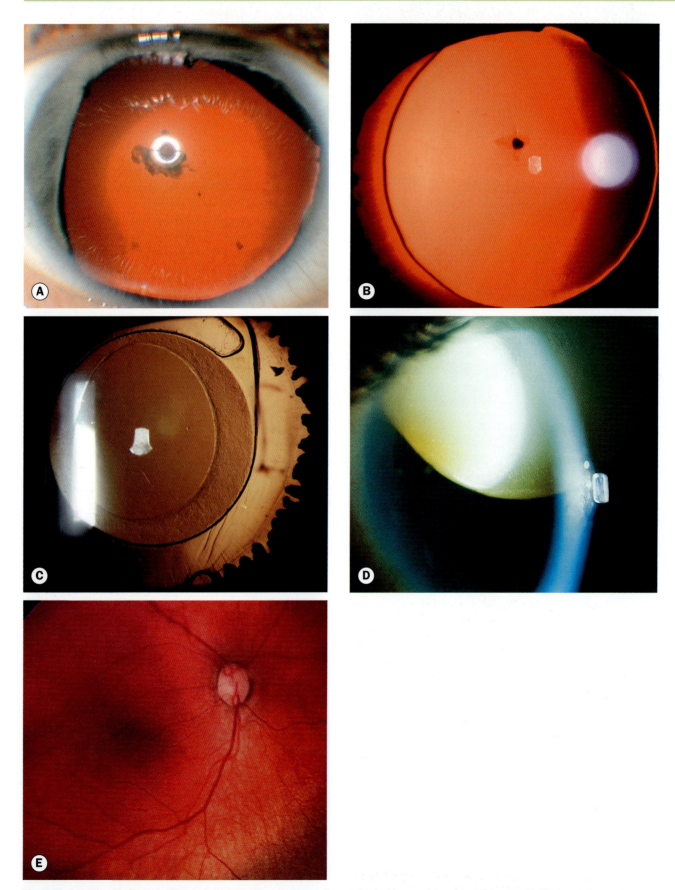

Fig. 10.92 Aniridia. **(A)** Partial; **(B)** total; **(C)** transillumination of pseudophakic eye showing silhouetted ciliary processes; **(D)** superior subluxation of cataractous lens; **(E)** foveal hypoplasia

(Courtesy of L MacKeen – fig. D)

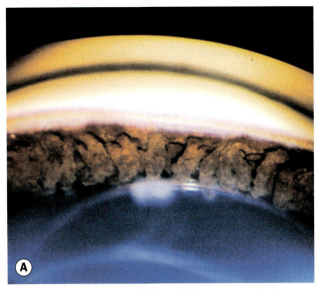

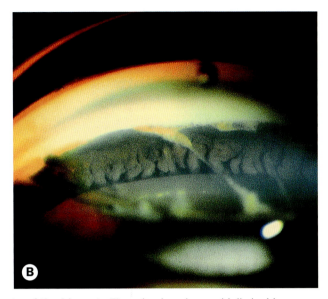

Fig. 10.93 Gonioscopy in aniridia. **(A)** Open angle showing remnants of the iris root; **(B)** angle closed synechially by iris rudiments

(Courtesy of R Curtis – fig. A)

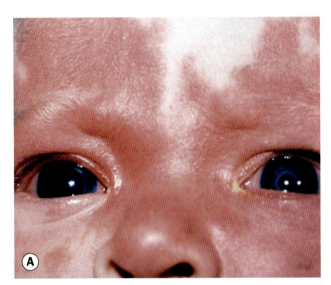

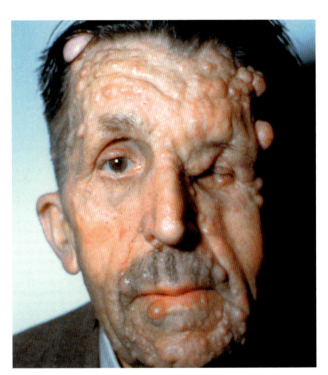

Fig. 10.95 Left facial hemiatrophy and multiple neurofibromas in neurofibromatosis type 1

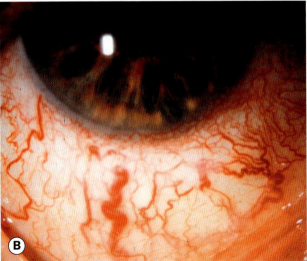

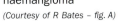

Fig. 10.94 Glaucoma in Sturge–Weber syndrome. **(A)** Bilateral naevus flammeus and buphthalmos; **(B)** episcleral haemangioma

(Courtesy of R Bates – fig. A)

GLAUCOMA IN PHACOMATOSES

Sturge–Weber syndrome

Introduction

Sturge–Weber syndrome (encephalotrigeminal angiomatosis) is a congenital, sporadic phacomatosis (see Ch. 1). Glaucoma ipsilateral to the facial haemangioma develops in about 30%, and in 60% of these IOP elevation occurs before the age of 2 years and may result in buphthalmos (Fig. 10.94A). In the remainder, glaucoma may develop at any time from infancy to adulthood. The pathogenesis is uncertain; putative mechanisms include trabeculodysgenesis in infants and raised episcleral venous pressure associated with arteriovenous communication in an episcleral haemangioma (Fig. 10.94B) in older patients.

Treatment

- **Medical** treatment alone may be adequate.
- **Goniotomy** may be successful in eyes with angle anomalies.
- **Combined trabeculotomy–trabeculectomy** gives good results in early-onset cases, but carries a relatively high risk of choroidal effusion and suprachoroidal haemorrhage; other surgical options may be utilized.

Neurofibromatosis type 1

Neurofibromatosis is a disorder that primarily affects cell growth of neural tissues. Inheritance is AD with irregular penetrance and variable expressivity (see Ch. 19). Glaucoma is relatively rare and, when present, usually unilateral and congenital. About 50% of patients with glaucoma have an ipsilateral plexiform neurofibroma of the upper eyelid, or facial hemiatrophy (Fig. 10.95). Various mechanisms have been identified, including congenital angle anomaly.

CLASSIFICATION

The Standardization of Uveitis Nomenclature (SUN) Working Group guidance on uveitis terminology, endorsed by the International Uveitis Study Group (IUSG), categorizes uveitis anatomically (Fig. 11.1):

- **Anterior**: the anterior chamber is the primary site of inflammation.
- **Intermediate**: primarily vitreous inflammation; includes pars planitis.
- **Posterior**: retina and/or choroid.
- **Panuveitis**: all uveal structures are involved.

An IUSG clinical classification based on aetiology is also in use:

- **Infectious**: bacterial, viral, fungal, parasitic, others.
- **Non-infectious**: with and without a known systemic association.
- **Masquerade**: neoplastic and non-neoplastic.

The SUN Working Group guidance includes the following descriptions relating to the timing of inflammatory activity:

- **Onset**: sudden or insidious.
- **Duration**: limited (3 months or less) or persistent.
- **Clinical course**: acute (of sudden onset and limited duration), recurrent (repeated episodes separated by untreated inactive periods), or chronic (persistent duration, with relapse less than 3 months after discontinuation of treatment). Remission is defined as inactivity (no visible cells) for 3 months or longer.

ANTERIOR UVEITIS

Introduction

Anterior uveitis is inflammation involving the anterior uveal tract – the iris and the anterior part (pars plicata) of the ciliary

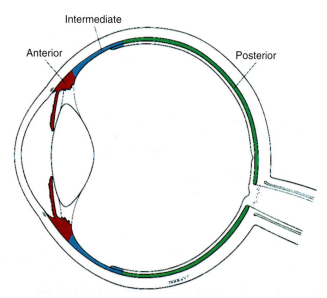

Fig. 11.1 Anatomical classification of uveitis

Intermediate

Anterior

Posterior

Table 11.1 Systemic associations of anterior uveitis

Idiopathic	No detectable systemic association – around 50%
Infectious	Varicella zoster – usually current or past ophthalmic shingles Tuberculosis Syphilis Lyme disease Miscellaneous systemic viral infections
Non-infectious	HLA-B27 positivity – around 20% of AAU – with or without manifestations of HLA-B27-related systemic disease (see text) Juvenile idiopathic arthritis Sarcoidosis Behçet disease Tubulointerstitial nephritis and uveitis syndrome Systemic lupus erythematosus Multiple sclerosis Drug-induced (see Ch. 20)
Masquerade	Neoplastic, e.g. lymphoma, anterior segment melanoma Non-neoplastic, e.g. juvenile xanthogranuloma

body – and is the most common form of uveitis. Iritis refers to inflammation primarily involving the iris, and iridocyclitis to involvement of both the iris and anterior ciliary body; in practice these are interchangeable as they cannot be distinguished clinically.

Acute anterior uveitis (AAU) is the most common presentation, of which HLA-B27-related and idiopathic forms make up the largest proportion. Aetiology in these cases is uncertain, but may involve cross-reactivity with particular microbial antigens in genetically predisposed individuals. AAU can be a feature of a wide variety of ocular conditions such as trauma (including surgery), lens-related inflammation and herpes simplex infection, or can be secondary to inflammation elsewhere in the eye, such as bacterial keratitis and scleritis. AAU can also be the presenting clinical scenario, without accompanying intermediate or posterior uveitis, in a range of systemic conditions including chronic inflammatory disorders such as sarcoidosis.

Chronic anterior uveitis (CAU) is less common than AAU. It is more commonly bilateral, and associated systemic disease is more likely. Granulomatous inflammatory signs (see below) are often present.

Surveys of systemic associations of anterior uveitis vary in their findings; Table 11.1 lists important possibilities, but is not exhaustive.

The prognosis is usually good in most idiopathic and HLA-B27-related AAU provided management is adequate. Outcomes are more variable in CAU and in cases where there is an underlying ocular or systemic disorder.

Clinical features

- **Symptoms** in AAU consist of the rapid onset of unilateral pain, photophobia, redness and watery discharge, sometimes preceded by mild ocular discomfort for a few days. Blurring of vision is related to severity. As recurrent disease is very common, especially with the idiopathic and HLA-B27-related types, there will often be a history of previous similar episodes. CAU may be of insidious or acute onset, and can be asymptomatic until the development of complications such as cataract.
- **Visual acuity** is variably impaired depending on the severity of inflammation and the presence of complications. It is frequently only mildly reduced in AAU.
- **'Ciliary injection'** (perilimbal injection, ciliary flush or just 'injection') is circumcorneal conjunctival hyperaemia with a violaceous (purplish) hue due to involvement of deeper blood vessels (Fig. 11.2A), and is typically seen in anterior uveitis of acute onset. Ciliary injection is characteristically absent in some forms of CAU, and occasionally AAU.
- **Miosis** due to pupillary sphincter spasm (Fig. 11.2B) predisposes to the formation of posterior synechiae (see below).

Table 11.2 Standardization of Uveitis Nomenclature (SUN) Working Group grading of anterior chamber cells (1 mm by 1 mm slit beam)

Grade	Cells in field
0	<1
0.5+	1–5
1+	6–15
2+	16–25
3+	26–50
4+	>50

- **Anterior chamber cells** (Fig. 11.2C) are a dependable indicator of inflammatory activity. Grading (SUN Working Group) is performed by estimating the number of cells in a 1 mm by 1 mm slit beam field, employing adequate light intensity and magnification (Table 11.2). This must be performed before pupillary dilatation, which can lead to shedding of pigment cells into the aqueous. Inflammatory cells are commonly also seen in the anterior vitreous.
- **Hypopyon** (Fig. 11.2D) refers to a whitish purulent exudate composed of myriad inflammatory cells in the inferior part

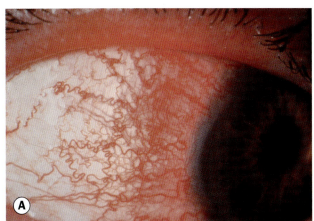

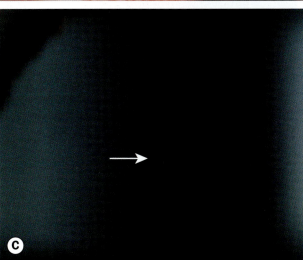

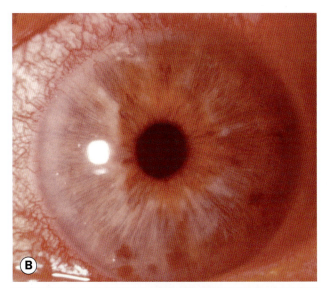

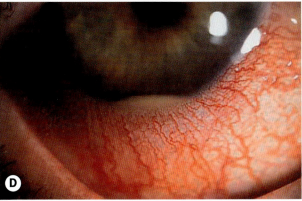

Fig. 11.2 Signs of acute anterior uveitis. **(A)** Ciliary injection; **(B)** miosis; **(C)** anterior chamber cells in mild anterior uveitis; **(D)** hypopyon

of the anterior chamber (AC), forming a horizontal level under the influence of gravity. Hypopyon is common in HLA-B27-associated AAU (see below), when a high fibrin content makes it immobile and slow to absorb. In patients with Behçet disease the hypopyon contains minimal fibrin and so characteristically shifts according to the patient's head position.

- **Keratic precipitates (KP)** are deposits on the corneal endothelium (Fig. 11.3A) composed of inflammatory cells such as lymphocytes, plasma cells and macrophages (Fig. 11.3B). They are usually concentrated inferiorly, often in a triangular pattern with the apex pointing up (Arlt triangle) under the influence of gravity and aqueous convection currents; a notable exception is Fuchs uveitis syndrome

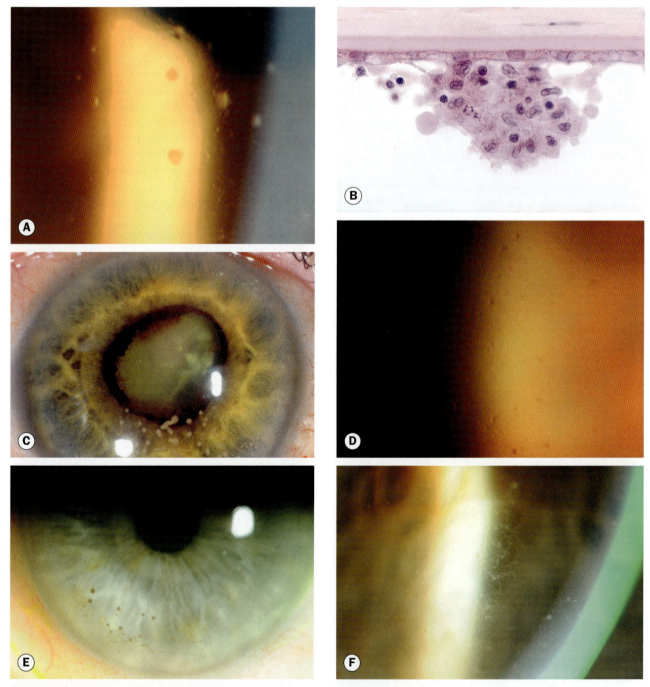

Fig. 11.3 Keratic precipitates (KP). **(A)** Highly magnified view of fresh KP in early anterior uveitis; **(B)** histology showing typical aggregate of inflammatory cells on the corneal endothelium; **(C)** large 'mutton fat' keratic precipitates; **(D)** stellate KPs in Fuchs uveitis syndrome; **(E)** old pigmented granulomatous KP; **(F)** endothelial cellular 'dusting' and early KP formation

(Courtesy of J Harry and G Misson, from Clinical Ophthalmic Pathology, *Butterworth-Heinemann 2001 – fig. B)*

(FUS), in which they are diffusely distributed. Their characteristics indicate the probable type of uveitis: typically smaller in the non-granulomatous inflammation typical of AAU, and medium to large in (classically chronic) granulomatous inflammation in which cell types may include epithelioid and multinucleated cells. Large greasy-appearing granulomatous KP are said to have a 'mutton fat' appearance (Fig. 11.3C). KP are small to medium and adopt a star-shaped ('stellate' – Fig. 11.3D) or filamentous morphology in FUS. KP usually resolve as acute inflammation subsides: long-standing non-granulomatous KP may become pigmented; granulomatous KP may become pigmented (Fig. 11.3E) and/or assume a 'ground glass' appearance. Endothelial dusting by numerous individual cells precedes the formation of true KP aggregates (Fig. 11.3F).

- **Aqueous flare** is haziness of the normally clear fluid in the anterior chamber, reflecting the presence of protein due to breakdown of the blood–aqueous barrier. Based on work in children with juvenile idiopathic arthritis-associated CAU, it is now thought that in most or all patients the presence of flare indicates active inflammation with a resultant higher risk of complications over the longer term. Flare may be graded clinically using a slit lamp to assess the degree of interference with visualization of iris and lens (Table 11.3). When available, laser flare photometry gives greater objectivity.
- **Fibrinous exudate** in the anterior chamber (Fig. 11.4) is common in severe AAU, and as with hypopyon is often seen with HLA-B27-related inflammation.
- **Iris nodules**: Koeppe nodules are located on the pupillary margin (Fig. 11.5A), and may be the site of posterior synechiae formation (see below). They can occur in both granulomatous and non-granulomatous anterior uveitis. Busacca nodules involve the iris stroma (Figs 11.5B and C) and are a feature of granulomatous uveitis. Yellowish nodules can develop from dilated iris vessels (roseolae) in syphilitic uveitis. Iris 'pearls' may be seen in lepromatous chronic anterior uveitis. Iris crystals (Russell bodies), thought to consist of immunoglobulin deposits, are a rare finding in some cases of chronic uveitis (Fig. 11.5D), including FUS.
- **Posterior synechiae (PS)** are inflammatory adhesions between the pupil margin and the anterior lens capsule (Figs 11.6A and B), and may be particularly likely to form at the

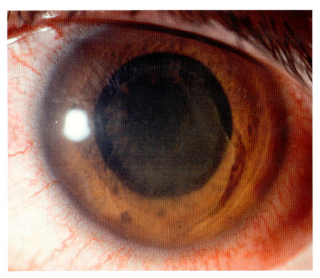

Fig. 11.4 Fibrinous exudate

location of a Koeppe nodule. They can develop rapidly, and to prevent their formation initial prophylaxis with a mydriatic agent is routine in all but very mild AAU. Once established, every attempt must be made to break PS (Fig. 11.6C) before they become permanent.

- **Iris atrophy** may offer useful diagnostic clues. Diffuse stromal atrophy is seen in FUS, and patchy or sectoral atrophy can occur in herpetic uveitis (Fig. 11.7); both patterns may be seen in both simplex and zoster-related inflammation, though the latter is said to more commonly give a sectoral pattern.
- **Heterochromia iridis** refers to a difference in colour between the iris of the two eyes, best seen in daylight. In the context of uveitis, heterochromia characteristically occurs in FUS; see also Table 11.6.
- **Iris neovascularization (rubeosis iridis)** can occur, particularly in chronic inflammation. The process tends to be less acute than with a primary vascular cause such as central retinal vein occlusion. Abnormal iris vessels are very common in FUS, but do not cause synechial angle closure. Iris neovascularization may also occur in posterior uveitis, particularly when retinal perfusion is compromised. New iris vessels may be difficult to differentiate from dilated normal vessels (sometimes called 'pseudorubeosis'); normal vessels course radially in contrast to the irregular distribution of neovascularization. Fluorescein angiography may show leakage from new vessels, though this can also be seen with dilated normal vessels, particularly in the presence of active inflammation.
- **Intraocular pressure (IOP)** may be reduced as the result of impairment of aqueous secretion by the ciliary epithelium, or elevated due to a variety of mechanisms (see 'Inflammatory glaucoma' in Chapter 10), including therapeutic steroids.
- **Posterior segment examination** should always be performed to detect a masquerading cause of anterior uveitis (e.g.

Table 11.3 SUN Working Group slit lamp grading scheme for anterior chamber flare

Grade	Description
0	None
1+	Faint
2+	Moderate (iris and lens details clear)
3+	Marked (iris and lens details hazy)
4+	Intense (fibrin or plastic aqueous)

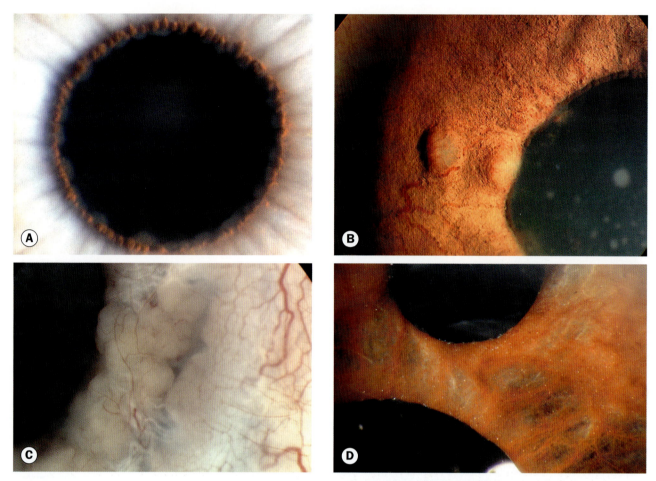

Fig. 11.5 Iris nodules in anterior uveitis. **(A)** Koeppe nodules in Fuchs uveitis syndrome; **(B)** Busacca and Koeppe nodules; **(C)** very large nodule in sarcoid uveitis; **(D)** iris crystals (Russell bodies) in chronic syphilitic uveitis
(Courtesy of C Barry – fig. A; C. Pavesio – figs B and C; S Chen – fig. D)

retinal detachment, tumour), primary intermediate or posterior segment inflammation, and complications of anterior uveitis such as cystoid macular oedema.

Investigation

Investigations are often negative, with no clear underlying cause determined in many patients. Rather than performing a battery of screening tests, investigation is tailored to each patient, directed by clinical features. Sometimes a likely cause may be obvious, such as severe anterior uveitis following intraocular surgery when endophthalmitis will lead the differential diagnosis list. In most cases, a careful review for systemic symptoms is essential to detect any clues to underlying disease, with referral to a specialist physician for further assessment where appropriate. Many associations of uveitis can present with a wide range of systemic features.

Investigation is generally not indicated in the following circumstances:

- A single episode of unilateral mild/moderate (no hypopyon) non-granulomatous AAU with no ocular or systemic suggestion of underlying disease.

- Typical clinical features of a specific entity for which investigation is not usually indicated (e.g. FUS).
- A systemic diagnosis compatible with the clinical features (e.g. sarcoidosis) has already been confirmed.

Situations in which investigation of anterior uveitis is generally appropriate include:

- Recurrent AAU.
- Severe AAU.
- Bilateral AAU.
- Anterior uveitis that is persistent, chronic or resistant to treatment.
- Granulomatous inflammatory signs (note that granulomatous conditions may give non-granulomatous AAU).
- Associated intermediate or posterior uveitis.
- Ocular or systemic clinical features suggesting underlying disease.
- Some authorities advocate routine syphilis serology for all uveitis patients at first presentation; a history of high-risk sexual behaviour in particular must prompt this.
- Repeating targeted previously negative investigations several years later is sometimes fruitful.

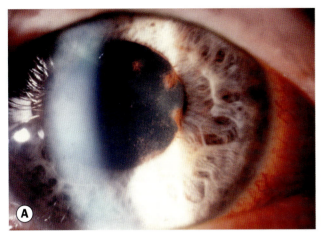

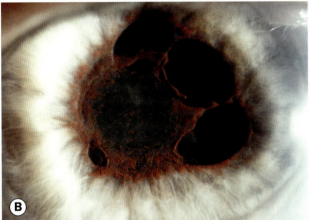

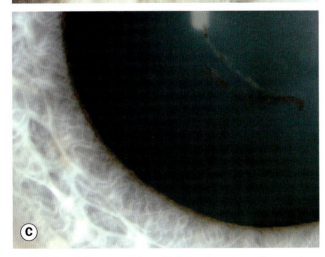

Fig. 11.6 Posterior synechiae. **(A)** Adhesions in active acute anterior uveitis; **(B)** extensive synechiae and pigment on the lens following severe acute anterior uveitis; **(C)** recently broken synechiae in a patient with HLA-B27-associated acute anterior uveitis

The following investigations should be considered:

- **HLA tissue typing (HLA-B27).** The major histocompatibility complex (MHC) is a group of genes involved in white cell–antigen interaction and other immune functions, including the encoding of cell surface glycoproteins. In humans the MHC, found on chromosome 6, is called the

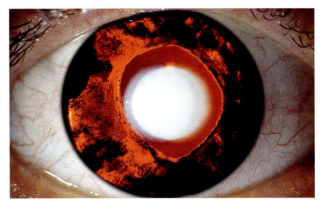

Fig. 11.7 Extensive iris atrophy following herpes zoster ophthalmicus – predominantly sectoral pattern
(Courtesy of C Barry)

human leukocyte antigen (HLA) system. HLA typing is used to determine organ transplantation compatibility and can also indicate predisposition to particular diseases. It has conventionally been performed by serological antigen identification, but increasingly involves analysis of DNA. HLA-B27 is a common (e.g. 6–8% of Caucasians in the USA, 0.5% of patients of Japanese ethnic origin) cell surface protein that presents peptides to T cells. The phenotype has a very strong association with acute anterior uveitis, ankylosing spondylitis and some other inflammatory conditions such as reactive arthritis (Reiter syndrome), psoriatic arthritis and arthritis in inflammatory bowel disease. It is present in 50% of patients with AAU who are otherwise fit and well, and 90% of patients with AAU who have an associated spondyloarthropathy, notably ankylosing spondylitis. Many HLA-B27 subtypes have been identified and their significance is subject to ongoing investigation. HLA types associated with ocular inflammatory disease are listed in Table 11.4. HLA-B27 testing should be performed in any adult or child with recurrent or chronic non-granulomatous anterior uveitis.

- **Syphilis serology**
  - Treponemal antibody tests such as the ELISA (enzyme-linked immunosorbent assay) are highly sensitive and specific, but take around 3 months to become positive.

Table 11.4 Examples of HLA associations with uveitis

HLA type	Associated disease
HLA-B27	Recurrent acute anterior uveitis
HLA-A29	Birdshot retinochoroidopathy
HLA-B51 and HLA B5	Behçet syndrome
HLA-B7 and HLA-DR2	(Presumed) ocular histoplasmosis syndrome
HLA-DR4	Sympathetic ophthalmitis
HLA-DR4	Vogt–Koyanagi–Harada syndrome

○ Non-specific titratable cardiolipin antibody tests such as the rapid plasma reagin (RPR) or venereal disease research laboratory (VDRL) are more commonly positive in early infection, and are used to help monitor disease activity; they become negative over time, typically in treated disease. False-positive results can occur.

○ Both categories of test should be performed when screening for ocular syphilis.

○ Clinical features suggesting a diagnosis of syphilis should prompt urgent referral to a physician specializing in infectious or sexually transmitted diseases.

- **Serum angiotensin-converting enzyme (ACE):** a non-specific test that indicates the presence of a granulomatous disease such as sarcoidosis, tuberculosis and leprosy. Elevation occurs in up to 80% of patients with acute sarcoidosis but may be normal during remissions. In children serum ACE levels tend to be higher and diagnostically less useful. Vigorous exercise can elevate ACE.

- **Lysozyme** is a group of enzymes found in polymorphonuclear neutrophils and numerous secretions including tears. It has a strong antibacterial action, mediating breakdown of the bacterial cell wall. Serum lysozyme assay is generally slightly less sensitive and specific than serum ACE in the diagnosis of sarcoidosis, but performing both tests may increase sensitivity and specificity.

- **Erythrocyte sedimentation rate (ESR) and C-reactive protein (CRP):** acute-phase reactants that are probably of limited value, but may be elevated in a range of systemic inflammatory disorders.

- **Complete blood count:** leukocytosis may raise suspicion of infection and, exceptionally, haematological malignancy. Eosinophilia may occur in parasitic infection.

- **Lyme disease:** serology may be considered, particularly in endemic areas. Serology for other infectious diseases such as **brucellosis** and **leptospirosis** can be requested if relevant risk factors are present (e.g. endemic region).

- **Antinuclear antibody (ANA):** limited use, except in children. In those with juvenile idiopathic arthritis (JIA) its presence is associated with a higher risk of CAU; cases of possible subclinical JIA have been reported in ANA-positive children with CAU.

- **Antineutrophil cytoplasmic antibody (ANCA):** limited use in anterior uveitis unless associated with scleritis and/or peripheral ulcerative keratitis, when cytoplasmic ANCA (c-ANCA) testing should be considered as evidence of Wegener granulomatosis.

- **Interferon-gamma release assay** (e.g. QuantiFERON-TB Gold™) blood test for tuberculosis.

- **HIV serology:** indicated for selected patients, usually those in whom an opportunistic infection has been diagnosed or is suspected.

- **Sacroiliac joint X-ray** may show evidence of sacroiliitis in ankylosing spondylitis and other seronegative spondyloarthropathies.

- **Chest X-ray** may show evidence of sarcoidosis or tuberculosis; a high level of suspicion for both of these treatable conditions (as well as syphilis) should always be adopted, particularly if inflammation is granulomatous.

- **Ocular imaging**
  ○ B-scan ultrasonography, if the posterior segment view is compromised by very small pupils or opaque media.
  ○ Optical coherence tomography (OCT) may reveal posterior segment complications such as cystoid macular oedema and epiretinal membrane.
  ○ Fundus autofluorescence (FAF) may demonstrate suspected posterior segment pathology as the lesions of several inflammatory conditions, such as multiple evanescent white dot syndrome (MEWDS), which may give mild anterior chamber inflammation, are often shown more effectively than on clinical examination.
  ○ Fluorescein angiography (FA) is useful in some cases of anterior uveitis such as the confirmation or exclusion of suspected posterior segment pathology, e.g. vasculitis, white dot syndromes, or identifying macular ischaemia as the cause of reduced vision if no macular abnormality is visible on OCT.
  ○ Indocyanine green angiography (ICGA) is rarely indicated in anterior uveitis, but might be used to look for subtle associated choroidal pathology.
  ○ Ultrasound biomicroscopy (UBM) is particularly indicated in cases of hypotony, and may demonstrate pathology such as subtle choroidal effusion, cyclodialysis cleft and cyclitic membrane.

- **Aqueous tap:** historically rarely performed in anterior uveitis, but viral causes are now recognized as being more frequent than previously realized. Herpesviruses (including cytomegalovirus) and rubella in particular should be considered in clinically suspicious cases, especially unexplained hypertensive uveitis and cases relatively unresponsive to topical steroids. An aqueous humour sample may be sent for polymerase chain reaction (PCR) analysis for evidence of viral genetic material, and for microscopy, culture and antibody assay; PCR may also help to exclude propionibacter infection in chronically inflamed pseudophakic eyes.

- **Iris biopsy** is rarely performed.

- **Vitreous biopsy** tends to be confined to the investigation of obscure posterior segment inflammation and suspected infectious endophthalmitis.

- **Conjunctival biopsy:** sampling of tissue such as a suspected granuloma or infiltrative lesion is occasionally indicated.

- **Referral to a specialist physician with resultant further investigation.** This is vital when systemic disease is suspected. For instance, if respiratory symptoms are present, a chest physician may arrange additional testing such as a high resolution computed tomography (CT) chest scan, a whole-body gallium scan (sarcoidosis), a purified protein derivative skin test for tuberculosis (negative test is a diagnostic indicator in sarcoidosis), and bronchoscopy with lavage/biopsy. Similarly neurological referral may lead to a cranial magnetic resonance imaging (MRI) and lumbar puncture, and gastroenterological referral to endoscopy.

Treatment

For patients with a treatable cause of inflammation such as an infection, specific treatment (see individual topics) is given either instead of or in addition to the general anti-inflammatory measures discussed below. Review frequency is set according to the severity and chronicity of inflammation; patients with severe inflammation may need to be seen within a day or two of initiating treatment. Those with mild recurrent idiopathic AAU may not need to be seen for several weeks after treatment is commenced.

- **Topical steroids**
  - Prednisolone 1% or dexamethasone 0.1% is commonly utilized as a first choice. Other preparations, of varying availability geographically, include difluprednate 0.05% (may be administered at a lower frequency), loteprednol etabonate 0.2% and 0.5% (moderate to marked potency but a lower tendency to elevate IOP), betamethasone, prednisolone 0.5%, fluorometholone and rimexolone; the latter three are of moderate to lower potency. The selection of topical steroid preparation can be modified according to severity and other factors such as a known tendency to IOP elevation. Steroid ointment (e.g. betamethasone) may be instilled at bedtime to supplement the drops. Additional anti-inflammatory treatment (see below) is necessary in some cases.
  - Treatment of AAU initially involves instillation at a frequency appropriate to the severity of inflammation, typically starting with one drop hourly in moderate to severe cases. Once the inflammation is controlled the instillation frequency should be carefully tapered; a commonly adopted regimen might consist of:
    - one drop hourly for 3 days, then
    - every two hours for 3 days, then
    - four times a day for 1 week, then
    - three times a day for 1 week, then
    - twice a day for 1 week, then
    - once a day for 1 week and stop; treatment is often discontinued by 5–6 weeks.

    Periodic review is undertaken as appropriate during the treatment course, with further assessment a week or two after cessation, following which the patient can be discharged but cautioned to re-attend urgently should symptoms recur.
  - Treatment of CAU is generally targeted at complete suppression of inflammation, with no anterior chamber cellular activity or flare – the latter is now thought to be an indicator of active inflammation in most or all cases. Even low-grade ongoing activity is associated with a greater incidence of complications that outweighs the risk of complications from treatment. Exacerbations are initially treated in the same way as AAU, though with more gradual tapering and typically a maintenance regimen; Fuchs uveitis syndrome is an exception to this approach.
  - Common complications of topical steroids include transient elevation of IOP in susceptible individuals

('steroid responders'); long-term treatment may lead to permanent IOP elevation with glaucomatous damage. Cataract can be induced, but is less common than with systemic steroid administration; the risk increases with dose and duration of therapy. Corneal complications are uncommon; they include secondary infection with bacteria and fungi, recrudescence of herpes simplex keratitis, and corneal melting. Systemic side effects are rare with topical steroids, but may occur following prolonged administration, particularly in children, in whom measures to reduce systemic absorption such as medial canthal pressure and blotting away of overspill from the eyelids following instillation should be discussed.

- **Cycloplegic agents.** These are used in AAU and in exacerbations of CAU to prevent the formation of posterior synechiae (PS), to break down recently formed synechiae and to promote comfort by relieving spasm of the pupillary and ciliary muscle. Commonly used anticholinergic agents in order of increasing potency and duration of action include cyclopentolate (duration 12–24 hours), homatropine and atropine (10–14 days). In the acute stage, phenylephrine 2.5% or 10% may be used to supplement anticholinergics and break PS. In mild or chronic anterior uveitis, a cycloplegic can be instilled at bedtime to prevent difficulties with accommodation during the day. In children, care should be taken to avoid systemic toxicity; a range of systemic adverse effects have occurred including seizures. Prolonged uniocular cycloplegia may induce amblyopia in the susceptible age group.

- **Mydricaine® No. 2.** This is a preparation containing adrenaline and atropine that is used to try to break fresh PS when drops are ineffective; it also contains local anaesthetic to improve comfort. Constituent quantities vary according to manufacturer but 0.3 ml containing 0.12 mg adrenaline, 1 mg atropine and 6 mg procaine is typical. It is usually administered by subconjunctival injection; division between the four conjunctival quadrants may enhance the effect. An alternative to injection is insertion of a cotton pledget soaked in Mydricaine into the superior and inferior fornices for 5 minutes. Serious cardiovascular events have been reported following injection (a transient sinus tachycardia is common), and the patient should be monitored after injection. Mydricaine No. 1 is a paediatric version that may also be effective in adults.

- **Tissue plasminogen activator (TPA).** In severe fibrinous anterior uveitis 12.5–25 µg of TPA in 0.1 ml injected into the anterior chamber (intracamerally) with a 30-gauge needle under topical anaesthesia will dissolve dense fibrinous exudate and may break down recently formed PS. Antiseptic precautions similar to those for intravitreal injection should be taken.

- **Subconjunctival steroid** can be administered in severe cases or to patients in whom poor compliance is likely. For example, betamethasone sodium phosphate solution (4 mg in 1 ml) can be given alone or in a combined preparation with betamethasone acetate suspension for a sustained effect (e.g. Celestone, 6 mg in 1 ml).

- **Regional steroid injection.** The use of an inferior approach ('orbital floor') or posterior sub-Tenon (Fig. 11.8) injection of depot steroid preparations (e.g. triamcinolone acetonide, methylprednisolone acetate) is common in the treatment of posterior segment inflammation, but is generally reserved in anterior uveitis patients for the treatment of cases complicated by cystoid macular oedema (CMO), and for patients noncompliant with topical administration. Periocular injections may also be administered at the time of surgery, and may rarely be used to supplement systemic therapy or when systemic steroids are contraindicated. The peak action is at about four weeks, with a maximum duration of action of around 3 months. Complications include subconjunctival haemorrhage, globe penetration, refractory elevation of IOP (up to 25%), cataract, ptosis, eyelid haemorrhage, eyelid ischaemic necrosis, retrobulbar haemorrhage, subdermal fat atrophy, extraocular muscle paresis, optic nerve injury, retinal and choroidal vascular occlusion and cutaneous hypopigmentation; systemic adverse effects are rare but can occur. Table 11.5 gives injection procedures; there is no clear evidence of the superiority of one route over the other, but advocates suggest there may be a lower risk of ocular perforation, of raised IOP and of ptosis with the orbital floor approach. Utilizing a plastic intravenous cannula via a superior sub-Tenon route has been described and is thought to offer a lower risk of perforation.
- **Intraocular steroids.** Intravitreal triamcinolone acetonide (4 mg in 0.1 ml, i.e. one-tenth of the orbital dose) is occasionally used in anterior uveitis for CMO unresponsive to other forms of therapy (see Fig. 13.34E), and rarely may be considered at the time of intraocular surgery in high risk anterior uveitis patients. Complications include elevation of IOP, cataract, endophthalmitis (sterile or infectious),

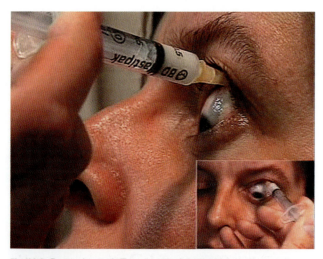

Fig. 11.8 Posterior sub-Tenon steroid injection
(Courtesy of C Pavesio)

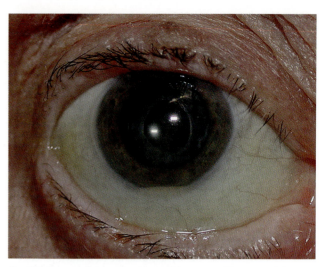

Fig. 11.9 Pseudohypopyon formed by crystalline steroid following intravitreal triamcinolone injection
(Courtesy of S Chen)

haemorrhage, retinal detachment and pseudohypopyon (Fig. 11.9). Slow-release intravitreal implants may occasionally be indicated.

- **Systemic steroids** are very rarely required for anterior uveitis but may be needed where the response to less aggressive treatment is inadequate. They are sometimes given as a short course prior to intraocular surgery as prophylaxis against worsening inflammation, having the advantage of rapid cessation of effect in comparison with depot peri- or intraocular steroid injection, but have major potential adverse effects.
- **Non-steroidal anti-inflammatory drugs (NSAIDs)** such as naproxen and tolmetin may be effective in CAU and can be used long-term under appropriate specialist physician supervision.
- **Antimetabolites** such as methotrexate are generally not required in the treatment of anterior uveitis, though may be necessary in exceptional patients such as juvenile idiopathic arthritis-associated CAU when other measures fail to control inflammation, or as a steroid-sparing measure.

UVEITIS IN SPONDYLOARTHROPATHIES

The spondyloarthropathies are a group of disorders featuring HLA-B27 positivity and enthesitis as common factors. There is often a family history of one or more of the group, which comprises ankylosing spondylitis, undifferentiated spondyloarthropathy, psoriatic arthritis, reactive arthritis (Reiter syndrome) and spondyloarthropathy with inflammatory bowel disease (ulcerative colitis and Crohn disease). They are often referred to as seronegative spondyloarthropathies, in that rheumatoid factor is not present and the pathophysiological basis differs. The American Uveitis Society has recently endorsed the use of biological blockers such as infliximab for second-line systemic immunosuppression in vision-threatening chronic uveitis.

Table 11.5 Procedure for inferior transseptal and posterior sub-Tenon regional steroid injection

Route	Technique
Inferior transseptal ('orbital floor') injection	A topical anaesthetic such as tetracaine (amethocaine) is instilled to prevent stinging by the antiseptic agents
	The skin of the lower eyelid and maxillary area is cleaned with an antiseptic agent such as an alcohol swab or povidone-iodine 5%
	The vial containing the steroid is shaken
	1 ml steroid (triamcinolone acetonide or methylprednisolone acetate 40 mg/ml) is drawn up into a 2 ml syringe and the drawing-up needle replaced with a 25-gauge 5/8 inch (16 mm) needle
	The patient is asked to maintain gaze straight ahead
	The needle is inserted through the skin (some practitioners inject via the conjunctiva), at approximately the junction of the outer third and inner two-thirds of the lower orbital rim, entering close to the bony margin whilst clearing the margin itself
	The needle is slowly advanced tangentially to (or, anatomy permitting, away from) the globe in similar fashion to a peribulbar local anaesthetic block up to the needle hub
	The skin may be indented to ensure the needle tip is sufficiently posterior to deposit the steroid away from the anterior subconjunctival area
	The tip may be felt to engage the bony orbital floor, and/or to pierce the orbital septum; as with the superior injection technique, the needle can be moved from side to side to ensure the sclera has not been engaged
	The plunger is slightly withdrawn and, if no blood enters the syringe, the full 1 ml is slowly injected and the needle carefully withdrawn
	Special care is required in a patient with a large eye (e.g. myopia) to avoid penetration of the globe
Posterior sub-Tenon approach	A topical anaesthetic such as tetracaine (amethocaine) is instilled
	A small cotton pledget impregnated with tetracaine, lidocaine (lignocaine) 2% gel or an alternative is placed into the superior fornix at the site of injection for 2 minutes
	The vial containing the steroid is shaken
	1 ml steroid (triamcinolone acetonide methylprednisolone acetate or 40 mg/ml) is drawn up into a 2 ml syringe and the drawing-up needle replaced with a 25-gauge 5/8 inch (16 mm) needle
	The patient is asked to look in the direction opposite to the superotemporal injection site
	The bulbar conjunctiva is penetrated with the tip of the needle, bevel towards the globe, slightly on the bulbar side of the fornix
	The needle is slowly inserted posteriorly, following the contour of the globe, keeping it as close to the globe as possible. In order not to penetrate the globe accidentally, wide side-to-side motions are made as the needle is being inserted and the limbus watched; movement of the limbus means that the sclera has been engaged
	When the needle has been advanced to the hub the plunger is slightly withdrawn and, if no blood enters the syringe, the full 1 ml is slowly injected
	A method utilizing a plastic intravenous cannula introduced via the same route following conjunctival incision and limited blunt dissection has been described

Ankylosing spondylitis

Introduction

Ankylosing spondylitis (AS) is characterized by inflammation, calcification and finally ossification of ligaments and capsules of joints with resultant bony ankylosis of the axial skeleton. It more commonly affects males, of whom 90% are HLA-B27-positive.

Systemic features

- **Presentation** is commonly in the third to fourth decades with the insidious onset of pain and stiffness in the lower back or buttocks.
- **Spondyloarthritis** causes progressive limitation of spinal movements; eventually the spine may become fixed in flexion (Fig. 11.10A). Spinal stenosis and fractures may occur.
- **Enthesitis** is characterized clinically by inflammation and pain at ligamentous attachments to bone.
- **Cardiac complications** are rare.
- **Radiology** of the sacroiliac joints shows juxta-articular osteoporosis in the early stages, followed by sclerosis and bony obliteration of the joint (Fig. 11.10B). Calcification of spinal ligaments gives rise to a 'bamboo spine'. Radiological changes often predate clinical symptoms.

Ocular features

- **AAU** is by far the most common ocular association, and occurs in about 25% of patients with AS; 25% of males with AAU will have AS. Either eye is frequently affected at different times but bilateral simultaneous involvement is rare. There is often no correlation between the severity and activity of eye and joint involvement. Chronicity occurs in a

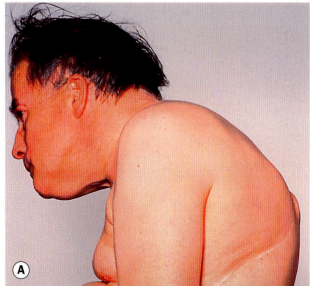

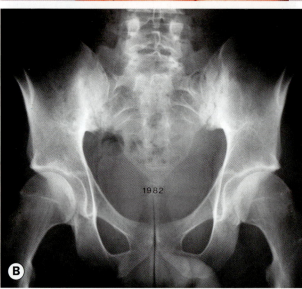

Fig. 11.10 Ankylosing spondylitis. **(A)** Fixed flexion deformity of the spine; **(B)** sclerosis and bony obliteration of the sacroiliac joints

(Courtesy of MA Mir, from Atlas of Clinical Diagnosis, Saunders 2003 – fig. A)

arthritis. Around 75% of patients are positive for HLA-B27. A range of infective agents can trigger the syndrome, which develops in 1–3% of men after non-specific urethritis, and around 4% of individuals after enteric infections caused by a range of organisms including *Shigella*, *Salmonella* and *Campylobacter*. *Chlamydia pneumoniae* respiratory infection and others may also precede ReA.

Systemic features

- **Presentation** is with the acute onset of malaise, with fever and dysuria 1–4 weeks after a linked infection in a patient aged between 20 and 40, with arthritis that may be preceded by conjunctivitis. A variety of other features may be present, though not always the defining triad.
- **Peripheral oligoarthritis** is acute, asymmetrical and migratory; 2–4 joints tend to be involved, most commonly the knees, ankles and toes.
- **Spondyloarthritis** affects about 50% of patients, manifesting with low back pain. This sometimes becomes chronic.
- **Enthesitis** manifests with plantar fasciitis, Achilles tenosynovitis, bursitis and calcaneal periostitis; reactive bone formation in the latter may result in a calcaneal spur.
- **Mucocutaneous lesions** include painless mouth ulceration, circinate balanitis and keratoderma blennorrhagica – skin lesions resembling psoriasis – involving the palms and soles (Fig. 11.11).
- **Genitourinary involvement** includes cervicitis, prostatitis and epididymitis.
- **Aortitis** occurs in 1–2%.

Ocular features

The eye is involved in 50% of cases with a urogenital inciting infection and 75% of enteric ReA syndrome.

- **Conjunctivitis** is very common; it classically follows urethritis but precedes arthritis. The inflammation is usually

few patients. HLA-B27-positive ankylosing spondylitis patients tend to have worse disease across a range of parameters, including earlier onset and greater intensity of inflammation with an increased frequency of complications.
- **Other ocular features** include scleritis, episcleritis, keratitis and mechanical ptosis.

Reactive arthritis

Introduction

Reactive arthritis (ReA, also known as Reiter syndrome) is characterized by a triad of non-specific urethritis, conjunctivitis and

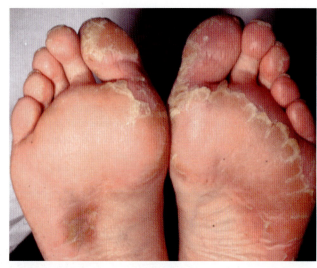

Fig. 11.11 Keratoderma blennorrhagica in reactive arthritis (Reiter syndrome)

mild, bilateral and mucopurulent with a papillary and/or follicular reaction. Spontaneous resolution occurs within 7–10 days and treatment is not required. Some patients develop peripheral corneal infiltrates.

- **AAU** occurs in 20%.
- **Episcleritis** sometimes occurs.

Psoriatic arthritis

Introduction

Up to 40% of patients with psoriasis develop arthritis. The arthritis is more common in whites than other racial groups and affects both sexes equally. There is a first-degree family history in 40% or more, and many genetic markers have been identified.

Systemic features

- **Presentation** of psoriatic arthritis is usually in middle age – later than skin features.
- **Skin.** There are multiple types of psoriasis. Plaque-type, the most common form, is characterized by well-demarcated raised silvery inflamed plaques (Fig. 11.12A) on the scalp, trunk, arms and legs. Psoriatic erythroderma features widespread exfoliative skin changes with associated inflammation, and pustular psoriasis inflamed but non-infectious pustules limited or generalized in distribution.
- **Nail changes (dystrophy)** include pitting, transverse depression and onycholysis (Fig. 11.12B).
- **Arthritis** is typically asymmetrical and involves the distal interphalangeal joints (sausage digits). Some patients develop enthesitis.

Ocular features

AAU occurs in approximately 7%; conjunctivitis, marginal corneal infiltrates and secondary Sjögren syndrome may occur but are uncommon.

FUCHS UVEITIS SYNDROME

Introduction

Fuchs uveitis syndrome (FUS), also known as Fuchs heterochromic iridocyclitis or cyclitis (FHC), is a chronic non-granulomatous condition diagnosed at an average of 40 years old. There is no gender or racial predilection. The cause is uncertain, but there is evidence that implicates the rubella virus. Signs in toxoplasmosis can be similar, and *T. gondii* has also been suspected as a cause. It is possible that most of the anterior chamber activity is due to blood–aqueous barrier breakdown rather than inflammation.

Clinical features

Detection is often incidental; findings are usually unilateral (90–95%).

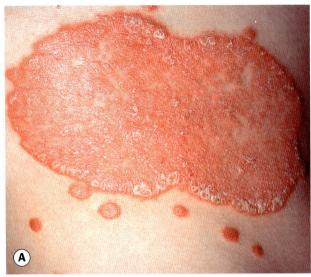

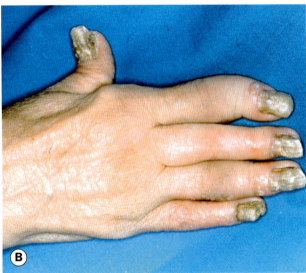

Fig. 11.12 Psoriasis. **(A)** Skin plaques; **(B)** arthritis and severe nail dystrophy

- **Symptoms.** Gradual blurring due to cataract is a common presentation, as are persistent floaters; heterochromia (see next) may be noted.
- **Heterochromia iridis** (Table 11.6) is demonstrated most effectively in daylight; most commonly the affected eye is hypochromic (Fig. 11.13A). Its quality is determined by the relative degrees of atrophy of the stroma and posterior pigment epithelium. It may be absent or subtle, particularly in brown eyes. In blue eyes, stromal atrophy allows the posterior pigmented layer to show through and become the dominant pigmentation, so that the eye sometimes becomes hyperchromic.
- **Posterior synechiae** are absent, except occasionally following cataract surgery.
- **Anterior chamber** shows faint flare and usually only mild cellular activity, though exacerbations can sometimes be marked. The eye is virtually always white, even during exacerbations.

Table 11.6 Causes of heterochromia iridis

Hypochromic
Idiopathic congenital
Horner syndrome, particularly if congenital
Waardenburg syndrome
Hyperchromic
Unilateral use of a topical prostaglandin analogue for
    glaucoma
Oculodermal melanocytosis (naevus of Ota)
Ocular siderosis
Diffuse iris naevus or melanoma
Sturge–Weber syndrome
Hypo- or hyperchromic
Fuchs uveitis syndrome
Other chronic anterior uveitides

- **Keratic precipitates** are characteristically stellate and grey–white in colour; they are located diffusely over the entire corneal endothelium (Fig. 11.13B and see Fig. 11.3D).
- **Iris nodules** (30%) on the pupillary border (Koeppe – Fig. 11.13C and see Fig. 11.5A) or occasionally in the stroma (Busacca). Tiny crystals (Russell bodies) may be present on the iris surface (see Fig. 11.5D).
- **Iris atrophy** is diffuse with loss of crypts; the iris appears smooth, with a prominent sphincter pupillae and sometimes blood vessels (see Fig. 11.13C); pigment epithelial atrophy can be demonstrated by retroillumination (Fig. 11.13D).
- **Iris vessels.** Fine irregular iris surface vessels (see Fig. 11.13C) are commonly present.
- **Vitritis.** Opacities in the anterior gel may be dense.
- **Cataract** is extremely common; a posterior subcapsular morphology is seen initially.
- **Glaucoma** is typically a later manifestation but is occasionally advanced at diagnosis. It develops in up to 60% of involved eyes. Several mechanisms are suspected.
- **Gonioscopy** may show fine radial angle vessels or small irregular peripheral anterior synechiae (Fig. 11.13E); the vessels are typically the source of the haemorrhage sometimes seen on incision into the anterior chamber (Amsler sign).
- **Fundus:** peripheral choroiditis foci/scarring have been reported. There may be an increased incidence of retinal dialysis. Macular oedema essentially does not occur, except following surgery.

Investigation

Diagnosis is clinical, though investigation may be necessary to exclude alternative conditions.

Treatment

- **Long-term monitoring** is indicated to detect glaucoma and other complications.
- **Topical steroids** may be used short-term for moderate/severe exacerbations, but are generally not thought to be helpful in the management of chronic low-grade inflammation.

- **Cataract surgery** carries a higher risk of complications. Poor mydriasis and the possibility of postoperative hyphaema, increased inflammation, worsening of glaucoma control and zonular dehiscence should be taken into account. Preoperative topical or systemic steroids are used by some practitioners.
- **Glaucoma** can be difficult to control medically. The place of laser trabeculoplasty is undefined, but is probably ineffective if PAS are present. Options include a glaucoma drainage device or trabeculectomy with mitomycin-C enhancement.
- **Pars plana vitrectomy** may be considered for visually problematic vitreous opacification.

UVEITIS IN JUVENILE IDIOPATHIC ARTHRITIS

Introduction

Juvenile idiopathic arthritis (JIA) is by far the most common systemic disease associated with childhood anterior uveitis; the prevalence is about 1:1000. It is defined as arthritis of unknown aetiology that begins before the age of 16 years and persists for at least 6 weeks; up to 50% of children affected have persistently active disease after 10 years. It may result from exposure to one or more unknown antigens in genetically predisposed individuals.

Clinical features

- **Arthritis.** JIA is classified by the International League of Associations for Rheumatology (ILAR, 2004 revision), according to the extent of joint involvement during the first 6 months:
  - Oligoarticular is the most common form. Four or fewer joints are involved, the knees most commonly, followed by the ankles and wrists. Girls are affected five times as often as boys, with a peak age of onset around 2 years. Some patients subsequently develop polyarthritis. About 75% of children are antinuclear antibody (ANA) positive, a strong risk factor for uveitis, which is common, affecting about 20% of children in this group.
  - Polyarticular (rheumatoid factor negative) affects five or more joints, typically both small and large joints symmetrically. The female:male ratio is about 3:1; the disease may commence at any age throughout childhood. Systemic features such as fever and rash may occur but are milder than in the systemic onset form (see below). About 40% of children are ANA-positive. Uveitis occurs in 5–10% of cases.
  - Polyarticular (rheumatoid factor positive) again affects five or more joints, and may resemble adult rheumatoid arthritis; there is a very low risk of uveitis.
  - Systemic, also known as Still (Still's) disease. Systemic features such as fever, episodic erythematous maculopapular rash, lymphadenopathy and hepatosplenomegaly may precede arthritis. The disease

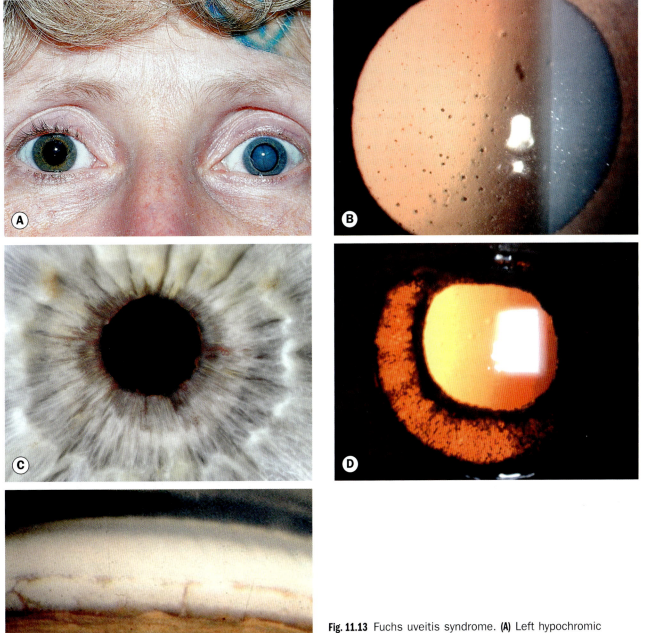

Fig. 11.13 Fuchs uveitis syndrome. **(A)** Left hypochromic heterochromia and cataract; **(B)** diffuse stellate keratic precipitates; **(C)** Koeppe nodules, stromal atrophy and prominent blood vessels including neovascularization; **(D)** band-like posterior pigment layer atrophy seen on retroillumination; **(E)** angle vessels and small peripheral anterior synechiae

(Courtesy of C Pavesio – fig. B; C Barry – fig. C)

occurs with equal frequency in boys and girls and may occur at any age throughout childhood. The majority are negative for ANA, and uveitis is rare.
  o Enthesitis-related, psoriatic and undifferentiated are three other forms under the ILAR classification; the first two have a relatively high risk of uveitis, risk in the latter is variable but often low.

- Anterior uveitis is a key cause of morbidity in JIA. It is particularly common in oligoarticular JIA, and relatively frequent in several other types. Progression to blindness has been high in historical data but shows a declining trend in recent years associated with improved screening and management. Arthritis usually antedates the diagnosis of uveitis.

○ Presentation. The uveitis of JIA is particularly dangerous because it is invariably asymptomatic and must generally be detected by screening with slit lamp examination. Even during acute exacerbations with +4 aqueous cells, it is rare for patients to complain, although a few report an increase in vitreous floaters. Often uveitis may not be suspected until the parents recognize complications such as strabismus, or an abnormal appearance of the eyeball due to band keratopathy or cataract.

○ Injection is usually absent even in the presence of severe uveitis.

○ Inflammation is chronic and non-granulomatous. Both eyes are affected in 70%; when bilateral, the severity of inflammation is usually symmetrical. During acute exacerbations, the entire endothelium shows 'dusting' by many hundreds of cells, but hypopyon is absent.

○ Posterior synechiae are common in long-standing undetected cases.

○ Band keratopathy and cataract (Fig. 11.14) are extremely common in severe cases.

○ Other serious complications include glaucoma (common), amblyopia, maculopathy (cystoid macular oedema, epiretinal membrane), cyclitic membrane and phthisis.

○ Prognosis. In about 10% the uveitis is mild, with never more than +1 aqueous cells, and persists for less than 12 months. About 15% of patients have one attack lasting less than 4 months, the severity of inflammation varying from +2 to +4 aqueous cells. In 50% of cases, the uveitis is moderate to severe and persists for more than 4 months, and in 25%, the uveitis is very severe, lasts for several years and responds poorly to treatment. The presence of complications at initial examination appears to be an important risk factor for the development of subsequent complications, regardless of therapy.

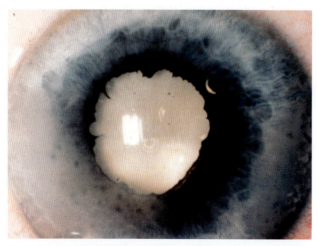

Fig. 11.14 Band keratopathy, posterior synechiae and mature cataract in chronic anterior uveitis associated with juvenile idiopathic arthritis

Investigation

- **Systemic diagnosis and management** should be performed by a physician familiar with the management of JIA, typically a paediatric rheumatologist.
- **Antinuclear antibody (ANA).** Positivity denotes an increased risk of uveitis.
- **HLA-B27 testing** is useful in differential diagnosis (see above) and if present may indicate an increased risk of uveitis.
- **Rheumatoid factor.** is also useful in differential diagnosis.
- **Screening.** There has been a shift in recommendation towards long-term 3–4 monthly review intervals in all higher-risk categories. Review should continue in most cases until the age of 12 years.
  - ○ Initial examination within 6 weeks of first diagnosis of JIA. Delayed early examination is an important cause of morbidity.
  - ○ Visual symptoms or a suspicion of ocular signs (synechiae, cataract, band keratopathy) should lead to urgent ophthalmological referral and slit lamp examination within a week.
  - ○ Initial 2-monthly examinations for 6 months may be considered for all newly diagnosed oligoarticular, psoriatic, polyarticular and enthesitis-related patients, regardless of ANA status, followed by 3–4 monthly intervals.
  - ○ Polyarticular: every 3–4 months; some guidelines reduce the interval to 6-monthly after a number of years. Higher-risk factors that might be taken into account in deciding whether to alter the interval include the presence of ANA, onset before 7 years of age and female gender.
  - ○ Systemic onset and polyarticular RF-positive patients: most authorities recommend at least an initial screening examination, with some guidelines suggesting annual review.
  - ○ Missed appointments must be effectively detected and patients rebooked.
  - ○ Information for parents should include an emphasis on the importance of compliance with screening, as well as the need to seek urgent advice should there be any cause for concern such as visual symptoms, ocular redness or clouding, or abnormal pupils.
  - ○ Self-monitoring. At eventual discharge from screening, patients should be warned to self-monitor by checking the monocular vision at least once a week; the risk of uveitis has not entirely disappeared by this age. They should also attend an optometrist annually for an eye examination. Selected patients such as those with learning difficulties may require ongoing ophthalmological screening.
- **Differential diagnosis**: investigations as appropriate. Particular considerations in children include:
  - ○ Idiopathic juvenile chronic iridocyclitis: otherwise healthy patients with juvenile CAU; also generally asymptomatic until complications occur.

○ Other types of juvenile arthritis and uveitis including juvenile reactive arthritis, juvenile inflammatory bowel disease-associated arthritis.

○ Juvenile sarcoidosis: rare; pulmonary involvement is less common than in adults; may be granulomatous and involve the posterior segment.

○ Lyme disease usually presents with intermediate uveitis in conjunction with significant anterior uveitis.

○ Intermediate uveitis: 20% of all cases of paediatric uveitis.

○ Neonatal-onset multisystem inflammatory disease is a rare, idiopathic, chronic relapsing disease that predominantly involves the skin, joints and the central nervous system. About 50% of children develop recurrent anterior uveitis. The absence of posterior synechiae and no tendency to glaucoma and cataract formation are characteristic.

○ Masquerade syndromes such as anterior segment involvement by retinoblastoma.

○ Familial juvenile systemic granulomatosis (Blau syndrome), is a rare autosomal dominant disorder characterized by childhood onset of granulomatous disease of skin (panuveitis and multifocal choroiditis), eyes and joints.

Treatment

The aim of treatment should be the suppression of all active inflammation.

- **Topical steroids** are effective in most cases (80%); acute exacerbations require very frequent instillation.
- **Mydriatic agents** may be required for exacerbations to prevent synechiae formation. A relatively short-acting preparation such as cyclopentolate should be used and discontinued as early as possible, particularly in monocular treatment of younger children susceptible to the development of amblyopia.
- **Periocular steroids.**
- **Oral steroids.**
- **Non-steroidal anti-inflammatory drugs (NSAIDs).**
- **Systemic immunosuppressive agents** will be required in resistant cases (e.g. methotrexate, infliximab, adalimumab, ciclosporin) and should be managed by a specialist ophthalmologist, typically in collaboration with a paediatric rheumatologist. Doses required are often low.

UVEITIS IN BOWEL DISEASE

Ulcerative colitis

Introduction

Ulcerative colitis (UC) is an idiopathic chronic relapsing inflammatory disease, involving the rectum and extending proximally to involve part or all of the large intestine. The disease is characterized by contiguous surface ulceration of the bowel mucosa with the development of crypt abscesses and pseudopolyps (Fig. 11.15A).

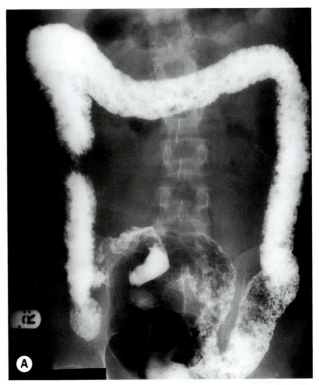

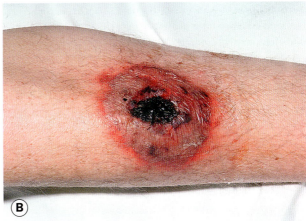

Fig. 11.15 Ulcerative colitis. **(A)** Barium enema shows pseudopolyposis, lack of haustral markings and straightening of the ascending colon; **(B)** pyoderma gangrenosum

Long-standing disease carries an increased risk of carcinoma of the colon. A genetic predisposition is thought to be important; inflammatory bowel disease is more common in patients with other autoimmune diseases such as ankylosing spondylitis, psoriasis and multiple sclerosis.

Systemic features

- **Presentation** is in the second to third decades with bloody diarrhoea, lower abdominal cramps, urgency and tenesmus. Constitutional symptoms include tiredness, weight loss, malaise and fever.
- **Cutaneous lesions** include oral aphthous ulceration, erythema nodosum and pyoderma gangrenosum (Fig. 11.15B).

- **Arthritis** is typically asymmetrical and involves large joints of the legs; sacroiliitis and ankylosing spondylitis (AS) may develop in HLA-B27-positive patients.
- **Hepatic disease** may be in the form of autoimmune hepatitis, sclerosing cholangitis and cholangiocarcinoma.
- **Thrombosis** may affect both arteries and veins.

Ocular features

- **AAU** occurs in about 5% and may coincide with exacerbations of colitis. As expected, uveitis is more common in patients with associated arthritis, AS and HLA-B27 positivity.
- **Other ocular features**: conjunctivitis, episcleritis and scleritis may all be more common than in the general population.

Crohn disease

Introduction

Crohn disease (CD) is an idiopathic chronic relapsing disease characterized by multifocal full-thickness granulomatous inflammation of the intestinal wall. It most frequently involves the terminal ileum and colon but in contrast to UC any area of the gastrointestinal tract, including the mouth, may be affected. There is strong evidence for a genetic aetiological component such as mutations in the *CARD15* (previously *NOD2*) gene. Infective agents almost certainly play a role.

Systemic features

- **Presentation** is typically in the second–third decades with abdominal pain and diarrhoea. Weight loss, fever, vomiting, oral aphthous ulceration and perirectal lesions such as abscesses and fistulae may occur.
- **Cutaneous lesions** include erythema nodosum and pyoderma gangrenosum (see Fig. 11.15B).
- **Anaemia** is common.
- **Hepatic disease** may occur.
- **Skeletal** features include finger clubbing, acute peripheral arthritis, sacroiliitis and ankylosing spondylitis (especially if HLA-B27-positive).

Ocular features

AAU occurs in about 3%; dry eye, conjunctivitis and scleritis may be more common than in the general population.

Whipple disease

Introduction

Whipple disease (intestinal lipodystrophy) is a rare chronic gastrointestinal inflammatory condition caused by infection with the bacterium *Tropheryma whipplei*. It occurs mainly in white middle-aged men and when diagnosed (duodenal biopsy; DNA detection in blood, ocular and other fluids) can be cured with antibiotics.

Systemic features

Inflammatory bowel disease with malabsorption; joint, cardiac and central nervous system (CNS) involvement is common.

Ocular features

- **Uveitis.** Keratitis, anterior uveitis, vitritis, retinitis with retinal haemorrhages, cotton-wool spots and potentially vascular occlusion, and multifocal choroiditis.
- **Neuro-ophthalmic** manifestations can be varied, e.g. gaze palsy, nystagmus, ophthalmoplegia, papilloedema and optic atrophy. Oculomasticatory myorhythmia is characteristic.

UVEITIS IN RENAL DISEASE

Tubulointerstitial nephritis and uveitis

Introduction

Tubulointerstitial nephritis and uveitis (TINU) is an uncommon disorder of immune origin characterized by a combination of acute tubulointerstitial nephritis and uveitis. It typically occurs in adolescent girls; renal disease usually precedes uveitis.

Systemic features

Presentation is with constitutional symptoms, proteinuria, anaemia, hypertension and renal failure. The response to systemic steroid therapy is good and renal function usually returns to normal within a few months without complication.

Ocular features

- **Bilateral non-granulomatous (occasionally granulomatous) anterior uveitis** that usually responds well to topical steroids. Disc and macular oedema may occur. Many cases are relapsing and some require systemic steroids or immunosuppressive therapy.
- **Intermediate, posterior or panuveitis** may occur.

IgA nephropathy

IgA nephropathy (Berger disease) is a relatively common kidney disease in which immunoglobulin A is deposited in the glomerular mesangium. Presentation is usually at age 16–35 with recurrent haematuria, often associated with an upper respiratory tract infection, but may be asymptomatic. AAU and other ocular inflammatory phenomena may occur but are uncommon.

INTERMEDIATE UVEITIS

Introduction

Intermediate uveitis (IU) is a chronic, relapsing disease of insidious onset in which, according to the SUN Working Group, the vitreous is the primary site of inflammation as determined clinically.

It incorporates pars planitis, posterior cyclitis and hyalitis. The diagnosis is essentially clinical; IU may be idiopathic (at least half) or associated with a systemic disease, and systemic investigations are routinely performed, especially in the presence of suggestive findings and/or in older individuals. Pars planitis (PP) is the term used for a subset of IU in which there is snowbanking and/or snowball formation (see below), but only if the inflammation is idiopathic – that is, with no identifiable underlying infection or systemic disease – otherwise the term intermediate uveitis is reverted to. IU accounts for up to 15% of all uveitis cases and about 20% of paediatric uveitis. A minority of patients have a benign course, with spontaneous resolution within several years. In other patients the disease is more severe and prolonged with episodic exacerbations. IU associated with systemic disease has a variable course.

Clinical features

- **Symptoms.** Presentation is with the insidious onset of blurred vision, often accompanied by vitreous floaters; there is usually no pain or redness. Though initial symptoms are often unilateral, objective findings are typically present asymmetrically in both eyes.
- **Visual acuity** is variably affected depending on inflammatory activity and complications, particularly CMO. The disease may last as long as 15 years and preservation of vision will depend largely on control of macular disease. In follow-up of up to 4 years, 75% of patients maintain a visual acuity of 6/12 or better.
- **Anterior uveitis.** In PP there may be a few cells and small scattered KP which occasionally have an inferior linear distribution. In other forms of IU, anterior uveitis and its associated findings such as PS can be more prominent, especially in children, and in sarcoidosis and Lyme disease.
- **Vitreous.** Vitreous cells with anterior predominance (Fig. 11.16A) are universal, with vitreous condensation and haze (Table 11.7) in more severe cases (Fig. 11.16B). Snowballs are whitish focal collections of inflammatory cells and exudate, usually most numerous in the inferior vitreous (Fig. 11.17A).
- **Peripheral periphlebitis** (Fig. 11.17B) is common, particularly in MS. Careful examination of a normal fellow eye in apparently unilateral disease may reveal mild vascular sheathing.
- **Snowbanking** (Figs 11.17C) is characterized by a grey–white fibrovascular and/or exudative plaque that may occur in any or all quadrants, but is most frequently found inferiorly.

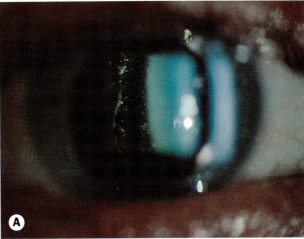

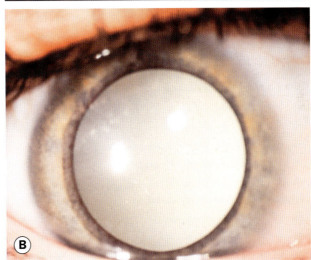

Fig. 11.16 Vitreous inflammatory activity. **(A)** Mild; **(B)** severe

Table 11.7 Grading of vitreous haze

Haze severity	Grading
Good view of nerve fibre layer (NFL)	0
Clear disc and vessels but hazy NFL	+1
Disc and vessels hazy	+2
Only disc visible	+3
Disc not visible	+4

- **Neovascularization** may occur, particularly in the retinal periphery (often associated with snowbanks) and on the optic nerve head; the latter usually resolves when activity is controlled. This can sometimes lead to vitreous haemorrhage, retinal detachment and cyclitic membrane formation. Focal peripheral retinal vasoproliferative tumours (see Ch. 12) are uncommon. Vitreous haemorrhage is more common in children.
- **Optic disc swelling** is common, especially in younger patients.
- **CMO** occurs in up to half of patients and is the major cause of impaired visual acuity.
- **Macular epiretinal membrane** formation is common.
- **Cataract** can be caused by steroid treatment or by the inflammation itself; both are probably contributory in the majority of patients.
- **Glaucoma** may occur in eyes with prolonged inflammation, particularly if receiving long-term steroid therapy.
- **Retinal detachment** is generally uncommon, but as it can progress to hypotony and phthisis in advanced cases,

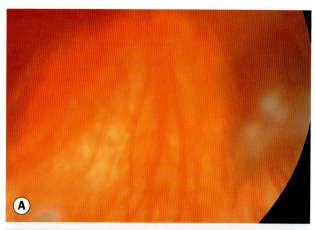

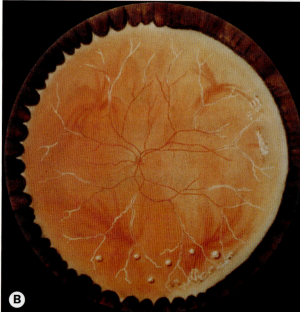

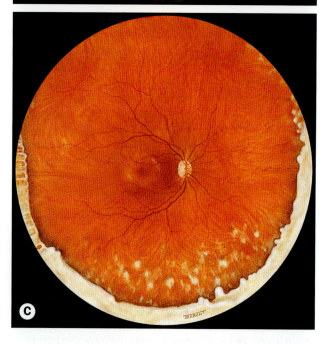

Fig. 11.17 Intermediate uveitis. **(A)** Snowballs; **(B)** peripheral periphlebitis and snowballs; **(C)** inferior snowbanking and snowballs

(Courtesy of CL Schepens, ME Hartnett and T Hirose, from Schepens' Retinal Detachment and Allied Diseases, *Butterworth-Heinemann, 2000 – fig. B)*

prevention should be a major goal of management. The aetiology may be tractional, rhegmatogenous and occasionally exudative. Retinoschisis has also been described.

Investigation

Inflammatory markers such as ESR and/or CRP should be checked, together with a complete blood count, as they may raise suspicion of a systemic inflammatory process. OCT is key to excluding subtle CMO, and FA will help in assessing severity. Other investigations are targeted at the exclusion of an underlying cause as below.

- **Multiple sclerosis.** Enquiry should be made in all patients about neurological symptoms, noting that IU may precede other symptoms of demyelination. MS should be suspected in patients aged 20–50; it is twice as common in women. Granulomatous AAU may occur. Cranial MRI imaging should be performed if any suspicion is raised.
- **Sarcoidosis.** A review of systems should include respiratory function. Sarcoid-associated IU is relatively uncommon and as with MS may antedate the onset of systemic disease. The presence of associated granulomatous anterior uveitis should arouse suspicion. A serum ACE level and chest X-ray should be performed in all adult patients.
- **Lyme disease-associated** IU is often associated with severe anterior uveitis. Serology should be performed if residence in or a visit to an endemic area is elicited.
- **Syphilis serology** – treponemal and cardiolipin antibody tests – should be performed.
- **Tuberculosis** is an uncommon association that may give respiratory symptoms and be demonstrated on chest X-ray. Tuberculin skin and/or blood (e.g. QuantiFERON™) testing should be performed prior to steroid treatment in the presence of any suspicion.
- **Other conditions** that may give vitritis mimicking IU include Fuchs uveitis syndrome, intraocular lymphoma (older patients), *Toxocara* granuloma, Whipple disease, endogenous *Candida* endophthalmitis (risk factors such as IV drug use) and toxoplasmosis. These will commonly be suspected on the basis of the history and specific clinical findings.

Treatment

An identified infection or other underlying disease should be treated specifically, supplemented by anti-inflammatory measures below as appropriate. Many authorities aim to abolish all active inflammation regardless of whether vision has been affected;

factors such as the presence of peripheral neovascularization may prompt earlier intervention.

- **Topical steroids** do not reach the posterior segment in high concentrations so have only a limited role, and are used principally to treat any anterior uveitic component. It has been proposed that in mild intermediate uveitis a course of frequent topical steroid of a few weeks' duration may exert some benefit and identify individuals at high risk of IOP elevation without committing to the extended action of depot injection.
- **Regional steroid injection.** Orbital floor or posterior sub-Tenon injection as described for anterior uveitis. Depending on severity, injection is performed 4–6 times at intervals of 2–4 weeks, accompanied by careful IOP monitoring.
- **NSAID.** If inflammation persists after regional injection, an agent such as naproxen 500 mg twice daily can be commenced.
- **Cryotherapy** (double freeze–thaw) to the pars plana and retinal periphery under peribulbar anaesthesia can be highly effective if inflammation is steroid-resistant, and may be appropriate prior to systemic steroids. It can be associated with transiently increased vitritis and other complications including retinal detachment, cataract, vitreous and anterior chamber haemorrhage, epiretinal membrane formation and hypotony. A repeat application may be needed after several months. Some authorities reserve cryotherapy for peripheral neovascularization with haemorrhage.
- **Peripheral retinal laser** adjacent to snowbanking and/or to ischaemic areas on FA is an alternative to cryotherapy, and may be as effective with a lower rate of complications.
- **Intraocular steroid.** Intravitreal triamcinolone has shown benefit, but the effect is of relatively short duration. Slow-release implants have demonstrated promising results.
- **Systemic steroids.** This modality is preferred over regional steroid by some practitioners if symptomatic inflammation is bilateral, though others prefer to avoid systemic steroids in most cases, proceeding directly to immunosuppressive chemotherapeutic agents. A large dose of 1–2 mg/kg/day is commenced, tapered slowly over months according to response. Familiarity with precautions to be taken, contraindications to and potential adverse effects of steroids is essential before prescribing; optimally steroids should be prescribed in conjunction with a specialist physician, such as a rheumatologist.
- **Immunosuppressive agents.** Mycophenolate, methotrexate, tacrolimus, ciclosporin and others are alternatives in steroid-resistant inflammation or as steroid-sparing agents. One or more of these may be available as local sustained-release preparations in the near future.
- **Other agents** demonstrating efficacy in refractory and other patients include interferon-beta (in MS-related IU), the anti-tumour necrosis factor infliximab, intravitreal bevacizumab and others.
- **Pars plana vitrectomy** typically substantially reduces inflammatory intensity and recurrence, though the mechanism is imperfectly understood. It may be particularly indicated in patients with tractional retinal detachment, epiretinal membrane, refractory CMO, dense vitreous opacity, vitreous haemorrhage or substantial peripheral neovascularization.
- **Cataract and glaucoma** are managed medically and surgically as indicated.

VOGT–KOYANAGI–HARADA (VKH) SYNDROME

Introduction

VKH is an idiopathic multisystem autoimmune disease featuring inflammation of melanocyte-containing tissues such as the uvea, ear and meninges. VKH predominantly affects Hispanic, Japanese and pigmented individuals; it is associated with HLA-DR1 and HLA-DR4 across different racial groups. VKH is sometimes subdivided into Vogt–Koyanagi disease, characterized mainly by skin changes and anterior uveitis, and Harada disease, in which neurological features and exudative retinal detachments predominate.

Clinical features

- **Prodromal phase** lasting a few days: neurological (meningitis and rarely encephalopathy with cranial nerve paresis and other focal lesions) and auditory manifestations (tinnitus, vertigo and deafness). Cranial nerve palsies and optic neuritis may occur.
- **Acute uveitic phase.** Bilateral granulomatous anterior and multifocal posterior uveitis with diffuse choroidal infiltration, Dalen–Fuchs nodules (see also sympathetic ophthalmitis below), vitritis, papillitis and exudative retinal detachments (Fig. 11.18 and see Fig. 11.21). Ciliary effusion with iris-lens diaphragm rotation can occur.

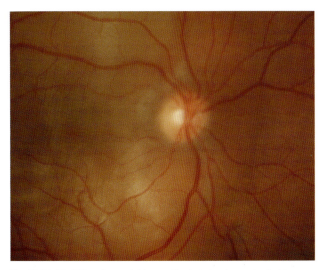

Fig. 11.18 Multifocal exudative retinal detachments in the acute uveitic phase of Vogt–Koyanagi–Harada syndrome
(Courtesy of C Barry)

- **Convalescent phase** follows several weeks later: localized alopecia, poliosis and vitiligo (Fig. 11.19); depigmented fundus appearance ('sunset glow' fundus – Fig. 11.20) and depigmented limbal lesions (Sugiura sign) in pigmented, especially Japanese, patients.
- **Chronic recurrent phase** is characterized by smouldering anterior uveitis with exacerbations. Recurrent posterior uveitis is much less common.
- **Diagnostic criteria** for VKH are set out in Table 11.8; in complete VKH, criteria 1–5 must be present, in incomplete VKH, criteria 1–3 and either 4 or 5 must be present, and in probable VKH (isolated ocular disease), criteria 1–3 must be present.
- **Ocular complications** include choroidal neovascularization, subretinal fibrosis, preretinal and disc new vessels and vitreous haemorrhage, cataract and glaucoma.
- **Prognosis** is very variable, and is partly dependent on aggressive control in the early stages. Neurological and

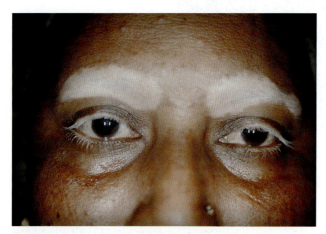

Fig. 11.19 Vitiligo and poliosis in Vogt–Koyanagi–Harada syndrome
(Courtesy of U Raina)

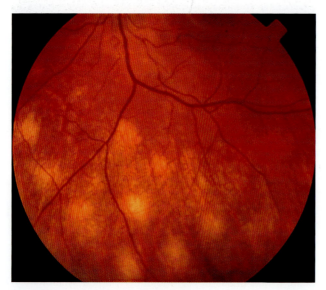

Fig. 11.20 'Sunset glow' fundus

Table 11.8 Modified diagnostic criteria for Vogt-Koyanagi–Harada syndrome

1. Absence of a history of penetrating ocular trauma
2. Absence of other ocular disease entities
3. Bilateral uveitis
4. Neurological and auditory manifestations
5. Integumentary findings, not preceding onset of central nervous system or ocular disease, such as alopecia, poliosis and vitiligo

auditory manifestations tends to resolve but skin, lash and hair changes usually persist.

Investigation

Systemic manifestations should be investigated and managed by an appropriate specialist.

- **Lumbar puncture** if diagnosis uncertain; CSF shows a transient lymphocytic pleocytosis, and melanin-containing macrophages.
- **FAF** demonstrates areas of serous detachment (Fig. 11.21A).
- **OCT** (Fig. 11.21B) allows quantification of subretinal fluid.
- **Ultrasonography** shows diffuse choroidal thickening and excludes posterior scleritis; UBM can be used to demonstrate ciliary effusions.
- **FA** of the acute phase shows multifocal hyperfluorescent dots at the level of the retinal pigment epithelium (RPE; Fig. 11.21C) followed by subretinal pooling (Fig. 11.21D). The chronic phase shows RPE window defects.
- **ICGA** during the acute phase of the disease shows regularly distributed hypofluorescent spots, most of which remain hypofluorescent during the late phase, when diffuse hyperfluorescence over the posterior pole is also shown. ICGA is useful for monitoring.

Treatment

High dose (1–2 mg/kg/day) oral prednisolone, tapered over 3–6 months; this may be preceded by intravenous methylprednisolone pulse therapy (500–1000 mg/day). Topical steroids and cycloplegics are used for anterior uveitis. Steroid-resistant patients may require immunosuppressives; biological blockers such as infliximab show promise.

SYMPATHETIC OPHTHALMITIS

Introduction

Sympathetic ophthalmitis (SO) is a bilateral granulomatous panuveitis occurring after penetrating trauma; uveal prolapse may have been a feature of the trauma. Less frequently the condition occurs following intraocular surgery, usually multiple vitreoretinal procedures. Presentation in trauma-induced cases is between 2 weeks and 3 months after initial injury in 65%. The incidence is probably 0.2–0.5% after injury and 0.01% following intraocular surgery.

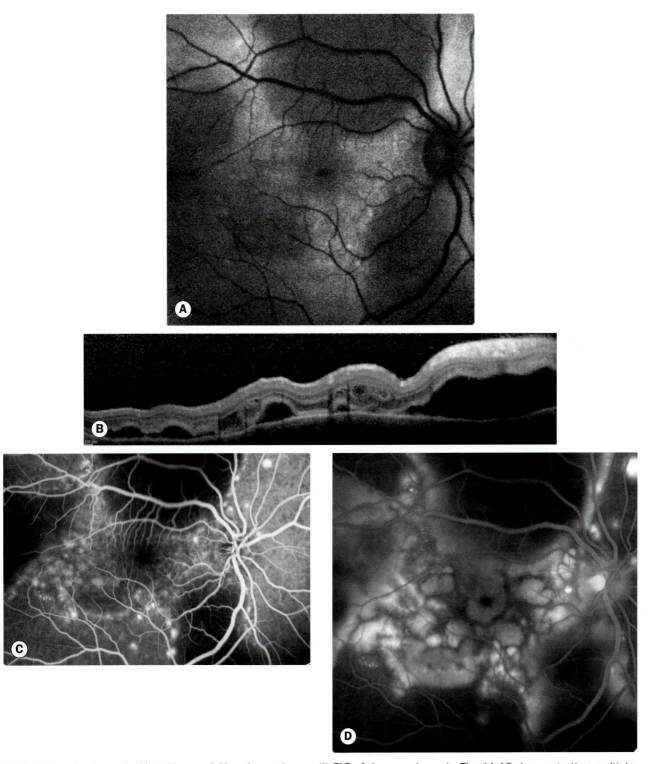

Fig. 11.21 Imaging in ocular Vogt–Koyanagi–Harada syndrome. **(A)** FAF of the eye shown in Fig. 11.18 demonstrating multiple exudative detachments; **(B)** OCT; **(C)** FA – multiple hyperfluorescent leaking spots in venous phase; **(D)** pooling of dye within detached areas in late FA images

(Courtesy of C Barry)

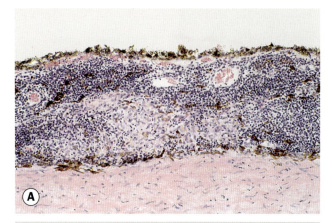

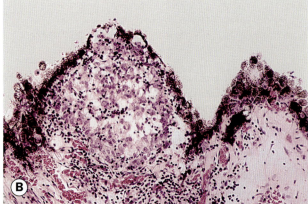

Fig. 11.22 Histology of sympathetic ophthalmitis. **(A)** Infiltration of the choroid by lymphocytes and scattered aggregations of epithelioid cells, many of which contain fine granules of melanin; **(B)** Dalen–Fuchs nodule – a granuloma situated between Bruch membrane and the retinal pigment epithelium

(Courtesy of J Harry)

Histopathology shows a diffuse lymphocytic infiltration of the choroid. Scattered aggregates of epithelioid cells are seen, many of which contain fine granules of melanin (Fig. 11.22A). Dalen–Fuchs nodules, which also occur in Vogt–Koyanagi–Harada syndrome (see above) are granulomas located between Bruch membrane and the RPE (Fig. 11.22B).

Clinical features

- **Symptoms.** There is a history of causative trauma; the exciting eye is frequently red and irritable (Fig. 11.23A). The sympathizing eye develops irritation, blurred vision, photophobia and loss of accommodation.
- **Anterior uveitis** develops in both eyes; this may be mild or severe and is usually granulomatous (Fig. 11.23B). The severity of inflammation may be markedly asymmetrical.
- **Fundus**: multifocal choroidal infiltrates develop in the midperiphery (Fig. 11.23C), with sub-RPE infiltrates corresponding to Dalen–Fuchs nodules. Exudative retinal detachment, vasculitis and optic disc swelling may all manifest. As inflammation settles, residual chorioretinal scarring may confer a 'sunset glow' appearance similar to VKH.

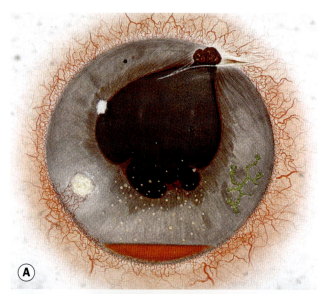

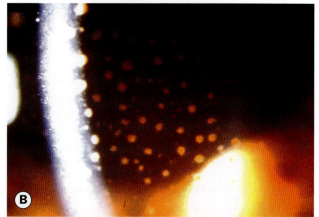

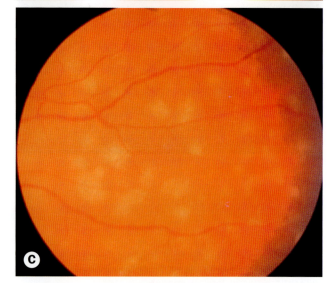

Fig. 11.23 Sympathetic ophthalmitis. **(A)** The exciting eye; **(B)** large keratic precipitates in the sympathizing eye; **(C)** multifocal choroidal infiltrates

(Courtesy of W Wykes – fig. A)

- **Systemic manifestations** similar to those in VKH can occur but are uncommon.
- **Prognosis** depends on the severity and location of disease and the response to treatment. With aggressive therapy 75% of sympathizing eyes retain a visual acuity of better than 6/60. Long-term follow-up is mandatory because relapses occur in 50% of cases, and may be delayed for several years.

Investigation

- **OCT** is useful for quantifying and monitoring change.
- **B-scan ultrasonography** may demonstrate choroidal thickening.
- **FA** shows multiple foci of leakage at the level of the RPE, with subretinal pooling in the presence of exudative retinal detachment.
- **ICGA** shows hypofluorescent spots in active disease, which resolve with treatment.
- **Ultrasound** may show choroidal thickening and exudative retinal detachment.

Treatment

- **Enucleation** of a severely injured eye in the first week or so following injury has historically been considered effective in preventing or reducing the severity of SO, but there is some evidence that little useful effect is exerted, particularly with modern standards of surgical repair. It may be considered for an injured eye with a hopeless visual prognosis. Evisceration has conventionally been viewed as inadequate, though recent evidence has raised the possibility of a protective effect provided all uveal tissue is removed.
- **Steroids** are the basis of treatment. High dose oral prednisolone is given for several months, and gradually tapered according to response. Initiation with intravenous methylprednisolone may be used in some cases. Supplementary topical steroids and cycloplegics may be given to target anterior uveitis, and peri- and intraocular steroids, including slow-release intravitreal implants, may facilitate reduced systemic treatment.
- Immunosuppressives such as azathioprine, ciclosporin and methotrexate can be used in resistant cases or as steroid-sparing agents. Biological blockers (e.g. infliximab, adalimumab) may be considered.

LENS-INDUCED UVEITIS

Introduction

Lens-induced or phacogenic (previously phacoanaphylactic) uveitis results from an immune response to lens proteins following exposure due to incomplete cataract extraction, trauma or rarely capsular degeneration in a mature cataract (Fig. 11.24). The most commonly encountered modern scenario is that of retained lens fragments following phacoemulsification, either in the posterior segment after posterior capsular rupture or zonular dehiscence, or

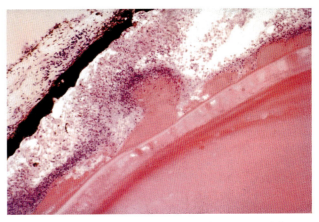

Fig. 11.24 Lens-induced uveitis – exposed lens material producing an inflammatory reaction
(Courtesy of J Harry and G Misson, from Clinical Ophthalmic Pathology, Butterworth-Heinemann, 2001)

an overlooked piece of nucleus or soft lens matter settling in the anterior chamber (see also Chapter 9). Differential diagnosis is from bacterial endophthalmitis, which is usually more severe; in doubtful cases management should be as for infection.

Clinical features

- **Symptoms.** Variable pain, photophobia, redness and blurring, usually with a history of recent (complicated or uncomplicated) cataract surgery and uncommonly of injury.
- **Anterior uveitis** is granulomatous and may be mild, moderate or severe.
- **Corneal oedema** is common adjacent to an anterior chamber lens fragment.
- **IOP** is frequently elevated.
- **Lens fragments** may be visible in the anterior or posterior segment.
- **Vitritis** of variable severity is usually present if lens fragments lie within the vitreous cavity.
- **Lens injury** may be evident in cases associated with trauma.
- **Complications** include CMO, glaucoma, epiretinal membrane and, rarely, more severe sequelae such as retinal detachment and cyclitic membrane.

Investigation

OCT, B-scan and biomicroscopic ultrasonography may be indicated.

Treatment

Treatment involves steroids, the route and intensity dependent on clinical circumstances, with surgical removal of all lens material from the anterior chamber or via pars plana vitrectomy as required. Small lens fragments in the posterior segment can often be managed conservatively and will absorb slowly over months. Cycloplegia and IOP-lowering treatment are commonly indicated. Penetrating or (uncommonly) blunt ocular injury should be managed concomitantly as appropriate, including removal of the damaged lens.

SARCOIDOSIS

Introduction

Sarcoidosis is a chronic disorder of unknown cause, manifesting with non-caseating granulomatous inflammatory foci. It can affect essentially any organ system, but the lungs and lymph nodes are the most commonly involved. It more frequently (10:1) affects patients of black than white ethnicity but is more common in colder climates. It is one of the most common systemic associations of uveitis.

Systemic features

- **Presentation.** Respiratory symptoms (cough, shortness of breath on exertion) and constitutional symptoms (malaise, arthralgia) each occur in about 50% of patients. Löfgren syndrome is an acute presentation carrying a very good prognosis, characterized by the triad of erythema nodosum (see below), bilateral hilar lymphadenopathy (Fig. 11.25A) on chest X-ray, and polyarthralgia, usually seen in women. A minority of patients are asymptomatic (incidentally abnormal chest X-ray). Diagnosis may be made as the result of investigation of extrapulmonary inflammation such as uveitis.
- **Lung** disease ranges from mild parenchymal infiltration to severe pulmonary fibrosis.
- **Skin** lesions are seen in about 25% of patients and can include erythema nodosum (tender erythematous plaques typically involving the shins – Fig. 11.25B), lupus pernio (indurated violaceous lesions involving exposed parts of the body such as the nose, cheeks, fingers and ears – Fig. 11.25C) and granulomatous papules or macules.
- **Neurological** disease is rare; meningitis and cranial nerve palsies may occur. Pituitary involvement can lead to hormonal abnormalities.

- **Cardiac involvement** is relatively uncommon (5% clinically), but is critically important as it may lead to arrhythmia and sudden death.
- **Lymphadenopathy.** Enlargement of superficial nodes is sometimes the initial clinical manifestation.

Ocular features

Ocular inflammation occurs in 25–70% of sarcoid patients depending on ethnicity; granulomatous anterior uveitis is the most common manifestation. Blindness can occur if not adequately managed. AAU typically affects patients with acute-onset sarcoidosis. CAU, typically granulomatous, tends to affect older patients with chronic pulmonary disease. The International Workshop on Ocular Sarcoidosis (IWOS), reporting in 2009, identified seven key signs in the diagnosis of intraocular sarcoidosis:

1. '**Mutton fat' KPs** (Fig. 11.26A) **and/or small granulomatous KPs and/or iris nodules** (Koeppe and/or Busacca – Fig. 11.26B).
2. **Trabecular meshwork (TM) nodules** (Fig. 11.26C) **and/or tent-shaped PAS.**
3. **Vitreous opacities: snowballs** (Fig. 11.26D) **and/or 'strings of pearls'.**
4. **Multiple chorioretinal peripheral lesions** (active and/or atrophic – Fig. 11.27). Choroidal lesions are uncommon and vary in appearance: multiple small pale-yellow infiltrates, sometimes with a punched-out appearance (Figs 11.27A and B) are the commonest; they are often most numerous inferiorly. Multiple large confluent infiltrates are less common (Fig. 11.27C). Multifocal choroiditis (Fig. 11.27D) carries a guarded visual prognosis even after resolution of activity, as a result of secondary choroidal neovascularization associated with macular or peripapillary chorioretinal scarring. Retinal granulomas may also occur, seen as discrete small yellow–white lesions (Fig. 11.27E).

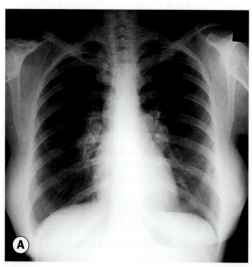
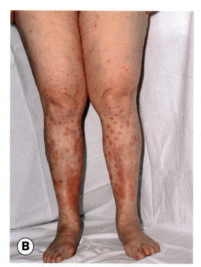
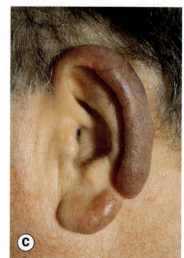

Fig. 11.25 Sarcoidosis. **(A)** Bilateral hilar lymphadenopathy; **(B)** erythema nodosum; **(C)** lupus pernio
(Courtesy of MA Mir, from Atlas of Clinical Diagnosis, Saunders 2003 – fig. C)

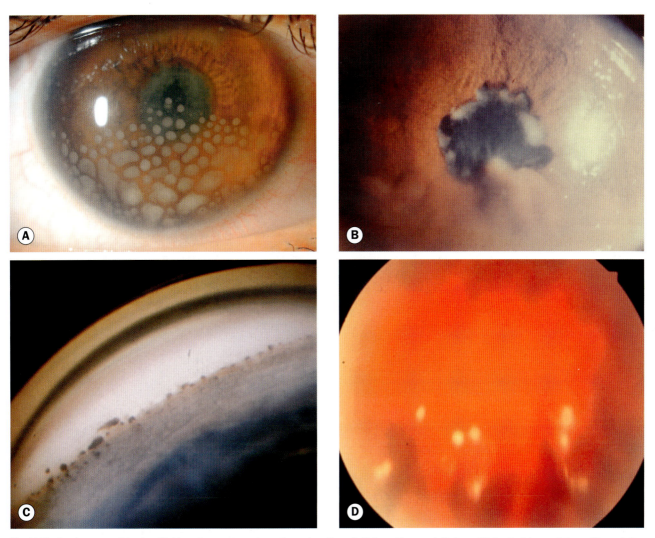

Fig. 11.26 Ocular sarcoidosis. **(A)** Very large granulomatous 'mutton fat' keratic precipitates; **(B)** large iris nodules; **(C)** nodular involvement of the trabecular meshwork; **(D)** snowballs
(Courtesy of J Salmon – fig. B)

5. **Nodular and/or segmental periphlebitis (± 'candle wax drippings') and/or retinal macroaneurysm in an inflamed eye.** Periphlebitis appears as yellowish or grey-white perivenous sheathing. Perivenous exudates referred to as 'candle wax drippings' (en taches de bougie) are typical of severe sarcoid periphlebitis (Fig. 11.28A). Occlusive periphlebitis (Fig. 11.28B) is uncommon, but peripheral retinal neovascularization may develop secondary to retinal capillary dropout. In black patients it may be mistaken for proliferative sickle-cell retinopathy.

6. **Optic disc nodule(s)/granuloma(s)** (Fig. 11.29) **and/or solitary choroidal nodule.** Solitary choroidal nodules are less common than multiple lesions in sarcoidosis. Focal optic nerve granulomas do not usually affect vision. Persistent disc oedema is a frequent finding in patients with retinal or vitreous involvement, and papilloedema due to CNS involvement may occur in the absence of other ocular manifestations.

7. **Bilaterality.**

8. Other ocular manifestations include **conjunctival nodules** resembling those of follicular conjunctivitis, **lacrimal gland infiltration** (Fig. 11.30) and **dry eye, eyelid skin nodules, orbital and scleral lesions**. Complications are those typically seen in idiopathic uveitis, including cataract, glaucoma, posterior and peripheral anterior synechiae, band keratopathy, vitreous haemorrhage, maculopathy (cystoid macular oedema, epiretinal membrane, choroidal neovascularization), retinal detachment and phthisis.

Investigation

In addition to the acquisition of histopathological evidence, IWOS judged the following five investigations to be of significant value in the diagnosis of ocular sarcoidosis in patients having a compatible uveitis:

1. **Negative tuberculin skin test in a BCG-vaccinated patient or in a patient having had a positive tuberculin skin test**

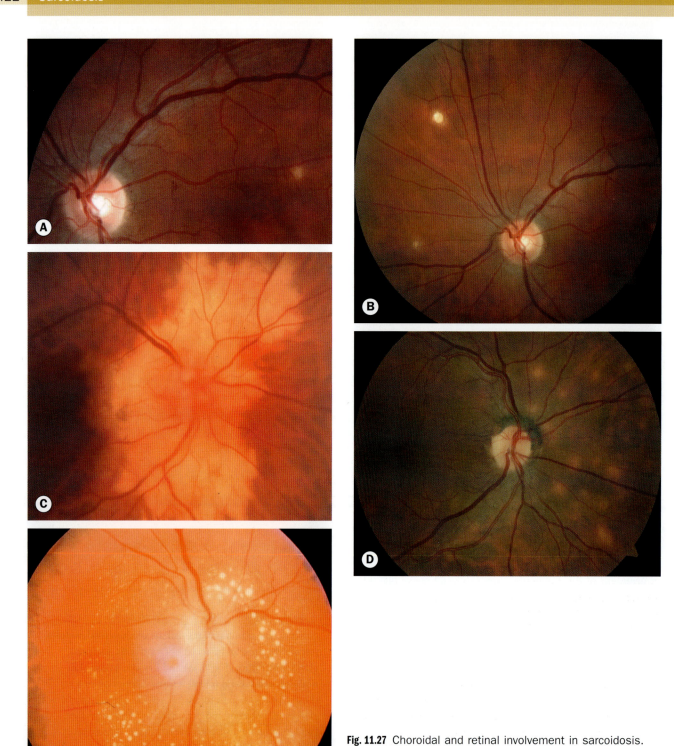

Fig. 11.27 Choroidal and retinal involvement in sarcoidosis. **(A)** Small choroidal granulomata; **(B)** same eye as (A) showing lesion with a punched-out appearance; **(C)** confluent choroidal infiltration; **(D)** multifocal choroiditis; **(E)** multiple small retinal granulomata

previously. A tuberculin skin test is negative in most sarcoid patients; a strongly positive reaction to one tuberculin unit makes a diagnosis of sarcoidosis highly unlikely.

2. **Elevated serum ACE levels and/or elevated serum lysozyme** as described for investigation of AAU.

3. **Chest X-ray showing bilateral hilar lymphadenopathy (BHL).** Chest radiography is abnormal in 90%.

4. **Abnormal liver enzyme tests.**

5. **Chest CT scan in patients with a negative chest X-ray result.** High-resolution CT scanning is of considerably greater value than standard resolution imaging.

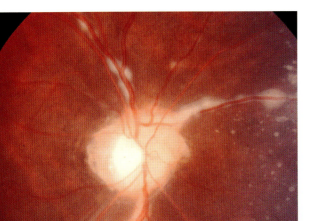

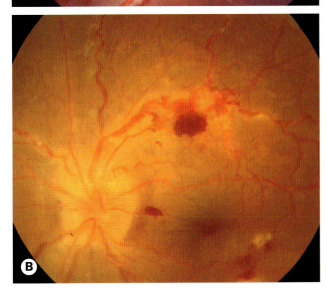

Fig. 11.28 Periphlebitis in sarcoidosis. **(A)** 'Candle wax drippings'; **(B)** occlusive periphlebitis and disc oedema
(Courtesy of P Morse – fig. A; C Pavesio – fig. B)

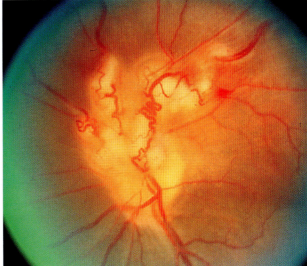

Fig. 11.29 Involvement of the optic nerve head in sarcoidosis – granulomata and periphlebitis
(Courtesy of J Donald M Gass, from Stereoscopic Atlas of Macular Diseases, *Mosby 1997)*

PET scanning and occasionally whole-body gallium scanning.

- **Calcium and vitamin D** levels may be abnormal depending on disease pattern and level of activity.
- **Hypercalciuria** is common.
- **Pulmonary function testing.**
- **Bronchoalveolar lavage fluid (BALF)** shows characteristic changes; CD4/CD8 T cell ratios are a key indicator.
- **Induced sputum analysis** correlates strongly with BALF, and is a noninvasive technique.

Four diagnostic levels were defined by the IWOS for ocular sarcoidosis:

1. **Definite ocular sarcoidosis**: biopsy-supported diagnosis in the presence of a compatible uveitis.
2. **Presumed ocular sarcoidosis**: biopsy not done but chest X-ray shows BHL with a compatible uveitis.

Other investigations are discussed below:

- **Fibreoptic bronchoscopy** with biopsy; histopathological confirmation of sarcoidosis is almost always required before starting treatment; the lung is a common site from which to establish this in the presence of clinical or investigational evidence of pulmonary disease, though a more easily accessible superficial lesion should be chosen if available.
- **Thoracic endosonography** (endobronchial or oesophageal) with needle aspiration has been shown in a large trial to be a more sensitive technique than bronchoscopic biopsy.
- **Miscellaneous biopsy sites** include superficial lymph nodes or skin lesions, conjunctival nodules and lacrimal glands (up to 75% of enlarged glands are positive). If the eye is involved, vitreous biopsy is very useful (e.g. CD4/CD8 ratio).
- **Other imaging modalities** include MRI cardiac and CNS imaging (MRI is less useful than CT for thoracic evaluation),

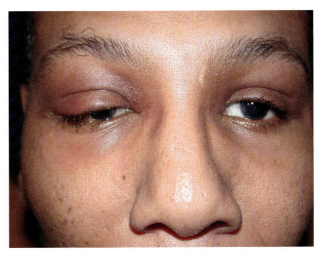

Fig. 11.30 Lacrimal gland enlargement in sarcoidosis

3. **Probable ocular sarcoidosis:** biopsy not done, no BHL on chest X-ray but ≥3/7 of the intraocular signs above and ≥2/5 positive laboratory tests.

4. **Possible ocular sarcoidosis:** lung biopsy negative but ≥4/7 signs and ≥2/5 positive laboratory tests.

It is critical that alternative causes of uveitis are adequately excluded by appropriate assessment and investigation.

Treatment

Corticosteroids have conventionally been the major treatment modality in ocular and systemic sarcoidosis, though alternative immunosuppressives are being used more commonly, particularly as steroid-sparing agents and in refractory disease. Treatment should be initiated aggressively to prevent sight-threatening complications.

- **Treatment of anterior and intermediate uveitis** is approached in a stepwise fashion as for idiopathic inflammation.
- **Posterior uveitis** generally requires systemic steroids and occasionally immunosuppressive agents such as methotrexate, azathioprine, ciclosporin and tumour necrosis factor (TNF) inhibitors (e.g. adalimumab).
- **Peripheral retinal neovascularization** can be treated with scatter photocoagulation to ischaemic areas demonstrated by FA.
- **Cystoid macular oedema** may respond to a topical NSAID.
- **Cataract and glaucoma** may require treatment; inflammation should be suppressed prior to surgery, preferably for at least 3 months in the case of cataract surgery.

BEHÇET DISEASE

Introduction

Behçet disease (BD) is an idiopathic, multisystem syndrome characterized by recurrent aphthous oral ulcers, genital ulceration and uveitis. Vasculitis is a key pathogenetic component and may involve small, medium and large veins and arteries. Mortality is around 5% at 5–10 years, typically due to cardiovascular or CNS complications. BD probably has an autoimmune basis, and may be precipitated by exposure to an infectious agent with subsequent cross-reaction. The disease typically affects patients from Turkey, the Middle and Far East (the ancient 'Silk Road' route), with a lower prevalence in Europe and North America. It is strongly associated with HLA-B51; the ethnic groups with a higher prevalence of BD also have a higher rate of HLA-B51 positivity. The peak age of onset is the third decade; reported gender prevalence varies with ethnicity.

Systemic features

The International Study Group for Behçet Disease (ISGBD), reporting in 1990, established criteria for diagnosis: recurrent oral ulceration (Fig. 11.31A) characterized by oral ulcers at least three times in a 12-month period, plus at least two of genital ulceration,

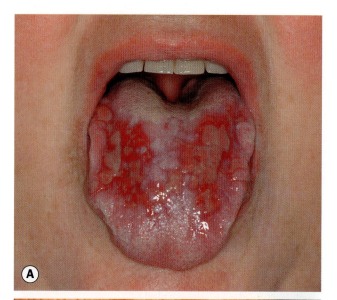

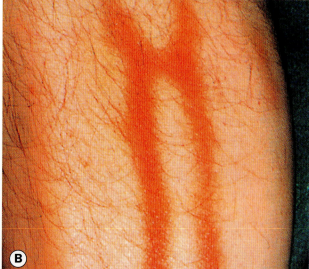

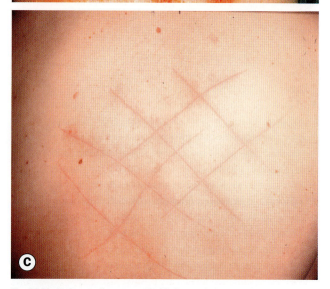

Fig. 11.31 Behçet disease. **(A)** Major aphthous ulceration; **(B)** superficial thrombophlebitis; **(C)** dermatographia
(Courtesy of MA Mir, from Atlas of Clinical Diagnosis, *Saunders 2003 – fig. B)*

ocular inflammation, characteristic skin lesions (erythema nodosum – see Fig. 11.25B, pseudofolliculitis, acneiform nodules, papulopustular lesions) and a pathergy reaction: pustule 24–48 hours after a sterile needle prick (>95% specific, but often negative in European and North American patients).

Presentation does not always conform to the criteria above. Additional features include:

- **Vascular lesions.** Aneurysms, including pulmonary and coronary, and venous thrombosis/thrombophlebitis (Fig. 11.31B).
- **Arthritis** occurs in 30%, though arthralgia is more common.
- **Dermatographia** (Fig. 11.31C), similar to the pathergy reaction, indicates skin hypersensitivity and consists of the formation of erythematous lines following stroking or scratching.
- **Neurological manifestations** (5%) such as meningoencephalitis of the brainstem, dural sinus thrombosis and cerebral aneurysms.
- **Gastrointestinal inflammation**, especially ileocaecal.
- **Hepatic and renal lesions** are relatively uncommon.

Ocular features

Ocular inflammation occurs in about 70%, and tends to be more severe in men; it is the presenting manifestation in about 10%. Signs are virtually always bilateral eventually. Relapsing/remitting acute onset panuveitis with retinal vasculitis and often spontaneous resolution even without treatment is the classical pattern of eye involvement; retinal vascular disease (vasculitis and occlusion) is the main cause of visual impairment.

- **AAU**, often bilateral, is typical. It is not granulomatous. A transient mobile hypopyon in a relatively white eye (Fig. 11.32A) is characteristic.
- **Vitritis** may be severe; it is universal in eyes with active posterior segment disease.
- **Retinitis.** Transient superficial white infiltrates (Fig. 11.32B) that heal without scarring may be seen during acute systemic disease. There may be deeper more diffuse retinitis similar in appearance to viral inflammation. Exudative detachments can also occur. Inflammatory deposits analogous to KPs may be seen on the inferior peripheral retina.

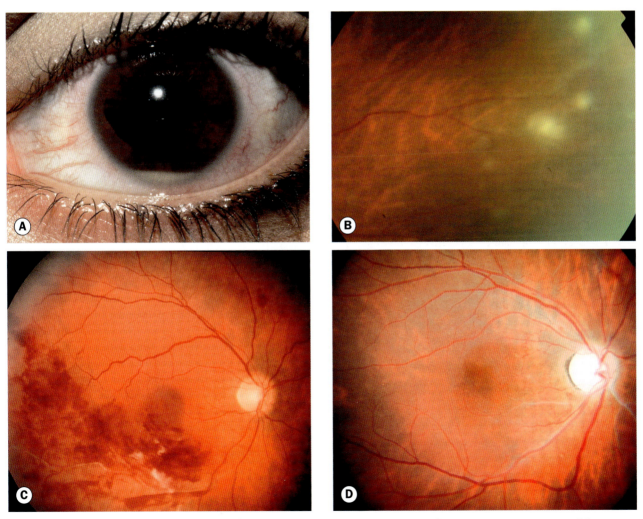

Fig. 11.32 Ocular lesions in Behçet disease. **(A)** Hypopyon in a white eye; **(B)** retinal infiltrates; **(C)** occlusive vasculitis; **(D)** end-stage disease

(Courtesy of A Dick – fig. C)

- **Retinal vasculitis** – arteritis as well as phlebitis, in contrast to pure venous involvement in sarcoidosis – can manifest with sheathing, perivascular haemorrhages and occlusion (Fig. 11.32C). Vascular leakage may give rise to diffuse retinal oedema and CMO.
- **Optic disc hyperaemia and oedema.** Raised intracranial pressure can also cause optic disc swelling and optic atrophy in BD.
- **Disc and retinal neovascularization** may be seen as a response to inflammation and ischaemia.
- **Uncommon manifestations** include conjunctivitis, conjunctival ulcers, episcleritis, scleritis and ophthalmoplegia from neurological involvement.
- **End-stage disease** is characterized by optic atrophy, retinal atrophy and gliosis, and sheathing, attenuation and ghosting of affected vessels (Fig. 11.32D); the vitreous tends to clear. Other complications include posterior synechiae, cataract, glaucoma and, uncommonly, retinal detachment and phthisis. Severe visual loss in males of up to two-thirds of patients at 10 years has been reported, but is probably much lower with aggressive management; the rate in women is about half that in men.

Investigation

- **HLA-B51** (see above).
- **Pathergy test** (see above).
- **Inflammatory markers** (e.g. ESR, CRP, complement levels, white cell count) may be elevated.
- **Thrombophilia screening** is appropriate in some patients to exclude other causes of thrombosis.
- **FA** delineates ischaemic areas and aids detection of posterior segment inflammation and monitoring of disease activity.
- **Laser flare photometry** of the anterior chamber correlates well with FA in determining the level of inflammatory activity.
- **Superficial lesion biopsy**, synovial fluid aspiration and lumbar puncture may be used to help rule out alternative diagnoses.
- **Systemic imaging** may include brain MRI/magnetic resonance angiography (MRA), CT/computed tomography angiography (CTA) and conventional angiography to identify ischaemia.

Treatment

Immunosuppressants are the mainstay of treatment; availability and expense may limit therapeutic options in many regions.

- **Topical steroids** alone may be adequate if – rarely – there is no trace of posterior segment involvement.
- **Systemic steroids and azathioprine** (2.5 mg/kg/day) in combination are recommended for the initial management of posterior uveitis in European League Against Rheumatism (EULAR) 2008 BD guidelines. Steroids should be tapered only slowly. Topical and/or regional steroids may also be used; there may be a high rate of ocular hypertension with intravitreal steroid injection. Azathioprine may have a role in prophylaxis.

- **Ciclosporin** (2–5 mg/kg/day) or infliximab, in combination with azathioprine and systemic steroids, is recommended by EULAR for severe eye disease (> 2 lines reduction in visual acuity and/or retinal vasculitis or macular involvement); a recent study recommended a single infliximab infusion as initial treatment of posterior uveitis. Hypertension, nephrotoxicity and neurotoxicity are concerns with ciclosporin, which should be avoided in patients with CNS involvement unless it is determined that severe eye disease warrants the risk. Infliximab may lead to activation of tuberculosis, and screening-positive patients should receive prophylactic treatment (e.g. isoniazid). Intravitreal administration is a novel alternative route of administration for infliximab.
- **Infliximab** or **adalimumab** should be considered early for vision-threatening Behçet disease (American Uveitis Society recommendation).
- **Interferon-alfa** (6 million IU per day subcutaneously initially, gradually tapered) with or without steroids is a EULAR-recommended alternative to the ciclosporin/infliximab/azathioprine/steroid regimen above for severe disease; it should not be used in combination with azathioprine (risk of myelosuppression).
- **Anticoagulants** are not recommended.

PARASITIC UVEITIS

Toxoplasmosis

Introduction

Toxoplasmosis is caused by *Toxoplasma gondii*, an obligate intracellular protozoan. It is estimated to infest at least 10% of adults in northern temperate countries and more than half of adults in Mediterranean and tropical countries. The cat is the definitive host, with intermediate hosts including mice, livestock, birds and humans. Oocysts are excreted in cat faeces and then ingested by intermediate hosts (Fig. 11.33), including via contaminated water supplies. Cat litter disposal with subsequent transfer to food is a well-known potential mode of infection in humans (though indoor cats have a low rate of toxoplasmosis infestation). The bradyzoite is an inactive stage lying dormant within cysts in tissues such as the eye, brain and skeletal muscle, and consumption of undercooked meat (or eggs) from an intermediate host can lead to infestation. Bradyzoite cysts (Fig. 11.34) can rupture to release tachyzoites, the proliferating active form, stimulating an inflammatory reaction. Conceptually it may be helpful to think of an acute phase and a long-term chronic phase of infection; during the latter new retinochoroidal scars may form asymptomatically over the course of years or decades. A critical mode of human infection is transplacental haematogenous spread to the fetus in a pregnant woman with active (not inactive latent) toxoplasmosis – this is usually primary infection in an immunocompetent host but occasionally reactivation of latent infection, the latter predominantly in the immunocompromised.

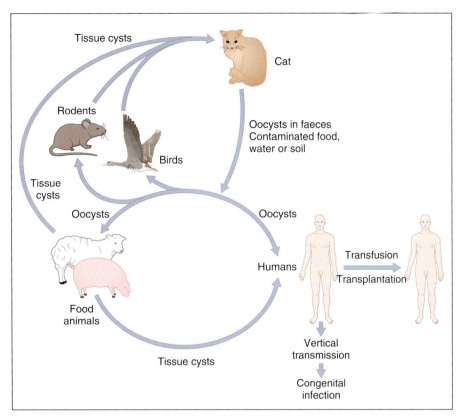

Fig. 11.33 Life cycle of *Toxoplasma gondii*

Occasionally infection may be transmitted via organ transplantation or blood transfusion.

Systemic features

- **Congenital toxoplasmosis.** The mother is often symptom-free or has only mild constitutional manifestations. The severity of fetal involvement is related to the duration of gestation at the time of maternal infection, tending to be more severe in early pregnancy, when fetal death may result (10% of all congenital toxoplasmosis). Neurological and visceral involvement may be very severe, but many cases are

subclinical, especially in later pregnancy. Retinochoroiditis may occur in over 75%, leaving scars that are commonly a later incidental finding (Fig. 11.35).

- **Postnatal childhood acquisition** probably accounts for over 50% of cases of childhood toxoplasmosis; as with adults, in immunocompetent patients this is usually subclinical. Ocular lesions are probably common, but may not develop for years after the initial infection.

- **Acquired toxoplasmosis in immunocompetent adults** is subclinical in 80–90%. Cervical lymphadenopathy, fever, malaise and pharyngitis are common features in symptomatic patients, but more serious systemic manifestations are rare. Early retinitis may occur in up to 20%.

- **Toxoplasmosis in immunocompromised patients** may be acquired or result from reactivation of pre-existing disease. As well as the constitutional symptoms occurring in the immunocompetent, meningoencephalitis, pneumonitis, retinochoroiditis and a range of other features can occur.

Ocular features

Toxoplasmosis constitutes 20–60% of all posterior uveitis. Reactivation at previously inactive cyst-containing scars is the rule in the immunocompetent, although a minority represent new infection. More than half of quiescent retinal lesions will have been acquired from postnatal infection. Recurrent episodes of inflammation are common and occur when the cysts rupture and release hundreds of tachyzoites into normal retinal cells. First

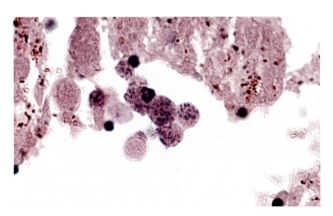

Fig. 11.34 *Toxoplasma gondii* tissue cysts containing bradyzoites
(Courtesy of J Harry)

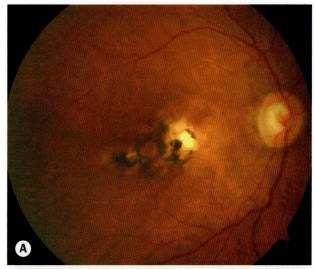

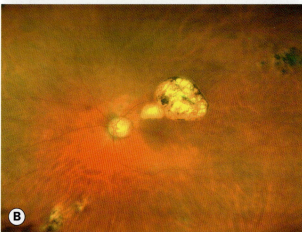

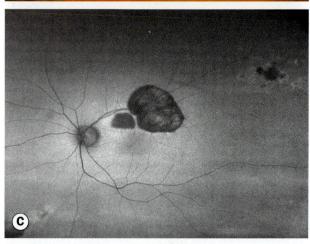

Fig. 11.35 Retinochoroidal scars in congenital toxoplasmosis. **(A)** Macular lesion; **(B)** multiple peripheral scars on wide-field imaging; **(C)** wide-field autofluorescence image of the eye in **(B)**

(Courtesy of S Chen – figs B and C)

presentation with symptomatic ocular infection occurs at an average age of 29 years, perhaps due to decreasing specific immunity. Ocular involvement from congenital infection may only be detected later in life with the incidental discovery of typical retinochoroidal scars, though occasionally macular or optic nerve damage may impair vision in childhood. Pregnancy may provoke the recurrence of ocular toxoplasmosis in the mother, during which it may be resistant to treatment.

- **Symptoms.** Unilateral acute or subacute onset of floaters, blurring and photophobia.
- **'Spill-over' anterior uveitis** is common. It may be granulomatous or resemble Fuchs uveitis syndrome; elevated IOP may develop.
- **A single inflammatory focus** of fluffy white retinitis or retinochoroiditis associated with a pigmented scar ('satellite lesion') is typical (Fig. 11.36A). Lesions tend to involve the posterior pole.
- *De novo* **foci** not associated with an old scar, and multiple lesions (Fig. 11.36B) are relatively uncommon in the immunocompetent but occur more frequently in the immunocompromised.
- **Vitritis** may be severe and impair fundus visualization. 'Headlight in the fog' is the classic description of a white retinal inflammatory nidus viewed through vitritis (Fig. 11.36C).
- **Vasculitis** may be arterial, but is more commonly venous.
- **Optic disc oedema** is common.
- **Extensive and fulminant retinal involvement** is generally confined to the immunocompromised, in whom it may be bilateral and difficult to distinguish from viral retinitis.
- **Retinochoroiditis may be absent** in the acute phase of acquired disease, with activity consisting of anterior uveitis, vitritis and retinal vasculitis; typical retinal scars may form later.
- **Neuroretinitis** similar to that seen in cat-scratch disease is rare, and may be a marker of acutely acquired rather than reactivated infection.
- **Punctate outer retinal toxoplasmosis** is an atypical manifestation featuring clusters of small (25–75 μm diameter) grey–white lesions.
- **Visual loss.** Causes of permanently reduced vision (around 25% of eyes) include macular inflammatory lesions (Figs 11.37A and B) and oedema, optic nerve involvement (Figs 11.37C), vascular occlusion (Figs 11.38A and B), serous, rhegmatogenous and tractional retinal detachment (Figs 11.38C and D), and late secondary choroidal neovascularization (Figs 11.38E and F).
- **Healing** in immunocompetent hosts usually occurs spontaneously within 6–8 weeks, although vitreous opacities take longer to clear. The inflammatory focus is replaced by a sharply demarcated atrophic scar that develops a pigmented border (Fig. 11.39).
- **Recurrence.** The average number of recurrent attacks per patient is 2.7; within five years more than half of patients may experience a further episode.

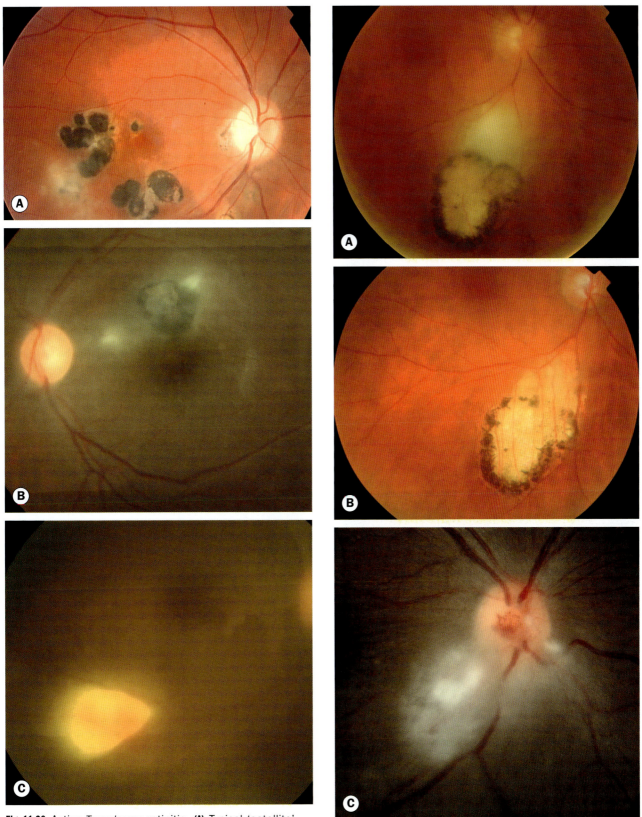

Fig. 11.36 Active *Toxoplasma* retinitis. **(A)** Typical 'satellite' lesion adjacent to an old scar; **(B)** two small foci; **(C)** severe vitreous haze and 'headlight in the fog' appearance of lesion

(Courtesy of S Chen – fig. A; C Pavesio – figs B and C)

Fig. 11.37 Common complications of *Toxoplasma* retinitis. **(A)** Macular involvement, at presentation and **(B)** following treatment; **(C)** juxtapapillary lesion involving the optic nerve head

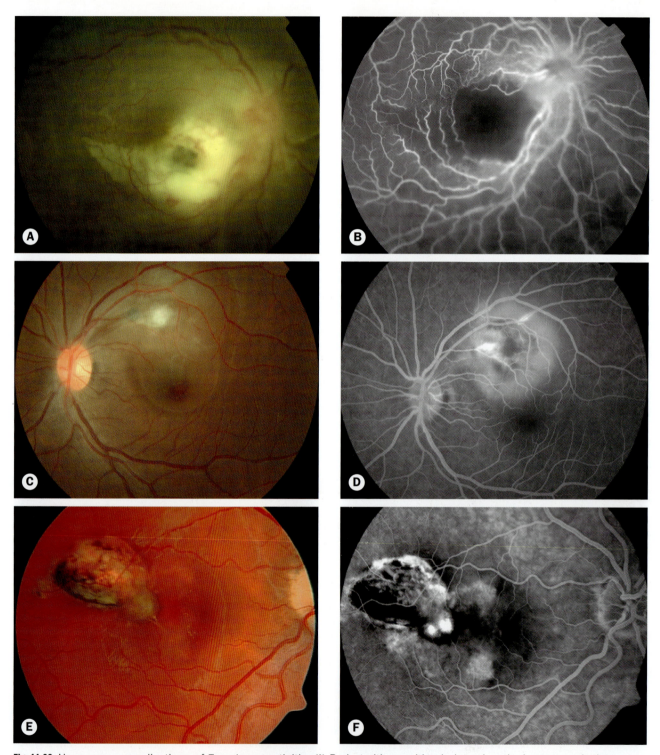

Fig. 11.38 Uncommon complications of *Toxoplasma* retinitis. **(A)** Periarteritis resulting in branch retinal artery occlusion; **(B)** FA shows extensive non-perfusion at the posterior pole; **(C)** serous macular detachment; **(D)** FA of (C) shows hyperfluorescence due to pooling of dye; **(E)** choroidal neovascularization adjacent to an old scar; **(F)** FA of (E) shows corresponding hyperfluorescence

(Courtesy of C Pavesio – figs A–D; P Gili – figs E and F)

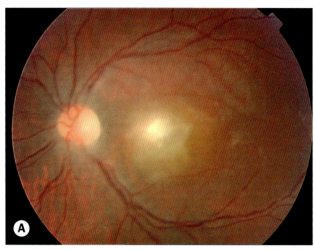

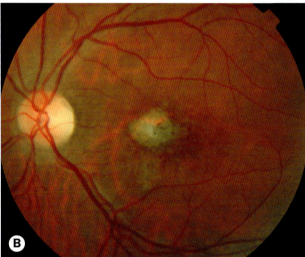

Fig. 11.39 Progression of *Toxoplasma* retinitis. **(A)** Moderate activity; **(B)** 3 months later, following antibiotic treatment *(Courtesy of S Chen)*

Investigation

Diagnosis is usually based on clinical examination findings.

- **Serology.** *Toxoplasma* IgG antibodies are detectable in the serum within 1–2 weeks of initial infection, and indicate exposure to the organism at some point in the past, providing circumstantial evidence to support clinical suspicion. However, community seroprevalence is high – at least a third of individuals in most communities. Positivity to IgM antibodies usually means that infection has been acquired within the last year, and so helps to distinguish between acute (newly acquired) and chronic infection; it is a critical test if newly acquired infection is suspected during pregnancy. Occasionally IgM is positive due to persistence or reactivation following earlier infection.

- **PCR testing** of intraocular fluid is variably sensitive (16–67%) but highly specific and can be diagnostic in clinically uncertain cases. Aqueous and vitreous probably give similar yields.

- **Ocular fluid antibody assessment.** Calculating the ratio (Goldmann–Witmer coefficient) of specific IgG in aqueous humour to that in serum seems to be a reasonably sensitive (48–90%) investigation.

- **Imaging.** Macular OCT will demonstrate any macular oedema if vitritis is not preventative. B-scan ultrasonic imaging can be used to exclude retinal detachment in the presence of severe vitritis. FAF (see Fig. 11.35C) may facilitate monitoring of inflammatory activity.

Treatment

Evidence for the efficacy of current regimens is limited; eradication of the parasite has not been demonstrated but parasite activity and multiplication may be reduced, with a decrease in size of the eventual retinochoroidal scar. The agents used have potential for significant morbidity, and as spontaneous resolution generally occurs, treatment is not administered in every case. Clear indications include a sight-threatening lesion involving the macula, papillomacular bundle, optic nerve head or a major blood vessel, for severe vitritis and in the immunocompromised. Treatment of congenital toxoplasmosis in neonates with antimicrobials for one year may reduce the frequency of subsequent development of retinochoroidal scars.

- **Prednisolone** (1 mg/kg) is given initially and tapered according to clinical response, but should always be used in conjunction with a specific anti-*Toxoplasma* agent, most frequently pyrimethamine combined with sulfadiazine ('classic' or 'triple' therapy, sometimes supplemented with clindamycin). Some authorities start steroids only after 24–48 hours of antimicrobial therapy. Systemic steroids should be avoided or used with extreme caution in immunocompromised patients.

- **Pyrimethamine** is a folic acid antagonist that is believed to be highly effective. It is administered as a loading dose of 75–100 mg for 1–2 days followed by 25–50 mg daily for 4 weeks in combination with oral folinic (not folic) acid 5 mg three times a week to retard thrombocytopenia, leukopenia and folate deficiency. Weekly blood counts should be performed. In acquired immunodeficiency syndrome (AIDS) pyrimethamine is avoided or used at a lower dosage because of possible pre-existing bone marrow suppression and the antagonistic effect of zidovudine when the drugs are combined.

- **Sulfadiazine** 1 g four times daily for 3–4 weeks is usually given in combination with pyrimethamine. Side effects of sulfonamides include renal stones, allergic reactions and Stevens–Johnson syndrome.

- **Intravitreal therapy** with clindamycin (1 mg) and dexamethasone (400 μg) may be as effective as triple therapy in reactivated infection; two to three injections (two-weekly intervals) may be required. It may be preferred in recurrent infection in pregnancy, but would not generally be used in isolation in the immunocompromised, and in newly acquired (IgM-positive) infection systemic therapy has apparently superior efficacy. Depot steroid intra- and periocular preparations such as triamcinolone should be avoided as uncontrolled progression has been reported.

- **Azithromycin** 250–500 mg daily shows evidence of reducing the rate of recurrence of retinochoroiditis and its use in combination with pyrimethamine, folinic acid and prednisolone is a promising newer regimen. Clarithromycin may be a good alternative to azithromycin.
- **Co-trimoxazole** (trimethoprim 160 mg/sulfamethoxazole 800 mg) twice daily in combination with prednisolone is a lower-cost and better-tolerated option that might not be quite as effective as classic therapy.
- **Clindamycin** 300 mg four times daily may be added to triple therapy (see above) or used instead of pyrimethamine. Pseudomembranous colitis is a potential adverse effect.
- **Atovaquone** theoretically attacks encysted bradyzoites, but does not seem to prevent recurrence *in vivo*; dosing is 750 mg two to four times daily.
- **Topical steroid and mydriatic** may be given for anterior uveitis.
- **Antimicrobial maintenance therapy** is used in immunocompromised patients.
- **Pregnancy.** Treatment of recurrent ocular toxoplasmosis during pregnancy should be chosen carefully and only started if clearly necessary; management should be multidisciplinary. Several of the drugs discussed above have the potential to harm the fetus. Intravitreal therapy (see above) for reactivated disease, or systemic treatment with azithromycin, clindamycin and possibly prednisolone may be appropriate. Specific treatment to prevent transmission to the fetus is not generally given except in newly acquired infection, when urgent specialist management is appropriate; spiramycin alone or in combination is commonly chosen.
- **Vitrectomy** may be performed in selected cases.

Toxocariasis

Introduction

Toxocariasis is caused by infestation with a common intestinal ascarid (roundworm) of dogs, *Toxocara canis*; puppies are more commonly infected than adult dogs, and are also more likely to spread the organism. The feline variant – *Toxocara cati* – may also be causative. Human infestation is by ingestion of soil or food contaminated with ova shed in canine faeces; young children are at particular risk from the soil of parks and playgrounds. Once ingested, ova develop into larvae, which penetrate the intestinal wall and travel to various organs such as the liver, lungs, skin, brain and eyes, with resultant inflammation (Fig. 11.40).

Clinical features

- **Asymptomatic** infestation is common.
- **Visceral toxocariasis (VT)**, also known as visceral larva migrans (VLM) is systemic infection of variable severity that usually occurs in a child aged 2–7 years. Fever, abdominal pain, pneumonitis, lymphadenopathy, hepatomegaly and myocarditis are some of the possible features. Spontaneous

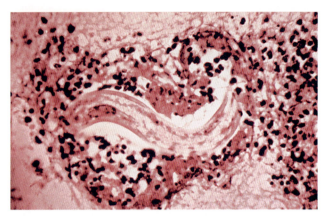

Fig. 11.40 *Toxocara canis* larva surrounded by an inflammatory tissue reaction

(Courtesy of CA Hart and P Shears, from Color Atlas of Medical Microbiology, *Mosby 2004)*

recovery is usual; death is very rare, and usually occurs in individuals hypersensitive to parasitic antigens.

- **Covert toxocariasis** is associated with mild systemic symptoms.
- **Ocular toxocariasis (OT)** (ocular larva migrans – OLM) generally occurs independently of VLM, and is associated with a lower parasitic load. It is typically unilateral, and in around two-thirds causes some degree of permanent visual impairment. In contrast to VT, it tends to occur in older children and adults.
  - Chronic endophthalmitis (Fig. 11.41) typically presents with leukocoria, strabismus, floaters or unilateral visual loss. Features may include anterior uveitis, vitritis, chorioretinitis, papillitis and a fundus granuloma (see below). A dense greyish-white exudate, similar to the snowbanking seen in pars planitis, may involve the peripheral retina and pars plana. Complications include tractional retinal or ciliary body detachment with hypotony leading to phthisis bulbi; the visual prognosis is often poor.
  - Posterior pole or peripheral granuloma without inflammation (Fig. 11.42) classically presents in an older child or adult with unilateral impaired vision or as an incidental finding. A 1–2 disc diameter-sized round yellow-white granuloma is present in the posterior fundus or periphery. Vitreoretinal traction may lead to complications due to macular distortion and/or retinal detachment.
  - Chorioretinal scar (Fig. 11.43).
  - Diffuse unilateral subacute neuroretinitis (DUSN). See below.

Investigation

It is particularly important to distinguish a *Toxocara* granuloma from retinoblastoma. Other helminthic organisms can give similar clinical manifestations.

- **Full blood count.** Eosinophilia may be present, particularly in VLM, and can become chronic.

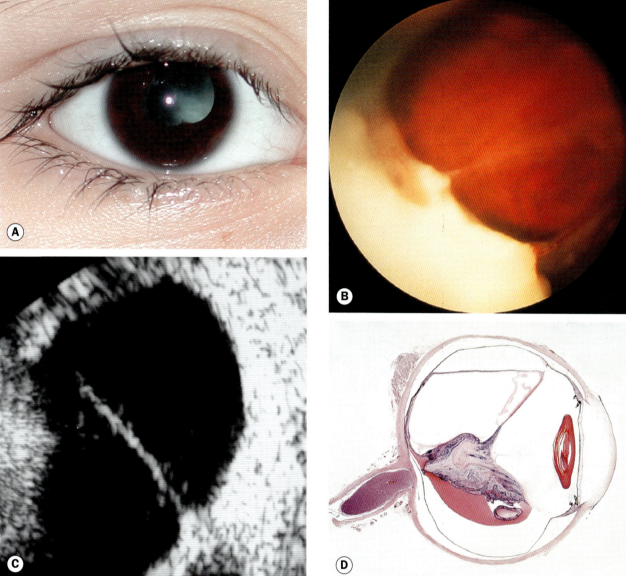

Fig. 11.41 Chronic *Toxocara* endophthalmitis. **(A)** Leukocoria; **(B)** peripheral exudation and vitreoretinal traction bands; **(C)** ultrasonography shows a vitreoretinal traction band; **(D)** a pathological specimen shows an inflammatory mass and total retinal detachment

(Courtesy of N Rogers – figs A and C; S Lightman – fig. B; J Harry and G Misson, from Clinical Ophthalmic Pathology, Butterworth-Heinemann 2001 *– fig. D)*

- **Hypergammaglobulinaemia** especially IgE.
- **Serology.** Antibodies to *Toxocara canis* are detectable in only about 50% of ocular cases. Positivity is common in the general population (14% overall in the USA).
- Ultrasonography may be useful if the media are hazy.
- Aqueous or vitreous sampling for eosinophilia, antibody detection and PCR.
- Biopsy of a granuloma of the skin or elsewhere for larvae is sometimes possible.

Ocular treatment

- **Prevention** by good hygiene practices and deworming of pets.

- **Steroids.** Topical, regional and systemic as indicated.
- **Anthelmintic agents** such as mebendazole and thiabendazole can be considered in OT, noting that worm death may promote inflammation.
- **Vitrectomy** for sight-threatening tractional sequelae.

Onchocerciasis

Introduction

Onchocerciasis, which affects the eyes and skin, is the second most common cause of infectious blindness in the world. It is endemic in areas of Africa and other regions, and disease is particularly

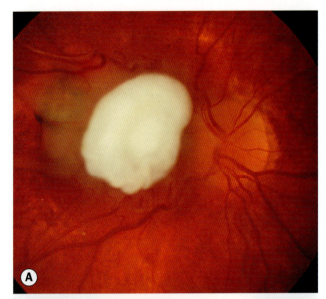

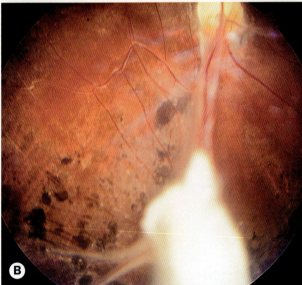

Fig. 11.42 *Toxocara* granuloma. **(A)** Juxtapapillary granuloma; **(B)** peripheral granuloma with a vitreous band extending to the disc

(Courtesy of J Donald M Gass, from Stereoscopic Atlas of Macular Diseases, *Mosby 1997 – fig. A)*

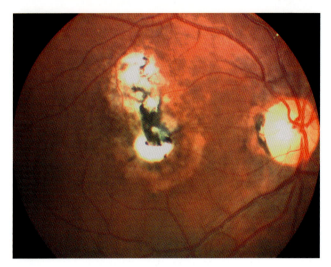

Fig. 11.43 Chorioretinal *Toxocara* scar at the macula

serology, tear or urine antigen detection (oncho-dipstick) and PCR of lesion fluid.

Clinical features

- **Systemic features** are principally dermatological and include pruritus, a maculopapular rash (onchodermatitis – Fig. 11.45A) involving the buttocks and extremities, and areas of hypo- and hyperpigmentation on the shins ('leopard skin' – Fig. 11.45B); scratching of itchy areas leads to lichenification. Onchocercomata are non-tender subcutaneous nodules (Fig. 11.45C) that enclose 2–3 adult worms. Severe lymphadenopathy can occur, with secondary lymphoedema. Eosinophilia is typical.
- **Live microfilariae** may be seen in the cornea, vitreous and suspended in the anterior chamber after the patient has

severe in savanna regions, where in some areas more than 50% of older adults are blind from the condition. Chronic onchocerciasis shortens lifespan by reducing resistance to other diseases. The parasitic helminth *Onchocerca volvulus* is causative; the vector is the *Simulium* blackfly, which breeds in fast-flowing water, hence the colloquial term 'river blindness'. Larvae are transmitted when the fly bites to obtain blood; they migrate to subcutaneous sites to form onchocercomas, where microfilariae are produced by adult worms (Fig. 11.44). Degenerating microfilariae excite an intense inflammatory reaction accounting for most of the clinical manifestations of the disease. The rickettsia *Wolbachia* lives symbiotically in adult worms and microfilaria and is important for microfilarial production. Diagnosis is by skin-snip biopsy,

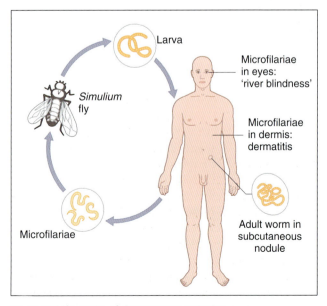

Fig. 11.44 Life cycle of *Onchocerca volvulus*

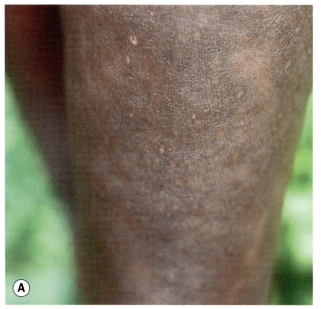

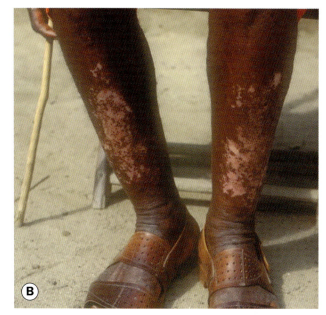

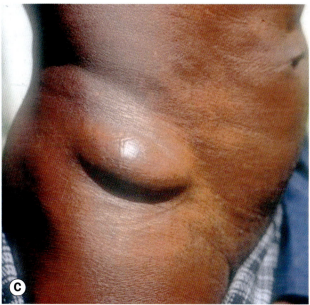

Fig. 11.45 Onchocerciasis systemic features. **(A)** Maculopapular rash; **(B)** 'leopard skin'; **(C)** subcutaneous nodule (onchocercoma)

(Courtesy of C Gilbert)

postured face-down for a few minutes followed by immediate slit lamp examination.

- **Anterior uveitis** is an early feature. Pear-shaped pupillary dilatation may be seen, and is due to posterior synechiae.
- **Keratitis.** Punctate keratitis (snowflake opacities) affects a third of patients and consists of infiltrates surrounding dead microfilariae; initial lesions are most commonly located at 3 and 9 o'clock in the anterior third of the stroma (Fig. 11.46A). Slowly progressing sclerosing keratitis may eventually involve the entire cornea (Fig. 11.46B).
- **Chorioretinitis** is usually bilateral and predominantly involves the temporal fundus, sparing the macula until late. Widespread choroidal sclerosis and atrophy can ensue (Fig. 11.46C). A perpetuating autoimmune response is

hypothesized for progressive longer-term chorioretinopathy that may persist after control of infection.

- **Optic neuritis** may be acute.

Treatment

- **Ivermectin** (supplied in many countries by Merck at no charge) kills microfilariae (but not adult worms) and is given at least annually for many years. It has been effective in substantially reducing transmission rates and morbidity, and no recent new cases have been reported in many communities. Ivermectin occasionally precipitates inflammation, so prophylactic prednisolone may be considered in patients with visible anterior chamber

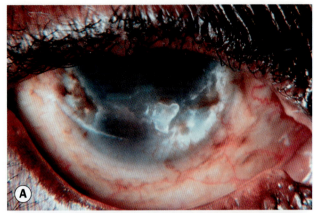

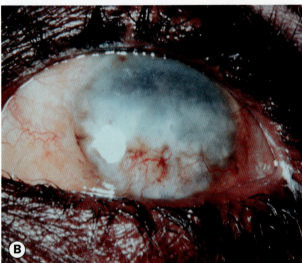

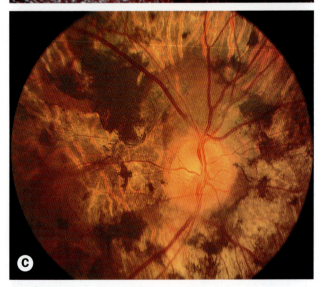

Fig. 11.46 Ocular onchocerciasis. **(A)** Moderate and **(B)** advanced corneal scarring; **(C)** choroidal pigment clumping and chorioretinal atrophy

(Courtesy of S Tuft – figs A and B)

microfilariae. Ivermectin may cause toxic encephalopathy in patients with *Loa loa* infection.

- **Moxidectin** is a newer drug that may be superior to ivermectin.
- **Doxycycline** 100–200 mg per day for six weeks targets *Wolbachia*, indirectly preventing microfilarial embryogenesis and substantially reducing numbers for an extended period. It also has some effect on adult worms, and may be a useful adjunct to ivermectin or moxidectin.
- **Suramin** is effective against adult worms. It is given intravenously.
- **Steroids**. Anterior uveitis is responsive.

Cysticercosis

Introduction

Cysticercosis refers to infection by *Cysticercus cellulosae*, the larval form of the pork tapeworm *Taenia solium*. Ingesting cysts of *T. solium* in undercooked pork leads to intestinal tapeworm development (taeniasis); the infested human then sheds eggs that lead to larval infection (cysticercosis) when ingested by the same or another individual. Inflammation develops in response to antigens released by dead organisms.

Clinical features

- **Systemic disease** may involve the lungs, muscle and CNS (neurocysticercosis). MRI and CT imaging are effective at demonstrating cysts; plain X-rays may show calcified cysts. Serology and stool analysis are useful for diagnosis.
- **Ocular features** include cysts of the conjunctiva and occasionally the orbit and eyelids. The anterior chamber may show a free-floating cyst (Fig. 11.47A). Larvae entering the subretinal space can cause exudative retinal detachment (Fig. 11.47B); they can also pass into the vitreous where released toxins can incite an intense vision-threatening inflammatory reaction.

Treatment

Systemic steroids to control inflammation are combined with surgical removal of the larvae from the anterior chamber, vitreous and subretinal space. Anthelmintic agents such as albendazole may be appropriate in systemic disease, but should be used with caution under specialist guidance, and often with steroid co-administration.

Diffuse unilateral subacute neuroretinitis (DUSN)

Introduction

DUSN is a clinical syndrome due to the presence of a single motile subretinal nematode such as *Toxocara canis*, *Baylisascaris procyonis* and *Ancylostoma caninum*. Misdiagnosis (e.g. multifocal

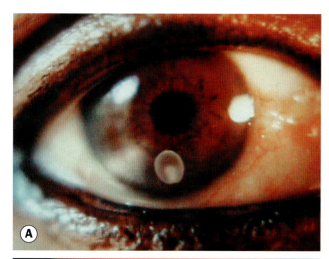

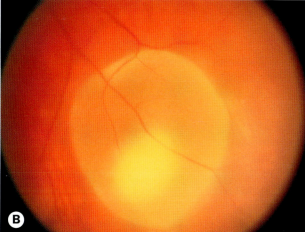

Fig. 11.47 Ocular cysticercosis. **(A)** Anterior chamber cyst; **(B)** subretinal cyst with overlying exudative retinal detachment

(Courtesy of A Pearson)

choroiditis) is common as the worm is often small and may be overlooked.

Clinical features

- **Presentation** is with insidious monocular visual decrease; diagnosis is essentially clinical. Electroretinography (ERG) is subnormal, even in early disease.
- **Acute disease.** Crops of grey–white outer retinal lesions (Fig. 11.48A), vitritis, papillitis and retinal vasculitis.
- **End-stage disease.** Optic atrophy, retinal vascular attenuation and diffuse RPE degeneration (Fig. 11.48B).

Treatment

Photocoagulation (200 μm, 0.2–0.5 s, 150–300 mW) is the treatment of choice when a worm can be visualized (<50%); if necessary a slit beam or very light laser burns are first used to shepherd (sometimes lure) the photosensitive nematode away from the fovea. Systemic albendazole (400 mg for 30 days) or vitrectomy may be appropriate in some cases. Steroid cover may be prudent with all treatment modalities.

VIRAL UVEITIS

Uveitis in human immunodeficiency virus infection

Introduction

Human immunodeficiency virus infection/acquired immuno-deficiency syndrome (HIV/AIDS) is transmitted by unprotected sexual intercourse (heterosexual contact overall globally but sex between men in wealthier countries), via contaminated blood or needles, and vertically from mother to child transplacentally, during birth or breastfeeding. HIV depletes CD4+ T cells, which are vital to the initiation of the immune response to pathogens. Although there is currently no cure or vaccine, the progression of disease can be slowed radically by combination drug therapy: highly active antiretroviral therapy (HAART). Prophylaxis against opportunistic infections may also be instituted.

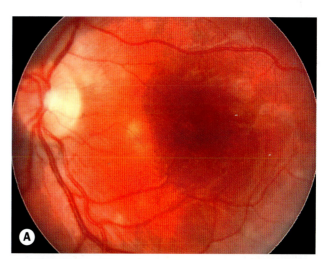

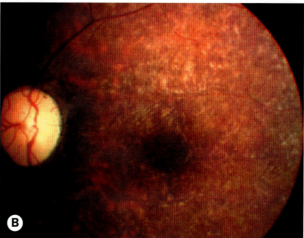

Fig. 11.48 Diffuse unilateral subacute neuroretinitis. **(A)** Active lesions; **(B)** end-stage disease

(Courtesy of J Donald M Gass, from Stereoscopic Atlas of Macular Diseases, *Mosby 1997 – fig. A; C de A Garcia – fig. B)*

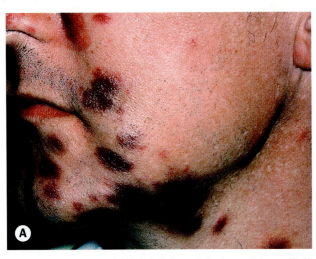

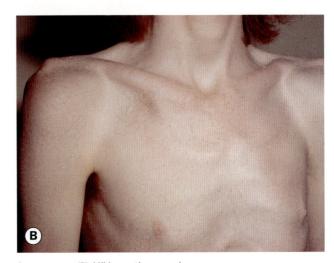

Fig. 11.49 Examples of AIDS-defining clinical conditions. **(A)** Kaposi sarcoma; **(B)** HIV wasting syndrome

Systemic features

- **Stages of infection**: (1) a flu-like illness may occur 2–4 weeks after infection, sometimes including a rash; (2) clinical latency is a predominantly asymptomatic period of several (average 8) years, sometimes with minor clinical features such as persistent generalized lymphadenopathy; (3) AIDS develops in about half of HIV-infected patients within 10 years and is defined as HIV infection with either a CD4$^+$ T count <200 cells/μl or the development of one or more AIDS-defining conditions.
- **AIDS-defining clinical conditions** include particular opportunistic infections such as respiratory or oesophageal candidiasis, *Pneumocystis jirovecii* pneumonia, cryptosporidiosis and cytomegalovirus retinitis, specific tumours including Kaposi sarcoma (Fig. 11.49A) and certain lymphomas, and other manifestations such as HIV wasting syndrome (Fig. 11.49B) and progressive multifocal leukoencephalopathy.

Ocular features

- **Eyelid.** Blepharitis, Kaposi sarcoma, multiple molluscum lesions and herpes zoster ophthalmicus.
- **Orbit.** Cellulitis (e.g. aspergillosis, contiguous sinus infection), B-cell lymphoma.
- **Conjunctiva.** Kaposi sarcoma, squamous cell carcinoma and microvasculopathy (up to 80%).
- **Cornea.** Keratoconjunctivitis sicca and an increased incidence of keratitis, e.g. herpes simplex and zoster, and fungal.
- **Anterior uveitis** associated with ocular infections, or (commonly) with drug toxicity, e.g. rifabutin, cidofovir.
- **HIV-related retinal microangiopathy.** Retinal microangiopathy is the most frequent retinopathy in patients with AIDS, developing in up to 70% of patients. It is associated with a declining CD4$^+$ count and higher plasma HIV-RNA levels and is a marker for increased cytomegalovirus (CMV) retinitis risk. Postulated causes include immune complex deposition, HIV infection of the retinal vascular endothelium, and abnormalities of flow. It manifests with cotton-wool spots and/or retinal haemorrhages (Fig. 11.50) and sometimes capillary abnormalities such as microaneurysms. In contrast to CMV retinitis, lesions are usually asymptomatic and almost invariably disappear spontaneously after several weeks.
- **Other viral retinitis**: cytomegalovirus retinitis (most common), progressive retinal necrosis, acute retinal necrosis.
- **Protozoal**: toxoplasmic retinochoroiditis, often atypical.
- **Fungal**: *Pneumocystis* choroiditis, *Histoplasma* chorioretinitis, cryptococcal choroiditis, candidiasis.
- **Bacterial**: syphilis, tuberculosis.
- **Neoplastic**: B-cell intraocular lymphoma.
- **Neuro-ophthalmological.** Usually secondary to meningitis or encephalopathy due to an opportunistic infection (e.g. toxoplasmosis, cryptococcosis, neurosyphilis) or neoplastic process (e.g. CNS lymphoma).

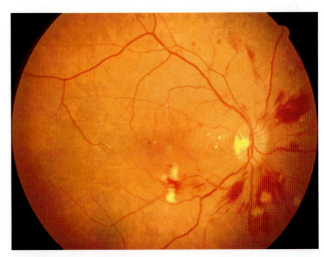

Fig. 11.50 HIV microangiopathy

Cytomegalovirus retinitis

Introduction

Infection with cytomegalovirus (CMV), a herpesvirus, is very common in the general population, causing no or minimal constitutional symptoms in most healthy individuals. CMV retinitis is seen in patients immunocompromised from a variety of causes; it is a common opportunistic ocular infection in patients with AIDS, in whom it may represent reactivation of latent infection. Without treatment, severe visual loss is essentially inevitable. Since the advent of HAART the incidence and severity have declined, though the prevalence remains high, partly due to increasing survival rates in AIDS patients, in whom systemic steroid therapy may be a risk factor. There is a very strong association with a low $CD4^+$ count.

Systemic features

Severe involvement of a range of organs including the lungs, CNS and skin can occur in the immunocompromised.

Ocular features

- **Presentation** is with reduced vision from macular involvement or with floaters from vitritis. One eye is usually affected initially, progressing to both eyes in 50% of patients if untreated. Indolent retinitis (see below) frequently starts in the periphery without symptoms and progresses over weeks.
- **Anterior uveitis** can occur but is usually mild with little or no injection; it is considered separately later in this chapter.
- **Cataract** is a common later-stage finding.
- **Vitritis** is typically mild, except in immune recovery (see below).
- **Retinitis.** The characteristic appearance is of one or two areas of dense white retinal infiltration associated prominently with flame-shaped retinal haemorrhages ('pizza pie' or 'Margherita pizza'), beginning peripherally (centrally in 10%) and extending along the course of the vascular arcades. Peripheral areas tend to appear granular, with fewer rounder haemorrhages and little vasculitis. Indolent (more peripheral and less aggressive – Fig. 11.51A) and fulminant (Fig. 11.51B) clinical patterns have been distinguished.
- **Optic neuritis** (Fig. 11.51C) may result from direct spread or from primary involvement.
- **Retinal necrosis** is evident in areas where active inflammation has settled, leaving irregular pigmentation, atrophy and holes frequently leading to retinal detachment (Fig. 11.51D), a major cause of visual morbidity (up to 50%).
- **Frosted branch angiitis (FBA)** describes marked vascular sheathing that occurs in about 6% (see Fig. 11.51D); this appearance is seen in other conditions, and the term is also used for a distinct idiopathic disorder (primary FBA).

- **Immune recovery uveitis (IRU).** This is a cause of limited visual outcome in CMV retinitis, thought to be due to a rejuvenated immune response against residual viral antigen following immune reconstitution with HAART. Manifestations can be severe, progressing to phthisis in some cases.

Treatment

Close liaison with an infectious disease physician is critical.
- **HAART** is the mainstay of management, restoring the patient's innate ability to suppress CMV activity. Discontinuation of antiviral treatment is considered when the $CD4^+$ count reaches >100–150 cells/μl.
- **Valganciclovir** is a pro-drug of ganciclovir that is taken orally and is as effective for both induction (900 mg twice daily for up to 3 weeks) and maintenance (900 mg daily). Neutropenia is a common side effect due to bone marrow suppression, but can be effectively treated with filgrastim (granulocyte colony-stimulating factor).
- **Ganciclovir, foscarnet and cidofovir** given intravenously were formerly key therapeutic agents, but substantial side effects have largely led to their relegation to reserve status.
- **Ganciclovir slow-release intravitreal implant** (Fig. 11.52) is now less commonly used but still has utility in situations such as intolerance of systemic treatment. It is as effective as intravenous therapy, and the duration of efficacy is 8 months. Intravitreal injection of other agents such as fomivirsen and cidofovir may occasionally be indicated.
- **Vitrectomy** with endolaser demarcation and silicone oil tamponade is successful in around 75% of CMV-related retinal detachments.
- **Steroids** may be required for IRU, though intravitreal and systemic administration should be used with caution.
- **Screening** of patients with low CD4 counts: 3-monthly < 50/μl, 6-monthly 50–100/μl, yearly if >100/μl.

Progressive retinal necrosis

Introduction

Progressive retinal necrosis (PRN; also known as progressive – or posterior – outer retinal necrosis, PORN) is a rare but devastating necrotizing retinitis usually caused by varicella zoster virus (VZV); other herpesviruses have been implicated. It occurs predominantly in AIDS, but may be associated with other immunocompromised states, particularly drug-induced. The prognosis is always extremely guarded, with no perception of light the outcome in more than half of affected eyes.

Ocular features

- **Presentation** is with rapidly progressive unilateral or bilateral visual loss.
- **Anterior uveitis and vitritis** are minimal, in contrast to CMV retinitis and ARN (see below).

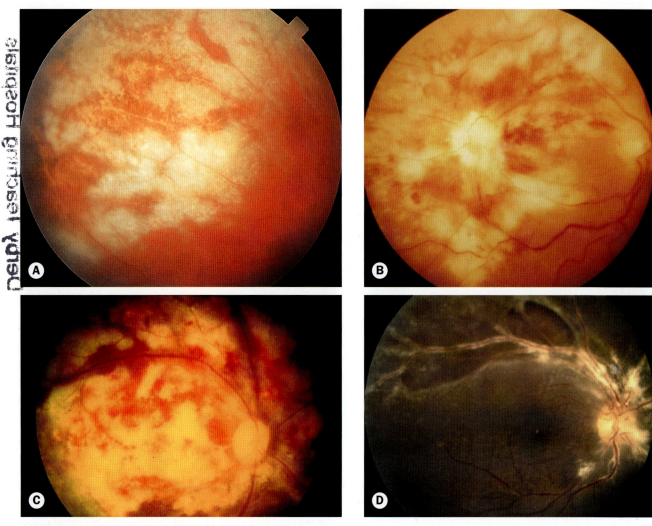

Fig. 11.51 Cytomegalovirus retinitis. **(A)** Indolent retinitis with typical granular appearance; **(B)** fulminating disease; **(C)** advanced disease involving the optic nerve head; **(D)** large posterior retinal tear with shallow localized detachment – there is vascular sheathing reminiscent of frosted branch angiitis

(Courtesy of C Barry – fig. D)

- **Retinitis.** Three stages are recognized:
  - ○ Early. Multifocal homogeneous yellow–white deep retinal infiltrates. The macula may be involved at an early stage, often giving a cherry-red spot (Fig. 11.53A).
  - ○ Established/middle. The signs typically spread rapidly around the retina, with very extensive full-thickness necrosis (Fig. 11.53B). Signs of vasculitis are absent or mild, and significant haemorrhage is uncommon. As inflammation clears, perivenular lucency is seen.
  - ○ Late. Scarring is plaque-like and characterized as 'cracked mud'. Rhegmatogenous retinal detachment (RRD) is very common, as is optic atrophy.

Investigation

Vitreous and/or aqueous PCR assay for viral DNA; antibody assay is less effective.

Treatment

Immune rescue with HAART together with aggressive antiviral therapy, e.g. intravitreal and intravenous ganciclovir and foscarnet. Vitreoretinal surgery for retinal detachment often yields poor results.

Acute retinal necrosis

Introduction

Acute retinal necrosis (ARN) is a rare but devastating necrotizing retinitis. It typically affects otherwise healthy individuals, but tends to be caused by herpes simplex virus (HSV) in younger and VZV in older patients; other herpesviruses are suspected. The prognosis is relatively poor, with more than half of patients eventually achieving only 6/60 as a result of retinal and optic nerve ischaemia or RRD.

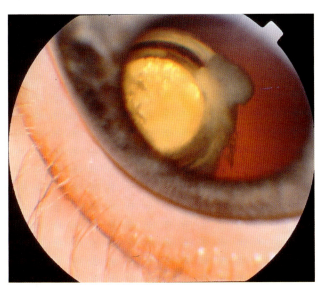

Fig. 11.52 Slow-release ganciclovir implant used in the treatment of cytomegalovirus retinitis – there is an associated localized lens opacity

(Courtesy of S Milewski)

- **Systemic features.** ARN has been reported following and occurring simultaneously with HSV encephalitis and herpetic skin infection.
- **Ocular features.** Presentation is initially unilateral with blurred vision and floaters. Pain is usually a feature. The American Uveitis Society defines criteria for diagnosis:
  1. Prominent anterior uveitis and vitritis (panuveitis). Episcleritis and scleritis may occur.
  2. One or more discrete foci of peripheral retinal necrosis. Deep yellow-white infiltrates with well-defined borders are seen (Figs 11.54A, B and C). Retinal haemorrhages can occur, but are generally less prominent than in CMV retinitis. The acute lesions resolve after 6–12 weeks, leaving behind necrotic retina with hyperpigmented borders. Secondary RRD is a major cause of visual morbidity.
  3. Circumferential spread of retinal involvement. Posterior pole involvement is late. Optic neuritis is sometimes a feature.
  4. Occlusive retinal vasculitis including arteritis. Preretinal neovascularization can develop and may lead to vitreous haemorrhage.
  5. Rapid progression of disease in the absence of treatment.

Investigation

Vitreous and/or aqueous PCR assay for viral DNA; antibody assay is less effective.

Treatment

- **Aciclovir**: intravenously (10 mg/kg every 8 hours) for 10–14 days and then orally 800 mg five times daily for 6–12 weeks. This may hasten resolution of the acute retinal lesions and

dramatically reduces the risk of second eye involvement. Long-term therapy is occasionally required.
- **Oral valaciclovir or famciclovir** may be substituted for oral aciclovir, with similar outcomes but better tolerability.
- **Intravitreal ganciclovir or foscarnet** may enhance the prognosis.
- **Systemic steroids** may be started 24 hours after initiation of antiviral therapy, especially in severe cases.
- **Laser retinopexy** around necrotic areas may be used to try to prevent RRD but is controversial.
- **Vitrectomy** for RRD, commonly with silicone oil tamponade.

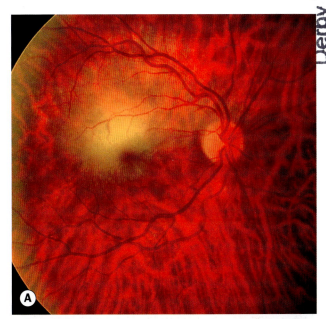

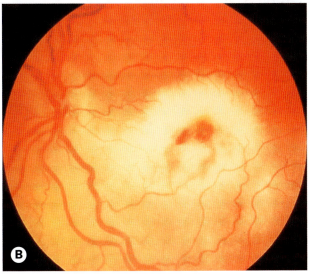

Fig. 11.53 Progressive retinal necrosis. **(A)** Early macular involvement; **(B)** established disease resulting from confluence of multiple foci – there is little or no haemorrhage

(Courtesy of J Donald M Gass, from Stereoscopic Atlas of Macular Diseases, *Mosby 1997 – fig. A; B Bodaghi – fig. B)*

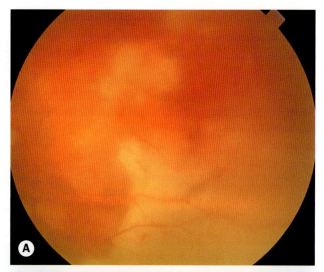

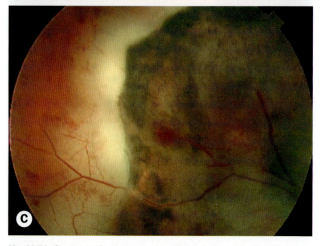

Fig. 11.54 Acute retinal necrosis. **(A)** Peripheral infiltrates with well-defined borders – there is vitreous haze, and a few perivascular haemorrhages; **(B)** advanced disease reaching the posterior pole; **(C)** full-thickness retinal necrosis

(Courtesy of S Kheterpal – fig. A; C Barry – fig. B)

Herpes simplex anterior uveitis

Introduction

Anterior uveitis may occur with or without active corneal disease (see Ch. 6). Patchy and occasionally sectoral iris atrophy that includes the pigment epithelium (Fig. 11.55A) is common, as is elevated IOP. The pupil may be larger than its fellow. As in Fuchs uveitis syndrome, KPs may be fine, stellate and diffusely distributed across the cornea, but can also be large and grouped. There is often a past history of herpes simplex keratitis, cold sores and sometimes genital herpes. Recurrent episodes of herpetic iritis involve the same eye in almost all patients. Distinguishing herpetic from cytomegalovirus iridocyclitis (see below) can be difficult.

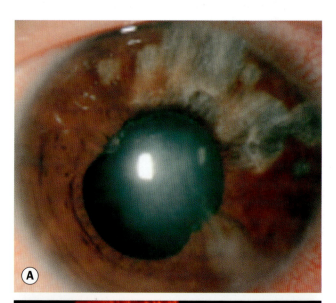

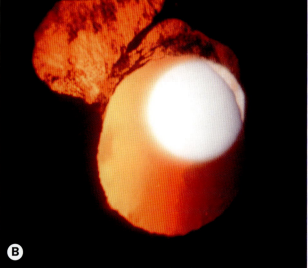

Fig. 11.55 (A) Iris atrophy in herpes simplex anterior uveitis; **(B)** sectoral iris atrophy in herpes zoster anterior uveitis

Treatment

Topical steroids (e.g. prednisolone acetate 1% four times daily) and a topical cycloplegic, in concert with an oral antiviral (e.g. aciclovir 400 mg five times a day; famciclovir or valaciclovir may be superior). Steroids may be delayed and used with caution if active epithelial disease is present, when a topical antiviral may be added. Raised IOP is treated as necessary.

Varicella zoster virus (VZV) anterior uveitis

Introduction

Anterior uveitis of variable severity occurs in around 50% of patients with herpes zoster ophthalmicus (HZO), and is generally of onset 1–3 weeks after the acute skin rash (occasionally in patients with HZO without dermatitis – zoster sine herpete). Zoster-associated iridocyclitis may be recurrent, when diagnosis is usually straightforward due to a past history of ipsilateral HZO. As with herpes simplex, signs may be of granulomatous inflammation, sectoral iris atrophy is often present (Fig. 11.55B), corneal sensation may be reduced and IOP raised. PCR analysis of aqueous is indicated exceptionally. Anterior segment inflammation can occur in primary VZV infection (chicken pox), particularly in the immunocompromised; neuroretinitis is rare. Uveitis has been reported following VZV vaccination.

Treatment

Topical steroids and mydriatics, in addition to standard systemic antiviral treatment of shingles. Systemic steroids are required rarely (e.g. optic neuritis). All patients with HZO must be monitored by an ophthalmologist dependent on severity, e.g. up to weekly for at least 6 weeks to detect occult ocular inflammation, and subsequently possibly long-term to detect late complications. Persistence or recurrence of anterior uveitis may respond to a week-long course of aciclovir 800 mg five times a day, and long-term systemic antiviral prophylactic treatment may be considered for repeated recurrence. VZV vaccination offers protection against shingles. See also Chapter 6.

Cytomegalovirus anterior uveitis

Introduction

Cytomegalovirus (CMV) iridocyclitis in the immunocompetent is now thought to be more common than previously realized, albeit still less prevalent than HSV- and VZV-related inflammation. It may be recurrent or chronic, and unilateral or bilateral. Elevated IOP is very common, and CMV has been reported as a cause of Posner–Schlossman (see Ch. 10) and Fuchs uveitis syndromes. Little or no ciliary injection, very limited flare, few cells, corneal endotheliitis, KP of a range of morphology and sectoral iris atrophy have been reported. Posterior synechiae are rare. A key

diagnostic indicator, in some cases only, may be a failure to respond to aciclovir and/or steroids; PCR and antibody assay of an aqueous sample should be considered if there is clinical suspicion.

Treatment

Oral valganciclovir in proven infection, which sometimes requires long-term continuation. IOP elevation may be persistent.

Rubella

Rubella (German measles) is a common childhood infection, and usually follows a benign and short-lived course. However, transplacental transmission of virus to the fetus from an infected mother can lead to congenital abnormalities of multiple organ systems, with severity generally worse the earlier in gestation infection occurs. Latent rubella virus may cause chronic anterior uveitis relatively unresponsive to steroids, and has been implicated in the causation of Fuchs uveitis syndrome. Reported ocular features of congenital rubella include cataract, anterior uveitis, 'salt and pepper' pigmentary retinopathy (Fig. 11.56), glaucoma and microphthalmos.

Measles

Congenital infection with the measles virus can cause spontaneous abortion or congenital systemic and ocular anomalies including cataract and retinopathy. Infection acquired in childhood typically features conjunctivitis and epithelial keratitis; occasionally retinitis with macular and disc oedema can occur. Subacute sclerosing panencephalitis (SSPE) is a late complication of measles infection, manifesting with chronic progressive neurodegenerative and usually fatal disease of childhood caused by the measles virus. Posterior uveitis (Fig. 11.57) is common, and may be the presenting feature.

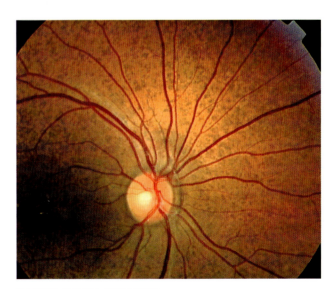

Fig. 11.56 Rubella retinopathy

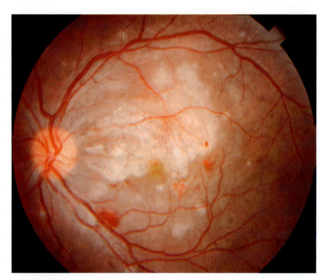

Fig. 11.57 Retinal involvement in subacute sclerosing panencephalitis
(Courtesy of Z Bashshur)

Mumps

Iridocyclitis and interstitial keratitis are rare complications of mumps.

Vaccinia

Smallpox vaccination using the vaccinia virus has been resumed for some groups as a result of the perceived risk of bioterrorism. Though rare, a range of anterior segment manifestations has been described, both from autoinoculation in vaccines and in close contacts.

FUNGAL UVEITIS

Presumed ocular histoplasmosis syndrome (POHS)

Introduction

Histoplasma capsulatum infection occurs following inhalation of the yeast form of this dimorphic fungus, and can lead to the systemic mycosis histoplasmosis – pulmonary involvement is the most common feature. It is common in AIDS. POHS is relatively common in areas of endemic histoplasmosis (e.g. the Mississippi river valley in the USA), implicating *H. capsulatum* in its aetiology. This is reinforced by data from skin antigen testing, but has not been established with certainty and it is possible that other causative factors, including alternative infective agents, may be involved. It is believed most likely that eye disease represents an immune-mediated response to microbial antigen, rather than immediate damage due to active infection.

Ocular features

Sixty per cent have bilateral signs.
- **Presentation.** POHS is usually asymptomatic unless macular choroidal neovascularization supervenes; signs may be discovered at a routine eye examination.
- **Classic triad:** (i) multiple white atrophic chorioretinal 'histo' spots about 200 μm in diameter (Fig. 11.58A); (ii) peripapillary atrophy (Fig. 11.58B); (iii) vitritis is absent. Linear midperipheral scars (Fig. 11.58C) also occur (5%).
- **Choroidal neovascularization** (CNV) is a late manifestation occurring in less than 5% of affected eyes. It is usually associated with a pre-existing macular histo spot. Associated subretinal fluid and haemorrhage lead to a fall in vision (Fig. 11.59).
- **Acute chorioretinitis** is almost always asymptomatic and rarely identified, but discrete oval–round whitish lesions <400 μm in diameter that may develop into classic punched-out histo spots have been described.

Investigation

Skin antigen testing was of limited utility and may have worsened POHS in some cases; it is no longer routinely available.
- **HLA testing.** POHS is associated with HLA-B7 and DRw2.
- **Serological testing** is helpful if positive, but is usually negative in the absence of systemic mycosis.
- **FA and OCT** when CNV is suspected.

Treatment

Spontaneous regression of CNV may occasionally occur, but without treatment 60% of eyes with CNV have a final visual acuity of less than 6/60.
- **Intravitreal anti-vascular endothelial growth factor (VEGF) injection** for CNV.
- **Amsler grid testing** of the fellow eye at least weekly, particularly if a macular histo spot is present (25% risk of CNV). Any role for antioxidant supplements is undefined.

Pneumocystis choroiditis

The fungus *Pneumocystis jirovecii*, a pulmonary commensal, is a major cause of mortality in uncontrolled AIDS. Systemic antimicrobial prophylaxis has replaced pulmonary-only preventative treatment with inhaled pentamidine, and along with immune reconstitution has dramatically reduced the incidence of *Pneumocystis* choroiditis. Multiple slowly progressing deep round yellow–orange lesions (Fig. 11.60), commonly bilateral, are characteristic. There is minimal vitritis, and visual loss is often negligible.

Cryptococcal choroiditis

Cryptococcus neoformans, a dimorphic yeast, enters the body through inhalation, and can spread to the eye in the bloodstream or from the CNS via the optic nerve. As with pneumocystosis, cryptococcosis was formerly responsible for much morbidity, but

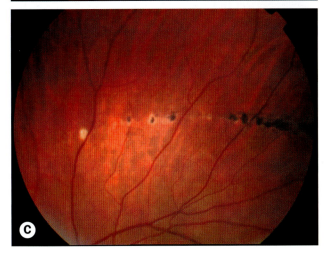

Fig. 11.58 Presumed ocular histoplasmosis syndrome. **(A)** Peripheral 'histo' spots; **(B)** circumferential peripapillary atrophy and 'histo' spots; **(C)** linear streaks

Endogenous *Candida* endophthalmitis

Introduction

Candida (usually the commensal *C. albicans*) can be introduced into the eye from the external environment by trauma or surgery or can spread from fungal keratitis, but endogenous infection is an important alternative route. Risk factors for metastatic spread include intravenous drug abuse, a septic focus associated with an indwelling catheter, chronic lung disease such as cystic fibrosis, general debilitation and diabetes. It is relatively uncommon in AIDS.

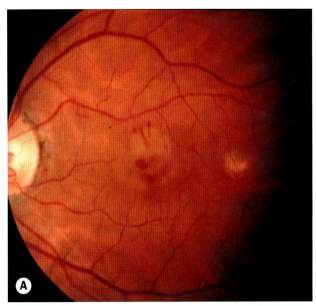

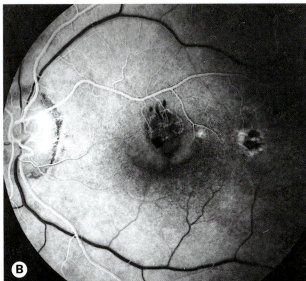

Fig. 11.59 Choroidal neovascularization in presumed ocular histoplasmosis. **(A)** The fovea shows a focal area of oedema and a few small haemorrhages, and a small histo spot temporally; **(B)** FA arterial phase shows a choroidal neovascular membrane just above the fovea

(Courtesy of S Milewski)

clinically significant infection is now much less common since the advent of more effective therapy for AIDS. Ocular involvement may occur directly (e.g. multifocal choroiditis – Fig. 11.61) with vasculitis and exudate or more commonly indirectly with papilloedema and ocular motility dysfunction.

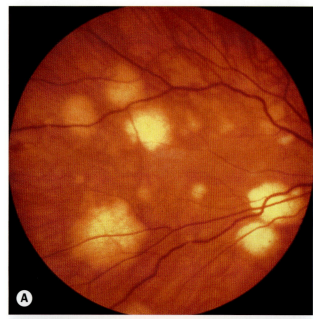

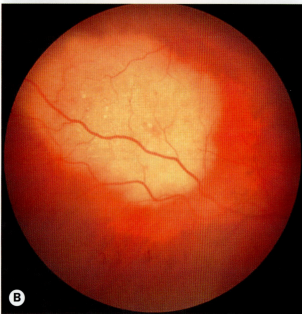

Fig. 11.60 Choroidal pneumocystosis. **(A)** Multifocal choroidal lesions; **(B)** large coalescent lesion
(Courtesy of S Mitchell – fig. A)

Clinical features

- **Presentation.** Systemic candidiasis may already have been diagnosed; up to a third of patients with untreated candidaemia will develop ocular involvement. Peripheral fundus lesions may cause little or no visual disturbance while central lesions or severe vitritis will manifest earlier. Progression is typically much slower than bacterial endophthalmitis. Bilateral involvement is common.
- **Anterior uveitis** is uncommon or mild in early disease but may become prominent later.

- **Vitritis.** May be marked (Fig. 11.62A), with fluffy 'cotton ball' (Fig. 11.62B) or 'string of pearls' colonies, sometimes progressing to abscess formation.
- **Chorioretinitis:** one or more small creamy white lesions with overlying vitritis (Fig. 11.62C). Retinal necrosis (Fig. 11.62D) may lead to retinal detachment, with severe proliferative vitreoretinopathy.

Investigation

- **Vitreous biopsy** (preferably using a vitreous cutter rather than a needle) to identify the organism (PCR and culture) and identify sensitivities.
- **Systemic investigation,** e.g. blood and urine cultures.

Treatment

- **Antifungal treatment.** The agent should be chosen with local microbiological specialist guidance. Infectious Diseases Society of America guidelines suggest intravenous amphotericin-B in combination with oral flucytosine, but resistance is a concern. Voriconazole orally or intravenously has a broad spectrum of antifungal action with low reported resistance and high ocular penetration; adjunctive intravitreal treatment may be given (100 μg in 0.1 ml), with serial injections probably needed.
- **Pars plana vitrectomy** should be considered at an early stage, especially for severe or unresponsive disease; as well as providing a substantial culture specimen, it reduces fungal and antigen load, facilitates therapeutic agent penetration and clears the ocular media.

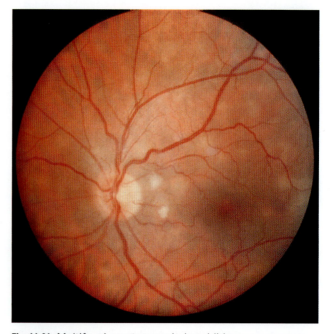

Fig. 11.61 Multifocal cryptococcal choroiditis
(Courtesy of A Curi)

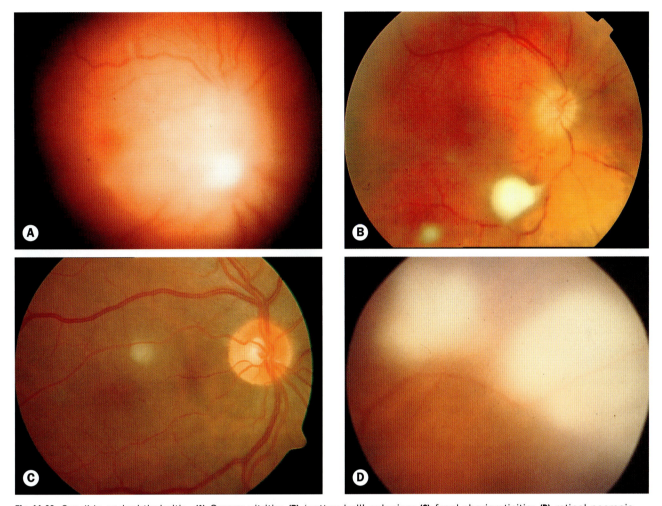

Fig. 11.62 *Candida* endophthalmitis. **(A)** Severe vitritis; **(B)** 'cotton ball' colonies; **(C)** focal chorioretinitis; **(D)** retinal necrosis

Aspergillus endophthalmitis

Aspergillus species are common environmental fungi, but cause disease in humans less commonly than *Candida*. Spores undergo airborne spread, and risk factors for infection include intravenous drug abuse, chronic lung disease, organ transplantation, and blood disorders; neutropenia may be of particular importance. Iridocyclitis and vitritis are common. Yellowish retinal and subretinal infiltrates tend towards macular involvement (Fig. 11.63) at an earlier stage than *Candida* infection; the disease progresses more rapidly, and the visual outcome is often worse. Occlusive retinal vasculitis is common. Systemic assessment is critical; endocarditis presents a particular risk. Investigation and treatment is similar to that of *Candida* endophthalmitis.

Coccidioidomycosis

Coccidioides immitis acquired by inhalation usually causes a mild pulmonary infection, but wider systemic involvement can occur,

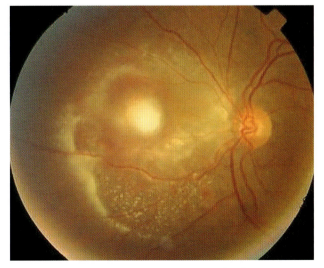

Fig. 11.63 Macular disease in *Aspergillus* infection
(Courtesy of A Curi)

and reinfection can lead to chronic lung disease. Ocular features include severe granulomatous anterior uveitis and multifocal choroiditis. Investigation and treatment is similar to that of *Candida* endophthalmitis.

BACTERIAL UVEITIS

Tuberculosis

Introduction

Tuberculosis (TB) is a chronic granulomatous infection usually caused in humans by *Mycobacterium tuberculosis*. TB is primarily a pulmonary disease but may spread by the bloodstream to other sites; ocular involvement commonly occurs without clinically overt systemic disease. Immune deficiency is a risk factor, when atypical mycobacteria such as *M. avium* may cause disease.

Ocular features

- **Anterior uveitis** is common and is usually granulomatous; iris nodules may be present. Broad posterior synechiae may be formed.
- **Vitritis** is very common, and may be secondary to anterior, intermediate or posterior primary foci. Macular complications include cystoid oedema and epiretinal membrane formation.
- **Choroidal granuloma (tubercle)**: focal elevated dome-shaped lesions (Fig. 11.64A) that may be unilateral or bilateral and solitary or multiple; extensive infiltration may occur in AIDS (Fig. 11.64B). A very large abscess-like tubercle is termed a tuberculoma.
- **Choroiditis** independent of tubercles, typically multifocal and in a centrifugally spreading serpiginous pattern (serpiginoid), has increasingly been recognized (Fig. 11.65). Choroiditis that tracks retinal vessels may have reasonably specificity for TB.
- **Retinal vasculitis** is preferentially venous. Retinal haemorrhages are common. Vascular occlusion with extensive ischaemia (Fig. 11.66) and preretinal or disc neovascularization can occur. It is hypothesized that at least some cases of Eales disease (see Ch. 13) represent a hypersensitivity reaction to TB.
- **Other manifestations include** reddish-brown eyelid nodules (lupus vulgaris), conjunctivitis, phlyctenulosis, interstitial keratitis, scleritis, exudative retinal detachment and optic neuropathy including neuroretinitis.

Investigation

The diagnosis is often clinical, taking into account evidence of previous TB exposure and other negative investigations.
- **Systemic** assessment by an appropriate specialist. Newer investigations include sputum testing with PCR and the interferon-gamma release assay (IGRA) blood test; this is approximately as sensitive as skin testing (80% in active

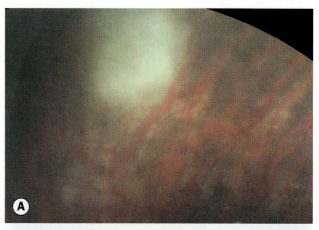

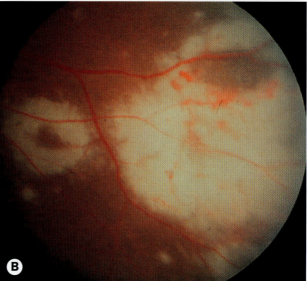

Fig. 11.64 Tuberculous choroiditis. **(A)** Choroidal granuloma; **(B)** diffuse infiltration in a patient with AIDS
(Courtesy of C de A Garcia – fig. B)

disease) but has the advantage of being independent of previous BCG vaccination. HIV status must be determined. Chest X-ray, CT, positron emission tomography (PET)/CT are among other tests that may be considered.
- **Ocular.** Aqueous or vitreous sampling rarely yields demonstrable (smear – acid-fast bacilli on Ziehl–Neelsen staining – or culture – Lowenstein–Jensen medium) mycobacteria; PCR is highly specific but of variable sensitivity. OCT is useful for macular evaluation. Fluorescein angiography may be helpful in establishing whether choroiditis is active, as well as confirming preretinal neovascularization and demonstrating ischaemia. FAF allows activity staging, lesions becoming progressively hypoautofluorescent with healing.

Treatment

- **Prolonged multi-drug therapy** (often four initially) should be prescribed and monitored by a specialist with experience in systemic TB management. If ethambutol is used,

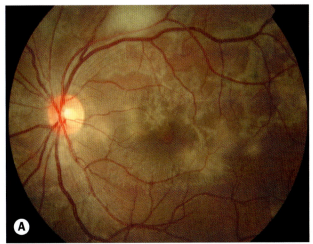

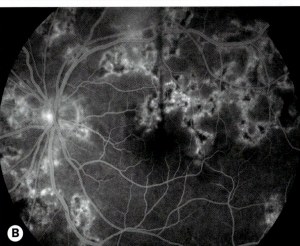

Fig. 11.65 Serpiginoid tuberculous choroiditis. **(A)** Clinical appearance – a granuloma is seen superiorly; **(B)** FA shows corresponding areas of hyper- and hypofluorescence
(Courtesy of C Pavesio)

monitoring for optic neuropathy should take place; rifabutin can cause anterior uveitis. Non-adherence to treatment is common.
- **Topical and systemic steroids** may be used concomitantly to reduce inflammation-induced damage, particularly in the early weeks of treatment, when they may retard paradoxical worsening of the fundus appearance.
- **Laser** may be applied to ischaemic retina to treat preretinal neovascularization.

Acquired syphilis

Introduction

Syphilis is caused by the spirochaete bacterium *Treponema pallidum*. In adults the disease is usually sexually acquired when organisms enter through a skin or mucous membrane abrasion; transmission by kissing, blood transfusion or percutaneous injury is rare. Transplacental infection of the fetus can also occur, when

the mother has become infected during or shortly before pregnancy (congenital syphilis – see Ch. 6).

Systemic features

The natural history of untreated syphilis is variable.
- **Primary syphilis** is characterized by a painless ulcer (chancre), commonly on the genitalia or anus.
- **Secondary syphilis** consists of a maculopapular rash (Fig. 11.67A) and other systemic features.
- **Latent syphilis.**
- **Tertiary syphilis** occurs in about 40% of untreated cases and is characterized by cardiovascular manifestations such as aortitis, neurosyphilis and gummatous infiltration (Fig. 11.67B) of bone and viscera.

Ocular features

- **Anterior uveitis** occurs in about 4% of patients with secondary syphilis; it may be granulomatous or

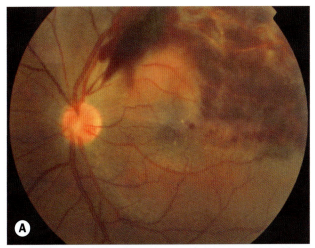

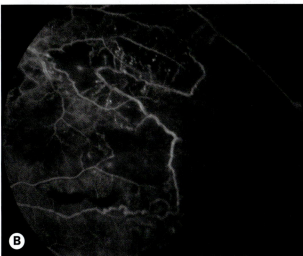

Fig. 11.66 Occlusive tuberculous periphlebitis. **(A)** Superior retinal branch occlusion; **(B)** FA shows extensive hypofluorescence due to capillary non-perfusion
(Courtesy of C Pavesio)

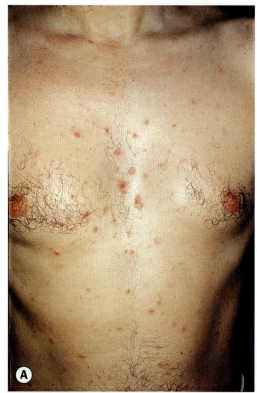

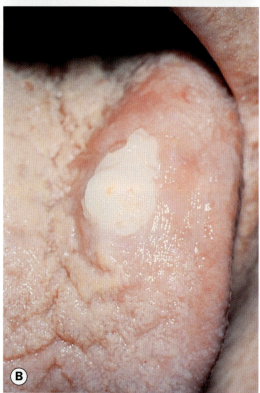

Fig. 11.67 Acquired syphilis. **(A)** Maculopapular rash in secondary disease; **(B)** gummatous infiltration of the tongue in tertiary disease

(Courtesy of RT Emond, PD Welsby and HA Rowland, from Colour Atlas of Infectious Diseases, Mosby 2003 – fig. B)

non-granulomatous and is bilateral in 50%. Roseolae (Fig. 11.68A) are dilated iris capillaries that may develop into yellowish nodules. IOP may be elevated.

- **Chorioretinitis** is often multifocal (Fig. 11.68B), bilateral and associated with vitritis; exudative retinal detachment can ensue.
- **Acute syphilitic posterior placoid chorioretinopathy (ASPPC)** is characterized by large pale-yellowish subretinal lesions in the posterior pole (Fig. 11.68C); it is thought to be due to retinal pigment epithelial infection and occurs more commonly in the immunocompromised.
- **Retinitis** has a 'ground glass' appearance; associated vasculitis may be occlusive and involve both arteries and veins.
- **Optic neuritis and neuroretinitis** (Fig. 11.68D).
- **Other features** include conjunctivitis, episcleritis and scleritis, intermediate uveitis, glaucoma, cataract and miscellaneous neuro-ophthalmic features related to CNS involvement including Argyll Robertson pupils (see Ch. 19).

Investigation

- **Serology** is the mainstay and is discussed under 'Anterior uveitis' earlier in this chapter.
- **Systemic assessment** by an appropriate specialist, including lumbar puncture to rule out neurosyphilis. HIV status should be established.
- **Aqueous and/or vitreous sampling** for PCR is sometimes indicated, such as when HIV positivity makes serology less reliable.

Treatment

This should be under the supervision of an infectious diseases specialist, but generally consists of an extended course of parenteral penicillin. Alternatives may be required, for instance in penicillin allergy, but are less effective, and parallel confirmatory allergen testing and desensitization may be considered. Topical and systemic steroids may be given in conjunction with antibiotics to ameliorate inflammatory damage. The Jarisch–Herxheimer reaction is a systemic response to treponemal antigens released on commencement of therapy, and may include progression of ocular signs.

Lyme disease

Introduction

Lyme disease (borreliosis), like syphilis, is caused by a spirochaete. The responsible organism, *Borrelia burgdorferi*, is transmitted through tick bites; deer are important vectors (Fig. 11.69A). An adult tick (Fig. 11.69B) can be distinguished from a head louse by the tick having eight legs – it is an arachnid – and the louse six (though larval ticks have only six). The disease is endemic in regions of North America, Europe and Asia, but can be difficult to diagnose. Several days after a bite an annular skin lesion, erythema chronicum migrans (Fig. 11.69C) forms at the site in 60–80%, often accompanied by constitutional symptoms (stage 1).

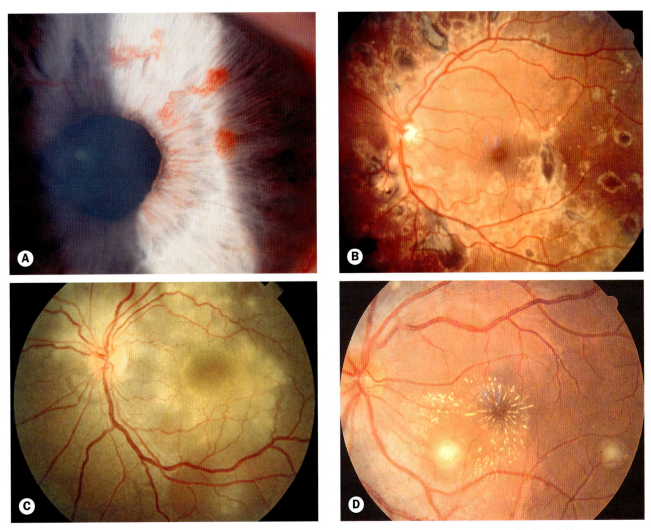

Fig. 11.68 Ocular syphilis. **(A)** Roseolae; **(B)** old multifocal chorioretinitis; **(C)** acute posterior placoid chorioretinitis; **(D)** neuroretinitis
(Courtesy of J Salmon – fig. B; C de A Garcia – fig. C)

Neurological (e.g. cranial nerve palsies, meningitis), cardiac (4–8% e.g. arrhythmia) and other manifestations may follow within a few weeks. Late (stage 3) complications include chronic arthritis of large joints, polyneuropathy and encephalopathy. Some patients develop chronic symptoms that may not respond to antibiotics.

Ocular features

These are varied; they tend to occur in established stage 2 and stage 3 (late) disease.

- **Uveitis** is relatively uncommon but can be anterior (granulomatous or non-granulomatous), intermediate (the most common), or posterior including multifocal choroiditis, vasculitis and neuroretinitis.
- **Other manifestations** include early (stage 1) transient conjunctivitis, bilateral stromal keratitis, episcleritis (Fig. 11.70), scleritis, orbital myositis, optic neuritis, papilloedema and ocular motor and facial nerve palsy (up to 25% of facial nerve palsy in endemic areas).

Investigations

Serology should be performed at least a month after infection; false positives can occur. PCR of CSF or synovial fluid is performed in appropriate cases. Diagnosis relies on a combination of clinical features and positive serology. Co-infection with other tick-borne diseases is possible.

Treatment

Treatment of early acute disease is highly effective and involves oral doxycycline (not children or in pregnancy), amoxicillin or erythromycin. Untreated, many patients with early or asymptomatic disease will experience no further problems. Patients with established disease, including ocular, may require extended intravenous penicillin or ceftriaxone. Keratitis and uveitis may need steroid treatment; systemic steroids should not be given without concomitant antibiotics. Appropriate personal protection (clothing, insect repellent) should be adopted in endemic areas to reduce

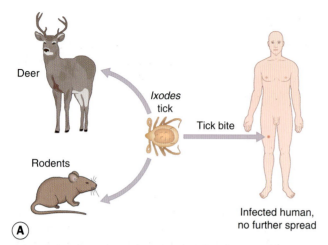

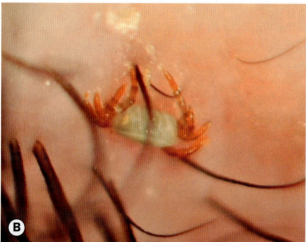

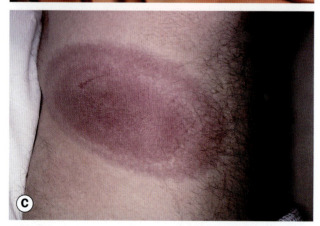

Fig. 11.69 Lyme disease. **(A)** Transmission; **(B)** tick attached to eyelid; **(C)** severe erythema chronicum migrans
(Courtesy of RT Emond, PD Welsby and HA Rowland, from Colour Atlas of Infectious Diseases, *Mosby 2003 – fig. C)*

the risk of tick bite. A Lyme disease vaccine is available, but does not offer complete or prolonged protection.

Brucellosis

Brucellosis is caused by the Gram-negative bacteria *Brucella melitensis* and *B. abortus*. It is usually transmitted from animals to man through milk products or uncooked meat. A variety of constitutional and ocular (20%) features are reported, the latter including chronic anterior and posterior uveitis, papilloedema and retinal haemorrhages. Investigation should include serology and blood culture. Treatment is with a combination of two antibiotics, e.g. streptomycin and doxycycline, with adjunctive steroids if required. Patients with known brucellosis should undergo ophthalmic examination.

Endogenous bacterial endophthalmitis

Introduction

Roth spots develop in about 1% of cases of bacteraemia, but no frank ocular infection occurs in the great majority of cases. A wide range of organisms can be responsible – Gram-positives predominate in North America and Europe and Gram-negatives in eastern Asian. Risk factors include debilitating disease of many types as well as other factors such as intravenous drug abuse; spread can occur from any potential focus such as an indwelling catheter or septic joint. Patients are usually systemically unwell, and mortality is relatively high – 5–10%. The prognosis is poorer than with postoperative endophthalmitis.

Ocular features

Diagnosis is frequently delayed. The main distinction is from endogenous fungal endophthalmitis.
- **Symptoms**: blurred vision, pain and redness.
- **Signs** are broadly similar to those of postoperative endophthalmitis (see Chapter 9), though retinal infiltrates may be an early feature, reflecting the route of infection (Fig. 11.71).

Investigation

The search for a septic focus (blood and urine cultures, septic arthritis, endocarditis, lumbar puncture etc.) should be in collaboration with an appropriate physician and involve a search.

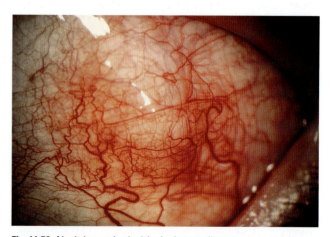

Fig. 11.70 Nodular episcleritis in Lyme disease
(Courtesy of P Watson)

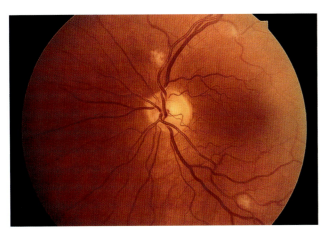

Fig. 11.71 Retinal infiltrates in endogenous bacterial endophthalmitis

Aqueous and vitreous samples should be taken for microscopy and culture.

Treatment

- **Systemic infection** is treated with intravenous antibiotics according to clinical suspicion and local microbiological advice. Broad spectrum empirical treatment may be necessary.
- **Endophthalmitis** is treated with intravitreal and an oral fluoroquinolone; the place of systemic steroids is undefined. Pars plana vitrectomy may improve prognosis in some patients.

Cat-scratch disease

Introduction

Cat-scratch disease (bartonellosis) is caused by *Bartonella henselae*, a Gram-negative rod. Infection is usually mediated transmitted by the scratch (or bite) of an apparently healthy cat, though feline contact is not always described. One or more red papules at the site of inoculation are followed by fever and regional lymphadenopathy (Fig. 11.72), though general symptoms are frequently absent; severe systemic disease occasionally occurs. The visual prognosis is usually reasonable.

Ocular features

The eyes are affected in 5–10%: neuroretinitis (see Ch. 19) is the most common manifestation and consists of disc oedema with macular exudate in a star conformation (see Fig. 19.12B); intermediate uveitis, focal retinochoroiditis, vasculitis, and conjunctivitis with a 2–4 mm conjunctival granuloma (Parinaud oculoglandular syndrome) may also be seen. Both eyes are involved in a minority.

Investigation

Includes serology for *B. henselae*.

Treatment

Oral antibiotics, e.g. co-trimoxazole, azithromycin, rifampicin or ciprofloxacin (avoided in children). Steroids have been used in some cases. Treatment is not usually given for mild systemic symptoms alone.

Leprosy

Introduction

Leprosy (Hansen disease) is a chronic granulomatous infection caused by *Mycobacterium leprae* and *M. lepromatosis*. The mode of spread remains uncertain, though nasal secretions have been implicated. Infection is thought to lead to a chronic immune response that leads to the peripheral neuropathy that is the primary pathogenetic mechanism. Genetic factors are probably important – only 5% of the general population is thought to be vulnerable to leprosy on substantial contact with the organism.

Systemic features

- **Tuberculoid ('paucibacillary' in WHO classification).** One or more hypopigmented macules and anaesthetic skin patches.
- **Borderline (multibacillary).** The most common form. Similar to tuberculoid, but more numerous and extensive lesions.
- **Lepromatous (multibacillary).** Widespread cutaneous thickening with leonine facies (Fig. 11.73A), peripheral plaques and nodules, upper respiratory tract involvement

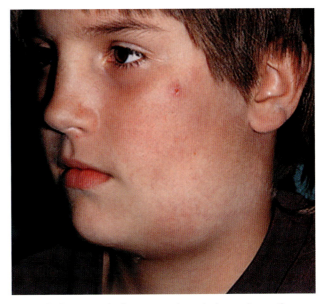

Fig. 11.72 Cat-scratch disease – ulcerated papule on the cheek caused by a cat scratch 2 weeks previously, with enlargement of submandibular lymph nodes

(Courtesy of BJ Zitelli and HW Davis, from Atlas of Pediatric Physical Diagnosis, *Mosby 2002)*

- **Miosis and iris atrophy** (Figs 11.74B and C) result from impaired dilator pupillae innervation.
- **Other features**: episcleritis and scleritis, retinal pearls, uveal effusion, cataract, glaucoma, decreased corneal sensation, facial nerve palsy, eyelid deformities and phthisis bulbi.

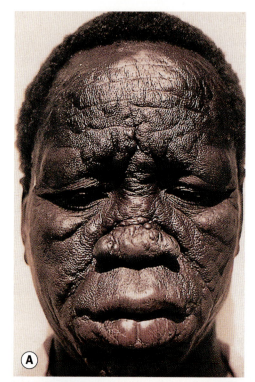

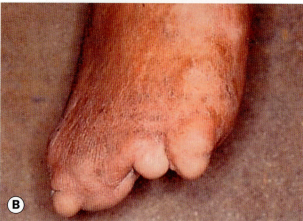

Fig. 11.73 Lepromatous leprosy. **(A)** Leonine facies; **(B)** loss of digits due to sensory neuropathy

(Courtesy of RT Emond, PD Welsby and HA Rowland, from Colour Atlas of Infectious Diseases, *Mosby 2003 – fig. A; CD Forbes and WF Jackson, from* Color Atlas and Text of Clinical Medicine, *Mosby 2003 – fig. B)*

and peripheral nerve lesions facilitating trauma that may result in shortening and loss of digits (Fig. 11.73B).

Ocular features

Ocular signs are principally due to direct bacterial invasion.

- **Anterior uveitis**: chronic and low-grade; classically 'plasmoid' (prominent fibrin).
- **Iris pearls** (pathognomonic): usually under 0.5 mm in diameter (Fig. 11.74A).
- **Keratitis**: thickened, beaded corneal nerves, punctate subepithelial lesions, pannus and vascularization.

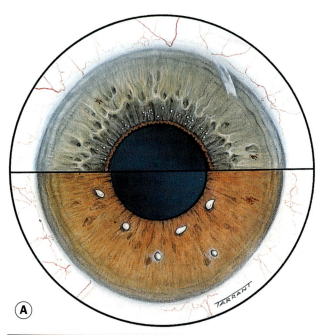

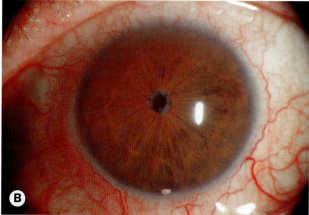

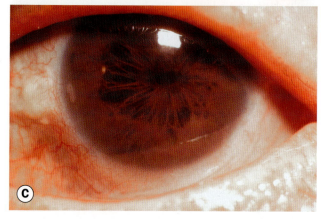

Fig. 11.74 Lepromatous chronic anterior uveitis. **(A)** Iris pearls; **(B)** miosis; **(C)** iris atrophy

Investigation

Skin, and occasionally ocular, specimens show acid-fast bacilli. The lepromin test distinguishes between tuberculoid and lepromatous leprosy.

Treatment

- **Systemic.** Combination regimens of extended duration with antibiotics such as dapsone, rifampicin and clofazimine. BCG vaccination offers some protection.
- **Ocular.** Anterior uveitis is treated with steroids. Specific complications are addressed as indicated.

MISCELLANEOUS IDIOPATHIC CHORIORETINOPATHIES

The conditions described below are uncommon inflammatory disorders principally involving the posterior segment. Their aetiology is unknown or incompletely understood. Other entities may present with similar clinical manifestations, and it is critical to exclude alternative diagnoses including infection and neoplasia. The 'white dot syndromes' (Table 11.9) constitute a subgroup with some features in common; there is variation between sources in the list of conditions falling into this category.

Central serous chorioretinopathy is considered in Chapter 14.

Multiple evanescent white dot syndrome (MEWDS)

Introduction

MEWDS is an uncommon idiopathic disease typically occurring in young adult females; 25–50% describe a preceding viral-like illness. Subsequent progression to AZOOR (see below) has been reported in some patients.

Clinical features

- **Presentation.** Common: painless monocular blurring (6/9–6/60) and photopsia; less common: floaters, scotomata, dyschromatopsia.
- **Subtle posterior vitritis** in 50%.
- **Posterior pole lesions.** Numerous small (100–300 μm) ill-defined deep grey-white patches sparing the fovea, which has a characteristic orange granular appearance and a dulled reflex (Figs 11.75A and B).
- **Optic disc oedema** is occasionally present.

Table 11.9 The white dot syndromes

Multiple evanescent white dot syndrome
Acute posterior multifocal placoid pigment epitheliopathy
Birdshot chorioretinopathy
Punctate inner choroidopathy
Serpiginous choroidopathy
Multifocal choroiditis and panuveitis
Subretinal fibrosis and uveitis

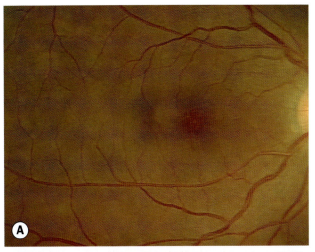
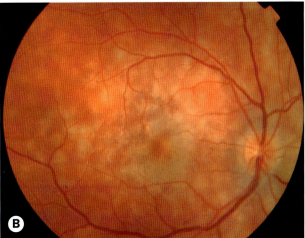

Fig. 11.75 Multiple evanescent white dot syndrome. **(A)** Foveal granularity and peripheral macular lesions; **(B)** numerous macular lesions
(Courtesy of P Gili – fig. A; Moorfields Eye Hospital – fig. B)

- **Recovery** occurs over weeks, often leaving subtle residual signs. Recurrence occasionally (10%) occurs.

Investigation

- **Visual fields.** The blind spot may be enlarged; may show other scotomata.
- **OCT** may show inner-segment/outer-segment junction disruption.
- **FAF.** Hyperautofluorescent spots corresponding to the macular lesions are visible during active inflammation; FAF has been used to demonstrate subclinical lesions in patients with only foveal granularity (Figs 11.76A and B).
- **FA** shows subtle early hyperfluorescence of the dots with late staining (Fig. 11.76C); occasionally vessel wall and disc staining may be seen.
- **ICGA** shows hypofluorescent spots (Fig. 11.76D) that are often more numerous than visible clinically or on FA.
- **ERG** shows a transiently reduced a-wave amplitude. Electrooculography (EOG) and visual evoked response (VER) abnormalities may be present.

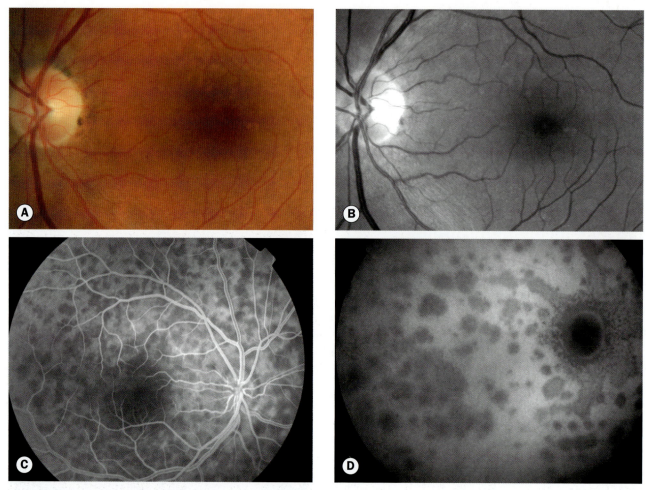

Fig. 11.76 Multiple evanescent white dot syndrome. **(A)** Resolving lesions superior and temporal to the fovea; **(B)** appearance on fundus autofluorescence; **(C)** FA arteriovenous phase shows subtle hyperfluorescent spots; **(D)** ICGA
(Courtesy of Moorfields Eye Hospital – figs C and D)

Treatment

This is generally not required, except for rare cases complicated by choroidal neovascularization.

Acute idiopathic blind spot enlargement syndrome (AIBSE)

AIBSE is a rare condition reported in young to middle-aged women. Features include photopsia and decreased vision, with blind spot enlargement and mild disc swelling. Recovery to normal or near-normal without treatment is usual. Some authorities believe that AIBSE is not distinct from MEWDS.

Acute posterior multifocal placoid pigment epitheliopathy (APMPPE)

Introduction

APMPPE is an uncommon idiopathic inflammatory disorder. It affects young to middle-aged adults of both genders equally. There is often a viral prodrome, and it is speculated to occur as a result of cell-mediated immunity to viral antigen. Associated cerebral vasculitis is relatively common and can cause stroke. Erythema nodosum and other systemic manifestations of vasculitis have been reported. The clinical picture of APMPPE can be mimicked by other entities such as sarcoidosis and tuberculosis.

Clinical features

- **Symptoms.** Subacute moderate visual impairment; central/paracentral scotomata; photopsia is frequent. The fellow eye is affected within a few days or weeks. Headache and other neurological symptoms are common and can commence many months after ocular disease onset.
- **Anterior uveitis and vitritis** are usually very mild.
- **Fundus.** Multiple large deep yellow–white placoid lesions, initially at the posterior pole (Fig. 11.77A). Within weeks the majority fade, with residual RPE disturbance of varying severity. Subretinal macular fluid may be seen. Vasculitis and papillitis are rare.
- **Prognosis.** In 25% of patients recovery is to only 6/15 or worse, with recurrence in up to 50%.

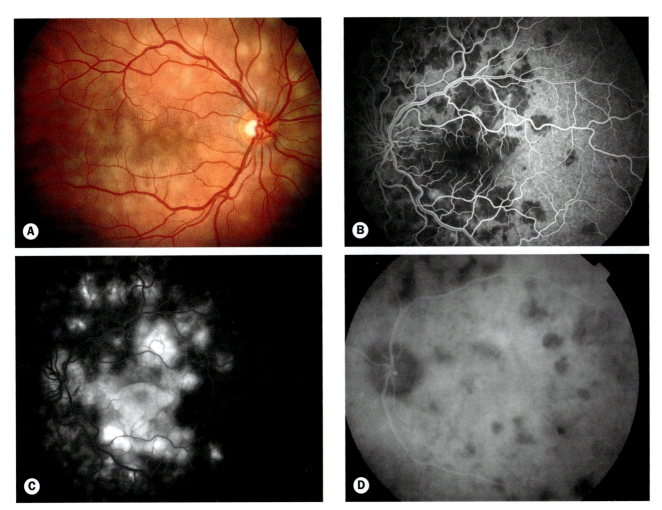

Fig. 11.77 (A) Acute posterior multifocal placoid pigment epitheliopathy; **(B)** FA early venous phase shows dense foci of hypofluorescence; **(C)** FA late phase shows hyperfluorescence; **(D)** ICGA shows focal hypofluorescence
(Courtesy of C Barry)

Investigation

Alternative diagnoses should be excluded.

- **HLA-B7 and HLA-DR2** are associated in a substantial proportion of patients.
- **OCT** for macular assessment.
- **FA** of active lesions shows early dense hypofluorescence and late staining (Figs 11.77B and C).
- **ICGA** demonstrates non-perfusion of the choriocapillaris (Fig. 11.77D).
- **CNS imaging** and lumbar puncture should be performed in patients with neurological symptoms.

Treatment

Steroids should be considered, especially for macular involvement. Steroids and possibly ciclosporin may be given for cerebral vasculitis. Patients should be instructed to seek medical advice urgently if neurological symptoms occur.

Serpiginous choroidopathy

Introduction

Serpiginous choroidopathy (choroiditis) is usually bilateral, though asymmetrical. It typically occurs in middle age, affects men more frequently than women, and is associated with HLA-B7. The disease is generally recurrent over years, with a relatively poor prognosis. TB uveitis can give a similar clinical picture ('serpiginoid').

Clinical features

- **Symptoms.** Initially unilateral blurring of central vision, scotoma or metamorphopsia.
- **Anterior uveitis and vitritis** are common but usually mild.
- **Fundus.** Active lesions (Fig. 11.78A) are grey–white and may remain active for several months before becoming scalloped and atrophic. The disease typically starts around the optic

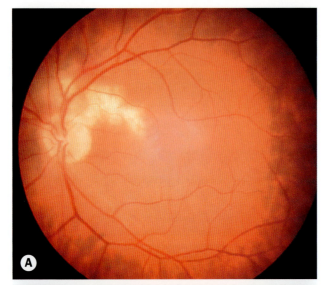

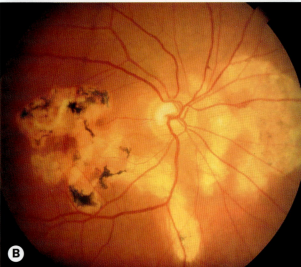

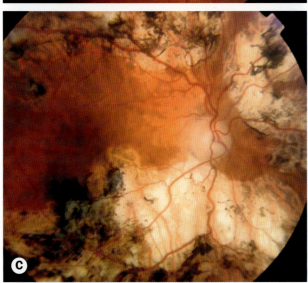

Fig. 11.78 Serpiginous choroidopathy. **(A)** Early active disease; **(B)** extension around the macula in typical snake-like fashion; **(C)** advanced scarring

(Courtesy of R Bates – fig. B)

disc and extends gradually (Fig. 11.78B), though a variant starting at the central macula (5%) is recognized. Recurrence is usually contiguous with or adjacent to existing areas, eventually resulting in extensive chorioretinal atrophy (Fig. 11.78C).

- **Complications.** CNV (15–35%), subretinal fibrosis, preretinal neovascularization.

Investigation

TB should be excluded, especially in endemic areas.
- **FA** of active lesions shows early hypofluorescence and late hyperfluorescence.
- **ICGA** of active lesions reveals marked hypofluorescence throughout all phases of the angiogram.

Treatment

Oral or intravenous steroids may control activity; a variety of immunosuppressives and infliximab may be effective, alone or in combination.

Relentless placoid chorioretinitis (RPC)

This refers to a rare entity showing features of both APMPPE and serpiginous choroiditis, and is also referred to as ampiginous choroiditis.

Persistent placoid maculopathy (PPM)

This rare condition features lesions similar to those of the macular variant of serpiginous choroidopathy, but which generally behave in a more benign fashion unless complicated by CNV (common).

Acute macular neuroretinopathy (AMN)

AMN is a rare self-limited condition that typically affects healthy young adult females. The disease may affect one or both eyes and may be preceded by a flu-like illness. Symptoms consist of decreased vision and paracentral scotomata. Red–brown wedge-shaped lesions are observed in a flower petal arrangement around the centre of the macula (Fig. 11.79), corresponding to the scotomata. FA is normal or shows faint hypofluorescence. Symptoms and signs fade slowly over months, with visual recovery.

Acute zonal occult outer retinopathy (AZOOR)

The acute zonal outer retinopathies (AZOR) are a group of rare conditions characterized by acute onset of loss of one or more zones of visual field, often temporal, in one or both eyes of young or middle-aged females, some of whom have an antecedent viral-like illness; photopsia and mild vitritis are frequent, and subtle vasculitis is sometimes seen. The mechanism is undefined as yet. Acute zonal occult outer retinopathy (AZOOR) is the most common of the AZOR syndromes, and is characterized by minimal fundoscopic signs early in the disease course; the other postulated

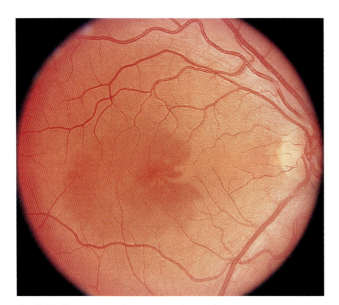

Fig. 11.79 Acute macular neuroretinopathy
(Courtesy of A Agarwal, from Gass' Atlas of Macular Diseases, *Elsevier, 2012)*

members of the group have more evident findings. Field loss may progress; in 50% stabilization occurs within 6 months but recovery is infrequent. Later findings include RPE clumping and vascular attenuation in the involved area (Fig. 11.80) and peripapillary region, although the fundus may remain normal. OCT, FA, ICGA and FAF may demonstrate abnormalities. ERG is important for diagnosis, characteristically showing a-wave and b-wave amplitude reduction and delayed 30 Hz flicker – that is, cones tend to be affected more than rods. EOG shows absence or severe

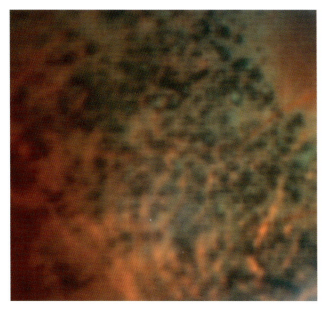

Fig. 11.80 Later retinal pigment epithelial changes in acute zonal occult outer retinopathy
(Courtesy of C Pavesio)

reduction of the light rise. Final visual acuity is 6/12 in at least one eye in most cases. Recurrence is sometimes seen.

Punctate inner choroidopathy (PIC)

Introduction

PIC typically affects young myopic women. Both eyes are frequently sequentially involved. It has similarities with MCP (see next) but involvement is predominantly macular. It is sometimes categorized with MCP (and possibly SFU – below) as 'pseudo-POHS'.

Clinical features

- **Symptoms.** Blurring, floaters and photopsia.
- **Anterior uveitis and vitritis** are usually absent or very mild.
- **Fundus.** Several small yellow–white macular spots with fuzzy borders at the level of the inner choroid and retina (Fig. 11.81A), sometimes with an overlying serous sensory retinal detachment. These evolve into sharply demarcated atrophic scars with little pigmentation, similar to the histo spots of POHS.
- **Prognosis.** Guarded; central vision may be compromised by a lesion at the fovea or, commonly, by CNV (up to 40% – Figs 11.81A and B).

Investigation

FA shows early hyperfluorescence and late staining of lesions, and demonstrates CNV (Figs 11.81C and D).

Treatment

This is usually reserved for CNV, though steroids may be considered for a foveal lesion.

Multifocal choroiditis and panuveitis (MFC, MCP)

Introduction

MCP is an uncommon, usually bilateral but asymmetrical, chronic/recurrent disease that typically affects young and middle-aged adult females. Severity and prognosis are very variable. Along with PIC and SFU (see below), it is sometimes termed pseudo-POHS.

Clinical features

- **Symptoms.** Blurring, floaters and photopsia.
- **Anterior uveitis** (50%).
- **Vitritis.**
- **Fundus.** Multiple discrete, ovoid, yellowish-grey lesions 50–350 μm in diameter at the posterior pole and/or periphery, sometimes with linear clusters and/or streaks.

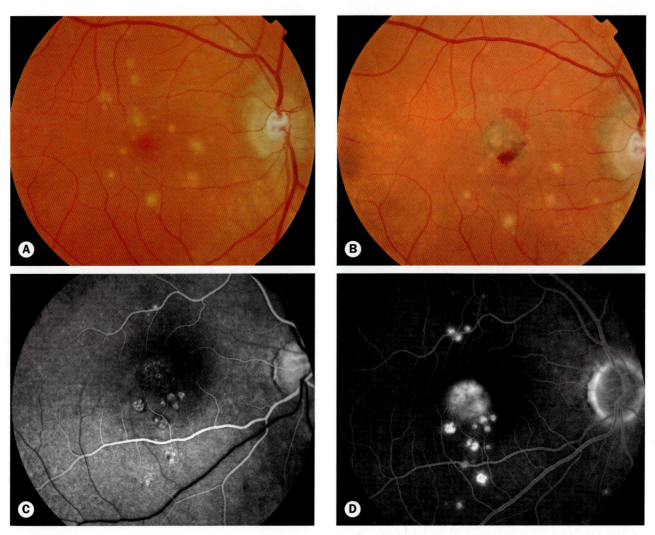

Fig. 11.81 Punctate inner choroidopathy. **(A)** Active lesions – there is also a suspicion of choroidal neovascularization immediately superior to the fovea; **(B)** the same eye as **(A)** 2 weeks later, showing clear choroidal neovascularization; **(C)** FA arterial phase of a different eye shows several hyperfluorescent spots with hypofluorescent edges inferior to the fovea and lacy hyperfluorescence at the fovea indicating choroidal neovascularization; **(D)** FA late phase of eye in **(C)** showing discrete hyperfluorescent spots and intense hyperfluorescence at the fovea

(Courtesy of S Chen – figs A and B; M Westcott – figs C and D)

Inactive lesions have sharply defined margins and pigmented borders resembling POHS (Fig. 11.82A). Peripapillary atrophy may be seen. The course is prolonged with the development of new lesions and recurrent inflammatory episodes. CNV (Figs 11.82B and C) occurs in 25–35%, CMO and subretinal fibrosis resembling SFU (see below) can develop.

- **Optic disc** oedema and blind spot enlargement may be present.

Investigation

- **Visual fields** may show large defects not corresponding with examination findings.
- **FA.** Early hypofluorescence and late hyperfluorescence. Old inactive lesions show window defects.

- **ICGA** shows hypofluorescent acute lesions which may not be clinically apparent. Old lesions remain hypofluorescent throughout.
- **ERG** remains normal until there is advanced retinal atrophy.

Treatment

Systemic and local steroids. Steroid-resistant patients require immunosuppressive therapy. CNV is treated with steroids and anti-VEGF agents.

Progressive subretinal fibrosis and uveitis syndrome (SFU)

SFU, also known as diffuse subretinal fibrosis, is an extremely rare chronic condition. It typically affects myopic young women,

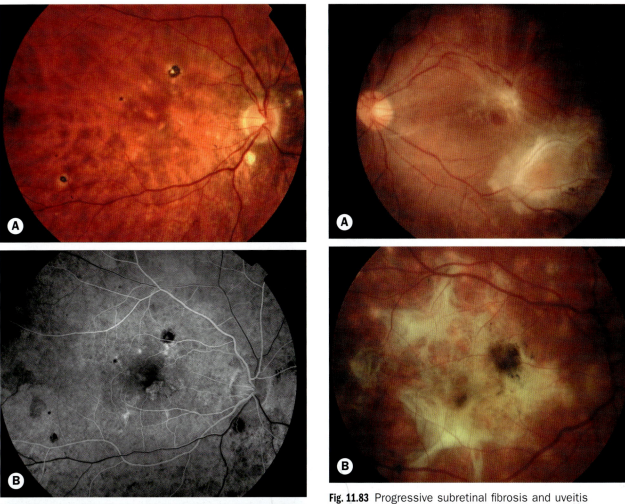

Fig. 11.83 Progressive subretinal fibrosis and uveitis syndrome. **(A)** Early and **(B)** advanced disease

Fig. 11.82 Choroidal neovascularization in multifocal choroiditis with uveitis. **(A)** Inactive lesions; **(B)** early venous phase fluorescein angiogram showing variable hypo- and hyperfluorescence of the lesions and lacy hyperfluorescence at the fovea indicating choroidal neovascularization; **(C)** late phase showing hyperfluorescence at the fovea due to leakage from choroidal neovascularization

(Courtesy of Moorfields Eye Hospital)

causing gradual blurring of vision in one then both eyes. Anterior uveitis and vitritis accompanies subretinal mounds at the posterior pole and midperiphery (Fig. 11.83A) progressing to widespread subretinal fibrosis (Fig. 11.83B). Steroids may be effective early in the disease, but the prognosis is poor. Some experts view SFU as part of a spectrum with MFC/MCP and PIC.

Birdshot retinochoroidopathy

Introduction

Birdshot retinochoroidopathy is an uncommon idiopathic chronic bilateral disease predominantly affecting middle-aged women.

Clinical features

- **Symptoms.** Insidious impairment of central vision associated with photopsia and floaters.
- **Vitritis** is prominent.

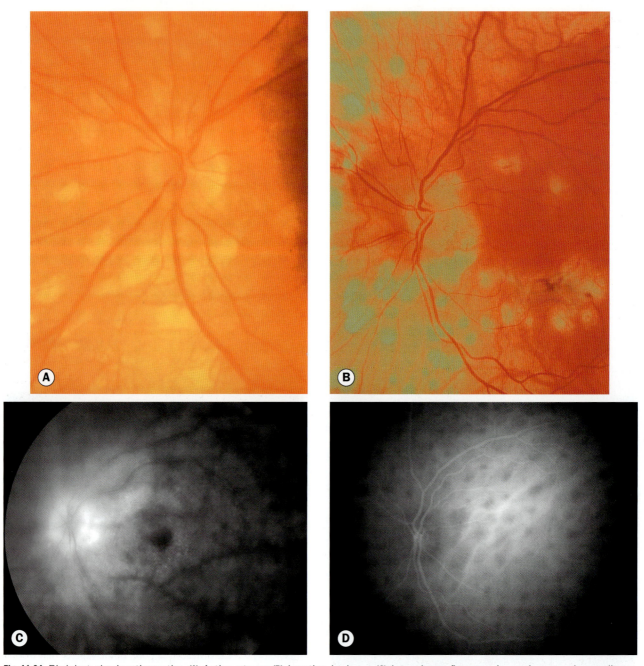

Fig. 11.84 Birdshot chorioretinopathy. **(A)** Active stage; **(B)** inactive lesions; **(C)** late phase fluorescein angiogram shows disc and vessel leakage, vessel wall staining and cystoid macular oedema; **(D)** early phase indocyanine green angiogram shows numerous hypofluorescent lesions

(Courtesy of C Barry – figs A and B; P Gili – fig. C)

- **Fundus.** Multiple ill-defined ovoid cream-coloured choroidal patches, less than one disc diameter in size, in the posterior pole and midperiphery (Fig. 11.84A). The lesions often appear to radiate outward from the disc but usually spare the macula itself. Inactive lesions consist of well-delineated atrophic spots (Fig. 11.84B). CMO, epiretinal membrane and CNV may develop.

- **Prognosis.** About one-third of patients have an eventual best visual acuity of less than 6/60.

Investigation

- **HLA-A29**: over 95% of patients are positive.
- **OCT** will confirm macular oedema.

- **Autofluorescence** will generally show more numerous hypoautofluorescent lesions than are seen on examination.
- **FA** shows extensive vascular leakage, with disc and vessel staining and CMO (Fig. 11.84C); lesions are initially hypofluorescent with later staining.
- **ICGA**: lesions are more numerous; they are hypofluorescent during the early and intermediate phases (Fig. 11.84D) and isofluorescent later.
- **ERG** is normal in early disease but with time shows rod and cone abnormalities.

Treatment

Systemic and intraocular steroids are reasonably effective in many patients, as are a variety of immunosuppressants and biological blockers such as infliximab.

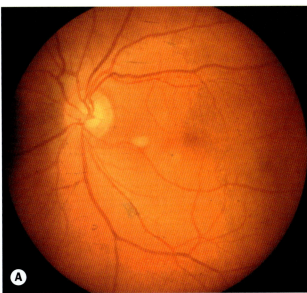

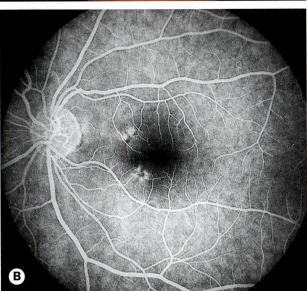

Fig. 11.85 (A) Acute retinal pigment epitheliitis; **(B)** FA venous phase shows corresponding focal hyperfluorescence
(Courtesy of M Prost)

Acute retinal pigment epitheliitis (ARPE)

ARPE (Krill disease) is a rare, idiopathic, self-limited condition of the RPE; it is unilateral in 75% of cases. Presentation is in young adults with mild disturbance of central vision; 1–2 weeks after the onset of symptoms the macula shows 2–4 discrete clusters of subtle small (one-fourth disc diameter) grey spots at the level of the RPE, surrounded by hypopigmented yellow haloes (Fig. 11.85A). Over 6–12 weeks the lesions resolve and vision returns to normal. Recurrences are uncommon. OCT shows hyper-reflectivity at the photoreceptor outer segment layer. FA may be normal, or the spots may show a hypofluorescent centre with a hyperfluorescent halo (Fig. 11.85B). The EOG is subnormal. Treatment is not required.

(Unilateral) acute idiopathic maculopathy (AIM)

AIM (UAIM) is a rare, self-limited condition that is most frequently unilateral and may be preceded by a flu-like illness. Patients are young adults who describe sudden marked reduction in central vision. A viral prodrome is common, and associated systemic infections have been noted. An irregularly yellow or grey exudative retinal detachment is seen at the macula (Figs 11.86A and B); small haemorrhages and papillitis may be associated. Within a few weeks the exudative changes resolve; a bull's eye appearance (Fig. 11.86C) may develop following resolution and can be associated with persistent visual loss. OCT shows hyper-reflectivity at the photoreceptor outer segment layer and RPE thickening; FAF shows stippled hyperautofluorescence that becomes hypofluorescent; FA shows early irregular mild hyperfluorescence at the detachment, with subsequent intense staining (Fig. 11.86D). Treatment is not given.

Acute multifocal retinitis

Acute multifocal retinitis is a very rare self-limited condition that may be preceded by a flu-like illness; it may be an atypical presentation of cat-scratch disease. It causes sudden onset mild visual loss in young adults; multiple areas of retinitis are seen posterior to the equator (Fig. 11.87), along with mild vitritis, disc oedema and sometimes a macular star. Recovery occurs over 2–4 months. Treatment as for cat-scratch disease may be considered.

Solitary idiopathic choroiditis (SIC)

SIC is a rare entity that presents with mild visual loss or is asymptomatic. A discrete post-equatorial dull-yellow choroidal elevation with ill-defined margins is seen (Fig. 11.88); vitritis is present during active disease. Contiguous subretinal fluid and a macular star may be present. With healing the lesion develops a better-defined margin with resolution of subretinal fluid and exudation. Treatment of a vision-threatening lesion is with systemic steroids.

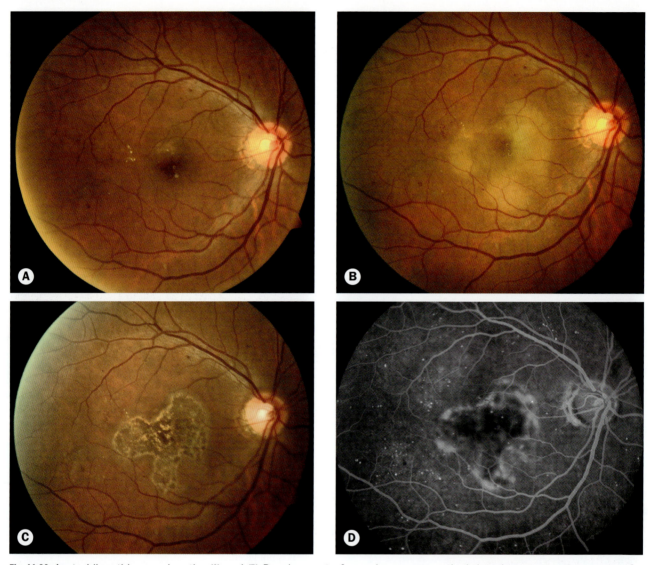

Fig. 11.86 Acute idiopathic maculopathy. **(A)** and **(B)** Development of macular sensory retinal detachment over the course of a month; **(C)** bull's eye appearance after a further month; **(D)** FA showing hyperfluorescence of subretinal fluid
(Courtesy of S Chen)

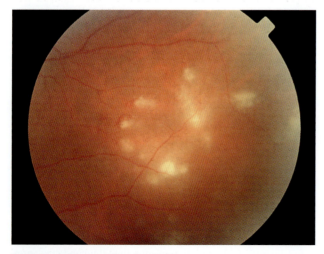

Fig. 11.87 Acute multifocal retinitis
(Courtesy of S Milewski)

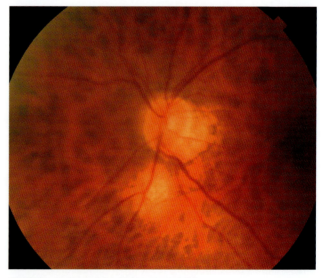

Fig. 11.88 Solitary idiopathic choroiditis
(Courtesy of S Chen)

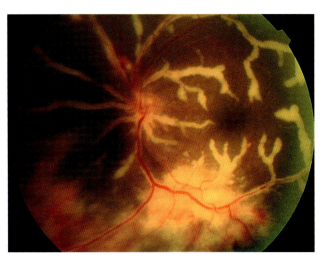

Fig. 11.89 Frosted branch angiitis
(Courtesy of J Donald Gass, from Stereoscopic Atlas of Macular Diseases, *Mosby 1997)*

Frosted branch angiitis (FBA)

FBA describes a characteristic fundus picture, usually bilateral, and may represent a specific entity (primary) or a common pathway in response to multiple stimuli. Secondary FBA may be associated with infectious retinitis, notably cytomegalovirus retinitis, and other conditions such as lymphoma and leukaemia. Primary (idiopathic) FBA is rare and typically affects children and young adults, in whom presentation is with bilateral visual loss (6/30 to PL), floaters and/or photopsia. There may be a viral prodrome. Florid sheathing of retinal arterioles and venules is seen (Fig. 11.89); anterior uveitis, vitritis and retinal oedema are common. Treatment is with systemic steroids, though some authorities believe the prognosis, which is usually good in the primary form, is unaffected.

Idiopathic retinal vasculitis, aneurysms and neuroretinitis syndrome (IRVAN)

Idiopathic retinal vasculitis, aneurysms and neuroretinitis syndrome is a rare entity that typically affects one or both eyes of healthy young women. Fundus signs consist of arteritis and multiple aneurysmal dilatations of arteriolar branches and on the optic nerve head, together with anterior uveitis and vitritis.

Disc oedema and a macular star (neuroretinitis) are common. Marked macular and circumpapillary exudative retinopathy can develop (Fig. 11.90A); the vascular changes are demonstrated very

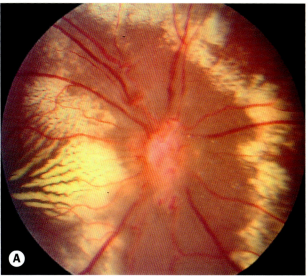

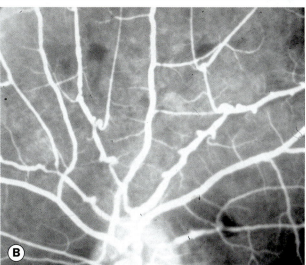

Fig. 11.90 Idiopathic retinal vasculitis, aneurysms and neuroretinitis syndrome. **(A)** Circinate pattern of hard exudates surrounding the disc. There is also venous irregularity and obscuration of the optic nerve head; **(B)** FA showing multiple aneurysms at arteriolar bifurcations and marked variation in arteriolar calibre
(Courtesy of J Donald Gass, from Stereoscopic Atlas of Macular Diseases, *Mosby 1997 – fig. A; RF Spaide, from* Diseases of the Retina and Vitreous, *WB Saunders 1999 – fig. B)*

well on FA (Fig. 11.90B). Extensive peripheral capillary nonperfusion may lead to preretinal neovascularization, and early panretinal photocoagulation should be considered. Intravitreal anti-VEGF treatment and steroids have been associated with good results in some patients and may be given in combination.

BENIGN EPIBULBAR TUMOURS

Conjunctival naevus

Introduction

A conjunctival naevus is the most common melanocytic conjunctival tumour; the overall risk of malignant transformation is less than 1%. Treatment by excision is usually for cosmesis, but sometimes for irritation or a suspicion of malignancy. The histological appearance is similar to that of cutaneous naevi, but as there is no conjunctival dermis, subepithelial and stromal replace dermal in the nomenclature:

- **Compound** naevi are characterized by the presence of naevus cells at the epithelial–subepithelial junction and within the subepithelial stroma, often with epithelial inclusions such as cysts and goblet cells (Fig. 12.1A).
- **Subepithelial** lesions are confined subepithelially.
- **Junctional** naevi consist of nests of naevus cells at the epithelial–subepithelial junction (Fig. 12.1B). They are uncommon.

Clinical features

- **Symptoms.** The lesion is typically initially noticed in the first or second decade.
- **Signs**
  - A solitary slightly or moderately elevated pigmented or partially pigmented lesion of variable size, most frequently juxtalimbal; over half contain small cysts (Figs 12.1C and D).
  - Naevi are mobile over the underlying sclera.
  - The extent of pigmentation is variable; absence is relatively common (Fig. 12.1E).
  - The plica, fornix and caruncle (Fig. 12.1F) are uncommon locations.
  - Naevi may become inflamed, especially in children and adolescents, and this may be mistaken for malignant change.
- **Signs of potential malignancy**
  - An unusual site such as the palpebral or forniceal conjunctiva.
  - Prominent feeder vessels.
  - Sudden growth or increase in pigmentation.
  - Development after the second decade.

Conjunctival papilloma

Conjunctival papillomata are strongly associated with human papillomavirus infection, especially types 6 and 11. Histopathologically they consist of a fibrovascular core covered by an irregular proliferation of non-keratinized stratified squamous epithelium containing goblet cells (Fig. 12.2A).

Clinical features

Lesions are sessile (wide base and flattish profile – Figs 12.2B and C) or pedunculated (frond-like – Fig. 12.2D), and are frequently located in the juxtalimbal area, fornix or the caruncle. They are usually solitary but may be multiple.

Large lesions may cause irritation, interfere with lid closure or encroach onto the cornea.

Treatment

Small lesions may resolve spontaneously. Large lesions are treated by excision, sometimes with cryotherapy to the base and the surrounding area. Options for recurrences include subconjunctival interferon alfa, carbon dioxide laser vaporization, topical mitomycin C and oral cimetidine.

Limbal dermoid

A limbal dermoid is a choristoma (a mass of histologically normal tissue in an abnormal location) consisting of a mass of collagenous tissue containing dermal elements; it is covered by stratified squamous epithelium (Fig. 12.3A). Presentation is in early childhood, with a smooth, yellowish, soft subconjunctival mass commonly located at the inferotemporal limbus, often with protruding hair (Fig. 12.3B). Lesions are occasionally very large and may virtually encircle the limbus (Fig. 12.3C). Treatment is indicated for cosmesis, chronic irritation, dellen formation and amblyopia from astigmatism or involvement of the visual axis. Small dermoids can undergo simple excision, but lamellar keratosclerectomy may be required for large lesions.

Systemic associations

- **Goldenhar syndrome** (oculoauriculovertebral spectrum – Fig. 12.3D) is usually sporadic.
  - Systemic features include hypoplasia of the malar, maxillary and mandibular regions, macrostomia and microtia, preauricular and facial skin tags, hemivertebrae (usually cervical), mental handicap, cardiac, renal and central nervous system (CNS) anomalies.
  - Ocular features, apart from dermoids, include upper lid notching or coloboma, microphthalmos and disc coloboma.
- **Treacher Collins syndrome** (see Ch. 1).
- **Linear naevus sebaceus of Jadassohn.**
  - Systemic features include warty or scaly cutaneous lesions, infantile spasms, CNS anomalies and developmental delay.
  - Ocular features, apart from dermoids, include ptosis, cloudy cornea, lid colobomas, fundus colobomas and microphthalmos.

Dermolipoma

A dermolipoma is similar in composition to a solid dermoid but also contains fatty tissue. Presentation tends to be in adult life as a soft yellowish subconjunctival mass near the outer canthus (Fig. 12.4A). The surface is usually keratinized, and in common with a dermoid, may exhibit hairs. Occasionally the lesion may extend into the orbit or anteriorly towards the limbus. Treatment is generally avoided due to the possibility of complications such as

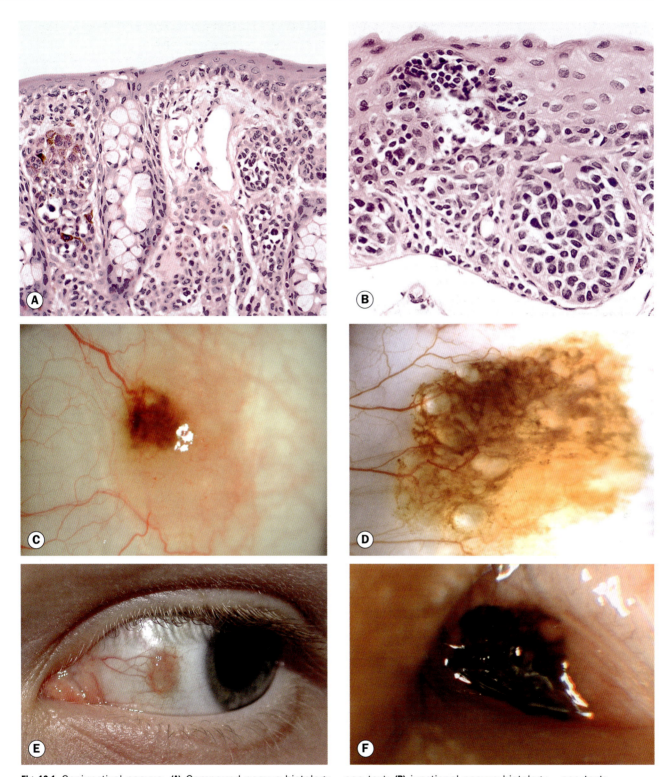

Fig. 12.1 Conjunctival naevus. **(A)** Compound naevus histology – see text; **(B)** junctional naevus histology – see text; **(C)** partially pigmented naevus; **(D)** cystic pigmented naevus; **(E)** non-pigmented naevus **(F)** caruncular location

(Courtesy of J Harry – fig. A; J Harry and G Misson, from Clinical Ophthalmic Pathology, Butterworth-Heinemann 2001 – fig. B; S Chen – figs D and E)

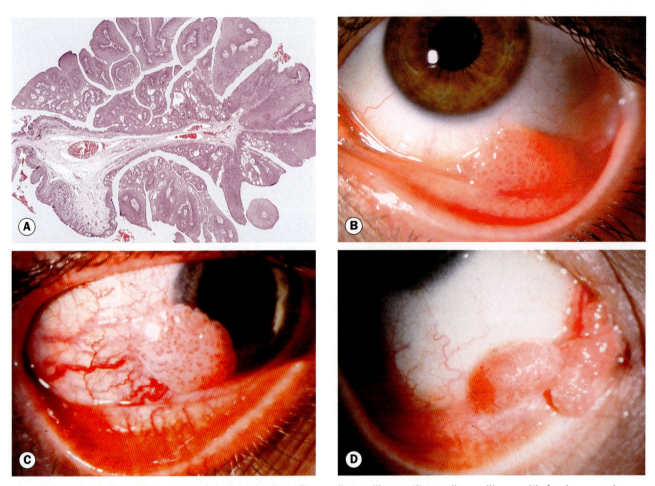

Fig. 12.2 Conjunctival papilloma. **(A)** Histology – see text; **(B)** sessile papilloma; **(C)** sessile papilloma with feeder vessels; **(D)** pedunculated papillomata

(Courtesy of J Harry – fig. A)

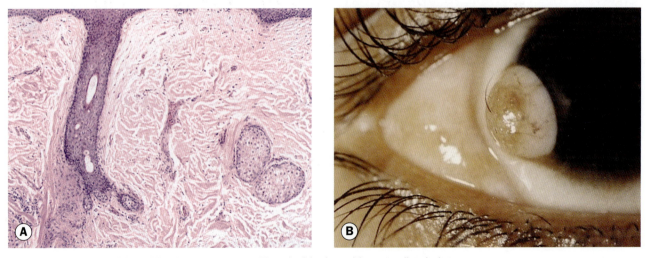

Fig. 12.3 Limbal dermoid. **(A)** Histology – see text; **(B)** typical lesion with protruding hair;

Continued

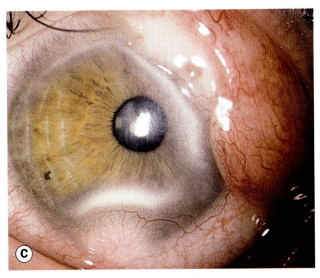

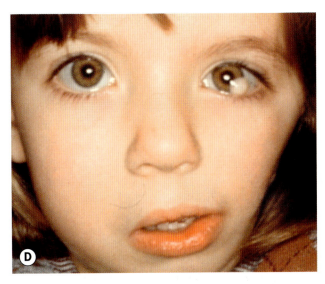

Fig. 12.3, Continued **(C)** complex dermoid; **(D)** Goldenhar syndrome
(Courtesy of J Harry and G Misson, from Clinical Ophthalmic Pathology, Butterworth-Heinemann 2001 – fig. A; U Raina – fig. B)

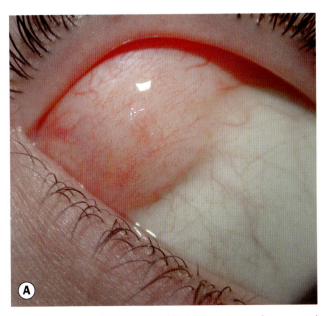

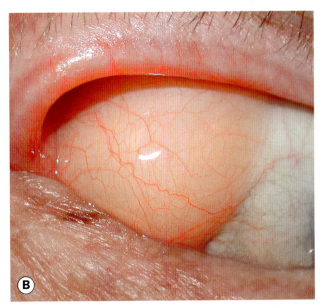

Fig. 12.4 (A) Dermolipoma; **(B)** orbital fat prolapse for comparison
(Courtesy of A Pearson)

scarring, ptosis, dry eye and ocular motility problems. In selected cases, debulking the anterior portion may improve cosmesis with lower risk. It is critical to distinguish a dermolipoma from a prominent lacrimal gland lobe and from orbital fat prolapse (Fig. 12.4B); lymphoma can also present in a similar fashion.

Pyogenic granuloma

A pyogenic granuloma is a fibrovascular proliferative response to a conjunctival insult such as surgery or trauma, or in association with a chalazion or foreign body incarceration. Histology shows granulation tissue with both acute and chronic inflammatory cells and a proliferation of small blood vessels; the term pyogenic granuloma is a misnomer as the lesion is neither pyogenic nor

granulomatous. Presentation is typically a few weeks after surgery for chalazion, strabismus or enucleation, with a rapidly growing dark pink fleshy conjunctival mass (Fig. 12.5A). Treatment with topical steroids is often successful; resistant cases require excision. The differential diagnosis includes suture granuloma, which can often be large and mistaken for a malignant lesion (Fig. 12.5B) and Tenon capsule granuloma or cyst.

Miscellaneous benign epibulbar tumours

- **Epibulbar telangiectasia** (Fig. 12.6A) may be associated with Sturge–Weber syndrome.

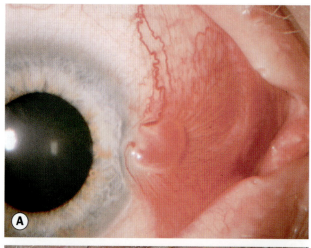

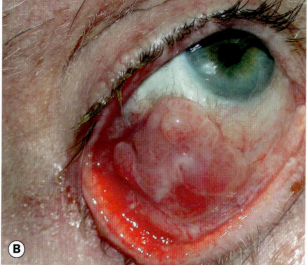

Fig. 12.5 (A) Pyogenic granuloma; **(B)** suture granuloma
(Courtesy of R Curtis – fig. A; Courtesy of S Chen – fig. B)

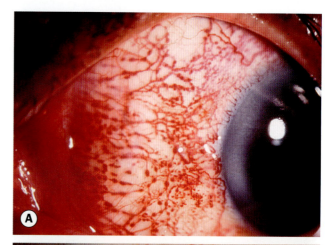

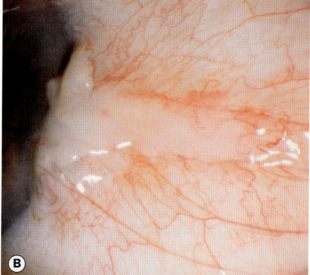

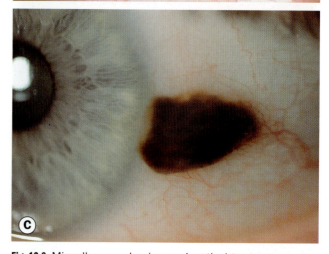

- **Reactive pseudoepitheliomatous hyperplasia** is a rapidly growing white juxtalimbal hyperkeratotic nodule (Fig. 12.6B) that develops secondary to irritation.
- **Melanocytoma** is a rare congenital lesion. It manifests as a slowly enlarging black lump (Fig. 12.6C) that cannot be moved freely over the globe.

Benign melanosis

Benign conjunctival epithelial melanosis (conjunctival hypermelanosis) is a normal variant, more common in darker-skinned individuals (over 90% of blacks, 5% of whites) due to the presence of excess melanin within basal layer conjunctival epithelial melanocytes. Melanocyte numbers are normal, that is, there is no melanocytic hyperplasia. It may have a protective effect against neoplasia. Benign melanosis appears during the first few years of life, and becomes static by early adulthood; both eyes are affected but involvement may be asymmetrical. Areas of flat, patchy, brownish pigmentation may be seen throughout the conjunctiva but are often concentrated at the limbus (Fig. 12.7A) and around

Fig. 12.6 Miscellaneous benign conjunctival tumours.
(A) Epibulbar telangiectasia in Sturge–Weber syndrome;
(B) reactive pseudoepitheliomatous hyperplasia;
(C) melanocytoma

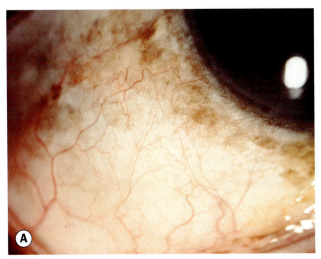

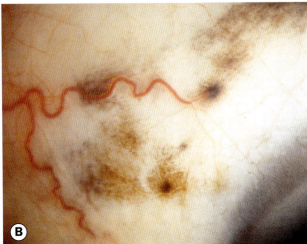

Fig. 12.7 Epithelial (racial) melanosis. **(A)** Juxtalimbal involvement; **(B)** at site of perforating vessel and nerve

perforating branches of vessels or nerves as they enter the sclera (Fig. 12.7B). The pigmented epithelium moves freely over the surface of the globe. A variant is seen in which small cysts are present.

MALIGNANT AND PREMALIGNANT EPIBULBAR TUMOURS

Primary acquired melanosis/ conjunctival melanocytic intra-epithelial neoplasia

Introduction

Approximately 75% of conjunctival melanomas (see below) arise in areas of melanocytic hyperplasia. Recent trends in the description of pigmented conjunctival lesions have led to controversy relating to terminology. Some classifications have historically used the term primary acquired melanosis (PAM) to encompass both

benign epithelial melanosis (see above) and melanocytosis/ melanocytic hyperplasia (with and without atypia), whilst others have restricted its use to the latter category. To avoid this ambiguity, the term conjunctival melanocytic intra-epithelial neoplasia (C-MIN) may be preferred for lesions exhibiting proliferation of melanocytes, with PAM reserved for clinical description before a histological diagnosis has been established. The differential diagnosis includes conjunctival naevus, benign melanosis, congenital ocular melanocytosis (see below), secondary pigmentation in Addison disease and pigmented squamous cell carcinoma.

- **PAM without cellular atypia or with mild atypia** is a benign intraepithelial proliferation of epithelial melanocytes (Fig. 12.8A) with little or no risk of malignant transformation.
- **PAM with severe atypia** can be regarded as melanoma *in situ* that has a substantial chance of progression to invasive melanoma over several years. The risk is higher the greater the extent of the lesion, measured in clock hours. Severe atypia is present in only a small minority of PAM.
- **C-MIN** is graded from 0 to 10 according to degree of atypia and spread, 0 corresponding to an absence of any melanocyte proliferation or atypia (i.e. melanosis only) and 5 to conjunctival melanoma *in situ*.

Diagnosis

- **Symptoms.** A pigmented area is noticed on the surface of one or both (10%) eyes at a median age of 56 years, usually in a white individual.
- **Signs**
  - Uni- or multifocal flat areas of irregular golden-brown to dark chocolate-coloured epithelial pigmentation, typically involving the limbus and interpalpebral region (Figs 12.8B and C). PAM *sine pigmento* has been reported.
  - Because any part of the conjunctiva may be affected, it is important to evert the eyelids (Fig. 12.8D); C-MIN may also extend onto the cornea.
  - Transformation to melanoma may be suggested by the appearance of nodular areas.
- **Investigation.** Careful documentation with drawing and/or photography of lesions undergoing observation is important. Immunohistochemical analysis of biopsied lesions is performed.
- **Treatment**
  - Observation of small (less than one clock hour) lesions may be appropriate; some advocate excision biopsy of every lesion.
  - Excision biopsy is generally preferred to incisional biopsy if possible (see under conjunctival melanoma below for surgical approach).
  - Double freeze–thaw cryotherapy may be administered to the excision site, and/or following histological confirmation of C-MIN postoperative topical mitomycin C, e.g. four cycles of 0.04% four times daily for 7 days separated by 3-week intervals, with punctum plugs *in situ* to reduce the risk of punctal stenosis and increase drug–surface contact time.

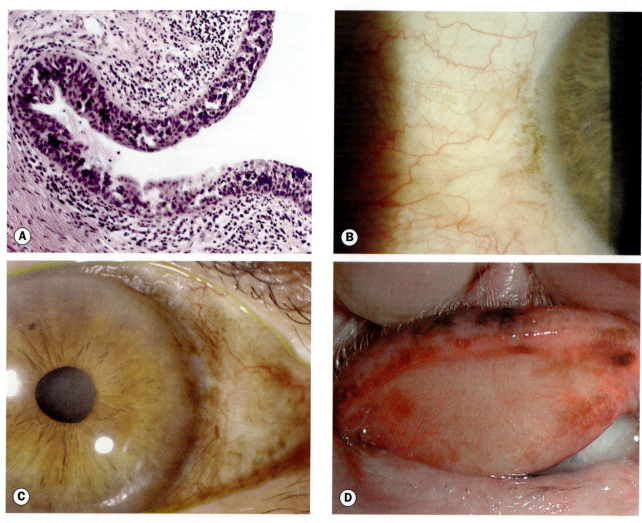

Fig. 12.8 Primary acquired melanosis (PAM). **(A)** Histology shows intraepithelial proliferation of conjunctival epithelial melanocytes; **(B)** small area of PAM; **(C)** more extensive PAM; **(D)** tarsal PAM associated with lentigo maligna of the eyelid
(Courtesy of J Harry and G Misson, from Clinical Ophthalmic Pathology, *Butterworth-Heinemann 2001 – fig. A; C Barry – fig. C; D Selva – fig. D)*

○ Amniotic membrane grafting may be necessary for large excision sites.

○ Larger lesions: mapping incisional biopsies can be accompanied by cryotherapy to all pigmented areas or topical mitomycin C as above.

○ Long-term follow-up is mandatory in all cases.

○ Corneal involvement: alcohol-mediated epitheliectomy followed by topical mitomycin C.

Conjunctival melanoma

Conjunctival melanoma is rare, accounting for about 2% of all ocular malignancies. Around 75% arise from an area of PAM, about 25% from a pre-existing junctional or compound naevus and rarely *de novo*. Presentation is often in the sixth decade, though patients with the rare dysplastic naevus syndrome develop multiple melanomas at a considerably younger age. The differential diagnosis includes naevus, ciliary body melanoma with extraocular extension, melanocytoma and pigmented conjunctival squamous carcinoma. The overall mortality is up to 19% at 5 years

and 30% at 10 years. Metastasis occurs in 20–30%; the main sites are regional lymph nodes, lung, brain and liver. Factors associated with a worse prognosis include caruncular, forniceal or lid margin location and tumour thickness of 2 mm or more.

Diagnosis

● **Appearance.** A black or grey vascularized nodule that may be fixed to the episclera. The limbus is a common site, but a melanoma may arise anywhere in the conjunctiva (Fig. 12.9A). Association with PAM/C-MIN is very common (Fig. 12.9B).

● **Amelanotic tumours** may give rise to diagnostic difficulty (Fig. 12.9C).

● **B-scan ultrasonography** may be helpful in characterization of the lesion.

● **Systemic screening** consists of regular general examination, liver function testing and ultrasound, chest X-ray and possibly whole body positron emission tomography/computed tomography (PET/CT) imaging where available.

● **Histology** shows melanomatous cellular atypia with invasion of the subepithelial stroma (Fig. 12.9D).

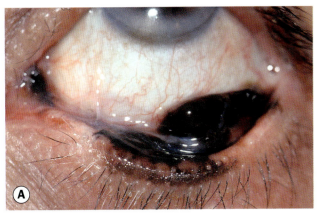

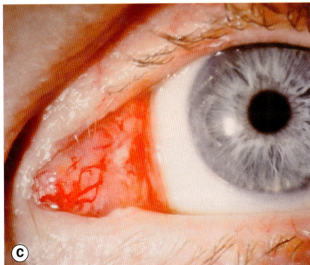

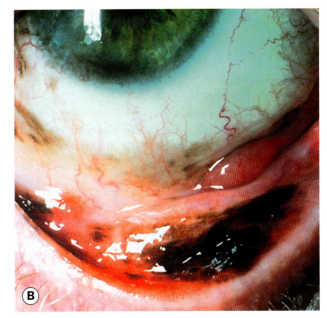

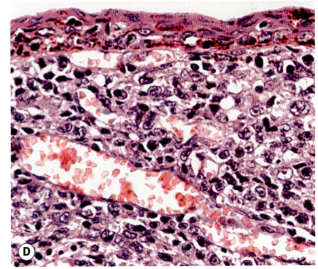

Fig. 12.9 Conjunctival melanoma. **(A)** Conjunctival melanoma extending into the eyelid; **(B)** multifocal melanoma arising from PAM; **(C)** amelanotic melanoma; **(D)** histology showing melanoma cells within the epithelium and subepithelial stroma
(Courtesy of C Barry – fig. A; J Harry – fig. D)

- **Sentinel lymph node biopsy** may be helpful in staging, though its place has not yet been fully defined.

Treatment

- Circumscribed lesions are treated by excision with a wide margin. As tumour seeding can occur during excision, contact with the tumour itself should be avoided and fresh instruments used to close the conjunctival defect.
- Adjunctive radiotherapy is routinely administered by some authorities, even if histology suggests that excision is complete; cryotherapy to the bed and surrounding tissue is an alternative. Proton beam radiotherapy can be applied if the caruncle or fornix is involved.

- Diffuse melanoma associated with extensive PAM/C-MIN is treated by excision of localized nodules with mitomycin C or cryotherapy to the diffuse component.
- Orbital recurrences are treated by local resection and radiotherapy. Exenteration may not improve survival and is therefore reserved for patients with extensive and aggressive disease when the eye cannot be preserved.
- The drug vemurafenib improves survival in patients with metastatic disease when the BRAF V600E mutation is present (50% of primary and metastatic conjunctival melanomas).
- Multifocal disease, non-limbal tumour location, tumour margin involvement and lack of adjunctive treatment are associated with a greater likelihood of recurrence.

Ocular surface squamous neoplasia

Introduction

Ocular surface squamous neoplasia (OSSN) describes a spectrum of benign, pre-malignant and malignant slowly progressive epithelial lesions of the conjunctiva and cornea. Older adults are usually affected unless a predisposing systemic condition is present. Risk factors include ultraviolet light exposure, a pale complexion, ciclosporin, smoking, petroleum product exposure, acquired immunodeficiency syndrome (AIDS) and xeroderma pigmentosum. Human papilloma virus infection (especially type 16) has been implicated in some cases. Metastatic disease is extremely rare.

Diagnosis

- **Symptoms.** A visible mass in one eye, sometimes accompanied by conjunctivitis-type symptoms.
- **Signs** are variable and clinical correlation with histological severity is unreliable. Most tend to develop within the interpalpebral fissure, particularly at the limbus, although any part of the conjunctiva or cornea may be involved. The lesion may appear fleshy, gelatinous, leukoplakic or papillomatous, superficial or feeder vessels may be prominent or the appearance may be avascular (Figs 12.10A–C). Intraocular extension is uncommon.
- **Investigations** include ultrasonic biomicroscopy (UBM) or anterior segment optical coherence tomography (OCT) to estimate the depth of invasion, exfoliative cytology and impression cytology.
- **Histology** shows the following spectrum; the first two are sometimes termed conjunctival–corneal intraepithelial neoplasia (CCIN):
  - Conjunctival epithelial dysplasia. Dysplastic cells are confined to the basal epithelial layers.
  - Carcinoma *in situ*. Dysplastic cells involve the full thickness of the epithelium.
  - Squamous cell carcinoma. Invasion of the underlying stroma (Fig. 12.10D).

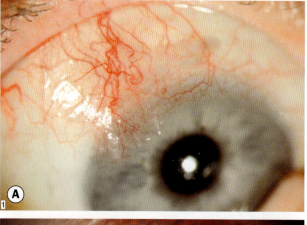

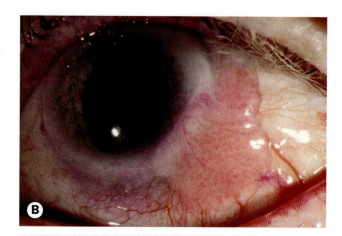

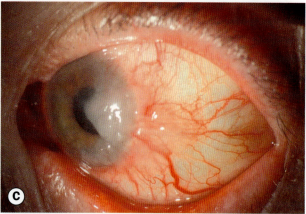

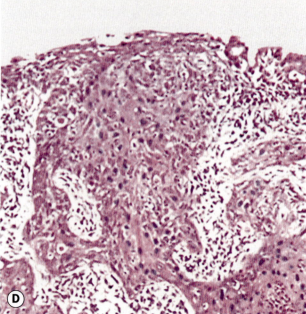

Fig. 12.10 Ocular surface squamous neoplasia. **(A)** Relatively small lesion; **(B)** larger gelatinous lesion stained with rose Bengal; **(C)** leukoplakic lesion; **(D)** histology of squamous cell carcinoma shows downward proliferation of irregular dysplastic epithelium with infiltration of subepithelial tissue

(Courtesy of B Damato – fig. C; J Harry – fig. D)

Treatment

- **Excision** with 2–4 mm margins and assessment for completeness of clearance, often with intraoperative frozen section, has been the conventional standard approach. Complete histological excision is associated with recurrence of 5–33%. Adjunctive measures reduce recurrence and include cryotherapy, brachytherapy or topical chemotherapy.
- **Topical chemotherapy.** Traditionally used as adjunctive treatment, this may also be employed as a primary modality to avoid the scarring and stem cell damage associated with extensive excision, to reduce tumour size prior to excision, or to treat recurrence. Agents include mitomycin C, 5-fluorouracil and interferon alfa-2b eye drop regimens; the latter two tend to be better tolerated.

Lymphoproliferative lesions

Introduction

The most common conjunctival lymphoproliferative lesion is reactive lymphoid hyperplasia, a proliferation of both B and T cells with germinal follicle formation. Conjunctival lymphoma may arise *de novo*, by extension from orbital lymphoma or associated with systemic lymphoma at diagnosis (up to 30%). Most conjunctival lymphomas are of B cell origin, arising from mucosa-associated lymphoid tissue (MALT) and tending to be indolent.

Diagnosis

- **Symptoms.** Painless swelling, redness or irritation; this is often bilateral, when systemic disease is more likely. Other possible symptoms include ptosis and diplopia.
- **Signs.** A slowly growing salmon-pink or flesh-coloured mobile infiltrate is seen on the epibulbar surface or in the fornices (Figs 12.11A and B). Rarely, a diffuse lesion may mimic chronic conjunctivitis.
- **Biopsy** is taken to confirm diagnosis; the uninvolved eye should also be biopsied (inferior fornix).
- **Investigation** for systemic involvement.

Treatment

- **Systemic disease** is treated as indicated, when local conjunctival measures may not be required.
- **External beam radiotherapy.**
- **Other options** include chemotherapy, excision of small lesions with adjuvant treatment, cryotherapy and intralesional injections of interferon alfa-2b or rituximab.

Kaposi sarcoma

Kaposi sarcoma is a slowly growing tumour that is typically found in patients with AIDS, but occasionally in the elderly and when there is long-term immunosuppression. A vascular bright red or

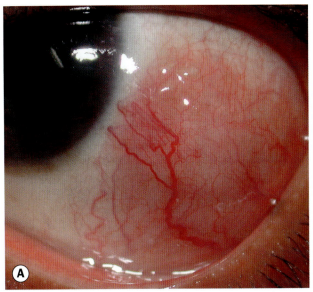

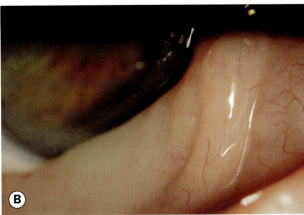

Fig. 12.11 Conjunctival lymphoproliferative lesions. **(A)** Epibulbar lymphoma; **(B)** large conjunctival lymphoma

purplish plaque or nodule is seen (Fig. 12.12), sometimes resembling (or associated with) conjunctival haemorrhage. Histology reveals a proliferation of spindle-shaped cells, vascular channels and inflammatory cells. If treatment is necessary, systemic AIDS therapy should be optimized, with local radiotherapy, excision and local or systemic chemotherapy as additional options.

IRIS TUMOURS

Iris naevus

Iris naevi consist of a proliferation of melanocytes in the superficial iris stroma, and appear as a circumscribed solitary flat or variably elevated pigmented lesion (Figs 12.13A–D). The normal iris architecture is disrupted. A diffuse naevus characteristically occurs in congenital ocular melanocytosis and in iris naevus (Cogan–Reese) syndrome (see Ch. 10). The malignant transformation rate

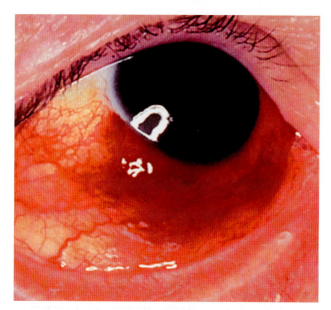

Fig. 12.12 Conjunctival Kaposi sarcoma

is up to 8% over 15 years; risk factors include young age (under 40), inferior location, bleeding from the lesion, diffuse iris involvement, feathery margins and ectropion uveae. Observation should be life-long and involve documentation by slit lamp examination and photography. Review should also include serial fundus examination, as iris naevus is a marker for all forms of uveal melanoma.

Iris freckle (ephelis)

Iris freckles (ephelides) are superficial lesions that are smaller than naevi, with no elevation or distortion (Fig. 12.14A and see Fig. 12.13A), and show increased melanocyte pigmentation but with a normal number of cells.

Brushfield spots

These are small whitish peripheral iris speckles arranged in a concentric ring (Fig. 12.14B), occurring particularly in Down syndrome though also as a normal finding in lighter irides. They consist of a focal mildly hyperplastic focus surrounded by a ring of hypoplasia and have no malignant potential (see also Ch. 9).

Lisch nodules

These are small well-defined nodules (Figs 12.14C and D) found in both eyes of virtually all patients with neurofibromatosis type 1 (see Ch. 19).

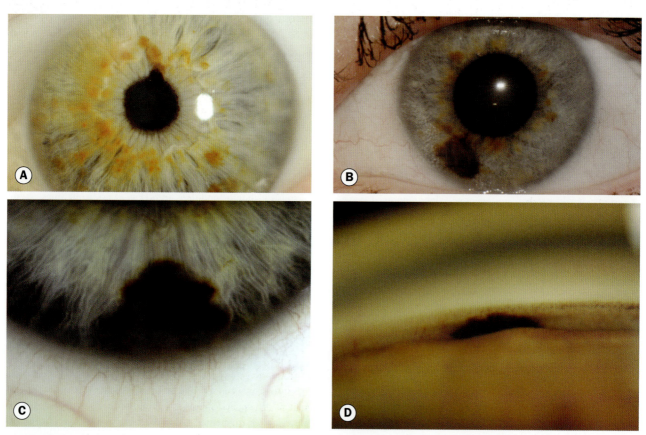

Fig. 12.13 Iris naevus. **(A)** Small lesion with mild ectropion uveae – freckles are also present; **(B)** larger naevus; **(C)** suspicious naevus with prominent associated vessels; **(D)** anterior chamber angle naevus
(Courtesy of C Barry – fig. B)

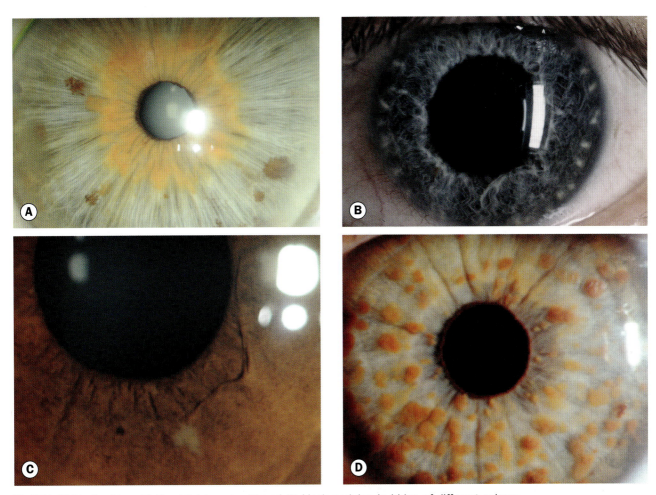

Fig 12.14 (A) Iris freckles; **(B)** Brushfield spots; **(C)** and **(D)** Lisch nodules in irides of different colours
(Courtesy of R Bates – fig. B)

Iris melanoma

Introduction

About 8% of uveal melanomas arise in the iris. The prognosis is comparatively good – only about 5% of patients develop metastasis within 10 years of treatment. Conditions associated with or predisposing to uveal melanomas include fair skin and lighter iris colour, numerous and/or atypical (dysplastic) cutaneous naevi, iris or choroidal naevi, congenital ocular and oculodermal melanocytosis (naevus of Ota) and uveal melanocytoma. Chronic sunlight exposure and arc welding are environmental risk factors. Presentation is typically in middle age, a decade earlier than ciliary body and choroidal melanoma.

Diagnosis

- **Symptoms.** Enlargement of a pre-existing naevus is typical, noticed either by the patient or at a routine eye examination. Signs indicative of malignant transformation include growth (Fig. 12.15) and the development of prominent blood vessels (see Fig. 12.13C).

- **Signs**
  - A pigmented (Fig. 12.16A) or non-pigmented (Fig. 12.16B) nodule at least 3 mm in diameter and 1 mm thick, typically located in the inferior half of the iris and often associated with surface blood vessels.
  - Pupillary distortion, ectropion uveae and occasionally localized cataract may be seen, although these can also occur with naevi.
  - Growth is usually slow, with extension across the iris surface.
  - The angle and anterior ciliary body may be infiltrated; extrascleral extension is rare (Fig. 12.16C).
  - Complications include hyphaema, cataract and glaucoma.
- **Histology** in the majority shows diffusely infiltrating spindle cells (see below) of low-grade malignancy (Fig. 12.16D). A minority contain an epithelioid cell component and can be more aggressive.
- **Ultrasound biomicroscopy** is used to rule out ciliary body involvement.
- **Fine-needle aspiration biopsy** may be employed prior to major surgical intervention.
- **Systemic investigation** should be carried out.

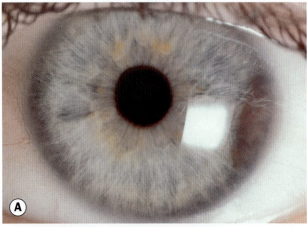

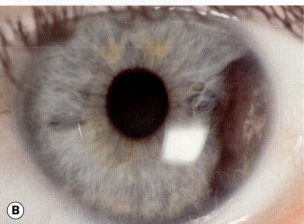

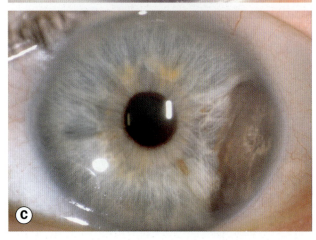

Fig. 12.15 Iris melanoma enlarging over several years
(Courtesy of C Barry)

Treatment

- **Sector iridectomy** for small tumours, and iridocyclectomy for tumours invading the angle.
- **Radiotherapy** with a radioactive plaque (brachytherapy) or external irradiation with a proton beam.
- **Enucleation** may be required for diffusely growing tumours, if radiotherapy is not possible.
- **Monitoring** for recurrence and metastasis.

Metastatic tumours

Metastasis to the iris (Figs 12.17A and B) is rare and is characterized by one or more fast-growing white, pink or yellow masses that may be associated with anterior uveitis and occasionally hyphaema. Breast and lung cancer and melanoma of the skin are among the most common types.

Miscellaneous iris tumours

- **Juvenile xanthogranuloma** is a rare idiopathic granulomatous disease of early childhood that involves the skin, muscle, stomach, salivary glands and other organs. Iris involvement is characterized by a localized or diffuse yellow lesion (Fig. 12.18A) that may be associated with spontaneous hyphaema or, less commonly, anterior uveitis and glaucoma. Treatment is with topical steroids.
- **Leiomyoma** is an extremely rare benign tumour arising from smooth muscle. The appearance is similar to that of an amelanotic melanoma (Fig. 12.18B).
- **Melanocytoma** is a darkly pigmented nodular mass with a mossy, granular surface, most frequently occupying the peripheral iris (Fig. 12.18C). It may undergo spontaneous necrosis resulting in seeding of the iris stroma and chamber angle, with elevation of intraocular pressure.
- **Vascular tumours** of various types have been described, the most common being racemose haemangioma (arteriovenous communication), typically seen as a large ectatic vessel and/ or bunch of grapes (Figs 12.18D and E).

IRIS CYSTS

Iris cysts are rare lesions. Anterior segment OCT and ultrasound biomicroscopy are especially useful to differentiate some lesions from ciliary body tumours.

- **Primary epithelial cysts**
  - Cysts arise from the iris or iridociliary pigment epithelium.
  - Three-quarters are in the peripheral iris, where they appear as a smooth dome-shaped bulging (Fig. 12.19A) best seen on gonioscopy (Fig. 12.19B). Mid-zone lesions again appear as a bulge in the iris – the wall may be manifest on pupillary dilatation. At the pupillary margin (least common), cysts appear darkly pigmented and often elongated.
  - They may rarely dislodge to float freely in the anterior chamber or vitreous (Fig. 12.19C).
  - The vast majority are asymptomatic and innocuous. Rarely, large cysts may obstruct vision and require collapse with photocoagulation.
- **Primary stromal cysts** may be congenital (more aggressive) or acquired.
  - Solitary unilateral structure with a smooth translucent anterior wall lying on or within the iris (Fig. 12.19D). Contained debris may be visible.
  - May remain stable for many years before enlarging; can sometimes rupture.

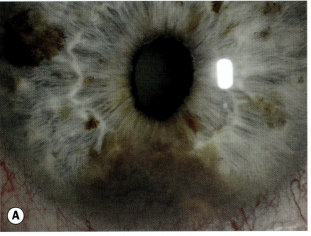

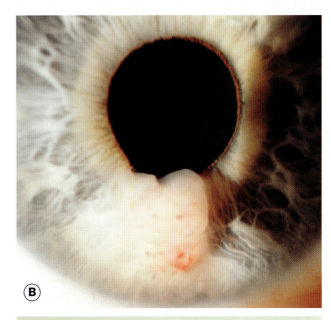

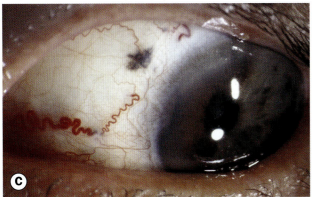

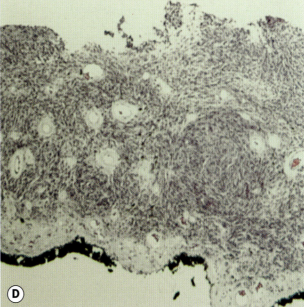

Fig. 12.16 Iris melanoma. **(A)** Typical iris melanoma; **(B)** amelanotic tumour; **(C)** angle invasion and extrascleral extension; **(D)** histology shows infiltration of the entire thickness of the stroma

(Courtesy of C Barry – figs A and C; J Harry and G Misson, from Clinical Ophthalmic Pathology, Butterworth-Heinemann 2001 – fig. D)

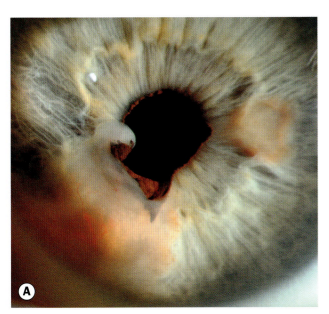

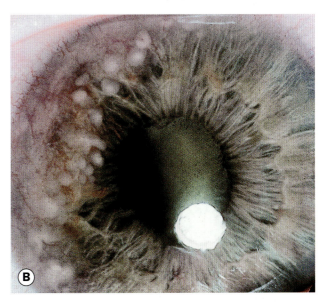

Fig. 12.17 Iris metastasis. **(A)** Metastasis from breast; **(B)** multiple small deposits

(Courtesy of P Saine – fig. A; B Damato – fig. B)

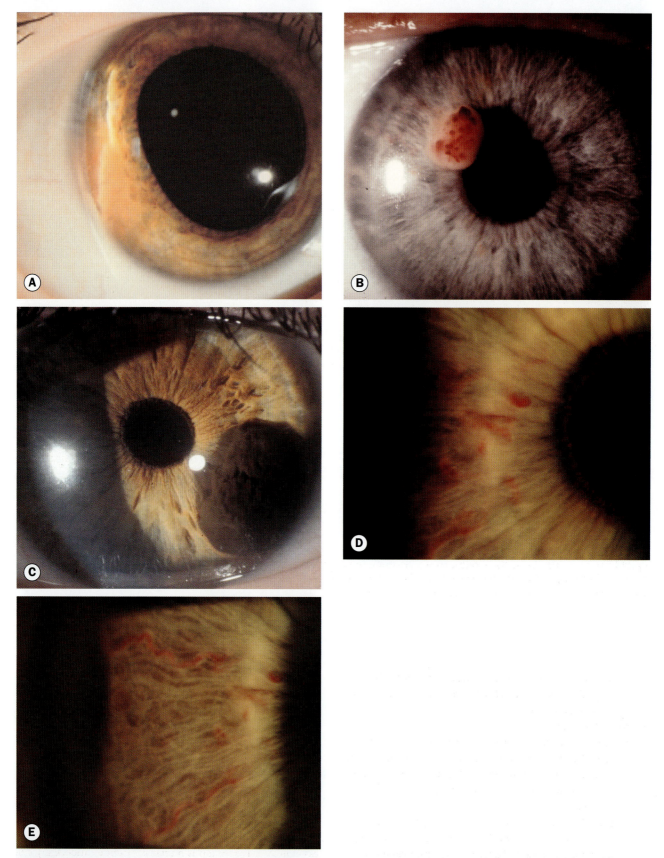

Fig. 12.18 (A) Juvenile iris xanthogranuloma; **(B)** leiomyoma; **(C)** melanocytoma; **(D)** racemose haemangioma; **(E)** supplying and draining vessels for lesion in **(D)**

(Courtesy of BJ Zitelli and HW Davis, from Atlas of Pediatric Physical Diagnosis, *Mosby 2002 – fig. A; B Damato – fig. B)*

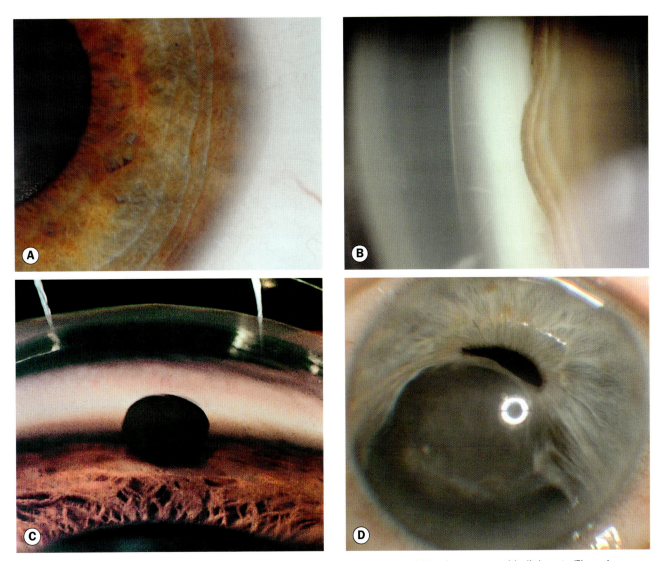

Fig. 12.19 Primary iris cysts. **(A)** Subtle dome-shaped elevation of the peripheral iris due to an epithelial cyst; **(B)** gonioscopy of lesion in **(A)**; **(C)** dislodged epithelial cyst in the angle; **(D)** very large stromal cyst

(Courtesy of Centre for Eye Health, Sydney – fig. A; J McAllister – fig. D)

○ Most congenital cysts require treatment by aspiration or surgical excision. Ethanol-induced sclerosis may avoid the need for excision.

- **Secondary cysts**
  ○ Traumatic cysts (Fig. 12.20A) occur following deposition of epithelial cells from the conjunctiva or cornea onto the iris after penetrating or surgical trauma. They frequently enlarge, leading to corneal oedema, anterior uveitis and glaucoma.
  ○ Extended use of long-acting miotics may be associated with usually bilateral small, multiple cysts located along the pupillary border (Fig. 12.20B). Their development can be prevented by the concomitant use of topical phenylephrine 2.5%.
  ○ Parasitic cysts are extremely rare.

CILIARY BODY TUMOURS

Ciliary body melanoma

Introduction

Ciliary body melanomas comprise around 12% of all uveal melanomas. Risk factors are as for iris melanoma. Presentation is usually in the sixth decade with visual symptoms, although occasionally discovery is incidental; diagnosis may be delayed as the lesion is easily missed. Distinction is principally from an iridociliary cyst though uveal effusion syndrome may cause diagnostic difficulty that can be resolved by imaging. Other ciliary body tumours are extremely rare and include melanocytoma, medulloepithelioma,

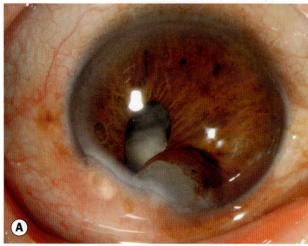

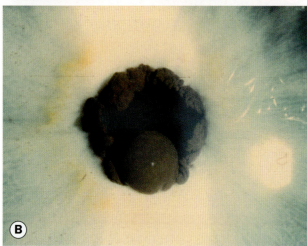

Fig. 12.20 Secondary iris cysts. **(A)** Traumatic cyst; **(B)** pupillary border cysts due to miotic therapy
(Courtesy of S Chen – fig. A; R Bates – fig. B)

metastases, adenocarcinoma, adenoma, neurolemmoma and leiomyoma.

Diagnosis

- **Signs**
  - A large tumour may be visualized with pupillary dilatation (Fig. 12.21A).
  - Overlying prominent episcleral (sentinel) vessels (Fig. 12.21B).
  - Erosion through the iris root may mimic iris melanoma, extraocular extension through scleral vessels a conjunctival melanoma (Fig. 12.21C).
  - Displacement of the lens (Fig. 12.21D) may cause astigmatism, subluxation or cataract.
- **Investigations**
  - Three-mirror contact lens examination and binocular indirect ophthalmoscopy.
  - Gonioscopy to detect angle invasion.
  - Ultrasonic biomicroscopy.

- Biopsy involving excisional, incisional or fine-needle aspiration techniques may be helpful in selected cases. Genetic profiling may help to determine the likelihood of metastasis (see choroidal melanoma).
- Investigation for systemic involvement, particularly hepatic.

Treatment

- **Iridocyclectomy** or sclerouvectomy for small or medium-sized tumours involving no more than one-third of the angle. Complications include retinal detachment, vitreous haemorrhage, cataract, lens subluxation, hypotony and incomplete resection.
- **Radiotherapy** by brachytherapy or proton beam irradiation.
- **Enucleation** may be necessary for large tumours.
- **Systemic treatment** is indicated when metastatic disease is evident.

Medulloepithelioma

Medulloepithelioma (previously known as diktyoma) is a rare embryonal neoplasm that arises from the inner layer of the optic cup and can be benign or malignant. Presentation is usually in the first decade with visual loss, pain, photophobia, leukocoria, or proptosis in advanced cases. A white, pink, yellow or brown ciliary body, retrolental or anterior chamber mass is seen (Figs 12.22A and B). Enucleation may be required.

TUMOURS OF THE CHOROID

Choroidal naevus

Choroidal naevi are present in 5–10% of Caucasians but are rare in darker-skinned races. Growth occurs mainly during the pre-pubertal years and is extremely rare in adulthood. For this reason clinically detectable growth should raise a suspicion of malignancy. The lifetime risk of malignant transformation is up to 1% from tertiary centre data. Histologically, the tumour is composed of a proliferation of spindle cell melanocytes within the choroid (Fig. 12.23A). It is vital to identify features suggesting a greater likelihood of malignancy; as with cutaneous melanoma, early treatment is associated with a substantially lower risk of metastasis. An extended period without any change provides no guarantee that progression will not occur in the future, as sudden enlargement of naevi has been documented following many years of stability.

Diagnosis

- **Symptoms**. The great majority are asymptomatic and detected on routine examination.
- **Signs**
  - Usually post-equatorial, oval or circular, brown to slate-grey lesion with indistinct feathery margins (Figs 12.23B and C).
  - Overlying drusen are typical.

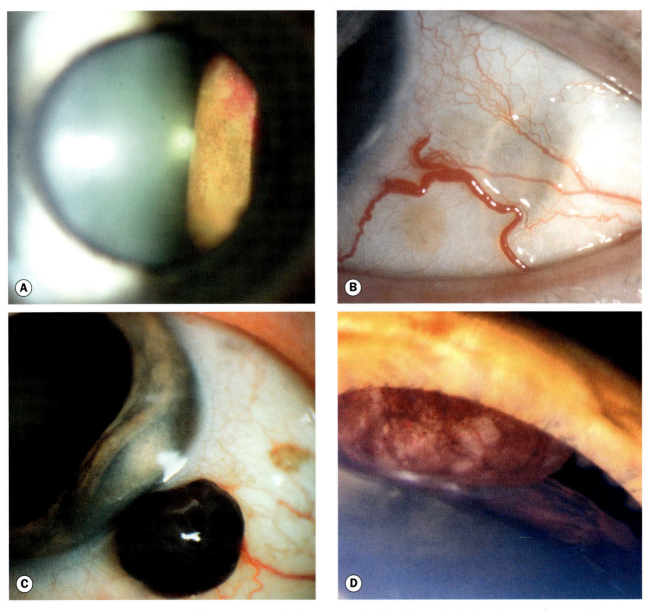

Fig. 12.21 Ciliary body melanoma. **(A)** Tumour seen on fundoscopy; **(B)** 'sentinel' vessels in the same quadrant as the tumour; **(C)** extraocular extension; **(D)** pressure on the lens
(Courtesy of B Damato – fig. B; R Curtis – fig. D)

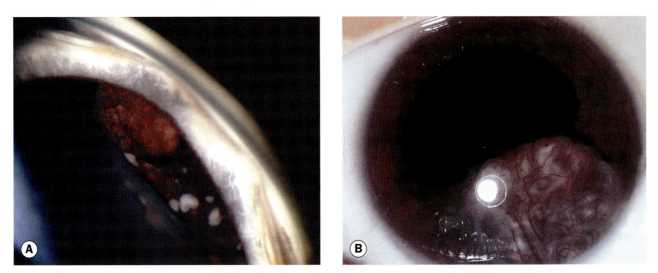

Fig. 12.22 Medulloepithelioma. **(A)** Cystic brown ciliary body mass; **(B)** anterior segment involvement
(Courtesy of R Curtis – fig. A)

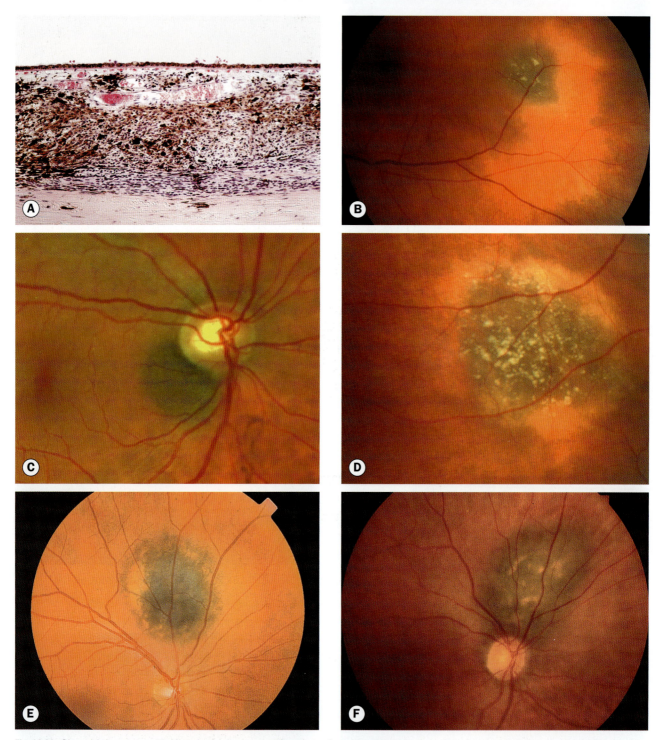

Fig. 12.23 Choroidal naevus. **(A)** Histology shows proliferation of melanocytes in the choroid, sparing the choriocapillaris; **(B)** typical small flat naevus with feathery edges, overlying drusen and a subtle broad halo; **(C)** peripapillary naevus; **(D)** naevus with overlying drusen and distinct halo; **(E)** and **(F)** overlying orange pigment

(Courtesy of J Harry – fig. A)

- ○ A depigmented halo is very common (Fig. 12.23D).
- ○ Amelanotic lesions can occur.
- • **Features suspicious of early melanoma**
  - ○ The presence of overlying orange pigment (lipofuscin – Figs 12.23E and F).
  - ○ The presence of associated subretinal fluid.

- ○ Acoustic hollowness on ultrasonography (US).
- ○ Symptoms such as photopsia, blurred vision.
- ○ Thickness greater than 2 mm; diameter over 5 mm.
- ○ Absence of drusen.
- ○ Margin within 3 mm of the optic disc.
- ○ The absence of a halo.

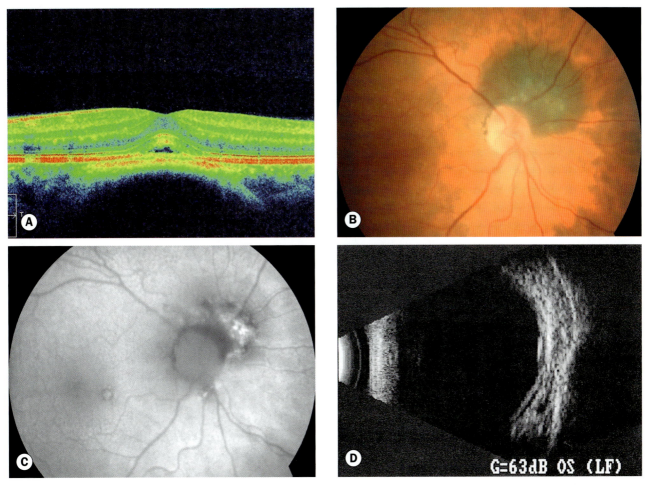

Fig 12.24 Imaging of choroidal naevi. **(A)** OCT; **(B)** and **(C)** colour photograph and fundus autofluorescence image of peripapillary naevus showing dramatic hyperautofluorescence of subtle orange pigment; **(D)** B-scan ultrasonography

(Courtesy of M Karolczak-Kulesza – fig. D)

- **Investigations**
  - Photographic documentation.
  - OCT (Fig. 12.24A) is useful for measurement of lesion thickness as well as the detection of subtle associated fluid (a high-risk factor). Secondary retinal changes tend to be more marked overlying a melanoma than a naevus.
  - Fundus autofluorescence (FAF) (Fig. 12.24B and C) can demonstrate subtle orange pigment that may not be easily discernible clinically; naevi may have patchy increased autofluorescence, but the appearance of intense diffuse or even confluent hyperautofluorescence is a useful diagnostic indicator of melanoma.
  - Fluorescein angiography (FA) is not helpful in distinguishing a melanoma from a naevus.
  - Ultrasonography (US) (Fig. 12.24D) shows a localized flat or slightly elevated lesion with high internal acoustic reflectivity; a hollow acoustic appearance is a risk factor for progression. Lesion thickness should be measured.

Treatment

- **Baseline** fundus photography and ultrasonography or OCT, with indefinite regular review.
- **Review interval** is determined by level of suspicion:
  - No suspicious features: 6 months until stability established (e.g. one year), then annual review.
  - One or two suspicious features: 4–6 months.
  - Three or more suspicious features: consider referral for ocular oncology subspecialist assessment.
- **Growth.** If growth is documented (Figs 12.25A and B) or highly suspicious features are present, the lesion should generally be regarded as a melanoma and managed accordingly.

Choroidal melanoma

Choroidal melanoma is the most common primary intraocular malignancy in adults and accounts for 80% of all uveal

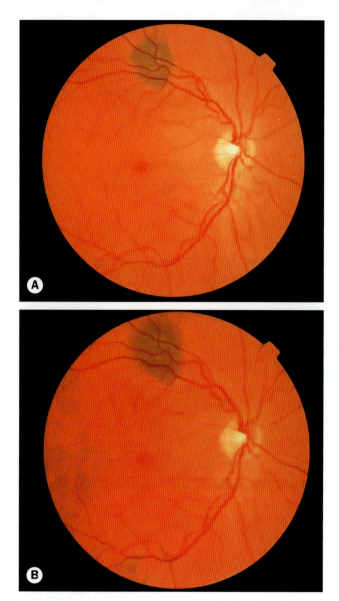

Fig 12.25 Naevus growth over 5 years
(Courtesy of S Chen)

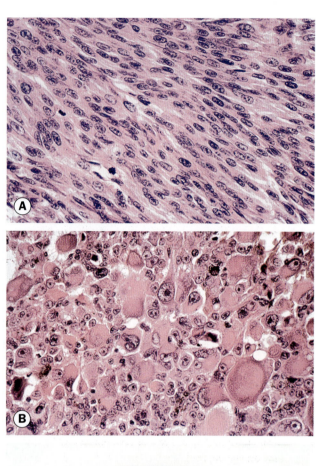

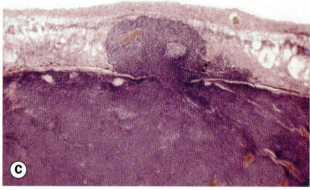

Fig. 12.26 Histology of choroidal melanoma. **(A)** Spindle cells – tightly arranged fusiform cells with indistinct cell membranes and slender or plump oval nuclei; **(B)** epithelioid cells – large pleomorphic cells with distinct cell membranes, large vesicular nuclei with prominent nucleoli, and abundant cytoplasm; **(C)** penetration of Bruch membrane in a 'collar stud' fashion

(Courtesy of J Harry – figs A and B; J Harry and G Misson, from Clinical Ophthalmic Pathology, Butterworth-Heinemann 2001 – fig. C)

melanomas, but is still relatively uncommon. Predisposing factors are as for iris melanoma (above). Presentation peaks at around the age of 60 years. Histopathologically, spindle (Fig. 12.26A) and epithelioid (Fig. 12.26B) cell types are seen, the former being arranged in bundles and having a better prognosis; epithelioid cells are larger and more pleomorphic with more frequent mitotic figures. Tumour composition is commonly exclusively spindle cell or a mixture of spindle and epithelioid. Lesions may penetrate Bruch membrane and the retinal pigment epithelium (RPE) with herniation into the subretinal space, classically assuming the shape of a collar stud (Fig. 12.26C). Scleral channel and vortex vein invasion can lead to orbital spread. Metastasis is commonly to the liver, bone and lung; only about 1–2% of patients have detectable metastases at the time of presentation. Mortality is up to 50% at 10 years; adverse prognostic factors include particular histological features (e.g. large numbers of epithelioid cells, mitotic activity), larger tumour dimensions, tumour genetic characteristics (e.g. somatic mutations in the tumour suppressor gene *BAP1*, present in nearly 50% of uveal melanomas, imply a greater chance of metastasis), extrascleral extension and anterior location.

Diagnosis

- **Symptoms** are often absent, with a tumour detected by chance on routine fundus examination; a range of visual disturbance can occur depending on tumour characteristics.
- **Signs**
  - A solitary elevated subretinal grey-brown (Fig. 12.27A) or rarely amelanotic (Fig. 12.27B) dome-shaped mass; diffuse infiltration is uncommon.
  - About 60% are located within 3 mm of the optic disc (Fig. 12.27C) or fovea.
  - Clumps of overlying orange pigment are common (Fig. 12.27D).
  - If the tumour breaks through the Bruch membrane it acquires a 'collar stud' (see Figs 12.26C and Fig. 12.29C) appearance.
  - Associated haemorrhage and subretinal fluid (Fig. 12.27E) are common; the latter may become bullous (Fig. 12.27F), and mask the underlying lesion.
  - Other signs can include sentinel vessels (Fig. 12.28), choroidal folds, inflammation, rubeosis iridis, secondary glaucoma and cataract.

Differential diagnosis

- **Pigmented lesions**
  - A choroidal naevus usually exhibits numerous surface drusen, without serous retinal detachment and little if any orange pigment.
  - Melanocytoma is deeply pigmented and usually located at the optic disc.
  - Congenital hypertrophy of the RPE is flat, is often grey–black and has a well-defined margin with lacunae.
  - Haemorrhage in the subretinal or suprachoroidal space, for example from choroidal neovascularization or retinal artery macroaneurysm.
  - Metastatic cutaneous melanoma has a smooth surface, a light brown colour, indistinct margins, extensive retinal detachment and often a past history of malignancy.
- **Non-pigmented lesions**
  - Circumscribed choroidal haemangioma is typically posterior, pink, dome-shaped and has a smooth surface.
  - Metastasis is often associated with exudative retinal detachment.
  - Solitary choroidal granuloma, e.g. sarcoidosis, tuberculosis.
  - Posterior scleritis, which can present with a large elevated lesion, but in contrast to melanoma pain is a common feature.
  - Large elevated choroidal neovascular lesion, which can be eccentrically located, usually in the temporal pre-equatorial region; typically associated with exudate and fresh haemorrhage, both of which rarely accompany a melanoma.
  - Prominent vortex vein ampulla is characterized by a small, smooth, brown, dome-shaped lesion, which disappears with pressure on the eye.

Investigation

Examination is sufficient for diagnosis in the majority of cases.

- **FA** is of limited diagnostic value because there is no pathognomonic pattern. The most common findings are an intrinsic tumour ('dual') circulation (Fig. 12.29A), mottled fluorescence during the arteriovenous phase and late diffuse leakage and staining. FA may, however, be useful in the differential diagnosis of simulating lesions.
- **US** is used to measure lesion dimensions and to detect tumours through opaque media and exudative retinal detachment; it may also demonstrate extraocular extension. The characteristic findings are internal homogeneity with low to medium reflectivity, choroidal excavation (Fig. 12.29B) and orbital shadowing; a basal acoustically quiet zone referred to as 'acoustic hollowing' is typical and is due to the greater tissue homogeneity in this region. A 'collar stud' configuration (Fig. 12.29C) is almost pathognomonic when present.
- **FAF.** Intense diffuse or confluent hyperautofluorescence, if present, is a useful diagnostic indicator of melanoma.
- **OCT** measures dimensions and may demonstrate associated subretinal fluid, often before clinically apparent. Secondary retinal changes are often evident overlying the lesion.
- **Indocyanine green angiography (ICGA)** usually shows hypofluorescence throughout the study and provides more information than FA about the extent of the tumour, due to lower interference from the RPE.
- **Magnetic resonance imaging (MRI)** (Fig. 12.29D) is useful to demonstrate extraocular extension and may be of some help in differential diagnosis.
- **Biopsy** is useful when the diagnosis cannot be established by less invasive methods. It may be performed either with a fine needle or using the 25-gauge vitrectomy system, the latter providing a larger sample.
- **Genetic tumour analysis** is becoming increasingly important in management, particularly with regard to prognosis; metastasis occurs almost exclusively with certain genetic profiles.
- **Systemic investigation** is directed principally towards detecting metastatic spread, though it may also be used to search for a primary tumour elsewhere if choroidal metastasis is likely. Liver function testing and ultrasonography are mainstays. Chest radiography rarely shows lung secondaries in the absence of liver disease. The comparative value of whole body PET/CT imaging is not fully defined; it has greater sensitivity for detecting metastatic disease, particularly extrahepatic lesions, but involves a substantial ionizing radiation dose.

Treatment

Treatment is performed to avoid the development of a painful and unsightly eye whilst conserving as much useful vision as possible. The extent to which ocular treatment influences survival is not yet defined, though there is some evidence that in general the risk of metastasis is lower with smaller earlier tumours. Management is individualized based on the characteristics of the particular

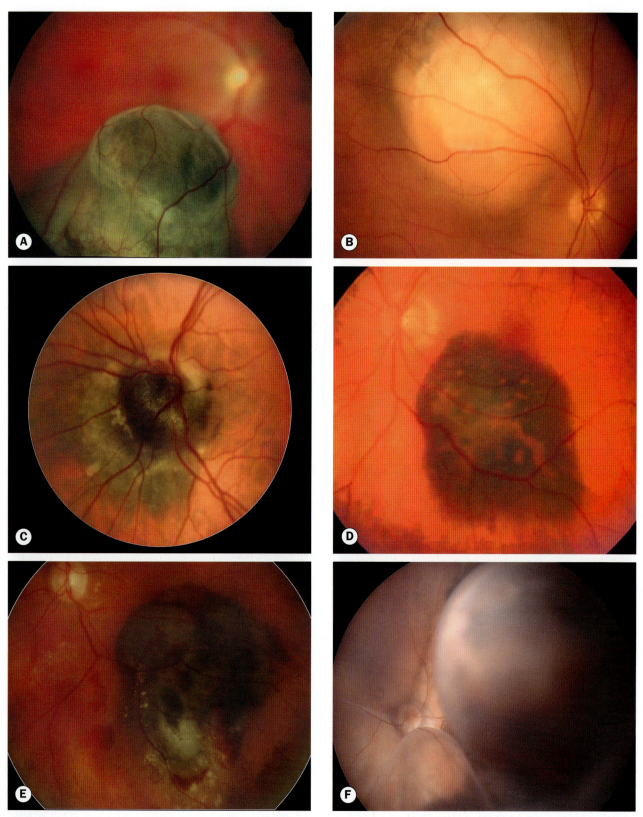

Fig. 12.27 Choroidal melanoma. **(A)** Typical pigmented melanoma; **(B)** amelanotic lesion; **(C)** melanoma of the optic disc; **(D)** overlying orange pigment; **(E)** associated haemorrhage and exudation; **(F)** extensive subretinal fluid with bullous detachment

(Courtesy of C Barry – figs A, C and E; B Damato – figs D and F)

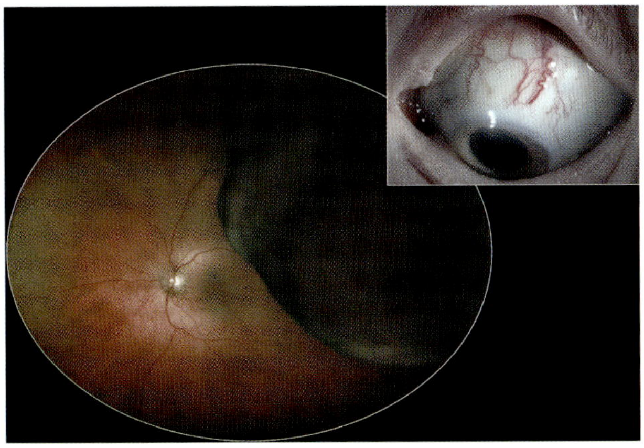

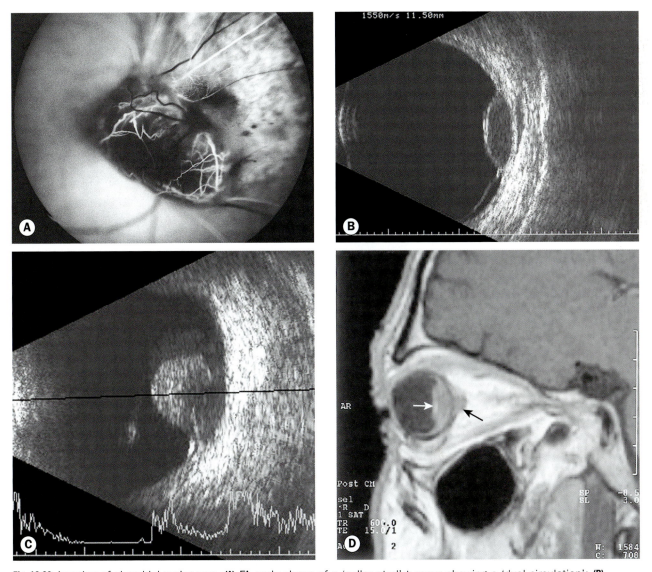

Fig. 12.28 Choroidal melanoma with overlying sentinel vessels

(Courtesy of C Barry)

tumour and the patient (e.g. general health, age, preferences, state of fellow eye).

- **Brachytherapy** (episcleral plaque radiotherapy) may be used for tumours less than 20 mm in basal diameter and up to 10 mm thick in which there is a reasonable chance of salvaging vision. Survival is similar to that following enucleation. A plaque is sutured to the sclera (Fig. 12.30A) for several days according to dosage requirement; regression begins about 1–2 months after treatment and continues over several years, leaving a flat or dome-shaped pigmented scar (Figs 12.30B and C). Complications include cataract, papillopathy (with or without disc neovascularization) and radiation retinopathy. Release of cytokines by the irradiated tumour can also cause retinopathy and other complications ('toxic tumour syndrome') that may need to be treated

Fig. 12.29 Imaging of choroidal melanoma. **(A)** FA early phase of a 'collar stud' tumour showing a 'dual circulation'; **(B)** B-scan of a dome-shaped tumour shows choroidal excavation; **(C)** B-scan of a 'collar stud' tumour; **(D)** T1-weighted MRI shows a choroidal melanoma (white arrow) and extraocular extension (black arrow)

(Courtesy of B Damato – figs A and B; S Milewski – fig. C; M Karolczak-Kulesza – fig. D)

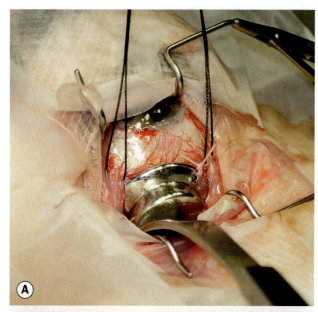

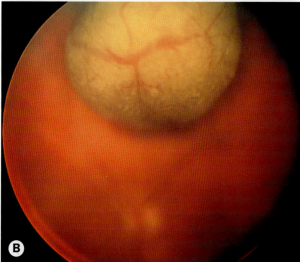

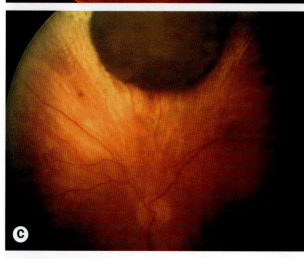

Fig. 12.30 Brachytherapy for choroidal melanoma.
(A) Placement of plaque; **(B)** amelanotic tumour prior to treatment; **(C)** smaller pigmented lesion following treatment

(Courtesy of S Chen – fig. A; C Barry – figs B and C)

specifically (e.g. endo/exoresection, intravitreal steroid/anti-VEGF).

- **External beam radiotherapy.** Fractionated irradiation with charged particles such as protons achieves a high dose in the tumour with relative sparing of adjacent tissues, and is used for tumours unsuitable for brachytherapy either because of large size or posterior location. Targeting is aided by suturing radio-opaque tantalum markers to the sclera. Regression is slower than with brachytherapy, but survival is comparable. Intraocular complications are similar, but extraocular complications such as loss of lashes, eyelid depigmentation and keratitis may be seen.

- **Stereotactic radiotherapy** uses multiple collimated beams from different directions, either concurrently or sequentially, so that only the tumour receives a high dose of radiation. It is relatively effective, though there may be a comparatively high complication rate.

- **Transpupillary thermotherapy (TTT)** uses an infrared laser beam to induce tumour cell death by hyperthermia rather than coagulation. Indications include the treatment of a small tumour when radiotherapy is inappropriate due to poor general health. It can be used as an adjunct to radiotherapy, particularly for vision-threatening exudation. Tumour response is gradual, the lesion first becoming darker and flatter, and eventually disappearing to leave bare sclera. Complications include retinal traction, retinal tear formation with rhegmatogenous detachment, vascular occlusion and neovascularization. Local recurrence is common, especially if the tumour is thick, amelanotic or involves the disc margin.

- **Trans-scleral choroidectomy.** This is a technically difficult procedure that may be used for carefully selected tumours that are too thick for radiotherapy but less than about 16 mm in diameter. Complications include retinal detachment, hypotony, wound dehiscence and local tumour recurrence.

- **Enucleation.** Indications include large tumour size, optic disc invasion, extensive involvement of the ciliary body or angle, irreversible loss of useful vision, and poor motivation to keep the eye. It is essential to perform ophthalmoscopy after surgical draping to ensure that the correct eye is removed. Manipulation of the eye should be kept to a minimum. Orbital recurrence is rare if there is no extraocular tumour spread or if any such extension is completely excised.

- **Systemic chemotherapy** has not been shown to be of benefit in cases where there is no evidence of metastatic spread.

Circumscribed choroidal haemangioma

Circumscribed choroidal haemangioma (CCH) consists of a mass of varying-sized vascular channels within the choroid (Fig. 12.31A). It is not associated with systemic disease. It may be dormant throughout life or may give rise to symptoms, usually in early adulthood, as a result of exudative retinal detachment. Slow enlargement can occur over many years.

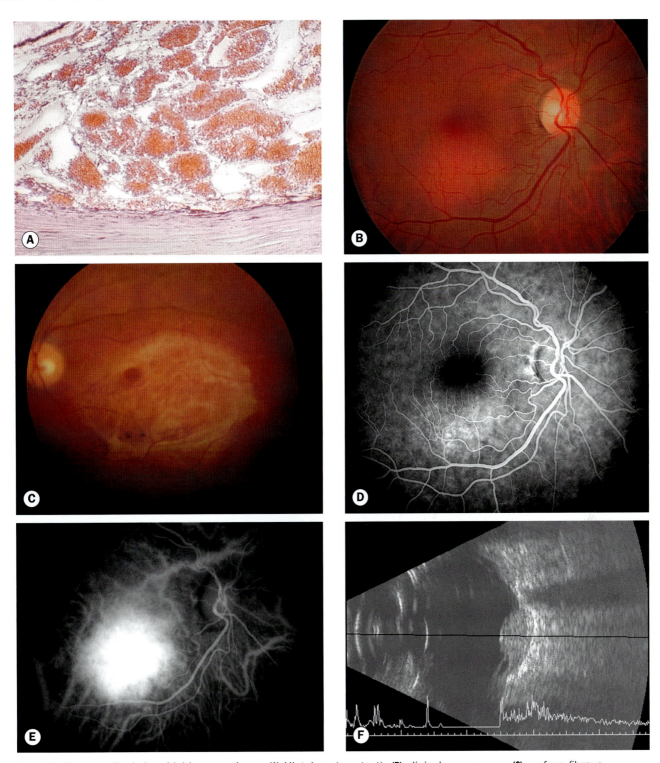

Fig. 12.31 Circumscribed choroidal haemangioma. **(A)** Histology (see text); **(B)** clinical appearance; **(C)** surface fibrous metaplasia; **(D)** FA early phase shows hyperfluorescence; **(E)** ICGA shows early hyperfluorescence; **(F)** B-scan shows an acoustically solid lesion with a sharp anterior surface and high internal reflectivity

(Courtesy of J Harry – fig. A; P Gili – figs B, D and E; B Damato – figs C and F)

Diagnosis

- **Signs**
  - An oval orange mass at the posterior pole with indistinct margins that blend with the surrounding choroid (Fig. 12.31B); median base diameter is 6 mm and median thickness 3 mm.
  - Subretinal fluid is usually present in symptomatic cases.
  - Complications include surface fibrous metaplasia (Fig. 12.31C), cystoid retinal degeneration, RPE degeneration and subretinal fibrosis.
- **OCT.** The overlying retina may be normal or show sub- and intraretinal fluid, retinoschisis and atrophy.
- **FA** reveals early spotty hyperfluorescence (Fig. 12.31D) and late diffuse but intense hyperfluorescence.
- **ICGA** provides useful diagnostic information, with strongly hyperfluorescent tumour vessels evident in the arterial phase (Fig. 12.31E), with diffuse hypofluorescence later.
- **FAF.** The lesion itself shows little or no intrinsic autofluorescence. Associated overlying orange pigment and (fresh) subretinal fluid show hyperautofluorescence, with RPE hyperplasia and atrophy giving hypoautofluorescence.
- **US** shows an acoustically solid lesion (high internal reflectivity) with a well-defined anterior surface (Fig. 12.31F).
- **MRI.** The tumour is iso- or hyperintense to the vitreous in T1-weighted images and isointense in T2-weighted images, with marked enhancement by gadolinium.

Treatment

The following may be used if vision is threatened. The superiority of any particular approach has not been established.

- **Photodynamic therapy (PDT)** using the same parameters as for choroidal neovascularization. Treatment may need to be repeated after a few months if subretinal fluid persists.
- **TTT** for lesions not involving the macula.
- **Photocoagulation** using a conventional thermal laser or micropulse treatment may be effective.
- **Radiotherapy** may be used for resistant lesions.
- **Intravitreal anti-VEGF therapy** typically reduces serous retinal detachment and can be used in combination with other modalities.
- **Oral propranolol** may be of benefit, particularly for associated exudative retinal detachment, but does not seem to consistently reduce tumour size.

Diffuse choroidal haemangioma

Diffuse choroidal haemangioma usually affects over half of the choroid and enlarges very slowly. It occurs almost exclusively in patients with Sturge–Weber syndrome ipsilateral to the naevus flammeus (see Ch. 1). The fundus has a diffuse deep red colour that is most marked at the posterior pole (Fig. 12.32A). Localized areas of thickening, simulating a circumscribed haemangioma, may be present within the larger lesion. B-scan ultrasonography shows diffuse choroidal thickening (Fig. 12.32B). Complications include secondary retinal cystoid degeneration and exudative

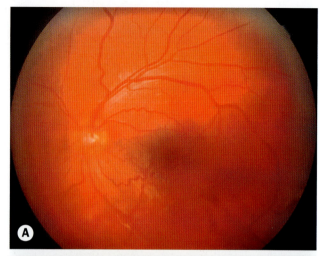

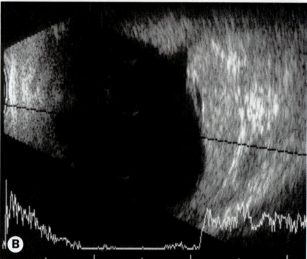

Fig. 12.32 (A) Diffuse choroidal haemangioma; **(B)** B-scan shows diffuse choroidal thickening
(Courtesy of B Damato – fig. B)

retinal detachment; neovascular glaucoma can ensue if exudative detachment is not treated. Treatment of vision-threatening cases involves PDT or low-dose radiotherapy.

Optic disc melanocytoma

Melanocytoma (magnocellular naevus) is a rare, distinctive, unilateral, heavily pigmented congenital hamartoma seen most frequently in the optic nerve head but that may arise anywhere in the uvea. Histology shows large deeply pigmented polyhedral or spindle cells with small nuclei. In contrast to choroidal melanoma, melanocytomas are relatively more common in dark-skinned individuals and have a female predominance. Most cases are asymptomatic, the condition being detected on routine ophthalmoscopy (mean age 50 years). The tumour is generally stationary, and treatment is not required except in the very rare event of malignant transformation. Other complications include spontaneous tumour necrosis, optic nerve compression and retinal vein obstruction.

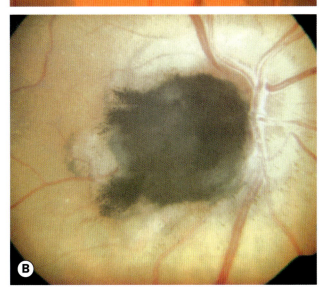

Fig. 12.33 Melanocytoma. **(A)** and **(B)** The same lesion at baseline and 11 years later

(Courtesy of S Chen)

Diagnosis

- A dark brown or black, flat or slightly elevated lesion with feathery edges that may extend over the edge of the disc (Figs 12.33A and B).
- Occasionally a large tumour occupies most of the disc surface and may lead to pigment dispersion into the vitreous.
- A relative afferent pupillary defect may be present, even if visual acuity (VA) is good.
- FA shows persistent dense hypofluorescence due to masking.

Choroidal osteoma

Choroidal osteoma is a rare benign ossifying tumour that has a strong female preponderance; patients are often young adults.

Both eyes are affected in about 10–20%. Histology shows mature cancellous bone, with overlying RPE atrophy. Presentation is in the second–third decades. Masquerading lesions include osseous metaplasia in association with a choroidal haemangioma, and sclerochoroidal calcification, the latter characterized by multiple geographical yellow–white fundus lesions that usually involve both eyes of an older adult.

Diagnosis

- **Symptoms.** Gradual visual impairment if the macula is involved by the tumour itself, or occasionally more rapid deterioration secondary to choroidal neovascularization.
- **Signs**
  - Initially orange, maturing lesions appear yellow–white; they are flat or minimally elevated with well-defined, scalloped margins near the disc or at the posterior pole (Figs 12.34A–D).
  - Spider-like fine vessels and bone-spicule RPE changes may develop (Fig. 12.34B).
  - Slow growth may occur over several years (Figs 12.34C and D).
  - Spontaneous resorption and decalcification may rarely occur.
  - The visual prognosis is poor if the lesion involves the fovea.
- **OCT** demonstrates overlying retinal changes, with enhanced depth imaging showing a lattice pattern in calcified tumour similar to the appearance of cancellous bone.
- **FA** manifests early, irregular, diffuse mottled hyperfluorescence and late staining (Fig. 12.35A).
- **FAF** shows mainly isoautofluorescence in calcified areas and hypoautofluorescence in decalcified regions.
- **ICGA** shows early hypofluorescence (Fig. 12.35B) and late staining. The tumour appears larger than on clinical examination.
- **US** shows a highly reflective anterior surface and orbital shadowing (Fig. 12.35C).
- **CT** demonstrates a dense plaque-like opacity at the level of the choroid (Fig. 12.35D).

Metastatic tumours

The choroid is by far the most common (90%) site for uveal metastases. The most frequent primary sites are the breast and bronchus. A choroidal secondary may be the initial presentation of a bronchial carcinoma, whereas a past history of breast cancer is the rule in patients with breast secondaries. Other less common primary sites include the gastrointestinal tract, kidney and skin (melanoma). The prostate is an extremely rare primary site. Survival is generally poor, with a median of 8–12 months.

Diagnosis

- **Symptoms.** Visual impairment may occur due to macular involvement by the lesion itself or associated exudative retinal detachment. A minority are discovered incidentally.

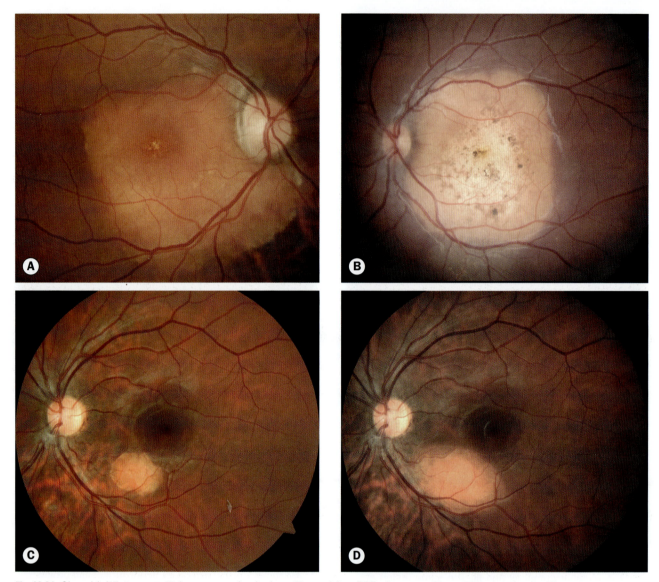

Fig. 12.34 Choroidal osteoma. **(A)** Large macular lesion; **(B)** overlying RPE changes; **(C)** and **(D)** growth over 5 years
(Courtesy of S Chen)

- **Signs**
  - The most common appearance is a fast-growing yellowish slightly elevated placoid lesion with indistinct margins, typically at the posterior pole and often multifocal and bilateral (10–30% – Figs 12.36A and B); overlying pigmentary changes are fairly common (Fig. 12.36C).
  - Melanoma secondaries are usually pigmented.
  - Secondary exudative retinal detachment is frequent and may occur in eyes with relatively small lesions.
- **US** may be useful in detection, particularly to demonstrate a lesion underlying exudative retinal detachment. A placoid tumour shows diffuse choroidal thickening; a larger dome-shaped lesion shows moderately high internal acoustic reflectivity (Fig. 12.36D).
- **OCT** shows overlying RPE thickening and photoreceptor irregularity, with subretinal fluid when present. Enhanced depth imaging OCT shows choriocapillaris thinning overlying the tumour.
- **FA** shows early hypofluorescence and diffuse late staining, but in contrast to choroidal melanoma a dual circulation is not seen.
- **ICGA** usually shows hypofluorescence through the study and may show additional deposits not evident on clinical examination or FA.
- **Biopsy** by fine needle aspiration or using a 25-gauge vitrectomy system may be appropriate when the primary site is unknown.
- **Systemic investigation** is directed at locating the primary tumour, if unknown, and other metastatic sites. The list below is not exhaustive.
  - Full history and physical examination.
  - Mammography.
  - Chest radiography and sputum cytology.

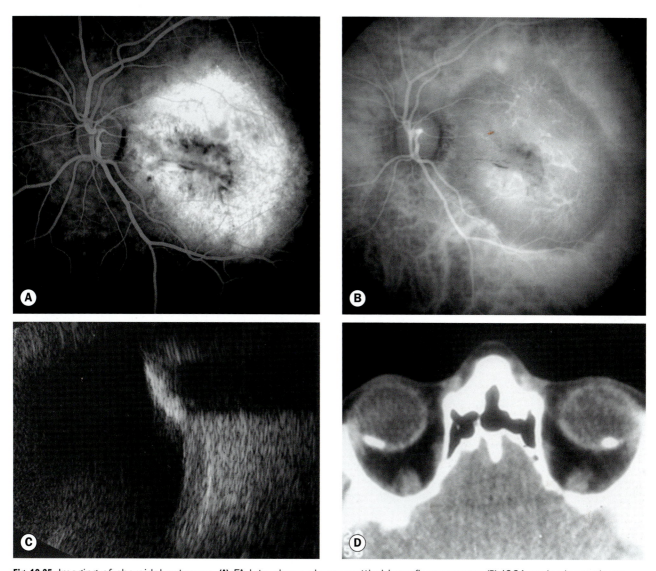

Fig. 12.35 Imaging of choroidal osteoma. **(A)** FA late phase shows mottled hyperfluorescence; **(B)** ICGA early phase shows hypofluorescence; **(C)** B-scan shows a highly reflective anterior surface and orbital shadowing; **(D)** axial CT demonstrates bilateral lesions with similar consistency to bone

(Courtesy P Gili – figs A and B)

○ Liver function tests.
○ Abdominal or whole body scans.
○ Faecal occult blood.
○ Urinalysis for red blood cells.
○ Abdominal ultrasound.
○ Whole-body imaging, e.g. PET/CT, MRI.

Treatment

- **Observation**, if the patient is asymptomatic or receiving systemic chemotherapy, which may also be beneficial for choroidal metastases.
- **Radiotherapy**, either external beam or brachytherapy, typically for solitary lesions.
- **TTT** is useful for small tumours with minimal subretinal fluid.

- **Anti-VEGF treatment** may lead to regression of metastases in some cases, as well as addressing secondary phenomena such as subretinal fluid accumulation. It is probably more effective in small early lesions.

NEURAL RETINAL TUMOURS

Retinoblastoma

Introduction

Retinoblastoma is rare, occurring in up to 1:18 000 live births, but is the most common primary intraocular malignancy of childhood and accounts for about 3% of all childhood cancers. After uveal

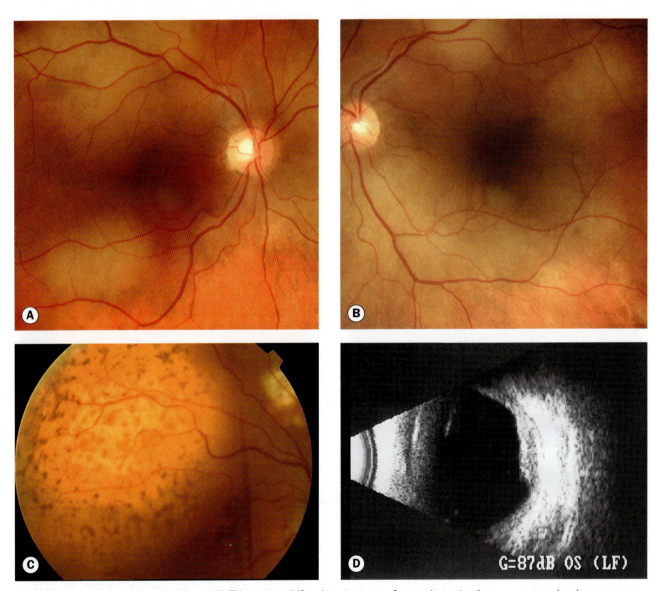

Fig. 12.36 Choroidal metastasis. **(A)** and **(B)** Bilateral multifocal metastases from a breast primary – regression in response to systemic chemotherapy is beginning in the left eye; **(C)** overlying pigmentary stippling; **(D)** B-scan showing moderate internal reflectivity

(Courtesy of C Barry – figs A and B; B Damato – fig. C)

melanoma, it is the second most common malignant intraocular tumour. Survival rates are over 95% in specialized centres, with preservation of vision in a majority of eyes, but are much lower in the developing world. Tumours are composed of small basophilic cells (retinoblasts) with large hyperchromatic nuclei and scanty cytoplasm. Many retinoblastomas are undifferentiated but varying degrees of differentiation are characterized by the formation of structures known as rosettes (Flexner–Wintersteiner, Homer–Wright and fleurettes – Fig. 12.37A). Growth (Fig. 12.37B) may be endophytic (into the vitreous) with seeding of tumour cells throughout the eye, or exophytic (into the subretinal space) leading to retinal detachment, or mixed, or the retina may be diffusely infiltrated. Optic nerve invasion (Fig. 12.37C) may occur, with spread of tumour along the subarachnoid space to the brain. Metastatic spread is to regional nodes, lung, brain and bone.

Genetics

The genetics of retinoblastoma are often highlighted as a paradigm illustrating the genetic basis of cancer. The tumour suppressor gene in which mutations predisposing to retinoblastoma occur is *RB1*; over 900 different mutations have been reported to date. The size of a gene deletion tends to correlate with aggressive retinoblastoma behaviour. Mutations in *RB1* or associated genes in a common pathway are also disrupted in many sporadic tumours. Modifier genes for retinoblastoma have also been identified and may constitute therapeutic targets.

- **Heritable** (hereditary, germline) retinoblastoma accounts for 40%. In heritable retinoblastoma one of the pair of alleles of *RB1* is mutated in all the cells in the body. When a further mutagenic event ('second hit' according to the 'two-hit'

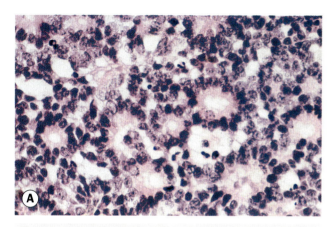

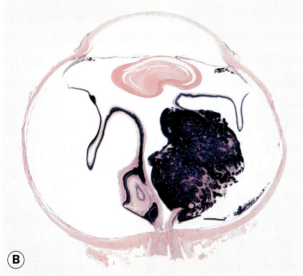

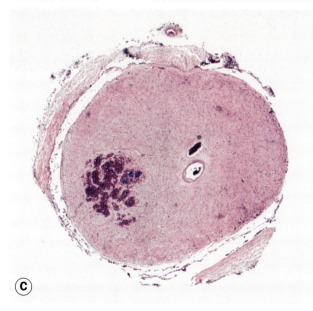

Fig. 12.37 Pathology of retinoblastoma. **(A)** well-differentiated tumour showing abundant Flexner–Wintersteiner rosettes; **(B)** whole eye section showing both endophytic and exophytic growth; **(C)** transverse section of the cut end of an optic nerve demonstrating an area of tumour infiltration
(Courtesy of J Harry)

hypothesis proposed by Knudson) affects the second allele, the cell may then undergo malignant transformation. Because of the presence of the mutation in all cells, a large majority of these children develop bilateral and multifocal tumours. Heritable retinoblastoma patients also have a predisposition to non-ocular cancers such as pinealoblastoma ('trilateral retinoblastoma', which occurs in up to 10%, usually before the age of 5), osteosarcomas, soft tissue sarcomas and melanomas; each of these tends to occur in a particular age group. The risk of a second malignancy is about 6% but this increases five-fold if external beam irradiation has been used to treat the original tumour, the second tumour tending to arise within the irradiated field.

- **Non-heritable** (non-hereditary, somatic) retinoblastoma. The tumour is unilateral, not transmissible and does not predispose the patient to second non-ocular cancers. If a patient has a solitary retinoblastoma and no positive family history, this is almost certainly (but not conclusively) non-heritable so that the risk in each sibling and the patient's offspring is about 1%. Ninety per cent of children with unilateral retinoblastoma will have the non-hereditary form.

- **Screening of at-risk family members.** Germline mutations are autosomal dominant and so transmitted to 50%, but because of incomplete penetrance only 40% of offspring will be affected. Detection of mutations in *RB1* has approached 95% in recent years. Once identified in a particular child, the same mutation can be sought in siblings, its presence confirming their high-risk status. Siblings at risk of retinoblastoma should be screened by prenatal ultrasonography, by ophthalmoscopy soon after birth and then regularly until the age of 4 or 5 years. Early diagnosis correlates with a higher chance of preserving vision, salvaging the eye and preserving life. If a child has heritable retinoblastoma, the risk to siblings is 2% if the parents are healthy, and 40% if a parent is affected. It is important that all family members, including the parents, are examined for the presence of retinoblastoma-associated eye lesions (retinomas, calcified retinal scars, phthisis).

Clinical features

- **Presentation** is within the first year of life in bilateral cases and around 2 years of age if the tumour is unilateral. Careful enquiry about a family history of ocular tumours is critical.
  - Leukocoria (white pupillary reflex) is the commonest presentation (60%) and may first be noticed in family photographs (Fig. 12.38A).
  - Strabismus is the second most common (20%); fundus examination is therefore mandatory in all cases of childhood squint.
  - Painful red eye with secondary glaucoma, which may occasionally be associated with buphthalmos (Fig. 12.38B).
  - Poor vision.
  - Inflammation or pseudoinflammation (Figs 12.38C and D).

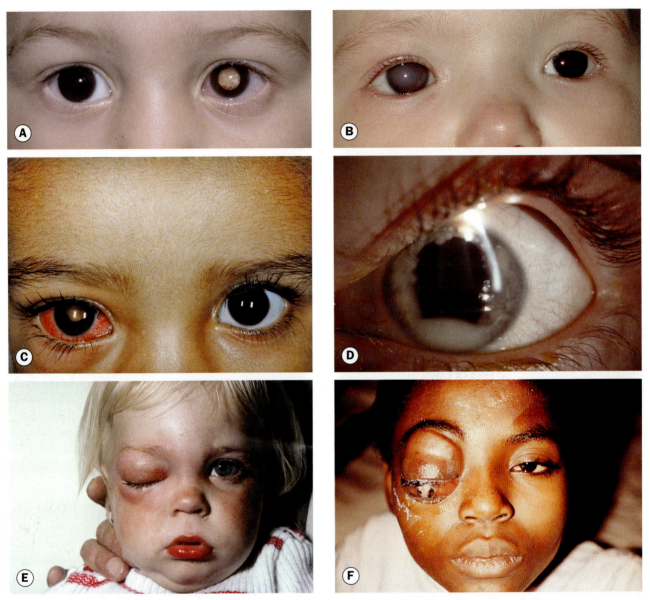

Fig. 12.38 Presentation of retinoblastoma. **(A)** Leukocoria; **(B)** secondary glaucoma and buphthalmos; **(C)** red eye due to uveitis; **(D)** iris nodules and pseudohypopyon; **(E)** orbital inflammation; **(F)** orbital invasion
(Courtesy of C Barry – fig. A; N Rogers – fig. B; U Raina – fig. C)

○ Routine examination of a patient known to be at risk.
○ Orbital inflammation mimicking orbital or preseptal cellulitis may occur with necrotic tumours (Fig. 12.38E).
○ Orbital invasion or visible extraocular growth may occur in neglected cases (Fig. 12.38F).
○ Metastatic disease involving regional lymph nodes and brain before the detection of ocular involvement is rare.
• **Signs**
○ An intraretinal tumour is a homogeneous, dome-shaped white lesion (Fig. 12.39A) that becomes irregular, often with white flecks of calcification.
○ An endophytic tumour projects into the vitreous as a white mass that may 'seed' into the gel (Figs 12.39B).

○ An exophytic tumour forms multilobular subretinal white masses and causes overlying retinal detachment (Figs 12.39C and D).

Investigation

• **Red reflex testing** with a direct ophthalmoscope is a simple screening test for leukocoria that is easily employed in the community.
• **Examination under anaesthesia** includes the following:
○ General examination for congenital abnormalities of the face and hands.
○ Tonometry.
○ Measurement of the corneal diameter.

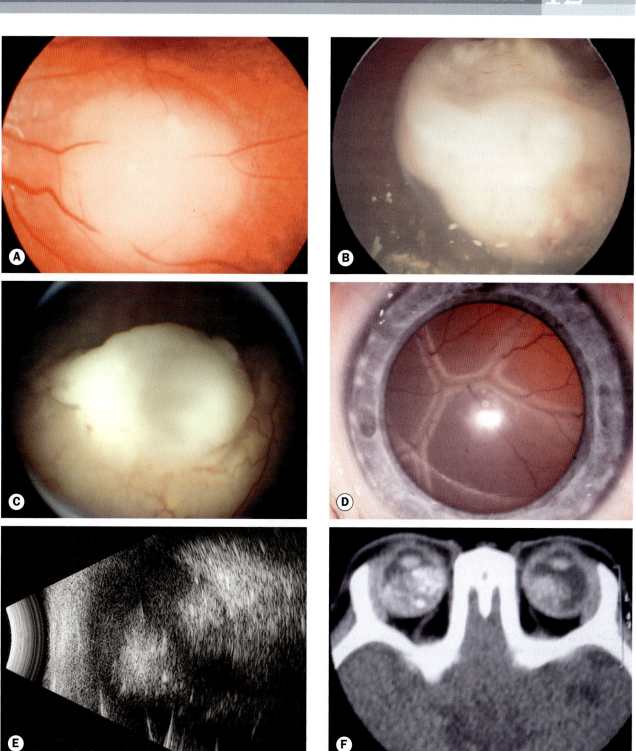

Fig. 12.39 Retinoblastoma. **(A)** Intraretinal tumour; **(B)** endophytic tumour with vitreous seeding; **(C)** mixed endophytic and exophytic growth; **(D)** total retinal detachment; **(E)** B-scan shows echoes from calcification; **(F)** axial CT shows bilateral tumours with calcification

(Courtesy of B Dixon-Romanowska – fig. B; L MacKeen – fig. C; K Nischal – fig. F)

○ Anterior chamber examination with a hand-held slit lamp.
○ Ophthalmoscopy, documenting all findings with colour drawings or photography.
○ Cycloplegic refraction.

- **US** is used mainly to assess tumour size. It also detects calcification (Fig. 12.39E) within the tumour and is helpful in the exclusion of simulating lesions such as Coats disease.
- **Wide-field photography** (portable if necessary) is useful for both surveying and documentation, and offers particular advantages in the management of retinoblastoma.
- **CT** also detects calcification (Fig. 12.39F) but entails a significant dose of radiation so is avoided by many practitioners. Plain X-rays may be used to detect calcification in resource-poor regions.
- **MRI** does not detect calcification but is useful for optic nerve evaluation, detection of extraocular extension and pinealoblastoma, and to aid differentiation from simulating conditions.
- **Systemic assessment** includes physical examination and MRI scans of the orbit and skull as a minimum in high-risk cases. If these indicate the presence of metastatic disease then bone scans, bone marrow aspiration and lumbar puncture are also performed.
- **Genetic studies** on tumour tissue and blood samples from the patient and relatives.

Treatment

The approach to management is collaborative between the ophthalmologist, paediatric oncologist, ocular pathologist, geneticist, allied health professionals and parents. Treatment is highly individualized.

- **Chemotherapy** is a mainstay of treatment in most cases, and may be used in conjunction with local treatments (focal consolidation – see below). Intravenous carboplatin, etoposide and vincristine (CEV) are given in three to six cycles according to the grade of retinoblastoma. Single- (carboplatin alone) or dual-agent therapy has also given favourable results in some circumstances, such as bridging therapy to allow deferral of more aggressive measures. Selective ophthalmic artery infusion has shown promising outcomes and study is ongoing. Intravitreal melphalan seems to be effective for vitreous seeding, though carries a very small risk of extraocular dissemination. Sub-Tenon carboplatin injection is now less commonly used given the availability of effective alternatives. Chemoreduction may be followed by focal treatment with cryotherapy or TTT to consolidate tumour control.
- **TTT** achieves focal consolidation following chemotherapy, or is sometimes used as an isolated treatment. Focal techniques such as TTT and cryotherapy exert both a direct effect and probably increase susceptibility to the effects of chemotherapy.

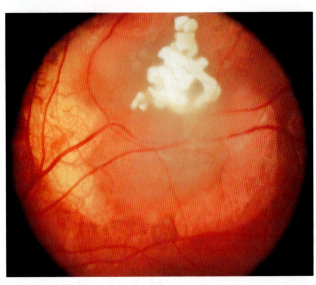

Fig. 12.40 Retinoblastoma – regression after brachytherapy

- **Cryotherapy** using a triple freeze–thaw technique is useful for pre-equatorial tumours without either deep invasion or vitreous seeding.
- **Brachytherapy** using a radioactive plaque can be utilized for an anterior tumour if there is no vitreous seeding, and in other circumstances such as resistance to chemotherapy (Fig. 12.40).
- **External beam radiotherapy** is avoided if possible, particularly in patients with heritable retinoblastoma because of the risk of inducing a second malignancy; retinoblastoma is highly radiation-sensitive, however. Adverse effects include cataract, radiation neuropathy, radiation retinopathy and hypoplasia of the bony orbit.
- **Enucleation** is generally indicated if there is neovascular glaucoma, anterior chamber infiltration, optic nerve invasion or if a tumour occupies more than half the vitreous volume. It is also considered if chemoreduction fails and is useful for diffuse retinoblastoma because of a poor visual prognosis and a high risk of recurrence with other modalities. Enucleation should be performed with minimal manipulation and it is imperative to excise a section of optic nerve to at least 10 mm.
- **Extraocular extension**
  ○ Adjuvant chemotherapy consisting of a 6-month course of CEV is given subsequent to enucleation at some centres if there is retrolaminar or massive choroidal spread.
  ○ External beam radiotherapy is indicated when there is tumour extension to the cut end of the optic nerve at enucleation, or extension through the sclera.
- **Review.** Careful review at frequent intervals is generally required following treatment, in order to detect recurrence or the development of a new tumour, particularly in heritable disease.

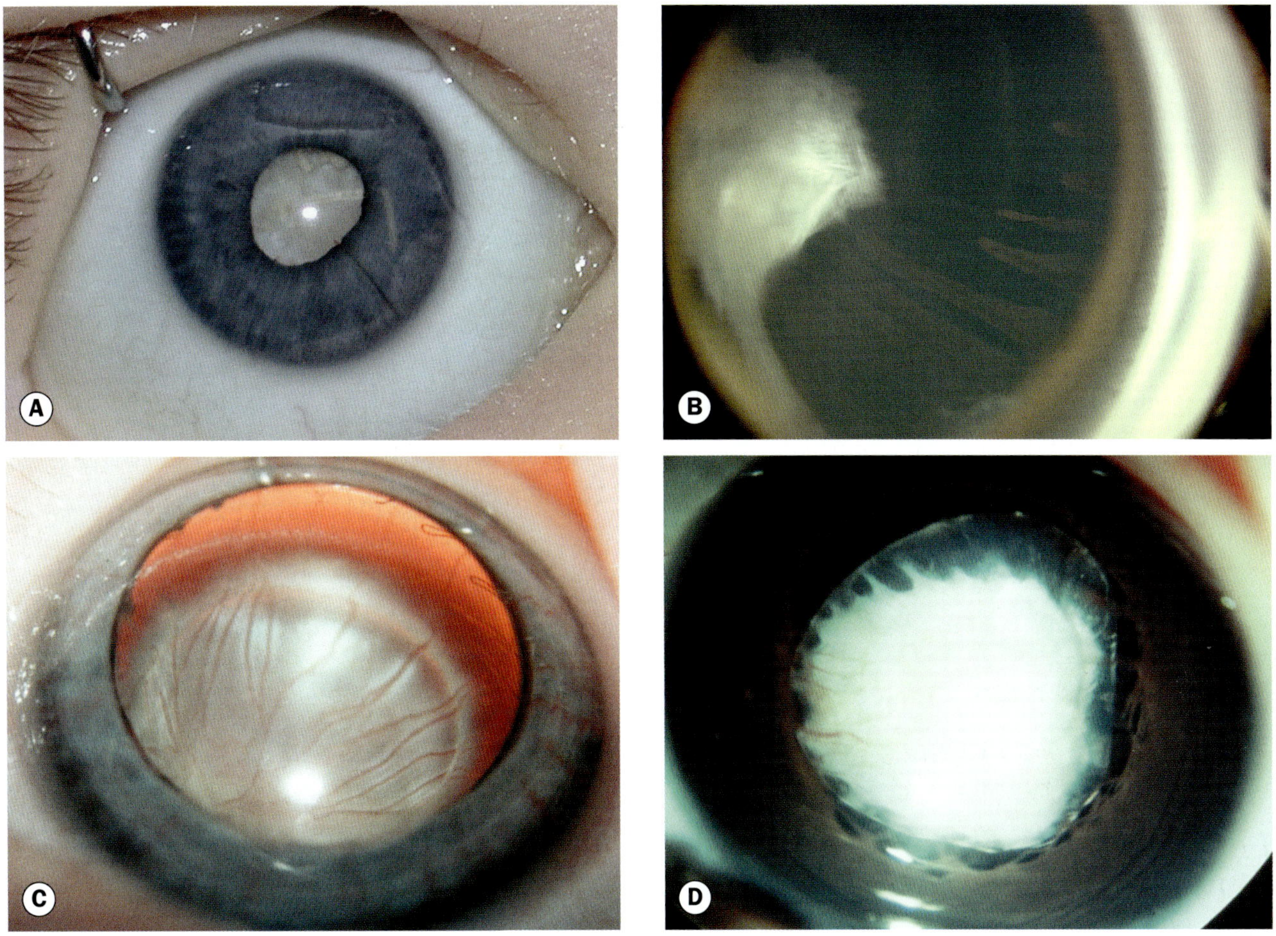

Fig. 12.41 Persistent anterior fetal vasculature. **(A)** Leukocoria with secondary cataract; **(B)** retrolental mass with elongated ciliary processes; **(C)** retrolental vessels and less dense fibrosis; **(D)** dense plaque with secondary lens changes
(Courtesy of S Chen – fig. A; Hospital for Sick Children, Toronto – fig. B; K Nischal – figs C and D)

Differential diagnosis

- **Persistent anterior fetal vasculature** (persistent hyperplastic primary vitreous – see also Ch. 17) is confined to the anterior segment and often involves the lens.
  - Presentation is with leukocoria (Fig. 12.41A) involving a retrolental mass into which elongated ciliary processes are inserted (Fig. 12.41B).
  - The size and density of the retrolental fibrovascular tissue is variable (Fig. 12.41C).
  - Complications include cataract (Fig. 12.41D) and angle-closure glaucoma.
  - Early lens and vitreoretinal surgery may preserve useful vision in some cases.
- **Persistent posterior fetal vasculature** is confined to the posterior segment and the lens is usually clear.
  - Presentation is with leukocoria, strabismus or nystagmus.
  - A dense fold of condensed vitreous and retina extends from the optic disc to the ora serrata (Fig. 12.42).
  - Treatment is not effective.
- **Coats disease** is almost always unilateral, more common in boys and tends to present later than retinoblastoma (see Ch. 13).

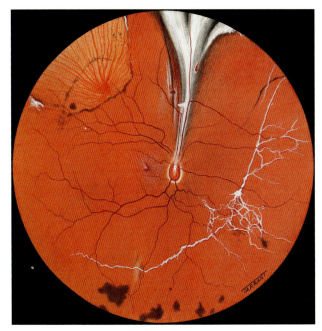

Fig. 12.42 Persistent posterior fetal vasculature

- **Retinopathy of prematurity**, if advanced, may cause retinal detachment and leukocoria. Diagnosis is usually straightforward because of the history of prematurity and low birth weight (see Ch. 13).
- **Toxocariasis**. Chronic *Toxocara* endophthalmitis (see Ch. 11) may cause a cyclitic membrane and a white pupil. A granuloma at the posterior pole may resemble an endophytic retinoblastoma.
- **Uveitis** may mimic the diffuse infiltrating type of retinoblastoma seen in older children. Conversely, retinoblastoma may be mistaken for uveitis, endophthalmitis or orbital cellulitis.
- **Vitreoretinal dysplasia** is caused by faulty differentiation of the retina and vitreous that results in a detached dysplastic retina forming a retrolental mass with leukocoria (Fig. 12.43). Other features include microphthalmos, shallow

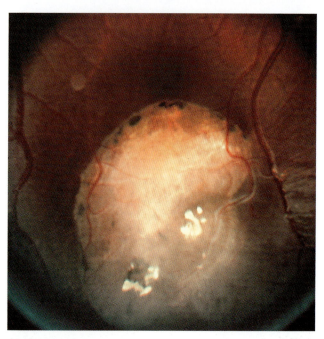

Fig. 12.44 Retinoma

anterior chamber and elongated ciliary processes. Dysplasia may occur in isolation or in association with systemic abnormalities:
  - Norrie disease is an X-linked recessive disorder in which affected males are blind at birth or early infancy. It is caused by mutations in the *NDP* gene. Systemic features include cochlear deafness and mental retardation.
  - Incontinentia pigmenti is an X-linked dominant condition that is lethal *in utero* for boys. Mutations have been found in the *NEMO* gene. It is characterized by a vesiculobullous rash on the trunk and extremities that with time is replaced by linear pigmentation. Other features include malformation of teeth, hair, nails, bones and CNS.
  - Walker–Warburg syndrome is an autosomal recessive condition characterized by absence of cortical gyri and cerebellar malformations that may be associated with hydrocephalus and encephalocele. Neonatal death is common and survivors suffer severe developmental delay. Apart from vitreoretinal dysplasia other ocular features include Peters anomaly, cataract, uveal coloboma, microphthalmos and optic nerve hypoplasia.
- **Other tumours**
  - Retinoma (retinocytoma) is a variant of retinoblastoma that generally exhibits benign behaviour but has a genetic profile indicating premalignancy – rarely, a retinoma can undergo late transformation into a rapidly growing retinoblastoma. It manifests as a smooth whitish dome-shaped lesion, which typically involutes spontaneously to a calcified mass associated with RPE alteration and chorioretinal atrophy (Fig. 12.44).
  - Retinal astrocytoma, which may be multifocal and bilateral (see below).

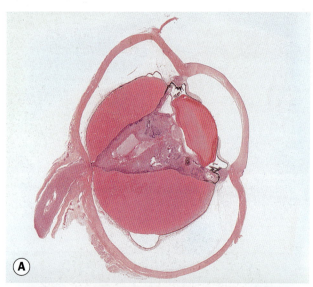

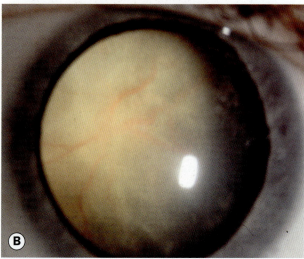

Fig. 12.43 Vitreoretinal dysplasia. **(A)** Pathological specimen; **(B)** clinical appearance

(Courtesy of J Harry and G Misson, from Clinical Ophthalmic Pathology, *Butterworth-Heinemann 2001 – fig. A)*

Retinal astrocytoma

Introduction

Astrocytoma (astrocytic hamartoma) of the retina and optic nerve head is rare; it frequently does not threaten vision or require treatment. Most are endophytic, protruding into the vitreous, but exophytic subretinal tumours can occur. Astrocytomas may be encountered as incidental solitary lesions in normal individuals but are most frequently seen in tuberous sclerosis (see below) and occasionally in association with neurofibromatosis type 1 and retinitis pigmentosa. About 50% of patients with tuberous sclerosis have one or more astrocytomas, which may be bilateral.

Diagnosis

- **Symptoms.** Most tumours are asymptomatic and detected on screening for tuberous sclerosis; isolated lesions unassociated with known systemic disease are usually found at a routine eye examination.
- **Signs.** A yellowish or white semitransparent plaque, nodule or mulberry-like lesion, often semitransparent in its periphery and calcified centrally (Fig. 12.45A).
- **Lesions can be large** (Fig. 12.45B) and/or have a cystic component (Fig. 12.45C); growth with vision-threatening complications can occur.
- **OCT** shows a granular hyper-reflective appearance of the retinal layers with relative sparing of underlying RPE.

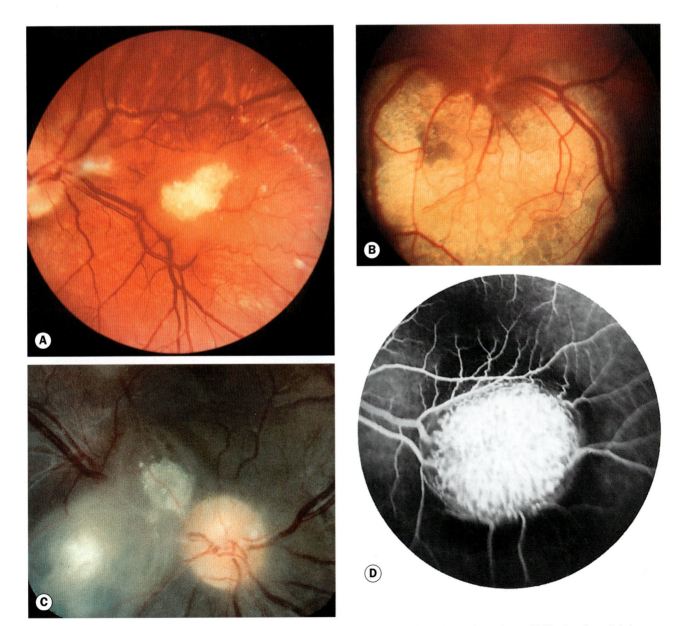

Fig. 12.45 Astrocytoma. **(A)** Yellowish mulberry-like lesion; **(B)** large diffuse lesion; **(C)** cystic variant; **(D)** FA showing staining
(*J Donald M Gass, from* Stereoscopic Atlas of Macular Diseases, *Mosby 1997 – fig. D*)

- **FAF** findings depend on the individual lesion's characteristics; typically hyperautofluorescence is seen in calcified areas with hypoautofluorescence elsewhere.
- **FA** shows a prominent superficial vascular network within the tumour in the arterial phase followed by late leakage and staining (Fig. 12.45D).
- **Systemic assessment.** With an isolated astrocytoma discovered incidentally in an older patient, the likelihood of the presence of forme fruste tuberous sclerosis is low. However, the option of genetic testing and systemic investigation may be offered.

Tuberous sclerosis

Tuberous sclerosis (Bourneville disease) is an autosomal dominant phacomatosis characterized by the development of hamartomas in multiple organ systems from all primary germ layers. The classic triad of epilepsy, mental retardation and adenoma sebaceum is present in only a minority of patients, but is diagnostic. About 60% of cases are sporadic and 40% are autosomal dominant.

- **Cutaneous signs**
  - Adenoma sebaceum, consisting of fibroangiomatous red papules with a butterfly distribution around the nose and cheeks (Fig. 12.46A), is universal.
  - Ash leaf spots are hypopigmented macules on the trunk, limbs and scalp (Fig. 12.46B). In infants with sparse skin pigmentation they are best detected using ultraviolet light, under which they fluoresce (Wood lamp).
  - Shagreen patches consist of diffuse thickening over the lumbar region.
  - Subungual hamartomas (Fig. 12.46C).
  - Skin tags (molluscum fibrosa pendulum).
  - Café-au-lait spots.
- **Neurological features**
  - Intracranial paraventricular subependymal astrocytic nodules and giant cell astrocytic hamartomas.
  - Learning difficulties.
  - Seizures.
- **Visceral tumours**
  - Renal angiomyolipomas and cysts.
  - Cardiac rhabdomyomas.
  - Pulmonary lymphangiomatosis.
- **Ocular features** apart from fundus astrocytomas include patchy iris hypopigmentation and atypical iris colobomas.

RETINAL VASCULAR TUMOURS

Capillary haemangioma

Introduction

Retinal capillary haemangioma is a rare sight-threatening tumour that may occasionally occur in isolation, although about 50% of patients with solitary lesions and virtually all patients with multiple lesions have von Hippel–Lindau disease (VHL – see below).

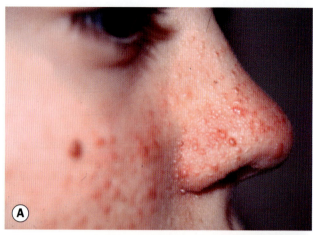
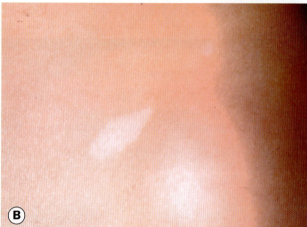
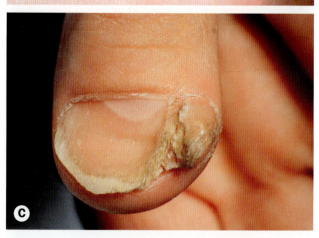

Fig. 12.46 Tuberous sclerosis. **(A)** Adenoma sebaceum; **(B)** ash leaf spot; **(C)** subungual hamartoma
(Courtesy of K Nischal – fig. A; MA Mir, from Atlas of Clinical Diagnosis, Mosby 2003 – fig. B)

The prevalence of retinal tumours in VHL is approximately 60%. Vascular endothelial growth factor (VEGF) is important in the development of retinal lesions, which are composed of capillary-like vascular channels between large foamy cells. The median age at haemangioma diagnosis in patients with VHL is earlier (18 years) than in those without VHL (31 years).

Diagnosis

- **Symptoms.** Tumours may be detected by screening of those at risk or because of symptoms due to macular exudates or retinal detachment.
- **Signs**
  - Early tumours appear as small red oval or round lesions located between an arteriole and venule (Fig. 12.47A).
  - A well-established tumour is seen as a round orange-red mass, usually located in the superior or inferior temporal periphery with dilatation and tortuosity of the supplying artery and draining vein extending from the optic disc (Fig. 12.47B).

- A juxtapapillary site is common (Figs 12.47C and D); lesions are often on the temporal side of the disc, so that leakage can rapidly threaten the fovea.
- **Complications**
  - Leakage with exudate formation and/or haemorrhage.
  - Fibrotic bands, which can progress to tractional or rhegmatogenous retinal detachment.
  - Vitreous haemorrhage, secondary glaucoma and phthisis bulbi.
- **FA** shows early hyperfluorescence and late leakage (Figs 12.48A and B).

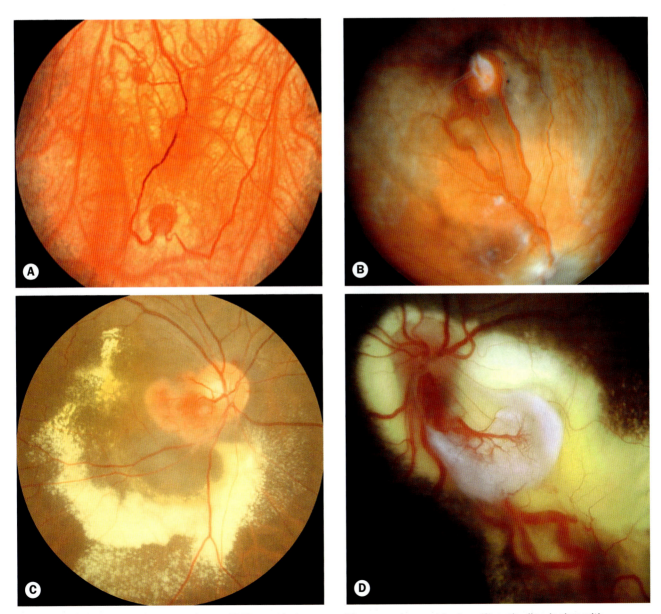

Fig. 12.47 Retinal capillary haemangioma. **(A)** Two early tumours; **(B)** more advanced lesion; **(C)** optic disc lesion with associated macular exudation; **(D)** very large optic disc lesion in von Hippel–Lindau syndrome
(Courtesy of B Damato – fig. B; C Barry – fig. C; S Chen – fig. D)

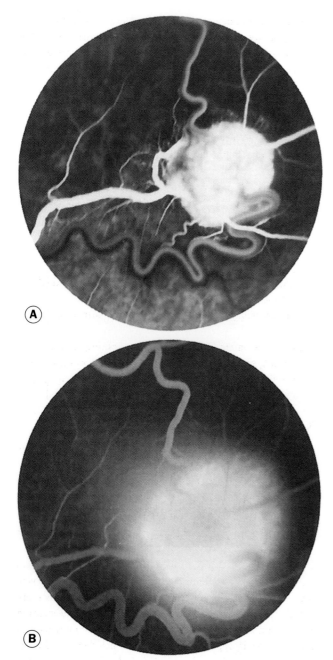

Fig. 12.48 FA of retinal capillary haemangioma. **(A)** Early filling; **(B)** late leakage

(Courtesy of J Donald M Gass, from Stereoscopic Atlas of Macular Diseases, *Mosby 1997)*

Treatment

- **Observation** is advised for asymptomatic juxtapapillary haemangiomas without exudation, because these may remain inactive for many years and because of the high risk of iatrogenic visual loss. Early peripheral lesions are not usually left untreated because they are relatively easy to ablate.
- **Laser photocoagulation** of small lesions. After closing the feeder vessels, the tumour is treated with low-energy, long duration burns. Multiple sessions may be needed.

- **Cryotherapy** for larger peripheral lesions, especially those with exudative retinal detachment. Vigorous treatment of a large lesion may cause extensive but usually temporary exudative retinal detachment.
- **Brachytherapy** for lesions too large for cryotherapy.
- **Vitreoretinal surgery** may be required for non-absorbing vitreous haemorrhage, epiretinal fibrosis or tractional retinal detachment. If appropriate, the tumour may be destroyed by endolaser photocoagulation or surgical removal.
- **Other modalities** include photodynamic therapy (PDT), which avoids damage to adjacent tissues, and anti-VEGF agents. These may be particularly appropriate for juxtapapillary tumours, which are otherwise virtually untreatable without visual loss.

Von Hippel–Lindau disease

Inherited VHL is autosomal dominant; about 20% are sporadic. It is caused by a mutation in the *VHL* tumour suppressor gene on chromosome 3.

- **Clinical features**
  - CNS haemangioma involving the cerebellum (Fig. 12.49A), spinal cord, medulla or pons affects about 25% of patients with retinal tumours.
  - Phaeochromocytoma.
  - Renal carcinoma (Fig. 12.49B) and pancreatic islet cell carcinoma.
  - Cysts of the testes, kidneys, ovaries, lungs, liver and pancreas.
  - Polycythaemia, which may be the result of factors released by a cerebellar or renal tumour.
  - Endolymphatic sac tumours develop in the inner ear in 10%, with consequent hearing and balance difficulties.
- **Screening** is vital; it is impossible to predict which patients with retinal haemangiomas will harbour systemic lesions. Relatives should also be screened because of the dominant inheritance pattern of the disease. The following screening protocol should be regularly performed in patients with established VHL and relatives at risk.
  - Annual physical examination, retinal examination from age 2 to 5 years (6-monthly from ages 10 to 30 years), renal ultrasonography from age 15 years, 24-hour urine collection for estimation of vanillyl mandelic acid and catecholamine levels from age 2 to 5 years to detect phaeochromocytoma.
  - Audiometry should be performed if there are any hearing or balance problems.
  - Two-yearly abdominal and brain MRI scans from the age of 15; if CNS lesions are symptom-free, treatment may not be required.
  - It is thought safe to discontinue screening at around age 60 years if no abnormality has been identified.
  - Genetic testing is indicated in all patients with suspected VHL and in first- and second-degree relatives. With modern techniques the likelihood of finding a mutation approaches 100%, and once a mutation has been

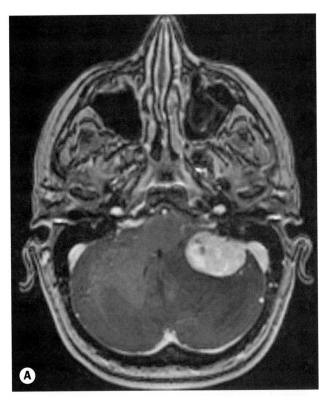

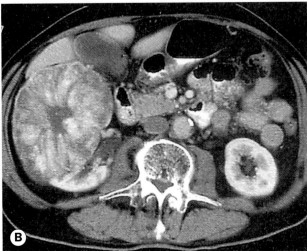

Fig. 12.49 Tumours in von Hippel–Lindau syndrome. **(A)** Axial MRI shows a cerebellar haemangioma; **(B)** axial CT of the abdomen shows a renal carcinoma

(Courtesy of CD Forbes and WF Jackson, from Atlas and Text of Clinical Medicine, *Mosby 2003 – fig. B)*

identified in the proband (initial subject) its presence can be confirmed or refuted in family members. Screening is unnecessary if the mutation is absent.

Cavernous haemangioma

Introduction

Cavernous haemangioma of the retina and optic nerve head is a rare unilateral congenital hamartoma. It is usually sporadic but occasionally can be inherited as autosomal dominant with incomplete penetrance in combination with lesions of the skin and CNS. Mutations in several different genes have been implicated. Histopathology shows multiple thin-walled dilated channels with surface gliosis.

Diagnosis

- **Symptoms** may occur secondary to vitreous haemorrhage. More frequently the lesions are detected by chance.
- **Signs**
  - Clusters of saccular aneurysms resembling a 'bunch of grapes' (Fig. 12.50A and B), with associated greyish fibrous tissue.
  - Because of sluggish flow of blood, the red cells may sediment and separate from plasma, giving rise to 'menisci' or fluid levels within the lesion.
  - A lesion occasionally involves the optic nerve head (Fig. 12.50C).
  - Haemorrhage and epiretinal membrane formation can occur.
- **OCT** demonstrates the aneurysmal vessels (Fig. 12.50D).
- **FA** highlights the sedimentation of erythrocytes and shows delayed filling in the venous phase and lack of leakage (Fig. 12.50E).

Treatment

Rarely, vitrectomy may be necessary for non-absorbing vitreous haemorrhage but photocoagulation should be avoided as it may precipitate haemorrhage and enlargement of the tumour.

Congenital retinal arteriovenous communication (racemose haemangioma)

A congenital arteriovenous communication, the more severe forms of which are often termed racemose haemangioma, is a rare sporadic congenital malformation, with unilateral involvement in single or multiple sites of the same eye, most commonly temporally. Occasionally reported complications include haemorrhage, exudation and vascular occlusion, though the vision is commonly unaffected and the condition discovered at a routine examination. A visual field defect may be present. Some patients may harbour ipsilateral brain, facial bone and skin lesions (Wyburn-Mason syndrome), particularly those with more severe retinal changes.

- **Group 1** consists of an anastomosis with the interposition of an abnormal capillary or arteriolar plexus. A congenital retinal macrovessel is often present (Fig. 12.51A); this is an aberrant blood vessel, often larger than normal and usually a vein, located in the posterior pole; it may cross the fovea and horizontal raphe. Areas of capillary non-perfusion and foveal cysts may be seen. The anomaly is non-progressive and is usually associated with good vision.
- **Group 2.** Direct arteriovenous communication, without an intervening capillary bed. The intervening channels may be intermediate or large in size (Fig. 12.51B).

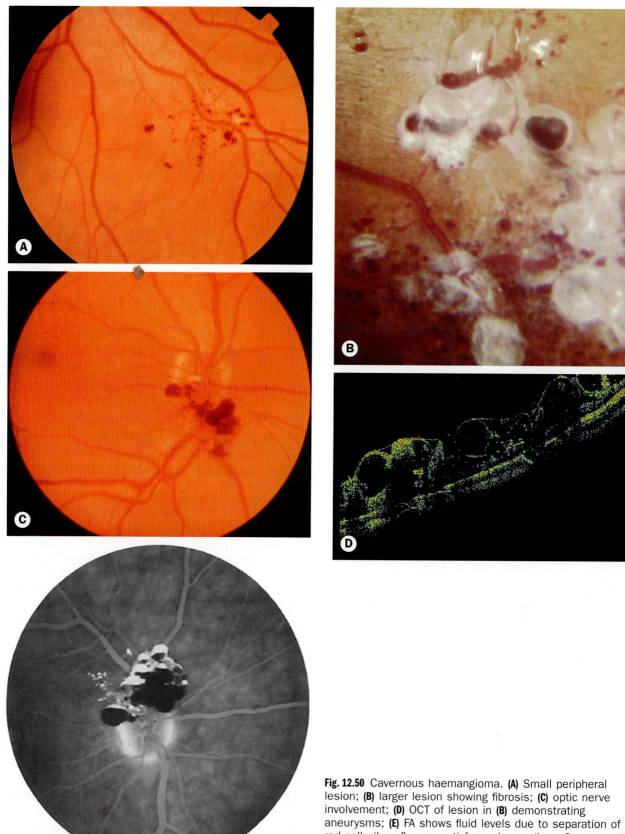

Fig. 12.50 Cavernous haemangioma. **(A)** Small peripheral lesion; **(B)** larger lesion showing fibrosis; **(C)** optic nerve involvement; **(D)** OCT of lesion in **(B)** demonstrating aneurysms; **(E)** FA shows fluid levels due to separation of red cells (hypofluorescent) from plasma (hyperfluorescent)

(Courtesy of S Chen – figs B and D; J Donald M Gass, from Stereoscopic Atlas of Macular Diseases, Mosby 1997 – fig. E)

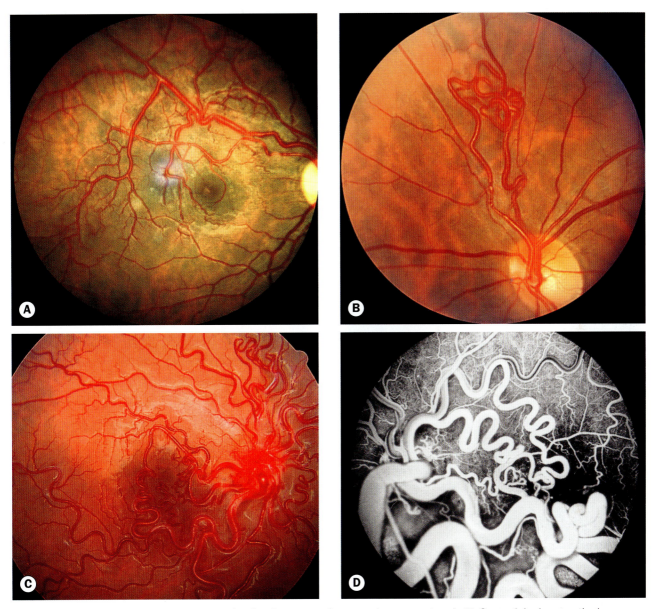

Fig. 12.51 Congenital arteriovenous communication (racemose haemangioma spectrum). **(A)** Group 1 lesion – retinal macrovessel; **(B)** group 2 – arteriovenous communication; **(C)** group 3 – typical racemose lesion with early sclerosis; **(D)** FA shows hyperfluorescence but absence of leakage

(Courtesy of C Barry – fig. B; J Donald M Gass, from Stereoscopic Atlas of Macular Diseases, *Mosby 1997 – fig. C)*

- **Group 3.** Many large-calibre tortuous anastomosing blood vessels that are often more numerous than normal, with venules and arterioles having a similar appearance. The changes extend from and are most evident in the region of the optic disc. With time the dilatation and tortuosity becomes more marked, and sclerosis may be seen (Fig. 12.51C); no leakage is seen on FA (Fig. 12.51D).

Vasoproliferative tumour

Retinal vasoproliferative tumour is a rare gliovascular lesion that can be primary (80%) or secondary to conditions such as intermediate uveitis, ocular trauma and retinitis pigmentosa. Secondary lesions may be multiple and occasionally bilateral depending on the underlying aetiology. Histology shows glial cells and a network of fine capillaries with some larger dilated vessels. Presentation is usually in the third–fifth decades, with blurring of vision due to macular exudation. A reddish-yellow globular vascular mass (Fig. 12.52A) is seen, most frequently in the inferotemporal periphery; retinal vessels may be seen entering the lesion posteriorly. Complications include subretinal exudation, exudative retinal detachment (Fig. 12.52B), macular oedema and fibrosis, and haemorrhage. Treatment with cryotherapy or brachytherapy induces regression of the tumour and exudation but the visual prognosis is guarded if there is maculopathy.

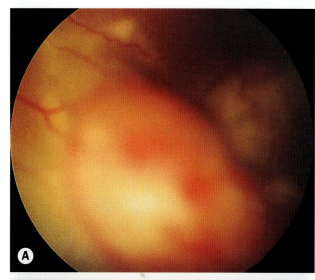

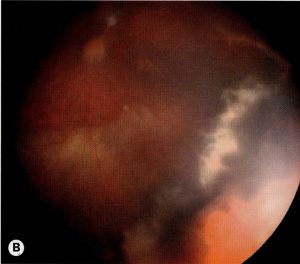

Fig. 12.52 Vasoproliferative tumour. **(A)** Globular vascular elevation; **(B)** lesion with associated retinal detachment *(Courtesy of B Damato)*

PRIMARY INTRAOCULAR LYMPHOMA

Introduction

Lymphoma is a group of conditions characterized by neoplastic proliferation of cells of the immune system typified by lymphadenopathy, constitutional symptoms and, occasionally, CNS involvement. The main classification and ocular manifestations are as follows:

- **Hodgkin disease** may cause anterior uveitis, vitritis and multifocal fundus lesions resembling chorioretinitis.
- **Non-Hodgkin lymphoma** can manifest with conjunctival involvement, orbital involvement, Mikulicz syndrome and uveal infiltration.
- **CNS B-cell lymphoma** may be associated with intermediate uveitis and sub-RPE infiltrates.

- **Primary vitreoretinal lymphoma (PVRL)** represents a subset of primary central nervous system lymphoma (PCNSL), a variant of extranodal non-Hodgkin lymphoma. The PCNSL cells are large, pleomorphic B lymphocytes with large multilobular nuclei, prominent nucleoli and scanty cytoplasm. The tumour arises from within the brain, spinal cord and leptomeninges, is aggressive and has a poor prognosis. About 20% of patients with PCNSL have ocular manifestations, which can precede or follow neurological involvement. Most patients with PVRL subsequently develop CNS symptoms, with a mean delay of 29 months. Most of those affected are older adults.
- **Primary uveal lymphoma** is a rare entity, usually of B-cell origin, that tends to follow an extended relatively benign course and will not be considered further in this section

Ocular features

- **Symptoms.** Unilateral floaters, blurred vision, red eye or photophobia. The symptoms frequently become bilateral after a variable interval.
- **Signs of PVRL**
  - Mild anterior uveitis with cells, flare and keratic precipitates.
  - Vitritis (Fig. 12.53A) may impede visualization of the fundus.
  - Large, often multifocal, subretinal infiltrates (Figs 12.53B–D).
  - Occasionally coalescence of sub-RPE deposits may completely encircle the fundus.
  - Other features include retinal vasculitis, vascular occlusion, exudative retinal detachment and optic atrophy.
  - Absence of cystoid macular oedema (CMO) is an important diagnostic indicator, since this is almost always present in true uveitic vitritis.

Neurological features

- **Symptoms.** An intracranial mass may cause headache, nausea, personality change, focal deficit or seizures; leptomeningeal disease may cause neuropathy, and spinal cord involvement may cause bilateral motor and sensory deficits.
- **Clinical neurological examination** may demonstrate abnormalities such as cranial nerve palsies, hemiparesis and ataxia.

Investigation

- **OCT** will confirm an absence of CMO in most cases, aiding differentiation from vitritis, and may demonstrate subretinal infiltrative lesions.
- **FA** shows blockage with a granular characteristic, due to the presence of sub-RPE accumulation of lymphomatous cells ('leopard skin spots').
- **US** may show vitreous debris, elevated subretinal lesions, retinal detachment and thickening of the optic nerve.

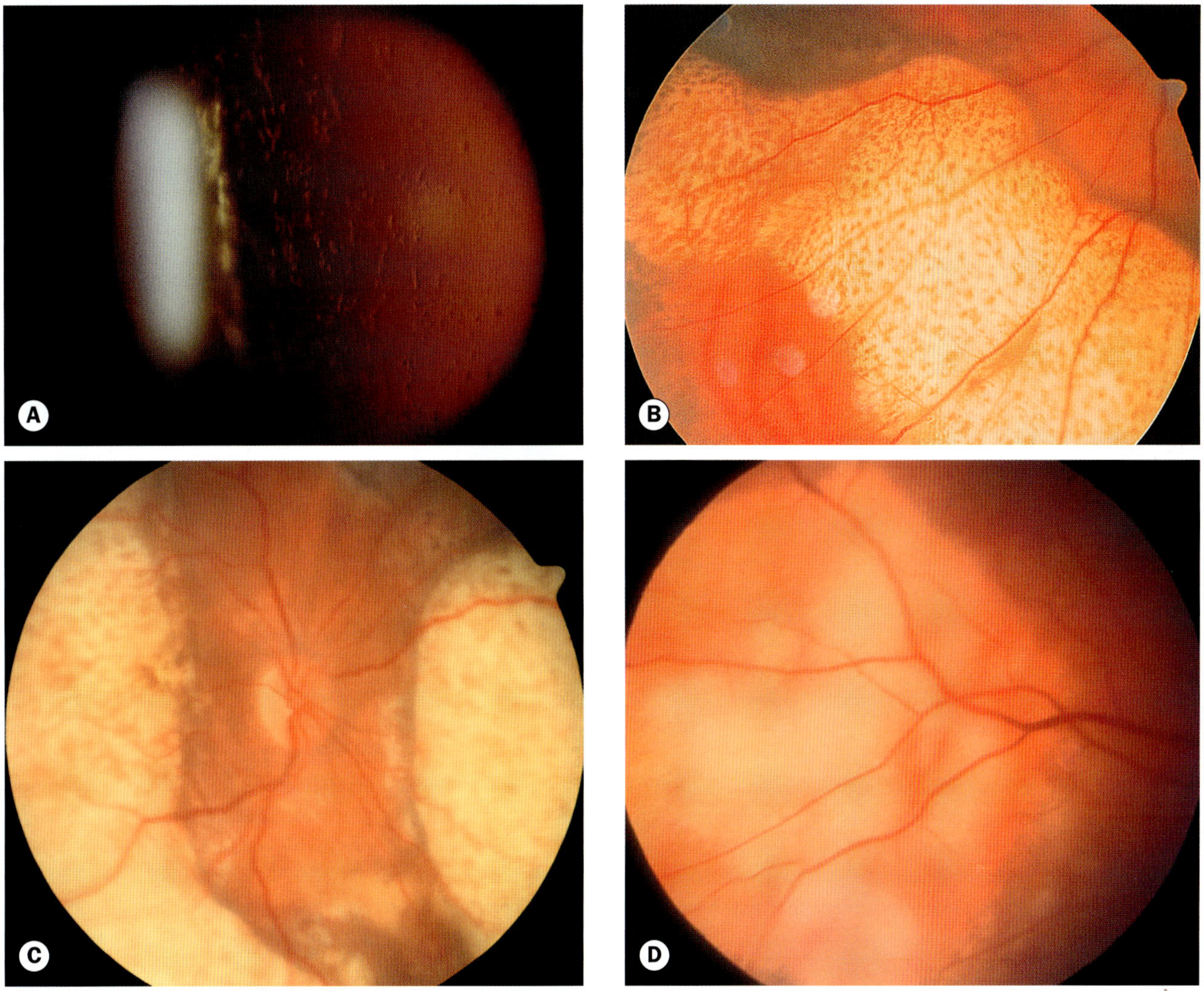

Fig. 12.53 Primary intraocular lymphoma. **(A)** Slit lamp photograph (retroillumination) showing vitreous cellular infiltrate; **(B)** and **(C)** extensive subretinal infiltration with overlying mottling; **(D)** multifocal subretinal infiltrates without mottling
(Courtesy of A Singh, H Lewis, A Schachat and D Peereboom, from Clinical Ophthalmic Oncology, *Saunders 2007 – fig. A; B Damato – fig. C)*

- **Cytology** of vitreous samples or subretinal nodules.
- **Immunohistochemistry** based on cell-surface markers allows identification of the lymphocytic proliferation, which is of a B-cell type in most patients.
- **MRI** of head and spine with gadolinium contrast may detect one or more intracranial tumours, diffuse meningeal or periventricular lesions, and/or localized intradural spinal masses; regular screening MRI scans of the CNS can be performed.
- **Lumbar puncture** may demonstrate malignant cells in the CSF in a minority of patients with abnormal MR imaging, but a positive result avoids the need for brain or eye biopsy.

Treatment

Treatment of both the eye and the brain is often indicated. Radiotherapy and chemotherapy are the mainstays, but an optimal algorithm has not been established. Treatment limited to the eye may not improve survival, but local treatment may be preferable if there is monocular disease and no evidence of involvement elsewhere.

- **Radiotherapy** has long been the first-line treatment for PVRL, but recurrence is common and complications such as radiation retinopathy and cataract can occur. It now tends to be reserved for some cases of bilateral disease but may be associated with lower recurrence rates than chemotherapy alone. It is better tolerated by younger patients.
- **Intravitreal** methotrexate is useful for recurrent disease, but close monitoring is needed to detect ocular complications and any recurrence.
- **Systemic chemotherapy** with a variety of agents such as methotrexate can prolong survival in patients with CNS disease. This can be given in combination with whole brain irradiation but neurotoxicity is a problem. A variety of methods have been developed to overcome the blood–brain barrier. Systemic treatment is usually effective for ocular

disease and this is preferred to ocular radiotherapy in some centres because in addition to avoiding radiation-induced complications it may improve survival. Monotherapy for primary intraocular lymphoma (PIOL) with ifosfamide or trofosfamide has also been successful.

- **Biologic agents involving** specific anti-B cell monoclonal antibodies (e.g. rituximab), may represent a useful alternative, but are generally given intravitreally because of poor penetration through the blood–brain barrier.

TUMOURS OF THE RETINAL PIGMENT EPITHELIUM

Congenital hypertrophy of the RPE

Introduction

Congenital hypertrophy of the retinal pigment epithelium (CHRPE) is an umbrella term encompassing three entities with distinct features and distinct implications.

Solitary (unifocal) CHRPE

- A flat or minimally elevated dark-grey or black (Fig. 12.54A), round, oval or larger scalloped-edged lesion with well-defined margins, usually located near the equator or in the peripheral fundus.
- A depigmented halo located just inside the margin (Fig. 12.54B), and depigmented lacunae (Fig. 12.54C) are common, particularly as a lesion matures; some lesions may become virtually totally depigmented.
- Median diameter is 4–5 mm but lesions can be much smaller or very large, especially in the far periphery (Fig. 12.54D), and may cause diagnostic difficulty unless the possibility of CHRPE is borne in mind.
- A posterior pole location is uncommon (2%).
- Histopathology shows densely packed RPE cells replete with large melanosomes – a combination of cellular hyperplasia and hypertrophy.
- Although formerly regarded as following a consistently stable course, a slight enlargement of the involved area over time is very common, and the development of a presumed adenomatous or adenocarcinomatous nodule arising within the lesion (see below) occurs in around 2%. Long-term review is therefore now advised.
- Solitary CHRPE does not have an association with increased gastrointestinal malignancy risk.

Grouped (multifocal) CHRPE

- Multiple lesions, much smaller than those of solitary CHRPE and without haloes or lacunae, orientated in a pattern simulating animal footprints ('bear-tracks' – Fig. 12.55A), often confined to one sector or quadrant of the fundus with the smaller spots located more centrally.
- There are typically several groups.

- Rarely the lesions may be depigmented ('polar bear tracks' – Fig. 12.55B).
- Only one eye is involved in almost all cases.
- The characteristic clinical appearance and monocular distribution serve to distinguish typical grouped CHRPE from the atypical multifocal variant associated with an increased risk of gastrointestinal malignancy (see below).

Atypical congenital hypertrophy of the RPE

- Multiple oval, spindle, comma- or fishtail-shaped lesions of very variable size associated with irregularly hypopigmented margins and perilesional areas (Figs 12.56A and B).
- Both eyes are involved.
- The lesions have a haphazard, not sectoral, distribution and may be pigmented, depigmented or heterogeneous.
- To emphasize the distinction with the CHRPE variants that are not associated with gastrointestinal malignancy, the alternative term 'retinal pigment epithelial hamartomas associated with familial adenomatous polyposis' (RPEH-FAP) has been proposed.
- **Systemic associations**
  - Familial adenomatous polyposis (FAP) is an autosomal dominant (AD) condition characterized by adenomatous polyps throughout the rectum and colon, which usually start to develop in adolescence. It results from a germline mutation in the gene *APC*; mutations falling within a certain codon range in this gene are associated with the presence of related CHRPE. Patients undergo regular colonoscopic screening with polyp excision. If untreated, virtually all patients with FAP develop carcinoma of the colorectal region by the age of 50 years. As a result of the dominant inheritance pattern, genetic testing and intensive survey of at-risk family members is imperative. Between 70 and 80% of patients with FAP have atypical CHRPE lesions, which are present at birth.
  - Gardner syndrome is characterized by FAP, osteomas of the skull, mandible and long bones, and cutaneous soft tissue tumours such as epidermoid cysts, lipomas and fibromas.
  - Turcot syndrome is an AD or autosomal recessive condition characterized by FAP and tumours of the CNS, particularly medulloblastoma and glioma.

Combined hamartoma of the retina and RPE

Introduction

Combined hamartoma of the retina and RPE is a rare lesion that is probably congenital. It may be more common in males. It typically occurs sporadically in normal individuals but sometimes in association with a systemic disorder, particularly neurofibromatosis type 2, which should be considered particularly in children or if bilateral lesions are present. Histopathology shows thickening

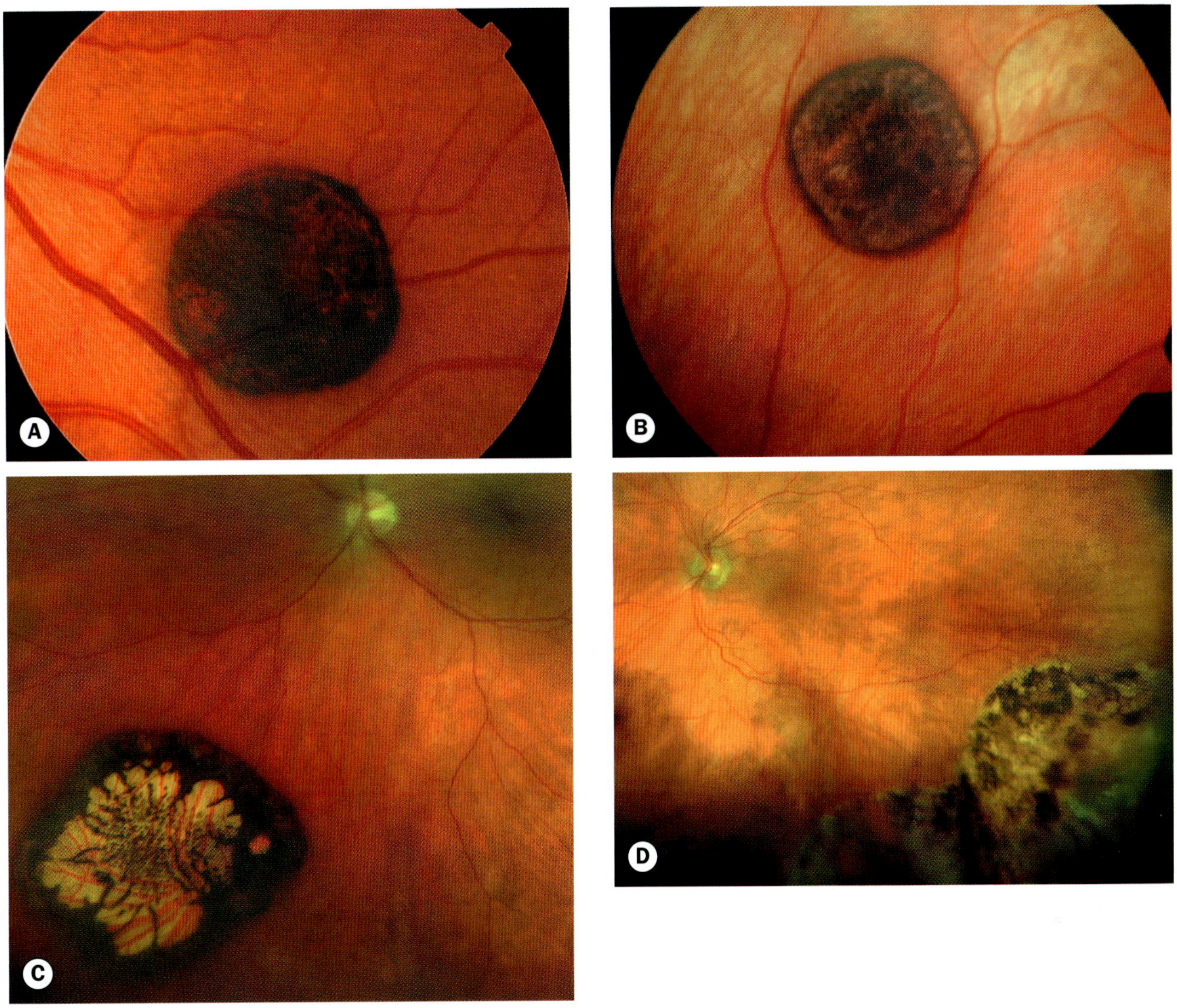

Fig. 12.54 Solitary CHRPE. **(A)** Heavily pigmented lesion; **(B)** partially depigmented lesion with halo; **(C)** large lesion with depigmented lacunae; **(D)** very large peripheral involvement
(Courtesy of S Chen – figs B and C)

of the RPE and sensory retina with prominent glial and vascular tissue.

Diagnosis

- **Symptoms.** The most common presentation is with decreased vision or strabismus in early childhood, though symptom onset in late childhood or early adulthood is also frequent.
- **VA** is 6/60 or worse in 40–50%, usually secondary to macular involvement.
- **Fundus**
  - Slightly elevated deep grey or brown – sometimes orange, yellow or green – pigmented lesion that blends into the adjacent RPE at its margins (Fig. 12.57A).
  - Superficial whitish epiretinal membrane (ERM) formation with retinal wrinkling. Occasionally vitreoretinal interface changes are marked (Fig. 12.57B), sometimes with focal tractional retinal detachment.
  - Tortuosity and prominence of overlying retinal vessels; there may be evident feeder and draining vessels.
  - The lesion is usually located at the posterior pole, often in a juxtapapillary or macular site; peripheral lesions (Fig. 12.57C) are uncommon. Dragging of the disc or macula may be present.
  - Uncommon findings include secondary macular oedema, exudation (Fig. 12.57D), choroidal and preretinal neovascularization, retinoschisis and retinal detachment.
- **OCT** will demonstrate associated epiretinal membrane formation; this has variously been reported as intrinsic to or distinct from the main lesion.
- **FA** shows early hyperfluorescence of the vascular abnormalities and blockage by pigment; the late phase may show leakage.

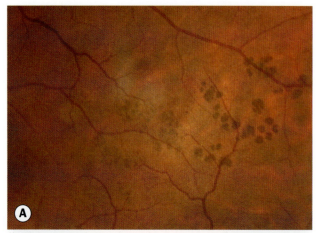

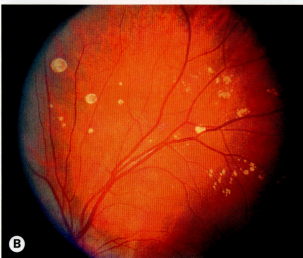

Fig. 12.55 Grouped CHRPE. **(A)** 'Bear-track' lesions; **(B)** 'polar bear track' lesions

(Courtesy of S Chen – fig. A; J Donald M Gass, from Stereoscopic Atlas of Macular Diseases, *Mosby 1997 – fig. B)*

Treatment

- **Monitoring** for complications.
- **Amblyopia therapy** is important in young children.
- **Specific treatment** for CNV and leakage where indicated.
- **Vitrectomy** for ERM has provided benefit in some cases.

Congenital simple hamartoma of the RPE

Congenital simple hamartoma of the RPE is a rare entity, usually incidentally diagnosed in asymptomatic children and young adults. It is typically a small (1.5 mm or less) jet-black nodular lesion, with well-defined margins, that appears to involve the full thickness of the retina and RPE and to protrude into the vitreous cavity (Fig. 12.58). A feeding artery and draining vein are generally seen. The lesion is typically located immediately adjacent to the foveola. VA is usually normal, but is occasionally impaired as a result of central foveal involvement or traction.

Adenoma and adenocarcinoma of the RPE

Adenoma of the RPE is an oval pigmented lesion that most commonly arises in the peripheral fundus, sometimes from an area of solitary CHRPE. Associated vitreous inflammatory cells and retinal exudation are frequently present. Associated prominent feeding and draining vessels may develop. The behaviour of an adenocarcinoma is thought to be similar to that of an adenoma. Most lesions are simply observed in the absence of vision-threatening complications, as metastasis has not been reported. Fine needle biopsy is sometimes required for diagnostic clarification.

Hyperplasia and migration of the RPE simulating uveal melanoma

Rare cases have been reported of massively proliferating RPE cells simulating a uveal melanoma, including by extraocular extension. True malignant tumours of the RPE are extraordinarily rare.

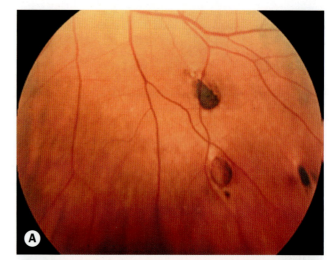

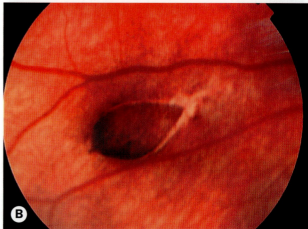

Fig. 12.56 (A) Atypical CHRPE; **(B)** characteristic depigmentation at one margin

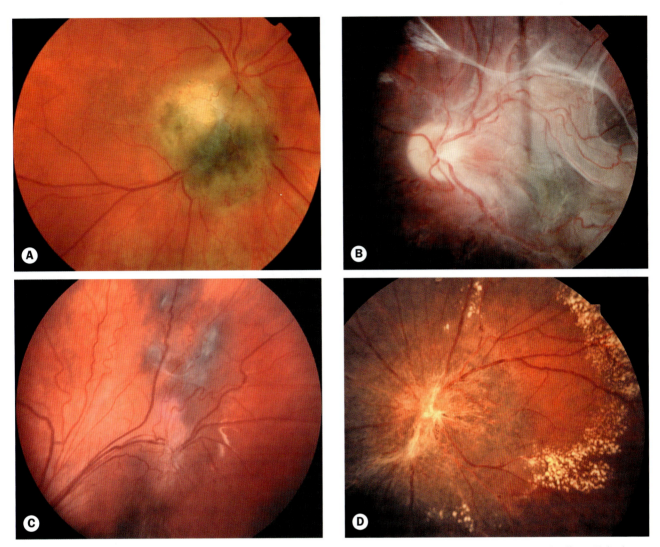

Fig. 12.57 Combined hamartoma of the retina and retinal pigment epithelium. **(A)** lesion obscuring the optic disc; **(B)** lesion with substantial preretinal glial component; **(C)** peripheral lesion; **(D)** larger peripapillary lesion with peripheral hard exudates

(Courtesy of S Chen – fig. A; S Milewski – fig. B)

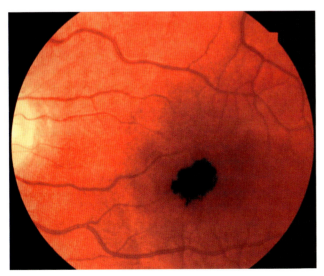

Fig. 12.58 Congenital simple hamartoma of the retinal pigment epithelium

PARANEOPLASTIC SYNDROMES

Paraneoplastic retinopathies are rare diseases that might be missed or misdiagnosed by the unwary observer. Many of the patients present with visual symptoms before the primary malignancy is diagnosed. It is therefore important for clinicians to be familiar with these syndromes in order to detect the underlying malignancy as early as possible.

Bilateral diffuse uveal melanocytic proliferation

Bilateral diffuse uveal melanocytic proliferation (BDUMP) is a very rare paraneoplastic syndrome occurring usually in patients with systemic, often occult, malignancy. It is characterized by the proliferation of benign melanocytes in the outer choroid often manifesting with multiple naevus-like choroidal lesions (Fig. 12.59), but a variety of other anterior and posterior ocular segment

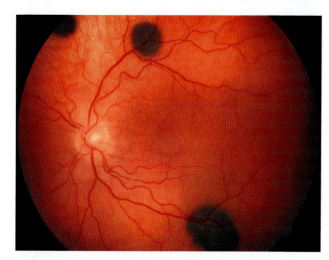

Fig. 12.59 Naevus-like lesions in diffuse uveal melanocytic proliferation
(Courtesy of A Leys)

features have been reported, including red-grey subretinal patches, rapid-onset cataract, episcleral and conjunctival lesions. Vision can be severely diminished. The mechanism is uncertain, but a circulating factor may be responsible in many cases. Detection of an occult primary malignancy might enable early treatment to enhance survival. Treatment of BDUMP itself is generally unrewarding – improvement with plasmapheresis has been reported – although successful treatment of the underlying primary tumour may be followed by regression of the BDUMP, but without improvement in vision.

Cancer-associated retinopathy

Cancer-associated retinopathy (CAR) is most frequently associated with small cell bronchial carcinoma. Visual symptoms precede the diagnosis of malignancy in half the cases, typically by several months but sometimes several years. Subacute visual loss occurs over weeks to months associated with photopsia; colour impairment, glare, photosensitivity and central scotoma are attributed to cone dysfunction. Night blindness, impaired dark adaptation, ring scotoma and peripheral field loss occur due to rod dysfunction. The fundus often appears normal on presentation, but attenuated arterioles, optic disc pallor and mild RPE changes develop as the disease progresses. The electroretinogram (ERG) is abnormal at an early stage under both photopic and scotopic conditions. As with BDUMP, CAR should prompt a thorough search for an underlying malignancy, though this is not always found and the condition is then regarded as an autoimmune retinopathy.

Melanoma-associated retinopathy

The presentation of melanoma-associated retinopathy (MAR) differs from CAR in that the visual symptoms usually arise after, rather than prior to, the diagnosis of cutaneous melanoma. There may be concurrent vitiligo. Autoantibodies from MAR sera react against bipolar cells in human retina; clinical and electrophysiological data also implicate bipolar cells as the target in MAR. Generally, symptoms and signs are less marked than in CAR. The ERG shows marked reduction of dark-adapted and light-adapted b-wave and preservation of a-wave (normal photoreceptor function), characteristic of bipolar cell dysfunction. The prognosis for vision is typically good.

Chapter 13

Retinal vascular disease

RETINAL CIRCULATION

Arterial system

- **The central retinal artery**, an end artery, enters the optic nerve approximately 1 cm behind the globe. It is composed of three anatomical layers:
  - ○ The intima, the innermost, is composed of a single layer of endothelium resting on a collagenous zone.
  - ○ The internal elastic lamina separates the intima from the media.
  - ○ The media consists mainly of smooth muscle.
  - ○ The adventitia is the outermost and is composed of loose connective tissue.
- **Retinal arterioles** arise from the central retinal artery. Their walls contain smooth muscle, but in contrast to arteries the internal elastic lamina is discontinuous.

Capillaries

Retinal capillaries supply the inner two-thirds of the retina, with the outer third being supplied by the choriocapillaris. The inner capillary network (plexus) is located in the ganglion cell layer, with an outer plexus in the inner nuclear layer. Capillary-free zones are present around arterioles (Fig. 13.1A) and at the fovea (foveal avascular zone – FAZ). Retinal capillaries are devoid of smooth muscle and elastic tissue; their walls consist of the following (Fig. 13.1B):

- **Endothelial cells** form a single layer on the basement membrane and are linked by tight junctions that form the inner blood–retinal barrier.
- **The basement membrane** lies beneath the endothelial cells with an outer basal lamina enclosing pericytes.
- **Pericytes** lie external to endothelial cells and have multiple pseudopodial processes that envelop the capillaries. Pericytes have contractile properties and are thought to participate in autoregulation of the microvascular circulation.

Venous system

Retinal venules and veins drain blood from the capillaries.

- **Small venules** are larger than capillaries but have a similar structure.
- **Larger venules** contain smooth muscle and merge to form veins.
- **Veins** contain a small amount of smooth muscle and elastic tissue in their walls and are relatively distensible. Their diameter gradually enlarges as they pass posteriorly towards the central retinal vein.

DIABETIC RETINOPATHY

Introduction

Ophthalmic complications of diabetes

- **Common**
  - ○ Retinopathy.
  - ○ Iridopathy (minor iris transillumination defects).
  - ○ Unstable refraction.
- **Uncommon**
  - ○ Recurrent styes.
  - ○ Xanthelasmata.
  - ○ Accelerated senile cataract.
  - ○ Neovascular glaucoma (NVG).
  - ○ Ocular motor nerve palsies.
  - ○ Reduced corneal sensitivity.
- **Rare.** Papillopathy, pupillary light-near dissociation, Wolfram syndrome (progressive optic atrophy and multiple neurological and systemic abnormalities), acute-onset cataract, rhino-orbital mucormycosis.

Prevalence

The reported prevalence of diabetic retinopathy (DR) in diabetics varies substantially between studies, even amongst contemporary populations in the same country, but is probably around 40%. It is more common in type 1 diabetes than in type 2 and sight-threatening disease is present in up to 10%. Proliferative diabetic

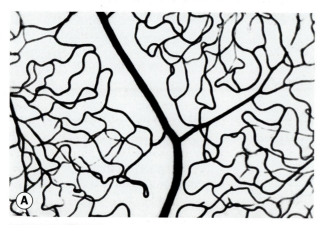

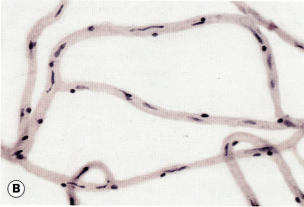

Fig. 13.1 Normal retinal capillary bed. **(A)** Periarteriolar capillary-free zone – flat preparation of Indian ink-injected retina; **(B)** endothelial cells with elongated nuclei and pericytes with rounded nuclei – trypsin digest preparation

(Courtesy of J Harry and G Misson, from Clinical Ophthalmic Pathology, *Butterworth-Heinemann 2001)*

retinopathy (PDR) affects 5–10% of the diabetic population; type 1 diabetics are at particular risk, with an incidence of up to 90% after 30 years.

Risk factors

- **Duration of diabetes** is the most important risk factor. In patients diagnosed with diabetes before the age of 30 years, the incidence of DR after 10 years is 50%, and after 30 years 90%. DR rarely develops within 5 years of the onset of diabetes or before puberty, but about 5% of type 2 diabetics have DR at presentation. It appears that duration is a stronger predictor for proliferative disease than for maculopathy.
- **Poor control of diabetes.** It has been shown that tight blood glucose control, particularly when instituted early, can prevent or delay the development or progression of DR. However, a sudden improvement in control may be associated with progression of retinopathy in the near term. Type 1 diabetic patients appear to obtain greater benefit from good control than type 2. Raised HbA1c is associated with an increased risk of proliferative disease.
- **Pregnancy** is sometimes associated with rapid progression of DR. Predicating factors include greater pre-pregnancy severity of retinopathy, poor pre-pregnancy control of diabetes, control exerted too rapidly during the early stages of pregnancy, and pre-eclampsia. The risk of progression is related to the severity of DR in the first trimester. If substantial DR is present, frequency of review should reflect individual risk, and can be up to monthly. Diabetic macular oedema usually resolves spontaneously after pregnancy and need not be treated if it develops in later pregnancy.
- **Hypertension**, which is very common in patients with type 2 diabetes, should be rigorously controlled (<140/80 mmHg). Tight control appears to be particularly beneficial in type 2 diabetics with maculopathy. Cardiovascular disease and previous stroke are also predictive.
- **Nephropathy**, if severe, is associated with worsening of DR. Conversely, treatment of renal disease (e.g. renal transplantation) may be associated with improvement of retinopathy and a better response to photocoagulation.
- **Other risk factors** include hyperlipidaemia, smoking, cataract surgery, obesity and anaemia.

Pathogenesis

DR is predominantly a microangiopathy in which small blood vessels are particularly vulnerable to damage from high glucose levels. Direct hyperglycaemic effects on retinal cells are also likely to play a role.

Many angiogenic stimulators and inhibitors have been identified; vascular endothelial growth factor (VEGF) appears to be of particular importance in the former category.

Classification

The classification used in the Early Treatment Diabetic Retinopathy Study (ETDRS – the modified Airlie House classification) is widely used internationally. An abbreviated version is set out in Table 13.1, in conjunction with management guidelines. The following descriptive categories are also in widespread use in clinical practice:

- **Background diabetic retinopathy (BDR)** is characterized by microaneurysms, dot and blot haemorrhages and exudates. These are generally the earliest signs of DR, and persist as more advanced lesions appear.
- **Diabetic maculopathy** strictly refers to the presence of any retinopathy at the macula, but is commonly reserved for significant changes, particularly vision-threatening oedema and ischaemia.
- **Preproliferative diabetic retinopathy (PPDR)** manifests with cotton wool spots, venous changes, intraretinal microvascular anomalies (IRMA) and often deep retinal haemorrhages. PPDR indicates progressive retinal ischaemia, with a heightened risk of progression to retinal neovascularization.
- **PDR** is characterized by neovascularization on or within one disc diameter of the disc (NVD) and/or new vessels elsewhere (NVE) in the fundus.
- **Advanced diabetic eye disease** is characterized by tractional retinal detachment, significant persistent vitreous haemorrhage and neovascular glaucoma.

Signs

Microaneurysms

Microaneurysms are localized outpouchings, mainly saccular, of the capillary wall that may form either by focal dilatation of the capillary wall where pericytes are absent, or by fusion of two arms of a capillary loop (Fig. 13.2A). Most develop in the inner capillary plexus (inner nuclear layer), frequently adjacent to areas of capillary non-perfusion (Fig. 13.2B). Loss of pericytes (Fig. 13.2C) may also lead to endothelial cell proliferation with the formation of 'cellular' microaneurysms (Fig. 13.2D). Microaneurysms may leak plasma constituents into the retina as a result of breakdown in the blood–retinal barrier, or may thrombose. They tend to be the earliest sign of DR.

- **Signs.** Tiny red dots, often initially temporal to the fovea (Fig. 13.3A); may be indistinguishable clinically from dot haemorrhages.
- **Fluorescein angiography (FA)** allows differentiation between dot haemorrhages and non-thrombosed microaneurysms. Early frames show tiny hyperfluorescent dots (Fig. 13.3B), typically more numerous than visible clinically. Late frames show diffuse hyperfluorescence due to leakage.

Retinal haemorrhages

- **Retinal nerve fibre layer haemorrhages** arise from the larger superficial pre-capillary arterioles (Fig. 13.4A) and assume their characteristic shape (Fig. 13.4B) because of the architecture of the retinal nerve fibre layer.

Table 13.1 Abbreviated Early Treatment Diabetic Retinopathy Study (ETDRS) classification of diabetic retinopathy

Category/description	Management
Non-proliferative diabetic retinopathy (NPDR)	
No DR	Review in 12 months
Very mild NPDR Microaneurysms only	Review most patients in 12 months
Mild NPDR Any or all of: microaneurysms, retinal haemorrhages, exudates, cotton wool spots, up to the level of moderate NPDR. No intraretinal microvascular anomalies (IRMA) or significant beading	Review range 6–12 months, depending on severity of signs, stability, systemic factors, and patient's personal circumstances
Moderate NPDR • Severe retinal haemorrhages (more than ETDRS standard photograph 2A: about 20 medium–large per quadrant) in 1–3 quadrants or mild IRMA • Significant venous beading can be present in no more than 1 quadrant • Cotton wool spots commonly present	Review in approximately 6 months Proliferative diabetic retinopathy (PDR) in up to 26%, high-risk PDR in up to 8% within a year
Severe NPDR The 4–2–1 rule; one or more of: • Severe haemorrhages in all 4 quadrants • Significant venous beading in 2 or more quadrants • Moderate IRMA in 1 or more quadrants	Review in 4 months PDR in up to 50%, high-risk PDR in up to 15% within a year
Very severe NPDR Two or more of the criteria for severe NPDR	Review in 2–3 months High-risk PDR in up to 45% within a year
Proliferative diabetic retinopathy (PDR)	
Mild–moderate PDR New vessels on the disc (NVD) or new vessels elsewhere (NVE), but extent insufficient to meet the high-risk criteria	Treatment considered according to severity of signs, stability, systemic factors, and patient's personal circumstances such as reliability of attendance for review. If not treated, review in up to 2 months
High-risk PDR • New vessels on the disc (NVD) greater than ETDRS standard photograph 10A (about ⅓ disc area) • Any NVD with vitreous haemorrhage • NVE greater than ½ disc area with vitreous haemorrhage	Treatment advised – see text Should be performed immediately when possible, and certainly same day if symptomatic presentation with good retinal view
Advanced diabetic eye disease See text for description	See text

- Intraretinal haemorrhages arise from the venous end of capillaries and are located in the compact middle layers of the retina (see Fig. 13.4A) with a resultant red 'dot/blot' configuration (Fig. 13.4C).
- Deeper dark round haemorrhages (Fig. 13.4D) represent haemorrhagic retinal infarcts and are located within the middle retinal layers (see Fig. 13.4A). The extent of involvement is a significant marker of the likelihood of progression to PDR.

Exudates

Exudates, sometimes termed 'hard' exudates to distinguish from the older term for cotton wool spots – 'soft' exudates, are caused by chronic localized retinal oedema; they develop at the junction of normal and oedematous retina. They are composed of lipoprotein and lipid-filled macrophages located mainly within the outer plexiform layer (Fig. 13.5A). Hyperlipidaemia may increase the likelihood of exudate formation.

- **Signs**
  - Waxy yellow lesions (Fig. 13.5B) with relatively distinct margins arranged in clumps and/or rings at the posterior pole, often surrounding leaking microaneurysms.
  - With time the number and size tend to increase (Fig. 13.5C), and the fovea may be involved.
  - When leakage ceases, exudates absorb spontaneously over a period of months, either into healthy surrounding capillaries or by phagocytosis.

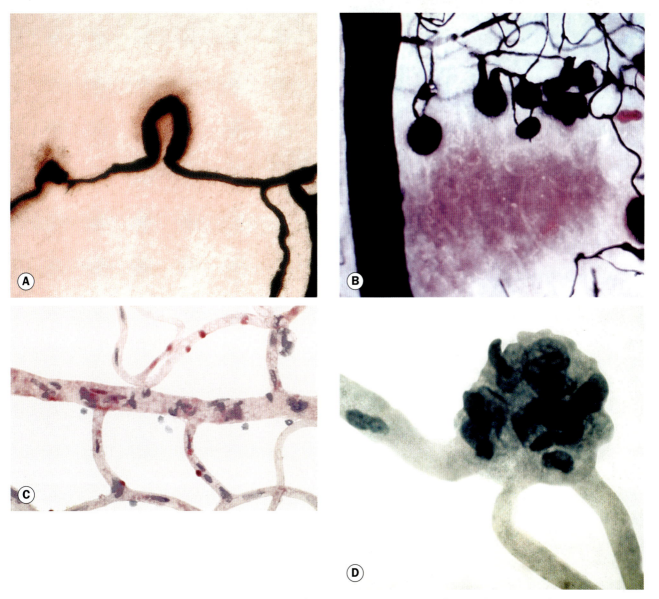

Fig. 13.2 Microaneurysms – histopathology. **(A)** Two arms of a capillary loop that may fuse to become a microaneurysm – flat preparation of Indian ink-injected retina; **(B)** an area of capillary non-perfusion and adjacent microaneurysms – flat preparation of Indian ink-injected retina; **(C)** eosinophilic (dark pink) degenerate pericytes – trypsin digest preparation; **(D)** microaneurysm with endothelial cell proliferation (cellular microaneurysm) – trypsin digest preparation

(Courtesy of J Harry and G Misson, from Clinical Ophthalmic Pathology, *Butterworth-Heinemann 2001 – figs A and C; J Harry – figs B and D)*

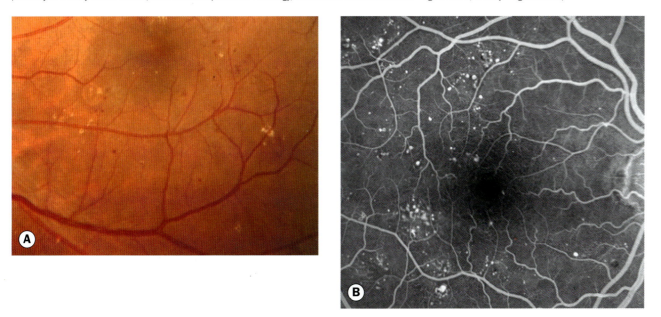

Fig. 13.3 Microaneurysms. **(A)** Microaneurysms and dot/blot haemorrhages at the posterior pole; **(B)** FA shows scattered hyperfluorescent spots in the posterior fundus

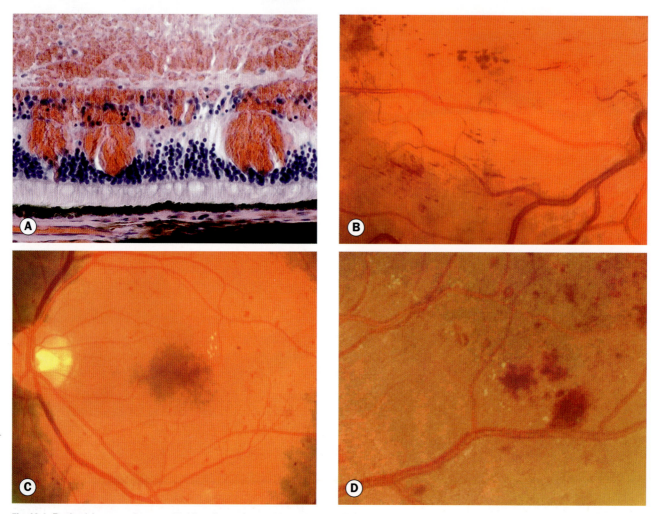

Fig. 13.4 Retinal haemorrhages. **(A)** Histology shows blood lying diffusely in the retinal nerve fibre and ganglion cell layers and as globules in the outer layers; **(B)** retinal nerve fibre layer (flame) haemorrhages; **(C)** dot and blot haemorrhages; **(D)** deep dark haemorrhages

(Courtesy of J Harry and G Misson, from Clinical Ophthalmic Pathology, *Butterworth-Heinemann 2001 – fig. A)*

    ○ Chronic leakage leads to enlargement and the deposition of crystalline cholesterol (Fig. 13.5D).
- **FA** will commonly show hypofluorescence only with large dense exudates, as although background choroidal fluorescence is masked, retinal capillary fluorescence is generally preserved overlying the lesions (Fig 13.6).

Diabetic macular oedema (DMO)

Diabetic maculopathy (foveal oedema, exudates or ischaemia) is the most common cause of visual impairment in diabetic patients, particularly type 2. Diffuse retinal oedema is caused by extensive capillary leakage, and localized oedema by focal leakage from microaneurysms and dilated capillary segments. The fluid is initially located between the outer plexiform and inner nuclear layers; later it may also involve the inner plexiform and nerve fibre layers, until eventually the entire thickness of the retina becomes oedematous. With central accumulation of fluid the fovea assumes a cystoid appearance – cystoid macular oedema (CMO) that is readily detectable on optical coherence tomography (OCT) (Fig. 13.7A) and assumes a central flower petal pattern on FA (Fig. 13.7B).

- **Focal maculopathy**: well-circumscribed retinal thickening associated with complete or incomplete rings of exudates (Fig. 13.8A). FA shows late, focal hyperfluorescence due to leakage, usually with good macular perfusion (Fig. 13.8B).
- **Diffuse maculopathy**: diffuse retinal thickening, which may be associated with cystoid changes; there are typically also scattered microaneurysms and small haemorrhages (Fig. 13.9A). Landmarks may be obscured by oedema, which may render localization of the fovea impossible. FA shows mid- and late-phase diffuse hyperfluorescence (Fig. 13.9B), and demonstrates CMO if present.

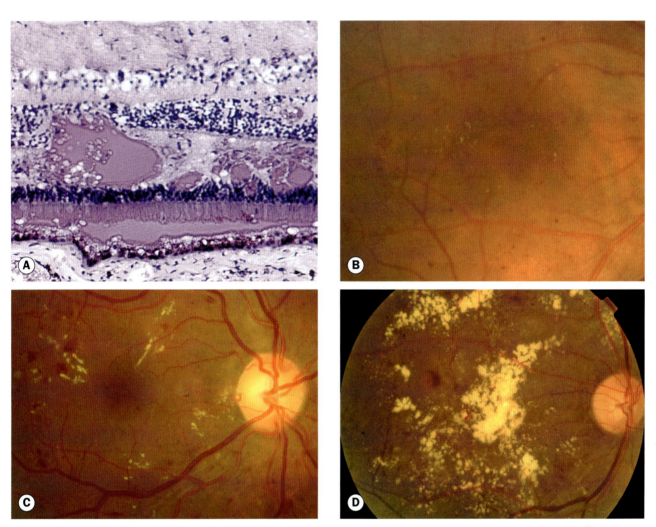

Fig. 13.5 Exudates. **(A)** Histology shows irregular eosinophilic deposits mainly in the outer plexiform layer; **(B)** small exudates and microaneurysms; **(C)** more extensive exudates, some associated with microaneurysms; **(D)** exudates involving the fovea, including central crystalline cholesterol deposition – focal laser has recently been applied superotemporal to the fovea

(Courtesy of J Harry – fig. A; S Chen – figs C and D)

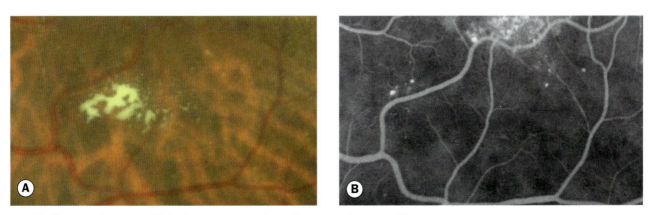

Fig. 13.6 FA of exudates. **(A)** Clinical appearance; **(B)** exudates not shown on FA

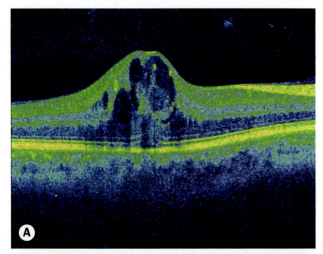

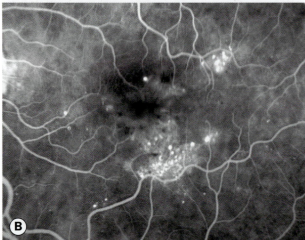

Fig. 13.7 Cystoid macular oedema. **(A)** OCT shows retinal thickening and cystoid spaces; **(B)** FA shows leaking microaneurysms and central diffuse hyperfluorescence with a flower-petal configuration – same patient as Fig. 13.6

Ischaemic maculopathy

- **Signs** are variable and the macula may look relatively normal despite reduced visual acuity. In other cases PPDR may be present.
- **FA** shows capillary non-perfusion at the fovea (an enlarged FAZ) and frequently other areas of capillary non-perfusion (Fig. 13.10) at the posterior pole and periphery.

Clinically significant macular oedema

Clinically significant macular oedema (CSMO) is detected on clinical examination as defined in the ETDRS (Fig. 13.11):

- Retinal thickening within 500 μm of the centre of the macula (Fig. 13.11, upper left).
- Exudates within 500 μm of the centre of the macula, if associated with retinal thickening; the thickening itself may be outside the 500 μm (Fig. 13.11, upper right).
- Retinal thickening one disc area (1500 μm) or larger, any part of which is within one disc diameter of the centre of the macula (Fig. 13.11, lower centre).

Cotton wool spots

Cotton wool spots are composed of accumulations of neuronal debris within the nerve fibre layer. They result from ischaemic disruption of nerve axons, the swollen ends of which are known as cytoid bodies, seen on light microscopy as globular structures in the nerve fibre layer (Fig. 13.12A). As cotton wool spots heal, debris is removed by autolysis and phagocytosis.

- **Signs.** Small fluffy whitish superficial lesions that obscure underlying blood vessels (Fig. 13.12B and C). They are clinically evident only in the post-equatorial retina, where the nerve fibre layer is of sufficient thickness to render them visible.

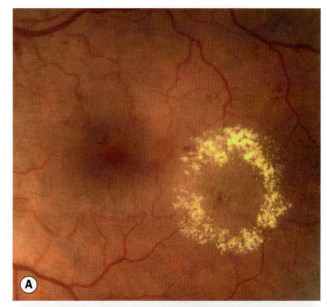

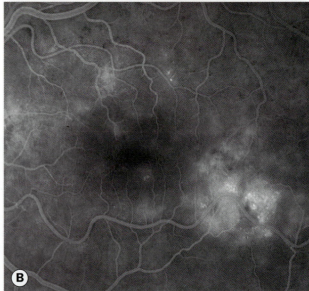

Fig. 13.8 Focal diabetic maculopathy. **(A)** A ring of hard exudates temporal to the macula; **(B)** FA late phase shows focal area of hyperfluorescence due to leakage corresponding to the centre of the exudate ring

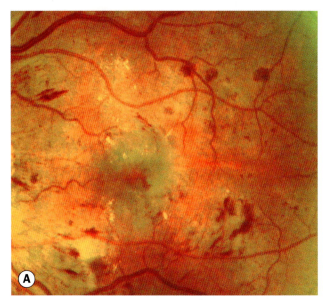

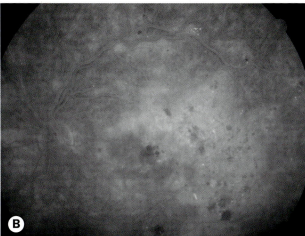

Fig. 13.9 Diffuse diabetic maculopathy. **(A)** Dot and blot haemorrhages – diffuse retinal thickening is present; **(B)** late-phase FA shows extensive hyperfluorescence at the posterior pole due to leakage
(Courtesy of S Chen – fig. B)

- **FA** shows focal hypofluorescence due to local ischaemia and blockage of background choroidal fluorescence.

Venous changes

Venous anomalies seen in ischaemia consist of generalized dilatation and tortuosity, looping, beading (focal narrowing and dilatation) and sausage-like segmentation (Fig. 13.13). The extent of the retinal area exhibiting venous changes correlates well with the likelihood of developing proliferative disease.

Intraretinal microvascular abnormalities

Intraretinal microvascular abnormalities (IRMA) are arteriolar–venular shunts that run from retinal arterioles to venules, thus bypassing the capillary bed and are therefore often seen adjacent to areas of marked capillary hypoperfusion (Fig. 13.14A).

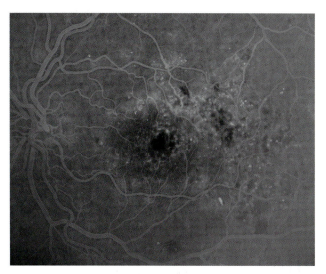

Fig. 13.10 Ischaemic diabetic maculopathy. FA venous phase shows hypofluorescence due to capillary non-perfusion at the central macula and elsewhere
(Courtesy of S Chen)

- **Signs**. Fine, irregular, red intraretinal lines that run from arterioles to venules, without crossing major blood vessels (Fig. 13.14B).
- **FA** shows focal hyperfluorescence associated with adjacent areas of capillary closure ('dropout') but without leakage.

Arterial changes

Subtle retinal arteriolar dilatation may be an early marker of ischaemic dysfunction. When significant ischaemia is present signs include peripheral narrowing, 'silver wiring' and obliteration, similar to the late appearance following a branch retinal artery occlusion.

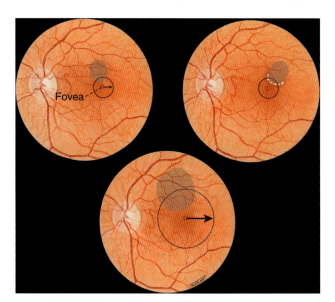

Fig. 13.11 Clinically significant macular oedema

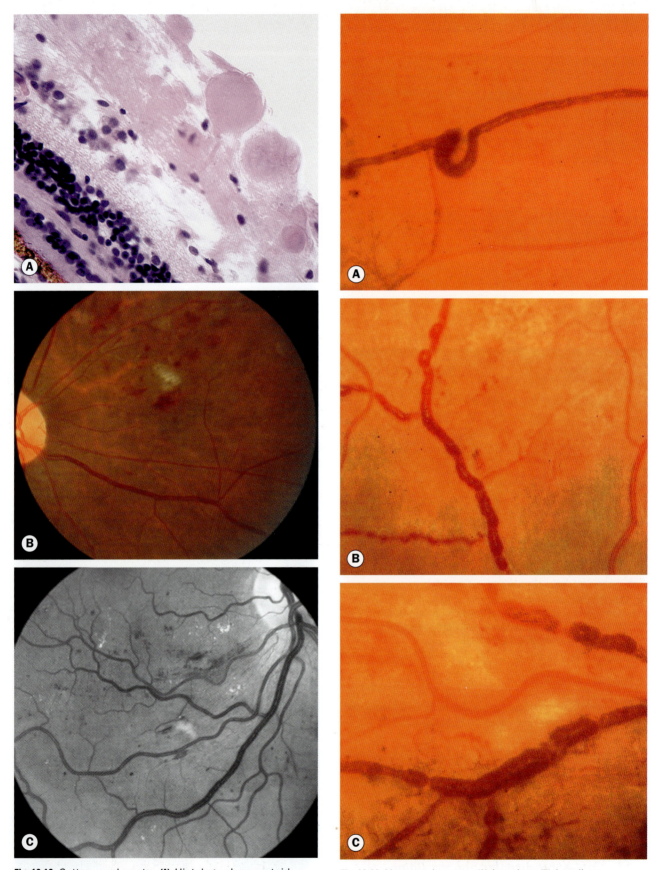

Fig. 13.12 Cotton wool spots. **(A)** Histology shows cytoid bodies in the retinal nerve fibre layer; **(B)** clinical appearance; **(C)** red-free photography showing differing appearance of cotton wool spots and haemorrhages, the latter appearing black – the smaller well-defined white lesions are exudates

(Courtesy of J Harry – fig. A)

Fig. 13.13 Venous changes. **(A)** Looping; **(B)** beading; **(C)** severe segmentation

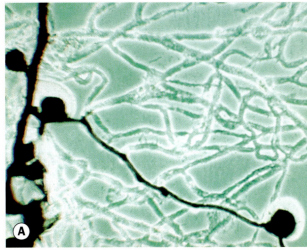

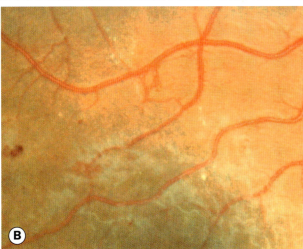

Fig. 13.14 Intraretinal microvascular abnormalities.
(A) Histology shows arteriolar-venular shunt and a few
microaneurysms within a poorly perfused capillary bed –
flat preparation of Indian ink-injected retina; phase
contrast microscopy; **(B)** clinical appearance
(Courtesy of J Harry – fig. A)

Proliferative retinopathy

It has been estimated that over one-quarter of the retina must be
non-perfused before PDR develops. Although preretinal new
vessels may arise anywhere in the retina, they are most commonly
seen at the posterior pole. Fibrous tissue, initially fine, gradually
develops in association as vessels increase in size.

- **New vessels at the disc** (NVD) describes neovascularization
  on or within one disc diameter of the optic nerve head (Fig.
  13.15).
- **New vessels elsewhere** (NVE) describes neovascularization
  further away from the disc (Fig. 13.16); it may be associated
  with fibrosis if long-standing.
- **New vessels on the iris** (NVI – Fig. 13.17), also known as
  rubeosis iridis, carry a high likelihood of progression to
  neovascular glaucoma (see Ch. 10).

- **FA** (see Fig. 13.15C) highlights neovascularization during the
  early phases of the angiogram and shows irregular expanding
  hyperfluorescence during the later stages due to intense
  leakage of dye from neovascular tissue. FA can be used to
  confirm the presence of new vessels (NV) if the clinical
  diagnosis is in doubt, and also delineates areas of ischaemic
  retina that might be selectively targeted for laser treatment.

Treatment

General

- **Patient education** is critical, including regarding the need to
  comply with review and treatment schedules in order to
  optimize visual outcomes.
- **Diabetic control** should be optimized.
- **Other risk factors**, particularly systemic hypertension
  (especially type 2 diabetes) and hyperlipidaemia should be
  controlled in conjunction with the patient's diabetologist.
- **Fenofibrate** 200 mg daily has been shown to reduce the
  progression of diabetic retinopathy in type 2 diabetics and
  prescription should be considered; the decision is
  independent of whether the patient already takes a statin.
- **Smoking** should be discontinued, though this has not been
  definitively shown to affect retinopathy.
- **Other modifiable factors** such as anaemia and renal failure
  should be addressed as necessary.

Treatment of diabetic macular oedema

Until recently laser photocoagulation was the mainstay of treatment for DMO, reducing the risk of visual loss by 50% overall
compared with observation. The availability of newer treatment
modalities and increasing evidence for their efficacy has dramatically altered the approach to management over recent years.
However, options should always be discussed fully with the
patient. In particular, patients with good vision who otherwise
meet criteria for treatment might prefer observation once the risks
of various interventions are taken into account.

- **Laser photocoagulation** (modified ETDRS focal/grid
  treatment).
  - Focal (Figs 13.18A and B). Diode or argon burns are
    applied to leaking microaneurysms 500–3000 μm from
    the foveola; spot size 50–100 μm, duration 0.05–0.1 s with
    sufficient power to obtain a greyish reaction beneath the
    microaneurysm.
  - Grid (Figs 13.18C–F). Burns are applied to macular areas
    of diffuse retinal thickening, treating no closer than
    500 μm from the foveola and 500 μm from the optic disc
    using a spot size of 50–100 μm and duration 0.05–0.1
    second, with power adjusted to give a mild reaction. A
    'modified' grid includes focal treatment to foci of leakage,
    usually microaneurysms.
- **Subthreshold micropulse diode laser.** This modality uses
  very short (microsecond order) laser pulse duration
  combined with a longer interval (e.g. 5% duty cycle)

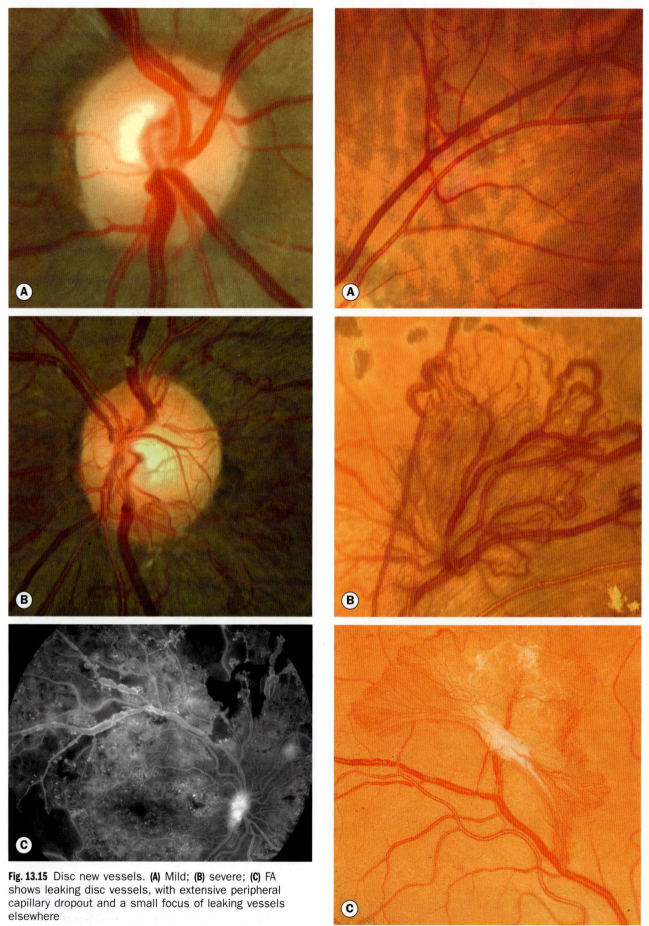

Fig. 13.15 Disc new vessels. **(A)** Mild; **(B)** severe; **(C)** FA shows leaking disc vessels, with extensive peripheral capillary dropout and a small focus of leaking vessels elsewhere

(Courtesy of S Chen – fig. B)

Fig. 13.16 New vessels elsewhere. **(A)** Mild; **(B)** severe; **(C)** associated with fibrosis

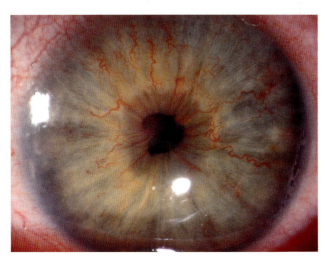

Fig. 13.17 New vessels on the iris (rubeosis iridis)
(Courtesy of C Barry)

allowing energy dissipation, minimizing collateral damage to the retina and choroid whilst stimulating the retinal pigment epithelium (RPE). Research to date indicates that similar results are achieved to those of conventional thermal laser.

- **Intravitreal anti-VEGF agents.** Following substantial clinical studies, intravitreal VEGF inhibitors (see also Ch. 14) have been adopted as a critical element of the management of diabetic maculopathy. Most current studies have looked at ranibizumab or bevacizumab.

- **Intravitreal triamcinolone.** In pseudophakic eyes intravitreal triamcinolone steroid injection followed by prompt laser is comparable to ranibizumab with regard to visual improvement and reducing retinal thickening. However, there is a significant risk of an elevation of intraocular pressure (IOP) and this must be monitored carefully. No benefit above laser has consistently been shown for phakic eyes, which have a substantially increased risk of cataract. Sustained-release intravitreal steroid implants have also demonstrated promising results.

- **Pars plana vitrectomy** (PPV – Fig. 13.19) may be indicated when macular oedema is associated with tangential traction from a thickened and taut posterior hyaloid (see Ch. 14 – vitreomacular traction syndrome). It has also been suggested that some eyes without a taut posterior hyaloid may also benefit from vitrectomy. Clinically, a taut thickened posterior hyaloid is characterized by an increased glistening of the pre-macular vitreous face. FA typically shows diffuse leakage and prominent CMO, but OCT is usually the definitive assessment. There are several other indications for PPV in the management of diabetic eye disease (see later).

- **Specific recommendations**
  - CSMO not involving the macular centre should be treated with photocoagulation (see Fig. 13.18), or with micropulse laser if available.
  - CSMO involving the macular centre but with normal or minimally affected vision, perhaps 6/9 or better, can

either undergo laser (micropulse may carry a lower risk of foveolar damage) or be observed if leakage arises very close to the fovea. If laser is performed, it is prudent to treat no closer than 500 μm from the perceived macular centre.
  - CSMO involving the macular centre and with reduced or reducing vision (6/9–6/90) and significant foveolar thickening on OCT should be considered for intravitreal anti-VEGF treatment, with initial induction using monthly injections for 3–6 months. An as-needed approach can subsequently be adopted. It is possible that combining anti-VEGF treatment with laser – probably deferred until completion of the induction phase – offers advantages, particularly in terms of reducing the frequency of injections, and investigation is ongoing.
  - Pseudophakic eyes with CSMO involving the macular centre and 6/9–6/90 vision should be considered for either the regimen above or intravitreal preservative-free triamcinolone followed soon afterwards by laser.
  - Options in resistant cases include intravitreal steroid: intravitreal triamcinolone – optimally preservative-free – or a sustained-release intravitreal steroid implant. Pars plana vitrectomy may be considered, particularly if vitreomacular traction is present.
  - Eyes with markedly reduced vision due to DMO generally have a poor prognosis, and optimal management is not determined. Depending on circumstances, observation or any of the interventions discussed above may be considered.

Laser treatment for proliferative retinopathy

Scatter laser treatment (panretinal photocoagulation – Fig. 13.20) continues to be the mainstay of PDR treatment, with intravitreal anti-VEGF injection and other modalities remaining adjunctive. The Diabetic Retinopathy Study (DRS) established the characteristics of high-risk proliferative disease and demonstrated the benefit of panretinal photocoagulation (PRP); for instance, severe NVD without haemorrhage carries a 26% risk of visual loss at 2 years that is reduced to 9% with PRP.

- **Informed consent.** Patients should be advised that PRP may occasionally cause visual field defects of sufficient severity to legally preclude driving a motor vehicle; they should also be made aware that there is some risk to central vision, and that night and colour vision may be affected.

- **Co-existent DMO.** If actual or imminent CSMO is also present, laser for this should preferably be carried out prior to PRP or at the same session; the intensity and amount of PRP should be kept to the lowest level likely to be effective, and may be spread over multiple sessions; adjunctive intravitreal steroid or an anti-VEGF agent may improve the outcome.

- **Lens.** A contact lens is used to provide a stable magnified fundus view. A panfundoscopic lens is now generally preferred to a three-mirror lens, as it is more difficult to inadvertently photocoagulate the posterior pole through

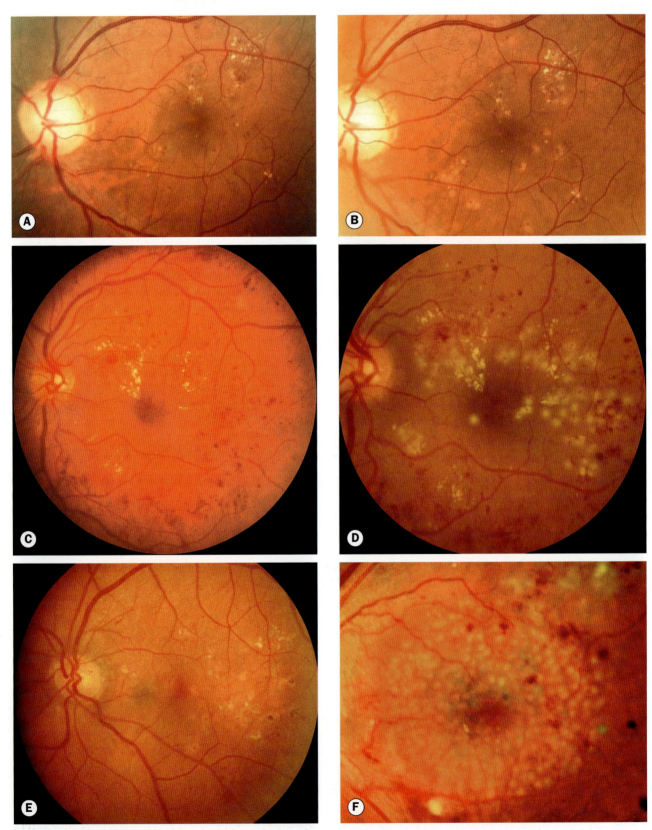

Fig. 13.18 Laser for clinically significant macular oedema. **(A)** Prior to focal laser treatment; **(B)** immediately following focal laser; **(C)** prior to modified macular grid laser treatment; **(D)** patient in (C) immediately post-grid laser; **(E)** appearance 2 months following a limited laser grid; **(F)** dense macular grid – the fovea is spared

(Courtesy of S Chen – figs A, B and F; R Bates – figs C–E)

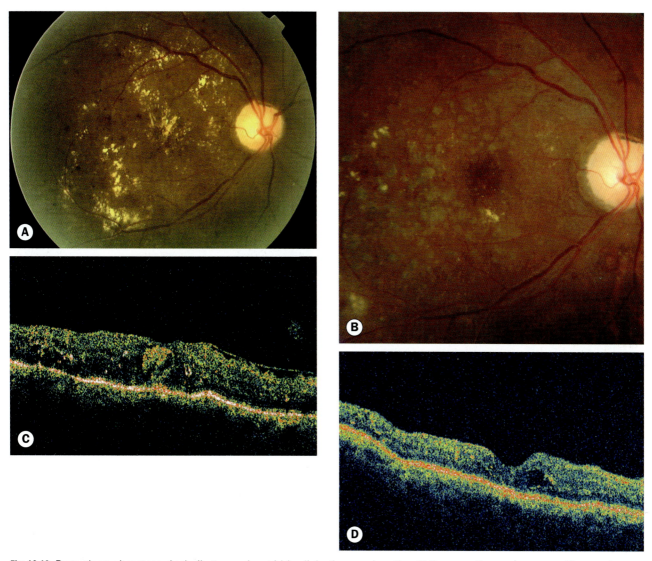

Fig. 13.19 Pars plana vitrectomy including macular grid in diabetic maculopathy. **(A)** Preoperative appearance; **(B)** appearance several weeks postoperatively; **(C)** and **(D)** pre- and postoperative macular OCT scans

(Courtesy of S Chen)

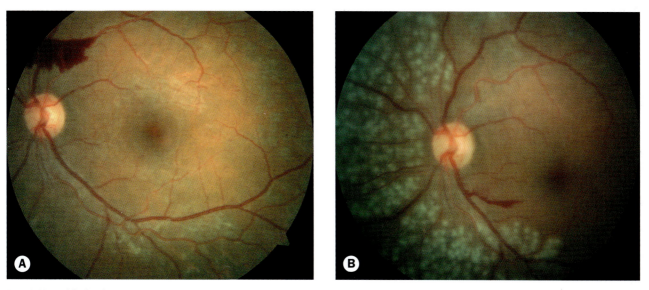

Fig. 13.20 **(A)** Limited panretinal photocoagulation, with fresh retrohyaloid haemorrhage; **(B)** more extensive treatment;

Continued

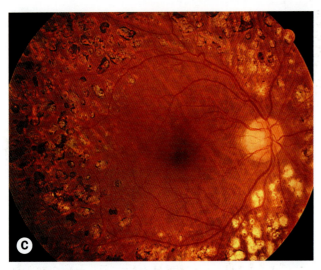

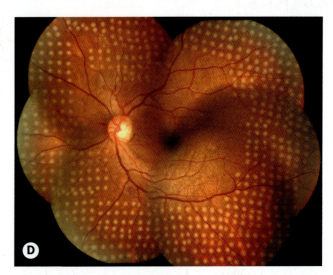

Fig. 13.20, Continued   (C) retinal appearance several weeks after laser; **(D)** composite image of 'pattern scan' multispot array treatment

(Courtesy of C Barry – fig. C; S Chen – fig. D)

the former. Some practitioners prefer to use a higher-magnification/smaller area contact lens (e.g. Mainster®, Area Centralis®) for the more posterior component of treatment. It is essential to constantly bear in mind that an inverted and laterally reversed image is seen.

- **Anaesthesia.** The amount of treatment it is possible to apply during one session may be limited by patient discomfort; this tends to be least at the posterior pole and greatest in the periphery and over the horizontal neurovascular bundles. It tends to worsen with successive sessions. Topical anaesthesia is adequate in most patients, although sub-Tenon or peribulbar anaesthesia can be administered if necessary.

- **Laser parameters**
  - Spot size. A retinal burn diameter of 400 µm is usually desired for PRP. The diameter selected at the user interface to achieve this depends on the contact lens used and the operator must be aware of the correction factor for the particular lens chosen. As an approximation, with panfundoscopic-type lenses the actual retinal spot diameter is twice that selected on the laser user interface; 200 µm is typically selected for PRP, equating to a 400 µm actual retinal diameter once relative magnification is factored in. With the Mainster and Area Centralis, the retinal diameter equates closely to the interface selection, so 400 µm may be selected.
  - Duration depends on the type of laser: 0.05–0.1 s was conventionally used with the argon laser, but newer lasers allow much shorter pulses to be used and 0.01–0.05 s (10–50 ms) is the currently recommended range. Multispot strategies available on some machines utilize a combination of short pulse duration (e.g. 20 ms), very short intervals and pre-programmed delivery arrays to facilitate the application of a large number of pulses in a short period (see Fig. 13.20D). True micropulse PRP is also under investigation and shows promising results. Shorter pulse duration seems to require a greater total

number of burns for an adequate response, and may be slower to achieve regression.
  - Power should be sufficient to produce only a light intensity burn.
  - Spacing. Burns should be separated by 1–1.5 burn widths.
  - Extent of treated area. The initial treatment session should consist of 1500 burns in most cases, though more may be applied if there is a risk of imminent sight loss from vitreous haemorrhage. The more extensive the treatment at a single session, the greater the likelihood of complications. Reported figures vary, but 2500–3500 burns are likely to be required for regression of mild PDR, 4000 for moderate PDR and 7000 for severe PDR. The number of burns offers only approximate guidance, as the effective extent of treatment is dependent on numerous variables.
  - Pattern of treatment. Treatment is generally restricted to the area outside the temporal macular vascular arcades; it is good practice to delineate a 'barrier' of laser burns temporal to the macula early in the procedure to help to reduce the risk of accidental macular damage. Many practitioners leave two disc diameters untreated at the nasal side of the disc, to preserve paracentral field. In very severe PDR it is advisable to treat the inferior fundus first, since any vitreous haemorrhage will gravitate inferiorly and obscure this area, precluding further treatment. Areas of vitreoretinal traction should be avoided.

- **Review** is dependent on PDR severity and the requirement for successive treatment applications; initial treatment should be fractionated over 2–3 sessions. Once an adequate number of burns have been applied review can be set for 4–6 weeks.

- **Indicators of regression** include blunting of vessel tips, shrinking and disappearance of NV, often leaving 'ghost' vessels or fibrosis (Fig. 13.21), regression of IRMA, decreased venous changes, absorption of retinal haemorrhages, disc pallor. Contraction of regressing vessels or associated

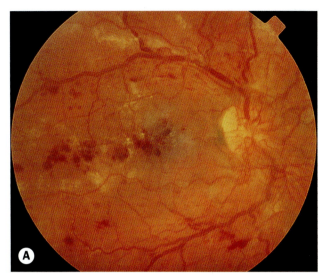 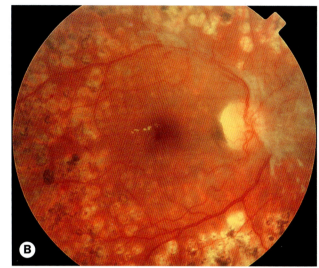

Fig. 13.21 Treatment of proliferative diabetic retinopathy. **(A)** Severe proliferative disease; **(B)** 3 months later the new vessels have regressed – there is residual fibrosis at the disc
(Courtesy of S Milewski)

induction of vitreous separation can precipitate vitreous haemorrhage. Significant fibrous proliferation can lead to tractional retinal detachment (see below). Patients should remain under observation, as recurrence can occur with a requirement for additional PRP.

VEGF inhibition for proliferative retinopathy

Intravitreal anti-VEGF injection has an adjunctive role in the treatment of PDR. Indication can include attempted resolution

of persistent vitreous haemorrhage (with prior B-scan ultrasonography to exclude retinal detachment) with the aim of avoiding vitrectomy, the initial treatment of rubeosis iridis (see below and Ch. 10) whilst a response to PRP is realized, and possibly the rapid control of very severe PDR to minimize the risk of haemorrhage.

Targeted retinal photocoagulation (TRP)

Wide-field fluorescein angiography allows accurate delineation of peripheral capillary non-perfusion (Fig. 13.22). Selective

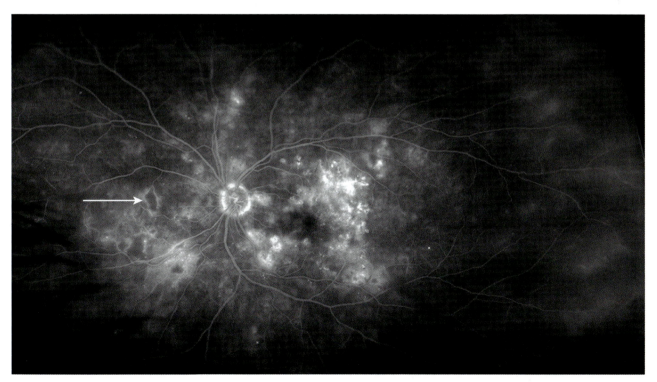

Fig. 13.22 Wide-field FA showing widespread areas of capillary non-perfusion – the arrow indicates a well-defined example
(Courtesy of S Chen)

treatment of these areas with scatter laser has been reported as effectively leading to regression of NV whilst minimizing potential complications.

Advanced diabetic eye disease

Advanced diabetic eye disease is a serious vision-threatening complication of DR that occurs in patients in whom treatment has been inadequate or unsuccessful. Occasionally, advanced disease is evident at, or prompts, presentation.

Clinical features

- **Haemorrhage** may be preretinal (retrohyaloid), intragel or both (Figs 13.23A and B). Intragel haemorrhages usually take longer to clear than preretinal because the former are usually more substantial. In some eyes, altered blood becomes compacted on the posterior vitreous face to form an 'ochre membrane'. Ultrasonography is used in eyes with dense vitreous haemorrhage to detect the possibility of associated retinal detachment.
- **Tractional retinal detachment** (Fig. 13.23C) is caused by progressive contraction of fibrovascular membranes over areas of vitreoretinal attachment. Posterior vitreous detachment in eyes with PDR is often incomplete due to the strong adhesions between cortical vitreous and areas of fibrovascular proliferation; haemorrhage often occurs at these sites due to stress exerted on NV.
- **Rubeosis iridis** (iris neovascularization – NVI) may occur in eyes with PDR, and if severe may lead to neovascular glaucoma (see Ch. 10). NVI is particularly common in eyes with severe retinal ischaemia or persistent retinal detachment following unsuccessful pars plana vitrectomy.

Indications for pars plana vitrectomy

Vitrectomy in diabetic retinopathy is typically combined with extensive endolaser PRP. Visual results depend on the specific indication for surgery and the severity of pre-existing disease.

- **Severe persistent vitreous haemorrhage** that precludes adequate PRP is the most common indication. In the absence of rubeosis iridis, vitrectomy has traditionally been considered within 3 months of the initial vitreous haemorrhage in type 1 diabetics and in most cases of bilateral haemorrhage. However, the outcome may be better with earlier surgery, and the availability of intravitreal anti-VEGF therapy may further modify the approach.
- **Progressive tractional RD** threatening or involving the macula must be treated without delay. However, extramacular tractional detachments may be observed, since they often remain stationary for prolonged periods.
- **Combined tractional and rhegmatogenous RD** should be treated urgently.
- **Premacular retrohyaloid haemorrhage** (Fig 13.24A), if dense and persistent should be considered for early vitrectomy because, if untreated, the internal limiting membrane or posterior hyaloid face may serve as a scaffold for subsequent fibrovascular proliferation and consequent tractional

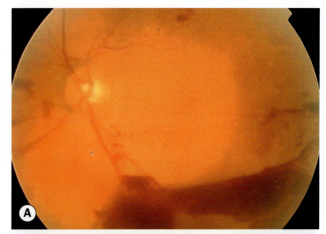

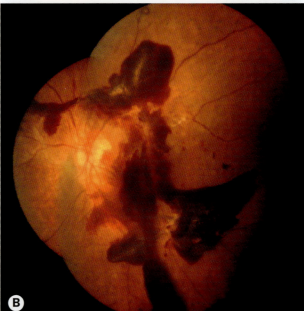

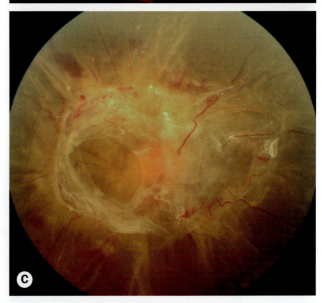

Fig. 13.23 Advanced diabetic eye disease. **(A)** Retrohyaloid and small amount of intragel haemorrhage; **(B)** more substantial intragel bleeding; **(C)** tractional retinal detachment
(Courtesy of S Chen – figs B and C)

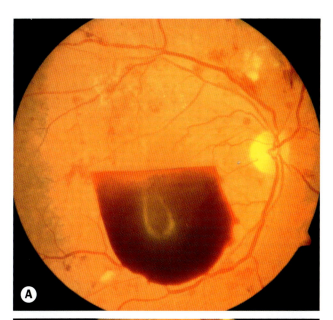

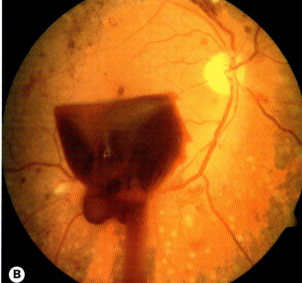

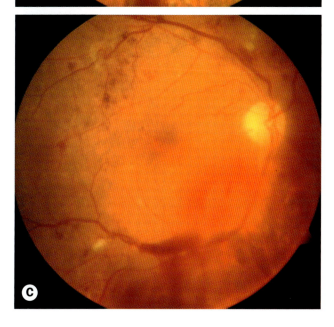

Fig. 13.24 Large premacular retrohyaloid haemorrhage. **(A)** Before and **(B, C)** after Nd:YAG laser hyaloidotomy
(Courtesy of S Chen)

macular detachment or macular epiretinal membrane formation. Dispersion with YAG laser (hyaloidotomy) is often successful (Figs 13.24B and C).

Diabetic papillopathy

Diabetic papillopathy (diabetic papillitis) has been speculated to be an uncommon variant of anterior ischaemic optic neuropathy, though is more commonly bilateral and tends to exhibit more diffuse disc swelling. The underlying pathogenesis is unclear but it may be the result of small-vessel disease. It occurs mainly in younger diabetics, and manifests with mild painless visual impairment that is unilateral in more than half of cases; bilateral disc swelling mandates the exclusion of raised intracranial pressure. Hyperaemic disc swelling is characteristic, and disc telangiectasia occasionally mistaken for neovascularization is present in many affected eyes (Fig. 13.25). Crowding of the fellow disc may be present. Resolution occurs over several months, often leaving mild disc pallor. Final visual acuity (VA) is 6/12 or better in 80%, subject to the effect of coexisting diabetic retinopathy. Distinction from retinal vein occlusion (RVO)-type papillophlebitis (see below) rests on the presence of more extensive retinal haemorrhages and venous congestion in the latter, but may not be

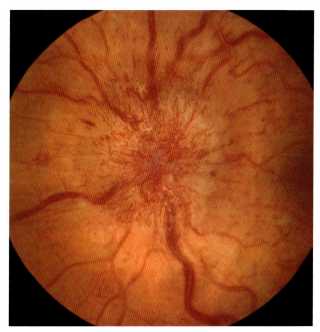

Fig. 13.25 Hyperaemic disc swelling and telangiectasia in diabetic papillopathy
(Courtesy of S Hayreh)

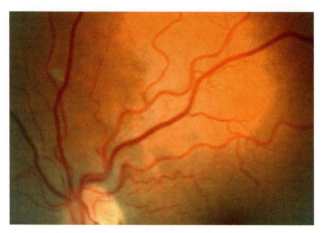

Fig. 13.26 Incidental finding of a single cotton wool spot – no positive findings on systemic investigation. A degree of vascular tortuosity may be an additional cardiovascular risk indicator

possible. Intravitreal anti-VEGF agents and steroids via various routes have been tried, with indeterminate benefit.

NON-DIABETIC RETINOPATHY

Up to 10% of individuals over the age of 40 without diabetes mellitus exhibit – usually very mild – retinopathic features such as microaneurysms, dot and blot haemorrhages and cotton wool spots (Fig. 13.26) that would be consistent with a diagnosis of diabetic retinopathy. Assuming that an alternative ocular cause such as RVO or idiopathic macular telangiectasia has been excluded, this 'non-diabetic' retinopathy tends to be associated with increased cerebro- and cardiovascular risk, and may be particularly prevalent in patients with known or incipient hypertension. There is evidence suggesting that it may be a marker of pre-clinical diabetes in some patients; higher venular calibre may also denote this. Appropriate management is undefined, though evaluation and optimal management of systemic vascular risk factors may be prudent. The signs commonly disappear spontaneously, and this is more likely in those with lower levels of cardiovascular risk.

RETINAL VENOUS OCCLUSIVE DISEASE

Introduction

Retinal vein thrombosis is strongly associated with age-related local and systemic factors. Typically, in branch retinal vein occlusion (BRVO) arteriolosclerotic thickening of a branch retinal arteriole is associated with compression of a venule at an arteriovenous crossing point, exacerbated by sharing an adventitial sheath. This leads to secondary changes that include endothelial cell loss, turbulent flow and thrombus formation. Similarly, the central retinal vein and artery possess a common sheath at crossing points posterior to the lamina cribrosa so that atherosclerotic changes of the artery may precipitate central retinal vein occlusion (CRVO).

Haematological pro-thrombotic factors are thought to be important in a minority, amplifying an atherosclerotic anatomical predisposition. Once venous occlusion has occurred, elevation of venous and capillary pressure with stagnation of blood flow ensues, resulting in retinal hypoxia, which in turn results in damage to the capillary endothelial cells, extravasation of blood constituents and liberation of mediators such as VEGF.

Risk factors

- **Age** is the most important factor; over 50% of cases occur in patients older than 65.
- **Hypertension** is present in two-thirds or more of RVO patients over the age of 50 years and in 25% of younger patients. It is most prevalent in patients with BRVO.
- **Hyperlipidaemia** is present in one-third or more of patients, irrespective of age.
- **Diabetes mellitus** is present in up to 15% of patients over 50 years of age overall. It is more prevalent in Asian and black patients, but uncommon in younger patients.
- **Glaucoma** and probably ocular hypertension are associated with a higher risk of CRVO and possibly BRVO.
- **Oral contraceptive pill.** In younger females the contraceptive pill is the most common underlying association, and probably should not be taken following RVO.
- **Smoking.** Current smoking may be associated with an increased incidence of RVO, though studies have shown inconsistent results.
- **Uncommon.** Dehydration, myeloproliferative disorders (e.g. myeloma, polycythaemia), thrombophilia (e.g. hyperhomocysteinaemia, antiphospholipid antibody syndrome, factor V Leiden mutation), inflammatory disease associated with occlusive periphlebitis (e.g. Behçet syndrome, sarcoidosis, Wegener granulomatosis), orbital disease and chronic renal failure.

Systemic assessment

The detection and management of associated systemic disease is aimed principally at reducing the risk of future vascular occlusive events, both ocular and systemic.

All patients

- **Blood pressure (BP).**
- **Erythrocyte sedimentation rate (ESR) or plasma viscosity (PV).**
- **Full blood count (FBC).**
- **Random blood glucose.** Further assessment for diabetes if indicated.
- **Random total and high-density lipoprotein (HDL) cholesterol.** Additional lipid testing may be considered.
- **Plasma protein electrophoresis.** To detect dysproteinaemias such as multiple myeloma.
- **Other tests.** Some authorities advocate routine investigation for systemic end-organ damage related to the cardiovascular risk factors commonly found in patients with RVO. This is

intended to help the prevention of further non-ocular damage, as well as facilitating systemic management to reduce the risk of recurrent ocular venous occlusion. Research is conflicting, some studies suggesting that cardio- and cerebrovascular mortality is not elevated above that of the general population in patients with RVO and others finding the converse.

- ○ Urea, electrolytes and creatinine to detect renal disease associated with hypertension; chronic renal failure is also a rare cause of RVO.
- ○ Thyroid function testing. There is a higher prevalence of thyroid disease in RVO patients.
- ○ Electrocardiography (ECG). Left ventricular hypertrophy is associated with hypertension.

Selected patients according to clinical indication

These tests might be considered in patients under the age of 50, in bilateral RVO, patients with previous thromboses or a family history of thrombosis, and some patients in whom investigation for the common associations is negative. Evidence of a causative link for many of these is limited.

- **Chest X-ray.** Sarcoidosis, tuberculosis, left ventricular hypertrophy in hypertension.
- **C-reactive protein (CRP).** Sensitive indicator of inflammation.
- **Plasma homocysteine level.** To exclude hyperhomocysteinaemia, for which there is reasonable evidence of an increased RVO risk.
- **'Thrombophilia screen'.** By convention this refers to heritable thrombophilias; tests might typically include thrombin time, prothrombin time and activated partial thromboplastin time, antithrombin functional assay, protein C, protein S, activated protein C resistance, factor V Leiden mutation, prothrombin G20210A mutation, lupus anticoagulant and anticardiolipin antibody (IgG and IgM); the last may be the most important of these.
- **Autoantibodies.** Rheumatoid factor, antinuclear antibody (ANA), anti-DNA antibody, antineutrophil cytoplasmic antibody (ANCA).
- **Serum angiotensin-converting enzyme (ACE).** Sarcoidosis.
- **Treponemal serology.** See Chapter 11.
- **Carotid duplex imaging** to exclude mimicking ocular ischaemic syndrome.

Branch retinal vein occlusion

Diagnosis

- **Symptoms** if the central macula is involved consist of the sudden painless onset of blurred vision and metamorphopsia. Peripheral occlusion may be asymptomatic.
- **VA** at presentation is very variable. Historically 50% of untreated eyes retain 6/12 or better in the long term, but about a quarter only achieve 6/60 or worse.

- **Iris** neovascularization (NVI) and neovascular glaucoma (NVG) are much less common in BRVO – 2–3% at 3 years – than in CRVO.
- **Fundus**
  - ○ Dilatation and tortuosity of the affected venous segment, with flame-shaped and dot/blot haemorrhages, principally in the retinal area drained by the thrombosed vein though an occasional haemorrhage may be identified elsewhere; cotton wool spots and retinal oedema may be absent but are often prominent (Fig. 13.27A).
  - ○ The superotemporal quadrant is most commonly affected.
  - ○ The site of occlusion may be identifiable as an arteriovenous crossing point.
  - ○ The acute features usually resolve within 6–12 months leaving venous sheathing and sclerosis, and variable persistent/recurrent haemorrhage (Fig. 13.27B); the severity of residual signs is highly variable.
  - ○ Collateral vessels may form near areas of limited capillary perfusion after weeks to months. They usually connect a poorly functioning to a normally functioning segment of the venous circulation, and typically appear as tortuous or looping channels. They may cross the horizontal raphe between the inferior and superior vascular arcades. The appearance of collaterals is associated with a better prognosis; ablation of collaterals should be avoided if laser is performed.
  - ○ Chronic macular oedema is the most common cause of persistent poor visual acuity after BRVO.
  - ○ Retinal neovascularization occurs in about 8% of eyes by three years; the risk is much higher in eyes with more than about 5 disc areas of non-perfusion on FA (over one-third of eyes). NVE are more common than NVD. NVE usually develop at the border of ischaemic retina drained by an occluded vein; they typically appear within 6–12 months but may develop at any time.
  - ○ Recurrent vitreous and preretinal haemorrhage, and occasionally tractional retinal detachment, can occur secondary to neovascularization.
- **FA** demonstrates peripheral and macular ischaemia (capillary non-perfusion, staining of vessel walls, vessel 'pruning' – small branches failing to fill – Fig. 13.27C), haemorrhage and oedema (Fig. 13.27D) with collateral vessels commonly forming in established cases (Fig. 13.27E). Venous filling is delayed. In late or subtle cases FA may be diagnostic.
- **OCT** allows quantification of macular oedema.

Management

Laser was formerly the standard of treatment for macular oedema in BRVO, but newer effective and relatively safe treatments are now available. However, the optimal regimen has not been ascertained, with investigation ongoing as to whether pharmacological treatments alone or in combination with laser, including novel modalities such as micropulse, carry the best risk/outcome profile.

- **Systemic assessment** should be carried out as above, with appropriate specialist referral when warranted.

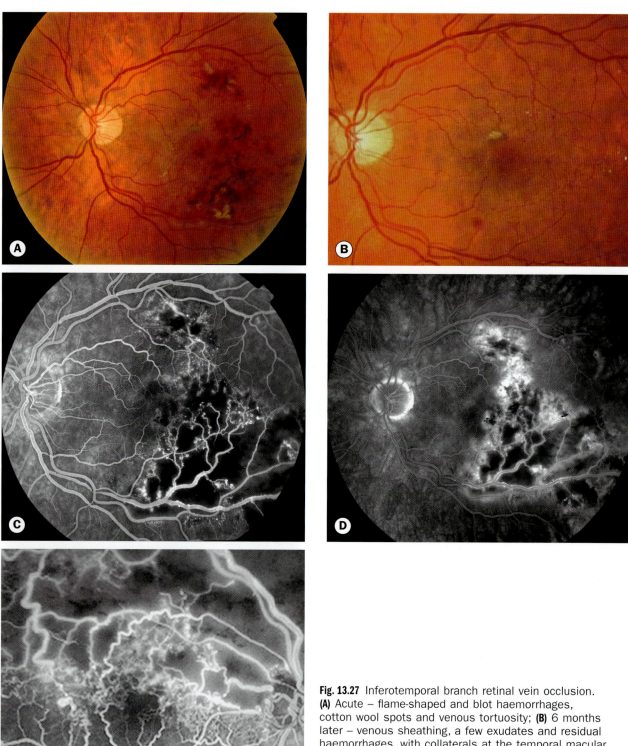

Fig. 13.27 Inferotemporal branch retinal vein occlusion.
(A) Acute – flame-shaped and blot haemorrhages, cotton wool spots and venous tortuosity; **(B)** 6 months later – venous sheathing, a few exudates and residual haemorrhages, with collaterals at the temporal macular edge; **(C)** early FA image of the acute occlusion principally showing capillary non-perfusion with some blockage by blood; **(D)** later image clearly demonstrates vessel wall staining, pruning and non-perfusion; **(E)** FA of chronic BRVO shows capillary non-perfusion, with tortuous superior–inferior collaterals temporally

(Courtesy of S Chen – figs A–D)

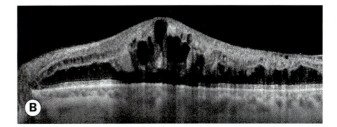

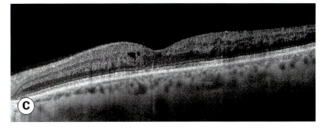

Fig. 13.28 Treatment of branch retinal vein occlusion. **(A)** Sector laser photocoagulation for neovascularization; **(B)** cystoid macular oedema before and **(C)** 4 weeks after bevacizumab intravitreal injection
(Courtesy of S Chen)

- **Observation** without intervention is usually indicated if visual acuity is 6/9 or better, or slightly worse but improving.
- **FA.** At 3 months, if visual acuity is 6/12 or worse, FA was conventionally performed to exclude substantial macular ischaemia prior to grid laser, though this may not be required before anti-VEGF treatment alone (see below).
- **NVE or NVD** are generally regarded as an indication for sector photocoagulation, though some authorities withhold treatment unless vitreous haemorrhage occurs because early intervention does not appear to affect the visual outcome. Burns of mild–moderate intensity, 400–500 μm actual diameter, 0.05 s duration and spaced one burn width apart are applied to the ischaemic area (Fig. 13.28A). FA can be used to confirm dubious NV if necessary, and to demonstrate ischaemic areas that might be specifically targeted with laser. Laser may be combined with 4–6 weekly intravitreal anti-VEGF injection.
- **NVI** is an indication for urgent sector PRP; secondary glaucoma is likely to be less aggressive than in CRVO. See Chapter 10 for the detailed management of NVG.
- **Intravitreal anti-VEGF agents** (Figs. 13.28B and C). These have been widely adopted for the treatment of macular oedema secondary to BRVO, and probably raise acuity more than laser (see below). There is also no requirement to wait for 3 months before commencing treatment. However, repeated injections are required. Combining intravitreal injections with laser may allow a reduction in the frequency of injections, but the optimal regimen is yet to be defined.
- **Intravitreal dexamethasone implant.** This confers visual improvement in BRVO substantially superior to observation alone. The treatment can be repeated after 4–6 months. Adverse effects include an increased glaucoma and cataract risk. As with anti-VEGF therapy, it may be used alone or in conjunction with laser.
- **Macular laser.** If visual acuity remains 6/12 or worse after 3–6 months due to macular oedema that is associated with

good central macular perfusion on FA, laser may be considered: 20–100 mild burns of diameter 50–100 μm and duration 0.01–0.05 s, concentrating on areas of leakage on FA; pulses at the shorter end of the duration range seem to inflict less damage to the retina whilst exerting an approximately comparable therapeutic effect. Treatment should not encroach within 0.5 disc diameters of the foveal centre. Retinal haemorrhages and blood vessels – especially collaterals – should not be treated. With the advent of intravitreal treatments, the threshold for macular laser has been raised, and it may be regarded as an adjunctive or combination modality.
- **Micropulse laser** may be as effective as conventional photocoagulation for macular oedema but inflicts considerably less retinal damage. Its onset of action is slower.
- **Intravitreal triamcinolone** in a preservative-free preparation is as effective as laser in eyes with macular oedema but has a less sustained effect and a relatively high rate of cataract formation and IOP elevation.
- **Periocular steroid injection** is less invasive than intravitreal, but almost certainly less effective.
- **Review** in cases that do not require early intervention should usually take place after 3 months and then at 3–6 monthly intervals for up to 2 years, principally to detect neovascularization.

Impending central retinal vein occlusion

Impending (partial) CRVO on average occurs in younger patients than those developing more severe occlusion; the prognosis is usually good but a proportion will deteriorate to ischaemic CRVO. The distinction between 'impending' and mild non-ischaemic CRVO (see below) is not clear, and may be artificial. Symptoms may be absent or consist of only minor or transient blurring that is characteristically worse on waking. On examination, there is mild retinal venous dilatation and tortuosity, with relatively few

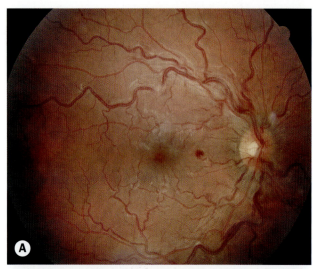

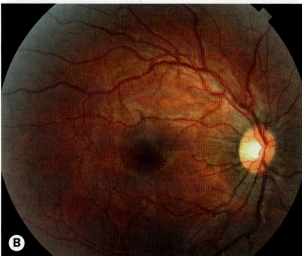

Fig. 13.29 Impending central retinal vein occlusion **(A)** before and **(B)** after spontaneous resolution

(Courtesy of S Chen)

small scattered dot and blot haemorrhages (Fig. 13.29); there may be mild macular oedema. Fundus autofluorescence (FAF) may reveal a fern-like perivenular appearance (see below), and FA generally demonstrates an impaired retinal circulation. Treatment is empirical, with lack of an established evidence base. Correcting any predisposing systemic conditions, avoiding dehydration, and lowering IOP to improve perfusion have been postulated. Antiplatelet agents, other anticoagulant measures and haemodilution are of no proven benefit, but may be considered in some cases.

Non-ischaemic central retinal vein occlusion

Diagnosis

Non-ischaemic CRVO, sometimes called 'venous stasis retinopathy' (also sometimes used to describe ocular ischaemic

syndrome – see later) is more common than the ischaemic form. Around a third will progress to ischaemic CRVO, often within months.

- **Symptoms.** A sudden painless monocular fall in vision.
- **VA** is impaired to a variable degree dependent on severity; eyes with initially good VA tend to have a good prognosis and vice versa; initial VA in the middle range (6/30–6/60) is an unreliable predictor of outcome. VA worse than 6/60 commonly indicates that substantial ischaemia is present. In cases that do not become ischaemic, vision returns to normal or near normal in about 50%.
- **Relative afferent pupillary defect (RAPD).** Absent or mild.
- **Fundus.** Signs are present in all quadrants.
  - Tortuosity and dilatation of all branches of the central retinal vein, with dot, blot and flame haemorrhages to a mild–moderate extent; cotton wool spots, optic disc and macular oedema are common but generally mild (Fig. 13.30A).
  - Patchy (or perivenular) ischaemic retinal whitening (PIRW) in a perivenular pattern at the posterior pole is an early sign occurring in younger patients with non-ischaemic CRVO (Fig. 13.30B).
  - Most acute signs resolve over 6–12 months; later findings are variable, depending on severity but may include: persistent scattered retinal haemorrhages; venous tortuosity, sheathing and sclerosis; epiretinal gliosis; macular pigmentary and atrophic changes; peripheral and optic disc collateral vessels (Fig. 13.30C).
  - The main cause of poor vision is chronic macular oedema and secondary atrophy.
  - Disc collaterals (see Fig. 13.30C) are common following CRVO, appearing as a small vascular loop on the optic nerve head. They are also known as optociliary shunts or retinochoroidal collaterals, and are thought to represent a compensatory circulation in response to impaired nerve perfusion; their development is believed to be associated with a markedly decreased risk of neovascularization. They can form in a range of conditions besides CRVO, including chronic glaucoma and chronic optic nerve compression.
- **FAF** in acute RVO may show a characteristic fern-like perivenular hypoautofluorescence due to masking of background signal by oedema; it corresponds to PIRW (see above) but is more commonly identifiable.
- **FA** shows delayed arteriovenous transit time, masking by haemorrhage, usually good retinal capillary perfusion and some late leakage (Fig. 13.30D).
- **OCT** is useful in the assessment of CMO, which is often mild in a non-ischaemic lesion (Fig. 13.30E).

Ischaemic central retinal vein occlusion

Ischaemic CRVO is characterized by substantially decreased retinal perfusion with capillary closure and retinal hypoxia. Macular ischaemia and NVG are the major causes of visual morbidity.

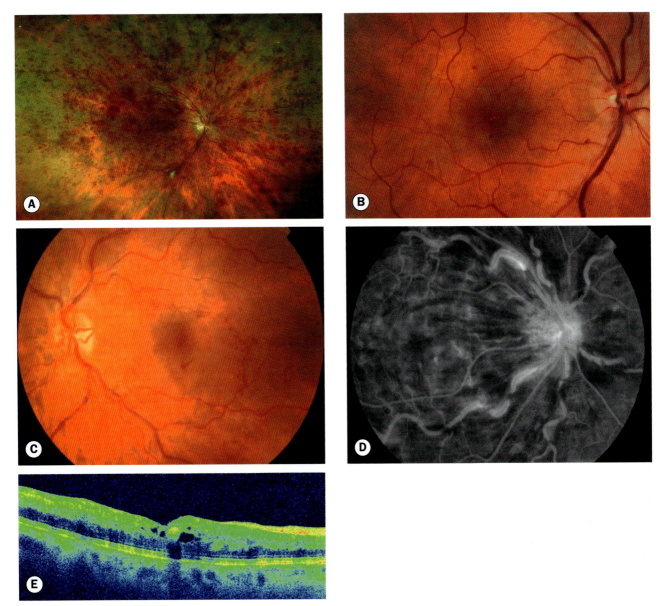

Fig. 13.30 Non-ischaemic central retinal vein occlusion (CRVO). **(A)** Acute – wide-field image showing venous tortuosity and dilatation, with moderate flame haemorrhages and at least one cotton wool spot; **(B)** young patient with mild non-ischaemic CRVO showing perivenular ischaemic retinal whitening (PIRW), particularly noticeable in the perifoveal region; **(C)** non-acute – disc collaterals and a few residual retinal haemorrhages; **(D)** FA late phase in a recent onset case shows masking by blood and staining of vessel walls but good capillary perfusion; **(E)** OCT showing mild cystoid macular oedema
(Courtesy of S Chen – figs A–C and E; Moorfields Eye Hospital – fig. D)

Diagnosis

- **Symptoms.** Sudden and severe monocular painless visual impairment. Occasionally presentation may be with pain, redness and photophobia due to neovascular glaucoma, a prior reduction in vision having passed unnoticed or been ignored.
- **VA** is usually CF or worse; the visual prognosis is generally extremely poor due to macular ischaemia.
- **RAPD** is present.
- **NVI.** Rubeosis iridis (Fig. 13.31A) develops in about 50% of eyes, usually between 2 and 4 months ('hundred-day

glaucoma'), and there is a high risk of neovascular glaucoma. The pupillary margin should be examined at each review prior to pharmacological mydriasis.
- **Gonioscopy.** Angle neovascularization (Fig. 13.31B) may occur in the absence of neovascularization at the pupillary margin. Routine gonioscopy should therefore be performed at each review, again prior to pupillary dilatation.
- **Fundus**
  ○ Severe tortuosity and engorgement of all branches of the central retinal vein. There are extensive deep blot and flame-shaped haemorrhages involving the peripheral and posterior retina and cotton wool spots are typically

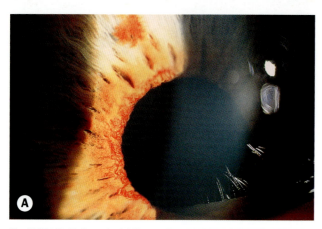
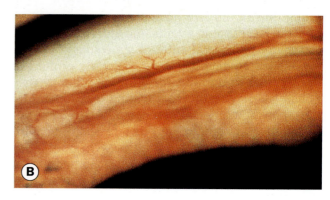

Fig. 13.31 (A) Rubeosis iridis at the pupillary border; **(B)** neovascularization of an open angle
(Courtesy of E Michael van Buskirk, from Clinical Atlas of Glaucoma, WB Saunders 1986 – fig. B)

prominent. There is usually optic disc swelling and hyperaemia (Fig. 13.32A).

○ Most acute signs resolve over 9–12 months. The macula may develop atrophic retinal and RPE changes, RPE hyperplasia, epiretinal membrane and chronic CMO. Rarely, subretinal fibrosis resembling that associated with exudative age-related macular degeneration may develop.

○ Retinal neovascularization occurs in about 5% of eyes – much less commonly than with BRVO, but severe vitreous haemorrhage can occur, obscuring vision and preventing retinal laser.

○ Optic disc collaterals (opticociliary shunts – see under non-ischaemic CRVO) are common and may protect the eye from anterior and posterior segment neovascularization; their development (Fig. 13.32B) probably indicates a dramatic reduction in the risk of this complication.

- **FA** shows a marked delay in arteriovenous transit time, masking by retinal haemorrhages, extensive areas of capillary non-perfusion and vessel wall staining and leakage (Figs 13.32C and D). The presence of more than 10 disc areas of retinal capillary non-perfusion is associated with a substantially increased risk of neovascularization.
- **OCT** enables quantification of CMO.
- **Electroretinogram (ERG)** is depressed and the extent of this has sometimes been used to assess neovascular risk.

Hemiretinal vein occlusion

Hemiretinal vein occlusion is regarded as a variant of CRVO by some authorities and may be ischaemic or non-ischaemic. It is less common than either BRVO or CRVO and involves occlusion of the superior or inferior branch of the central retinal vein (CRV). A *hemispheric* occlusion blocks a major branch of the CRV at or near the optic disc. The less common *hemicentral* occlusion involves one trunk of a dual-trunked CRV that has persisted in the anterior part of the optic nerve head as a congenital variant.

Prognosis depends on the severity of retinal ischaemia, but management has been less well studied than BRVO and CRVO. Extensive retinal ischaemia implies a risk of neovascular glaucoma and should be managed in the same way as ischaemic CRVO (see

below), otherwise management, particularly of macular oedema, may be as for BRVO.

Diagnosis

- **Symptoms.** A sudden onset altitudinal visual field defect (Fig. 13.33A).
- **VA** reduction is variable.
- **NVI** is more common than in BRVO but less than in CRVO.
- **Fundus** shows the features of BRVO, involving the superior or inferior retinal hemisphere (Fig. 13.33B). NVD may be more common than in either CRVO or BRVO.
- **FA** shows masking by haemorrhages, hyperfluorescence due to leakage and variable capillary non-perfusion (Fig. 13.33C).

Treatment of the complications of CRVO

The management of non-ischaemic CRVO is generally much less aggressive than ischaemic CRVO, so it is important to distinguish the two as far as possible.

- **Systemic assessment** as described above is essential, followed by appropriate systemic management (discussed below).
- **Treatment of macular oedema.** Treatment is generally indicated for VA worse than 6/9 and/or with significant central macular thickening (e.g. >250 μm) on OCT, but is unlikely to be of benefit if 6/120 or worse. Intravitreal anti-VEGF agents or dexamethasone implant are the current standard of care.

○ Intravitreal anti-VEGF agents (e.g. ranibizumab 0.5 mg) may initially be given monthly for 6 months and subsequently less intensively, with typically a two- to three-line gain in VA. As with age-related macular degeneration, initial research suggests that aflibercept may facilitate less frequent administration for an equivalent effect.

○ Intravitreal dexamethasone implant. The GENEVA trial of a sustained-release biodegradable dexamethasone intravitreal implant (Ozurdex®) showed substantial visual and anatomical (Figs 13.34A–D) improvement over the first 2 months following a single implantation, and

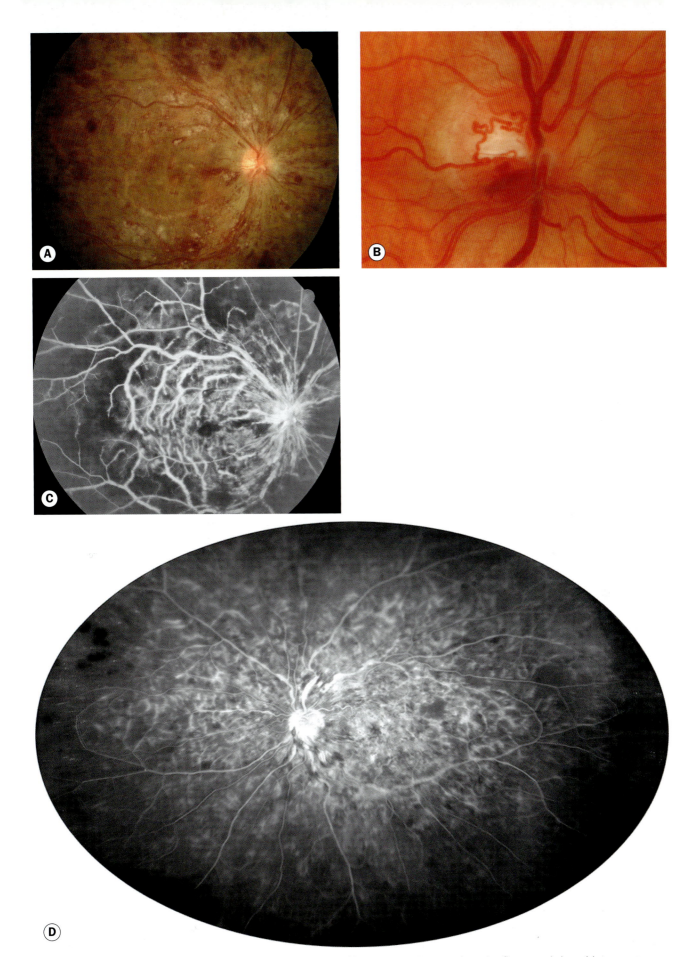

Fig. 13.32 Recent ischaemic central retinal vein occlusion. **(A)** Numerous cotton wool spots, flame and deep blot haemorrhages; **(B)** opticociliary shunt; **(C)** FA of (A) shows extensive hypofluorescence due to capillary non-perfusion; **(D)** wide-field FA showing extensive peripheral ischaemia

(Courtesy of S Chen – figs A, C and D; C Barry – fig. B)

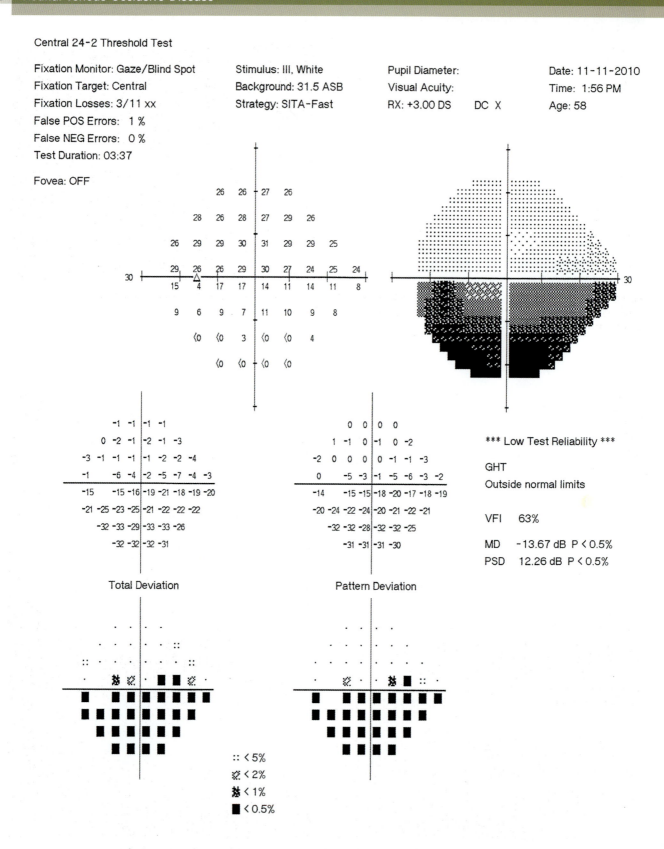

Central 24-2 Threshold Test

Fixation Monitor: Gaze/Blind Spot
Fixation Target: Central
Fixation Losses: 3/11 xx
False POS Errors: 1 %
False NEG Errors: 0 %
Test Duration: 03:37

Fovea: OFF

Stimulus: III, White
Background: 31.5 ASB
Strategy: SITA-Fast

Pupil Diameter:
Visual Acuity:
RX: +3.00 DS   DC X

Date: 11-11-2010
Time: 1:56 PM
Age: 58

Total Deviation

Pattern Deviation

*** Low Test Reliability ***

GHT
Outside normal limits

VFI   63%

MD   -13.67 dB P < 0.5%
PSD   12.26 dB P < 0.5%

:: < 5%
▧ < 2%
▨ < 1%
■ < 0.5%

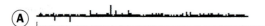

Fig. 13.33 (A) Inferior altitudinal visual field defect due to a superior hemiretinal vein occlusion;

Continued

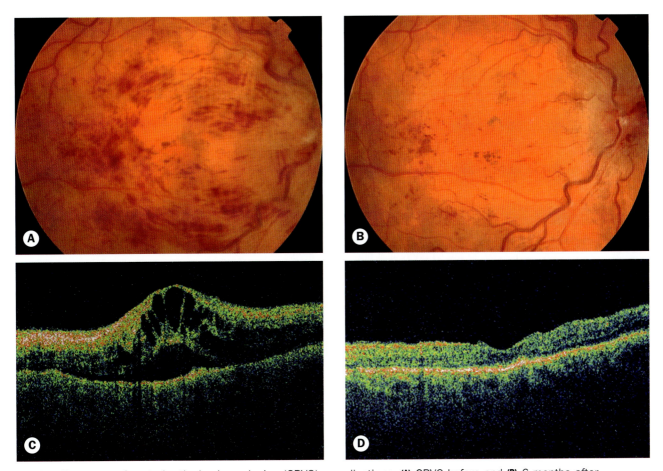

Fig. 13.33, Continued (B) inferior hemiretinal vein occlusion; **(C)** FA late phase shows extensive hypofluorescence due to capillary non-perfusion, with mild perivascular hyperfluorescence

(Courtesy of S Chen – fig. A; C Barry – figs B and C)

Fig. 13.34 Treatment of central retinal vein occlusion (CRVO) complications. **(A)** CRVO before and **(B)** 6 months after intravitreal dexamethasone implant; **(C)** and **(D)** corresponding macular OCT images;

Continued

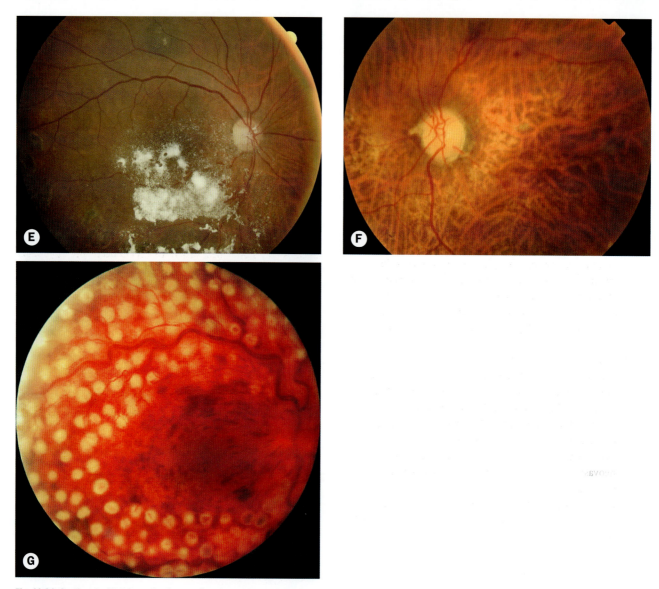

Fig. 13.34, Continued **(E)** triamcinolone after intravitreal administration; **(F)** a radial optic neurotomy incision site is visible on the nasal side of the optic nerve head; **(G)** panretinal photocoagulation

(Courtesy of S Chen – figs A–F)

although this declined to baseline by 6 months the treatment could then be repeated. As with triamcinolone, there was a slightly higher rate of IOP elevation and cataract. Administration within 90 days of CMO onset is likely to be associated with a better outcome. Treatment can be repeated after 4–6 months.

- Intravitreal triamcinolone (Fig. 13.34E). The SCORE study showed an improvement of three or more lines of vision at one year in over 25% of patients (versus 7% of controls) treated with an average of two injections of 1 mg triamcinolone, using a preservative-free preparation developed for intraocular use. There was a slightly higher rate of IOP elevation and cataract than with observation.
- Laser photocoagulation. Although macular oedema is anatomically improved, laser is typically not beneficial for visual outcome, except in some younger patients.

- Investigational treatments include chorioretinal anastomosis, vitrectomy with radial optic neurotomy (Fig. 13.34F) and local recombinant tissue plasminogen activator (rtPA) CRV infusion.

- **Treatment of neovascularization**
  - Panretinal photocoagulation (PRP) should be performed without delay in eyes with NVI or angle neovascularization. This initially involves placing 1500–2000 burns of 0.5–0.1 s duration, spaced one burn width apart, with sufficient energy to produce a pale to moderate reaction, avoiding areas of haemorrhage (Fig. 13.34G). Treatment may be fractionated, and further photocoagulation is commonly required.
  - Intravitreal anti-VEGF injections are commonly administered adjunctively every 6 weeks until the eye stabilizes, and lead to more rapid resolution of new

vessels than PRP alone. If intravitreal treatment is administered first, a delay of a few days is probably prudent to avoid contaminating the fresh injection site. VEGF inhibitors are likely to be of lower value if synechial angle closure is present.

- The management of NVG is discussed in Chapter 10.
- Vitreous haemorrhage may respond to intravitreal anti-VEGF – research is limited – but definitive treatment is with vitrectomy and endolaser.

- **Review**
  - Ischaemic CRVO. Where possible, patients with ischaemic CRVO should be seen monthly for 6 months with a view to the early detection of anterior segment neovascularization. Prophylactic PRP is generally not recommended even with marked ischaemia unless iris new vessels develop, though may be considered in patients unlikely to attend scheduled review. Subsequent monitoring should usually be for up to 2 years to detect significant ischaemia and macular oedema; once a disc collateral has developed, the risk of neovascularization is probably much lower.
  - Non-ischaemic CRVO. In a clearly non-ischaemic occlusion, initial follow-up should take place after 3 months. Structured arrangements for review of test results should be in place. The patient should be instructed to make contact if the vision deteriorates as this may indicate the development of significant ischaemia. Pain or redness, which may indicate neovascular glaucoma and occasionally inflammation without rubeosis, should also be reported. Subsequent review is dependent on the clinical picture and any treatment, with discharge from follow-up usually taking place at 18–24 months.

Systemic management in retinal vein occlusion

- **Control of systemic risk factors.** Although there is no conclusive evidence that vascular mortality is higher in RVO patients, independently important cardiovascular risk factors are very commonly identified during investigation following RVO. Addressing these as appropriate is critical, and as well as conferring systemic benefit this may also reduce the risk of the recurrence of retinal vein occlusion. Smoking should be strongly discouraged.
- **Antiplatelet therapy.** The role of aspirin or alternative antiplatelet agents in reducing the risk of further retinal venous occlusion is unclear and they are generally not prescribed unless systemically indicated.
- **Hormone replacement therapy (HRT).** The risk of HRT remains undefined. Most authorities would avoid commencing oestrogen-containing HRT following RVO, though depending on indication and other circumstances it may be appropriate to continue if already taking this. Appropriate expert advice should be obtained; the presence of other thrombophilia risk factors is associated with a

substantially increased risk of systemic venous thrombosis in conjunction with HRT.
- **Oral contraceptive pill.** This should probably be discontinued following RVO.
- **Others.** A range of systemic treatment modalities (e.g. isovolaemic haemodilution, plasmapheresis, recombinant tissue plasminogen infusion) has been employed to try to improve visual outcomes in RVO, but clear evidence for benefit is lacking. Dehydration should be avoided.

Papillophlebitis

Papillophlebitis is an uncommon poorly defined condition that typically affects individuals under the age of 50 years who may have a higher prevalence of hypertension and diabetes. Some or all cases may simply be a variant of CRVO occurring in younger people, though optic disc swelling or inflammation of the central retinal vein have been speculated as the initiating event in at least some instances. There is likely to be some diagnostic overlap with diabetic papillopathy. Papillophlebitis typically causes only mild to moderate reduction of vision with no RAPD, and has a generally good prognosis. Disc oedema is the dominant finding, and retinal haemorrhages and other signs such as cotton wool spots are predominantly peripapillary and confined to the posterior pole (Fig. 13.35). CMO may be present, and posterior or anterior segment neovascularization have been reported occasionally in concert with capillary non-perfusion on FA. It may be bilateral, when raised intracranial pressure must be ruled out. Investigation should probably be as for CRVO in a young individual; distinction from diabetic papillopathy may be difficult. Treatment with intravitreal anti-VEGF or steroid has been reported.

RETINAL ARTERIAL OCCLUSIVE DISEASE

Aetiology

The outer retina is supplied by the ciliary arteries via the choriocapillaris and the inner retina by the central retinal artery (CRA).

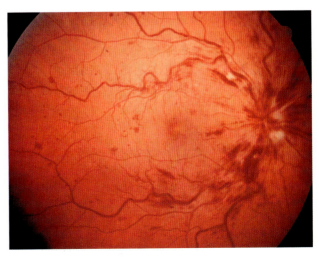

Fig. 13.35 Papillophlebitis

The ophthalmic artery gives rise to both the CRA – its first branch – and the ciliary arteries; the latter also supply the anterior segment via the rectus muscles. Atherosclerosis-related embolism and thrombosis are thought to be responsible for the majority of cases of retinal artery occlusion, but the proportion of cases due to each of these is unknown. Inflammation in or around the vessel wall (e.g. giant cell arteritis – GCA, systemic lupus erythematosus, Wegener granulomatosis, polyarteritis nodosa), vasospasm (e.g. migraine) and systemic hypotension contribute in a minority. The origin of emboli is most commonly an atheromatous carotid plaque; the ophthalmic artery is the first branch of the internal carotid artery, so embolic material has an easy route to the eye. Emboli can be refractile yellow–white cholesterol (Hollenhorst) plaques (Fig. 13.36A), greyish elongated fibrin-platelet aggregates (Fig. 13.36B), non-scintillating white calcific particles (Fig. 13.36C), and rarely vegetations from bacterial endocarditis, cardiac myxomatous material, fat and others. Thrombophilic disorders that may be associated with retinal artery occlusion (one-third of young patients) include hyperhomocysteinaemia, antiphospholipid antibody syndrome and inherited defects of various natural anticoagulants. Sickling haemoglobinopathies and Susac syndrome (retinocochleocerebral vasculopathy), a microangiopathy characterized by the triad of retinal artery occlusion, sensorineural deafness and encephalopathy, are other rare associations.

Systemic assessment

Following diagnosis and initial evaluation by an ophthalmologist many elements of the assessment may be carried out by a specialist stroke team. Urgent specialist vascular evaluation, typically within 24 hours, is rapidly becoming the standard of care following a retinal arterial event, including amaurosis fugax; the risk of a stroke is relatively high in the first few days after a transient ischaemic attack (TIA). The detection of atrial fibrillation is of particular importance as admission for anticoagulation may be indicated.

All patients

Many or most patients will already be aware of vascular risk factors and/or disease.

- **Smoking** should be enquired about.
- **Symptoms of GCA** (1–2% of central retinal artery occlusion – CRAO) such as headache, jaw claudication, scalp tenderness, limb girdle pain, weight loss and existing polymyalgia rheumatica (see Ch. 19). GCA is extremely unlikely under 55–60 years. It constitutes an ophthalmic emergency.
- **Pulse** should be palpated to detect arrhythmia, particularly atrial fibrillation.
- **Blood pressure.**
- **Cardiac auscultation** for a murmur.
- **Carotid auscultation** is of limited value as the absence of a bruit does not exclude significant stenosis.
- **ECG** to detect arrhythmia and other cardiac disease.
- **ESR or PV,** and **CRP** to identify possible GCA.

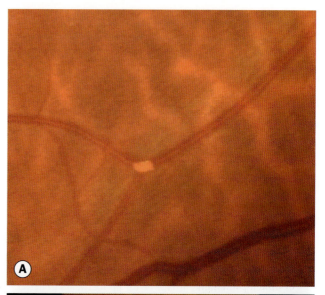

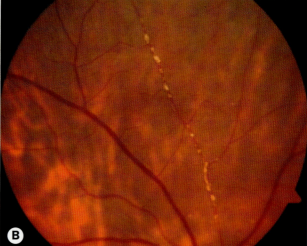

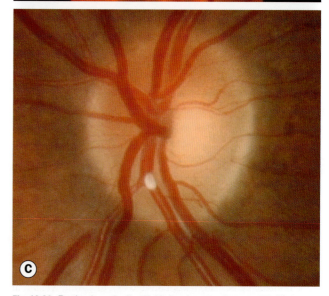

Fig. 13.36 Retinal emboli. **(A)** Hollenhorst plaque; **(B)** fibrin-platelet emboli; **(C)** calcific embolus at the disc
(Courtesy of L Merin – fig. A; S Chen – fig. B; C Barry – fig. C)

- **Other blood tests** include FBC (platelets may be raised in GCA), glucose, lipids, and urea and electrolytes, the latter to exclude derangement including dehydration.
- **Carotid duplex scanning** is a non-invasive screening test involving a combination of high-resolution real-time ultrasonography with Doppler flow analysis. If significant stenosis is present, surgical management may be considered.

Selected patients

The following additional tests can be considered on a targeted basis in some patients, particularly if younger and with no known cardiovascular risk factors, or there is an atypical clinical picture (Fig. 13.37).

- **Further carotid imaging** (see Ch. 19).
- **Cranial magnetic resonance imaging (MRI) or computed tomography (CT)** may be indicated to rule out intracranial or orbital pathology.
- **Echocardiography.** Usually performed in young patients or if there is a specific indication such as a history of rheumatic fever, known cardiac valvular disease, or intravenous drug use.
- **Chest X-ray.** Sarcoidosis, tuberculosis, left ventricular hypertrophy in hypertension.
- **24-hour ECG** to exclude intermittent arrhythmia.
- **Additional blood tests**
  - Fasting plasma homocysteine level to exclude hyperhomocysteinaemia.
  - 'Thrombophilia screen'. By convention refers to heritable thrombophilias, which have predominantly been implicated in venous rather than arterial thromboses.
  - Plasma protein electrophoresis to detect dysproteinaemias such as multiple myeloma.
  - Thyroid function tests, especially if atrial fibrillation is present; may be associated with dyslipidaemia.
  - Autoantibodies. Rheumatoid factor, anticardiolipin antibody, antinuclear antibody, anti-double stranded DNA antibodies, principally looking for vasculitis in younger patients.
  - Syphilis serology.
  - Blood cultures.

Amaurosis fugax

Amaurosis fugax is characterized by transient monocular loss of vision, often described as a curtain coming down over the eye; the absence of pain may be included in the definition. The Amaurosis Fugax Study Group divided the causes into five categories (embolic, hemodynamic, ocular, neurologic and idiopathic), but in clinical practice it is typically used to refer to transient visual loss of embolic origin. It is common for patients to be unaware of whether transient unilateral visual loss affects one eye or the ipsilateral hemifield of both, the latter indicating cerebral rather than more anterior ischaemia. Embolic visual loss, which may be complete, usually lasts a few minutes. Recovery is generally in the same pattern as the loss, although usually more gradual. Frequency of

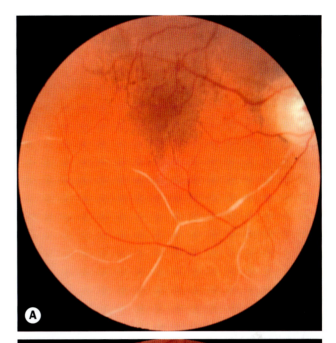

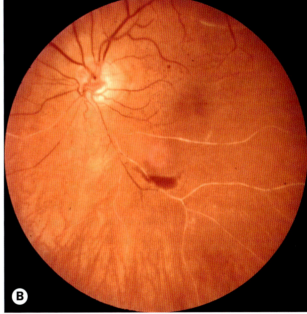

Fig. 13.37 (A) and **(B)** Multiple bilateral branch retinal artery occlusions in polyarteritis nodosa

attacks may vary from several times a day to once every few months. The attacks may sometimes be accompanied by an ipsilateral cerebral TIA, with contralateral neurological features. Investigation and systemic management of embolic-pattern amaurosis fugax is the same as that of retinal arterial occlusion and should be undertaken similarly urgently due to the high risk of stroke.

Branch retinal artery occlusion

- **Symptoms.** Sudden and profound painless altitudinal or sectoral visual field loss. Branch retinal artery occlusion

(BRAO) can sometimes go unnoticed, particularly if central vision is spared.

- **VA** is variable. In patients where central vision is severely compromised, the prognosis is commonly poor unless the obstruction is relieved within a few hours (see below).
- **RAPD** is often present.
- **Fundus** signs may be subtle (Figs 13.38A, B and D).
  ○ Attenuation of arteries and veins with sludging and segmentation of the blood column ('cattle trucking/boxcarring').
  ○ Cloudy white oedematous (ground glass) retina corresponding to the area of ischaemia.
  ○ One or more occluding emboli may be seen, especially at bifurcation points.
  ○ The affected artery is likely to remain attenuated. Occasionally, recanalization may leave absent ophthalmoscopic signs.
- **Visual field testing** confirms the defect, which rarely recovers.
- **FA** shows delay in arterial filling and hypofluorescence of the involved segment due to blockage of background fluorescence by retinal swelling (Figs 13.38C and E).
- **Review** in 3 months is warranted to review the appearance of the fundus, the visual fields, provide advice on prognosis and confirm that systemic management has been carried out appropriately.

Central retinal artery occlusion

- **Symptoms.** Sudden profound loss of vision, painless except in GCA.
- **VA** is severely reduced except if a cilioretinal artery supplying a critical macular area preserves central vision (see below). Absence of light perception usually indicates either GCA or ophthalmic artery occlusion. The prognosis is poor in all cases unless recovery occurs in the first few hours.
- **RAPD** is profound, sometimes total (amaurotic pupil).
- **Fundus** shows similar changes to BRAO but involving all retinal quadrants (Fig. 13.39A).
  ○ The orange reflex from the intact choroid stands out at the thin foveola, in contrast to the surrounding pale retina, giving rise to a 'cherry-red spot' appearance.
  ○ The peripapillary retina may appear especially swollen and opaque.
  ○ An occasional small haemorrhage is not unusual.
  ○ Emboli are visible in 20%, when Nd:YAG embolysis may be considered (see below).
  ○ In eyes with a cilioretinal artery part of the macula will remain of normal colour (Fig. 13.39B).
  ○ Retinal signs can sometimes be subtle; retinal oedema may take several hours to develop.
  ○ Over a few days to weeks the retinal cloudiness and 'cherry-red spot' gradually disappear although the arteries remain attenuated. Later signs include optic atrophy, vessel sheathing and patchy inner retinal atrophy and RPE changes (Fig. 13.39C).

○ Around 2% of eyes with CRAO develop retinal or disc neovascularization.
○ Rubeosis iridis may occur in up to about 1 in 5 eyes, typically earlier than in CRVO (4–5 weeks compared with 3 months, though sometimes later), and along with very poor vision may indicate ophthalmic artery occlusion.
- **OCT** may show a highly reflective embolic plaque within the superficial optic nerve head.
- **FA** shows a variable delay in arterial filling and masking of background choroidal fluorescence by retinal oedema. A patent cilioretinal artery will fill during the early phase (Fig. 13.39D).
- **Electroretinography** may be helpful to establish the diagnosis if in doubt, particularly to distinguish from optic nerve disease, typically when signs are subtle; a diminished b-wave is present.
- **Review.** The patient should be seen by an ophthalmologist after 3–4 weeks and a minimum of twice subsequently at monthly intervals in order to detect incipient neovascularization, particularly of the anterior segment. In this event, PRP should be performed as for ischaemic CRVO, and intravitreal injection of VEGF inhibitor might be considered. Appropriate systemic management is critical.

Cilioretinal artery occlusion

A cilioretinal artery is present in 15–50% of eyes, providing the central macula with a second arterial supply derived from the posterior ciliary circulation. Its main importance is that when present it may facilitate preservation of central vision following central retinal artery occlusion, provided the fovea is supplied.

- **Isolated.** This (Figs 13.40A and B) is rare; it may occur in young patients with an associated systemic vasculitis.
- **Combined with CRVO.** This (Fig. 13.40C) is not uncommon; occlusion is transient and the prognosis is better than in isolated cilioretinal artery occlusion.
- **Combined with anterior ischaemic optic neuropathy** (Fig. 13.40D), typically affects patients with GCA and carries a very poor prognosis.

Treatment of acute retinal artery occlusion

Retinal artery occlusion is an emergency because it causes irreversible visual loss unless the retinal circulation is re-established prior to the development of retinal infarction. Theoretically, timely dislodgement of thrombus or emboli may ameliorate subsequent visual loss. The following treatments may be tried in patients with occlusions of less than 24–48 hours' duration at presentation, though evidence of benefit is limited. The number of measures tried and the intensity of treatment should be tailored to the individual (more aggressive if lower duration of occlusion, good general health, monocularity; more aggressive systemic treatment may be avoided in the frail elderly); options, including the lack of

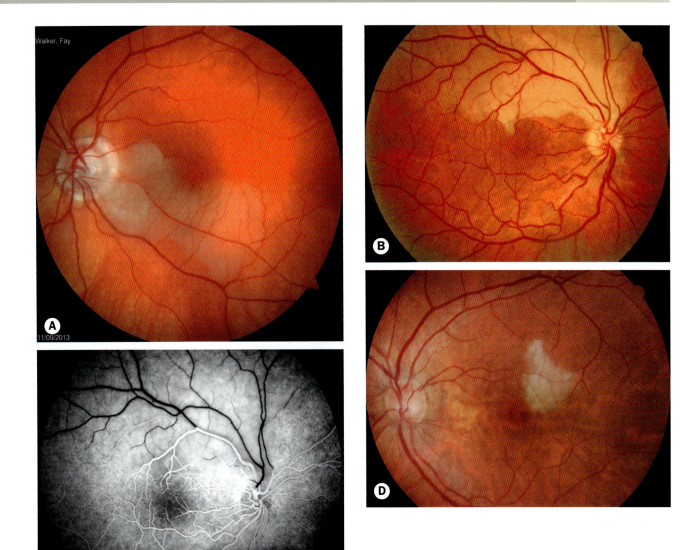

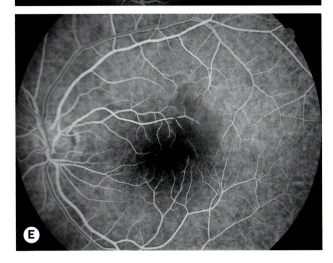

Fig. 13.38 Embolic branch retinal artery occlusions.
(A) Inferotemporal occlusion – embolus visible over the disc;
(B) superior branch retinal artery occlusion due an embolus
at the disc; **(C)** FA shows lack of arterial filling of the
involved artery and hypofluorescence of the involved
segment due to blockage of background fluorescence by
retinal swelling; **(D)** small macular branch artery occlusion;
(E) FA of (D)

(Courtesy of C Barry – figs B and C; S Chen – figs D and E)

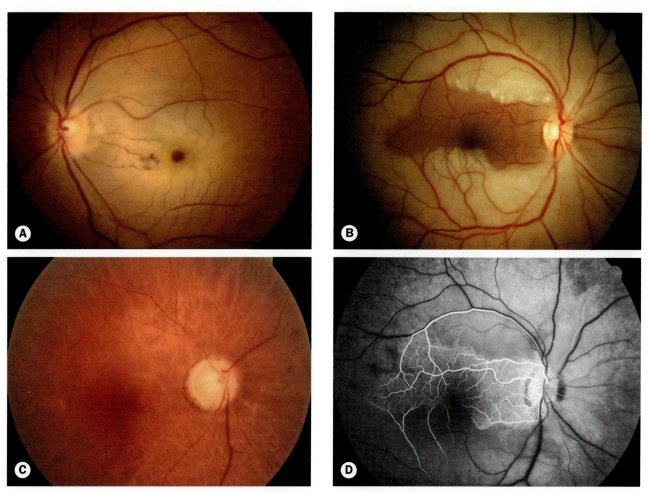

Fig. 13.39 Central retinal artery occlusion (CRAO). **(A)** Recent CRAO with a 'cherry-red spot' at the macula; **(B)** CRAO with a patent cilioretinal artery; **(C)** posterior pole appearance several months after onset; **(D)** FA shows blockage of background fluorescence by retinal oedema but normal perfusion of a sector of retina in the eye in (B)

(Courtesy of S Chen – fig. A; L Merin – figs B and D)

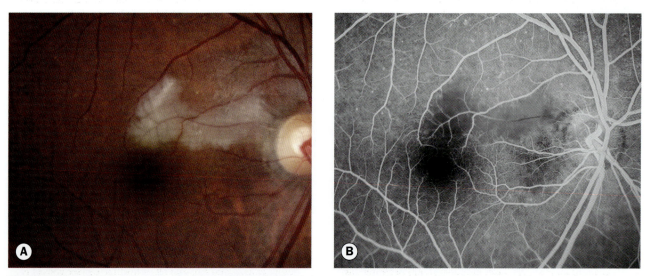

Fig. 13.40 Cilioretinal artery occlusion. **(A)** Isolated; **(B)** FA of the eye in (A) shows hypofluorescence in the affected area due to reduced filling and masking by retinal oedema;

Continued

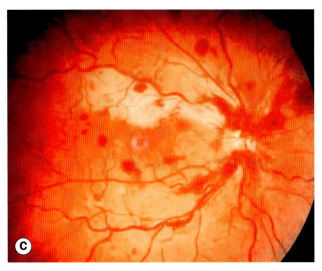
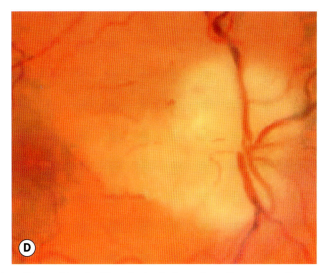

Fig. 13.40, Continued **(C)** combined with central retinal vein occlusion; **(D)** combined with anterior ischaemic optic neuropathy
(Courtesy of S Chen – figs A and B)

evidence for clear benefit and the risks, should be discussed before use.

- **Adoption of a supine posture** might improve ocular perfusion and should always be implemented.
- **Ocular massage** using a three-mirror contact lens (allows direct artery visualization). The aim is to mechanically collapse the arterial lumen and cause prompt changes in arterial flow, improving perfusion and potentially dislodging an embolus or thrombus. One described method consists of positive pressure for 10–15 seconds followed by release, continued for 3–5 minutes. Self-massage through closed eyelids can be continued by the patient.
- **Anterior chamber paracentesis** using a 27-gauge needle to withdraw 0.1–0.2 ml of aqueous is controversial but has been advocated by some authorities. Povidone-iodine 5% and topical antibiotic are instilled a few minutes prior to the procedure, with a short course of antibiotic afterwards. It may be prudent for ocular massage to be avoided following paracentesis.
- **Topical apraclonidine 1%, timolol 0.5% and intravenous acetazolamide 500 mg** to achieve a more sustained lowering of intraocular pressure.
- **Sublingual isosorbide dinitrate** to induce vasodilatation.
- **'Rebreathing'** into a paper bag in order to elevate blood carbon dioxide and respiratory acidosis has been advocated, as this may promote vasodilatation.
- **Breathing a high oxygen (95%) and carbon dioxide (5%) mixture,** 'carbogen', has been advocated for a possible dual effect of retarding ischaemia and vasodilatation.
- **Hyperosmotic agents.** Mannitol or glycerol have been used for their possibly more rapid IOP-lowering effect as well as increased intravascular volume.
- **Transluminal Nd:YAG laser embolysis/embolectomy** has been advocated for BRAO or CRAO in which an occluding embolus is visible; shots of 0.5–1.0 mJ or higher are applied

directly to the embolus using a fundus contact lens. Embolectomy has been said to occur if the embolus is ejected into the vitreous via a hole in the arteriole. The number of shots described in reports is extremely variable. The main complication is vitreous haemorrhage; pressure on the globe may curtail bleeding.

- **Thrombolysis.** Extrapolating from successful treatment of stroke and myocardial infarction, various strategies have been used to deliver thrombolytic agents to the ophthalmic artery, including local arterial (internal carotid and ophthalmic) and intravenous infusion. A recent large trial of local intra-arterial fibrinolysis with recombinant tissue plasminogen activator (rtPA) showed no benefit over conservative treatment that included isovolaemic haemodilution, with a nearly 40% adverse reaction rate in the rtPA group. It has been speculated that this may reflect very early loss of retinal viability, and perhaps the resistance to dissolution of embolic, versus thrombotic, obstruction.

Systemic management following retinal arterial occlusion

The risk of stroke is relatively high in the first few days following retinal artery occlusion or amaurosis fugax, and as discussed above, 'fast-track' referral to a specialist stroke clinic is advisable.

- **General risk factors** as discussed above should be addressed and smoking should be discontinued. Urgent referral to an appropriate physician is mandatory for significant cardiac arrhythmia.
- **Antiplatelet therapy** is commenced provided there are no contraindications; an immediate loading dose of 600 mg may be given; alternative/additional agents include dipyridamole and clopidogrel. If fibrinolysis (see above) is being considered, this should be discussed with a physician prior to starting antiplatelet treatment.

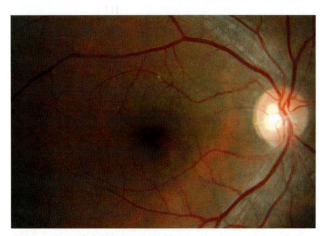

Fig. 13.41 Asymptomatic retinal embolus

- **Oral anticoagulation** (e.g. warfarin) may be prescribed for some patients, particularly those with atrial fibrillation.
- **Carotid endarterectomy** may be indicated in patients with symptomatic stenosis greater than 70%.

Asymptomatic retinal embolus

It is not uncommon to identify a retinal embolus on routine examination of an asymptomatic older patient (Fig. 13.41). This indicates a substantially increased risk of stroke and ischaemic heart disease, and management should consist of evaluation and treatment of risk factors discussed above. A higher threshold for carotid surgery is appropriate.

OCULAR ISCHAEMIC SYNDROME

Introduction

Ocular ischaemic syndrome (OIS) results from chronic ocular hypoperfusion secondary to severe (more than 90%) ipsilateral atherosclerotic carotid stenosis. It typically affects older patients and may be associated with diabetes, hypertension, cardio- and cerebrovascular disease. The male:female ratio is about 2:1. Five-year mortality is around 40%, most frequently from cardiac disease. OIS, along with non-ischaemic CRVO, is sometimes termed 'venous stasis retinopathy' but it may be prudent to avoid this term.

Diagnosis

OIS is unilateral in 80%. The signs are variable and may be subtle such that the condition is missed or misdiagnosed.

- **Symptoms.** Gradual loss of vision over weeks or months although occasionally loss may be sudden or intermittent (amaurosis fugax). Ocular and periocular pain may also be present (40%). Patients may notice unusually persistent after-images, or worsening of vision with sudden exposure to bright light ('bright light amaurosis fugax'), with slow adaptation. The prognosis for vision is often very poor, though patients with better acuity at presentation are more

likely to retain this. About 25% will deteriorate to light perception by the end of 1 year.
- **Anterior segment**
  - Diffuse episcleral injection and corneal oedema.
  - Aqueous flare with few cells (ischaemic pseudo-iritis).
  - Iris atrophy with a mid-dilated, poorly reacting pupil.
  - Rubeosis iridis is common, developing in up to 90%, and often progresses to neovascular glaucoma; the IOP may remain low due to poor ocular perfusion.
  - Cataract in advanced cases.
- **Fundus**
  - Venous dilatation, arteriolar narrowing, deep round and flame haemorrhages and occasionally disc oedema (Fig. 13.42A) and cotton wool spots.
  - Proliferative retinopathy with NVD and occasionally NVE.
  - Spontaneous arterial pulsation, most pronounced near the optic disc, is present in most cases or may be easily induced by exerting gentle pressure on the globe (digital ophthalmodynamometry).
  - Macular oedema can occur.
  - In diabetic patients retinopathy may be more severe ipsilateral to carotid stenosis.
- **FA.** Delayed choroidal filling and prolonged arteriovenous transit is the major feature; non-perfusion, vessel wall staining and retinal oedema may also be evident (Figs 13.42B–D).
- **Carotid imaging** may involve duplex ultrasonography, digital subtraction angiography, MR or CT angiography.

Management

- **Anterior segment inflammation** is treated with topical steroid and a mydriatic as appropriate.
- **Neovascular glaucoma** is managed medically or surgically (see Ch. 10).
- **Proliferative retinopathy** can be treated with PRP although the outcome is considerably less certain than in proliferative diabetic retinopathy. Intravitreal anti-VEGF agents may be beneficial.
- **Macular oedema** may respond to intravitreal steroid or anti-VEGF agents, or to carotid surgery.
- **Carotid surgery.** Endarterectomy or stenting may be performed to reduce the risk of stroke; it may be beneficial for proliferative retinopathy and neovascular glaucoma, and may help to stabilize vision. Endarterectomy cannot be performed where there is total obstruction, and in this situation extracranial–intracranial arterial bypass surgery is sometimes carried out. It should be noted that an increase in ocular perfusion following surgery can sometimes be associated with a rise in IOP and exacerbation of neovascularization. Surgery tends to be of greater benefit when performed before the onset of severe ocular ischaemia.
- **Investigation and management of cardiovascular risk factors** in conjunction with the appropriate medical specialists is essential. OIS is occasionally the only

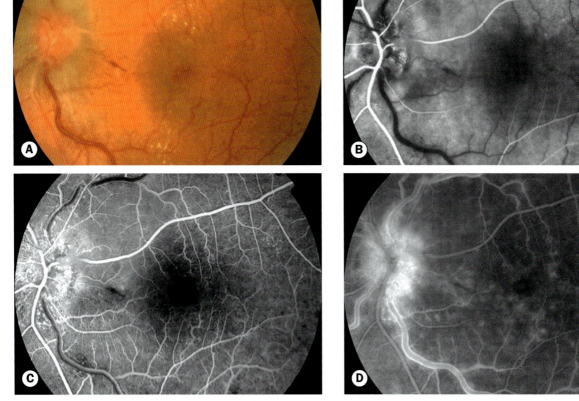

Fig. 13.42 Ocular ischaemic syndrome. **(A)** Venous dilatation, arteriolar narrowing, a few scattered flame haemorrhages and hard exudates, and disc oedema; **(B)** and **(C)** FA early phase shows delayed choroidal filling and prolonged arteriovenous transit; **(D)** FA late phase shows disc and perivascular hyperfluorescence, with spotty hyperfluorescence at the posterior pole due to leakage

(Courtesy of Moorfields Eye Hospital)

manifestation of marked systemic vascular disease. Full investigation should be carried out, broadly similar to that for retinal arterial occlusion.

HYPERTENSIVE EYE DISEASE

Retinopathy

The primary response of the retinal arterioles to systemic hypertension is vasoconstriction; this is less marked in older individuals due to involutional sclerosis conferring increased rigidity. Arteriolosclerosis refers to hardening and loss of elasticity of small vessel walls, manifested most obviously by arteriovenous (AV) nipping (nicking) at crossing points; its presence makes it probable that hypertension has been present for many years, even if the BP is currently controlled. Mild AV changes may be seen in the absence of hypertension. In sustained hypertension the inner blood–retinal barrier is disrupted, increased vascular permeability leading to flame-shaped retinal haemorrhages and oedema.

- **Grade 1.** Mild generalized retinal arteriolar narrowing (Fig. 13.43A).

- **Grade 2.** Focal arteriolar narrowing (Fig. 13.43B) and arteriovenous nipping (Fig. 13.43C). A 'copper wiring' opacified appearance of arteriolar walls may be seen (Fig. 13.43D).
- **Grade 3.** Grade 2 plus retinal haemorrhages (dot, blot, flame), exudates (chronic retinal oedema may result in the deposition of hard exudates around the fovea as a 'macular star' – Fig. 13.43E) and cotton wool spots.
- **Grade 4.** Severe grade 3 plus optic disc swelling (Fig. 13.43F); this is a marker of malignant hypertension.
- **Markers of preclinical systemic disease.**
  - ○ Reduced retinal arteriolar calibre (see Fig. 13.43A) is an early pre-hypertensive sign and if identified should prompt BP monitoring.
  - ○ Wider venular calibre is relatively specific for impaired glucose metabolism.
  - ○ Low arteriolar calibre and high venular calibre are both thought to be markers of preclinical cardiovascular disease.
  - ○ Increased venular tortuosity (Fig 13.44A) can be associated with chronic hypertension and pre-hypertension, though evidence on arteriolar tortuosity is

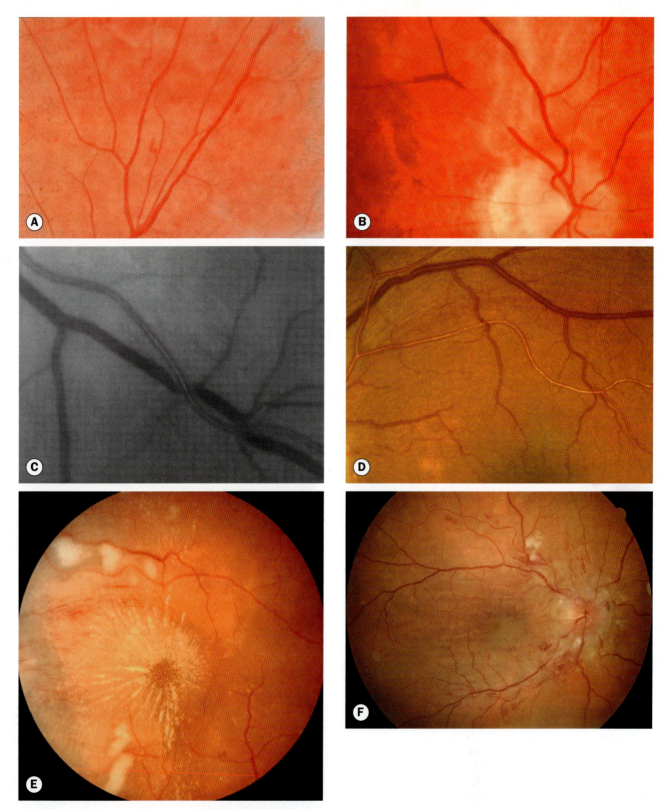

Fig. 13.43 Hypertensive retinopathy. **(A)** Generalized arteriolar attenuation; **(B)** focal arteriolar attenuation; **(C)** red-free photograph showing arteriovenous nipping; **(D)** 'copper wiring'; **(E)** grade 3 retinopathy with macular star; **(F)** grade 4 hypertensive retinopathy

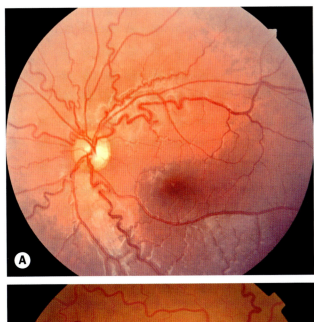

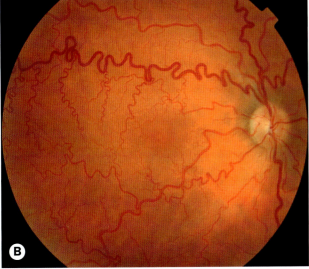

Fig. 13.44 Vascular tortuosity. **(A)** Selective venous tortuosity – the arterioles are unaffected; **(B)** mixed arteriolar and venular tortuosity

(Courtesy of S Chen – fig. B)

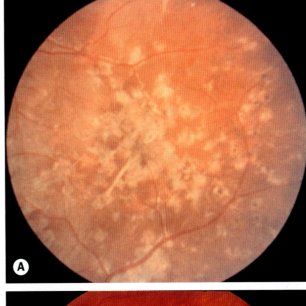

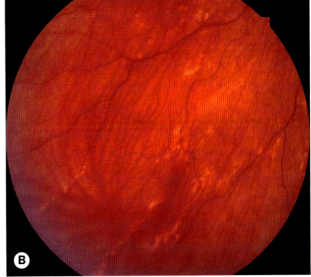

Fig. 13.45 Hypertensive choroidopathy. **(A)** Elschnig spots; **(B)** Siegrist lines

conflicting – straightening of arterioles has been reported in some studies. Numerous other causes of retinal vascular tortuosity (Fig. 13.44B) have been described, notably conditions associated with high and low vascular flow.

Choroidopathy

Hypertensive choroidopathy is rare but may occur as the result of an acute hypertensive crisis (accelerated hypertension) in young adults.

- **Elschnig spots** are focal choroidal infarcts seen as small black spots surrounded by yellow haloes (Fig. 13.45A).
- **Siegrist streaks** are flecks arranged linearly along choroidal vessels (Fig. 13.45B), and are indicative of fibrinoid necrosis associated with malignant hypertension.

- **Exudative retinal detachment**, sometimes bilateral, may occur in acute severe hypertension such as that associated with toxaemia of pregnancy.

SICKLE CELL RETINOPATHY

Sickling haemoglobinopathies

Sickling haemoglobinopathies are caused by one or more abnormal haemoglobins that induce red blood cells to adopt an anomalous shape (Fig. 13.46) under conditions of physiological stress such as hypoxia and acidosis, with resultant vascular occlusion. Mutant haemoglobin variants S and C can be found in combination with the normal adult haemoglobin A or, less commonly,

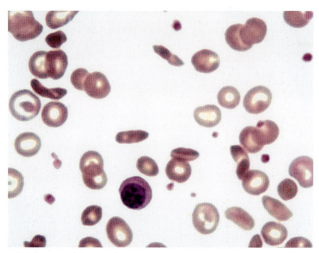

Fig. 13.46 Several sickle red cells and one nucleated red cell in a peripheral smear of a patient with homozygous (HbSS) sickle cell anaemia
(Courtesy of N Bienz)

with other mutant haemoglobin variants. Retinopathy can occur in sickle cell disease (homozygous for mutant haemoglobin S, i.e. SS), sickle cell C disease (SC – the most likely to develop severe retinopathy) and sickle cell-thalassaemia disease (S-Thal). It is rare in patients with sickle cell trait (SA – found in 10% of African-Americans), unless there is other co-existing systemic disease such as diabetes or an inflammatory disorder. Carbonic anhydrase inhibitors (CAI) should be avoided in sickling disorders as they can precipitate sickling and vascular occlusion.

Anterior segment

- **Conjunctiva.** Dark red corkscrew- or comma-shaped vessels that are typically transient.
- **Iris.** Patches of ischaemic atrophy, often extending from the pupillary edge to the collarette, and occasionally rubeosis.
- **Hyphaema** may be spontaneous or follow minor trauma. Careful IOP control (avoiding CAI) is critical to reduce the risk of RVO in the presence of a hyphaema.

Non-proliferative retinopathy

- **Venous changes.** Tortuosity (see Fig. 13.44) is very common and is thought to be due to peripheral arteriovenous shunting; RVO is uncommon, though is a risk with raised IOP.
- **Arteriolar changes.** Occlusions can involve branch, central or macular (Fig. 13.47A) vessels and if seen acutely may benefit from measures such as 100% oxygen and exchange transfusion. 'Silver wiring' of arterioles in the peripheral retina signifies previously occluded vessels. Corkscrewing of peripheral vessels may be seen.
- **Optic disc 'sign of sickling'.** Dark red blots on the disc surface due to small vessel occlusion.
- **'Salmon patches'.** Orange–red mid-peripheral superficial intraretinal haemorrhages (Fig. 13.47B) that may break

through to become preretinal or subretinal. The initiating event is thought to be a vascular occlusion. Salmon patches resolve to leave schisis cavities containing refractile deposits, 'black sunbursts' (see below) when the RPE is sufficiently stimulated, or a combination lesion.
- **Black sunbursts.** Patches of peripheral RPE hyperplasia and chorioretinal atrophy (Fig. 13.47C) that evolve from some salmon patches; the extent and morphology of pigmentation is variable, but an outer pale band is generally present.
- **Macular (retinal) depression sign.** An oval depression in the temporal macular retina due to retinal thinning following arteriolar occlusion, with irregularity of the light reflex. Vascular anomalies such as microaneurysms, and epiretinal membranes may occur.
- **Peripheral areas of whitening or darkening** (Fig. 13.47D).
- **Angioid streaks** (see Ch. 14) occur in up to 6%.

Proliferative retinopathy

Diagnosis

The development of proliferative retinopathy is usually insidious, with no symptoms unless vitreous haemorrhage or retinal detachment occurs.
- **Stage 1.** Peripheral arteriolar occlusion.
- **Stage 2.** Peripheral arteriovenous anastomosis (Fig. 13.48A) proximal to non-perfused areas.
- **Stage 3.** 'Sea fan' neovascularization (Fig. 13.48B) develops at the edge of perfused retina, usually with a single supplying arteriole and a single draining venule. Disc neovascularization may rarely occur.
- **Stage 4.** Vitreous haemorrhage from the new vessels (Fig. 13.48C).
- **Stage 5.** Rhegmatogenous retinal detachment caused by a retinal break associated with extensive fibrovascular proliferation (Fig. 13.48D). Tractional detachment may also occur.
- FA in stage 3 shows filling of sea fans and peripheral capillary non-perfusion (Fig. 13.48E) followed by leakage from the new vessels (Fig. 13.48F). Wide-field imaging is especially suited to evaluation of this condition.

Treatment

- **Observation** if vitreous haemorrhage has not occurred, particularly in middle-aged and older patients. Many neovascular complexes involute spontaneously (Fig. 13.49) as a result of auto-infarction or fibrotic strangulation, subsequently appearing as greyish fibrovascular lesions.
- **Laser or cryotherapy** ablation of peripheral non-perfused retina is probably the optimal approach, though ablation of neovascularization may also be used; ablation of feeder vessels is now rarely performed due to a high incidence of subsequent choroidal neovascularization.
- **Vitreoretinal surgery** may be required for tractional retinal detachment and/or persistent vitreous haemorrhage.

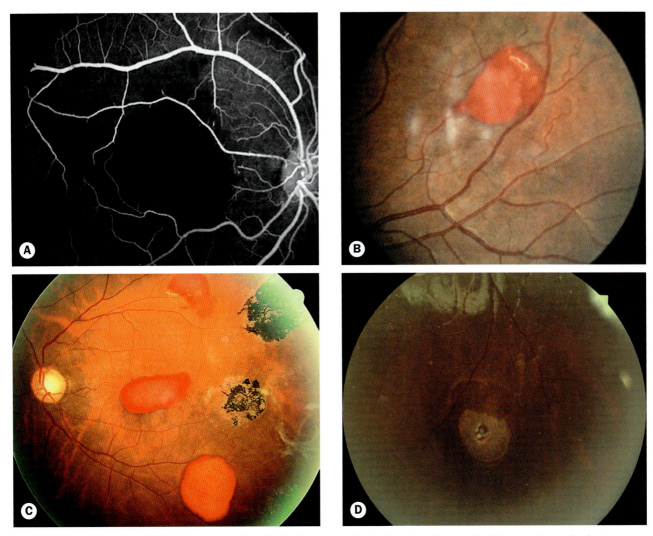

Fig. 13.47 Non-proliferative sickle-cell retinopathy. **(A)** FA shows macular ischaemia; **(B)** preretinal haemorrhage ('salmon patch'); **(C)** RPE hyperplasia ('black sunburst') and preretinal haemorrhages; **(D)** retinal hole and an area of whitening superiorly

(Courtesy of J Donald M Gass, from Stereoscopic Atlas of Macular Diseases, *Mosby 1997 – fig. B)*

Caution is required as anterior segment ischaemia, potentially severe, is very common following scleral explant application.

THALASSAEMIA RETINOPATHY

Thalassaemias are common gene disorders in which a mutation gives rise to abnormal haemoglobin with a consequent failure of normal red blood cell maturation. Ocular involvement occurs in patients with thalassaemia major and thalassaemia intermedia. Changes are caused by the disease itself as well as treatment with blood transfusions and iron chelating agents such as desferrioxamine. A major mechanism is tissue deposition of iron (siderosis) from the lysing of abnormal red cells. The ocular features predominantly affect the posterior segment and are non-proliferative, though vitreous haemorrhage has been reported. Visual dysfunction is rarely severe. Manifestations include cataract, a smooth featureless iris, vascular tortuosity, angioid streaks,

optic neuropathy and pigmentary retinal mottling, including pattern dystrophy-like macular changes. The fundus appearance may resemble that of pseudoxanthoma elasticum.

RETINOPATHY OF PREMATURITY

Introduction

Retinopathy of prematurity (ROP) affects premature low birth-weight infants; additional systemic illness is a risk factor. Early exposure to high ambient oxygen concentrations has been regarded as a key risk, but recent evidence questions its significance; it is likely that, in the early phase of ROP development, vessel growth is retarded by hyperoxia but that subsequently retinal hypoxia promotes anomalous vascularization. The retina has no blood vessels until the fourth month of gestation, when vascular complexes grow from optic disc hyaloid vessels towards

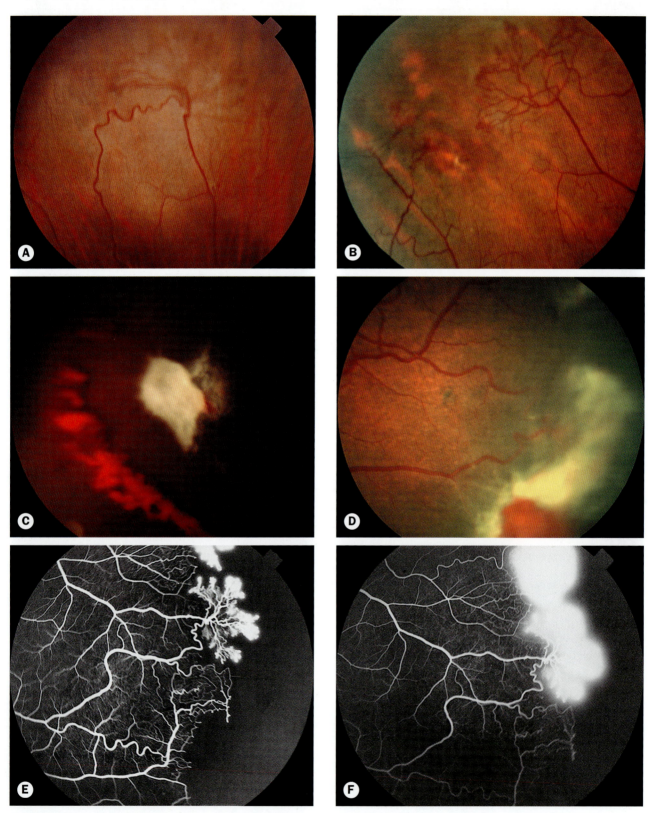

Fig. 13.48 Proliferative sickle cell retinopathy. **(A)** Peripheral arteriovenous anastomosis (mild neovascularization is also present); **(B)** 'sea fan' neovascularization; **(C)** haemorrhage from the new vessels; **(D)** extensive fibrovascular proliferation; **(E)** FA early phase shows filling of new vessels and extensive peripheral retinal capillary non-perfusion; **(F)** late phase shows leakage from the new vessels

(Courtesy of K Nischal – fig. A; R Marsh – figs B–D)

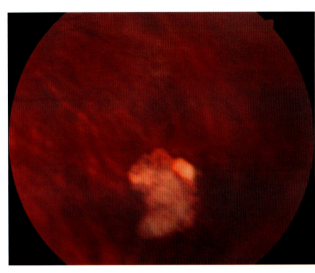

Fig. 13.49 Proliferative sickle retinopathy – spontaneous involution of a neovascular tuft

(Courtesy of R Marsh)

the periphery. The nasal retina is normally fully vascularized after 8 months of gestation, the temporal periphery at or by 1 month after delivery. Vascular endothelial growth factor (VEGF) is believed to play an important role in the vascularization process.

Active disease

The clinical findings in ROP are described as below according to the 2005 International Classification of Retinopathy of Prematurity (ICROP).

Location

Concentric zones centred on the optic disc are described (Fig. 13.50).

- **Zone I** is bounded by an imaginary circle, the radius of which is twice the distance from the disc to the centre of the macula. With a 28 dioptre binocular indirect lens, only zone I is seen if any part of the optic nerve head is visible.
- **Zone II** extends concentrically from the edge of zone I; its radius extends from the centre of the disc to the nasal ora serrata.
- **Zone III** consists of a residual temporal crescent anterior to zone II.

Staging

This describes the abnormal vascular response at the junction of immature avascular peripheral and vascularized posterior retina. Staging for the eye as a whole is determined by the most severe manifestation.

- **Stage 1** (demarcation line) is a thin, flat, tortuous, grey-white line running roughly parallel with the ora serrata. It is more prominent in the temporal periphery. There is abnormal branching or 'arcading' of vessels leading up to the line (Fig. 13.51A).

- **Stage 2** (ridge) arises in the region of the demarcation line, has height and width, and extends above the plane of the retina. Blood vessels enter the ridge and small isolated neovascular tufts may be seen posterior to it (Fig. 13.51B).
- **Stage 3** (extraretinal fibrovascular proliferation) extends from the ridge into the vitreous. It is continuous with the posterior aspect of the ridge, causing a ragged appearance as the proliferation becomes more extensive (Fig. 13.51C). The severity of stage 3 can be subdivided into mild, moderate and severe depending on the extent of extraretinal fibrous tissue infiltrating the vitreous. The highest incidence of this stage is around the post-conceptual age of 35 weeks.
- **Stage 4** (partial retinal detachment) is divided into extrafoveal (stage 4A – Fig. 13.51D) and foveal (stage 4B). The detachment is generally concave and circumferentially orientated. In progressive cases the fibrous tissue continues to contract and the detachment increases in height and extends anteriorly and posteriorly.
- **Stage 5** refers to total retinal detachment.
- **'Plus' disease** signifies a tendency to progression and is characterized by dilatation and tortuosity of blood vessels (Fig. 13.51E) involving at least two quadrants of the posterior fundus. Other features include failure of the pupil to dilate and vitreous haze. 'Pre-plus' disease is also described.
- **Aggressive posterior ('rush' disease)** is uncommon but if untreated usually progresses to stage 5, sometimes within a few days. It is characterized by its posterior location, prominence of plus disease and ill-defined nature of the retinopathy.

Type

Treatment guidelines at most centres have been revised based on the Early Treatment of Retinopathy of Prematurity (ETROP) clinical trial. The concept of 'threshold disease' formerly taken as the criterion for treatment has been superseded, with outcomes

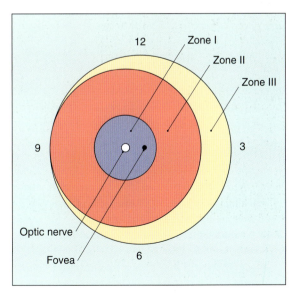

Fig. 13.50 Grading of retinopathy of prematurity according to location

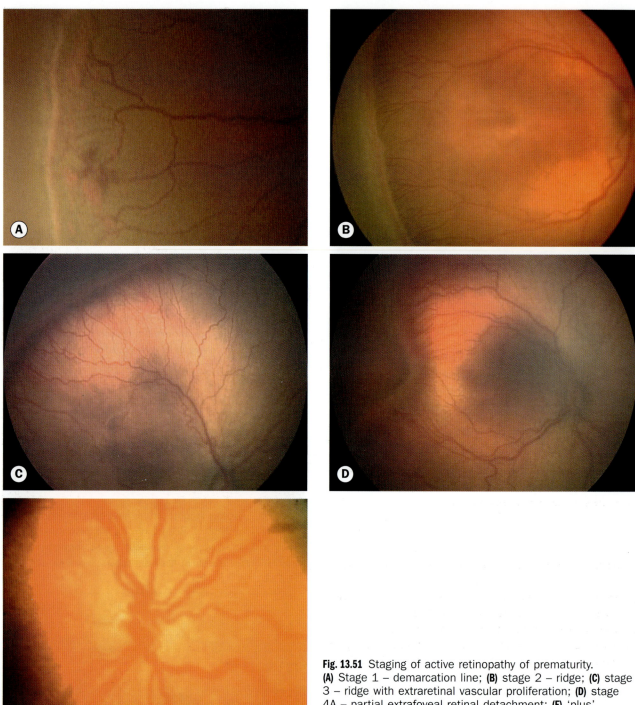

Fig. 13.51 Staging of active retinopathy of prematurity.
(A) Stage 1 – demarcation line; **(B)** stage 2 – ridge; **(C)** stage 3 – ridge with extraretinal vascular proliferation; **(D)** stage 4A – partial extrafoveal retinal detachment; **(E)** 'plus' disease
(Courtesy of L MacKeen – figs A, C and D; P Watts – fig. B)

improved by earlier intervention; the outcome after treatment varies depending on severity of disease; 30% of high-risk zone I ROP will have an unfavourable visual outcome.

- **Type 1.** Treatment is now recommended within 72 hours for type 1 disease.
  - ○ Any ROP stage in zone I when accompanied by plus disease.
  - ○ Stage 3 to any extent within zone I.
  - ○ Stage 2 or 3 in zone II, together with plus disease.

- **Type 2** disease requires observation.
  - ○ Stage 1 or 2 in zone I without plus disease.
  - ○ Stage 3 ROP within zone II without plus disease.

Screening

Formal criteria vary, but babies born at or before 30–32 weeks gestational age, or weighing 1500 g or less, should be screened for ROP; severe illness in other premature babies may also prompt screening. This may involve indirect ophthalmoscopy with a 28 D lens or a 2.2 panfunduscopic Volk lens and scleral depression, or a wide field retinal camera with careful oversight. Screening should begin 4–7 weeks postnatally. Subsequent review is at 1–3 week intervals, depending on the severity of the disease, continuing until retinal vascularization reaches zone III. The pupils in a premature infant can be dilated with 0.5% cyclopentolate and 2.5% phenylephrine. Topical anaesthetic is instilled, and a neonatal eyelid speculum used; monitoring, especially for apnoea, is prudent during and 24–48 hours after examination. About 10% of babies screened require treatment. Refractive error, strabismus and amblyopia are more common in children with ROP, and longer-term monitoring is required.

Treatment

- **Laser ablation** of avascular peripheral retina (Fig. 13.52) has largely replaced cryotherapy because visual and anatomical outcomes are superior.
- **Intravitreal anti-VEGF agents.** Bevacizumab has been used for the treatment of ROP, but an optimal regimen is yet to be established. Zone I disease is more likely to respond than zone II. Allowing retinal development to proceed normally without the destruction integral to laser treatment is a potential advantage. However, systemic complications and long-term effects in this age group are undetermined.
- **Pars plana vitrectomy** for tractional retinal detachment not involving the macula (stage 4A) can be performed successfully with respect to anatomical (90% success) and visual outcome. The visual outcome in stages 4B (e.g. 60%) and 5 (e.g. 20%) is typically disappointing even with successful anatomical reattachment.

Cicatricial disease

About 20% of infants with active ROP develop cicatricial complications, which range from innocuous to extremely severe. In general, the more advanced or the more posterior the proliferative disease at the time of involution, the worse the cicatricial sequelae. Findings range from moderate temporal vitreoretinal fibrosis and straightening of vascular arcades (Fig. 13.53A) with 'dragging' of the macula and disc (Fig. 13.53B), progressing to retrolental fibrovascular tissue that can lead to falciform retinal fold formation (Fig. 13.53C) and to retinal detachment (Fig. 13.53D), sometimes total (Fig. 13.53E) and known as 'retrolental fibroplasia'; the latter term has been used synonymously with ROP in the past. Secondary angle-closure glaucoma may develop due to progressive shallowing of the anterior chamber caused by forward displacement of the iris–lens diaphragm with anterior synechiae formation. Lensectomy and anterior vitrectomy may be tried, but the results are generally poor.

RETINAL ARTERY MACROANEURYSM

A retinal artery macroaneurysm is a localized dilatation of a retinal arteriole; it has a predilection for older hypertensive (75%) women.

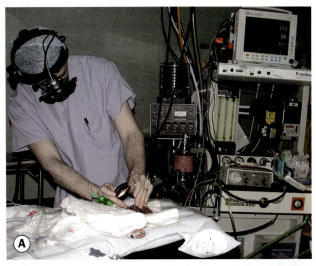

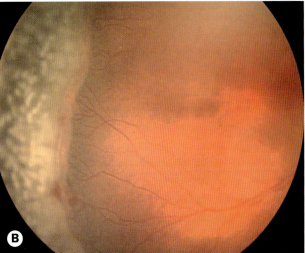

Fig. 13.52 Treatment of retinopathy of prematurity.
(A) Head-mounted binocular indirect ophthalmoscopy laser under general anaesthesia; **(B)** appearance immediately following laser photocoagulation for type 1 disease
(Courtesy of S Chen – fig. A; P Watts – fig. B)

Dyslipidaemia is also associated. 90% involve only one eye; they are usually solitary.

Diagnosis

- **Symptoms.** Insidious impairment of vision due to leakage involving the macula; sudden visual loss due to haemorrhage is less common.
- **Fundus.** A saccular arteriolar dilatation is typical, often at a bifurcation or an arteriovenous crossing on a temporal vascular arcade. The aneurysm may enlarge to several times the diameter of the vessel; there is associated retinal haemorrhage in 50%.
- **Course**
  ○ Chronic leakage. Persistent retinal oedema with exudate formation (Fig. 13.54A) is common and may affect central vision.

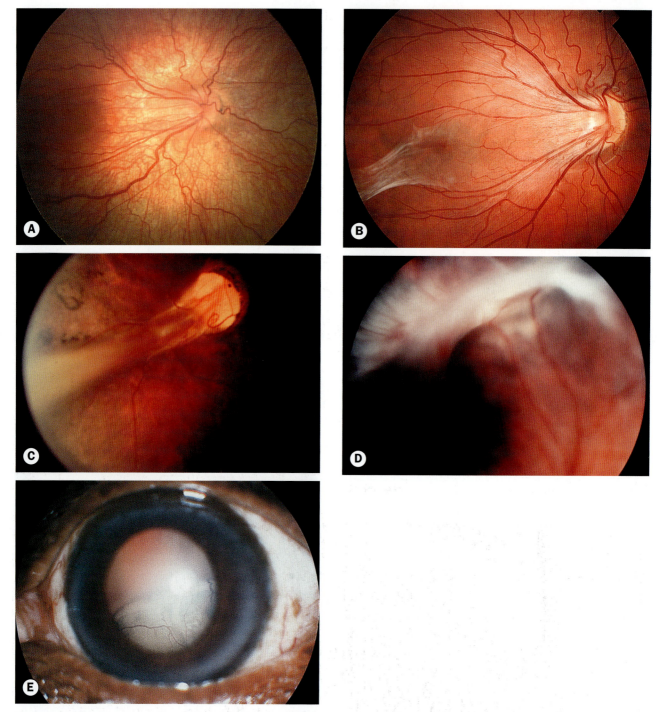

Fig. 13.53 Cicatricial retinopathy of prematurity. **(A)** Straightening of vascular arcades; **(B)** 'dragging' of the disc and macula; **(C)** falciform retinal fold; **(D)** retrolental fibrovascular tissue and partial retinal detachment; **(E)** total retinal detachment

○ Haemorrhage. Intra-, sub- (Fig. 13.54B) or preretinal (Fig. 13.54C) bleeding, in association with which the diagnosis may be overlooked. The prognosis for central visual function in those with submacular haemorrhage is generally poor.

○ Spontaneous involution following thrombosis and fibrosis is very common and may precede or follow the development of leakage or haemorrhage.

○ Other complications. Epiretinal membrane, choroidal neovascularization.

• **FA.** Uniform filling of the macroaneurysm is typical (Fig. 13.54D), with late leakage. Incomplete filling is due to thrombosis.

• **OCT** can demonstrate the lesion itself (Fig. 13.54E), but its main use is to document and monitor macular oedema, and less commonly subhyaloid haemorrhage (Fig. 13.54F).

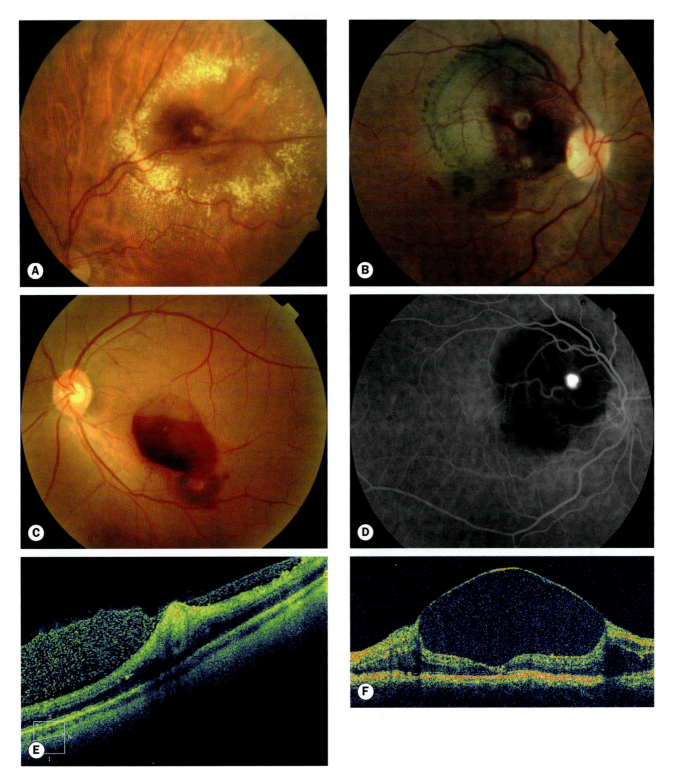

Fig. 13.54 Retinal artery macroaneurysm. **(A)** Associated with exudate; **(B)** sub- (darker) and intraretinal (brighter red) haemorrhage; **(C)** preretinal (retrohyaloid) haemorrhage; **(D)** FA early venous phase shows hyperfluorescence of the microaneurysm, which is surrounded by hypofluorescence due to masking by blood – same lesion as (B); **(E)** OCT of macroaneurysm with preretinal blood; **(F)** OCT of loculated subhyaloid haemorrhage

(Courtesy of S Chen)

- **Vascular risk factors** should be checked, especially blood pressure and serum lipids.

Treatment

- **Observation** is indicated in eyes with good visual acuity in which the macula is not threatened, and in those with mild retinal haemorrhage without significant oedema. In many cases macroaneurysms will spontaneously involute (Fig. 13.55), particularly following retinal or vitreous haemorrhage.
- **Laser** treatment (Figs 13.56A and B) may be considered if oedema or exudates threaten or involve the fovea, particularly if there is documented visual deterioration. Burns may be applied to the lesion itself, the surrounding area (to reduce the risk of arteriolar occlusion), or both; subthreshold laser may be as effective as standard photocoagulation. It may take several months for oedema and exudate to fully absorb.

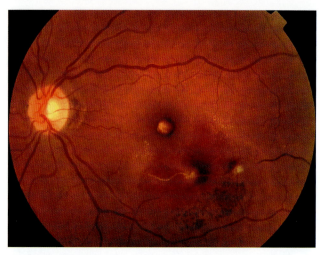

Fig. 13.55 Spontaneously involuted retinal artery macroaneurysms

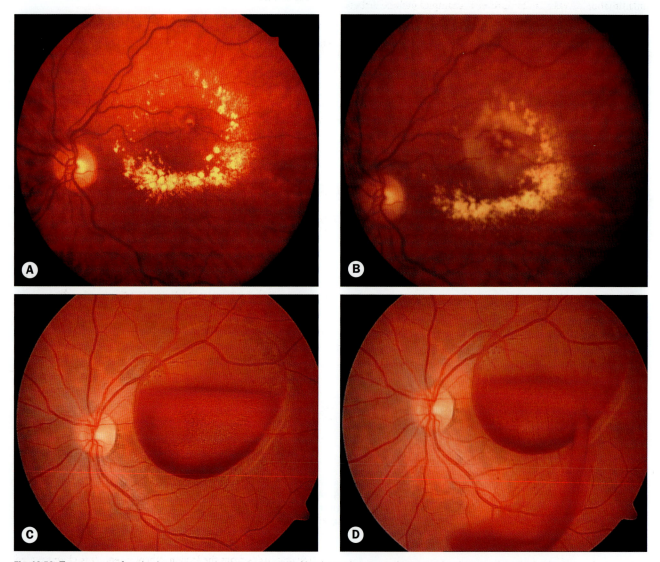

Fig. 13.56 Treatment of retinal artery macroaneurysm. **(A)** Hard exudates at the macula due to chronic leakage; **(B)** immediately following laser application; **(C)** large preretinal haemorrhage overlying the macula; **(D)** following YAG laser hyaloidotomy, showing blood dispersing into the vitreous

(Courtesy of P Gili – figs C and D)

- **Intravitreal bevacizumab** closed 95% of macroaneurysms in a case series, with resolution of macular oedema.
- **YAG laser hyaloidotomy** may be considered for a persistent premacular haemorrhage in order to disperse the blood into the vitreous cavity (Figs 13.56C and D), from where it may be absorbed more quickly.
- **Intravitreal gas injection** with face-down positioning may shift subretinal haemorrhage away from the macula. Adjunctive intravitreal recombinant tissue plasminogen activator (rtPA) may be used.
- **Vitrectomy** may be necessary for persistent vitreous haemorrhage.

PRIMARY RETINAL TELANGIECTASIA

Retinal capillary telangiectasia is relatively common. Most cases develop secondary to another retinal condition, typically involving inflammation or vascular compromise; examples include diabetic retinopathy and retinal venous occlusion. Primary retinal telangiectasia comprises a group of rare, idiopathic, congenital or acquired retinal vascular anomalies characterized by dilatation and tortuosity of retinal blood vessels, multiple aneurysms, vascular leakage and the deposition of hard exudates. Retinal telangiectasis involves the capillary bed, although the arterioles and venules may also be involved.

Idiopathic macular telangiectasia

This is described in Chapter 14.

Coats disease

Introduction

Coats disease is an idiopathic retinal telangiectasia that is generally of onset in early childhood. It is associated with intraretinal and subretinal exudation, and frequently exudative retinal detachment, without signs of vitreoretinal traction. About 75% of patients are male and 95% have involvement of only one eye. Presentation is most frequently in the first decade of life. Although it is not clearly inherited, a genetic predisposition may be involved as at least some patients have a somatic mutation in the *NDP* gene, which is also mutated in Norrie disease. It is now considered that Leber miliary aneurysms, previously regarded as a distinct condition, represents a generally milder form of the same disease, presenting later, in a more localized pattern, and carrying a better visual prognosis. Differential diagnosis from other causes of leukocoria in children, particularly retinoblastoma, is important. The prognosis is variable and dependent on the severity of involvement at presentation; younger children frequently have a more aggressive clinical course.

Diagnosis

- **Symptoms.** Unilateral visual loss, strabismus or leukocoria (Fig. 13.57A).

- **Fundus**
  - ○ Telangiectasia and fusiform focal aneurysmal arteriolar dilatations (Figs 13.57B and C), often initially in the inferior and temporal quadrants between the equator and ora serrata.
  - ○ Intra- and subretinal exudate (Fig. 13.57C), often affecting areas remote from the vascular abnormalities, particularly the macula. Progression to extensive exudative retinal detachment (Fig. 13.57D) may occur.
- **Complications** include rubeosis iridis, glaucoma, uveitis, cataract and phthisis bulbi.
- **FA** in mild cases shows early hyperfluorescence of telangiectases and aneurysmal dilatations (Fig. 13.57E) and late staining and leakage (Fig. 13.57F).
- **OCT** may be useful for the assessment of the macula in cooperative older children.

Treatment

- **Observation** in patients with mild, non-vision threatening disease and in those with a comfortable eye with total retinal detachment for whom there is no potential for restoration of useful vision.
- **Laser ablation** of points of leakage should be considered if progressive exudation is documented (Fig. 13.58). Multiple repeated treatments over an extended term are commonly required.
- **Anti-VEGF therapy.** Limited studies of anti-VEGF therapy have been carried out, but initial results are promising, including as an adjunct to laser. Long-term safety in childhood remains undetermined.
- **Intravitreal triamcinolone** (2–4 mg) has been used with good effect in eyes with total exudative retinal detachment.
- **Cryotherapy**, with a double freeze–thaw method, in eyes with extensive exudation or subtotal retinal detachment although this may result in marked reaction with increased leakage. Therefore, laser photocoagulation is still the preferred option if possible.
- **Vitreoretinal surgery** may be considered in eyes with significant tractional preretinal fibrosis or total exudative detachment; There is a poor visual prognosis but successful retinal re-attachment may prevent the development of neovascular glaucoma.
- **Enucleation** may be required in painful eyes with neovascular glaucoma.

EALES DISEASE

Introduction

Eales disease is an idiopathic occlusive peripheral periphlebitis. It is rare in Caucasians but is an important cause of visual morbidity in young males from the Indian subcontinent. It is characterized by three overlapping stages: inflammatory, occlusive and retinal neovascular, and is diagnosed principally by clinical examination. The visual prognosis is good in the majority of cases. Tubercular

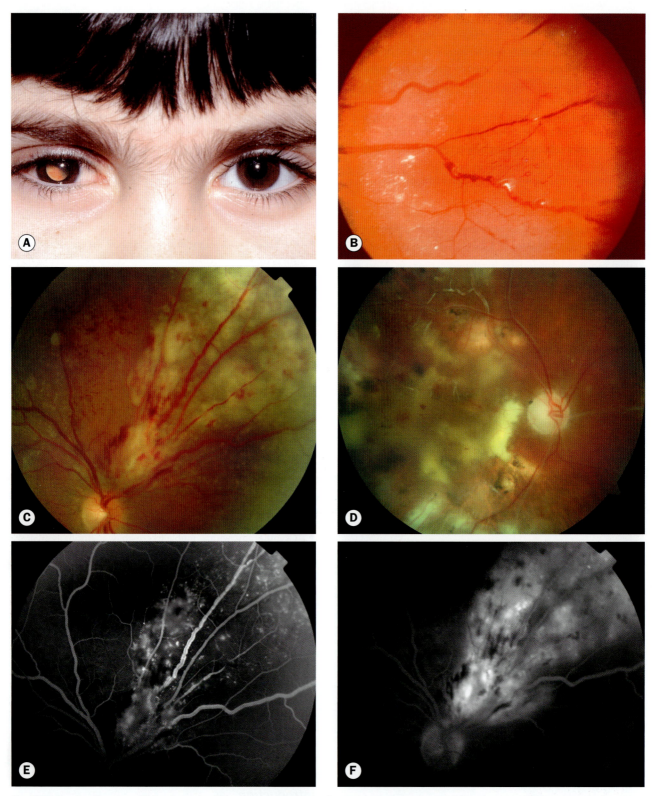

Fig. 13.57 Coats disease. **(A)** Leukocoria; **(B)** retinal telangiectasia and aneurysmal arteriolar changes; **(C)** progressively more extensive vascular abnormalities and exudation; **(D)** extensive exudative retinal detachment; **(E)** FA early phase of eye in (C) demonstrating telangiectasis and aneurysmal dilatations; **(F)** late-phase FA showing leakage

(Courtesy of S Chen – figs C, E and F)

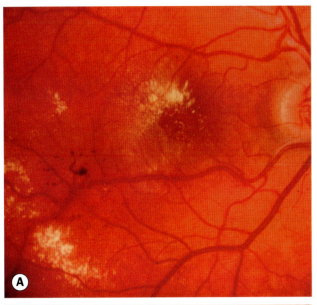

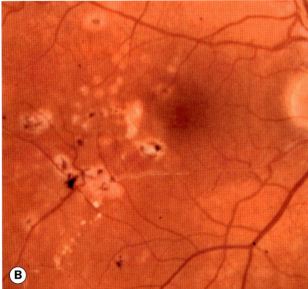

Fig. 13.58 (A) Exudates in relatively mild Coats disease;
(B) resolution several months after laser photocoagulation

protein hypersensitivity may be important in the aetiology, but
evidence is conflicting; some patients may have tubercular
vasculitis.

Diagnosis

- **Symptoms.** Floaters or sudden visual reduction due to
  vitreous haemorrhage.
- **Systemic neurological features** have been reported.
- **Mild anterior uveitis** is often present.
- **Fundus.** The condition is typically bilateral, though often
  asymmetrical.
  - Peripheral periphlebitis (Fig. 13.59A): sheathing,
    superficial retinal haemorrhages and sometimes cotton
    wool spots. Pigmented chorioretinal scars may be seen.

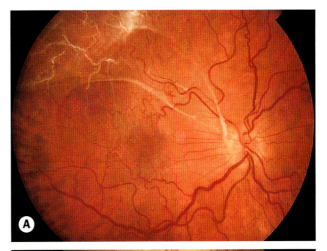

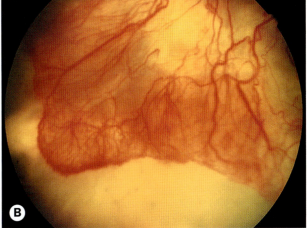

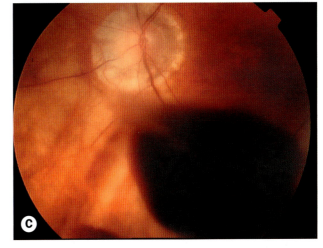

Fig. 13.59 Eales disease. **(A)** Peripheral vascular sheathing
and occlusion; **(B)** peripheral neovascularization;
(C) haemorrhage from new vessels

- Branch retinal vein occlusion.
- Peripheral capillary non-perfusion; microaneurysms,
  tortuosity, vascular shunts and neovascularization (Fig.
  13.59B) with recurrent vitreous haemorrhage (one-third
  of eyes – Fig. 13.59C) may develop at the junction of
  perfused and non-perfused retina. Disc new vessels can

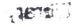

sometimes develop. The vitreous haemorrhage tends to be limited and to absorb over weeks, but can persist in some cases.
- ○ Macular involvement with the same changes can occur but is rare; macular oedema can develop.
- **Complications** include tractional retinal detachment, macular epiretinal membrane, neovascular glaucoma and cataract.
- **FA** will identify vasculitis and areas of non-perfusion; wide-field imaging is especially helpful.
- **Investigation** should be performed to rule out other causes of vasculitis (e.g. sarcoidosis, tuberculosis) and peripheral retinal neovascularization (e.g. haemoglobinopathies).

Treatment

- **Steroids.** Periocular, systemic, topical, and intravitreal steroids seem to be helpful in the inflammatory stage.
- **Antitubercular treatment.** This is strongly advocated by some authorities but is controversial. It may be considered in selected patients in combination with steroids, either to avoid reactivation of prior tubercular infection (e.g. strongly positive skin test, QuantiFERON®) or possibly when severe ocular inflammatory signs are present.
- **Scatter photocoagulation** or cryotherapy of non-perfused retina to reduce the neovascular stimulus.
- **Intravitreal VEGF inhibitors** may be helpful but research is ongoing.
- **Vitrectomy** for persistent vitreous haemorrhage, tractional detachment and macular epiretinal membrane.

RADIATION RETINOPATHY

Radiation retinopathy may develop following treatment of intraocular tumours by plaque therapy (brachytherapy) or external beam irradiation of sinus, orbital or nasopharyngeal malignancies. It is characterized by delayed retinal microvascular changes with endothelial cell loss, capillary occlusion and microaneurysm formation. Affected patients may also develop cataract and keratopathy (Fig. 13.60). There is some evidence that it is more likely to occur in genetically predisposed individuals. The interval between exposure and disease is variable and unpredictable, although commonly between 6 months and 3 years. There is a direct relationship with radiation dose.

- **Signs**
  - ○ Capillary occlusion with the development of telangiectasis and microaneurysms, best seen on FA (Figs 13.61A–C).
  - ○ Retinal oedema, exudate, cotton wool spots and haemorrhages (Figs 13.61D and E).
  - ○ Papillopathy (Fig. 13.61F); radiation optic neuropathy may occur but is less common as the nerve seems to be less sensitive than retinal vessels.
  - ○ Proliferative retinopathy.
- **Treatment** is frequently unsatisfactory. Options include laser, steroids and intravitreal anti-VEGF agents.

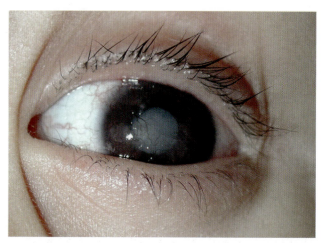

Fig. 13.60 Radiation keratopathy
(Courtesy of N Rogers)

- **Prognosis** depends on the severity of involvement. Poor prognostic features include papillopathy and proliferative retinopathy, which may result in vitreous haemorrhage and tractional retinal detachment.

PURTSCHER RETINOPATHY

Purtscher retinopathy may follow severe trauma, especially chest compressive and head injury, and involves occlusion and ischaemia associated with microvascular damage, and is thought to result from embolism and in some cases vascular occlusion by other mechanisms such as complement-mediated white blood cell aggregation. When it results from causes other than trauma (e.g. fat or amniotic fluid embolism, acute pancreatitis, pre-eclampsia, systemic vasculitides) it is sometimes referred to as 'Purtscher-like' retinopathy. Presentation is with sudden bilateral visual reduction, typically to 6/60 or less. Multiple unilateral or bilateral superficial white retinal patches – capillary bed infarcts known as Purtscher flecken – resembling large cotton wool spots (Fig. 13.62) are seen, often associated with superficial peripapillary haemorrhages, typical cotton wool spots and disc swelling. Elevated complement 5a levels may be diagnostic where there is no history of trauma. The acute fundus changes usually resolve within a few weeks, but only a small proportion will regain normal vision. Treatment of the underlying cause is not always possible.

VALSALVA RETINOPATHY

The Valsalva manoeuvre consists of forcible exhalation against a closed glottis, thereby creating a sudden increase in intrathoracic and intra-abdominal pressure (e.g. weight-lifting, blowing up balloons). The associated sudden rise in venous pressure may rupture perifoveal capillaries leading to pre-macular haemorrhage of varying severity (Fig. 13.63); vitreous haemorrhage may also occur. Treatment is with observation, or YAG laser membranotomy in some cases.

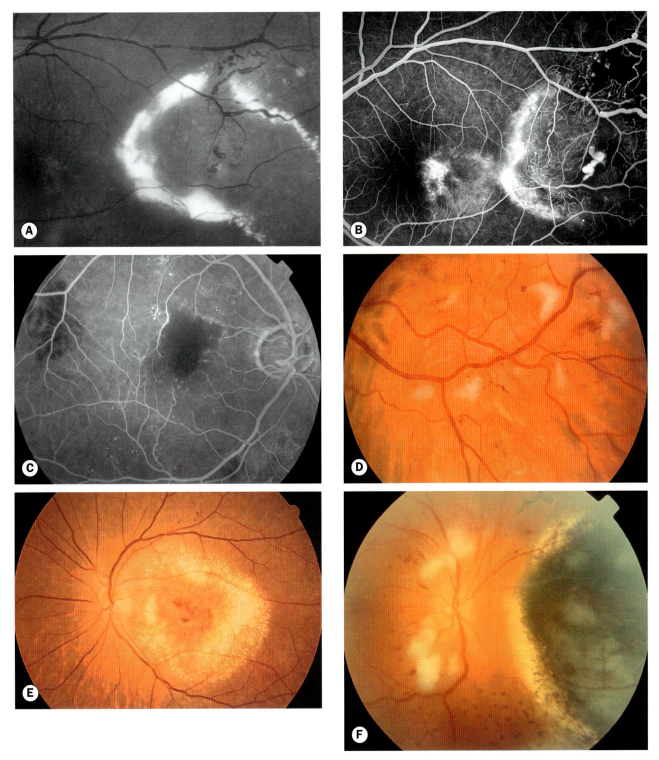

Fig. 13.61 Radiation retinopathy. **(A)** Red-free photograph and **(B)** FA of aneurysmal and telangiectatic lesions associated with retinal capillary non-perfusion and leakage with exudation; **(C)** more severe retinal capillary non-perfusion and microvascular abnormalities; **(D)** microvascular abnormalities, cotton wool spots and haemorrhages; **(E)** severe macular involvement; **(F)** papillopathy following treatment of a choroidal melanoma

(Courtesy of C Barry – figs A and B)

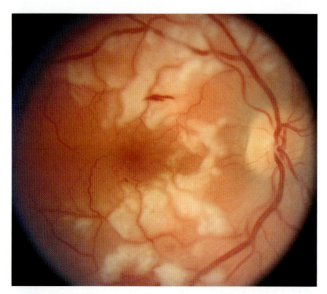

Fig. 13.62 Purtscher flecken in Purtscher retinopathy
(Courtesy of L Merin)

LIPAEMIA RETINALIS

Lipaemia retinalis is a rare condition characterized by creamy-white discoloration of retinal blood vessels (Fig. 13.64) in some patients with hypertriglyceridaemia; in mild examples only peripheral vessels are affected, but in extreme cases the fundus takes on a salmon colour. The visualization of high levels of chylomycrons in blood vessels accounts for the fundus appearance. Visual acuity is usually normal but electroretinogram amplitude may be decreased.

RETINOPATHY IN BLOOD DISORDERS

Leukaemia

Introduction

The leukaemias are malignancies of haematopoietic stem cells involving abnormal proliferation of white blood cells. The acute

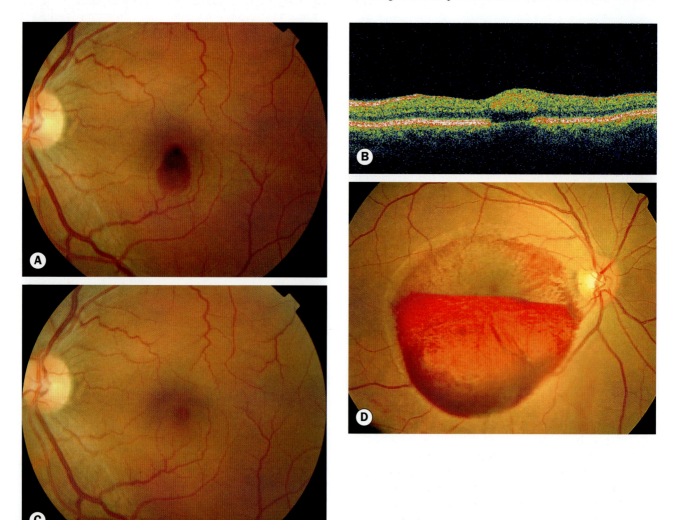

Fig. 13.63 Valsalva retinopathy. **(A)** Acute presentation; **(B)** macular OCT; **(C)** case in (A) 5 months later; **(D)** severe case
(Courtesy of S Chen – figs A–C; J Donald M Gass, from Stereoscopic Atlas of Macular Diseases, Mosby 1997 – fig. D)

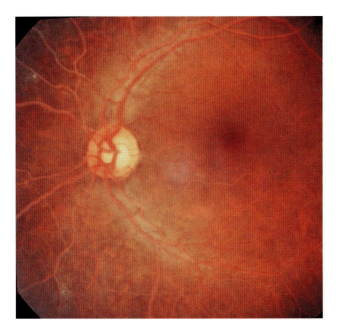

Fig. 13.64 Lipaemia retinalis

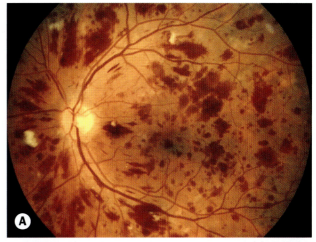

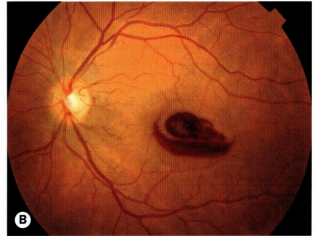

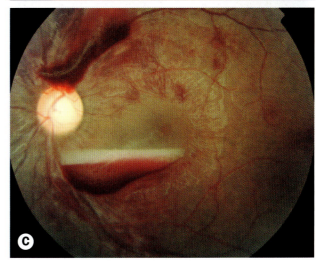

leukaemias are characterized by the replacement of bone marrow with immature (blast) cells. Chronic leukaemias are associated, at least initially, with well-differentiated (mature) leukocytes and occur almost exclusively in adults. The four major variants of leukaemia are:

- **Acute lymphocytic** (lymphoblastic) predominantly affects children, in whom there is around a 90% 5-year survival rate.
- **Acute myeloid** (myeloblastic) is most frequently seen in older adults.
- **Chronic lymphocytic** has a very chronic course, and many patients die from unrelated disease.
- **Chronic myelocytic** has a progressive clinical course and often a less favourable prognosis.

Ocular features

Ocular involvement is more commonly seen in the acute than the chronic forms and virtually any ocular structure may be involved. Primary leukaemic infiltration is fairly rare. Secondary changes such as those associated with anaemia, thrombocytopenia, hyperviscosity and opportunistic infections are more common and include intraocular bleeding, infection and vascular occlusion.

- **Fundus**
  - Retinal haemorrhages and cotton wool spots are common (Fig. 13.65).
  - Roth spots are retinal haemorrhages with white centres (Fig. 13.66), the whitish element thought to be composed of coagulated fibrin in most cases. They occur in acute leukaemias, and in a range of other conditions such as bacteraemia (classically subacute bacterial endocarditis), diabetes, hypertension and anaemia.
  - Peripheral retinal neovascularization is an occasional feature of chronic myeloid leukaemia (Fig. 13.67A).

Fig. 13.65 Retinal haemorrhages in leukaemia. **(A)** Numerous flame haemorrhages with cotton wool spots and Roth spots; **(B)** premacular bleed; **(C)** large retrohyaloid haemorrhage – a separate white cell layer is evident
(Courtesy of C Barry – fig. A; S Chen – figs B and C)

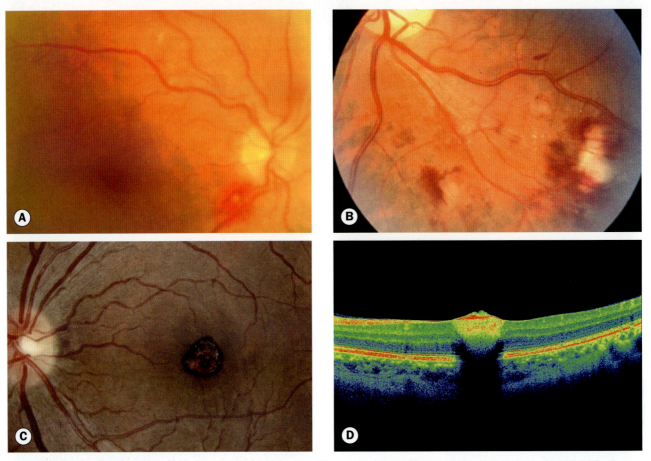

Fig. 13.66 Roth spots. **(A)** Typical appearance; **(B)** large lesion; **(C)** macular lesion in acute myeloid leukaemia; **(D)** OCT of lesion in (C)

(Courtesy of S Chen – figs C and D)

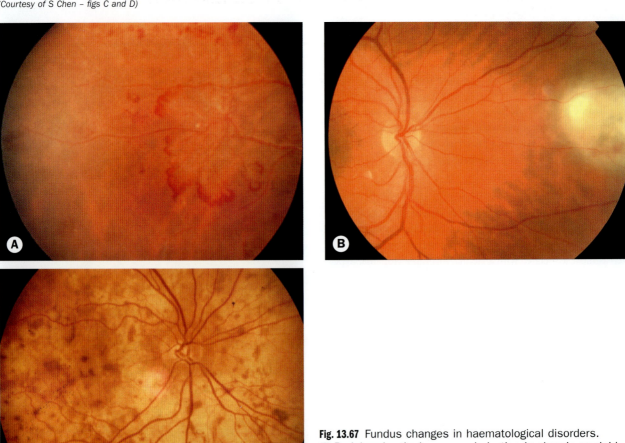

Fig. 13.67 Fundus changes in haematological disorders. **(A)** Peripheral retinal neovascularization in chronic myeloid leukaemia; **(B)** leukaemic chorioretinal deposit; **(C)** 'leopard skin' appearance due to choroidal infiltration in chronic leukaemia

(Courtesy of P Morse – fig. A)

○ Retinal and choroidal infiltrates may occur, most commonly posterior to the equator (Fig. 13.67B), and may masquerade as posterior uveitides; in chronic leukaemia they may give rise to a 'leopard skin' appearance (Fig. 13.67C).

○ Optic nerve infiltration may cause swelling and visual loss.

- **Other features**
  ○ Orbital involvement, particularly in children (Fig. 13.68).
  ○ Iris thickening, iritis and pseudohypopyon.
  ○ Spontaneous subconjunctival haemorrhage and hyphaema.
  ○ Cranial nerve palsies.

Anaemia

The anaemias are a group of disorders characterized by a decrease in the number of circulating red blood cells or in the amount of haemoglobin in each cell, or both. Retinal changes in anaemia are usually innocuous and rarely of diagnostic importance.

- **Retinopathy**
  ○ Retinal venous tortuosity is related to the severity of anaemia but may occur in isolation.

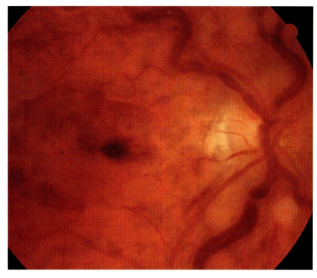

Fig. 13.69 Retinal haemorrhages, and gross venous dilatation and segmentation in hyperviscosity

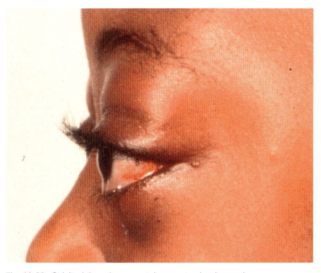

Fig. 13.68 Orbital involvement in acute leukaemia

○ Dot, blot and flame haemorrhages, cotton wool spots and Roth spots (see Fig. 13.66) are more common with co-existing thrombocytopenia.

- **Optic neuropathy** may occur in pernicious anaemia.

Hyperviscosity

The hyperviscosity states are a diverse group of rare disorders characterized by increased blood viscosity due to polycythaemia or abnormal plasma proteins.

- **Polycythaemia** is caused by the neoplastic proliferation of erythrocytes with increased bone marrow activity and hyperviscosity.
- **Waldenström macroglobulinaemia** is a malignant lymphoproliferative disorder with monoclonal IgM production, which most frequently affects elderly men.
- **Ocular features** include retinal haemorrhages and venous changes (Fig. 13.69), and occasionally retinal vein occlusion and conjunctival telangiectasia.

Chapter 14

Acquired macular disorders

INTRODUCTION

Anatomical landmarks

The macula (Fig. 14.1A) is a round area at the posterior pole, lying inside the temporal vascular arcades. It measures between 5 and 6 mm in diameter, and subserves the central 15–20° of the visual field. Histologically, it shows more than one layer of ganglion cells, in contrast to the single ganglion cell layer of the peripheral retina. The inner layers of the macula contain the yellow xanthophyll carotenoid pigments lutein and zeaxanthin in far higher concentration than the peripheral retina (hence the full name 'macula lutea' – yellow plaque).

- **The fovea** is a depression in the retinal surface at the centre of the macula (Figs 14.1B and C), with a diameter of 1.5 mm – about the same as the optic disc.
- **The foveola** forms the central floor of the fovea and has a diameter of 0.35 mm (see Fig. 14.1C). It is the thinnest part of the retina and is devoid of ganglion cells, consisting only of a high density of cone photoreceptors and their nuclei (Fig. 14.2), together with Müller cells.
- **The umbo** is a depression in the very centre of the foveola (see Fig. 14.1C) which corresponds to the foveolar light reflex (see Fig. 14.1A), loss of which may be an early sign of damage.
- **The foveal avascular zone** (FAZ – see Fig. 14.1C), a central area containing no blood vessels but surrounded by a

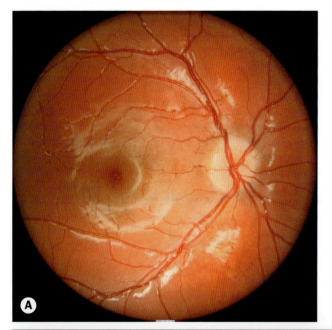

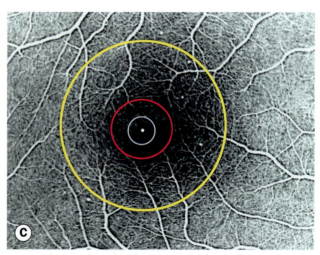

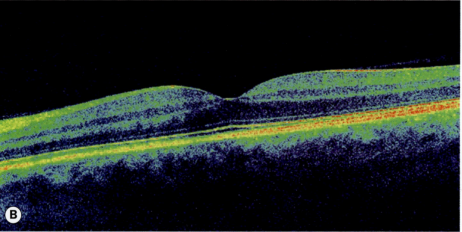

Fig. 14.1 Anatomical landmarks. **(A)** Normal foveolar (almost punctate central reflex) and macular (band-like reflex encircling the fovea) light reflexes; **(B)** OCT showing the foveal depression; **(C)** fluorescein angiogram – fovea (yellow circle), approximate extent of the foveal avascular zone (red circle), foveola (lilac circle), umbo (central white spot)
(Courtesy of S Chen – fig. B)

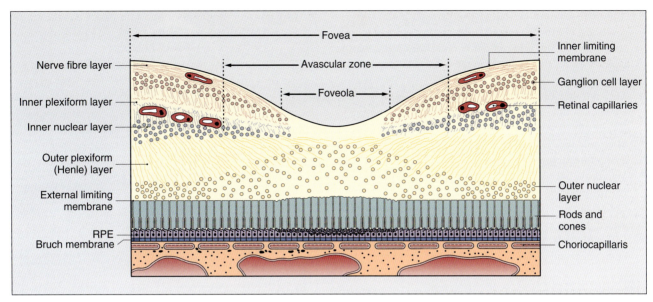

Fig. 14.2 Cross-section of the fovea (RPE = retinal pigment epithelium)

continuous network of capillaries, is located within the fovea but extends beyond the foveola. The exact diameter varies with age and in disease, and its limits can be determined with accuracy only by fluorescein angiography (average 0.6 mm).

Retinal pigment epithelium

- **Structure**
  - The retinal pigment epithelium (RPE) is composed of a single layer of cells that are hexagonal in cross-section. The cells consist of an outer non-pigmented basal element containing the nucleus, and an inner pigmented apical section containing abundant melanosomes.
  - The cell base is in contact with Bruch membrane, and at the cell apices multiple thread-like villous processes extend between the outer segments of the photoreceptors.
  - At the posterior pole, particularly at the fovea, RPE cells are taller and thinner, more regular in shape and contain more numerous and larger melanosomes than in the periphery.
- **Function**
  - RPE cells and intervening tight junctional complexes (zonula occludentes) constitute the outer blood–retinal barrier, preventing extracellular fluid leaking into the subretinal space from the choriocapillaris, and actively pumping ions and water out of the subretinal space.
  - Its integrity, and that of the Bruch membrane, is important for continued adhesion between the two, thought to be due to a combination of osmotic and hydrostatic forces, possibly with the aid of hemidesmosomal attachments.
  - Facilitation of photoreceptor turnover by the phagocytosis and lysosomal degradation of outer segments following shedding.

- Preservation of an optimal retinal milieu. Maintenance of the outer blood–retinal barrier is a key factor, as are the inward transport of metabolites (mainly small molecules such as amino acids and glucose) and the outward transport of metabolic waste products.
- Storage, metabolism and transport of vitamin A in the visual cycle.
- The dense RPE pigment serves to absorb stray light.

Bruch membrane

- **Structure.** The Bruch membrane separates the RPE from the choriocapillaris and on electron microscopy consists of five distinct elements:
  - The basal lamina of the RPE.
  - An inner collagenous layer.
  - A thicker band of elastic fibres.
  - An outer collagenous layer.
  - The basal lamina of the inner layer of the choriocapillaris.
- **Function.** The RPE utilizes Bruch membrane as a route for the transport of metabolic waste products out of the retinal environment. Changes in its structure are thought to be important in the pathogenesis of many macular disorders – for example, intact Bruch membrane may be important in the suppression of choroidal neovascularization (CNV).

CLINICAL EVALUATION OF MACULAR DISEASE

Symptoms

- **Blurred vision** and difficulty with close work may be an early symptom. Onset can be rapid in some conditions, such as CNV.

- **A positive scotoma**, in which patients complain of something obstructing central vision, is a symptom of more severe disease. This is in contrast to optic neuropathy, which typically causes a missing area in the visual field (negative scotoma).
- **Metamorphopsia** (distortion of perceived images) is a common symptom that is virtually never present in optic neuropathy.
- **Micropsia** (decrease in image size) is caused by spreading apart of foveal cones, and is less common.
- **Macropsia** (increase in image size) is due to crowding together of foveal cones, and is uncommon.
- **Colour** discrimination may be disturbed, but is generally less evident than in even relatively mild optic neuropathy.
- **Difficulties related to dark adaptation,** such as poor vision in dim light and persistence of after-images, may occur.

Visual acuity

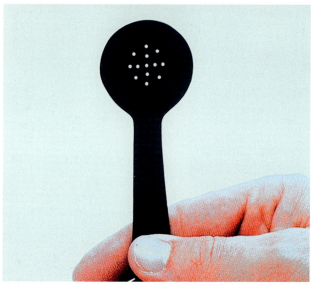

Fig. 14.4 Pinhole occluder

Snellen visual acuity

Distance visual acuity (VA) is directly related to the minimum angle of separation (subtended at the nodal point of the eye) between two objects that allow them to be perceived as distinct. In practice, it is most commonly carried out using a Snellen chart, which utilizes black letters or symbols (optotypes) of a range of sizes set on a white chart (Fig. 14.3), with the subject reading the chart from a standard distance. Distance VA is usually first measured using a patient's refractive correction, generally their own glasses or contact lenses. For completeness, an unaided acuity may also be recorded. The eye reported as having worse vision should be tested first, with the other eye occluded. It is important to push the patient to read every letter possible on the optotypes being tested.

- **Normal monocular VA** equates to 6/6 (metric notation; 20/20 in non-metric 'English' notation) on Snellen testing. Normal corrected VA in young adults is often superior to 6/6.
- **Best-corrected VA** (BCVA) denotes the level achieved with optimal refractive correction.
- **Pinhole VA:** a pinhole (PH) aperture compensates for the effect of refractive errors, and consists of an opaque occluder perforated by one or more holes of about 1 mm diameter (Fig. 14.4). However, PH acuity in patients with macular disease and posterior lens opacities may be worse than with spectacle correction. If the VA is less than 6/6 Snellen equivalent, testing is repeated using a pinhole aperture.
- **Binocular VA** is usually superior to the better monocular VA of each eye, at least where both eyes have roughly equal vision.

Very poor visual acuity

- **Counts (or counting) fingers** (CF) denotes that the patient is able to tell how many fingers the examiner is holding up at a specified distance (Fig. 14.5), usually 1 metre.
- **Hand movements (HM)** is the ability to distinguish whether the examiner's hand is moving when held just in front of the patient.
- **Perception of light (PL):** the patient can discern only light (e.g. pen torch), but no shapes or movement. Careful occlusion of a fellow seeing eye is necessary. If poor vision is due only to dense media opacity such as cataract, the patient should readily be able to determine the direction from which the light is being projected (Fig. 14.6).

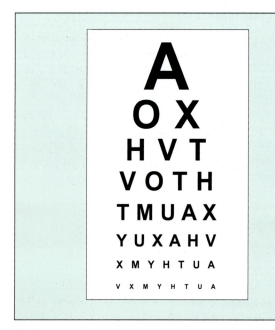

Fig. 14.3 Snellen visual acuity chart

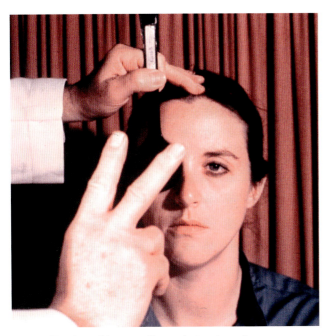

Fig. 14.5 Testing of 'counts fingers' visual acuity

LogMAR acuity

LogMAR charts address many of the deficiencies of the Snellen chart (Table 14.1), and are the standard means of VA measurement in research and increasingly in clinical practice.

- LogMAR is an acronym for the base-10 logarithm of the minimum angle of resolution, and refers to the ability to resolve the elements of an optotype. Thus, if a letter on the 6/6 (20/20) equivalent line subtends 5′ of arc, and each limb

Table 14.1 Comparison of Snellen and logMAR visual acuity testing

Snellen	LogMAR
Shorter test time	Longer test time
More letters on the lower lines introduces an unbalanced 'crowding' effect	Equal numbers of letters on different lines controls for 'crowding' effect
Fewer larger letters reduces accuracy at lower levels of VA	Equal numbers of letters on low and higher acuity lines increases accuracy at lower VA
Variable readability between individual letters	Similar readability between letters
Lines not balanced with each other for consistency of readability	Lines balanced for consistency of readability
6 m testing distance: longer testing lane (or a mirror) required	4 m testing distance on many charts: smaller testing lane (or no mirror) required
Letter and row spacing not systematic	Letter and row spacing set to optimize contour interaction
Lower accuracy and consistency so relatively unsuitable for research	Higher accuracy and consistency so appropriate for research
Straightforward scoring system	More complex scoring
Easy to use	Less user-friendly

of the letter has an angular width of 1′, an MAR of 1′ is needed for resolution. For the 6/12 (20/40) line, the MAR is 2′, and for the 6/60 (20/200) line it is 10′.

- The logMAR score is simply the base-10 log of the MAR, so as the log of the MAR value of 1′ is zero, 6/6 is equivalent to logMAR 0.00. The log of the 6/60 MAR of 10′ is 1, so 6/60 is equivalent to logMAR 1.00. The log of the 6/12 MAR of 2′ is 0.301, giving a logMAR score of 0.30. Scores better than 6/6 have a negative value.
- As letter size changes by 0.1 logMAR units per row and there are five letters in each row, each letter can be assigned a score of 0.02. The final score can therefore take account of every letter that has been read correctly and the test should continue until half of the letters on a line are read incorrectly.

LogMAR charts

- **The Bailey–Lovie** chart (Fig. 14.7).
  - Used at 6 m testing distance.
  - Each line of the chart comprises five letters and the spacing between each letter and each row is related to the width and the height of the letters. A 6/6 letter is 5′ in height by 4′ in width.

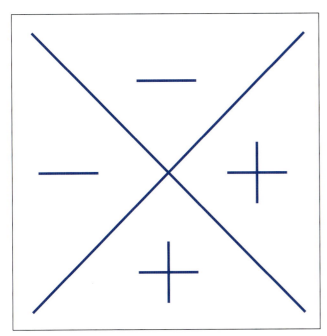

Fig. 14.6 Notation for the projection of light test (right eye); the patient cannot detect light directed from the superior and temporal quadrants

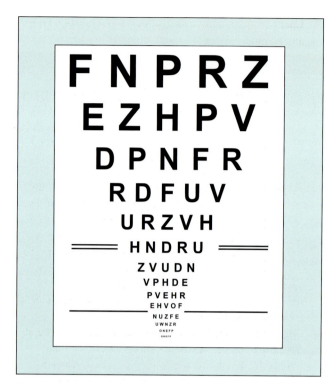

Fig. 14.7 Bailey–Lovie chart

○ The distance between two adjacent letters on the same row is equal to the width of a letter from the same row, and the distance between two adjacent rows is the same as the height of a letter from the lower of the two rows.

○ Snellen VA values and logMAR VA are listed to the right and left of the rows respectively.

• **Other charts** are available that are calibrated for 4 m. The Early Treatment Diabetic Retinopathy Study (ETDRS) charts utilize balanced rows comprising Sloan optotypes, developed to confer equivalent legibility between individual letters and rows. ETDRS letters are square, based on a 5 × 5 grid, i.e. 5′ × 5′ for the 6/6 equivalent letters at 6 m.

• **Computer charts** are available that present the various forms of test chart on display screens, including other means of assessment such as contrast sensitivity (see below).

Contrast sensitivity

• **Principles.** Contrast sensitivity is a measure of the ability of the visual system to distinguish an object against its background. A target must be sufficiently large to be seen, but must also be of high enough contrast with its background; a light grey letter will be less well seen against a white background than a black letter. Contrast sensitivity represents a different aspect of visual function to that tested by the spatial resolution tests described above, which all use high-contrast optotypes.

○ Many conditions reduce both contrast sensitivity and visual acuity, but under some circumstances (e.g. amblyopia, optic neuropathy, some cataracts, and

higher-order aberrations), visual function measured by contrast sensitivity can be reduced whilst VA is preserved.

○ Hence, if patients with good VA complain of visual symptoms (typically evident in low illumination), contrast sensitivity testing may be a useful way of objectively demonstrating a functional deficit. Despite its advantages, it has not been widely adopted in clinical practice.

• **The Pelli–Robson** contrast sensitivity letter chart is viewed at 1 metre and consists of rows of letters of equal size (spatial frequency of 1 cycle per degree) but with decreasing contrast of 0.15 log units for groups of three letters (Fig. 14.8). The patient reads down the rows of letters until the lowest-resolvable group of three is reached.

• **Sinusoidal (sine wave) gratings** require the test subject to view a sequence of increasingly lower contrast gratings.

Near visual acuity

Near vision testing can be a sensitive indicator of the presence of macular disease. A range of near vision charts (including logMAR and ETDRS versions) or a test-type book can be used. The book or chart is held at a comfortable reading distance and this is measured and noted. The patient wears any necessary distance correction together with a presbyopia correction if applicable (usually their own reading spectacles). The smallest type legible is recorded for each eye individually and then using both eyes together.

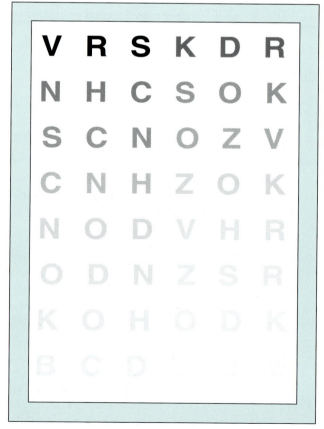

Fig. 14.8 Pelli–Robson contrast sensitivity letter chart

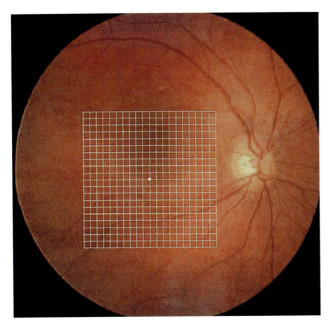

Fig. 14.9 Amsler grid superimposed on the macula; the central fixation dot of the grid probably does not coincide with the foveal anatomical centre in this image

(Courtesy of A Franklin)

Amsler grid

The Amsler grid evaluates the 20° of the visual field centred on fixation (Fig. 14.9). It is principally useful in screening for and monitoring macular disease, but will also demonstrate central visual field defects originating elsewhere. Patients with a substantial risk of CNV should be provided with an Amsler grid for regular use at home.

Charts

There are seven charts, each consisting of a 10 cm outer square (Figs 14.10 and 14.11).

- Chart 1 consists of a white grid on a black background, the outer grid enclosing 400 smaller 5 mm squares. When viewed at about one-third of a metre, each small square subtends an angle of 1°.
- Chart 2 is similar to chart 1 but has diagonal lines that aid fixation for patients with a central scotoma.
- Chart 3 is identical to chart 1 but has red squares. The red-on-black design aims to stimulate long wavelength foveal cones. It is used to detect subtle colour scotomas and desaturation in toxic maculopathy, optic neuropathy and chiasmal lesions.
- Chart 4 consists only of random dots and is used mainly to distinguish scotomas from metamorphopsia, as there is no form to be distorted.
- Chart 5 consists of horizontal lines and is designed to detect metamorphopsia along specific meridians. It is of particular use in the evaluation of patients describing difficulty reading.
- Chart 6 is similar to chart 5 but has a white background and the central lines are closer together, enabling more detailed evaluation.

- Chart 7 includes a fine central grid, each square subtending an angle of a half degree, and is more sensitive.

Technique

The pupils should not be dilated, and in order to avoid a photostress effect the eyes should not yet have been examined on the slit lamp. A presbyopic refractive correction should be worn if appropriate. The chart should be well illuminated and held at a comfortable reading distance, optimally around 33 cm.

1. One eye is covered.
2. The patient is asked to look directly at the central dot with the uncovered eye, to keep looking at this, and to report any distortion or waviness of the lines on the grid.
3. Reminding the patient to maintain fixation on the central dot, he or she is asked if there are blurred areas or blank spots anywhere on the grid. Patients with macular disease often report that the lines are wavy whereas those with optic neuropathy tend to remark that some of the lines are missing or faint but not distorted.
4. The patient is asked if he or she can see all four corners and all four sides of the square – a missing corner or border should raise the possibility of causes other than macular disease, such as glaucomatous field defects or retinitis pigmentosa.

The patient may be provided with a recording sheet and pen and asked to draw any anomalies (Fig. 14.12).

Pupils

The pupillary reactions to light are usually normal in eyes with macular disease, although extensive pathology such as a large area of CNV can give a relative afferent pupillary defect (RAPD). In

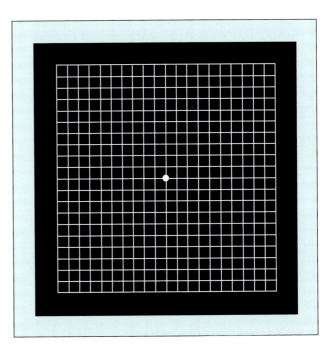

Fig. 14.10 Amsler grid chart

(Courtesy of A Franklin)

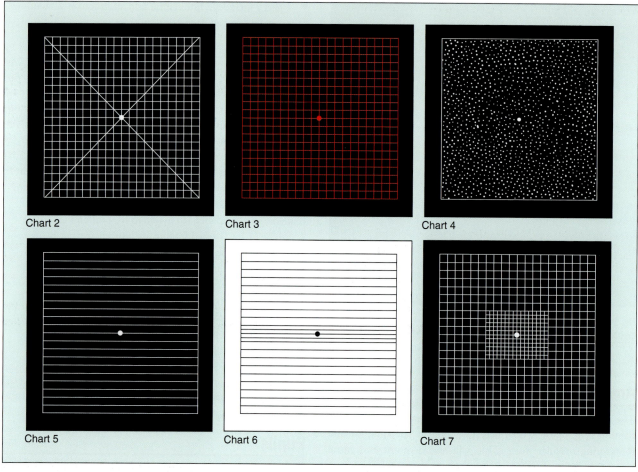

Fig. 14.11 Amsler charts 2–7
(Courtesy of A Franklin)

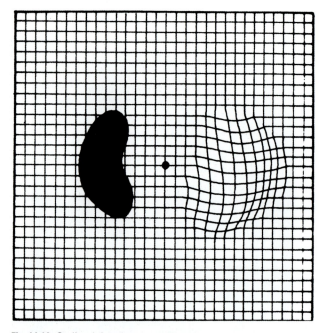

Fig. 14.12 Stylized Amsler recording sheet shows wavy lines indicating metamorphopsia, and a dense scotoma

contrast, an RAPD occurs in relatively mild cases of asymmetrical optic neuropathy.

Colour vision

Colour vision is commonly affected only in proportion to the decrease in visual acuity in macular disease, again in contrast to optic neuropathy where subtle colour desaturation is an early sign. Inherited retinal dystrophies such as cone dystrophy are an exception.

Plus lens test

A temporary hypermetropic shift may occur in some conditions due to an elevation of the sensory retina – the classic example is central serous chorioretinopathy (CSR). A +1.00 dioptre lens will demonstrate the phenomenon.

INVESTIGATION OF MACULAR DISEASE

Microperimetry

This is a newer investigative technique that has hitherto been used principally in research but may increasingly be incorporated into clinical practice. It measures sensitivity at finely spaced central retinal loci, including in patients with poor fixation, and uses a tracking system based on image registration to facilitate serial monitoring, allowing detection of subtle change.

Fundus fluorescein angiography

Introduction

Fluorescein angiography (FA) should be performed only if the findings are likely to influence management.

- **Fluorescence** is the property of certain molecules to emit light of a longer wavelength when stimulated by light of a shorter wavelength. The excitation peak for fluorescein is about 490 nm (in the blue part of the spectrum) – the wavelength of maximal absorption of light energy by fluorescein. Stimulated molecules will emit yellow–green light of about 530 nm (Fig. 14.13).
- **Fluorescein** (sodium fluorescein) is an orange water-soluble dye that, when injected intravenously, remains largely intravascular (>70% bound to serum proteins). It is excreted in the urine over 24–36 hours.
- **FA** involves photographic surveillance of the passage of fluorescein through the retinal and choroidal circulations following intravenous injection.
- **Outer blood–retinal barrier.** The major choroidal vessels are impermeable to both bound and free fluorescein. However, the walls of the choriocapillaris contain fenestrations through which unbound molecules escape into the extravascular space, crossing Bruch membrane but on reaching the RPE are blocked by intercellular complexes termed tight junctions or zonula occludentes (Fig. 14.14).
- **Inner blood–retinal barrier** is composed principally of the tight junctions between retinal capillary endothelial cells, across which neither bound nor free fluorescein can pass; the basement membrane and pericytes play only a minor role in this regard (Fig. 14.15A). Disruption of the inner

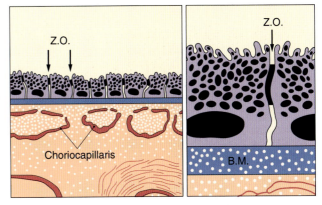

Fig. 14.14 The outer blood–retinal barrier (Z.O. = zonula occludentes; B.M. = Bruch membrane)

blood–retinal barrier permits leakage of both bound and free fluorescein into the extravascular space (Fig. 14.15B).

- **Filters** (Fig. 14.16)
  - Cobalt blue excitation filter. Incident white light from the camera is filtered so that blue light enters the eye, exciting the fluorescein molecules in the retinal and choroidal circulations.
  - Yellow–green barrier filter blocks any blue light reflected from the eye, allowing only yellow–green emitted light to pass.

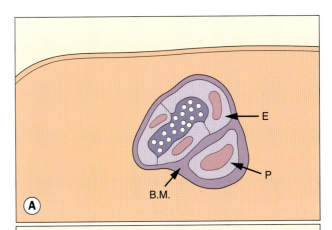

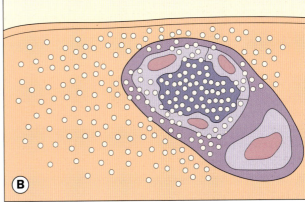

Fig. 14.15 Inner blood–retinal barrier. **(A)** Intact; **(B)** disrupted (E = endothelial cell; B.M. = basement membrane; P = pericyte)

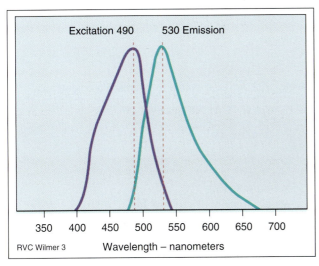

RVC Wilmer 3   Wavelength – nanometers

Fig. 14.13 Excitation and emission of fluorescein

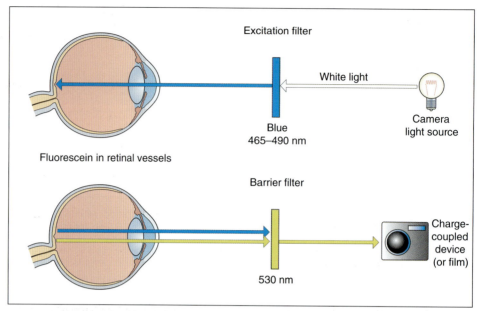

Fig. 14.16 Principles of fluorescein angiography

- **Image capture** in modern digital cameras uses a charge-coupled device (CCD). Digital imaging permits immediate picture availability, easy storage and access, image manipulation and enhancement. Modern devices also typically require a lower concentration of injected fluorescein to obtain high-quality images, with a correspondingly substantially lower incidence of adverse effects.
- **Contraindications**
  - Fluorescein allergy is an absolute contraindication, and a history of a severe reaction to any allergen is a strong relative contraindication. Preventative anti-allergy pre-treatment may be helpful in some cases.
  - Other relative contraindications include renal failure (a lower fluorescein dose is used), pregnancy, moderate–severe asthma and significant cardiac disease.
  - Allergy to iodine-containing media or seafood is not a clear contraindication to FA or to indocyanine green angiography (ICGA).

Technique

Facilities must be in place to address possible adverse events. This includes adequate staffing, a resuscitation trolley that includes drugs for the treatment of anaphylaxis, a couch (or reclining chair) and a receiver in case of vomiting; significant nausea and vomiting, and probably other adverse reactions, are now much less common with the lower fluorescein concentrations required by modern digital cameras.

- Adequate pharmacological mydriasis is important to obtain high-quality images; media opacity such as cataract may reduce picture quality.
- The procedure is explained and formal consent taken. It is important to mention common and serious adverse effects

(Table 14.2), particularly the invariable skin and urine staining. As noted above, adverse effects are generally now much less common.

- The patient should be seated comfortably in front of the fundus camera, and colour photographs, red-free (green incident light, to enhance red detail) and autofluorescence images taken as indicated.
- An intravenous cannula is inserted; a standard cannula is often preferred rather than a less secure 'butterfly' winged infusion set. After cannulation, the line should be flushed with normal saline to check patency and exclude extravasation.
- Fluorescein, usually 5 ml of a 10% solution, is drawn up into a syringe and injected over the course of 5–10 seconds, taking care not to rupture the cannulated vein (Fig. 14.17).
- Oral administration at a dose of 30 mg/kg is an alternative if venous access cannot be obtained or is refused; a 5 ml vial of 10% (100 mg/ml) sodium fluorescein contains 500 mg, and

Table 14.2 Adverse events in fluorescein angiography

Discoloration of skin and urine (invariable)
Extravasation of injected dye, giving a painful local reaction (treat with cold compress)
Nausea, vomiting (now rare with lower concentrations of fluorescein)
Itching, rash
Sneezing, wheezing
Vasovagal episode or syncope (usually due to anxiety but sometimes to ischaemic heart disease)
Anaphylactic and anaphylactoid reactions (1:2000 angiograms)
Myocardial infarction (extremely rare)
Death (1:220 000 in the largest study)

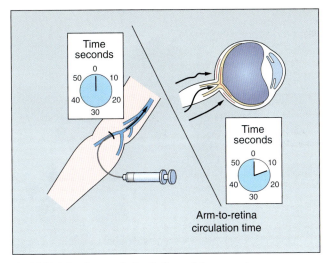

Fig. 14.17 Injection and circulation of fluorescein

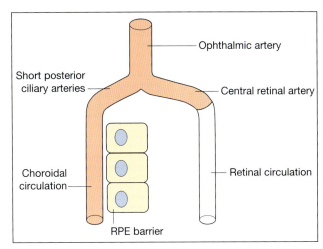

Fig. 14.18 Fluorescein access to the eye

pictures should be taken over 20–60 minutes following ingestion.

- Images are taken at 1–2 second intervals initially to capture the critical early transit phases, beginning 5–10 seconds after injection, tapering frequency through subsequent phases.
- With monocular pathology, control pictures of the opposite eye should be taken, usually after the initial transit phase has been photographed in the index eye.
- If appropriate, images may be captured as late as 10–20 minutes.
- Stereo images may be helpful to demonstrate elevation, and are usually taken by manually repositioning the camera sideways or by using a special device (a stereo separator) to adjust the image; these are actually 'pseudostereo', true stereo requiring simultaneous image capture from different angles.

Angiographic phases

Fluorescein enters the eye through the ophthalmic artery, passing into the choroidal circulation through the short posterior ciliary arteries and into the retinal circulation through the central retinal artery (Fig. 14.18); the choroidal circulation fills about 1 second before the retinal. Precise details of the choroidal circulation are typically not discernible, mainly because of rapid leakage of free fluorescein from the choriocapillaris; melanin in the RPE cells also blocks choroidal fluorescence. The angiogram consists of the following overlapping phases:

- **The choroidal** (pre-arterial) phase typically occurs 9–15 seconds after dye injection – longer in patients with poor general circulation – and is characterized by patchy lobular filling of the choroid due to leakage of free fluorescein from the fenestrated choriocapillaris. A cilioretinal artery, if present, will fill at this time because it is derived from the posterior ciliary circulation (Fig. 14.19A).
- **The arterial phase** starts about a second after the onset of choroidal fluorescence, and shows retinal arteriolar filling and the continuation of choroidal filling (Fig. 14.19B).

- **The arteriovenous (capillary) phase** shows complete filling of the arteries and capillaries with early laminar flow in the veins in which the dye appears to line the venous wall leaving an axial hypofluorescent strip (Fig. 14.19C). This phenomenon reflects initial drainage from posterior pole capillaries filling the venous margins, as well as the small-vessel velocity profile, with faster plasma flow adjacent to vessel walls where cellular concentration is lower.
- **The venous phase.** Laminar venous flow (Fig. 14.19D) progresses to complete filling (Fig. 14.19E), with late venous phase featuring reducing arterial fluorescence. Maximal perifoveal capillary filling is reached at around 20–25 seconds in patients with normal cardiovascular function, and the first pass of fluorescein circulation is generally completed by approximately 30 seconds.
- **The late (recirculation) phase** demonstrates the effects of continuous recirculation, dilution and elimination of the dye. With each succeeding wave, the intensity of fluorescence becomes weaker although the disc shows staining (Fig. 14.19F). Fluorescein is absent from the retinal vasculature after about 10 minutes.
- **The dark appearance of the fovea** (Fig. 14.20A) is caused by three factors (Fig. 14.20B):
  ○ Absence of blood vessels in the FAZ.
  ○ Blockage of background choroidal fluorescence due to the high density of xanthophyll at the fovea.
  ○ Blockage of background choroidal fluorescence by the RPE cells at the fovea, which are larger and contain more melanin and lipofuscin than elsewhere in the retina.

Causes of hyperfluorescence

- **Autofluorescent** compounds absorb blue light and emit yellow–green light in a similar fashion to fluorescein, but much more weakly. Autofluorescence can be detected on standard fundus photography with the excitation and barrier filters both in place; some modern digital cameras have

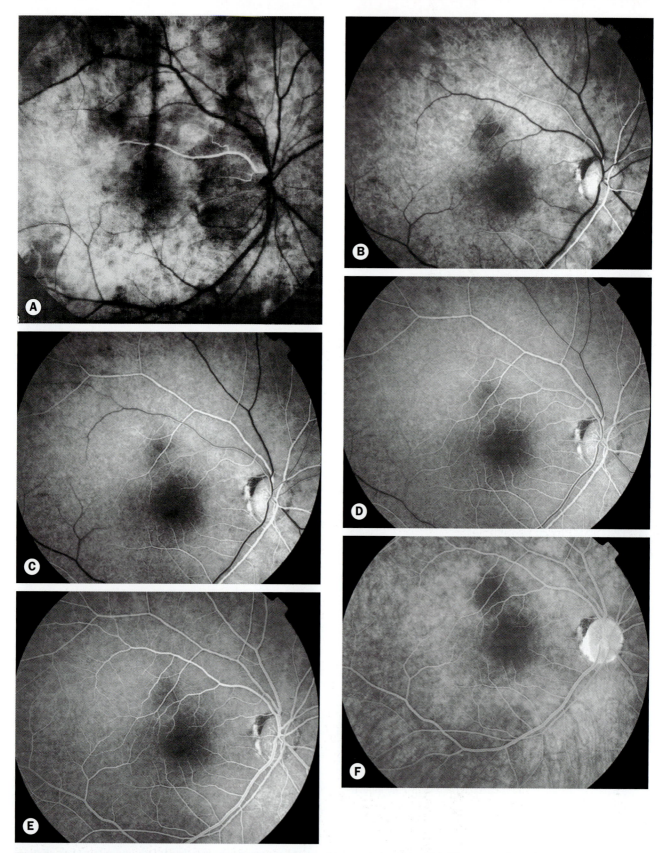

Fig. 14.19 Normal fluorescein angiogram. **(A)** Choroidal phase shows patchy choroidal filling as well as filling of a cilioretinal artery; **(B)** arterial phase shows filling of the choroid and retinal arteries; **(C)** arteriovenous (capillary) phase shows complete arterial filling and early laminar venous flow; **(D)** early venous phase shows marked laminar venous flow; **(E)** mid-venous phase shows almost complete venous filling; **(F)** late (recirculation) phase shows weaker fluorescence with staining of the optic disc

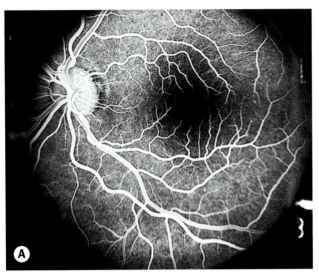

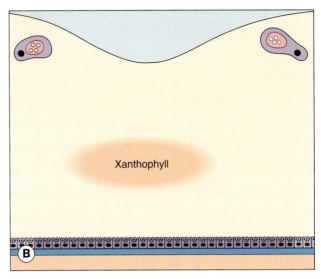

Fig. 14.20 (A) Dark appearance of the fovea on FA; **(B)** anatomical causative factors (see text)

enhanced autofluorescence detection capability, though imaging is most effective with scanning laser ophthalmoscopy. Autofluorescent lesions classically include optic nerve head drusen (Fig. 14.21) and astrocytic hamartoma, but with increased availability of

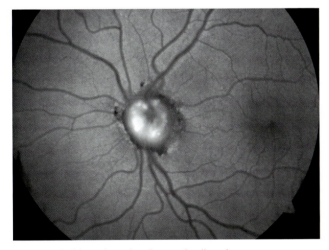

Fig. 14.21 FAF imaging showing optic disc drusen

high-sensitivity imaging, patterns associated with a wide range of posterior segment pathology have been characterized.

- **Pseudofluorescence** (false fluorescence) refers to non-fluorescent reflected light visible prior to fluorescein injection; this passes through the filters due to the overlap of wavelengths passing through the excitation then the barrier filters. It is more evident when filters are wearing out.
- **Increased fluorescence** may be caused by (a) enhanced visualization of normal fluorescein density, or (b) an increase in fluorescein content of tissues.
- **A window defect** is caused by atrophy or absence of the RPE as in atrophic age-related macular degeneration (Fig. 14.22A), a full-thickness macular hole, RPE tears and some drusen. This results in unmasking of normal background choroidal fluorescence, characterized by very early hyperfluorescence that increases in intensity and then fades without changing size or shape (Figs 14.22B and C).
- **Pooling** in an anatomical space occurs due to breakdown of the outer blood–retinal barrier (RPE tight junctions):
  - In the subretinal space, e.g. CSR (Fig. 14.23A). This is characterized by early hyperfluorescence, which, as the

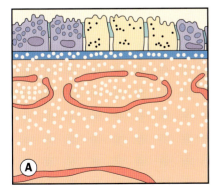

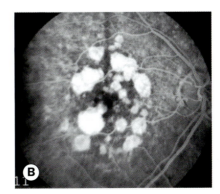

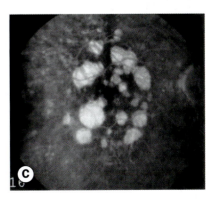

Fig. 14.22 Hyperfluorescence caused by window defects associated with dry age-related macular degeneration

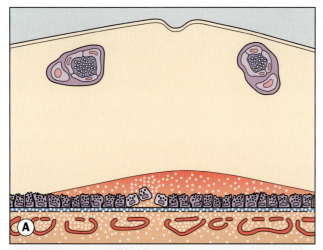

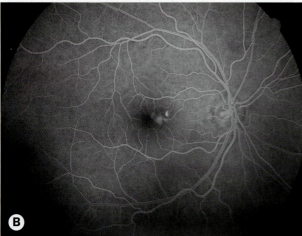

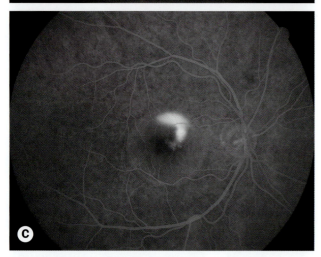

Fig. 14.23 Hyperfluorescence caused by pooling of dye in the subretinal space in central serous chorioretinopathy
(Courtesy of S Chen – figs B and C)

responsible leak tends to be only small (Fig. 14.23B), slowly increases in intensity and area, the maximum extent remaining relatively well defined (Fig. 14.23C).
   ○ In the sub-RPE space, as in pigment epithelial detachment (PED – Fig. 14.24A). This is characterized by

early hyperfluorescence (Fig. 14.24B) that increases in intensity but not in size (Fig. 14.24C).
- **Leakage** of dye is characterized by fairly early hyperfluorescence, increasing with time in both area and intensity. It occurs as a result of breakdown of the inner blood–retinal barrier due to:
  - Dysfunction or loss of existing vascular endothelial tight junctions as in background diabetic retinopathy (DR), retinal vein occlusion (RVO), cystoid macular oedema (CMO – Fig. 14.25A) and papilloedema.
  - Primary absence of vascular endothelial tight junctions as in CNV, proliferative diabetic retinopathy (Fig. 14.25B), tumours and some vascular anomalies such as Coats disease.
- **Staining** is a late phenomenon consisting of the prolonged retention of dye in entities such as drusen, fibrous tissue, exposed sclera and the normal optic disc (see Fig. 14.19F), and is seen in the later phases of the angiogram, particularly after the dye has left the choroidal and retinal circulations.

Causes of hypofluorescence

Reduction or absence of fluorescence may be due to: (a) optical obstruction (masking or blockage) of normal fluorescein density (Fig. 14.26) or (b) inadequate perfusion of tissue (filling defect).
- **Masking of retinal fluorescence.** Preretinal lesions such as blood will block all fluorescence (Fig. 14.27).
- **Masking of background choroidal fluorescence** allows persistence of fluorescence from superficial retinal vessels:
  - Deeper retinal lesions, e.g. intraretinal haemorrhages, dense exudates.
  - Subretinal or sub-RPE lesions, e.g. blood (Fig. 14.28).
  - Increased density of the RPE, e.g. congenital hypertrophy (Fig. 14.29).
  - Choroidal lesions, e.g. naevi.
- **Filling defects** may result from:
  - Vascular occlusion, which may involve the retinal arteries, veins or capillaries (capillary drop-out – Fig. 14.30A), or the choroidal circulation. FA is sometimes used to demonstrate optic nerve head filling defects as in anterior ischaemic optic neuropathy.
  - Loss of the vascular bed as in myopic degeneration and choroideremia (Fig. 14.30B).

Systematic approach to fluorescein angiogram analysis

A fluorescein angiogram should be interpreted methodically to optimize diagnostic accuracy.
1. Clinical findings, including the patient's age and gender, should be noted before assessing the images.
2. Note whether images of right, left or both eyes have been taken.
3. Comment on any colour and red-free images and on any pre-injection demonstration of pseudo- or autofluorescence.

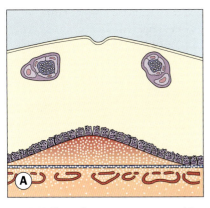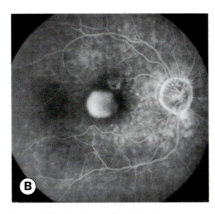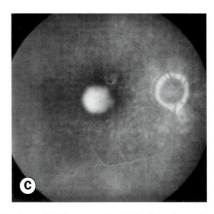

Fig. 14.24 Hyperfluorescence caused by pooling of dye in the sub-retinal pigment epithelium (RPE) space in RPE detachment

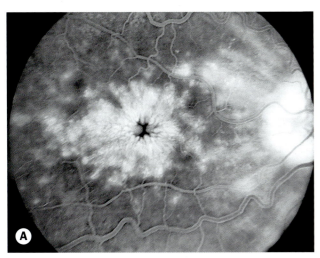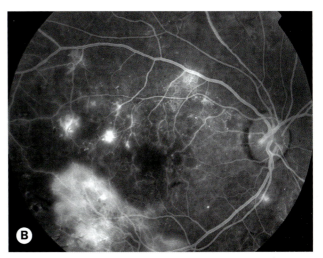

Fig. 14.25 Causes of hyperfluorescence due to leakage. **(A)** Cystoid macular oedema; **(B)** proliferative diabetic retinopathy showing leakage from extensive vessels on the inferior macular arcade
(Courtesy of P Gili – fig. A; S Chen – fig. B)

4. Looking at the post-injection images, indicate whether the overall timing of filling, especially arm-to-eye transit time, is normal.
5. Briefly scan through the sequence of images in time order for each eye in turn, initially concentrating on the eye with the

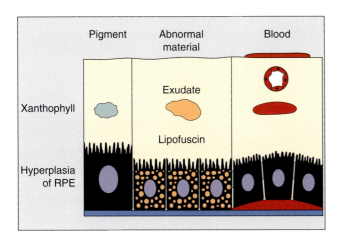

Fig. 14.26 Causes of blocked fluorescence

greatest number of shots as this is likely to be the one about which there is greater concern. On the first review, look for any characteristic major diagnostic, especially pathognomonic, features; examples might include a lacy filling pattern or a 'smokestack' (see later).
6. Go through the run for each eye in greater detail, noting the evolution of any major features found on the first scan and then providing a description of any other findings using the methodical consideration of the causes of hyper- and hypofluorescence set out above.

Indocyanine green angiography

Introduction

- **Advantages over FA.** Whilst FA is an excellent method of studying the retinal circulation, it is of limited use in delineating the choroidal vasculature, due principally to masking by the RPE. In contrast, the near-infrared light utilized in indocyanine green angiography (ICGA) penetrates ocular pigments such as melanin and xanthophyll,

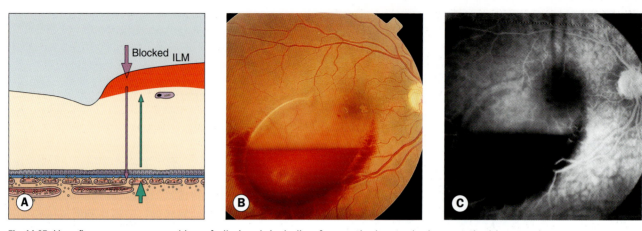

Fig. 14.27 Hypofluorescence – masking of all signal, including from retinal vessels, by preretinal haemorrhage (ILM = internal limiting membrane)

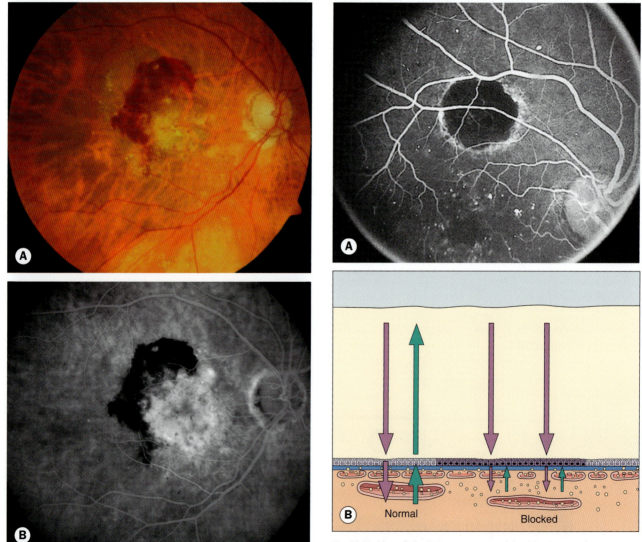

Fig. 14.28 Hypofluorescence – blockage by sub- and intraretinal haemorrhage, showing persistence of signal from retinal vessels

(Courtesy of S Chen)

Fig. 14.29 Hypofluorescence caused by blockage of background fluorescence by congenital hypertrophy of the retinal pigment epithelium

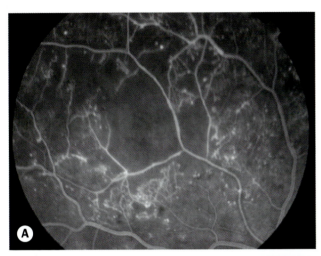

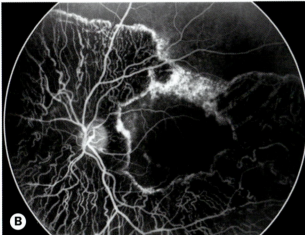

Fig. 14.30 Hypofluorescence caused by filling defects.
(A) Capillary drop-out in diabetic retinopathy;
(B) choroideremia

(Courtesy of C Barry – fig. B)

as well as exudate and thin layers of subretinal blood, making this technique eminently suitable. An additional factor is that about 98% of ICG molecules bind to serum protein (mainly albumin), considerably higher than the binding of fluorescein; therefore, as choriocapillaris fenestrations are impermeable to larger protein molecules, most ICG is retained within choroidal vessels. Infrared light is also scattered less than visible light, making ICGA superior to FA in eyes with media opacity.

- **Image capture.** ICG fluorescence is only 1/25th that of fluorescein so modern digital ICGA uses high-sensitivity videoangiographic image capture by means of an appropriately adapted camera. Both the excitation (805 nm) and emission (835 nm) filters are set at infrared wavelengths (Fig. 14.31). Alternatively, scanning laser ophthalmoscopy (SLO) systems provide high contrast images, with less scattering of light and fast image acquisition rates facilitating high quality ICG video.
- **The technique** is similar to that of FA, but with an increased emphasis on the acquisition of later images (up to about 45 minutes) than with FA. A dose of 25–50 mg in 1–2 ml water for injection is used.
- **Phases of ICGA:** (i) early – up to 60 seconds post-injection; (ii) early mid-phase – 1–3 minutes; (iii) late mid-phase – 3–15 minutes; and (iv) late phase – 15–45 minutes (Fig. 14.32).

Adverse effects

ICGA is generally better tolerated than FA.
- Nausea, vomiting and urticaria are uncommon, but anaphylaxis probably occurs with approximately equal incidence to FA.
- Serious reactions are exceptionally rare. ICG contains iodide and so should not be given to patients allergic to iodine or

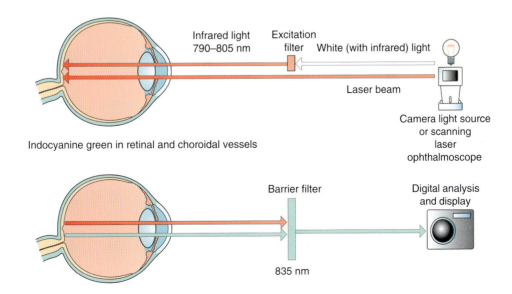

Fig. 14.31 Principles of indocyanine green angiography

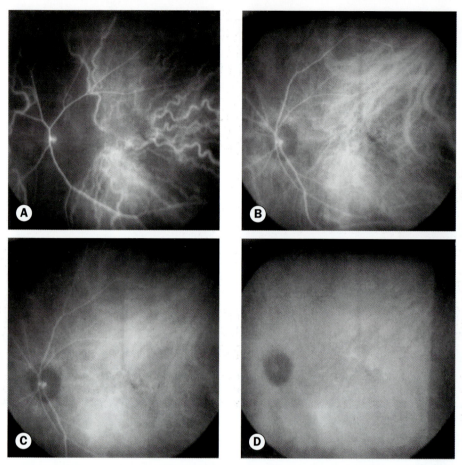

Fig. 14.32 Normal indocyanine green angiogram. **(A)** Early phase (up to 60 seconds post-injection) showing prominent choroidal arteries and poor early perfusion of the 'choroidal watershed' zone adjacent to the disc; **(B)** early mid-phase (1–3 minutes) showing greater prominence of choroidal veins as well as retinal vessels; **(C)** late mid-phase (3–15 minutes) showing fading of choroidal vessels but retinal vessels are still visible; diffuse tissue staining is also present; **(D)** late phase (15–45 minutes) showing hypofluorescent choroidal vessels and gradual fading of diffuse hyperfluorescence
(Courtesy of S Milewski)

possibly shellfish – iodine-free preparations such as infracyanine green are available.

- ICGA is relatively contraindicated in liver disease (excretion is hepatic), and as with FA in patients with a history of a severe reaction to any allergen, moderate or severe asthma and significant cardiac disease. Its safety in pregnancy has not been established.

Diagnosis

Examples of pathological images are shown under the discussion of individual conditions where relevant.

- **Hyperfluorescence**
  - A window defect similar to those seen with FA.
  - Leakage from retinal or choroidal vessels (Fig. 14.33), the optic nerve head or the RPE; this gives rise to tissue staining or to pooling.
  - Abnormal retinal or choroidal vessels with an anomalous morphology (see Fig. 14.33) and/or exhibiting greater fluorescence than normal.

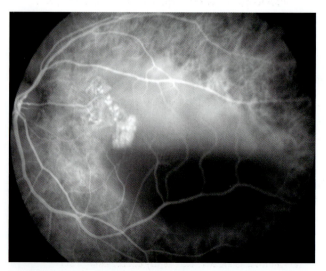

Fig. 14.33 ICGA image showing hyperfluorescence due to polyps and leakage in polypoidal choroidal vasculopathy
(Courtesy of S Chen)

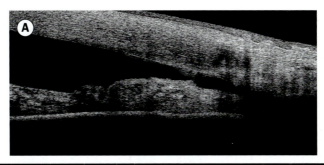

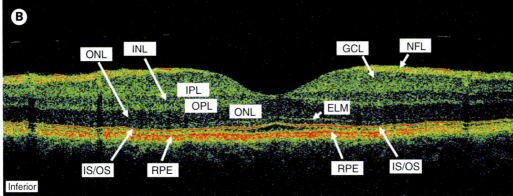

Fig. 14.34 OCT imaging. **(A)** Anterior chamber angle; **(B)** spectral-domain image of the macula: ELM = external limiting membrane; GCL = ganglion cell layer; INL = inner nuclear layer; IPL = inner plexiform layer; IS/OS = photoreceptor inner-segment/outer-segment junction; NFL = nerve fibre layer; ONL = outer nuclear layer; OPL = outer plexiform layer; RPE = retinal pigment epithelium

(Courtesy of J Fujimoto – fig. B)

- **Hypofluorescence**
  - ○ Blockage (masking) of fluorescence. Pigment and blood are self-evident causes, but fibrosis, infiltrate, exudate and serous fluid also block fluorescence. A particular phenomenon to note is that in contrast to its FA appearance, a pigment epithelial detachment appears predominantly hypofluorescent on ICGA.
  - ○ Filling defect due to obstruction or loss of choroidal or retinal circulation.

Indications

- **Polypoidal choroidal vasculopathy (PCV):** ICGA is far superior to FA for the imaging of PCV (see Fig. 14.33).
- **Exudative age-related macular degeneration (AMD).** Conventional FA remains the primary method of assessment, but ICGA can be a useful adjunct, particularly if PCV is suspected.
- **Chronic central serous chorioretinopathy** in which it is often difficult to interpret areas of leakage on FA. However, ICGA shows choroidal leakage and the presence of dilated choroidal vessels. Previously unidentified lesions elsewhere in the fundus are also frequently visible using ICGA.
- **Posterior uveitis.** ICGA can provide useful information beyond that available from FA in relation to diagnosis and the extent of disease involvement.

- **Choroidal tumours** may be imaged effectively but ICGA is inferior to clinical assessment for diagnosis.
- **Breaks in Bruch membrane** such as lacquer cracks and angioid streaks are more effectively defined on ICGA than on FA.
- If **FA is contraindicated**.

Optical coherence tomography

Introduction

Optical coherence tomography (OCT) is a non-invasive, non-contact imaging system providing high resolution cross-sectional images of the posterior segment. Imaging of the anterior segment (AS-OCT – Fig. 14.34A) has also been increasingly adopted. OCT is analogous to B-scan ultrasonography but uses near-infrared light interferometry rather than sound waves, with images created by the analysis of interference between reflected reference waves and those reflected by tissue. Most instruments in current use employ spectral/Fourier domain technology, in which the mechanical movement required for image acquisition in older 'time domain' machines has been eliminated and the information for each point on the A-scan is collected simultaneously, speeding data collection and improving resolution. Promising newer modalities include swept-source (SS) OCT that can acquire images at a much higher rate and with extremely high retinal element resolution and better imaging depth; choroidal definition is improving rapidly. So-called adaptive optics allows correction of higher-order optical aberrations to greatly improve resolution, and wide-field, intraoperative, functional and Doppler (blood flow measurement) OCT applications may all have clinical utility in the future.

Applications

- **Macula.** The diagnosis and monitoring of macular pathology has been revolutionized by the advent of OCT imaging, e.g. AMD, diabetic maculopathy, macular hole, epiretinal membrane and vitreomacular traction, CSR and retinal venous occlusion.
- **Glaucoma.** The widespread availability of OCT in ophthalmology suites for the assessment of medical retinal disease has contributed to its increased adoption as an adjunct to clinical and perimetric assessment in the management of glaucoma.
- **Retinal detachment.** Distinction of retinal detachment from retinoschisis.
- **Anterior segment OCT** has an expanding range of clinical applications such as suspected angle-closure glaucoma and corneal analysis (pachymetry, pre- and post-corneal refractive procedures, diagnosis and monitoring).

Normal appearance

High reflectivity structures can be depicted in a pseudo-colour image as red, intermediate as green-yellow and low reflectivity as blue-black. Fine retinal structures such as the external limiting membrane and ganglion cell layer can be defined (Fig. 14.34B). Detailed quantitative information on retinal thickness can be displayed numerically and in false-colour topographical maps; three-dimensional images can be constructed and different retinal layers studied in relief (Fig. 14.35).

Fundus autofluorescence

Imaging of fundus autofluorescence (FAF) using an enhanced fundus camera or scanning laser ophthalmoscopy permits visualization of accumulated lipofuscin in the retinal pigment epithelium. The scope of its place in the clinical management of macular degeneration and other conditions has not yet been clearly defined. It can be useful, for instance, to demonstrate more extensive macular disease than is visible clinically, in order either to determine the cause of unexplained poor visual acuity or to establish the reason for substantial visual symptoms despite good measured acuity. There is speculation that it may have greater utility in the future in the management of dry AMD once effective therapies become available. A key finding may be that FAF in patients with geographic atrophy (see below) shows distinct areas of autofluorescence at the leading edges of lesions that seems to precede retinal demise (Fig. 14.36); hyperautofluorescence is thought to commonly indicate retinal pigment epithelial stress. Autofluorescence is discussed further under 'Fluorescein angiography' above.

Wide-field imaging

Several wide-field (also referred to as ultrawide-field) high resolution imaging devices are now available. These are able to capture views of up to about 80% of the area of the retina in a single image; some have the facility of imaging FAF and FA (Fig. 14.37 and see especially Ch. 16), and can provide extremely useful additional information.

AGE-RELATED MACULAR DEGENERATION

Introduction

Age-related macular degeneration (AMD) is a degenerative disorder affecting the macula. It is characterized by the presence of specific clinical findings, including drusen and RPE changes, in the absence of another disorder. Later stages of the disease are associated with impairment of vision.

Classification

- **Conventionally,** AMD has been divided into two main types:
  - Dry (non-exudative, non-neovascular) AMD is the most common form, comprising around 90% of diagnosed disease. Geographic atrophy (GA) is the advanced stage of dry AMD; it has been authoritatively suggested that the term 'dry AMD' be used only to describe GA rather than earlier stages of AMD.
  - Wet (exudative, neovascular) AMD is much less common than dry, but is associated with more rapid progression to advanced sight loss. The main manifestations are CNV and PED, though in recent years at least two additional conditions, retinal angiomatous proliferation (RAP) and polypoidal choroidal vasculopathy (PCV), have been included under the umbrella of neovascular AMD by many authorities.
- A **recent expert consensus** committee has provided a clinical classification of AMD (Table 14.3).

Epidemiology

- AMD is the most common cause of irreversible visual loss in industrialized countries. In the USA, it is responsible for around 54% of severe sight loss (better eye worse than 6/60) in Caucasian, 14% in Hispanic and 4% in black individuals. The prevalence increases with age and symptoms are rare in patients under 50 years of age.
- In the UK, significant visual impairment (binocularly 6/18 or worse) from AMD affects about 4% of the population aged over 75 years and 14% of those over 90, with 1.6% over 75 having binocular acuity of less than 6/60.
- Patients with late AMD in one eye, or even moderate vision loss due to non-advanced AMD in one eye, have about a 50% chance of developing advanced AMD in the fellow eye within 5 years.

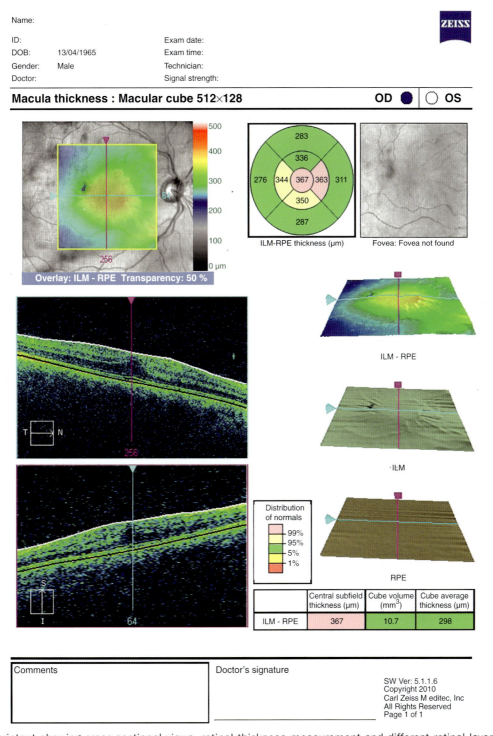

Fig. 14.35 OCT printout showing cross-sectional views, retinal thickness measurement and different retinal layers in a three-dimensional reconstruction in a patient with a macular epiretinal membrane and consequent loss of the foveal depression

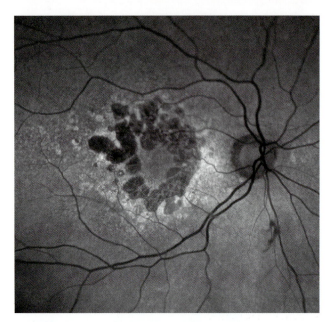

Fig. 14.36 Hyperautofluorescence edging areas of geographic atrophy

(Courtesy of S Chen)

Table 14.3 Clinical classification of age-related macular degeneration (AMD)

Category	Definition, based on presence of lesions within two disc diameters of the fovea in either eye
No apparent ageing changes	No drusen No AMD pigmentary abnormalities
Normal ageing changes	Only drupelets No AMD pigmentary abnormalities
Early AMD	Medium drusen (>63 μm but <125 μm) No AMD pigmentary abnormalities
Intermediate AMD	Large drusen (>125 μm) Any AMD pigmentary abnormalities
Late AMD	Neovascular AMD and/or any geographic atrophy

Pigmentary abnormalities: any definite hyper- or hypopigmentary abnormalities associated with medium or large drusen but not due to other known disease.

Drupelets: a newly proposed term for small drusen (<63 μm).

The size of drusen can be estimated by comparison with the approximately 125 μm diameter of a retinal vein at the optic disc margin.

Risk factors

AMD is multifactorial in aetiology, and is thought to involve a complex interaction between polygenic, lifestyle and environmental factors.

- **Age** is the major risk factor.
- **Race.** Late AMD is more common in white individuals than those of other races.

- **Heredity.** Family history is important; the risk of AMD is up to three times as high if a first-degree relative has the disease. Variants in many genes have been implicated in AMD risk and protection such as the complement factor H gene *CFH*, which helps to protect cells from complement-mediated damage, with several times the risk of AMD for homozygotes with a particular single nucleotide polymorphism (SNP), and

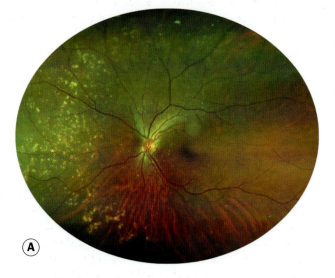

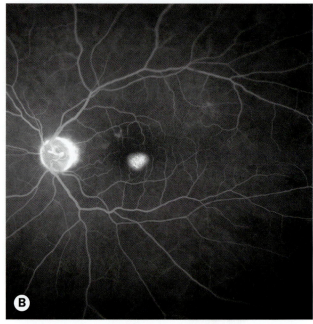

Fig. 14.37 Wide-field imaging. **(A)** Colour image of peripheral drusen; **(B)** FA in central serous chorioretinopathy

(Courtesy of S Chen)

the *ARMS2* gene on chromosome 10. Genes related to lipid metabolism are also thought to be important.

- **Smoking** roughly doubles the risk of AMD.
- **Hypertension** and other cardiovascular risk factors are likely to be associated.
- **Dietary factors.** High fat intake and obesity may promote AMD, with high antioxidant intake having a protective effect in some groups (see below).
- **Aspirin** may increase the risk of neovascular AMD. Though the evidence is limited, if an individual at high risk requires an antiplatelet agent it may be sensible to consider an alternative to aspirin.
- **Other factors** such as cataract surgery, blue iris colour, high sunlight exposure and female gender are suspected, but their influence remains less certain.

Drusen

Histopathology

Drusen (singular: druse) are extracellular deposits located at the interface between the RPE and Bruch membrane (Fig. 14.38A). The material of which they are composed has a broad range of constituents, and is thought to be derived from immune-mediated and metabolic processes in the RPE. Their precise role in the pathogenesis of AMD is unclear, but is positively associated with the size of lesions and the presence or absence of associated pigmentary abnormalities. Age-related drusen are rare prior to the age of 40, but are common by the sixth decade. The distribution is highly variable, and they may be confined to the fovea, may encircle it or form a band around the macular periphery. They may also be seen in the peripheral and mid-peripheral fundus (see Ch. 16).

Clinical features

There is a strong association between the size of drusen (Fig. 14.38B–E) and the risk of developing late AMD over a 5-year period.

- **Small drusen (drupelets),** sometimes termed 'hard' drusen, are typically well-defined white–yellow and by definition measure ≤63 μm – less than half the width of a retinal vein at the optic disc margin – in diameter. Their presence as the only finding probably carries little increased risk of visual loss, unless associated with pigmentary abnormalities.
- **Intermediate drusen** are fairly well-defined yellow–white focal deposits at the level of the RPE measuring between 63 μm and 125 μm. Without accompanying pigmentary abnormalities, they carry only a very small risk of progression to late AMD over 5 years, but this increases to over 10% if pigmentary abnormalities are present in both eyes.
- **Large drusen** are less well delineated yellow–white deep retinal lesions measuring over 125 μm in diameter; the term

'soft' drusen (see Fig. 14.38B) is sometimes used synonymously. As they enlarge and become more numerous (see Figs 14.38C and D), they may coalesce giving a localized elevation of the RPE, a 'drusenoid RPE detachment' – see below. The presence of large drusen in both eyes is associated with a 13% risk of progression to late AMD over 5 years, but with accompanying bilateral pigmentary abnormalities this rises to about 50%.

- **Dystrophic calcification** may develop in all types of drusen.
- **Pigmentary abnormalities.** Hyper- and hypopigmentation (see Fig. 14.38E) not due to other retinal disease is associated with a significantly higher likelihood of progression to late AMD with visual loss.

OCT

Medium-sized and large drusen are seen as hyper-reflective irregular nodules beneath the RPE, located on or within the Bruch membrane (Fig 14.38F).

Fluorescein angiography

FA findings depend on the state of the overlying RPE and on the affinity of the drusen for fluorescein. Hyperfluorescence can be caused by a window defect due to atrophy of the overlying RPE, or by late staining. Hypofluorescent drusen masking background fluorescence are hydrophobic, with a high lipid content, and tend not to stain.

Differential diagnosis

A number of conditions feature lesions similar to age-related drusen, and at least some may have a similar pathophysiological basis.

- **Doyne honeycomb retinal dystrophy** (malattia leventinese, autosomal dominant radial drusen) is an uncommon condition in which fairly characteristic drusen (Fig. 14.39A) appear during the second or third decades (see Ch. 15); the genetic basis has been established for the majority of cases.
- **Cuticular drusen**, also known as grouped early adult-onset or basal laminar drusen (not to be confused with basal laminar deposit and basal linear deposit in AMD – see dry AMD below), tend to be seen in relatively young adults. The lesions consist of small (25–75 μm) yellowish nodules (Fig. 14.39B) that tend to cluster and increase in number with time and can progress to serous PED. FA characteristically gives a 'stars in the sky' appearance (Fig. 14.39C). The condition has been linked to a variant of the *CFH* gene.
- **Type 2 membranoproliferative glomerulonephritis** is a chronic renal disease that occurs in older children and adults. A minority of patients develop bilateral diffuse drusen-like lesions. The *CFH* gene has again been implicated.

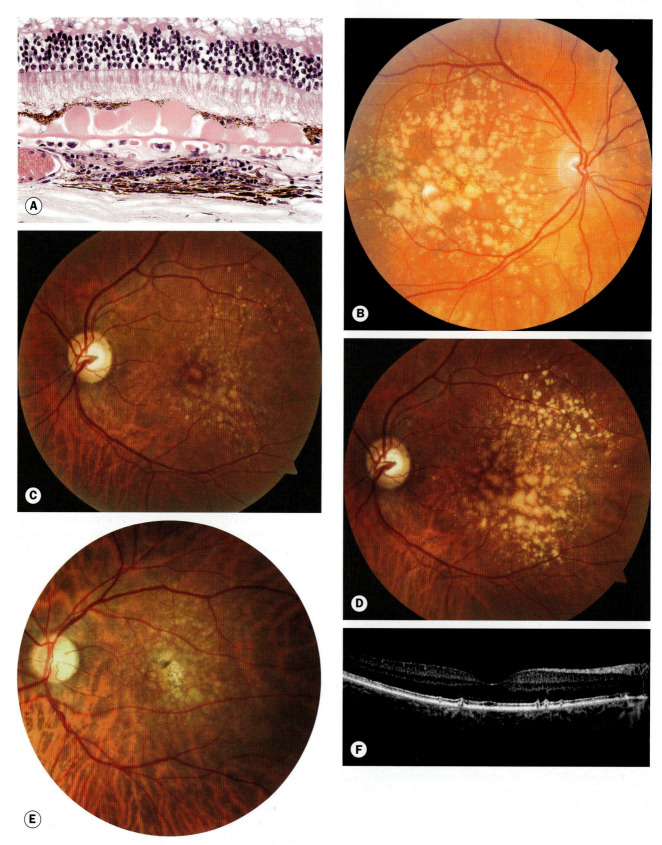

Fig. 14.38 Drusen. **(A)** Histopathology shows homogeneous eosinophilic deposits lying between the retinal pigment epithelium (RPE) and the inner collagenous layer of Bruch membrane; **(B)** mixed small, intermediate and large drusen; **(C)** initial image; and **(D)** same eye 4 years later showing increase in number and size of drusen; **(E)** drusen with associated pigmentary abnormalities; **(F)** OCT showing nodules associated with the RPE

(Courtesy of J Harry – fig. A; S Chen – figs B–E)

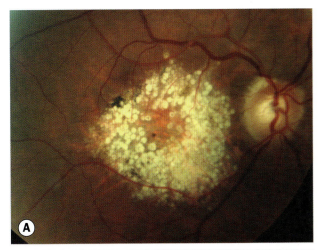

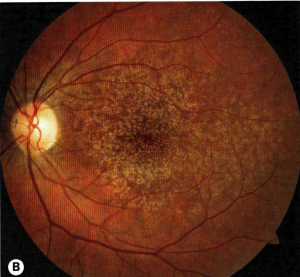

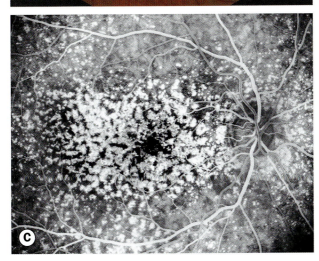

Fig. 14.39 (A) Doyne honeycomb retinal dystrophy;
(B) cuticular drusen; **(C)** FA shows hyperfluorescent
spots – 'stars in the sky' appearance

(Courtesy of S Chen – fig. A; C Barry – figs B and C)

Antioxidant supplementation

Introduction

There is substantial evidence, notably from the Age-Related Eye Disease Study (AREDS, now known as AREDS1) and the follow-up AREDS2, that taking high-dose antioxidant vitamins and minerals on a regular basis can decrease the risk of the development of advanced AMD in individuals with certain dry AMD features. The recommendation was made in AREDS1 that individuals aged over 55 should undergo examination for the following high-risk characteristics, and if one or more are present should consider antioxidant supplementation:

- Extensive intermediate- (≥63 μm to 125 μm) drusen.
- At least one large (≥125 μm) druse.
- GA in one or both eyes.
- Late AMD in one eye (greatest benefit in AREDS1).

In AREDS1 the reduction in risk of progression to advanced AMD at 10 years was in the order of 25–30% for those with the more advanced of these signs at baseline who took supplements; supplements did not discernibly reduce progression in those with early or no AMD at baseline.

AREDS2

The regimen used in AREDS1 consisted of vitamin C, vitamin E, the beta-carotene form of vitamin A, and 80 mg daily of zinc (with copper to prevent zinc-induced copper deficiency). However, high zinc doses are potentially associated with genitourinary tract problems, and there are data suggesting that 25 mg of zinc may be the maximal level that is absorbed. Beta-carotene almost certainly increases the incidence of lung cancer in current and former smokers. AREDS2 looked at adjusting the beta-carotene and zinc components, and also whether additional or alternative supplements could enhance outcomes. AREDS2 found:

- The carotenoids lutein and zeaxanthin are a safe alternative to beta-carotene, and are probably superior (possible 18% reduction in risk of advanced AMD above that conferred by the AREDS1 regimen).
- Lutein and zeaxanthin supplementation added to the original AREDS1 regimen was only associated with a statistically significantly reduced (26%) risk of AMD in patients in whom the dietary intake of these was not already high (self-described and blood testing); there was evidence that competition for absorption between different carotenoids may have prevented the demonstration of superiority in other patients. This group also showed a one-third reduction in the likelihood of cataract surgery.
- Adding omega-3 fatty acids to the regimen did not seem to enhance outcomes.
- Lowering the zinc dose did not lead to a statistically significant prognostic worsening, and is likely to be associated with a lower incidence of side-effects such as gastrointestinal and urinary problems.

- Recommended daily supplementation based on AREDS2:
  - Vitamin E (400 IU).
  - Vitamin C (500 mg).
  - Lutein (10 mg).
  - Zeaxanthin (2 mg).
  - Zinc (25–80 mg; the lower dose may be equally effective).
  - Copper (2 mg; this may not be required with the lower zinc dose).

Other considerations

- A liberal green leafy vegetable intake confers a lower risk of AMD, and for individuals with a strong family history of AMD and those with early AMD who do not meet the AREDS criteria, this may be a prudent lifestyle choice.
- Cessation of smoking should be advised.
- Protective measures against exposure to excessive sunlight should be considered.
- Some authorities consider that evidence still supports the regular consumption of oily fish.

Non-exudative (dry, non-neovascular) AMD

Diagnosis

- **Symptoms** consist of gradual impairment of vision over months or years. Both eyes are usually affected, but often asymmetrically. Vision may fluctuate, and is often better in bright light.
- **Signs** in approximately chronological order:
  - Numerous intermediate–large soft drusen; may become confluent.
  - Focal hyper- and/or hypopigmentation of the RPE (Fig. 14.40A and B).
  - Sharply circumscribed areas of RPE atrophy associated with variable loss of the retina and choriocapillaris (Fig. 14.40C).
  - Enlargement of atrophic areas, within which larger choroidal vessels may become visible and pre-existing drusen disappear (GA – Fig. 14.40D). Visual acuity may be severely impaired if the fovea is involved. Rarely, CNV may develop in an area of GA.
  - Drusenoid RPE detachment (see below).
- **OCT**
  - Drusen – see above.
  - Loss of RPE and morphological alterations of the overlying retina of increasing severity are seen in GA, including increased hyper-reflectivity initially in the outer retinal layers and eventual photoreceptor loss.
  - Outer retinal tubulations may be seen; these are thought to consist of degenerating photoreceptors aggregated into tubular structures that appear as roundish hyporeflective spaces (Fig. 14.40E), often around the margin of GA.
  - Outer retinal corrugations. This recently described phenomenon is an undulating hyper-reflective layer on

OCT thought to correspond to the histological finding of basal *laminar* deposit, a layer that accumulates between the RPE and the RPE basement membrane (the inner layer of the Bruch membrane) in AMD. Basal *linear* deposit is a distinct finding consisting of membranous debris laid down between the RPE basement membrane and the inner collagenous layer of the Bruch membrane that may progress focally to form drusen.

- **FA** of atrophic areas shows a window defect due to unmasking of background choroidal fluorescence (see Fig. 14.22), if the underlying choriocapillaris is still intact. Exposed sclera may exhibit late staining.

Management

- **Prophylaxis**
  - Antioxidant supplementation if indicated.
  - Risk factors should be addressed, e.g. smoking, ocular sun protection, cardiovascular, dietary.
- **An Amsler grid** should be provided for home use, with advice to self-test on a regular basis, perhaps weekly, and to seek professional advice urgently in the event of any change, when imaging (e.g. OCT, FA) should be performed to rule out progression to neovascular AMD. This might be of increased importance following cataract surgery.
- **Provision of low vision aids** and, for patients with significant visual loss, certification as visually impaired if available as this may facilitate access to social and financial support.
- **Experimental surgery**
  - Miniature intraocular telescope implantation may provide benefit in selected cases.
  - Retinal translocation surgery has had limited success.
  - Visual prostheses of various types are under investigation, but are likely to be adopted for severe retinal dystrophies initially.
- **Potential new therapies.** An extensive range of therapies shows promise for the treatment of dry AMD. Examples are:
  - Lampalizumab, a complement-inhibiting monoclonal antibody injected intravitreally on a monthly basis reduced progression of GA by 44%.
  - Visual cycle modulation: ameliorating the formation of cytotoxic products by reducing the rate of vitamin A processing; clinical trials (e.g. fenretinide, emixustat) are under way.
  - Photocoagulation of drusen leads to a substantial reduction in their extent, but does not seem to reduce the risk of progression to AMD. A newer modality using extremely short (nanosecond range) pulses of non-thermal laser energy may have a rejuvenating effect on the RPE and Bruch membrane.
  - Saffron (20 mg/day); preliminary evidence suggests a neuroprotective effect.
  - Others include subretinal stem cell transplantation, and intravitreal injection of a range of drugs including ciliary neurotrophic factor, steroid inserts and neuroprotective drugs including brimonidine.

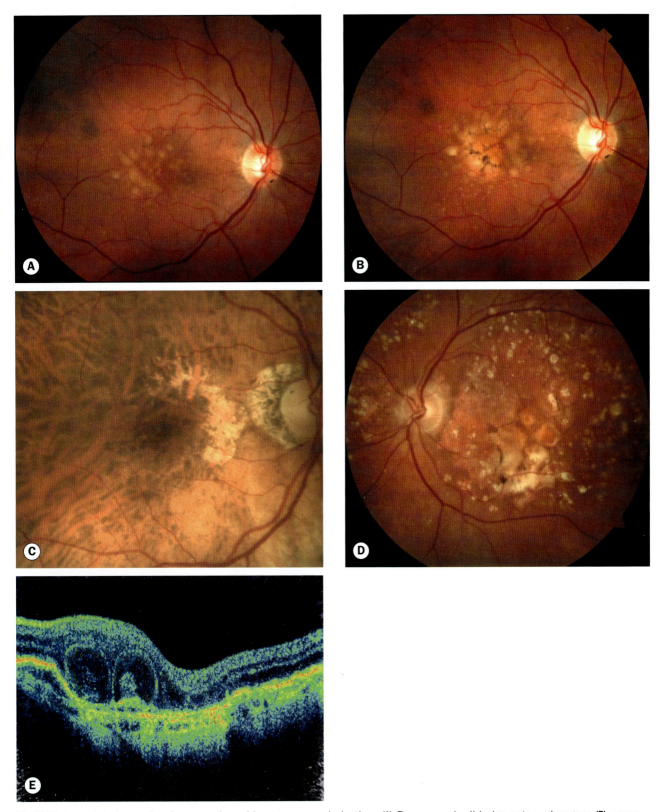

Fig. 14.40 Age-related macular degeneration without neovascularization. **(A)** Drusen and mild pigmentary changes; **(B)** same eye as (A) 4 years later with moderate retinal atrophy and pigmentary abnormalities; **(C)** small and intermediate drusen with geographic atrophy; **(D)** substantial geographic atrophy and pigmentary abnormalities; **(E)** OCT- outer retinal tubulations

(Courtesy of S Chen)

Retinal pigment epithelial detachment

Pathogenesis

Pigment epithelial detachment (PED) from the inner collagenous layer of Bruch membrane is caused by disruption of the physiological forces maintaining adhesion. The basic mechanism is thought to be the reduction of hydraulic conductivity of a thickened and dysfunctional Bruch membrane, thus impeding movement of fluid from the RPE towards the choroid. Immune-mediated processes may also be important. The different types are discussed below.

Serous PED

- **Symptoms.** Blurred central vision (sometimes induced hypermetropia) and metamorphopsia.
- **Signs**
  - An orange dome-shaped elevation with sharply delineated edges, often with a paler margin of subretinal fluid (Fig. 14.41A). Multiple lesions may occur.
  - An associated pigment band may indicate chronicity.
  - Associated blood, lipid exudation, chorioretinal folds or irregular subretinal fluid may indicate underlying CNV.

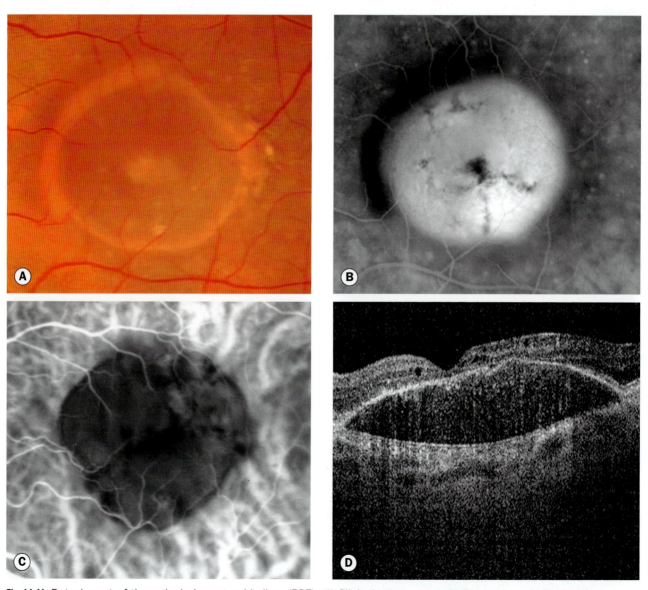

Fig. 14.41 Detachment of the retinal pigment epithelium (RPE). **(A)** Clinical appearance; **(B)** FA shows hyperfluorescence; **(C)** ICGA shows hypofluorescence with a faint ring of surrounding hyperfluorescence; **(D)** OCT shows separation of the RPE from Bruch membrane;

Continued

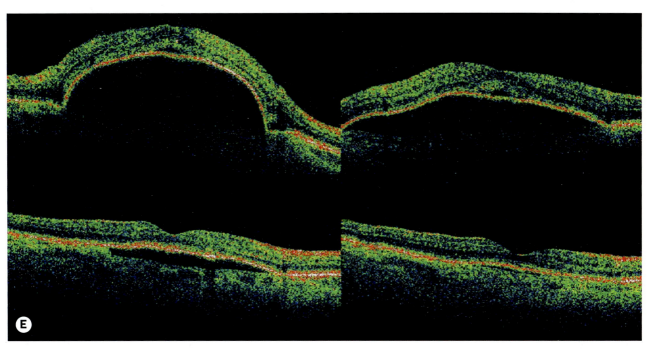

Fig. 14.41, Continued **(E)** gradual resolution of a pigment epithelial detachment with sequential monthly injections of bevacizumab

(Courtesy of P Gili – figs A and B; A Bolton – fig. C; S Chen – fig. E)

○ If no drusen are seen, polypoidal choroidal vasculopathy (PCV – see below) should be suspected.

- **FA:** a well demarcated oval area of hyperfluorescent pooling (Fig. 14.41B) that increases in intensity but not in area with time; an indentation (notch) may signify CNV.

- **ICGA:** an oval hypofluorescent area with a surrounding hyperfluorescent ring (Fig. 14.41C). Occult CNV (focal hot spot or diffuse plaque) is detected in over 90%.

- **OCT** shows separation of the RPE from the Bruch membrane by an optically empty area (Fig. 14.41D). CNV may be indicated by a notch between the main elevation and a second small mound.

- **Natural course**
  ○ Persistence with increasing atrophy and gradually worsening vision.
  ○ Patients aged over 60 have a worse prognosis (6/60 or less), but speed of deterioration varies.
  ○ Resolution leaving GA with visual loss (spontaneous resolution with relative preservation of vision is more common in younger patients).
  ○ RPE tear formation (see below) or haemorrhage from CNV can occur, with sudden visual loss.
  ○ Up to a third of eyes develop clinical CNV within 2 years, but the proportion is much higher angiographically.

- **Management**
  ○ Observation may be appropriate in clinically stable patients without readily detectable CNV, especially those younger than 60.
  ○ Intravitreal injection of vascular endothelial growth factor (VEGF) inhibitor may stabilize or improve vision

(Fig. 14.41E), and should be considered particularly when there is associated CNV; however, there is a 5–20% risk of RPE tear.
  ○ Combining photodynamic therapy (PDT) with intravitreal anti-VEGF or intravitreal triamcinolone injection (IVTA) can also be effective, though the RPE tear risk persists.

Fibrovascular PED

By definition (Macular Photocoagulation Study classification), fibrovascular PED represents a form of 'occult' CNV (see below).

- **Signs.** The PED is much more irregular in outline and elevation than serous PED.

- **OCT.** Less uniform than a serous PED; both fluid and fibrous proliferation are shown, the latter as irregular scattered reflections.

- **FA** shows markedly irregular granular (stippled) hyperfluorescence, with uneven filling of the PED, leakage and late staining.

- **ICGA** demonstrates CNV more effectively.

- **Management** is essentially as for serous PED with CNV.

Drusenoid PED

Drusenoid PED develops from confluent large soft drusen, and is often bilateral.

- **Signs.** Shallow elevated pale areas with irregular scalloped edges (Fig. 14.42A).

- **FA.** Early diffuse hypofluorescence with patchy relatively faint early hyperfluorescence, progressing to moderate irregular late staining (Fig. 14.42B).

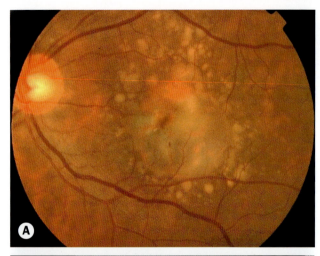

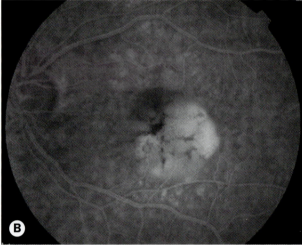

Fig. 14.42 Drusenoid detachment of the retinal pigment epithelium. **(A)** Clinical appearance; **(B)** FA late phase shows moderate hyperfluorescence due to staining

- **ICGA.** Hypofluorescence predominates.
- **OCT** shows homogeneous hyper-reflectivity within the PED, in contrast to optically empty serous PED. There is commonly no subretinal fluid.
- **Natural course.** The outlook is usually better than other forms of PED, with only gradual visual loss, though probably around 75% still progress to develop GA and 25% CNV by 10 years from diagnosis. Long-term stability is common: at 3 years, only about one-third will have GA or CNV.
- **Management.** Observation in most cases, with no evidence to support the efficacy of any intervention.

Haemorrhagic PED

Virtually every haemorrhagic PED has underlying CNV or poly-poidal choroidal vasculopathy (PCV): the latter should always be considered if no drusen are present.
- **Symptoms.** Sudden impairment of central vision.
- **Signs** (Fig. 14.43)

○ Elevated dark red dome-shaped lesion with a well-defined outline.
○ Blood may break through into the subretinal space, assuming a more diffuse outline and a lighter red colour.
- **FA.** Dense masking of background fluorescence, but overlying vessels are visible.
- **Management** of large haemorrhagic lesions is described below under 'Haemorrhagic AMD', but the prognosis for central vision is generally poor. CNV associated with a small haemorrhagic PED can be managed conventionally. Management of PCV is discussed separately.

Retinal pigment epithelial tear

An RPE tear may occur at the junction of attached and detached RPE. Tears may occur spontaneously, following laser (including PDT), or after intravitreal injection. Older patients and large irregular PEDs associated with CNV are at higher risk.
- **Symptoms.** Sudden fall in vision with foveal involvement.
- **Signs.** A crescent-shaped pale area of RPE dehiscence is seen, next to a darker area corresponding to the retracted and folded flap (Figs 14.44A and B).
- **OCT.** Loss of the normal dome shape of the RPE layer in the PED, with hyper-reflectivity of the folded RPE (Figs 14.44C and D).
- **FA** late phase shows hypofluorescence over the flap due to the thickened folded RPE, with adjacent hyperfluorescence, initially over the exposed choriocapillaris where the RPE is absent and later due to scleral staining. The two areas are often separated by a sharply defined border (Fig. 14.44E).
- **The prognosis** in subfoveal tears is poor. Good VA is usually maintained if the fovea is spared.

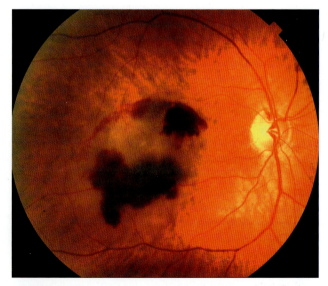

Fig. 14.43 Haemorrhagic detachment of the retinal pigment epithelium (RPE); subretinal blood is present in the lighter red areas and sub-RPE blood in the darker red areas
(Courtesy of S Chen)

Choroidal neovascularization (CNV)

Introduction

Choroidal neovascularization (CNV) consists of a blood vessel complex that extends through Bruch membrane from the choriocapillaris into the sub-RPE (type 1) or subretinal (type 2) space. It occurs in many different disorders, usually when Bruch membrane and/or RPE function has been compromised by a degenerative, inflammatory, traumatic or neoplastic process. AMD is the most common causative association, followed by myopic degeneration. The present discussion relates to CNV arising *de novo* as the primary lesion in neovascular AMD, but CNV may also develop secondary to retinal angiomatous proliferation and polypoidal choroidal vasculopathy (RAP and PCV – see below), both of which are considered by many practitioners to themselves be variants of neovascular AMD. The prognosis of untreated CNV is generally poor, with 'hand movements' VA a common outcome. Understanding of aetiopathogenesis has improved over recent years; the promotion and inhibition of blood vessel growth by cytokines is important, particularly vascular endothelial growth factor (VEGF), which binds to endothelial cell receptors, promoting proliferation and vascular leakage. The inhibitory mediators pigment epithelium-derived factor (PEDF) and complement factor H (CFH) are also thought to play key roles. Supplementary endothelial progenitor cells are thought to be recruited from systemic reservoirs, enhancing growth of the new vessel complex.

Clinical features

- **Symptoms**. Acute or subacute painless blurring of vision, usually with metamorphopsia. Haemorrhage may give a positive scotoma.
- **Signs**
  ○ The CNV itself may be identifiable as a grey–green or pinkish-yellow lesion (Fig. 14.45A).
  ○ Associated medium–large drusen are a typical finding in the same or fellow eye.
  ○ Localized subretinal fluid, sometimes with CMO.
  ○ Intra- and subretinal lipid deposition, sometimes extensive (Fig. 14.45B).
  ○ Haemorrhage (Fig. 14.45C) is common, e.g. subretinal, preretinal/retrohyaloid, vitreous.
  ○ There may be an associated serous, fibrovascular drusenoid or haemorrhagic PED.
  ○ Retinal and subretinal cicatrization ('disciform' scar) in an evolved or treated lesion (Fig. 14.45D).

Fluorescein angiography

FA was previously used to diagnose CNV and to plan and monitor the response to laser photocoagulation or PDT. Current indications include:

- Diagnosis of CNV prior to committing to anti-VEGF treatment; FA should usually be performed urgently on the basis of clinical suspicion.

- As an adjunct to diagnosis of an alternative form of neovascular AMD such as PCV and RAP.
- Exceptionally, localization for extrafoveal photocoagulation, or guidance for PDT.
- Monitoring is now predominantly with OCT.

Terminology used to describe CNV on FA is derived from the Macular Photocoagulation Study (MPS):

- **Classic CNV** (20%) fills with dye in a well-defined 'lacy' pattern during early transit (Fig. 14.46A), subsequently leaking into the subretinal space over 1–2 minutes (Fig. 14.46B), with late staining of fibrous tissue (Fig. 14.46C). Most CNV is subfoveal, extrafoveal being defined as ≥200 μm from the centre of the foveal avascular zone on FA.
- **Occult CNV** (80%) is used to describe CNV when its limits cannot be fully defined on FA (Fig. 14.47). Variants are fibrovascular PED (see above) and 'late leakage of an undetermined source' (LLUS).
- **Predominantly or minimally classic** CNV is present when the classic element is greater or less than 50% of the total lesion respectively.

Indocyanine green angiography

ICGA demonstrates CNV as a focal hyperfluorescent 'hot spot' (Fig. 14.48) or 'plaque'; benefits adjunctive to FA include:

- Increased sensitivity in the detection of CNV, e.g. if low-density haemorrhage, fluid or pigment preclude adequate FA visualization.
- The distinction of CNV from other conditions that may have a similar presentation, particularly PCV, RAP and CSR.
- The delineation of occult CNV may still have utility for combined modality treatment, and for patients who refuse intravitreal therapy.

Optical coherence tomography

OCT is critical in quantitative monitoring of the response to CNV treatment. It has to date been of limited assistance in the diagnosis of CNV, though ongoing technological refinements are likely to lead to increasing utility. Typically, CNV is shown as a thickening and fragmentation of the RPE and choriocapillaris. Subretinal and sub-RPE fluid, blood and scarring are demonstrated (Fig. 14.49). Outer retinal tubulations (see Fig. 14.40E) may be present, often in a branching pseudodendritic conformation.

Treatment with anti-VEGF agents

- **Principles.** Inhibitors of VEGF block its interaction with receptors on the endothelial cell surface and so retard or reverse vessel growth. They have become the predominant means of treatment for CNV, dramatically improving the visual prognosis. Intravitreal injection is the standard method of administration, notable risks including retinal detachment, damage to the lens, RPE tears and endophthalmitis. Sustained elevation of intraocular pressure (IOP) and sterile uveitis may also occur. Systemically, there

Text continued on p. 614

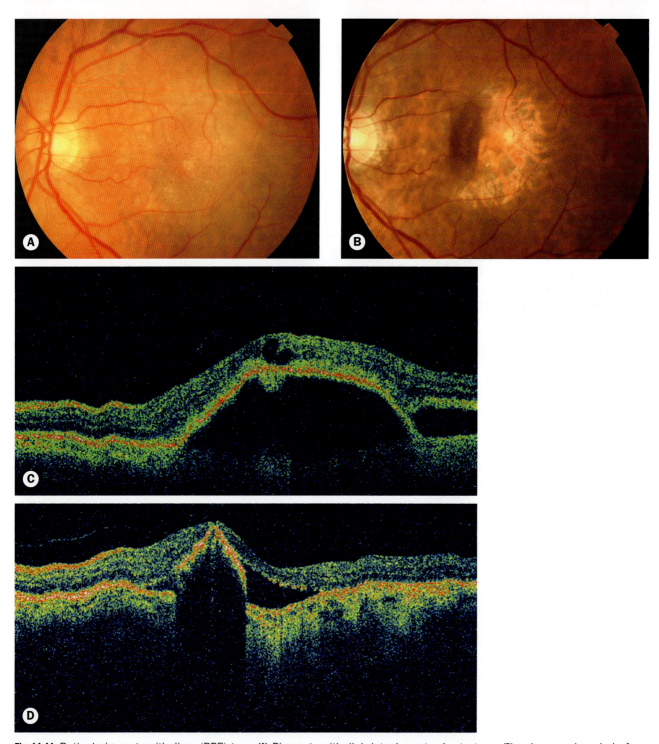

Fig. 14.44 Retinal pigment epithelium (RPE) tear. **(A)** Pigment epithelial detachment prior to tear; **(B)** pale area denuded of RPE with an adjacent darker area consisting of rolled-up RPE following a tear; **(C)** OCT prior to tear; **(D)** OCT following a tear shows corrugation of the elevated RPE and hyper-reflectivity of the rolled-up region;

Continued

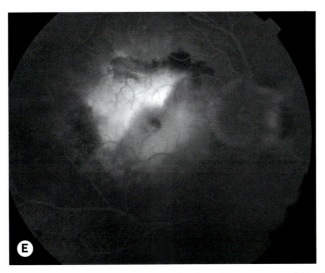

Fig. 14.44, Continued **(E)** FA late phase of a different eye shows relative hypofluorescence of the folded flap with adjacent hyperfluorescence where the RPE is absent

(Courtesy of S Chen – figs A–D; C Barry – fig. E)

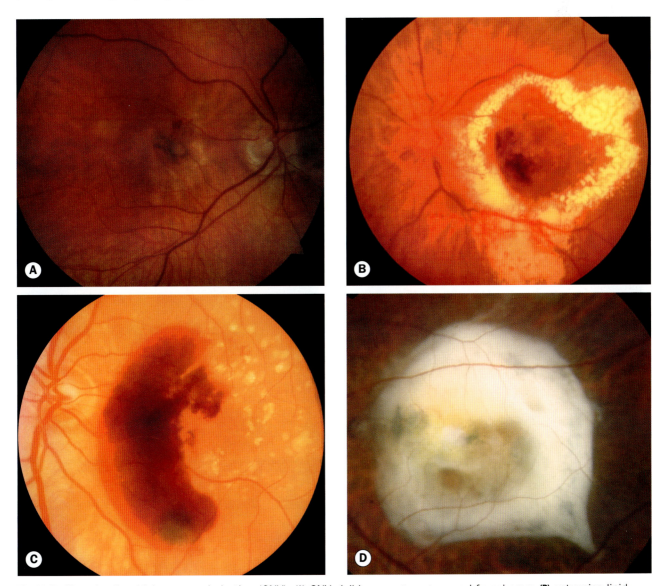

Fig. 14.45 Signs in choroidal neovascularization (CNV). **(A)** CNV visible as a grey–green subfoveal area; **(B)** extensive lipid deposition; **(C)** haemorrhage – intra- and subretinal; **(D)** 'disciform' scarring

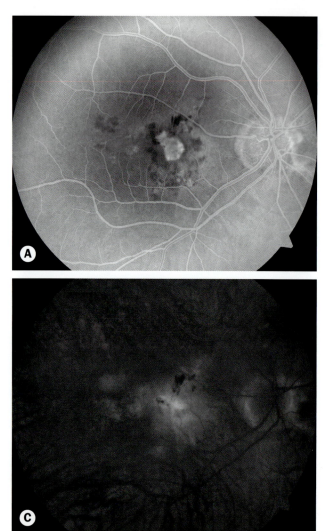

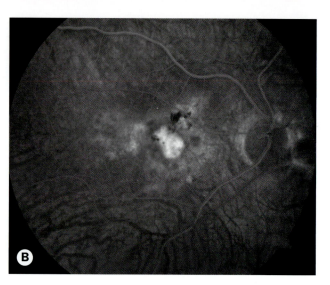

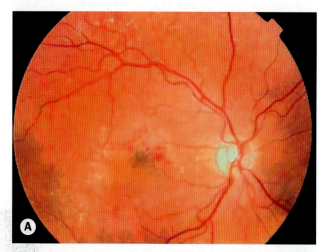

Fig. 14.46 FA of classic subfoveal choroidal neovascularization – the eye in Fig. 14.45A. **(A)** FA early venous phase – 'lacy' hyperfluorescent pattern; **(B)** late venous phase – more intense hyperfluorescence with leakage and staining; **(C)** persistent staining at 10 minutes

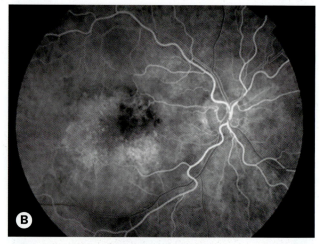

Fig. 14.47 FA of occult choroidal neovascularization. **(A)** Specks of blood at the fovea; **(B-D)** FA shows diffuse hyperfluorescence but the limits of the membrane cannot be defined

Continued

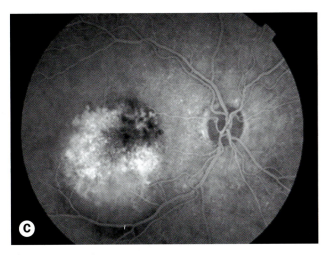
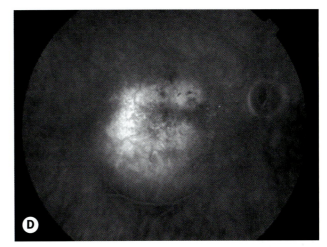

Fig. 14.47, Continued

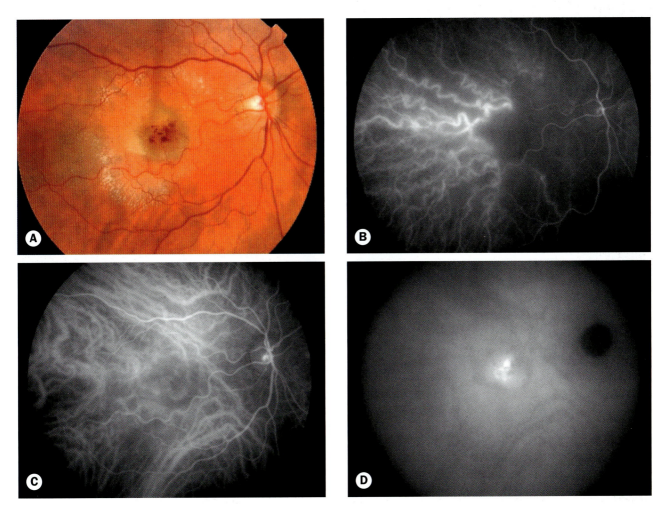

Fig. 14.48 ICGA of choroidal neovascularization (CNV). **(A)** Blood and fluid at the macula surrounded by hard exudates; **(B–D)** shows a small area of increasing hyperfluorescence ('hot spot') from underlying CNV

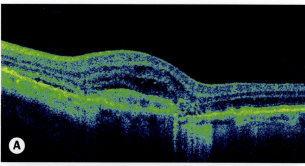
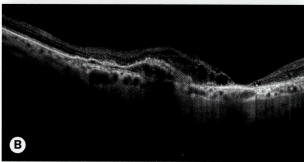

Fig. 14.49 OCT. **(A)** Choroidal neovascularization and subretinal fluid; **(B)** long-established lesion with secondary atrophic retinal changes

is a suspicion of a slightly increased incidence of stroke. All available anti-VEGF agents seem to have potential for benefit in a range of vascular eye diseases.

- **Indications.** All CNV subtypes respond to anti-VEGF therapy, but benefit is only likely in the presence of active disease; the presence of a mature fibrotic disciform scar with little or no fluid makes treatment extremely unlikely to be useful. Evidence for active CNV includes fluid or haemorrhage, leakage on FA, an enlarging CNV membrane, or deteriorating vision judged likely to be due to CNV activity. An eye with almost any level of vision may benefit, although better VA at the outset is associated with a better final VA and patients with only 'hand movements' should be assessed on an individual basis. It is likely that anti-VEGF agents have a reduced duration of action in vitrectomized eyes.

- **Aflibercept (Eylea®)** is a recombinant fusion protein that binds to VEGF-A, VEGF-B and placental growth factor (PlGF). After becoming commercially available, it was adopted rapidly into clinical practice, principally because the recommended maintenance regimen consists of one injection every 2 months in contrast to the monthly injections recommended with ranibizumab and bevacizumab (see below), though in some patients dosing is required more frequently than every 2 months. The standard dose is 2 mg in 0.05 ml; an induction course of three injections is given at monthly intervals.

- **Ranibizumab (Lucentis®).** Ranibizumab is a humanized monoclonal antibody fragment developed specifically for use in the eye, though is derived from the same parent mouse antibody as bevacizumab (see next). It non-selectively binds

and inhibits all isoforms of VEGF-A. The usual dose is 0.5 mg in 0.05 ml. Three main treatment strategies are adopted in AMD:

- ○ Regular monthly injection is the regimen adopted in initial major trials. Overall, around 95% of patients maintain vision regardless of lesion type, and 35–40% significantly improved, most markedly during the first 3 months. This regimen seems to offer a marginally better visual outcome, but may be associated with progression to geographic atrophy of slightly greater severity than less intensive administration and the long-term implications of this remain undetermined. There is a suggestion that systemic adverse events may, counterintuitively, be less common with regular monthly injections than discontinuous schedules.

- ○ Three initial monthly injections followed by monthly review with re-injection when deterioration occurs as assessed by VA (e.g. loss of 5 letters or more) and OCT (e.g. retinal thickness increase of 100 μm or more).

- ○ 'Treat and extend' entails administering three initial injections at monthly intervals and then gradually increasing the period between injections until deterioration is evident. If possible a tailored interval is determined for each patient.

- **Bevacizumab (Avastin®).** In contrast to ranibizumab, bevacizumab is a complete antibody originally developed to target blood vessel growth in metastatic cancer deposits. Its use for AMD and other indications is 'off label'; it is very much cheaper than ranibizumab and aflibercept. Clinical trial results suggest that it is approximately comparable to ranibizumab in efficacy and safety, though some assessments have suggested that the risk of serious systemic adverse events is marginally higher with bevacizumab than ranibizumab. Treatment strategies in AMD are similar to those used for ranibizumab. The dose of bevacizumab is usually 1.25 mg/0.05 ml.

- **Pegaptanib (Macugen®).** Pegaptanib sodium was the first anti-VEGF agent approved by regulatory authorities for ocular treatment; the results are similar to outcomes with PDT, and its use is now extremely limited.

- **Technique of intravitreal injection.** Various protocols are in use; a typical approach is set out in Table 14.4; this applies to ant-VEGF injection – there are slight differences for intravitreal steroid administration.

Patients can return to normal activity after 24 hours, but should be warned to seek advice urgently should they experience any deterioration in their vision or symptoms of inflammation.

Treatment with photodynamic therapy (PDT)

Verteporfin is a light-activated compound preferentially taken up by dividing cells including neovascular tissue. It is infused intravenously and then activated by diode laser to cause thrombosis. The main indication was previously subfoveal predominantly classic CNV with visual acuity of 6/60 or better. Severe adverse effects are rare. With the advent of anti-VEGF treatment, PDT is

Table 14.4 Technique of intravitreal injection

- The procedure and its risks should be explained to the patient and appropriate consent obtained.
- The environment should be appropriate, e.g. a dedicated 'clean room' with adequate illumination.
- The indication and the eye to be treated should be checked and the eye marked.
- It should be confirmed that anterior and posterior segment examination (including IOP) has been carried out recently to exclude contraindications.
- Confirmation should be obtained that a syringe of the drug to be injected is available.
- Bilateral injections are optimally administered at separate sessions to minimize risk, but if necessary different instruments and drug batches should be used.
- A surgical mask should be worn.
- Topical anaesthetic and mydriatic agents are instilled.
- Povidone-iodine 5% (chlorhexidine if allergic to iodine) is applied to the ocular surface and at least 3 minutes allowed prior to injection.
- Subconjunctival lidocaine 1% or 2% may be used to supplement the topical agent. Some practitioners prefer lidocaine gel, though concerns have been expressed regarding the possibility of microorganism retention within this.
- Hands are washed using a standard surgical procedure, and sterile gloves donned.
- The periocular skin, eyelids and lashes are cleaned with 5–10% povidone iodine.
- As for other forms of intraocular surgery, a sterile periocular drape may be advisable.
- The sterile pouch containing a pre-prepared syringe is opened, or a sterile syringe is used to draw up the appropriate volume of drug from a vial of ready-prepared drug. A needle (typically 30-gauge, 0.5 inch) on the syringe is primed to expel any air.
- A sterile speculum is placed in the eye.
- The patient is instructed to look away from the injection site – this is most commonly inferotemporal because of ease of access, though any quadrant can be used; the 3 and 9 o'clock positions are avoided because of the risk of neurovascular damage.
- A gauge is used to identify an injection site 3.5–4.0 mm posterior to the limbus (pars plana).
- Forceps can be used to stabilize the eye, and if wished to apply anterior traction to the conjunctiva so that the conjunctival hole does not overlie the scleral track.
- The needle is advanced perpendicularly through the sclera towards the centre of the eyeball, and the required volume of drug (usually 0.05 ml) injected into the vitreous cavity. Some practitioners make an attempt to 'step' the needle track.
- The needle is removed and discarded.
- It has become usual practice not to use post-injection antibiotics as there is a suggestion that serial use may increase the rate of infection by promoting bacterial resistance.
- Elevated IOP can occlude the central retinal artery, and it is important routinely to ensure this remains perfused after the procedure by checking the patient's vision (subjectively is adequate), directly visualizing the artery, or optimally by checking the IOP (particularly in glaucoma patients). If occlusion occurs, urgent paracentesis should be carried out; simply lying down may restore blood flow.
- A clear plastic eye shield may be used until the local anaesthetic has worn off, and during sleep for the first night or two, but practice varies.

now rarely used for CNV, but combination therapy (see below) and refusal of intravitreal treatment remain indications. Reduced-intensity regimens have been used with good effect in CSR.

Combination and other experimental therapies

Although anti-VEGF therapy has revolutionized the management of CNV, further investigation is attempting to achieve outcomes that are better still, particularly a reduction in the frequency of intravitreal injections. To date, regimens that include the combination of PDT with anti-VEGF treatment have not been shown to be superior to anti-VEGF treatment alone, but investigation is ongoing, including parallel inhibition of anti-VEGF agents with inhibition of other cytokines and with low-intensity macular radiotherapy. Sustained-release anti-VEGF systems, and gene therapy utilizing adenoviral vectors to facilitate the production of cytokines within the eye, are other avenues of potential therapeutic advantage.

Laser

Thermal argon or diode laser ablation of CNV is now rarely used, though may still be suitable for the treatment of small classic extrafoveal membranes well away from the macular centre, and possibly some cases of PCV and RAP.

Haemorrhagic AMD

The visual prognosis for most eyes with extensive subretinal or sub-RPE haemorrhage is relatively poor. Clinical trials assessing surgical drainage of extensive subretinal or sub-RPE haemorrhage with CNV excision did not show any significant improvement in prognosis, and rhegmatogenous retinal detachment was frequent. However, results superior to the untreated course have been reported for intravitreal anti-VEGF injection alone, and liquefaction of blood by intravitreal (or subretinal, requiring vitrectomy) recombinant tissue plasminogen activator (rtPA) and pneumatic displacement may be appropriate for large or thick haemorrhage. If the patient takes a coumarin anticoagulant, liaison with the prescribing physician is worthwhile to assess if this could reasonably be stopped – there is an association with massive macular haemorrhage. Antiplatelet drugs do not usually require discontinuation, though aspirin may be associated with a greater risk of CNV than other agents. Alternative pathology (e.g. PCV, macroaneurysm) that may be associated with extensive haemorrhage should always be considered.

RETINAL ANGIOMATOUS PROLIFERATION

Retinal angiomatous proliferation (RAP) may be a variant of neovascular AMD in which the major component of the neovascular complex is initially located within the retina. The process may originate within the deep retinal capillary plexus or within the choroid, in the latter case with the early formation of a retinal-choroidal anastomosis (RCA) without underlying type 1 CNV; the term 'type 3 neovascularization' has been suggested. The disease is frequently bilateral and symmetrical, and is probably substantially underdiagnosed; it may constitute 10–20% of neovascular AMD in Caucasians.

Diagnosis

- **Presentation** is similar to that of CNV but PED and exudate are more frequent. Haemorrhages are also more common and tend to be superficial and multiple.
- **Stage 1:** Intraretinal neovascularization (IRN). Dilated telangiectatic retinal vessels and small angiomatous lesions, typically accompanied by intra-, sub- and preretinal haemorrhage, oedema and exudate (Fig. 14.50A).
- **Stage 2:** Subretinal neovascularization (SRN) extends into the subretinal space associated with increasing oedema and exudate. A serous PED may be present.
- **Stage 3:** CNV. Perfusion is principally via the choroid, with RCA formation. CNV is clearly evident clinically or angiographically; a disciform scar will often form.
- **OCT** demonstrates neovascularization as a hyper-reflective area. Other features depend on the stage.
- **FA** is usually similar to occult or minimally classic CNV (Fig. 14.50B), but may show focal intraretinal hyperfluorescence.
- **ICGA** is diagnostic in most cases, showing a hot spot in mid and/or late frames (Fig. 14.50C), and frequently a perfusing retinal arteriole and draining venule ('hairpin loop' when linked).

Treatment

Anti-VEGF therapy shows encouraging results; favourable outcomes in combination with PDT have been reported. Limited success has been reported for other modalities, including PDT alone and photocoagulation of feeder vessels, though the latter may be used in resistant cases.

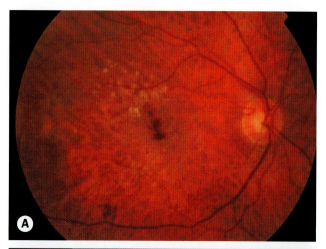

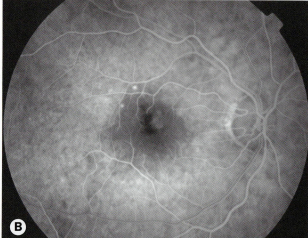

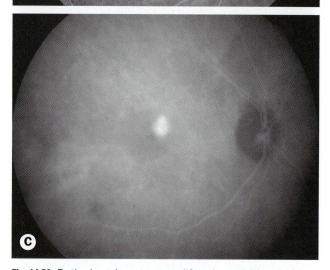

Fig. 14.50 Retinal angiomatous proliferation. **(A)** Macular drusen and a small intraretinal haemorrhage at the macula; **(B)** FA early venous phase shows faint hyperfluorescence from a small frond of intraretinal neovascularization; **(C)** ICGA late phase shows hyperfluorescence of the frond ('hot spot')
(Courtesy of Moorfields Eye Hospital)

POLYPOIDAL CHOROIDAL VASCULOPATHY

Introduction

Polypoidal choroidal vasculopathy (PCV), like RAP, is believed by many to be a variant of neovascular AMD. It is characterized by a branching vascular network of inner choroidal vessels with multiple terminal aneurysmal protuberances that appear to be the source of bleeding and exudation. It is more common in patients of African and East Asian ethnic origin than in whites and more common in women than men (5:1). The disease is often bilateral but tends to be asymmetrical. Overall, it is relatively common, and the presence of prominent haemorrhage should lead to the consideration of PCV, particularly if there is an absence of drusen and the patient is relatively young and Asian or black.

Diagnosis

- **Presentation** is usually in late middle age with the sudden onset of unilateral visual impairment.
- **Signs**
  - Terminal swellings are frequently visible as reddish-orange nodules beneath the RPE in the peripapillary or macular area (Fig. 14.51A), and less commonly the periphery.
  - Multiple recurrent serosanguineous retinal and RPE detachments (Fig. 14.51B).
  - Deterioration can be slow with intermittent bleeding and leakage, resulting in macular damage and visual loss; up to 50% may have a favourable outlook, with eventual spontaneous resolution of exudation and haemorrhage.
- **ICGA** is the key investigation in PCV.
  - Hyperfluorescent nodules and a network of large choroidal vessels with surrounding hypofluorescence appear in the early phase. The polyp-like swellings rapidly begin to leak (see Fig. 14.33 – same eye as Fig. 14.51A).
  - The previously darker surrounding region becomes hyperfluorescent by the late phase.
  - A cluster of grape-like lesions may carry a higher risk of severe visual loss.

Treatment

The favourable prognosis without treatment in a significant proportion of cases should be borne in mind, and asymptomatic polyps may be observed.

- Anti-VEGF agents appear to be less effective than in typical CNV, but may suppress leakage and bleeding.
- Combination anti-VEGF and PDT may be superior to anti-VEGF treatment alone; PDT may lead to regression of polyps and putatively an extended treatment effect, but carries an additional complication risk.
- Laser photocoagulation of feeder vessels or polyps may be effective in selected cases.

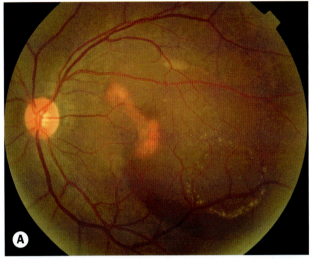

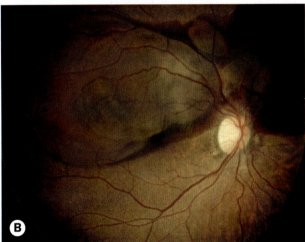

Fig. 14.51 Polypoidal choroidal vasculopathy. **(A)** Reddish-orange nodular terminal swellings with leakage; **(B)** serosanguineous retinal pigment epithelial detachment with associated subretinal fluid
(Courtesy of S Chen)

PERIPHERAL EXUDATIVE HAEMORRHAGIC CHORIORETINOPATHY

Peripheral exudative haemorrhagic chorioretinopathy (PEHCR) is an uncommon disorder affecting predominantly older women. It typically manifests with peripheral retinal haemorrhage, exudation and PED associated with CNV. It is bilateral in a substantial minority. The visual prognosis is often good, but the macula may be involved by extensive disease. The aetiology is unknown, though it may be a form of neovascular AMD; at least a proportion of cases share characteristics with polypoidal choroidal vasculopathy. Treatment for sight-threatening disease generally consists of intravitreal anti-VEGF injection.

IDIOPATHIC CHOROIDAL NEOVASCULARIZATION

Idiopathic CNV is an uncommon condition that affects patients under the age of 50 years and is usually unilateral. The diagnosis is one of exclusion of other possible associations of CNV in younger patients, such as angioid streaks, high myopia and chorioretinal inflammatory conditions such as presumed ocular histoplasmosis. The condition carries a better visual prognosis than that associated with AMD and in some cases spontaneous resolution may occur. Treatment is typically with an anti-VEGF agent.

VITREOMACULAR INTERFACE DISORDERS

Epiretinal membrane

Introduction

An epiretinal membrane (ERM) is a sheet-like fibrocellular structure that develops on or above the surface of the retina. Proliferation of the cellular component and contraction of the membrane leads to visual symptoms, primarily due to retinal wrinkling, obstruction and localized elevation with or without pseudocyst formation and CMO.

- **Idiopathic**
  - No apparent cause, such as previous retinal detachment, surgery, trauma or inflammation.
  - Residual vitreous tissue remains on the retinal surface following cortical separation in around 50% of eyes, with subsequent proliferation. The predominant cellular constituent is glial cells, probably derived from the indigenous posterior hyaloid membrane (PHM) cell population (laminocytes). ERM development can occur at any stage of posterior vitreous detachment (PVD); it is now believed that the process of PVD from initiation to completion often extends over the course of years.
  - About 10% are bilateral.
  - Tend to be milder than secondary ERMs.
- **Secondary**
  - Occur following retinal detachment surgery (most frequent cause of secondary ERM), retinal break, panretinal photocoagulation, retinal cryotherapy, retinal vascular disease, inflammation and trauma.
  - Binocularity is dependent on whether both eyes are affected by the causative factors.
  - Cell type more varied; pigment cells are prominent – thought to be derived from the RPE.

Diagnosis

- **Symptoms.** Blurring and metamorphopsia; mild cases are often asymptomatic.

- **Signs**
  - VA is highly variable, depending on severity.
  - An irregular translucent sheen (cellophane maculopathy) is present in early ERM, often best detected using green (red-free) light (Fig. 14.52A).
  - As the membrane thickens and contracts it becomes more obvious (macular pucker) and typically causes mild distortion of blood vessels (Fig. 14.52B).
  - Advanced ERM may give severe distortion of blood vessels, marked retinal wrinkling and striae and may obscure underlying structures (Fig. 14.52C).
  - Associated findings may include macular pseudohole (Fig. 14.52D), CMO, retinal telangiectasia and small haemorrhages.
- **Amsler grid** testing typically shows distortion.
- **OCT** shows a highly reflective surface layer associated with retinal thickening (Fig. 14.52E). Disruption of the inner-segment/outer-segment junction may be associated with a worse visual outcome following surgery. OCT is also useful to exclude significant vitreomacular traction (see later).
- **FA** has been superseded by OCT for routine assessment of ERM, but highlights vascular tortuosity and demonstrates any leakage. It is sometimes indicated to investigate the cause of an ERM, such as a prior retinal vein occlusion.

Treatment

- **Observation** if the membrane is mild and non-progressive. Spontaneous resolution of visual symptoms sometimes occurs, typically due to separation of the ERM from the retina as a previously incomplete PVD completes. CMO or tractional detachment may require fairly prompt surgery to minimize secondary degenerative change.
- **Surgical removal** of the membrane via vitrectomy to facilitate peeling usually improves or eliminates distortion (the main benefit), with an improvement in visual acuity of at least two lines in around 75% or more; in about a quarter VA is unchanged, and around 2% get worse. The surgical complications are principally those of vitrectomy. Removal of the internal limiting membrane (ILM) in concert with ERM peeling may be beneficial but remains controversial. Visual improvement commonly does not occur for several months postoperatively. Recurrence is rare.

Full-thickness macular hole

Introduction

Full-thickness macular hole (FTMH) is a relatively common cause of central visual loss, with a prevalence of approximately 3:1000; onset is most common in females aged 60–70. The risk of fellow eye involvement at 5 years is around 10%. The role of vitreomacular traction (VMT – see below) in the aetiology of macular hole has increasingly been defined over recent years; a new OCT-based classification has been published by the International

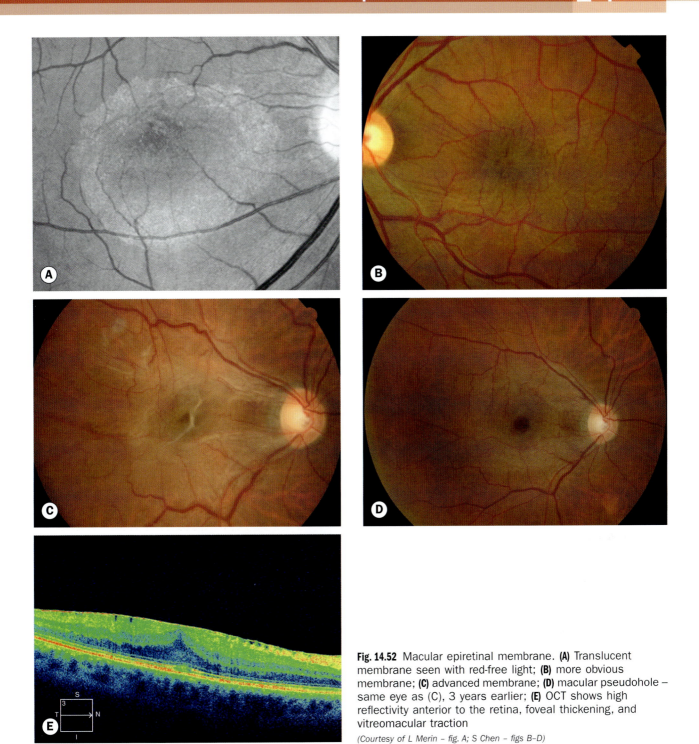

Fig. 14.52 Macular epiretinal membrane. **(A)** Translucent membrane seen with red-free light; **(B)** more obvious membrane; **(C)** advanced membrane; **(D)** macular pseudohole – same eye as (C), 3 years earlier; **(E)** OCT shows high reflectivity anterior to the retina, foveal thickening, and vitreomacular traction

(Courtesy of L Merin – fig. A; S Chen – figs B–D)

Vitreomacular Traction Study (IVTS) Group with the intention of replacing the older Gass clinical classification; both systems are discussed below, and vitreomacular traction is considered at greater length as a separate topic later in the chapter. Other causes of full-thickness macular hole include high myopia, which can lead to macular retinal detachment, and blunt ocular trauma. Lesions that may sometimes have a similar appearance include macular pseudohole and lamellar hole (see 'Vitreoretinal traction').

Clinical features

- **Symptoms.** Presentation of a full-thickness dehiscence may be with impairment of central vision in one eye, or as a relatively asymptomatic deterioration, first noticed when the fellow eye is occluded or at a routine sight test. Symptoms are absent or mild prior to the development of a full-thickness lesion; metamorphopsia may be present.

- **Signs and OCT features**
  - Stage 0 macular hole (IVTS: vitreomacular adhesion – VMA) was a term proposed originally to denote the OCT finding of oblique foveal vitreoretinal traction before the appearance of clinical changes.
  - Stage 1a: 'Impending' macular hole (IVTS: vitreomacular traction – VMT) appears as flattening of the foveal depression with an underlying yellow spot. Pathologically, the inner retinal layers detach from the underlying photoreceptor layer, often with the formation of a cyst-like schisis cavity. The differential diagnosis of a foveal yellow spot includes adult vitelliform macular dystrophy, solar and laser pointer retinopathy, and CMO.
  - Stage 1b: Occult macular hole (IVTS: vitreomacular traction – VMT) is seen as a yellow ring (Fig. 14.53A). With loss of structural support, the photoreceptor layer commonly undergoes centrifugal displacement (Fig. 14.54B).
  - Stage 2: Small full-thickness hole (IVTS: small or medium FTMH with VMT) consists of a full-thickness hole less than 400 μm in diameter (Fig. 14.53B and see Fig. 14.56B) at its narrowest point; the defect may be central, slightly eccentric or crescent-shaped. A dehiscence is present in the inner retina with persistent vitreofoveolar adhesion (Fig. 14.54C).
  - Stage 3: Full-size macular hole (IVTS: medium or large FTMH with VMT). A full-thickness hole greater than 400 μm in diameter, with a red base in which yellow–white dots may be seen. A surrounding grey cuff of subretinal fluid is usually present (Figs 14.53C and 14.54D), and an overlying retinal operculum (sometimes called a pseudo-operculum) may be visible. Visual acuity is commonly reduced to 6/60, but is occasionally better, particularly with eccentric fixation. Opercula (Fig. 14.54E) consist primarily of glial tissue and condensed vitreous cortex, though 40% contain photoreceptor elements. By definition, there is persistent parafoveal attachment of the vitreous cortex.
  - Stage 4: Full-size macular hole with complete PVD (IVTS: small, medium or large FTMH without VMT). The clinical appearance is indistinguishable from stage 3. The posterior vitreous is completely detached, often suggested (but not confirmed) by the presence of a Weiss ring. A significant proportion of idiopathic macular holes have an associated ERM.
  - Spontaneously resolved macular hole. Macular holes may heal spontaneously, often resuming a near-normal or even normal clinical and OCT appearance. A tiny outer

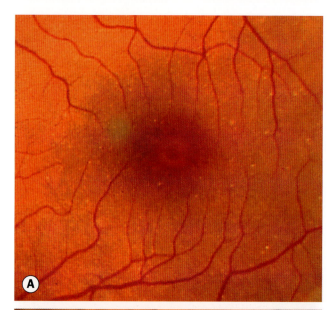

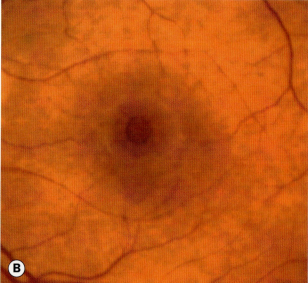

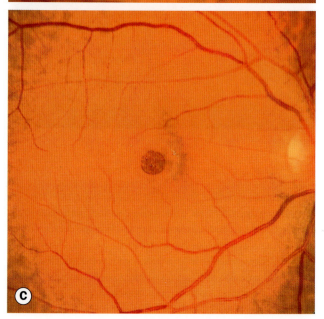

Fig. 14.53 Macular hole. **(A)** Occult – stage 1b; **(B)** small full-thickness – stage 2; **(C)** full-size – stage 3

(Courtesy of J Donald M Gass, from Stereoscopic Atlas of Macular Diseases, Mosby 1997 – fig. A; S Milenkov – fig. B; S Chen – fig. C)

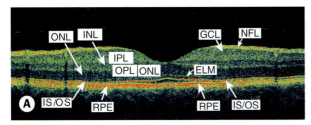
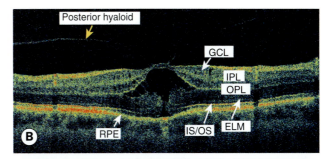
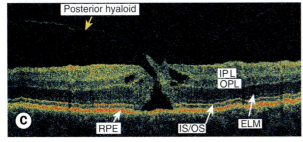
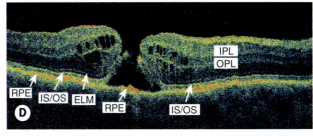
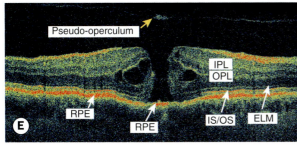
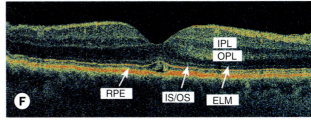

Fig. 14.54 High resolution OCT of full-thickness macular hole (FTMH). **(A)** Normal; **(B)** stage 1b – vitreomacular traction – shows attachment of the posterior hyaloid to the fovea, separation of a small portion of the sensory retina from the RPE in the foveolar region and intraretinal cystic changes; **(C)** eccentric stage 2 – small FTMH with vitreomacular traction (VMT) – shows attachment of the vitreous to the lid of the hole and cystic change; **(D)** stage 3 – medium or large FTMH with VMT – with intraretinal cystic spaces; **(E)** stage 4 – large FTMH with no VMT – shows a full-thickness macular hole with intraretinal cystic spaces and an overlying operculum (sometimes termed a pseudo-operculum); **(F)** stage 4 after surgical closure, showing outer retinal disturbance (ELM = external limiting membrane; GCL = ganglion cell layer; INL = inner nuclear layer; IPL = inner plexiform layer; IS/OS = photoreceptor inner-segment/outer-segment junction; NFL = nerve fibre layer; ONL = outer nuclear layer; OPL = outer plexiform layer; RPE = retinal pigment epithelium)

(Courtesy of J Fujimoto)

retinal – often inner-segment/outer-segment junction – or other subfoveolar defect may persist after spontaneous or surgical closure (Fig. 14.54F and see Fig. 14.56D); solar retinopathy commonly gives a similar appearance, as does scarring from several other conditions where the foveal centre is a focus of damage.

Investigation

- **Amsler grid** testing will usually show non-specific central distortion rather than a scotoma.
- **The Watzke–Allen test** is performed by projecting a narrow slit beam over the centre of the hole vertically and horizontally, preferably using a fundus contact lens. A patient with a macular hole will report that the beam is thinned or broken. Patients with other pathology usually see a distorted beam of uniform thickness.
- **OCT** is extremely useful in diagnosis and staging (see Fig. 14.54).

- **FAF** shows a markedly hyperfluorescent foveolar spot in stages 3 and 4, and punctate fluorescence in stage 2.
- **FA** in a full-thickness hole shows an early well-defined window defect (Fig. 14.55A) due to xanthophyll displacement and RPE atrophy. Late frames may show the surrounding subretinal fluid as a hyperfluorescent halo (Fig. 14.55B).

Treatment

- **Observation.** About 50% of stage 1 holes resolve following spontaneous vitreofoveolar separation, so these are managed conservatively. About 10% of full-thickness holes also close spontaneously, sometimes with marked visual improvement; spontaneous resolution is more common with smaller FTMH. Treatment is not usually given for spontaneously healed holes, though vitrectomy with ERM peeling is sometimes indicated.
- **Pharmacological vitreolysis** with ocriplasmin is a newer treatment that may be suitable for small earlier-stage holes. It is discussed under 'Vitreomacular traction' below.

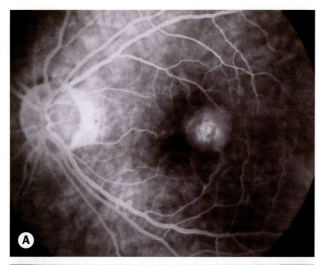

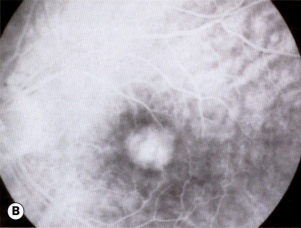

Fig. 14.55 FA of stage 4 macular hole. **(A)** Early-phase window defect with early surrounding pooling; **(B)** surrounding cuff of subretinal fluid demonstrated in later shots

- **Surgery** may be considered in stage 2 or greater holes and for some lamellar holes. Superior results are usually achieved in smaller lesions present for under 6 months, but substantial visual improvement has been reported in long-standing cases.
  - Operative treatment consists of vitrectomy, together with (i) peeling of the ILM facilitated by vital dye staining, (ii) relief of vitreomacular traction by either induction of a total PVD if not already present or removal of the perifoveal vitreous, and (iii) gas tamponade; the need for extended face-down positioning has been questioned.
  - The hole is closed in up to 100% of cases and visual improvement occurs over the course of months in 80–90% of eyes, with a final visual acuity of 6/12 or better in approximately 65%. Worsening of visual acuity occurs in up to 10% of eyes. Mild residual abnormality on OCT such as a defect in the inner-segment/outer-segment junction or other disturbance adjacent to the RPE (see Figs 14.54F and 14.56D) is common, and may also provide

a diagnostic indicator of a spontaneously healed macular hole or microhole.
  - Complications are essentially those of vitrectomy and the adjunctive procedures.

Macular microhole

Macular microhole refers to a small (<150 μm) full-thickness foveal retinal defect that in the current classification of vitreoretinal interface pathology (see below) is synonymous with a small full-thickness macular hole. Symptoms are often minimal and may consist of mild central blurring, metamorphopsia (distortion) or disturbed reading vision. Visual acuity is typically impaired less than with a larger FTMH, and the abnormality may not be noticed immediately. The full-thickness defect typically heals within a few weeks, and by the time of initial examination only a well-demarcated red spot (Fig. 14.56A) rather than a visibly full-thickness defect may be present. OCT demonstrates the defect, either full-thickness (Fig. 14.56B), or more commonly by the time of presentation involving only the outer retinal layers (Fig. 14.56C). A microhole (or healed larger macular hole – see Fig. 14.54F) may be represented by only a tiny focal defect in the inner-segment/outer-segment layer (Fig. 14.56D), a similar appearance to which can occur in other conditions such as solar retinopathy.

Vitreomacular traction

Introduction

Physiological PVD (see Ch. 16) usually proceeds gradually over an extended period to encompass complete separation from the macula and optic nerve head: complete PVD. If adhesion of the gel persists at the central macula, an anomalous PVD is present and can precede a range of macular conditions. An expert panel, the International Vitreomacular Traction Study Group, recently published a classification of vitreomacular interface disease based principally on OCT appearance in order to unify previously disparate terminology.

- **Vitreomacular adhesion (VMA)** refers to residual attachment of the vitreous within a 3 mm radius of the central macula in the presence of perifoveal vitreous separation; in most cases it constitutes a stage in a dynamic process of PVD so may not incur pathological sequelae. There is no distortion of the foveal contour or any secondary retinal changes. Focal VMA involves an area of attachment of ≤1500 μm diameter, broad VMA >1500 μm.
- **Vitreomacular traction (VMT)** is defined as the presence of retinal changes on OCT with evident perifoveal (within 3 mm) PVD. Distortion of the foveal surface contour and/or other structural retinal changes may be present (Figs 14.57A and B). Focal (Fig. 14.57C) and broad types are defined as for VMA. Concurrent VMT is associated with other macular disease, e.g. AMD, RVO, DR. Isolated VMT is unassociated with other macular disease.

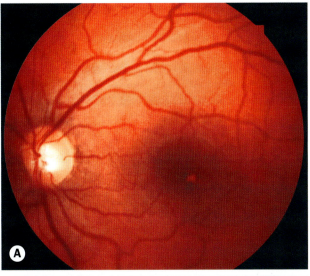
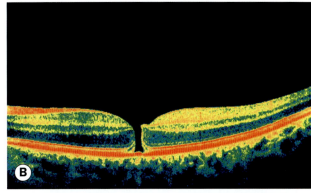
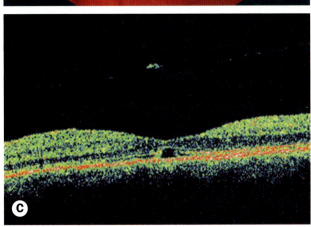
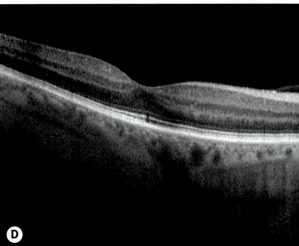

Fig. 14.56 Macular microhole (small full-thickness macular hole). **(A)** Small red foveal lesion; **(B)** full-thickness sensory retinal defect on OCT; **(C)** OCT showing outer retinal defect – a full-thickness defect was documented 3 weeks earlier in this eye, and a small operculum can be seen; **(D)** tiny focal inner/outer segment junction deficit

(Courtesy of M Lai, S Bressler, J Haller, from American Journal of Ophthalmology, *141:210–12 – fig. C)*

- **Full-thickness macular hole (FTMH).** A foveal lesion featuring interruption of all retinal layers from the internal limiting membrane to the RPE (see above). FTMH can be small (≤250 μm), medium (>250 to ≤400 μm) or large (>400 μm). Other considerations include (i) the status of the vitreous (with or without VMT) and (ii) the presence of an identifiable cause such as trauma.
- **Lamellar macular hole.** This is a partial-thickness defect of the inner retina at the fovea but maintenance of an intact photoreceptor layer. Its pathogenesis is incompletely defined, but may develop from anomalous PVD, sometimes following a foveal pseudocyst, or represent abortive FTMH formation in some patients. Classically, lamellar hole was described as a sequel to CMO.
- **Macular pseudohole.** This lesion mimics the clinical appearance of a FTMH, but is caused by distortion of the perifoveal retina into heaped edges by ERM, without any loss of retinal tissue, and near-normal foveal thickness; there is a central defect in the membrane. VMT may be present.

- **Epiretinal membrane (ERM).** ERM is independent of the IVTS classification, but a majority of eyes with broad VTS have an associated ERM. Vitreous remnants on the retinal surface following PVD provide a mechanism for the development of idiopathic ERM.

Diagnosis

- **Symptoms in VMT** include decreased vision, metamorphopsia, photopsia and micropsia, but are usually milder in lamellar holes and pseudoholes, and absent in VMA.
- **Signs** in VMT may include retinal surface thickening, wrinkling and distortion (Fig. 14.57D), foveal pseudocyst, CMO, macular schisis or detachment, and capillary leakage; the limit of the attached gel may be visible as a whitish band or reflex. Visible changes may be subtle. Both lamellar holes and pseudoholes can appear as a discrete reddish oval or round foveal spot.
- **OCT** is the key investigation; features are described above.

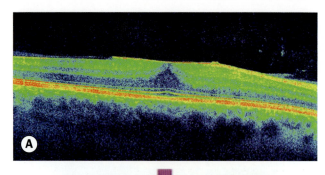

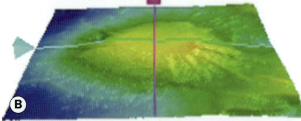

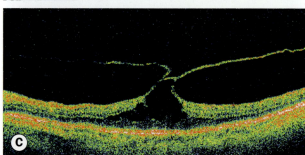

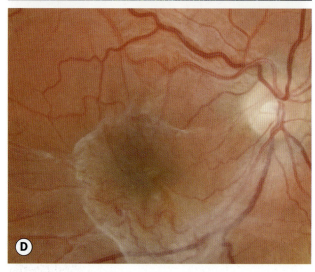

Fig. 14.57 Vitreomacular traction (VMT). **(A)** and **(B)** show an OCT of the same eye, in which the foveal contour is flattened and the foveal surface slightly elevated above the surrounding retina; **(C)** OCT of focal VMT; **(D)** VMT with retinal surface thickening and wrinkling and an associated epiretinal membrane – the area of vitreous attachment is demarcated by a whitish line that extends around the optic disc as well as the macula

Treatment

Treatment of FTMH and ERM is considered under separate topics above.

- **Observation.** Spontaneous separation occurs in a proportion of patients with VMT, and is probably more likely in milder cases; published figures vary. Observation is appropriate in patients with VMA and in many cases of VMT.
- **Pharmacological vitreolysis.** Intravitreal injection of ocriplasmin, a recombinant form of human plasmin, releases VMT in over 25% of eyes, and may close macular holes where VMT is present (40% versus 10% with placebo). Results are generally inferior to vitrectomy. Smaller areas of VMT and smaller macular holes have better outcomes; the presence of ERM is a poorer prognostic indicator for ocriplasmin treatment. Diffuse retinal dysfunction of uncertain mechanism, including substantially decreased acuity, has been reported as a rare side effect.
- **Pars plana vitrectomy** with peeling of the adherent area and any associated ERM usually gives good results in VMT. The benefit of vitrectomy for lamellar and pseudoholes is less clear-cut, but is probably greater if significant ERM is present.

CENTRAL SEROUS CHORIORETINOPATHY

Overview

Central serous chorioretinopathy (CSR) is an idiopathic disorder characterized by a localized serous detachment of the sensory retina at the macula secondary to leakage from the choriocapillaris through one or more hyperpermeable RPE sites. CSR typically affects one eye of a young or middle-aged Caucasian man; women with CSR tend to be older. Imperfectly defined risk factors include steroid administration (including intravitreal), Cushing syndrome, *Helicobacter pylori* infection, pregnancy, psychological stress and sleep apnoea syndrome.

Clinical features

- **Symptoms.** Unilateral blurring, metamorphopsia, micropsia and mild dyschromatopsia.
- **Signs**
  - VA is typically 6/9–6/18, but may improve with a weak convex lens due to acquired hypermetropia from retinal elevation.
  - Round or oval detachment of the sensory retina at the macula (Fig. 14.58A).
  - The subretinal fluid may be clear (particularly in early lesions) or turbid; precipitates may be present on the posterior retinal surface (see Fig. 14.60A).
  - One or more depigmented RPE foci (often small PEDs) of variable size may be visible within the neurosensory detachment; small patches of RPE atrophy (Fig. 14.58B) and hyperplasia elsewhere in the posterior pole may

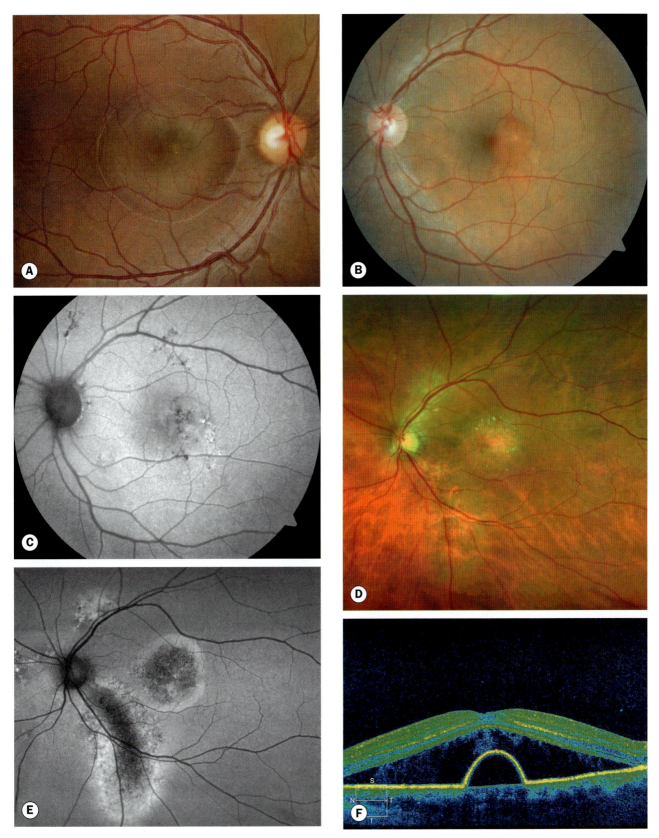

Fig. 14.58 Central serous chorioretinopathy (CSR). **(A)** Serous retinal and underlying pigment epithelial detachment; **(B)** small patches of pigmentary abnormality in a patient with resolving foveal CSR; **(C)** FAF of the same eye as (B) showing scarring from additional subclinical lesions; **(D)** chronic lesions, the inferior with a gravitational tract; **(E)** same eye as (C) on wide-field autofluorescence imaging; **(F)** OCT of the eye in (A) shows separation of the sensory retina from the retinal pigment epithelium and a smaller underlying pigment epithelial detachment

(Courtesy of S Chen – figs A, D–F)

indicate the site of previous lesions, and are typically seen easily on FAF imaging (Fig. 14.58C).

- ○ Chronic lesions may be associated with substantial underlying atrophic change (Fig. 14.58D); fluid can sometimes track downwards in a gravity-dependent fashion (gravitational tract), best shown on FAF imaging (Fig. 14.58E), and can occasionally progress to bullous CSR (see below).
- ○ The optic disc should be examined to exclude a congenital pit as the cause of a neurosensory detachment (see Ch. 19).
- **Course**
  - ○ Spontaneous resolution within 3–6 months, with return to near-normal or normal vision, occurs in around 80%; recurrence is seen in up to 50%.
  - ○ A substantial minority follow a chronic course lasting more than 12 months. Prolonged detachment is associated with gradual photoreceptor and RPE

degeneration and permanently reduced vision; multiple recurrent attacks may also give a similar clinical picture.
  - ○ CMO, CNV or RPE tears develop in a small minority.
- **Bullous CSR** is characterized by large single or multiple serous retinal and RPE detachments.

Investigation

- **Amsler grid** confirms metamorphopsia corresponding to the neurosensory detachment.
- **OCT** shows an optically empty neurosensory elevation. Other findings may include one or more smaller RPE detachments (Fig. 14.58F), precipitates on the posterior surface of detached retina, and thickened choroid. Degenerative changes may be seen in chronic or recurrent cases.
- **FA** shows an early hyperfluorescent spot that gradually enlarges (an 'ink blot' – Figs 14.59A and B) or, less

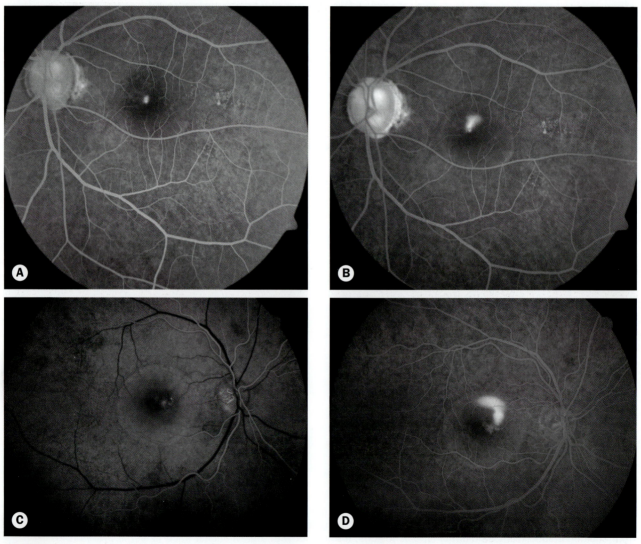

Fig. 14.59 FA of central serous chorioretinopathy. **(A)** and **(B)** 'Ink blot' appearance; **(C)** and **(D)** 'smokestack' appearance
(Courtesy of S Chen)

commonly, forms a vertical column ('smokestack' – Figs 14.59C and D) followed by diffusion throughout the detached area. An underlying PED may be demonstrated. Multiple focal leaks or diffuse areas of leakage can be evident, particularly in chronic or recurrent disease.

- **FAF** shows a focal decrease in fundus autofluorescence at the leakage site, and at sites of old lesions (see Figs 14.58C and E). A gravitational tract is sometimes seen.
- **ICGA.** The early phase may show dilated or compromised choroidal vessels at the posterior pole, and the mid-stage areas of hyperfluorescence due to choroidal hyperpermeability. Subclinical foci are commonly visible.

Management

- **Observation** is appropriate in many cases. All treatment modalities can be associated with RPE tear formation; this can also occur spontaneously.
- **Corticosteroid treatment** should be discontinued if possible, particularly in chronic, recurrent or severe cases.
- **Laser.** Micropulse diode laser to the RPE site of leakage has shown good results (Figs 14.60A and B) in several studies, and is associated with significantly less retinal damage on OCT than conventional photocoagulation.
- **PDT** at 30–50% of the dose used for CNV in conjunction with 50% light intensity typically leads to complete resolution, including in severe chronic cases, and is associated with a considerably lower incidence of significant choroidal ischaemia than higher-intensity regimens.
- **Intravitreal anti-VEGF agents** show some promise and may be used in conjunction with other treatments.
- **Others.** Case reports show benefit with a variety of agents including aspirin, beta-blockers, mifepristone and eplerenone, but controlled assessment is limited to date.

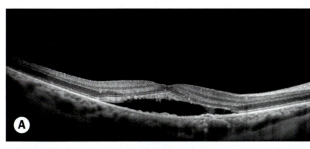

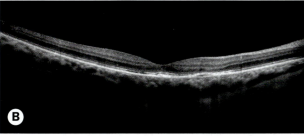

Fig. 14.60 Micropulse laser treatment of central serous chorioretinopathy. **(A)** Prior to treatment; **(B)** after successful treatment

IDIOPATHIC MACULAR TELANGIECTASIA

Idiopathic macular telangiectasia (IMT, MacTel) is a condition of unknown pathogenesis. It may be more common than previously believed and can be confused with DR, prior RVO and other causes of macular vascular changes. A family history is present in a small proportion of cases.

Type 1: aneurysmal telangiectasia

This may be closely related to Coats disease, or more specifically the milder form of Coats previously known as Leber miliary aneurysms; it generally involves only one eye, and both the peripheral retina and macula can be affected. Patients are typically middle-aged males.

- **Symptoms.** Mild to moderate blurring of vision in one eye.
- **Signs**
  - Telangiectasia and microaneurysms; early signs may be subtle and more readily detected on red-free photography (Fig. 14.61A).
  - Larger aneurysms form as the condition progresses.
  - Macular oedema, including cystoid changes.
  - Chronic leakage and lipid deposition (Fig. 14.61B).
- **OCT** demonstrates retinal thickening, CMO and localized exudative retinal detachment.
- **FA** shows telangiectasia and multiple capillary, venular and arteriolar aneurysms (Figs 14.61C and D) with late leakage and CMO (Fig. 14.61E). There is minimal non-perfusion.
- **Treatment** is with laser to points and areas of leakage, but can be technically difficult depending on the proximity of changes to the foveola. Intravitreal VEGF inhibitors may be effective.

Type 2: perifoveal telangiectasia

This bilateral form is more common than type 1, and usually has a worse visual prognosis. Males and females are equally affected; onset is in middle age. In contrast to type 1, findings are generally limited to the perifoveal area. Degeneration of Müller cells is thought to be an important pathogenic mechanism.

- **Symptoms.** Blurring in one or both eyes. Distortion may be a feature.
- **Signs**
  - Greyish loss of parafoveol retinal transparency extending up to one disc diameter from the foveola, initially temporal to (Fig. 14.62A) and later surrounding the fovea.
  - Fine superficial crystalline retinal deposits may be seen (Fig. 14.62B).
  - Parafoveal telangiectasia may not be visible clinically but can often be demonstrated more readily by red-free photography. Right-angled venules (Fig. 14.62C) are characteristic. The abnormal vessels can proliferate to subretinal neovascularization distinct from CNV but similar to retinal angiomatous proliferation – the proliferative stage of the condition.

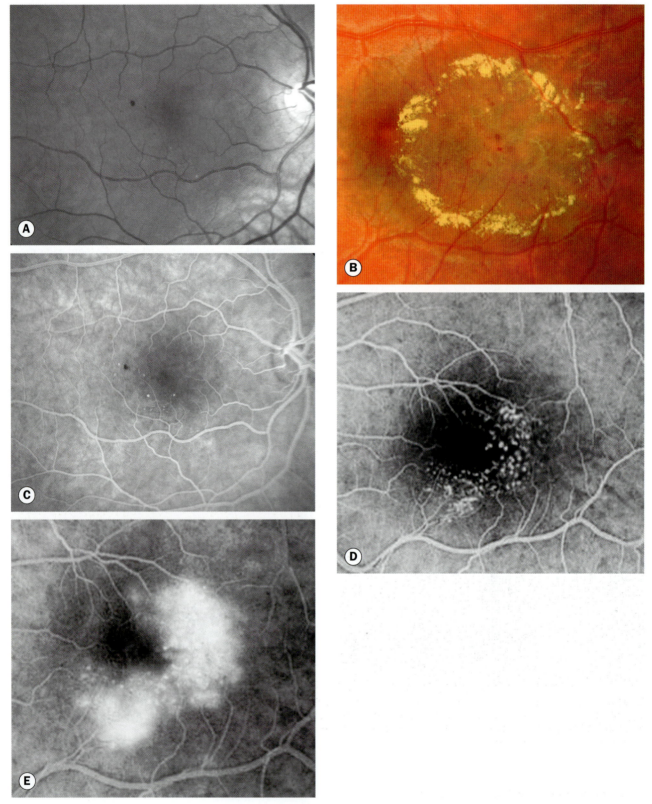

Fig. 14.61 Idiopathic macular telangiectasia type 1 – aneurysmal telangiectasia. **(A)** Early disease – red-free image; **(B)** aneurysms and telangiectasis surrounded by a ring of exudate; **(C)** FA of eye in (A) showing microaneurysms; **(D)** FA early phase of the eye in (B) shows telangiectasis temporal to the fovea; **(E)** FA late phase of eye in (B) and (D) showing leakage

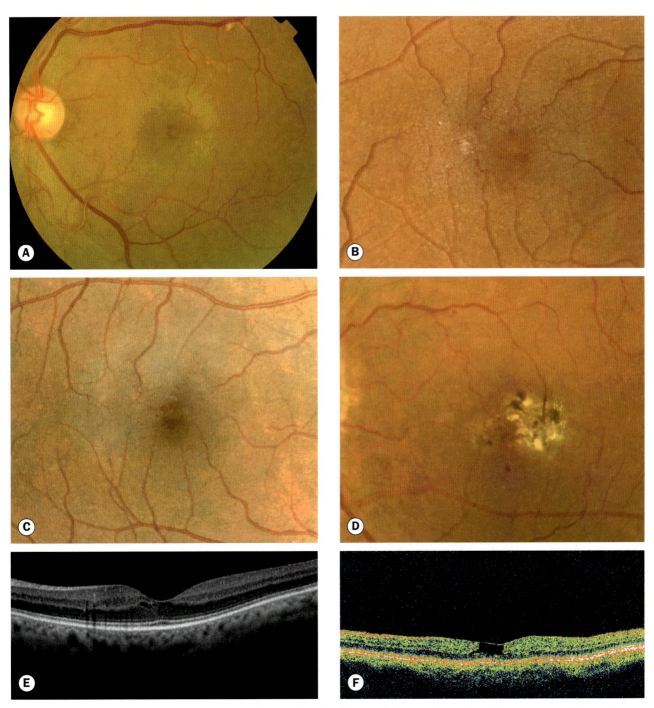

Fig. 14.62 Idiopathic macular telangiectasia type 2 – perifoveal. **(A)** Loss of temporal parafoveal transparency; **(B)** macular crystals and early telangiectasis; **(C)** telangiectasis with small parafoveal right-angled venules; **(D)** pigment plaques; **(E)** pseudocystic perifoveal spaces on OCT; **(F)** inner lamellar subfoveal cyst

(Courtesy of S Chen – figs A–D and F)

○ Foveal atrophy may simulate a lamellar hole.
○ Small RPE plaques (Fig. 14.62D) develop in many patients, often associated with the right-angled venules.
○ Aneurysms are uncommon but have been reported; lipid deposition does not tend to be a feature.
○ Visual acuity generally does not deteriorate to less than 6/60 unless CNV supervenes, although CNV in this condition tends to carry a better prognosis than in AMD.
● **OCT** findings are a key aid to diagnosis. The formation of hyporeflective inner retinal spaces of variable size (Fig. 14.62E), morphologically distinct from those seen in CMO, is characteristic in moderate though not early disease; an inner lamellar cyst that enlarges with progressive disease is

commonly seen underlying the fovea (Fig. 14.62F). Thinning and disruption of the photoreceptor layers is also very common, and may occur early. Pigment clumps are shown as intraretinal hyper-reflective plaques with posterior shadowing. Foveal thinning is common, but diffuse parafoveal retinal thickening is variably present. Hyper-reflective inner retinal dots corresponding to telangiectatic vessels are seen early on in many patients.

- **FAF** changes occur early in the disease course, and may precede clinically detectable signs. Central foveal hyperautofluorescence is a common early finding; this gradually increases in extent but in more advanced disease an area of well-demarcated central hypoautofluorescence develops. Retinal crystals and pigment clumping give hypoautofluorescence. Irregular central and peripheral areas of increased signal surrounding patches of decreased signal may be seen.
- **FA** in early disease shows bilateral perifoveal telangiectasia with early leakage from the abnormal vessels progressing to diffuse leakage, though without CMO. The cystoid spaces identifiable on OCT do not hyperfluoresce on FA. FA is also used to confirm CNV.
- **Macular pigment optical density** (MPOD) imaging shows a possibly pathognomonic pattern of oval reduction in density corresponding to the late distribution of hyperfluorescence on FA. MPOD is preserved from 6° outwards.
- **Treatment.** Intravitreal anti-VEGF agents decrease leakage on FA in the non-proliferative stage but are probably not helpful visually. They are likely to be useful in the proliferative stage, especially for CNV.

Occlusive telangiectasia

This extremely rare condition presents in late middle age and carries a poor visual prognosis. The manifestations relate to capillary occlusion rather than telangiectasia: progressive occlusion of parafoveal capillaries with marked aneurysmal dilatation of terminal capillaries.

CYSTOID MACULAR OEDEMA

Introduction

Cystoid macular oedema (CMO) results from the accumulation of fluid in the outer plexiform and inner nuclear layers of the retina with the formation of tiny cyst-like cavities (Fig. 14.63). Fluid may initially accumulate intracellularly in Müller cells, with subsequent rupture. Coalescence of smaller cavities may occur over time with subsequent progression to a foveal lamellar hole with irreversible impairment of central vision. CMO is a non-specific manifestation of any type of macular oedema. Causes include:

- **Ocular surgery and laser**, e.g. phacoemulsification, panretinal photocoagulation and miscellaneous other procedures.

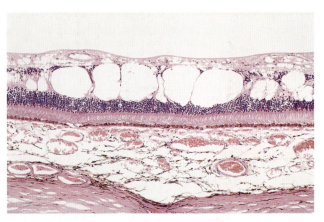

Fig 14.63 Histology of cystoid macular oedema shows cystic spaces in the outer plexiform and inner nuclear layer
(Courtesy of J Harry and G Misson, from Clinical Ophthalmic Pathology, *Butterworth-Heinemann 2001)*

- **Retinal vascular disease**, e.g. DR, RVO.
- **Inflammation**, e.g. intermediate uveitis, severe or chronic uveitis of any kind.
- **Drug-induced**, e.g. topical prostaglandin derivatives.
- **Retinal dystrophies**, e.g. retinitis pigmentosa.
- **Conditions involving vitreomacular traction**, e.g. ERM.
- **CNV**.
- **Fundus tumours**, e.g. retinal capillary haemangioma.
- **Systemic disease**, e.g. chronic renal failure.

Diagnosis

- **Symptoms** may include blurring, distortion and micropsia.
- **Signs**
  - Loss of the foveal depression, thickening of the retina and multiple cystoid areas in the sensory retina (Fig. 14.64A), best seen with red-free light using a fundus contact lens (Fig. 14.64B).
  - Optic disc swelling is sometimes present.
  - A lamellar hole may be visible.
  - Features of associated disease.
- **Amsler chart** demonstrates central blurring and distortion.
- **FA.** A petaloid pattern is seen due to dye accumulation in microcystic spaces in the outer plexiform layer (Fig. 14.64C).
- **OCT** shows retinal thickening with cystic hyporeflective spaces, and loss of the foveal depression (Fig. 14.64D). A lamellar hole may be demonstrated in advanced cases.

MICROCYSTIC MACULAR OEDEMA

Microcystic changes of the inner nuclear layer distinct from classic CMO can occur in eyes with optic neuritis and some other forms of optic neuropathy. It is believed to be caused by retrograde degeneration of the inner retinal layers that manifests with impaired fluid resorption.

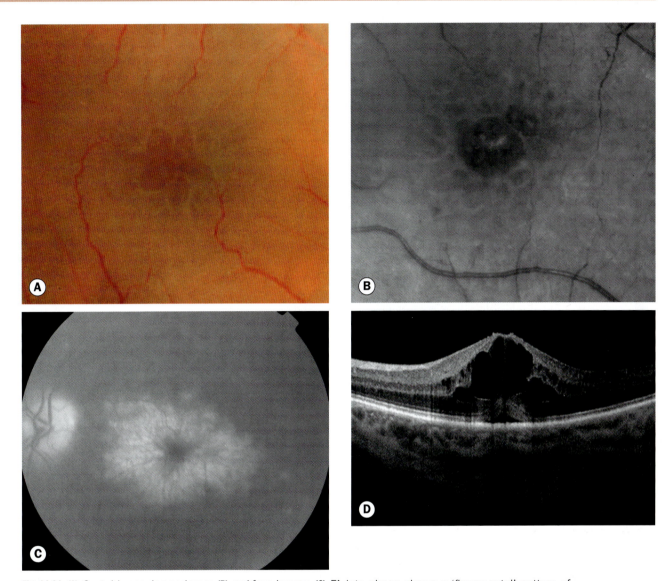

Fig. 14.64 (A) Cystoid macular oedema; **(B)** red-free image; **(C)** FA late phase shows a 'flower petal' pattern of hyperfluorescence; **(D)** OCT shows hyporeflective spaces within the retina, macular thickening and loss of the foveal depression

(Courtesy of J Donald M Gass, from Stereoscopic Atlas of Macular Diseases, Mosby 1997 – fig. A; P Gili – fig. B; S Chen – fig. C)

DEGENERATIVE MYOPIA

Introduction

Myopia is the result of complex hereditary and environmental factors; there is strong evidence for a causative association with long-term intensive near visual activity, particularly reading. A refractive error of more than −6 dioptres constitutes a common definition of high myopia, in which axial length is usually greater than 26 mm; it affects over 2% of an adult Western European or American population and may be as high as 10% in East Asians. Pathological or degenerative myopia is characterized by progressive anteroposterior elongation of the scleral envelope associated with a range of secondary ocular changes, principally thought to relate to mechanical stretching of the involved tissues. It is a

significant cause of legal blindness, with maculopathy the most common cause of visual loss. Various techniques such as scleral buckling and patching have been used to try to stem the progression of myopia or reinforce extremely thinned areas, but remain controversial. Table 14.5 lists systemic associations of myopia.

Table 14.5 Systemic associations of high myopia

Down syndrome
Stickler syndrome
Marfan syndrome
Prematurity
Noonan syndrome
Ehlers–Danlos syndrome
Pierre–Robin syndrome

Diagnosis

- **A pale tessellated** (tigroid) appearance is due to diffuse attenuation of the RPE with visibility of large choroidal vessels (Fig. 14.65A).

- **Focal chorioretinal atrophy** is characterized by patchy visibility of choroidal vessels, and often sclera (Fig. 14.65B).
- **Anomalous optic nerve head.** This may appear unusually small, large or anomalous with a 'tilted' conformation (Fig. 14.65C). Peripapillary chorioretinal atrophy is very common,

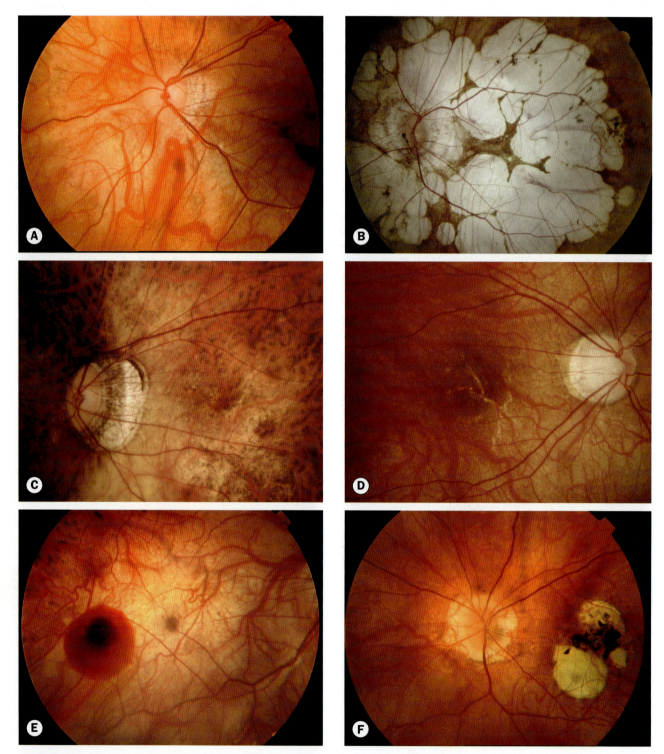

Fig. 14.65 High myopia. **(A)** Tessellated fundus; **(B)** focal chorioretinal atrophy and tilted disc; **(C)** tilted disc; **(D)** lacquer cracks; **(E)** 'coin' haemorrhage; **(F)** Fuchs spot

(Courtesy of S Chen – figs B–D)

most commonly as a temporal crescent of thinned or absent RPE.

- **Acquired optic disc pit** formation is not uncommon, and is thought to be due to expansion of the peripapillary region as the eye enlarges over time.
- **Lattice degeneration** (see Ch. 16).
- **Lacquer cracks** are ruptures in the RPE–Bruch membrane–choriocapillaris complex characterized by fine irregular yellow lines criss-crossing at the posterior pole (Fig. 14.65D) in around 5% of highly myopic eyes and can be complicated by CNV.
- **Subretinal 'coin' haemorrhages** (Fig. 14.65E) may develop from lacquer cracks in the absence of CNV.
- **A Fuchs spot** (Fig. 14.65F) is a raised, circular, pigmented lesion at the macula developing after a subretinal haemorrhage has absorbed.

- **A staphyloma** is a peripapillary or macular ectasia of the posterior sclera (Figs 14.66A and B) due to focal thinning and expansion present in about a third of eyes with pathological myopia. Associations include macular hole formation and 'dome-shaped macula', an overlying anterior bulge typically involving the retina, RPE and inner choroid best shown on OCT (Fig. 14.66C); it may be complicated by a foveal detachment.
- **(Peripapillary) intrachoroidal cavitation**, formerly described as peripapillary detachment of pathological myopia (PDPM), may occur adjacent to the nerve, commonly inferiorly. Clinically, it may be evident as a small yellowish-orange peripapillary area typically inferior to the disc (Fig. 14.66D); it can generally be identified on OCT (Figs 14.66E and F). Visual field defects are common and frequently mimic glaucoma.

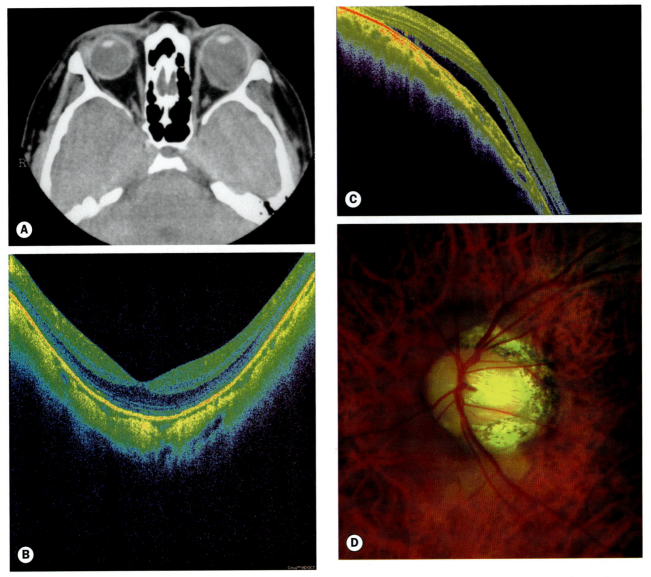

Fig. 14.66 High myopia. **(A)** axial CT shows a left posterior staphyloma; **(B)** staphyloma on OCT; **(C)** dome-shaped macula; **(D)** intrachoroidal cavitation (ICC) – orange peripapillary area inferior to the disc;

Continued

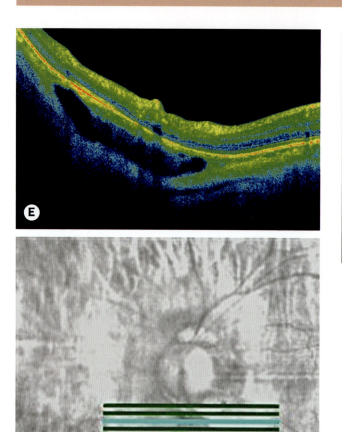

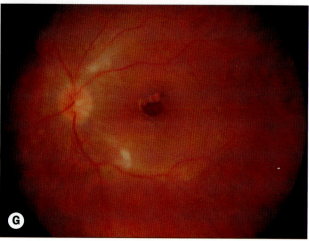

Fig. 14.66, Continued **(E)** OCT appearance of ICC; **(F)** central line indicates the plane of the image in (E); **(G)** shallow retinal detachment confined to the posterior pole, caused by a myopia-related macular hole

(Courtesy of S Chen – figs B–F; M Khairallah – fig. G)

- **Rhegmatogenous retinal detachment (RD)** is much more common in high myopia, the pathogenesis including increased frequency of PVD, lattice degeneration, asymptomatic atrophic holes, myopic macular holes (see below) and occasionally giant retinal tears.
- **CNV**
  - 10% of highly myopic eyes develop CNV.
  - The prognosis is better in younger patients with myopia-related CNV than in AMD.
  - Anti-VEGF therapy is generally the treatment of choice; a lower injection frequency may be needed than for AMD but RD risk is higher.
- **Macular retinoschisis** (foveoschisis) and macular retinal detachment without macular hole formation may occur in highly myopic eyes with posterior staphyloma, probably as a result of vitreous traction. Some cases are associated with intrachoroidal cavitation (see above). Retinoschisis may be mistaken clinically for CMO, and is better characterized by OCT than biomicroscopy.

- **Macular hole** may occur spontaneously or after relatively mild trauma, and is associated with the development of rhegmatogenous retinal detachment much more commonly than age-related idiopathic macular hole (Fig. 14.66G). Myopic macular retinoschisis and myopic macular hole may be part of the same pathological process. Vitrectomy may be effective for both, but the best surgical technique remains undefined.
- **Peripapillary detachment** is an innocuous yellow–orange elevation of the RPE and sensory retina at the inferior border of the myopic conus (anomalous optic nerve head complex).
- **Cataract.** Posterior subcapsular or early onset nuclear sclerotic.
- **Glaucoma.** There is an increased prevalence of primary open-angle glaucoma, pigmentary glaucoma and steroid responsiveness.
- **Amblyopia** is uncommon but may develop when there is a significant difference in myopia between the two eyes.

- **Dislocation of the lens** (natural or artificial) is a rare but well-recognized risk.

ANGIOID STREAKS

Introduction

Angioid streaks are crack-like dehiscences in brittle thickened and calcified Bruch membrane, associated with atrophy of the overlying RPE. Approximately 50% of patients with angioid streaks have a systemic association:

- **Pseudoxanthoma elasticum (PXE)**, a hereditary disorder of connective tissue in which there is progressive calcification, fragmentation and degeneration of elastic fibres in the skin, eye and cardiovascular system, is by far the most common association of angioid streaks (Grönblad–Strandberg syndrome). Patients develop a 'plucked chicken' appearance of the skin, most commonly on the neck, axillae and antecubital fossae. Approximately 85% of patients develop ocular involvement of variable severity, usually after the second decade of life.
- **Ehlers–Danlos syndrome** is a rare, usually autosomal dominant, disorder of collagen. There are 11 subtypes but only type 6 (ocular sclerotic) is associated with ocular features.
- **Paget disease** is a chronic, progressive metabolic bone disease characterized by excessive and disorganized resorption and formation of bone. Angioid streaks occur in only about 2%; it is thought that calcium binds to the elastin of Bruch membrane, imparting brittleness and fragility.
- **Haemoglobinopathies** occasionally associated with angioid streaks are numerous, including sickle-cell trait and disease and thalassaemias; in these the brittle Bruch membrane is thought to be due to iron deposition.
- **Miscellaneous other associations** have been reported.

Diagnosis

- **Signs**
  - Grey or dark red linear lesions with irregular serrated edges that intercommunicate in a ring-like fashion around the optic disc and radiate outwards from the peripapillary area (Fig. 14.67A). The streaks tend to increase in width and extent slowly over time.
  - 'Peau d'orange' (orange skin), also known as leopard skin, mottled yellowish speckling (Figs 14.67B and C) is common, particularly in cases associated with PXE.
  - Optic disc drusen are frequently (up to 25%) associated (Fig. 14.67D).
  - Scleral depression is relatively contraindicated in these eyes, due to the risk of further damage to the Bruch membrane leading to new angioid streaks or choroidal rupture.

- **Complications.** Though angioid streaks are typically asymptomatic at first, visual impairment occurs eventually in over 70% of patients.
  - CNV is by far the most common cause of visual loss.
  - Choroidal rupture may occur following relatively trivial trauma (Fig. 14.67E).
  - Foveal involvement by a streak.
- **Red-free photography** demonstrates the streaks.
- **FA** shows hyperfluorescent window defects due to RPE atrophy overlying the streaks, associated with variable associated hypofluorescence corresponding to RPE hyperplasia. FA is generally indicated only if CNV is suspected.
- **FAF.** Streaks are autofluorescent; they are often more extensive than clinically, which may confirm the diagnosis in subtle cases (Fig. 14.67F); peau d'orange is shown.

Treatment

Following systemic investigation where appropriate, usually via referral to an appropriate physician, observation is the approach in most cases. Patients should be warned against participating in contact sports and advised to use protective spectacles when necessary. CNV should usually be treated with intravitreal anti-VEGF agents, but commonly recurs or develops at a new site.

CHOROIDAL FOLDS

Introduction

Choroidal folds are parallel grooves or striae involving the inner choroid, Bruch membrane, the RPE and sometimes the retina (chorioretinal folds). They are likely to develop in association with any process that induces sufficient compressive stress within the choroid, Bruch membrane and retina. Primary mechanisms include choroidal congestion and scleral compression, and occasionally tissue contraction. Choroidal folds should be distinguished from retinal folds, which have a different pathogenesis (usually ERM). Causes include:

- **Idiopathic ('congenital')** folds may be present in healthy, often hypermetropic, individuals in whom visual acuity is typically unaffected. The folds are usually bilateral. A syndrome of idiopathic acquired hypermetropia with choroidal folds has been described – in these patients elevated intracranial pressure should always be excluded even without evident papilloedema (see next) although a constricted scleral canal causing optic disc congestion has been proposed as an alternative mechanism in some patients.
- **Papilloedema.** Choroidal folds may occur in patients with chronically elevated intracranial pressure, when they may be associated with reduction of visual acuity that may be permanent.
- **Orbital disease** such as retrobulbar tumours and thyroid ophthalmopathy may cause choroidal folds associated with impaired vision.

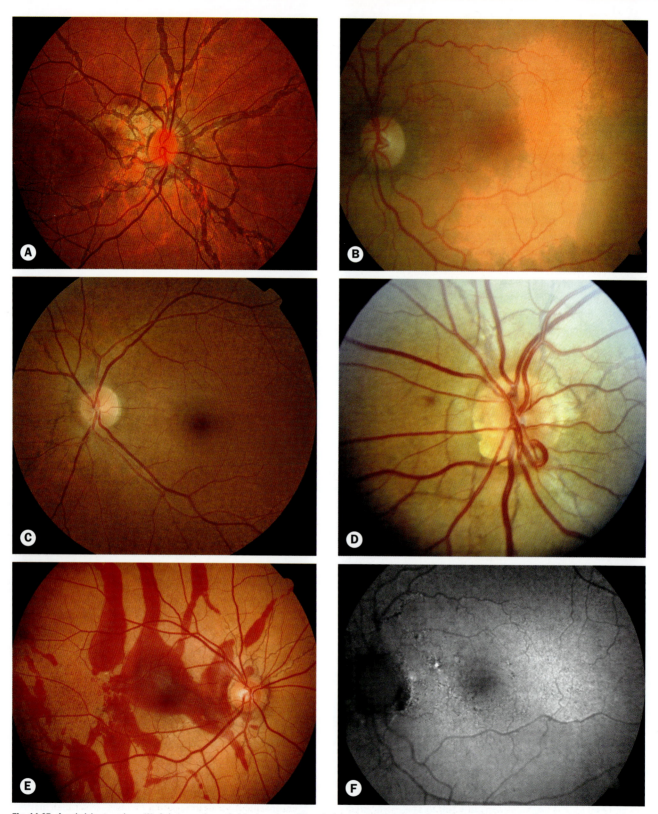

Fig. 14.67 Angioid streaks. **(A)** Advanced angioid streaks; **(B)** subtle angioid streaks around the optic disc, with 'peau d'orange' at the temporal macula; **(C)** angioid streaks with more marked peau d'orange; **(D)** angioid streaks and optic disc drusen; **(E)** subretinal haemorrhage caused by a traumatic choroidal rupture; **(F)** FAF imaging of the eye in (B), showing more extensive changes than evident clinically, including demonstration of the peau d'orange

(Courtesy of P Saine – fig. A; S Chen – figs C–E)

- **Ocular disease** such as choroidal tumours, inflammation such as posterior scleritis, scleral buckling for retinal detachment, and hypotony.

Diagnosis

- **Symptoms.** The effect on vision is variable and dependent on the cause; many patients are asymptomatic.
- **Signs**
  - Parallel lines, grooves or striae typically located at the posterior pole. The folds are usually horizontally orientated (Fig. 14.68A).

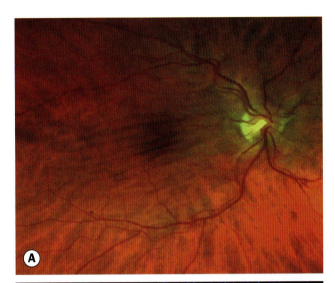

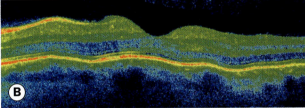

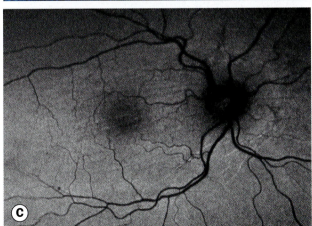

Fig. 14.68 Choroidal folds **(A)** Wide-field photograph; **(B)** OCT appearance; **(C)** FAF

(Courtesy of S Chen)

- The crest (elevated portion) of a fold is yellow and less pigmented as a result of stretching and thinning of the RPE and the trough is darker due to compression of the RPE.
  - Clinical examination should be directed towards the exclusion of optic disc swelling, as well as other ocular or orbital pathology.
- **OCT** allows differentiation between choroidal, chorioretinal and retinal folds (Fig. 14.68B).
- **FAF** effectively demonstrates the folds (Fig. 14.68C) and may show associated atrophy; if this is marked the appearance can be mistaken for angioid streaks.
- **FA** shows hyperfluorescent crests as a result of increased background choroidal fluorescence showing through the stretched and thinned RPE and hypofluorescent troughs due to blockage of choroidal fluorescence by the compressed and thickened RPE.
- **Supplementary imaging.** Ultrasound, computed tomography (CT) or magnetic resonance (MR) scanning of the orbits or brain may be indicated. In elevated intracranial pressure or acquired hypermetropia with choroidal folds, an enlarged perineural space may be noted on B-scanning and MR of the optic nerves.

HYPOTONY MACULOPATHY

Introduction

Maculopathy is common in eyes developing hypotony, defined as IOP less than 5 mmHg. The most common cause is excessive drainage following glaucoma filtration surgery, for which adjunctive antimetabolites confer a higher risk; other causes include trauma (cyclodialysis cleft, penetrating injury), chronic uveitis (by directly impairing ciliary body function and by tractional ciliary body detachment due to cyclitic membrane) and retinal detachment. Systemic causes of hypotony (usually bilateral) include dehydration, hyperglycaemia in uncontrolled diabetes, uraemia and treatment with hyperosmotic agents or carbonic anhydrase inhibitors. The development of secondary choroidal effusion may act to perpetuate the hypotony. With time the hypotonous process can itself lead to further damage, including sclerosis and atrophy of ciliary processes. Prolonged severe hypotony may lead to phthisis bulbi and loss of the eye. Treatment to restore normal IOP is directed according to cause.

Diagnosis

- **VA** is variably affected; delayed normalization of IOP may result in permanent visual impairment, though substantial improvement has been reported following reversal of hypotony after several years.
- **Fine retinal folds** radiating outwards from the foveola, which may also show CMO (Fig. 14.69).
- **Chorioretinal folds** may radiate outwards in branching fashion from the optic disc; these are due to scleral collapse with resultant chorioretinal redundancy.

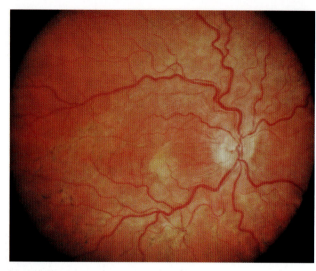

Fig. 14.69 Hypotony maculopathy showing cystoid macular oedema and retinal folds
(Courtesy of P Gili)

- **Miscellaneous.** A variety of other features may be present, related both to aetiology and secondary effects of hypotony, including a shallow anterior chamber, choroidal effusion, cataract, corneal decompensation, optic disc oedema, uveitis, wound leak or an unexpected filtering bleb adjacent to a wound (e.g. following cataract surgery), cyclodialysis cleft on gonioscopy, and retinal detachment.
- **Ultrasound biomicroscopy** may show a cyclitic membrane or cyclodialysis cleft if there is clinical reason to suspect this.

- **B-scan ultrasonography** will demonstrate choroidal effusions.
- **A-scan ultrasonography** or interferometry may show reduced axial length.

SOLAR RETINOPATHY

- **Pathogenesis.** Retinal injury results from photochemical effects of solar radiation after directly or indirectly viewing the sun (eclipse retinopathy).
- **Presentation** is within a few hours of exposure with impairment of central vision and a small central scotoma.
- **Signs**
  - VA is variable according to severity.
  - A small yellow or red foveolar spot (Fig. 14.70A) that fades within a few weeks.
  - The spot evolves to a sharply defined foveolar defect with irregular borders (Fig. 14.70B), or a lamellar hole.
- **OCT** shows foveal thinning with a focal hyporeflective area, the depth of which correlates with the extent of visual acuity loss but which generally includes the photoreceptor inner and outer segments (see Fig. 14.56C for similar appearance).
- **Treatment** is not available.
- **Prognosis** is good in most cases with improvement of visual acuity to normal or near-normal levels within 6 months; in a minority, significantly reduced vision persists.

FOCAL CHOROIDAL EXCAVATION

Focal choroidal excavation (FCE) is a recently described relatively common condition in which one or more areas of macular choroidal excavation are detected in one or both eyes of a patient, typically middle-aged and possibly more commonly Eastern

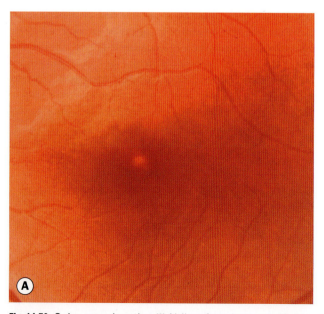

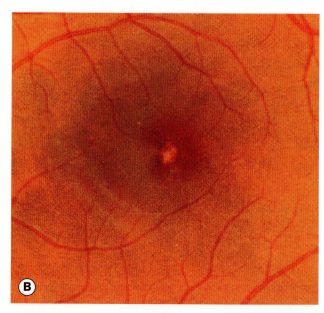

Fig. 14.70 Solar maculopathy. **(A)** Yellow foveolar spot; **(B)** foveolar defect

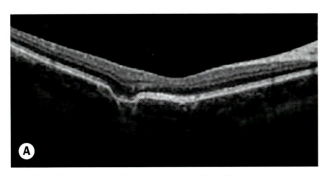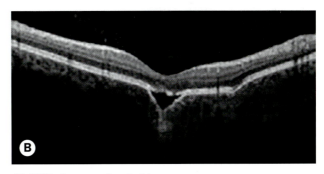

Fig. 14.71 Focal choroidal excavation. **(A)** OCT of conforming type; **(B)** OCT of nonconforming type
(Courtesy of J Chen and R Gupta, from Canadian Journal of Ophthalmology, *2012; 47: e56–8)*

Asian, without a history of ocular disease known to produce choroidal thinning. Vision is variably affected, and may be compromised by complications such as CNV, CSR and PCV. Overlying pigment epithelial disturbance or small yellowish-white deposits, sometimes vitelliform, are often seen clinically. On OCT, in 'conforming' FCE the overlying RPE and inner-segment/outer-segment junction follow the outwards indentation of the excavation (Fig. 14.71A); in contrast, in 'nonconforming' FCE the photoreceptor layers are disrupted and appear to be separated from the RPE (Fig. 14.71B).

Hereditary fundus dystrophies

INTRODUCTION

General

The hereditary fundus dystrophies are a group of disorders that commonly exert their major effect on the retinal pigment epithelium (RPE)–photoreceptor complex and the choriocapillaris to cause a range of visual impairment; the most common group of dystrophies is retinitis pigmentosa. Some dystrophies manifest in early childhood, others do not present until later in life. Isolated dystrophies have features confined to the eye, whilst syndromic dystrophies are part of a wider disease process that also affects tissues elsewhere in the body. Treatments such as gene therapy are being actively investigated, but are unlikely to be available imminently.

Anatomy

There are two types of retinal photoreceptor:
- **The rods** are the most numerous (120 million) and are of the densest concentration in the mid-peripheral retina. They are most sensitive in dim illumination and are responsible for night, motion sense and peripheral vision. If rod dysfunction occurs earlier or is more severe than cone dysfunction, it will result in poor night vision (nyctalopia) and peripheral field loss, the former usually occurring first.
- **The cones** are far fewer in number (6 million) and are concentrated at the fovea. They are most sensitive in bright light, and mediate day vision, colour vision, central and fine vision. Cone dysfunction therefore results in poor central vision, impairment of colour vision (dyschromatopsia) and occasionally problems with day vision (hemeralopia).

Inheritance

Most dystrophies are inherited, but sometimes a new mutation (allelic variant) can occur in an individual, and can subsequently be passed to future generations.
- **Autosomal dominant** (AD) dystrophies often exhibit variable expressivity, and tend to have a later onset and milder course than recessive disorders.
- **Recessive** dystrophies may be autosomal (AR) or X-linked (XLR). They generally have an earlier onset and a more severe course than AD conditions. In some cases female carriers of XLR conditions show characteristic fundus findings.
- **X-linked dominant** (XLD) conditions are very rare; they are typically lethal in boys (e.g. Aicardi syndrome).
- **Mitochondrial** DNA is inherited solely via the maternal line; retinal dystrophies associated with mitochondrial DNA variants are extremely rare and occur as part of a wider systemic disease. A maternal carrier will usually possess a mixture of mitochondria, only some of which contain the dysfunctional gene, and the presence and severity of a resultant dystrophy in offspring depends on the proportion of faulty mitochondria inherited.
- **Digenic** conditions are due to the combined effect of mutations in two different genes.

Classification

As well as division by inheritance pattern, dystrophies can be considered as generalized, in which the clinical effects involve the entire fundus (rod-cone or cone-rod, depending on which photoreceptor type is predominantly dysfunctional), or central (local, macular) in which only the macula is affected. They can also be classified according to the element that is the focus of the pathological process (e.g. photoreceptors, RPE or choroid), and by whether they are stationary (non-progressive) or progressive.

INVESTIGATION

Electroretinography

Introduction

The electroretinogram (ERG) measures retinal electrical activity; when stimulated by light of adequate intensity, ionic flow – principally sodium and potassium – is induced in or out of cells such that a potential is generated. The recording is made between an active electrode either in contact with the cornea or a skin electrode placed just below the lower eyelid margin, and a reference electrode on the forehead. The potential between the two electrodes is then amplified and displayed (Fig. 15.1). The normal ERG is predominantly biphasic (Fig. 15.2):
- **The a-wave** is an initial fast corneal-negative deflection generated by the photoreceptors.
- **The b-wave** is a subsequent slower positive large amplitude deflection. Although it is generated from Müller and bipolar cells, it is directly dependent on functional photoreceptors

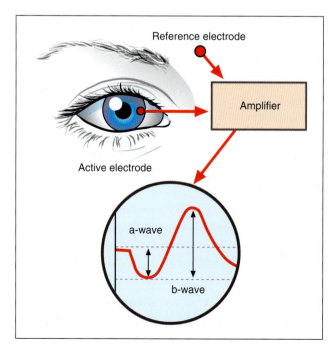

Fig. 15.1 Principles of electroretinography

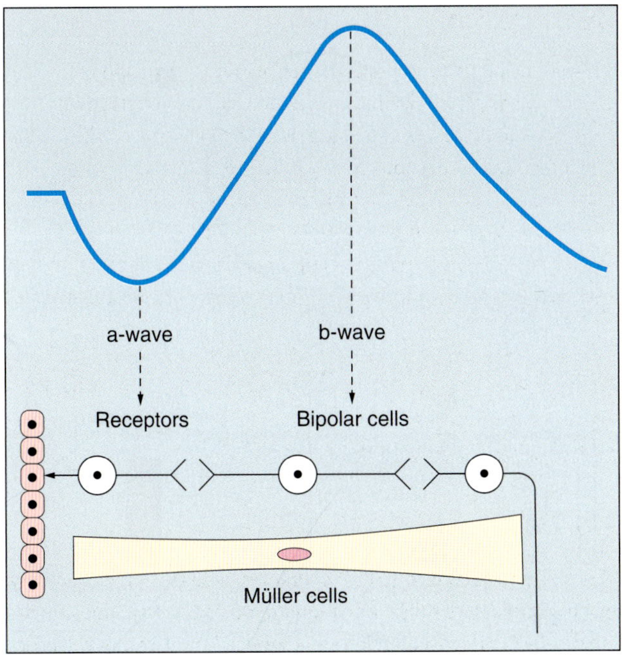

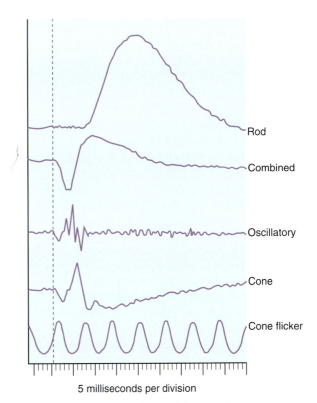

Fig. 15.2 Components and origins of the electroretinogram

and its magnitude makes it a convenient measure of photoreceptor integrity. Its amplitude is measured from the a-wave trough to the b-wave peak. It consists of b-1 and b-2 subcomponents; the former probably represents both rod and cone activity and the latter mainly cone activity, and it is possible to distinguish rod and cone responses with appropriate techniques. The b-wave is enhanced with dark adaptation and increased light stimulus.

- **The c-wave** is a third (negative) deflection generated by the RPE and photoreceptors.
- **Latency** is the interval to the commencement of the a-wave after the stimulus is applied.
- **Implicit time** is the interval from the stimulus to the b-wave peak.

Electroretinography is used for the diagnosis of a range of different retinal disorders on the basis of characteristic patterns of change, as well as monitoring of disease progress in dystrophies and other conditions such as some forms of uveitis (e.g. birdshot retinochoroidopathy) and drug toxicity (e.g. hydroxychloroquine).

Full-field ERG

A standard full-field ERG consists of five recordings (Fig. 15.3) taken during diffuse stimulation of the entire retinal area, and is used to assess generalized retinal disorders but may not detect localized pathology. The first three are elicited after 30 minutes of dark adaptation (scotopic), and the last two after 10 minutes of adaptation to moderately bright diffuse illumination (photopic). It may be difficult to dark-adapt children for 30 minutes and therefore dim light (mesopic) conditions can be utilized to evoke predominantly rod-mediated responses to low-intensity white or blue light stimuli.

- **Scotopic ERG**
  - Rod responses are elicited with a very dim flash of white or blue light, resulting in a large b-wave and a small or non-recordable a-wave.
  - Combined rod and cone responses are elicited with a very bright white flash, resulting in a prominent a-wave and b-wave.
  - Oscillatory potentials are elicited by using a bright flash and changing the recording parameters. The oscillatory wavelets occur on the ascending limb of the b-wave and are generated by cells in the inner retina.
- **Photopic ERG**
  - Cone responses are elicited with a single bright flash, resulting in an a- and a b-wave with subsequent small oscillations.
  - Cone flicker is used to isolate cones by using a flickering light stimulus at a frequency of 30 Hz to which rods cannot respond. It provides a measure of the amplitude and implicit time of the cone b-wave. Cone responses can be elicited in normal eyes up to 50 Hz, after which point individual responses are no longer recordable ('critical flicker fusion').

Multifocal ERG

Multifocal ERG is a method of producing topographical maps of retinal function (Fig. 15.4). The stimulus is scaled for variation in photoreceptor density across the retina. At the fovea, where the density of receptors is high, a lesser stimulus is employed than in the periphery where receptor density is lower. As with

Rod

Combined

Oscillatory

Cone

Cone flicker

5 milliseconds per division

Fig. 15.3 Normal electroretinographic recordings

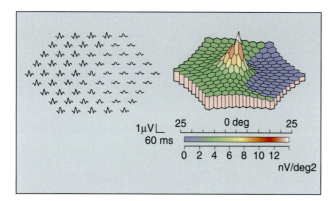

Fig. 15.4 Multifocal electroretinogram

conventional ERG, many types of measurements can be made. Both the amplitude and timing of the troughs and peaks can be measured and reported and the information can be summarized in the form of a three-dimensional plot which resembles the hill of vision. The technique can be used for almost any disorder that affects retinal function.

Focal ERG

Focal (foveal) ERG is used to assess macular disease.

Pattern ERG

A similar stimulus to that used in visual evoked potentials (see Ch. 19), pattern reversal, is used to target ganglion cell function, typically in order to detect subtle optic neuropathy.

Electro-oculography

The electro-oculogram (EOG) measures the standing potential between the electrically positive cornea and the electrically negative back of the eye (Fig. 15.5). It reflects the activity of the RPE and the photoreceptors. This means that an eye blinded by disease proximal to the photoreceptors will have a normal EOG. In general, diffuse or widespread disease of the RPE is needed to significantly affect the response. As there is much variation in EOG amplitude in normal subjects, the result is calculated by dividing the maximal height of the potential in the light ('light peak') by the minimal height of the potential in the dark ('dark trough'). This is expressed as a ratio (Arden ratio) or as a percentage. The normal value is greater than 1.85 or 185%.

Dark adaptometry

Dark adaptation (DA) is the phenomenon by which the visual system adapts to decreased illumination, and evaluation of this is particularly useful in the investigation of nyctalopia. The retina is exposed to an intense light for a time sufficient to bleach 25% or more of the rhodopsin in the retina. Following this, normal rods are insensitive to light and cones respond only to very bright stimuli. Subsequent recovery of light sensitivity can be monitored by placing the subject in the dark and periodically presenting spots of light of varying intensity in the visual field and asking the

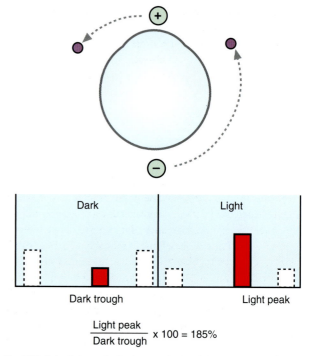

$$\frac{\text{Light peak}}{\text{Dark trough}} \times 100 = 185\%$$

Fig. 15.5 Principles of electro-oculography

subject if they are perceived. The threshold at which the subject just perceives a light is recorded, the flashes repeated at regular intervals and the increased sensitivity of the eye to light plotted: the sensitivity curve (Fig. 15.6).

- **The cone branch** of the curve represents the initial 5–10 minutes of darkness during which cone sensitivity rapidly improves. The rod photoreceptors are also recovering, but more slowly during this time.
- **The 'rod-cone' break** normally occurs after 7–10 minutes when cones achieve their maximum sensitivity, and the rods become perceptibly more sensitive than cones.
- **The rod branch** of the curve is slower and represents the continuation of improvement of rod sensitivity. After 15–30

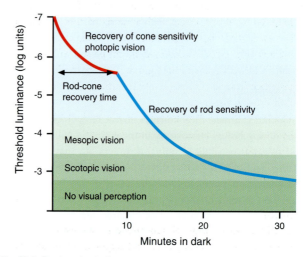

Fig. 15.6 Dark adaptation curve

minutes, the fully dark-adapted rods allow the subject to perceive a spot of light over 100 times dimmer than would be possible with cones alone. If the flashes are focused onto the foveola (where rods are absent), only a rapid segment corresponding to cone adaptation is recorded.

Colour vision testing

Introduction

Dyschromatopsia may develop in dystrophies prior to the impairment of other visual parameters; assessment of colour vision is also useful in the evaluation of optic nerve disease and in determining the presence of a congenitally anomalous colour defect. Colour vision depends on three populations of retinal cones, each with a specific peak sensitivity; blue (tritan) at 414–424 nm, green (deuteran) at 522–539 nm and red (protan) at 549–570 nm. Normal colour perception requires all these primary colours to match those within the spectrum. Any given cone pigment may be deficient (e.g. protanomaly – red weakness) or entirely absent (e.g. protanopia – red blindness). Trichromats possess all three types of cones (although not necessarily functioning perfectly), while absence of one or two types of cones renders an individual a dichromat or monochromat, respectively. Most individuals with congenital colour defects are anomalous trichromats and use abnormal proportions of the three primary colours to match those in the light spectrum. Those with red–green deficiency caused by abnormality of red-sensitive cones are protanomalous, those with abnormality of green-sensitive cones are deuteranomalous and those with blue–green deficiency caused by abnormality of blue-sensitive cones are tritanomalous. Acquired macular disease tends to produce blue–yellow defects, and optic nerve lesions red–green defects.

Colour vision tests

- **The Ishihara test** is designed to screen for congenital protan and deuteran defects, but is simple to use and widely available and so in practice is frequently used to screen for colour vision deficit of any type. It consists of a test plate followed by 16 plates, each with a matrix of dots arranged to show a central shape or number that the subject is asked to identify (Fig. 15.7A). A colour-deficient person will only be able to identify some of the figures. Inability to identify the test plate (provided visual acuity is sufficient) indicates non-organic visual loss.
- **The Hardy–Rand–Rittler test** is similar to the Ishihara, but can detect all three congenital colour defects (Fig. 15.7B).
- **The City University test** consists of 10 plates, each containing a central colour and four peripheral colours (Fig. 15.7C) from which the subject is asked to choose the closest match.
- **The Farnsworth–Munsell 100-hue test** is a sensitive but longer test for both congenital and acquired colour defects. Despite the name, it consists of 85 caps of different hues in

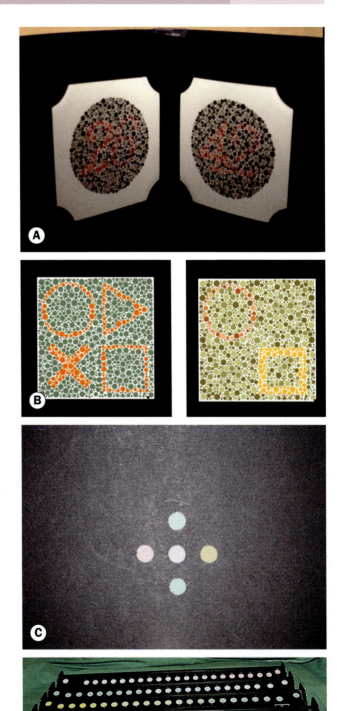

Fig. 15.7 Colour vision tests. **(A)** Ishihara; **(B)** Hardy–Rand–Rittler; **(C)** City University; **(D)** Farnsworth–Munsell 100-hue test

(Courtesy of T Waggoner – fig. B)

four racks (Fig. 15.7D); the subject is asked to rearrange randomized caps in order of colour progression, and the findings are recorded on a circular chart. Each of the three forms of dichromatism is characterized by failure in a specific meridian of the chart (Fig. 15.8).

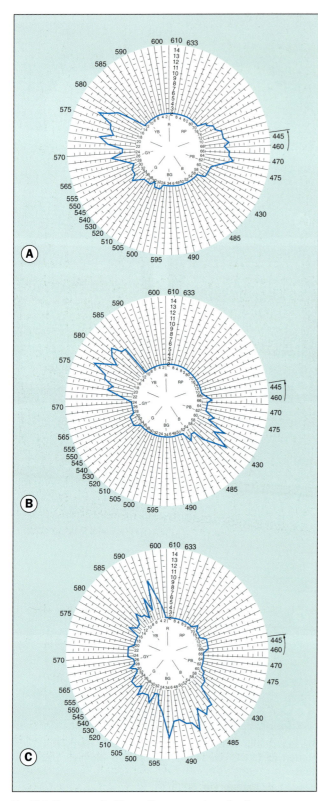

Fig. 15.8 Farnsworth–Munsell test results of colour deficiencies. **(A)** Protan; **(B)** deuteran; **(C)** tritan

GENERALIZED PHOTORECEPTOR DYSTROPHIES

Retinitis pigmentosa

Introduction

Retinitis pigmentosa (RP), or pigmentary retinal dystrophy, denotes a clinically and genetically diverse group of inherited diffuse retinal degenerative diseases initially predominantly affecting the rod photoreceptors, with later degeneration of cones (rod-cone dystrophy). It is the most common hereditary fundus dystrophy, with a prevalence of approximately 1:5000. The age of onset, rate of progression, eventual visual loss and associated ocular features are frequently related to the mode of inheritance; RP may occur as a sporadic (simplex) disorder, or be inherited in an AD, AR or XLR pattern. Many cases are due to allelic variation (mutation) of the rhodopsin gene. XLR is the least common but most severe form, and may result in complete blindness by the third or fourth decades, generally due to loss of function of a specific protein. AR disease can also be severe, and like XLR is commonly due to loss of function in a particular pathway. Sporadic cases may have a more favourable prognosis, with retention of central vision until the sixth decade or later. AD disease generally has the best prognosis. In 20–30% of cases, RP, often atypical (see below), is associated with a systemic disorder (syndromic RP); these conditions are usually of AR or mitochondrial inheritance. A similar clinical picture can be given by drug toxicity (see Ch. 20). Around 5% of RP belongs to the very early-onset severe type grouped together as Leber congenital amaurosis (see separate topic).

Diagnosis

The classic triad of findings comprises bone-spicule retinal pigmentation, arteriolar attenuation and 'waxy' disc pallor.

- **Symptoms.** Nyctalopia and dark adaptation difficulties are frequently presenting symptoms, but peripheral visual problems may be noticed; reduced central vision tends to be a later feature but can be involved earlier, including by complications such as cataract. Photopsia (flashing lights) is not uncommon. There may be a family history of RP, and a pedigree should be prepared.
- **Signs**
  - Visual acuity (VA) may be normal; contrast sensitivity is affected at an earlier stage than VA.
  - Bilateral mid-peripheral intraretinal perivascular 'bone-spicule' pigmentary changes and RPE atrophy associated with arteriolar narrowing (Figs 15.9A and B).
  - There is a gradual increase in density of the pigment with anterior and posterior spread, and a tessellated fundus appearance develops due to unmasking of large choroidal vessels (Fig. 15.9C).
  - Peripheral pigmentation may become severe, with marked arteriolar narrowing and disc pallor (Fig. 15.9D).

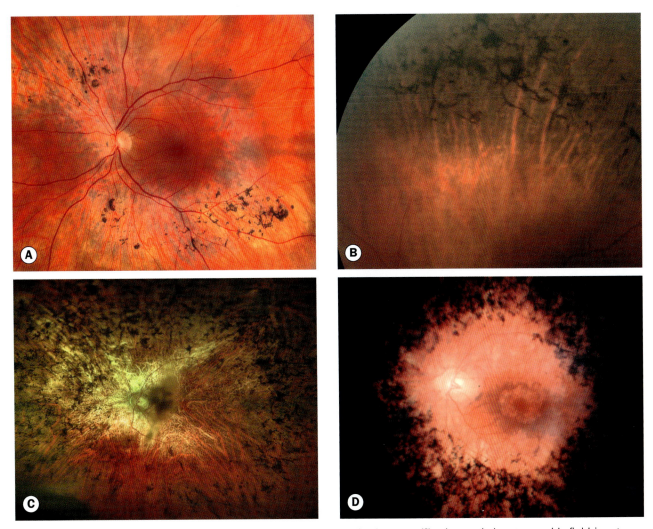

Fig. 15.9 Progression of retinitis pigmentosa. **(A)** and **(B)** relatively early changes; **(C)** advanced changes – wide-field image; **(D)** end-stage disease

(Courtesy of P Saine – fig. A; S Chen – figs B and C)

- The macula may show atrophy, epiretinal membrane (ERM) formation and cystoid macular oedema (CMO).
- Myopia is common.
- Optic disc drusen occur more frequently in patients with RP.
- Female carriers of the XLR form may have normal fundi or show a golden-metallic ('tapetal') reflex at the macula (Fig. 15.10A) and/or small peripheral patches of bone-spicule pigmentation (Fig. 15.10B).
- **Complications** include posterior subcapsular cataract (common in all forms of RP), open-angle glaucoma (3%), keratoconus (uncommon) and posterior vitreous detachment. Occasionally seen are intermediate uveitis and a Coats-like disease with lipid deposition in the peripheral retina and exudative retinal detachment.
- **Investigation**. Investigation for mimicking infectious conditions (e.g. syphilis) is sometimes warranted.
  - Full-field ERG is a sensitive diagnostic test. In early disease it shows reduced scotopic rod and combined

responses (Fig. 15.11); photopic responses reduce with progression, and eventually the ERG becomes extinguished. Multifocal ERG may provide more specific information.
  - EOG is subnormal, with absence of the light rise.
  - DA is prolonged; it may be useful in equivocal early cases.
  - Perimetry initially demonstrates small mid-peripheral scotomata that gradually coalesce, and may deteriorate to leave a tiny island of residual central vision (Fig. 15.12) that may subsequently be extinguished. Microperimetry (see Ch. 14), when available, is useful for central visual assessment.
  - Optical coherence tomography (OCT) will identify CMO.
  - Genetic analysis may identify the particular mutation responsible in an individual patient and facilitate genetic counseling, including the risk of transmission to offspring. It may also inform a decision on vitamin A supplementation.

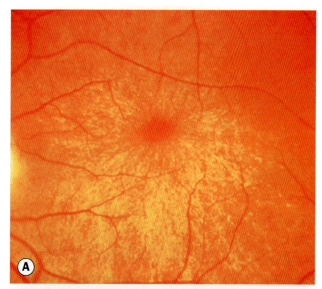

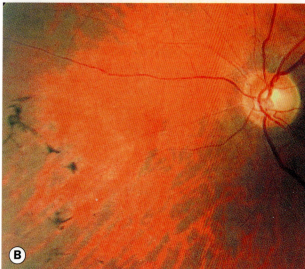

Fig. 15.10 Findings in carriers of X-linked retinitis pigmentosa. **(A)** 'Tapetal' reflex at the macula; **(B)** mild peripheral pigmentary changes

(Courtesy of D Taylor and CS Hoyt, from Pediatric Ophthalmology and Strabismus, Elsevier Saunders 2005 – fig. A)

Treatment

- Regular follow-up (e.g. annual) is essential to detect treatable vision-threatening complications, provide support and maintain contact in case of therapeutic innovation.
- No specific treatment is yet commercially available, but modalities such as gene therapy and retinal prostheses show promise for the future.
- Cataract surgery is generally beneficial.
- Low-vision aid provision, rehabilitation and social service access when appropriate.
- Smoking should be avoided.
- Sunglasses, 'nanometer-controlled' to block wavelengths up to about 550 nm, and with side-shielding, should be worn outdoors, and other light-protective strategies adopted.

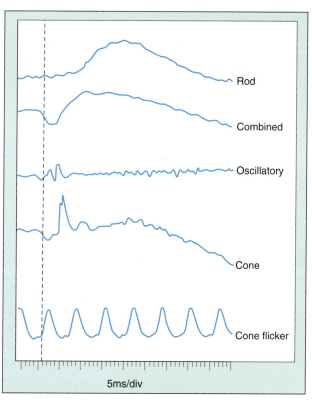

Fig. 15.11 ERG in early retinitis pigmentosa shows reduced scotopic rod and combined responses

Indoor amber spectacles blocking to 511–527 nm may improve contrast sensitivity and comfort.
- CMO in RP may respond to oral acetazolamide, and sometimes topical carbonic anhydrase inhibitors.
- High-dose vitamin A supplementation (e.g. palmitate 15 000 units per day) probably has a marginal benefit, but caution may be advisable in light of potential adverse effects, notably the increased risk of lung cancer flagged by the Age-Related Eye Disease Study (AREDS) in smokers taking beta-carotene (see Ch. 14), hepatotoxicity in susceptible subjects and worsening retinal function in some genetic subtypes of RP; it should be avoided in pregnancy or planned pregnancy. If supplementation is used, visual function should be carefully monitored during the early months of treatment, and regular vitamin A blood levels and liver function testing must be performed. Lutein, possibly with zeaxanthin, may be safer alternatives and the AREDS doses may be taken. Patients with mutations in gene *RHO1* may be more likely to benefit, but it should probably be avoided in patients with *ABCA4* mutations (see 'Stargardt disease'). Vitamin deficiencies should probably be addressed in all patients, though with caution, again particularly with *ABCA4* mutations.
- Several other drugs (e.g. calcium-channel blockers) have shown potential benefits but their efficacy and safety in RP have not been fully ascertained.
- Potentially (even mildly) retinotoxic medications should be avoided or used with caution. Candidates include erectile dysfunction drugs, isotretinoin and other retinoids,

Central 24-2 Threshold Test

Fixation Monitor: Gaze/Blind Spot   Stimulus: III, White   Pupil Diameter: 8.3 mm   Date: 05-03-2013

Fixation Target: Central   Background: 31.5 ASB   Visual Acuity: Time: 15:14

Fixation Losses: 0/14   Strategy: SITA-Fast   RX: +4.00 DS   DC X   Age:

False POS Errors: 0 %

False NEG Errors: N/A

Test Duration: 05:44

Fovea: OFF

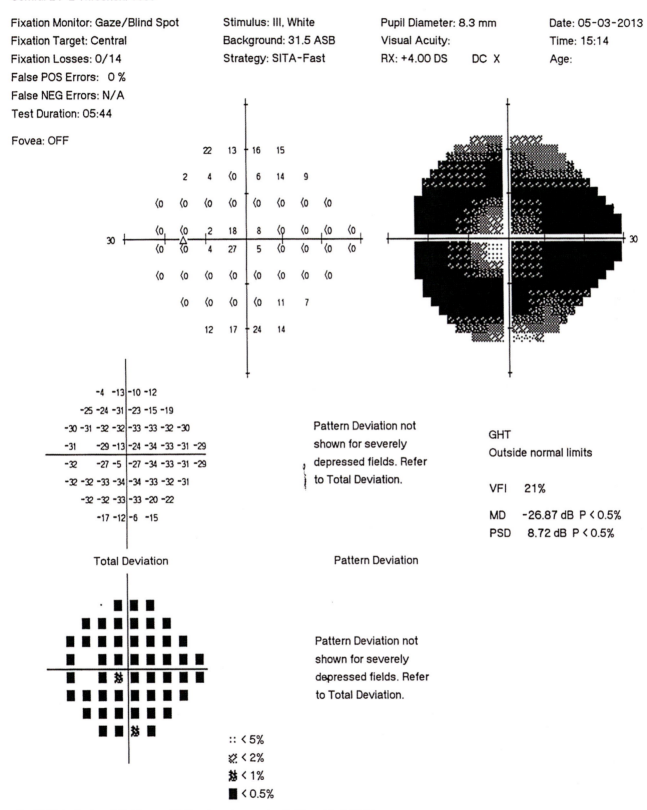

Pattern Deviation not shown for severely depressed fields. Refer to Total Deviation.

Total Deviation

Pattern Deviation

Pattern Deviation not shown for severely depressed fields. Refer to Total Deviation.

GHT
Outside normal limits

VFI   21%

MD   -26.87 dB P < 0.5%

PSD   8.72 dB P < 0.5%

:: < 5%

< 2%

< 1%

< 0.5%

Fig. 15.12 Left visual field constriction in advanced retinitis pigmentosa

(Courtesy of S Chen)

phenothiazines, hydroxychloroquine, tamoxifen and vigabatrin. Potentially neurotoxic drugs (see Ch. 20) should also be used with caution.

Atypical retinitis pigmentosa

Introduction

The term 'atypical RP' has conventionally been used to group together heterogeneous disorders clinically having features in common with typical pigmentary retinal dystrophy. The precise conditions included within this category vary between authors.

Atypical RP associated with a systemic disorder (syndromic RP)

- **Usher syndrome** (AR, genetically heterogeneous) accounts for about 5% of all cases of profound deafness in children, and about half of all cases of combined deafness and blindness. There are three major types, ranging from type I (75%), which features profound congenital sensorineural deafness and severe RP with an extinguished ERG in the first decade, to type III (2%), with progressive hearing loss, vestibular dysfunction and relatively late-onset pigmentary retinopathy. Systemic features are widely variable and can

include premature ageing, skeletal anomalies, mental handicap and early demise. There is often a 'salt and pepper' pattern of retinal pigmentation and optic atrophy.

- **Kearns–Sayre syndrome** (mitochondrial inheritance) is characterized by chronic progressive external ophthalmoplegia with ptosis (Fig. 15.13A) associated with other systemic problems, described in Ch. 19. The fundus usually has a salt and pepper appearance most striking at the macula; less frequent findings are typical RP or choroidal atrophy similar to choroideremia.
- **Bassen–Kornzweig syndrome** or abetalipoproteinaemia (AR) is a condition in which fat and fat-soluble vitamin (A, D, E, K) absorption is dysfunctional. There is a failure to thrive in infancy, with the development of severe spinocerebellar ataxia. A blood film shows 'thorny' red cells (acanthocytosis – Fig. 15.13B). The fundus exhibits scattered white dots followed by RP-like changes developing towards the end of the first decade; there may also be ptosis, ophthalmoplegia, strabismus and nystagmus. Vitamin supplementation and a low-fat diet are implemented.
- **Refsum disease** (AR) consists of genetically and clinically distinct infantile and adult forms. Phytanic acid accumulates throughout the body, with substantial and varied skin (Fig. 15.13C), neurological and visceral features. Retinal changes may be similar to RP or take on a salt and pepper

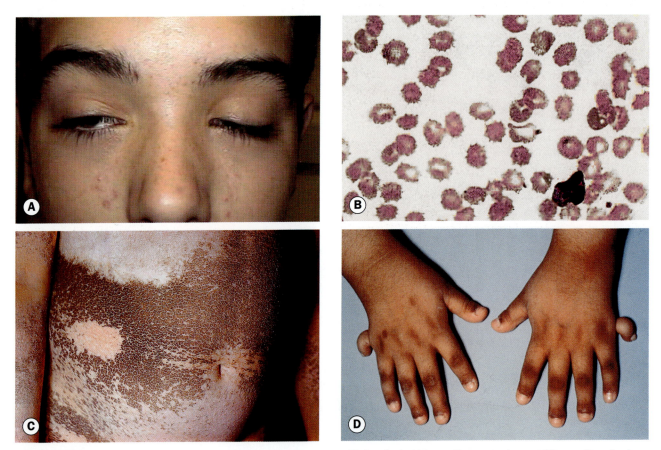

Fig. 15.13 Selected systemic associations of retinitis pigmentosa. **(A)** Ptosis in Kearns–Sayre syndrome; **(B)** acanthocytosis in Bassen–Kornzweig syndrome; **(C)** ichthyosis in adult Refsum disease; **(D)** polydactyly in Bardet–Biedl syndrome

appearance, and there may be other ocular features such as cataract and optic atrophy. A low phytanic acid diet can retard progression.

- **Bardet–Biedl syndrome** (genetically heterogeneous) can encompass a range of systemic abnormalities including polydactyly (Fig. 15.13D) and mental handicap. There is typically a bull's-eye maculopathy due to cone-rod dystrophy and less frequently typical RP, RP *sine pigmento* and retinitis punctata albescens. Almost 80% have severe changes by the age of 20 years.

Retinitis pigmentosa sine pigmento

RP *sine pigmento* is characterized by an absence or paucity of pigment accumulation (Fig. 15.14A), which may subsequently appear with time. Functional manifestations are similar to typical RP.

Retinitis punctata albescens

Retinitis punctata albescens (AR or AD) is characterized by scattered whitish-yellow spots, most numerous at the equator, usually sparing the macula, and associated with arteriolar attenuation (Fig. 15.14B). They are similar to the spots in fundus albipunctatus, and there is speculation and some genetic supporting evidence that the two clinical presentations are variants of the same disorder; the relative natural history of the two is yet to be completely defined. Nyctalopia and progressive field loss occur, in contrast to the benign prognosis believed to pertain in fundus albipunctatus, and the retinal findings may come to resemble those of retinitis pigmentosa.

Sector retinitis pigmentosa

Sector (sectoral) RP (AD) is characterized by involvement of inferior quadrants only (Fig. 15.14C). Progression is slow, and many cases are apparently stationary. Unilateral RP can also occur.

Leber congenital amaurosis

Leber congenital amaurosis (AR, genetically heterogeneous) is a severe rod-cone dystrophy that is the commonest genetically defined cause of visual impairment in children. The ERG is usually non-recordable even in early cases. Systemic associations include mental handicap, deafness, epilepsy, central nervous system and renal anomalies, skeletal malformations and endocrine dysfunction.

- **Presentation** is with blindness at birth or early infancy, associated with roving eye movements or nystagmus, and photoaversion.
- **Signs** are variable but may include:
  - Absent or diminished pupillary light reflexes.
  - The fundi may be normal in early life apart from mild arteriolar narrowing.
  - Initially mild peripheral pigmentary retinopathy (Fig. 15.15A), salt and pepper changes, and less frequently yellow flecks.
  - Severe macular pigmentation (Fig. 15.15B) or coloboma-like atrophy (Fig. 15.15C).

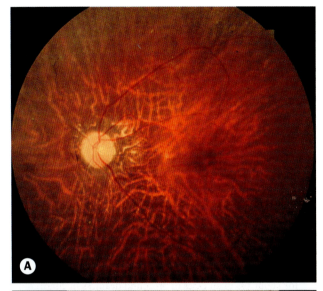

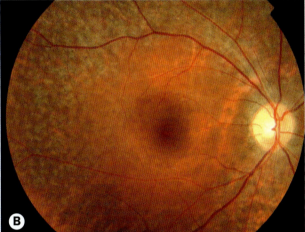

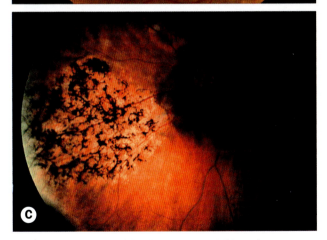

Fig. 15.14 Atypical retinitis pigmentosa. **(A)** *Sine pigmento*; **(B)** retinitis punctata albescens; **(C)** sectoral
(Courtesy of Moorfields Eye Hospital – fig. B)

  - Pigmentary retinopathy, optic atrophy and severe arteriolar narrowing in later childhood.
  - Oculodigital syndrome: constant rubbing of the eyes may cause orbital fat atrophy with enophthalmos (Fig. 15.15D), and subsequent keratoconus or keratoglobus.

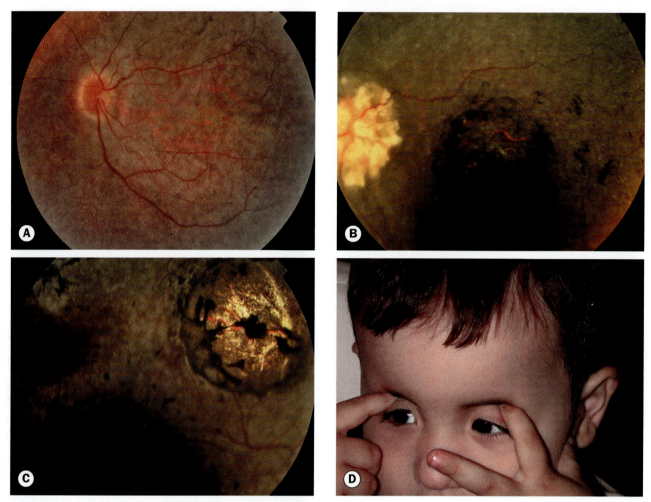

Fig. 15.15 Leber congenital amaurosis. **(A)** Mild pigmentary retinopathy; **(B)** macular pigmentation and optic disc drusen; **(C)** coloboma-like macular atrophy; **(D)** oculodigital syndrome
(Courtesy of A Moore – figs A–C; N Rogers – fig. D)

    ○ Other associations include strabismus, hypermetropia and cataract.
- **Treatment** should generally be as for retinitis pigmentosa; gene therapy offers some hope for the future.

Pigmented paravenous chorioretinal atrophy

Pigmented paravenous chorioretinal atrophy (predominantly AD) is usually asymptomatic and non-progressive. The ERG is normal. Paravenous bone-spicule pigmentation (Fig. 15.16) is seen, together with sharply outlined zones of chorioretinal atrophy that follow the course of the major retinal veins; changes may also encircle the optic disc. The optic disc and vascular calibre are usually normal.

Cone dystrophy

Introduction

Cone dystrophies are in most cases actually cone-rod dystrophies, with cones being affected earlier and more severely than the rods.

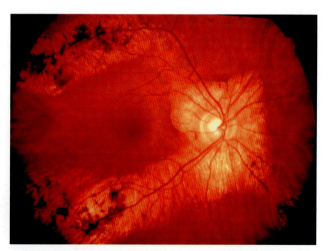

Fig. 15.16 Pigmented paravenous retinochoroidal atrophy
(Courtesy of C Barry)

They are much less common than rod-cone dystrophies. Most are sporadic, with some AD and XLR inheritance. Presentation is in early adulthood, with impairment of central vision rather than the nyctalopia of rod-cone dystrophy. The prognosis is commonly poor, with an eventual visual acuity of 6/60 or worse.

Diagnosis

- **Symptoms.** Gradual bilateral impairment of central and colour vision, which may be followed by photophobia.
- **Signs.** The features may evolve through the stages below.
  - The macula may be virtually normal or show non-specific central pigmentary changes (Fig. 15.17A) or atrophy.
  - A bull's-eye maculopathy (Figs 15.17B and C) is classically described but is not universal; causes of a bull's-eye appearance are given in Table 15.1.

Table 15.1 Other causes of bull's-eye macula

In adults
Chloroquine maculopathy
Advanced Stargardt disease
Cone and cone-rod dystrophy
Fenestrated sheen macular dystrophy
Benign concentric annular macular dystrophy
Clofazimine retinopathy

In children
Bardet–Biedl syndrome
Hallervorden–Spatz syndrome
Leber congenital amaurosis
Lipofuscinosis
Autosomal dominant cerebellar ataxia

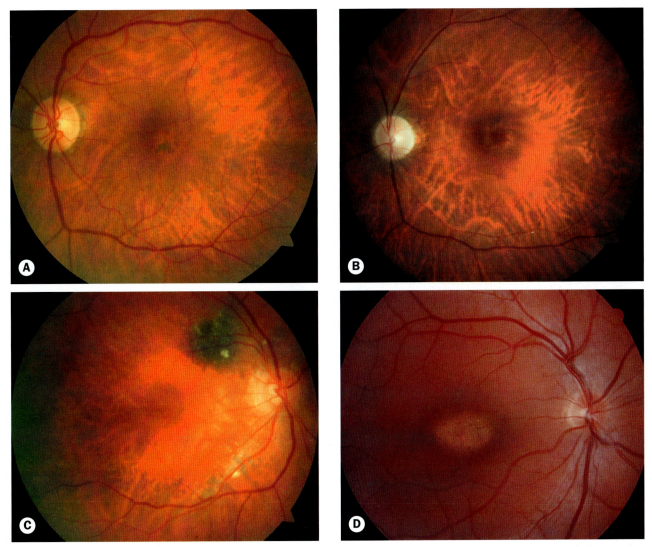

Fig. 15.17 Cone dystrophy. **(A)** Early pigment mottling; **(B)** and **(C)** bull's-eye macular appearances – a choroidal naevus is also present in (C); **(D)** central macular atrophy
(Courtesy of C Barry – fig. D)

○ Progressive RPE atrophy at the macula (Fig. 15.17D) with eventual geographic atrophy.

- **Investigation**
  ○ Fundus autofluorescence (FAF) is often the key diagnostic test, showing various annular patterns concentric with the fovea (Figs 15.18A–C).
  ○ ERG: photopic responses are subnormal or non-recordable and flicker fusion frequency is reduced, but rod responses are preserved until late (Fig. 15.18D).
  ○ EOG is normal to subnormal.
  ○ DA: the cone segment is abnormal; the rod segment is initially normal, but may become subnormal later.
  ○ Colour vision: severe deuteron–tritan defect out of proportion to visual acuity.
  ○ Fluorescein angiography (FA) shows a round hyperfluorescent window defect with a hypofluorescent centre (Fig. 15.18E).

Treatment

There is no specific treatment for cone dystrophies, but lutein, zeaxanthin and omega-3 fatty acids have been prescribed in some cases. General measures (e.g. minimizing phototoxicity) as for rod-cone dystrophies should be considered where applicable.

Stargardt disease/fundus flavimaculatus

Introduction

Stargardt disease (juvenile macular dystrophy) and fundus flavi-maculatus (FFM) are regarded as variants of the same disease, and together constitute the most common macular dystrophy. The condition is characterized by the accumulation of lipofuscin within the RPE. Three types are recognized: STGD1 (AR) is the most common, and is usually caused by mutation in the gene *ABCA4*; STGD3 (AD) and STGD4 (AD) are uncommon, and are related to different genes. Presentation is typically in childhood or adolescence, but sometimes later. The prognosis for the maculopathy is poor; once visual acuity drops below 6/12 it tends to worsen rapidly before stabilizing at about 6/60. Patients with flecks only in the early stages have a relatively good prognosis and may remain asymptomatic for many years until the development of macular disease.

Diagnosis

- **Symptoms.** Gradual impairment of central vision that may be out of proportion to examination findings; malingering may be suspected. There may also be complaints of reduced colour vision and impairment of dark adaptation.
- **Signs**
  ○ The macula may initially be normal or show non-specific mottling (Fig. 15.19A), progressing to an oval 'snail slime' (Fig. 15.19B) or 'beaten-bronze' appearance (Fig. 15.19C) and subsequently to geographic atrophy (Fig. 15.19D) that may

tend to a bull's-eye configuration (see Fig. 15.19C). A small proportion develop choroidal neovascularization (CNV).
  ○ Numerous yellow–white round, oval or pisciform (fish-shaped) lesions at the level of the RPE; these may be confined to the posterior pole (Fig. 15.19E) or extend to the mid-periphery.
  ○ New lesions develop as older ones become ill-defined and atrophic.

- **Investigation**
  ○ OCT will demonstrate flecks (Fig. 15.20A) and atrophy.
  ○ FAF shows a characteristic appearance with hyperautofluorescent flecks (Fig. 15.20B) and macular hypoautofluorescence (Fig. 15.20C), and may be key to the diagnosis in early cases.
  ○ Visual fields show central loss (Fig. 15.20D), and microperimetry can accurately document progression.
  ○ ERG: Photopic is normal to subnormal, scotopic may be normal.
  ○ EOG is commonly subnormal, especially in advanced cases.
  ○ FA: The classic feature is a 'dark choroid' due to masking of background choroidal fluorescence by diffuse RPE abnormality; the macula shows mixed hyper- and hypofluorescence (Fig. 15.20E). Fresh flecks show early hypofluorescence due to blockage, and late hyperfluorescence due to staining; old flecks show RPE window defects (Fig. 15.20F).
  ○ Indocyanine green angiography (ICGA) shows hypofluorescent spots, often more numerous than seen clinically.

Treatment

- General measures should be considered as for retinitis pigmentosa; protection from excessive high energy light exposure may be particularly important.
- Vitamin A supplementation is avoided as it may accelerate lipofuscin accumulation.
- Gene therapy and stem cell trials have been initiated and show promising results.

Bietti crystalline corneoretinal dystrophy

Bietti dystrophy (AR, *CYP4VZ* gene) is characterized by deposition of crystals in the retina and the superficial peripheral cornea. It is much more common in East Asians, particularly Chinese, than other ethnicities. The mechanism may be linked to an error in systemic lipid metabolism. The rate of progression is variable; specific treatment is not currently available.

- **Presentation.** Young adults with slowly progressive visual loss constitute the typical case.
- **Signs**
  ○ Superficial peripheral corneal crystals.
  ○ Numerous fine yellow–white crystals scattered throughout the posterior fundus (Fig. 15.21A) are followed by localized atrophy of the RPE and choriocapillaris at the macula.

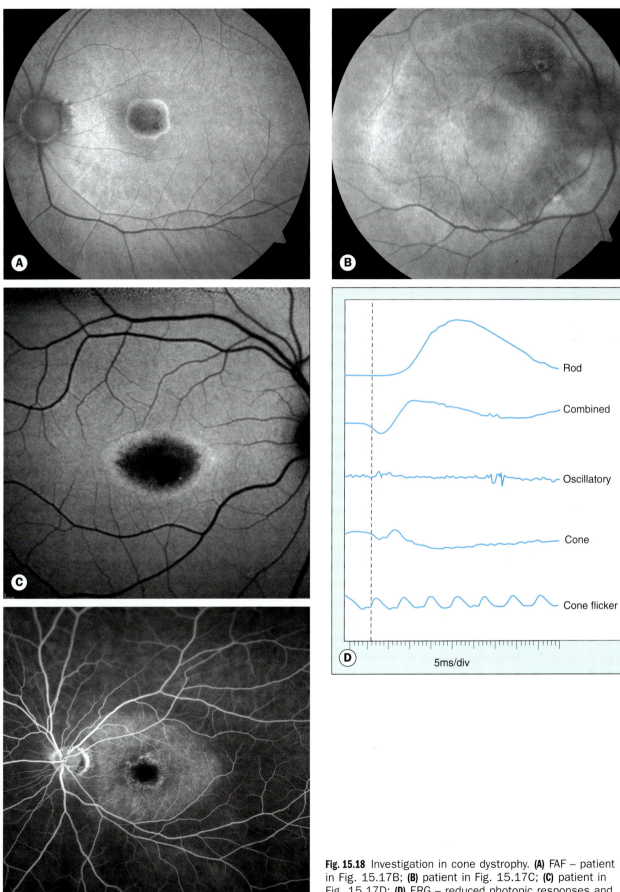

Fig. 15.18 Investigation in cone dystrophy. **(A)** FAF – patient in Fig. 15.17B; **(B)** patient in Fig. 15.17C; **(C)** patient in Fig. 15.17D; **(D)** ERG – reduced photopic responses and flicker fusion frequency; **(E)** wide-field fluorescein angiogram

(Courtesy of C Barry – fig. C; S Chen – fig. E)

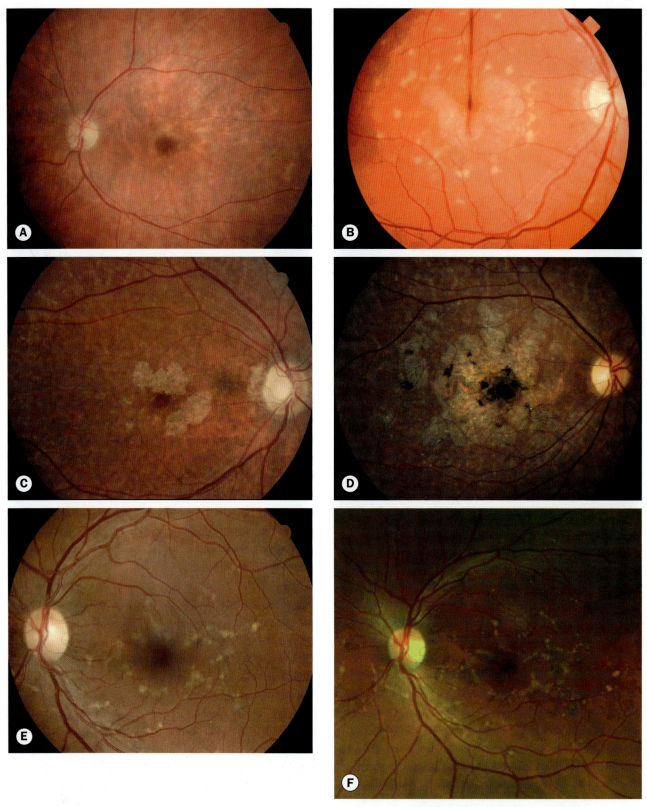

Fig. 15.19 Stargardt disease/fundus flavimaculatus. **(A)** Non-specific macular mottling; **(B)** 'snail slime' maculopathy surrounded by flecks; **(C)** quasi bull's-eye maculopathy surrounded by flecks – note the 'beaten-bronze' paramacular appearance; **(D)** geographic atrophy; **(E)** posterior pole flecks; **(F)** posterior pole flecks – wide-field image

(Courtesy of S Chen – figs A, C, D, E and F)

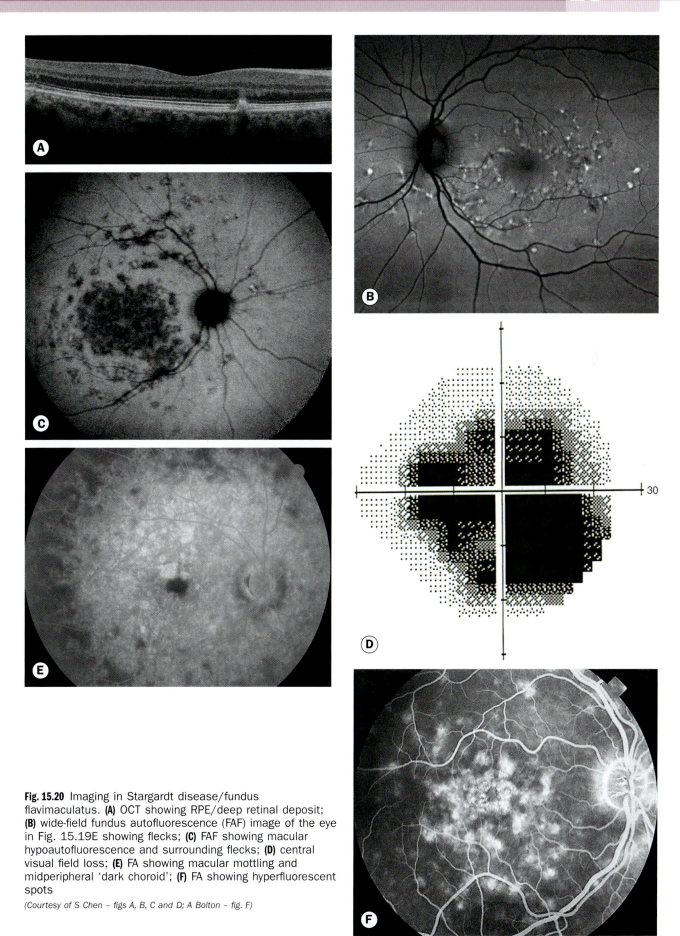

Fig. 15.20 Imaging in Stargardt disease/fundus flavimaculatus. **(A)** OCT showing RPE/deep retinal deposit; **(B)** wide-field fundus autofluorescence (FAF) image of the eye in Fig. 15.19E showing flecks; **(C)** FAF showing macular hypoautofluorescence and surrounding flecks; **(D)** central visual field loss; **(E)** FA showing macular mottling and midperipheral 'dark choroid'; **(F)** FA showing hyperfluorescent spots

(Courtesy of S Chen – figs A, B, C and D; A Bolton – fig. F)

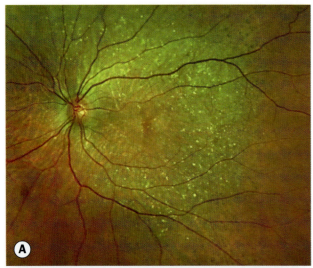

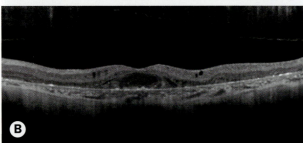

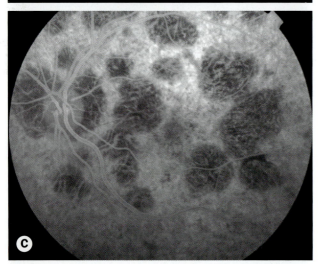

Fig. 15.21 Bietti corneoretinal crystalline dystrophy. **(A)** Wide-field image showing crystalline deposits; **(B)** OCT showing deposits and macular changes; **(C)** FA showing characteristic hypofluorescent patches

(Courtesy of C Barry – figs A and B)

  ○ Diffuse atrophy of the choriocapillaris subsequently develops, with a decrease in size and number of the crystals.
  ○ There is gradual confluence and expansion of the atrophic areas into the periphery, leading to diffuse chorioretinal atrophy in end-stage disease.

• **Investigation**
  ○ Visual fields show constriction.
  ○ OCT demonstrates the crystalline deposits and macular changes (Fig. 15.21B).
  ○ ERG is subnormal.
  ○ FA in moderate disease shows characteristic large hypofluorescent patches corresponding to choriocapillaris loss, with intact overlying retinal vessels (Fig. 15.21C); the patches become confluent over time.

Alport syndrome

Alport syndrome (predominantly XLR) is caused by mutations in several different genes, all of which encode particular forms of type IV collagen, a major basement membrane component. It is characterized by chronic renal failure, often associated with sensorineural deafness. There are scattered yellowish punctate flecks in the perimacular area (Fig. 15.22A), which are often subtle (Fig. 15.22B) and larger peripheral flecks, some of which may become confluent (Fig. 15.22C). The ERG is normal, and the prognosis for vision is excellent. Anterior lenticonus and posterior polymorphous corneal dystrophy may occasionally be seen.

Familial benign fleck retina

Familial benign fleck retina (benign flecked retina syndrome) is a very rare AR disorder. It is asymptomatic, so usually discovered by chance. Numerous diffusely distributed yellow–white polymorphous lesions spare the fovea and extend to the far periphery (Fig. 15.23). The flecks autofluoresce, and are probably composed of lipofuscin. The ERG is normal, and the prognosis excellent.

Congenital stationary night blindness

Introduction

Congenital stationary night blindness (CSNB) refers to a group of disorders characterized by infantile-onset nyctalopia but nonprogressive retinal dysfunction. The fundus appearance may be normal or abnormal.

With a normal fundus appearance

CSNB with a normal fundus appearance is sometimes classified into type 1 (complete) and type 2 (incomplete) forms that are generally due to mutations in different genes. The former is characterized by a complete absence of rod pathway function and essentially normal cone function clinically and on ERG, the latter by impairment of both rod and cone function. Mutations in numerous genes have been implicated, with XLR, AD and AR inheritance patterns; the AD form is usually associated with normal visual acuity, but many AR and XLR patients have poor vision with nystagmus, and often significant myopia.

With an abnormal fundus appearance

• **Oguchi disease** (AR). The fundus has an unusual golden-yellow colour in the light-adapted state (Fig. 15.24A), which

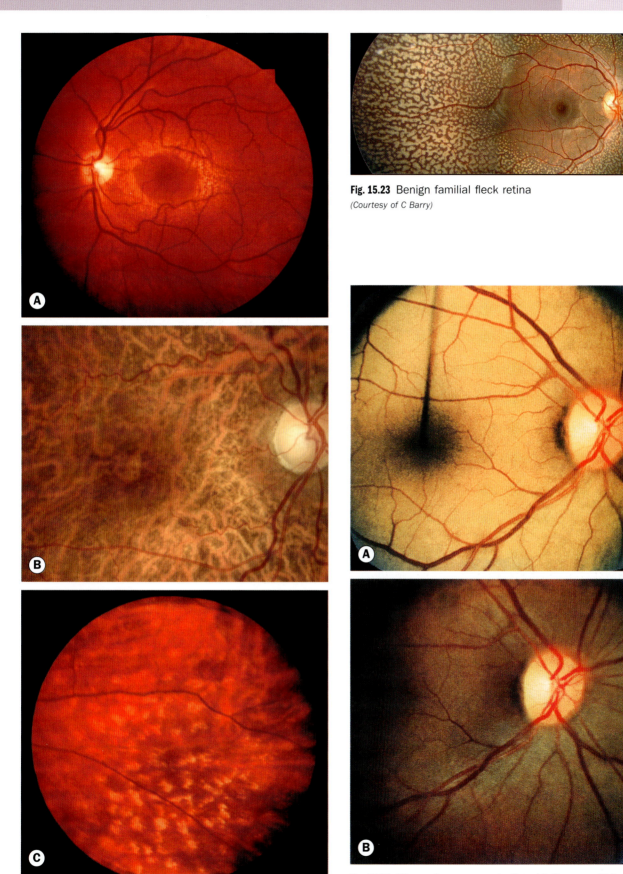

Fig. 15.23 Benign familial fleck retina

(Courtesy of C Barry)

Fig. 15.22 Alport syndrome. **(A)** Perimacular flecks; **(B)** subtle flecks; **(C)** peripheral flecks

(Courtesy of J Govan – figs A and C)

Fig. 15.24 Mizuo phenomenon in Oguchi disease. **(A)** In the light-adapted state; **(B)** in the dark-adapted state

(Courtesy of J Donald M Gass, from Stereoscopic Atlas of Macular Diseases, *Mosby 1997)*

becomes normal after prolonged dark adaptation (Mizuo or Mizuo–Nakamura phenomenon – Fig 15.24B). Rod function is absent after 30 minutes of dark adaptation but recovers to a near-normal level after a long period of dark adaptation.

- **Fundus albipunctatus** is an AR or AD condition that may be the same entity as retinitis punctata albescens (see earlier); they can both be caused by mutation in the *RLBP1* gene. The fundus shows a multitude of subtle, tiny yellow–white spots at the posterior pole (Fig. 15.25A), sparing the fovea – sometimes the macula – and extending to the periphery. In contrast to retinitis punctata albescens, the retinal blood vessels, optic disc, peripheral fields and visual acuity are believed to remain normal, though the natural history is not yet absolutely defined. Fluorescein angiography

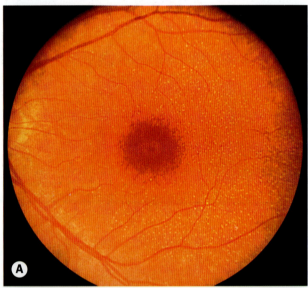

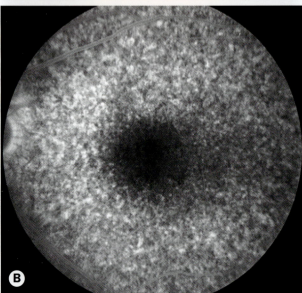

Fig. 15.25 Fundus albipunctatus. **(A)** Clinical appearance; **(B)** FA shows mottled hyperfluorescence
(Courtesy of C Barry)

shows mottled hyperfluorescence, indicating depigmentation of the RPE (Fig. 15.25B). The ERG is variably abnormal; both cones and rods may be affected.

Congenital monochromatism (achromatopsia)

This is a group of congenital disorders in which colours cannot be perceived and visual acuity is reduced, particularly in brightly illuminated environments (hemeralopia).

Rod monochromatism (complete achromatopsia)

In rod monochromatism (AR) visual acuity is poor, typically 6/60; there is congenital nystagmus and photophobia. Colour vision is totally absent, all colours appearing as shades of grey. The macula usually appears normal but may be hypoplastic. The photopic (cone) ERG is abnormal and the scotopic may also be subnormal.

Blue cone monochromatism (incomplete achromatopsia)

Blue cone monochromatism (XLR) features only slightly subnormal acuity at 6/6–6/9, but colour vision is completely absent. Nystagmus and photophobia are not typical features. There is a normal macula.

The ERG is normal except for the absence of cone responses to red and white light.

MACULAR DYSTROPHIES

Best vitelliform macular dystrophy

Introduction

Best vitelliform macular dystrophy (early- or juvenile-onset vitelliform macular dystrophy) is the second most common macular dystrophy, after Stargardt disease. It is due to allelic variation in the *BEST1* gene. Inheritance is AD with variable penetrance and expressivity. The prognosis is usually reasonably good until middle age, after which visual acuity declines in one or both eyes due to CNV, scarring or geographic atrophy.

Diagnosis

- **Signs.** There is gradual evolution through the following stages:
  - Pre-vitelliform is characterized by a subnormal EOG in an asymptomatic infant or child with a normal fundus.
  - Vitelliform develops in infancy or early childhood and does not usually impair vision. A round, sharply delineated ('sunny side up egg yolk') macular lesion between half a disc and two disc diameters in size develops within the RPE (Fig. 15.26A); the size of the

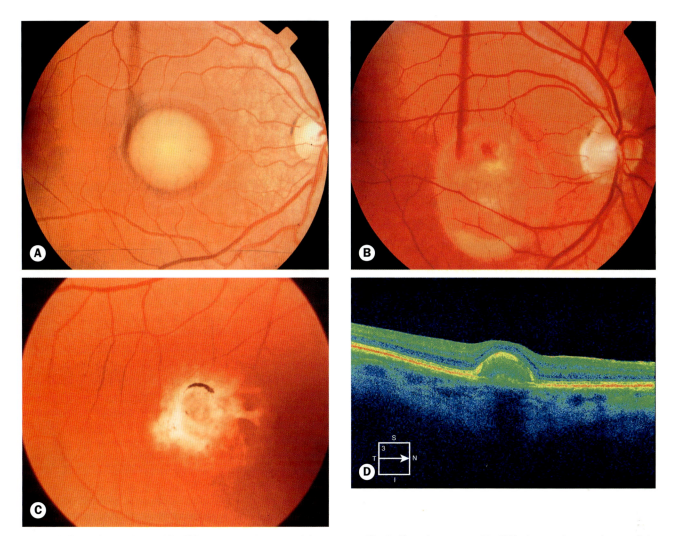

Fig. 15.26 Best dystrophy. **(A)** Vitelliform stage; **(B)** pseudohypopyon; **(C)** vitelliruptive stage; **(D)** OCT shows abnormal material within and anterior to the RPE

(Courtesy of S Chen – fig. D)

lesions and stage of development in the two eyes may be asymmetrical, and sometimes only one eye is involved initially. Occasionally the condition may be extramacular and multiple.

○ Pseudohypopyon may occur when part of the lesion regresses (Fig. 15.26B), often at puberty.

○ Vitelliruptive: the lesion breaks up and visual acuity drops (Fig. 15.26C).

○ Atrophic in which all pigment has disappeared leaving an atrophic area of RPE.

• **Investigation**

○ FAF: the yellowish material is intensely hyperautofluorescent (see Fig. 15.28C); hypoautofluorescent areas supervene in the later atrophic stages.

○ OCT shows material beneath, above and within the RPE (Fig. 15.26D).

○ FA shows corresponding hypofluorescence due to masking.

○ EOG is severely subnormal during all stages (Arden index less than 1.5), and is also abnormal in carriers with clinically normal fundi.

Multifocal vitelliform lesions without Best disease

Occasionally multifocal vitelliform lesions (Fig. 15.27), identical to those in Best dystrophy but distributed around the macular vascular arcades and optic disc, may become manifest in adult life and give rise to diagnostic problems. However, in these patients the EOG is normal and the family history is negative. Occasionally genetically confirmed Best dystrophy may present with multifocal lesions. The relationship between multifocal vitelliform lesions, juvenile vitelliform (Best) dystrophy and adult-onset vitelliform macular dystrophy is incompletely defined, though some cases of each are associated with mutations in the same genes.

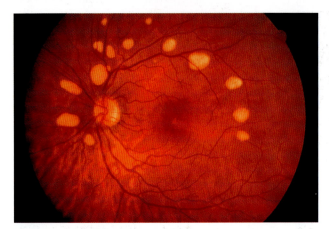

Fig. 15.27 Multifocal vitelliform lesions without Best disease
(Courtesy of C Barry)

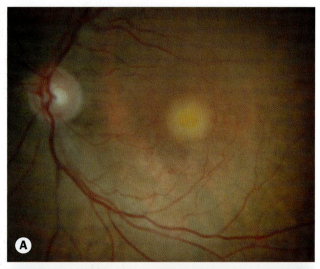

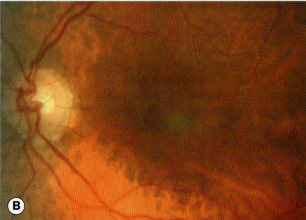

Adult-onset vitelliform macular dystrophy

Adult-onset vitelliform macular (foveomacular) dystrophy (AOVMD) is sometimes classified with juvenile-onset vitelliform macular dystrophy, but they are generally considered distinct entities; AOVMD may be a form of pattern dystrophy of the RPE (see next), and at least one family has been described with a combination of AOVMD and other pattern dystrophies. In contrast to juvenile Best disease, the foveal lesions are typically smaller, present later and generally do not evolve in a similar fashion. A minority of cases are caused by mutation in the *PRPH2* (*RDS*) or the *BEST1* gene.

- **Symptoms.** Often the condition is discovered by chance, but may present in late middle or old age with decreased central vision. The prognosis is very variable, though often the vision is reduced by one or more lines by presentation and mild deterioration occurs subsequently.
- **Signs.** A round or oval slightly elevated yellowish subfoveal deposit (Fig. 15.28A), generally smaller than the lesions of Best disease, is seen in one or both eyes. There may be central pigmentation, and numerous associated drusen are present in some cases. The material may persist, absorb, or break up and disperse at a late stage, leaving atrophy of very variable severity; choroidal neovascularization sometimes supervenes.
- **Investigation**
  - OCT shows hyper-reflective material associated with the RPE, similar to Best disease (see Fig. 15.26D).
  - FAF imaging shows intense hyperautofluorescence corresponding to the deposited material, which is typically much more obvious than on clinical examination (Fig. 15.28B and C); if atrophy supervenes, there is hypoautofluorescence.
  - FA shows central hypofluorescence surrounded by a small irregular hyperfluorescent ring.

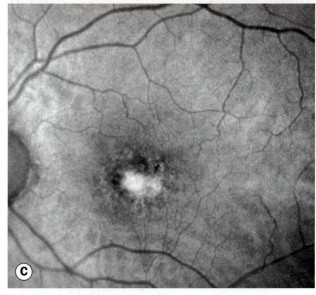

Fig. 15.28 (A) Adult-onset macular vitelliform dystrophy; **(B)** smaller lesion; **(C)** fundus autofluorescence image of the eye in (B) – the lesion is much more obvious

Pattern dystrophy of the retinal pigment epithelium

Pattern (patterned) dystrophy of the RPE encompasses several clinical appearances associated with the accumulation of lipofuscin at the level of the RPE and manifesting with yellow, whitish, grey or pigmented deposits at the macula in a variety of morphologies. All the described entities tend to have characteristics in common including typically AD (occasionally AR) inheritance, a slow course leading to mild to moderate foveal atrophy, and a normal ERG but occasionally an abnormal EOG. Symptoms often begin in early adulthood or later. The different clinical pictures are believed in many cases to represent variable expression of a single disorder, particularly as different forms of pattern dystrophy can affect siblings with the same mutation and even the two eyes in the same patient. Notably, a pattern dystrophy-like appearance can occur in response to a range of pathogenic stimuli.

- **Butterfly-shaped:** foveal yellow and melanin pigmentation, commonly in a spoke-like or butterfly wing-like conformation (Fig. 15.29A); drusen- or Stargardt-like flecks may be associated with any pattern dystrophy (Fig. 15.29B). FA shows central and radiating hypofluorescence with surrounding hyperfluorescence (Fig. 15.29C). More than one gene has been implicated.
- **Reticular (Sjögren):** a network of pigmented lines at the posterior pole.
- **Multifocal pattern dystrophy simulating fundus flavimaculatus:** multiple, widely scattered, irregular yellow lesions; they may be similar to those seen in fundus flavimaculatus (Fig. 15.30A). FA shows hyperfluorescence of the flecks; the choroid is not dark (Fig. 15.30B).
- **Macroreticular (spider-shaped):** initially pigment granules are seen at the fovea; reticular pigmentation develops that spreads to the periphery (Fig. 15.31).
- **Adult-onset vitelliform** – see above.
- **Fundus pulverulentus** is extremely rare. Macular pigment mottling develops.

North Carolina macular dystrophy

North Carolina macular dystrophy is a rare non-progressive condition. It was first described in families living in the mountains of North Carolina and subsequently in many unrelated families in other parts of the world. Inheritance is AD with complete penetrance but highly variable expressivity.

- **Grade 1** is characterized by yellow–white, drusen-like peripheral (Fig. 15.32A) and macular deposits that develop during the first decade but may remain asymptomatic throughout life.
- **Grade 2** is characterized by deep, confluent macular deposits (Fig. 15.32B). The long-term visual prognosis is guarded because some patients develop neovascular maculopathy (Fig. 15.32C) and subretinal scarring.
- **Grade 3** is characterized by coloboma-like atrophic macular lesions (Fig. 15.32D) associated with variable impairment of visual acuity.

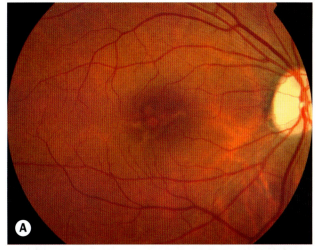

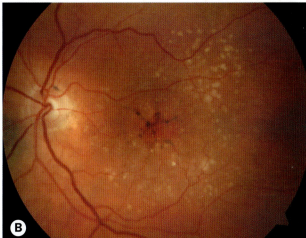

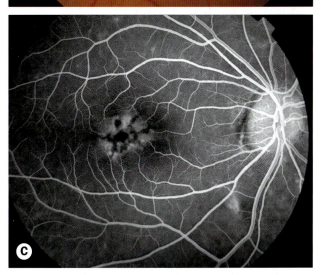

Fig. 15.29 Butterfly-shaped pattern dystrophy of the RPE. **(A)** Spokes of yellowish material and pigment radiating from the foveola; **(B)** associated with flecks; **(C)** FA of the eye in (A) showing central and spoke-like radiating hypofluorescence with surrounding hyperfluorescence *(Courtesy of Moorfields Eye Hospital – figs A and C)*

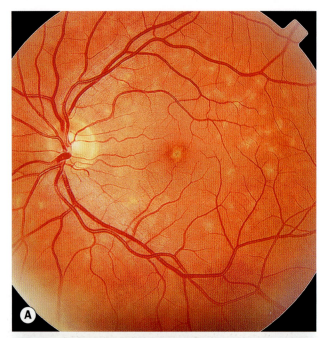

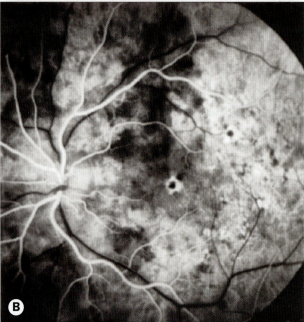

Fig. 15.30 (A) Multifocal pattern dystrophy simulating fundus flavimaculatus; **(B)** FA shows hyperfluorescence but the choroid is not dark
(Courtesy of S Milewski)

Familial dominant drusen

Familial dominant drusen (Doyne honeycomb choroiditis, malattia leventinese) is thought to represent an early-onset variant of age-related macular degeneration. Inheritance is AD with variable expressivity; mutations in the gene *EFEMP1* are responsible. Asymptomatic yellow–white, elongated, radially orientated drusen develop in the second decade; they may involve the disc margin and extend nasal to the disc (Fig. 15.33A). With age the lesions become increasingly dense and acquire a honeycomb pattern

(Fig. 15.33B). Visual symptoms may occur in the fourth to fifth decades due to RPE degeneration, geographic atrophy or occasionally CNV. The ERG is normal, but the EOG is subnormal in patients with advanced disease.

Sorsby pseudoinflammatory dystrophy

Sorsby pseudoinflammatory (hereditary haemorrhagic) macular dystrophy is a rare disorder that results in bilateral visual loss, typically in late middle age. Inheritance is AD with full penetrance but variable expressivity; allelic variation in the gene *TIMP3* is responsible. Early presentation may be in the third decade with nyctalopia, when confluent yellow–white drusen-like deposits may be seen along the arcades, nasal to the disc and in the mid-periphery (Fig. 15.34A), or in the fifth decade with sudden visual loss due to exudative maculopathy secondary to CNV (Fig. 15.34B) and subretinal scarring (Fig. 15.34C). Peripheral chorioretinal atrophy may occur by the seventh decade and result in loss of ambulatory vision. The ERG is initially normal but may be subnormal in later disease.

Concentric annular macular dystrophy

The prognosis is good in the majority of cases of (benign) concentric annular macular dystrophy, an AD disorder, although a minority develop progressive loss of acuity and nyctalopia. Presentation is in adult life with mild impairment of central vision; bull's-eye maculopathy is associated with slight vascular attenuation but a normal disc. A paracentral ring scotoma is present on visual field testing. FA shows an annular RPE window defect.

Central areolar choroidal dystrophy

Central areolar choroidal dystrophy, also termed central choroidal sclerosis, is a genetically heterogeneous (types 1–3 are described) but typically AD condition presenting in the third or fourth

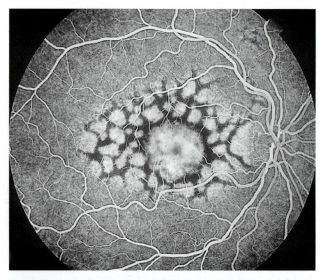

Fig. 15.31 FA of macroreticular pattern dystrophy
(Courtesy of RF Spaide, from Diseases of the Retina and Vitreous, WB Saunders 1999)

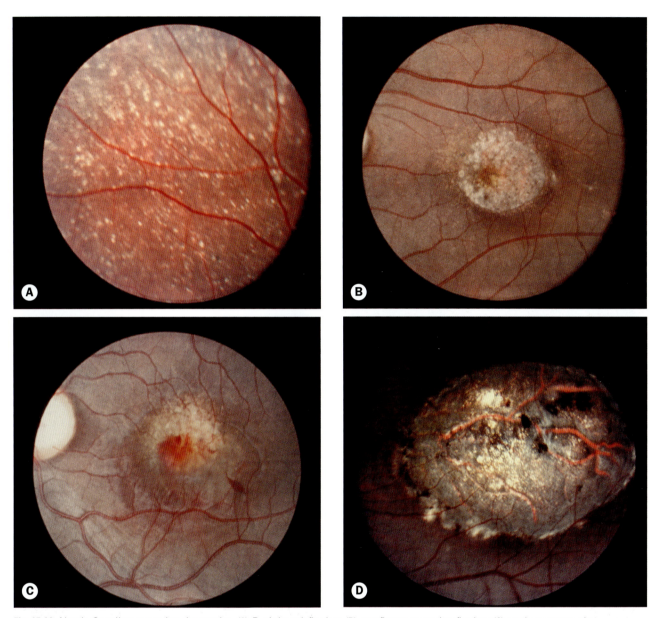

Fig. 15.32 North Carolina macular dystrophy. **(A)** Peripheral flecks; **(B)** confluent macular flecks; **(C)** early neovascular maculopathy; **(D)** coloboma-like macular lesion

(Courtesy of P Morse)

decades with gradual impairment of central vision. Non-specific foveal granularity progresses to well-circumscribed RPE atrophy and loss of the choriocapillaris (Fig. 15.35A), and subsequently slowly expanding geographic atrophy with prominence of large choroidal vessels (Figs 15.35B and C). The prognosis is poor.

Dominant cystoid macular oedema

Bilateral cystoid macular oedema (AD) commonly presents in adolescence with gradual impairment of central vision; treatment tends to be ineffective and geographic atrophy inevitably ensues.

Sjögren–Larsson syndrome

Sjögren–Larsson syndrome (AR) is a neurocutaneous disorder secondary to defective enzyme (fatty aldehyde dehydrogenase) activity, and is characterized by congenital ichthyosis and neurological problems. Presentation is with photophobia and poor vision, and glistening yellow–white crystalline deposits develop at the macula (Fig. 15.36), appearing during the first two years of life. Visual evoked potential testing is abnormal. Pigmentary retinopathy (50%), cataract and colobomatous microphthalmos may also occur.

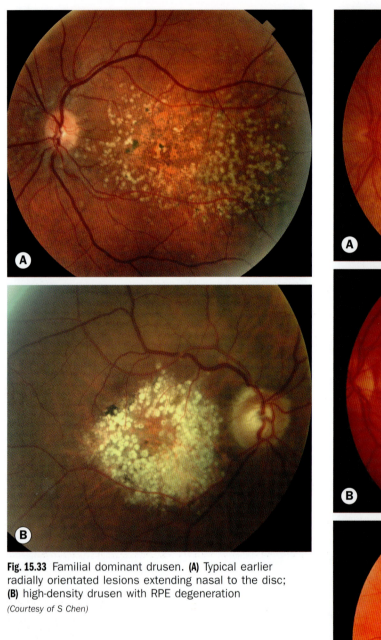

Fig. 15.33 Familial dominant drusen. **(A)** Typical earlier radially orientated lesions extending nasal to the disc; **(B)** high-density drusen with RPE degeneration
(Courtesy of S Chen)

Familial internal limiting membrane dystrophy

Presentation of this AD condition may be in middle age with reduced central vision; a glistening inner retinal surface is evident at the posterior pole (Fig. 15.37). The prognosis is poor.

Maternally inherited diabetes and deafness

Maternally inherited diabetes and deafness (MIDD) constitutes around 1% of all cases of diabetes, with inheritance via mitochondrial DNA. A majority of patients develop progressive dystrophic macular changes (Fig. 15.38), but vision is not usually affected. Some patients have other ocular features, such as pigmentary retinopathy and ptosis.

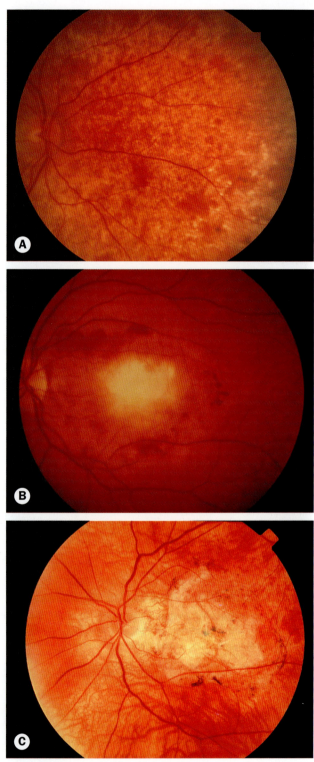

Fig. 15.34 Sorsby pseudoinflammatory macular dystrophy. **(A)** Confluent flecks nasal to the disc; **(B)** exudative maculopathy; **(C)** scarring in end-stage disease
(Courtesy of Moorfields Eye Hospital – fig. B)

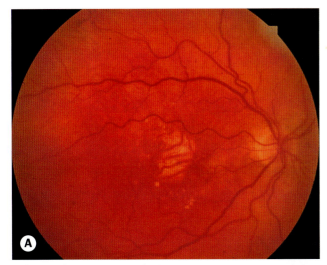

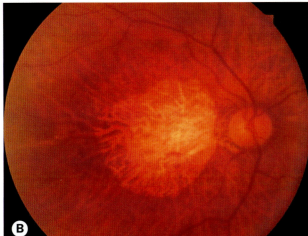

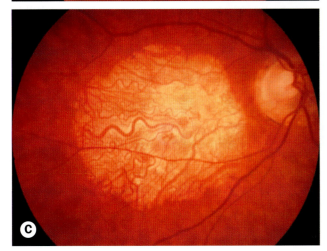

Fig. 15.35 Progression of central areolar choroidal dystrophy.
(A) Early; **(B)** intermediate; **(C)** end-stage

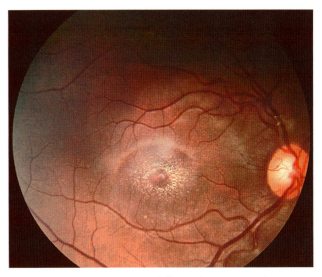

Fig. 15.36 Macular crystals in Sjögren–Larsson syndrome
(Courtesy of D Taylor and C S Hoyt, from Pediatric Ophthalmology and
Strabismus, *Elsevier Saunders 2005)*

GENERALIZED CHOROIDAL DYSTROPHIES

Choroideremia

Choroideremia (tapetochoroidal dystrophy) is a progressive
diffuse degeneration of the choroid, RPE and photoreceptors.
Inheritance is XLR, so that males are predominantly affected.
However, it is important to identify female carriers as 50% of their
sons will develop choroideremia and 50% of their daughters will
be carriers. The prognosis is very poor; although most patients
retain useful vision until the sixth decade, very severe visual loss

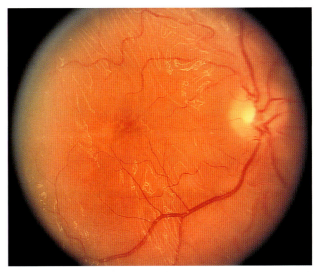

Fig. 15.37 Familial internal limiting membrane dystrophy
(Courtesy of J Donald M Gass, from Stereoscopic Atlas of Macular Diseases,
Mosby 1997)

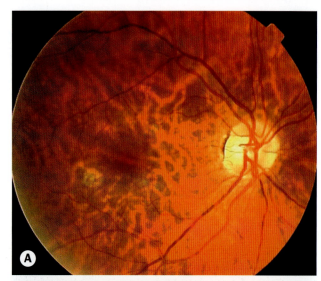

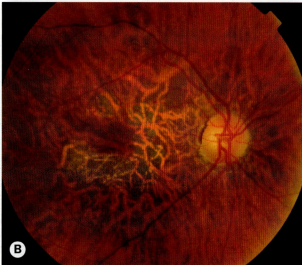

Fig. 15.38 Macular changes in maternally inherited diabetes and deafness. **(A)** Initial appearance; **(B)** 6 years later
(Courtesy of S Chen)

occurs thereafter. The gene responsible is *CHM*; a contiguous extended gene deletion leads to associated deafness and mental handicap.

- **Symptoms.** Nyctalopia, often beginning in adolescence, is followed some years later by reduced peripheral and central vision; clinically problematic disease occurs almost exclusively in males, but if present in females a number of genetic mechanisms can be responsible.
- **Signs**
  ○ Female carriers show mild, patchy peripheral RPE atrophy and mottling (Fig. 15.39A); acuity, fields and ERG are usually normal.
  ○ Males initially exhibit mid-peripheral RPE abnormalities that may, on cursory examination, resemble RP. Over time, atrophy of the RPE and choroid spreads peripherally and centrally (Fig. 15.39B). The end-stage appearance consists of isolated choroidal vessels coursing

over bare sclera, retinal vascular attenuation and optic atrophy. In contrast to primary retinal dystrophies, the fovea is spared until late (Fig. 15.39C).

- **Investigation**
  ○ ERG: scotopic is non-recordable; photopic is severely subnormal.
  ○ FA shows filling of the retinal and large choroidal vessels but not of the choriocapillaris. The intact fovea is hypofluorescent and is surrounded by hyperfluorescence due to an extensive window defect (Fig. 15.39D).
- **Treatment.** Early clinical trials of specific gene therapy for choroideremia, involving the introduction of functional copies of the faulty gene into the eye, have produced promising results.

Gyrate atrophy

Gyrate atrophy (AR) is caused by a mutation in the gene (*OAT*) encoding the main ornithine degradation enzyme, ornithine aminotransferase. Deficiency of the enzyme leads to elevated ornithine levels in the plasma, urine, cerebrospinal fluid and aqueous humour. The visual prognosis is generally poor, with legal blindness occurring around the age of 50 from geographic atrophy.

- **Symptoms.** Myopia and nyctalopia in adolescence, with a subsequent gradual worsening of vision.
- **Signs**
  ○ Mid-peripheral depigmented spots associated with diffuse pigmentary mottling may be seen in asymptomatic cases.
  ○ Sharply demarcated circular or oval areas of chorioretinal atrophy develop; these may be associated with numerous glistening crystals at the posterior pole (Fig. 15.40A).
  ○ Coalescence of atrophic areas and gradual peripheral and central spread (Fig. 15.40B).
  ○ The fovea is spared until late (Fig. 15.40C).
  ○ Extreme attenuation of retinal blood vessels.
  ○ Vitreous degeneration and early-onset cataract is common; CMO and ERM may also occur.
- **Investigation**
  ○ FA shows sharp demarcation between areas of choroidal atrophy and normal choriocapillaris.
  ○ ERG is subnormal is early disease and later becomes extinguished.
- **Treatment.** There are two clinically different subtypes of gyrate atrophy based on the response to pyridoxine (vitamin B_6), which may normalize plasma and urinary ornithine levels. Patients who are responsive to vitamin B_6 generally have a less severe and more slowly progressive clinical course than those who are not. Reduction in ornithine levels with an arginine-restricted diet is also beneficial.

Progressive bifocal chorioretinal atrophy

In progressive bifocal chorioretinal atrophy (AD), the implicated gene region overlaps with that responsible for North Carolina macular dystrophy but the two conditions are believed to be due

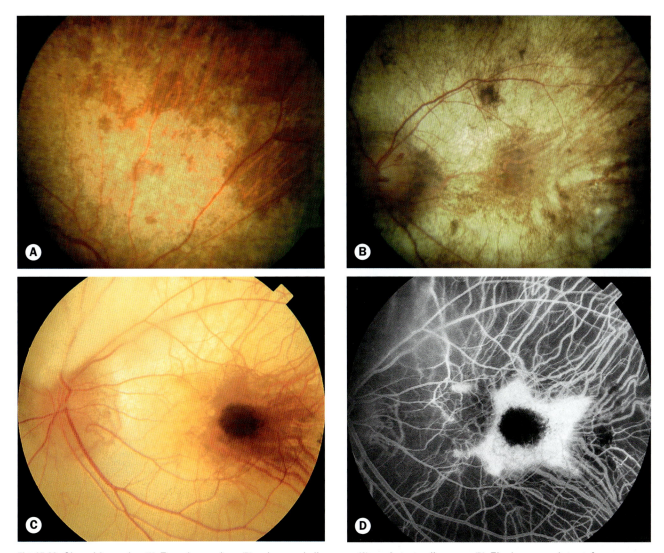

Fig. 15.39 Choroideremia. **(A)** Female carrier; **(B)** advanced disease; **(C)** end-stage disease; **(D)** FA shows an intact fovea
(Courtesy of S Chen – fig. B; S Milewski – figs C and D)

to different mutations. Dual foci of chorioretinal atrophy develop temporal and nasal to the disc, with inevitable macular involvement (Fig. 15.41). Nystagmus, myopia and retinal detachment may occur.

HEREDITARY VITREORETINOPATHIES

Juvenile X-linked retinoschisis

Introduction

Juvenile retinoschisis is characterized by bilateral maculopathy, with associated peripheral retinoschisis in 50%. The basic defect is mediated via the Müller cells, leading to splitting of the retinal nerve fibre layer from the rest of the sensory retina, in contrast to acquired (senile) retinoschisis in which splitting occurs at the outer plexiform layer. Inheritance is XLR, with the implicated gene in most cases designated *RS1*. The prognosis is often poor due to progressive maculopathy; visual acuity deteriorates during the first two decades, but may remain reasonably stable until the fifth or sixth decades before further deterioration.

Diagnosis

- **Symptoms.** Presentation in boys is usually between the ages of 5 and 10 years with reading difficulties. Less frequently squint or nystagmus occurs in infancy associated with advanced peripheral retinoschisis, often with vitreous haemorrhage. Carrier females are generally asymptomatic.
- **Signs**
  - The most common appearance is foveal schisis, appearing as spoke-like striae radiating from the foveola, associated with cystoid changes (Fig. 15.42A); over time the striae become less evident, leaving a blunted foveal reflex.

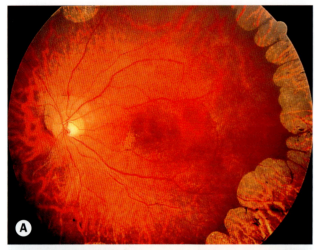

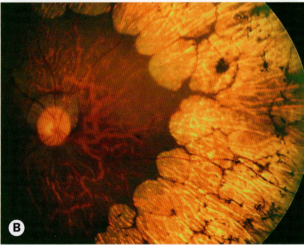

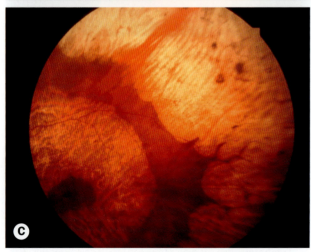

Fig. 15.40 Gyrate atrophy. **(A)** Early disease; **(B)** advanced disease; **(C)** end-stage disease with preservation of the fovea

○ Whitish drusen-like dots and pigment variation may be seen (Fig. 15.42B); the macula is occasionally normal.

○ Peripheral schisis predominantly involves the inferotemporal quadrant. It does not extend but secondary changes may occur; the inner layer, which

consists only of the internal limiting membrane and the retinal nerve fibre layer, may develop oval defects (Figs 15.42C and D) and in extreme cases the defects coalesce, leaving only retinal blood vessels floating in the vitreous ('vitreous veils') (Fig. 15.42E). Silvery peripheral dendritic figures (Fig. 15.42F), vascular sheathing and pigmentary changes are common, and retinal flecks and nasal dragging of retinal vessels may be seen.

○ Complications include vitreous and intra-schisis haemorrhage, neovascularization, subretinal exudation (Fig. 15.43A), and rarely rhegmatogenous or tractional retinal detachment and traumatic rupture of the foveal schisis (Fig. 15.43B).

- **Investigation**
  ○ OCT is useful for documenting maculopathy progression; cystic spaces in the inner nuclear and outer plexiform layers are commonly present (Fig. 15.44A), but the fovea may simply appear disorganized.
  ○ FAF shows variable macular abnormality, including spoke-like patterns and central hypoautofluorescence with surrounding hyperautofluorescence (Fig. 15.44B).
  ○ ERG is normal in eyes with isolated maculopathy. Eyes with peripheral schisis show a characteristic selective decrease in amplitude of the b-wave as compared with the a-wave on scotopic and photopic testing (Fig. 15.44C).
  ○ EOG is normal in eyes with isolated maculopathy but subnormal in eyes with advanced peripheral lesions.
  ○ FA of maculopathy may show mild window defects but no leakage, in contrast to CMO.

Treatment

- **Topical or oral carbonic anhydrase inhibitors** (e.g. dorzolamide three times daily) may reduce foveal thickness and improve visual acuity in some patients.

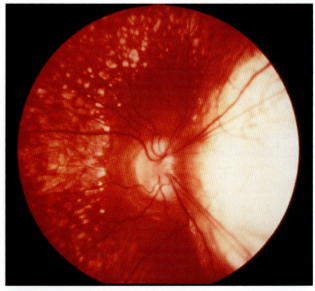

Fig. 15.41 Progressive bifocal chorioretinal atrophy
(Courtesy of Moorfields Eye Hospital)

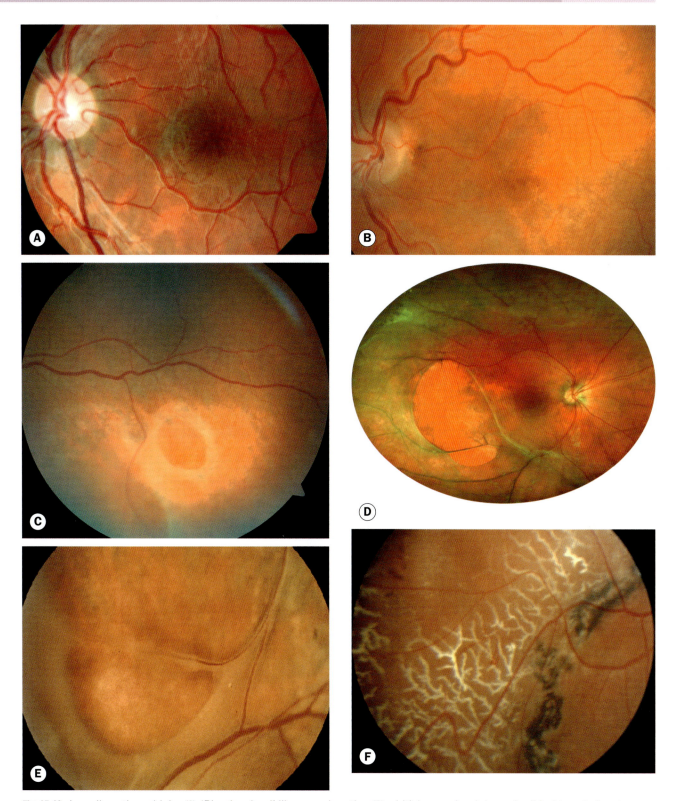

Fig. 15.42 Juvenile retinoschisis. **(A)** 'Bicycle wheel'-like maculopathy; **(B)** whitish macular dots and mild pigment change; **(C)** and **(D)** large, typically oval, inner leaf defects; **(E)** 'vitreous veils'; **(F)** peripheral dendritic lesions
(Courtesy of K Slowinski – fig. A; S Chen – fig. D; C Barry – fig. E; Moorfields Eye Hospital – fig. F)

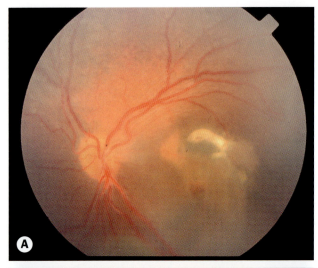

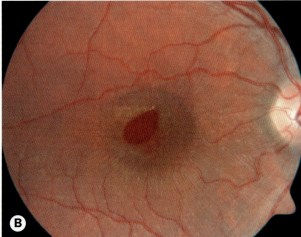

Fig. 15.43 Complications of juvenile retinoschisis. **(A)** Subretinal exudation; **(B)** traumatic hole in macular schisis

(Courtesy of G-M Sarra – fig. A; K Slowinski – fig. B)

- **Vitrectomy** may be required for vitreous haemorrhage or retinal detachment repair, but is technically challenging. As retinoschisis cavities are non-progressive, surgery is not performed purely to flatten these.
- **Gene therapy** is under investigation, with the aim of restoring normal function of the protein abnormality underlying retinoschisis.

Stickler syndrome

Stickler syndrome (hereditary arthro-ophthalmopathy) is a genetically heterogeneous disorder of collagen connective tissue. Inheritance is AD (STL1–STL3) or AR (STL4 and STL5) with complete penetrance but variable expressivity. Stickler syndrome is the most common inherited cause of retinal detachment in children. In general, the prognosis has been poor but may be improving with elevated standards of care.

- **Stickler syndrome type I (STL1 – membranous vitreous type)** is the most common form, and is the result of mutations in the *COL2A1* gene. The classic ocular and

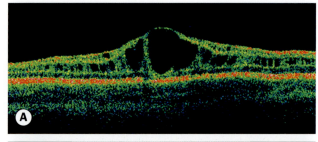

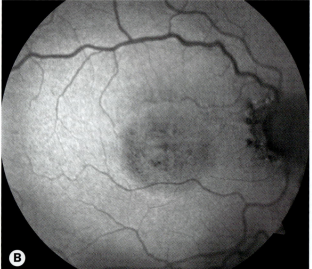

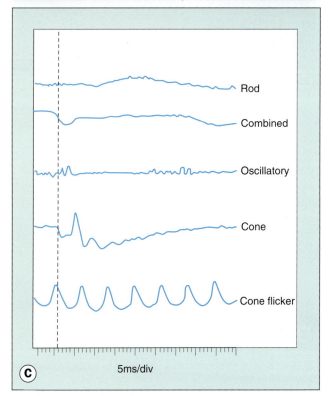

Fig. 15.44 Investigation in X-linked retinoschisis. **(A)** OCT showing cyst-like foveal changes; **(B)** fundus autofluorescence – central hypofluorescence with surrounding hyperfluorescence; **(C)** ERG showing selective decrease in b-wave amplitude

(Courtesy of J Talks – fig. A)

systemic features are present as originally described by Stickler, though there is also a solely or predominantly ocular (non-syndromic) form of STL1.

- **STL2 (beaded vitreous type)** is caused by mutations in the *COL11A1* gene. Patients have congenital non-progressive high myopia, sensorineural deafness and other features of Stickler syndrome type 1.
- **STL3 (non-ocular type)** is due to mutations in the *COL11A2* gene. Affected individuals have the typical systemic features, but no ocular manifestations.
- **STL4** and **STL5 (AR types)** are extremely rare.

Systemic features include mid-facial hypoplasia (Fig. 15.45A), Pierre-Robin-type features (micrognathia, cleft palate – Fig. 15.45B, and glossoptosis – backward displacement of the tongue), bifid uvula, mild spondyloepiphyseal dysplasia, joint hypermobility and early-onset osteoarthritis. Deafness may be sensorineural or caused by recurrent otitis media.

Diagnosis

The three characteristic ocular features are high myopia, vitreoretinal degeneration with an associated extremely high rate of retinal detachment, and cataract.

- **Signs**
  - In STL1 patients exhibit an optically empty vitreous, a retrolenticular membrane and circumferential equatorial

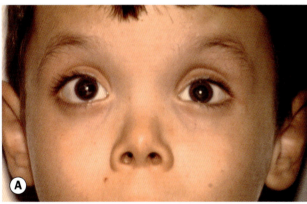

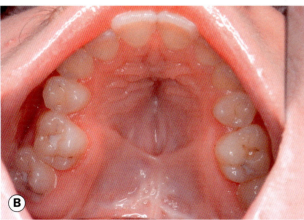

Fig. 15.45 Stickler syndrome. **(A)** Facial appearance; **(B)** cleft and high-arched palate
(Courtesy of K Nischal – fig. B)

membranes that extend a short way into the vitreous cavity (Fig. 15.46A and see Figs 15.47A and B).
  - In STL2 patients the vitreous has a fibrillary and beaded appearance.
  - Radial lattice-like degeneration associated with RPE hyperplasia, vascular sheathing and sclerosis (Figs 15.46B and C).
  - Retinal detachment develops in approximately 50% in the first decade of life, often as a result of multiple or giant tears that may involve both eyes.
  - Presenile cataract characterized by frequently non-progressive peripheral cortical wedge-shaped, fleck or lamellar opacities is common.
  - Ectopia lentis can occur, but is uncommon.
  - Glaucoma (5–10%) is associated with congenital angle anomaly.

Treatment

- Prophylactic 360° retinal laser or cryotherapy may reduce the incidence of retinal detachment, but as a minimum regular screening with prophylactic treatment of retinal breaks is essential. Long-term review of all patients is mandatory.
- Retinal detachment repair is challenging, with proliferative vitreoretinopathy particularly common. Vitrectomy is generally indicated. Re-detachment may occur later.
- Cataract in Stickler is often visually inconsequential, particularly when early. If surgery is required, a careful preoperative retinal evaluation with treatment of breaks should be performed. Vitreous loss and postoperative retinal detachment are relatively common.
- Glaucoma treatment may be required; if early-onset and presumably related to angle anomaly, management is generally as for congenital glaucoma (see Ch. 10).

Wagner syndrome

Wagner syndrome (VCAN-related vitreoretinopathy) is a rare condition having some features in common with Stickler syndrome, but no association with systemic abnormalities; erosive vitreoretinopathy is now known to be the same disorder. Inheritance is AD and mutations in the gene *VCAN* can be responsible. Severity is variable, with up to 50% developing retinal detachment, often before the age of 15.

- **Signs**
  - Patients tend to have low to moderate myopia.
  - The key abnormal finding is an optically empty vitreous cavity (Fig. 15.47A) lacking structural elements, and it is thought this leads to reduced 'scaffolding' support for the retina.
  - The peripheral retinal vasculature is deficient.
  - Greyish-white avascular strands and membranes extend into the vitreous cavity and there may be a circumferential ridge-like condensation of the gel at or anterior to the retinal periphery (Fig. 15.47B).
  - Peripheral retinal changes including progressive chorioretinal atrophy (Fig. 15.47C) occur and nyctalopia

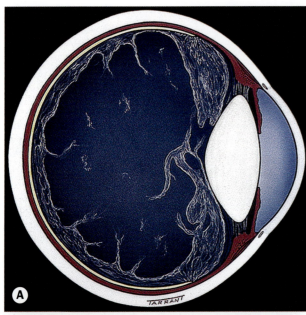

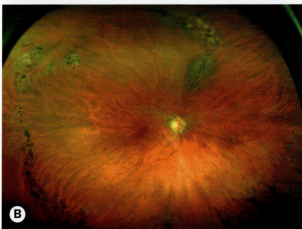

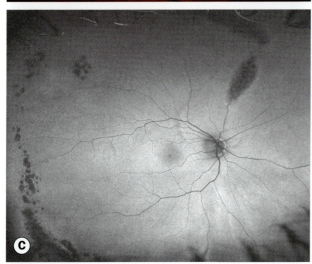

Fig. 15.46 Stickler syndrome. **(A)** Vitreous liquefaction and membranes; **(B)** radial lattice degeneration and pigmentary changes – wide-field image; **(C)** wide-field autofluorescence image of eye in (B)

(Courtesy of S Chen – figs B and C)

is commonly troublesome; the visual fields gradually constrict.

○ Cataract is common in younger adults, and glaucoma can develop.

- **Investigation.** FA shows non-perfusion due to choriocapillaris loss (Fig. 15.47D). The ERG may initially be normal, but later shows a reduction of scotopic b-wave amplitudes and diffuse cone-rod loss.

- **Treatment.** Retinal breaks and detachment are treated as they occur, but extensive prophylaxis is avoided.

Familial exudative vitreoretinopathy

Familial exudative vitreoretinopathy (Criswick–Schepens syndrome) is a slowly progressive condition characterized by failure of vascularization of the temporal retinal periphery, similar to that seen in retinopathy of prematurity. Inheritance is AD and rarely XLR or AR, with high penetrance and variable expressivity; four genes in a common pathway have been implicated. Presentation is in childhood; the prognosis is frequently poor, especially with early aggressive onset.

- **Signs**
  ○ High myopia may be present.
  ○ Stage 1: peripheral avascularity. There is abrupt termination of retinal vessels at the temporal equator. Vitreous degeneration and peripheral vitreoretinal attachments are associated with areas of 'white without pressure'. Vascular straightening (Fig. 15.48A) may be present.
  ○ Stage 2: peripheral vascular tortuosity and telangiectasia (Fig. 15.48B) progresses to preretinal fibrovascular proliferation (Figs 15.48C and D), with or without subretinal exudation (Fig. 15.48E).
  ○ Stage 3: tractional and/or rhegmatogenous macular-sparing retinal detachment, with or without exudation.
  ○ Stages 4 and 5 are macula-involving (Fig. 15.48F) and total retinal detachment, respectively.
  ○ Vitreous haemorrhage, cataract and neovascular glaucoma can occur.

- **Investigation.** Wide-field FA is invaluable (Fig. 15.49) in confirming the diagnosis, ensuring accurate targeting and completeness of ablation of avascular retina, and identifying asymptomatic cases with subtle features.

- **Treatment.** Relatives should be screened.
  ○ Lifelong monitoring is required.
  ○ Laser ablation of avascular retina is recommended, usually once neovascularization has occurred.
  ○ Vitrectomy for retinal detachment is challenging but often successful.
  ○ Intravitreal anti-VEGF treatment can be useful as a temporizing measure.

Enhanced S-cone syndrome and Goldmann–Favre syndrome

The human retina has three cone photoreceptor types: short-wave sensitivity (S), middle-wave sensitivity (M) and long-wave

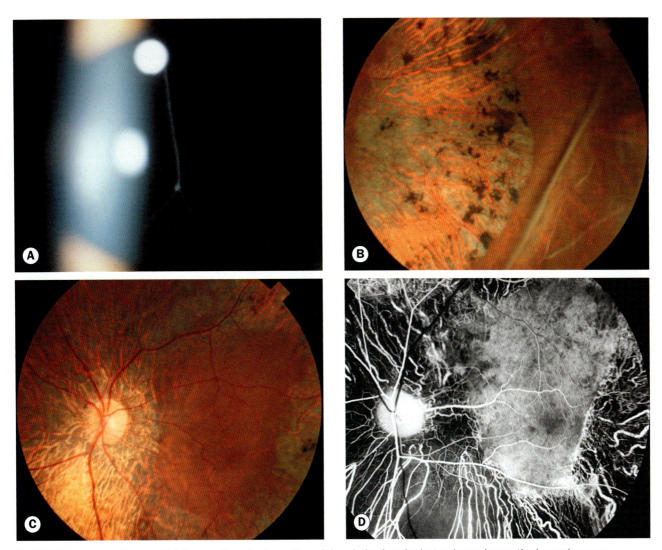

Fig. 15.47 Wagner syndrome. **(A)** Vitreous liquefaction; **(B)** peripheral chorioretinal atrophy and preretinal membranes; **(C)** progressive chorioretinal atrophy; **(D)** FA shows gross loss of the choriocapillaris
(Courtesy of E Messmer)

sensitivity (L). Most inherited retinal dystrophies exhibit progressive attenuation of rods and all classes of cones. However, enhanced S-cone syndrome is characterized by hyperfunction of S-cones and severe impairment of M- and L-cones, with non-recordable rod function. Goldmann–Favre syndrome represents a severe variant. Inheritance is AR with variable expressivity; the gene implicated is *NR2E3*. Presentation is with nyctalopia in childhood, and sometimes hemeralopia (reduced vision in bright light). Pigmentary changes along the vascular arcades or mid-periphery may be associated in more advanced cases with round pigment clumps (Fig. 15.50A). Macular changes may include cystoid maculopathy (without fluorescein leakage) and schisis (Fig. 15.50B). Vitreous degeneration and peripheral retinoschisis can occur. The prognosis for central and peripheral vision is poor in many patients, particularly by late middle age, and there is no treatment other than supportive measures.

Snowflake vitreoretinal degeneration

This rare AD condition (gene *KCNJ13*) has some similarities to Wagner syndrome; retinal detachment is less common, and the prognosis is usually very good.

- **Signs** (Fig. 15.51)
  - Stage 1 shows extensive areas of 'white without pressure' in patients typically under the age of 15 years.
  - Stage 2 shows snowflake-like yellow–white crystalline deposits in areas of 'white with pressure' in patients between 15 and 25.
  - Stage 3 manifests with vascular sheathing and pigmentation posterior to the area of snowflake degeneration in patients between 25 and 50.
  - Stage 4 is characterized by increased pigmentation, gross vascular attenuation, areas of chorioretinal atrophy, and

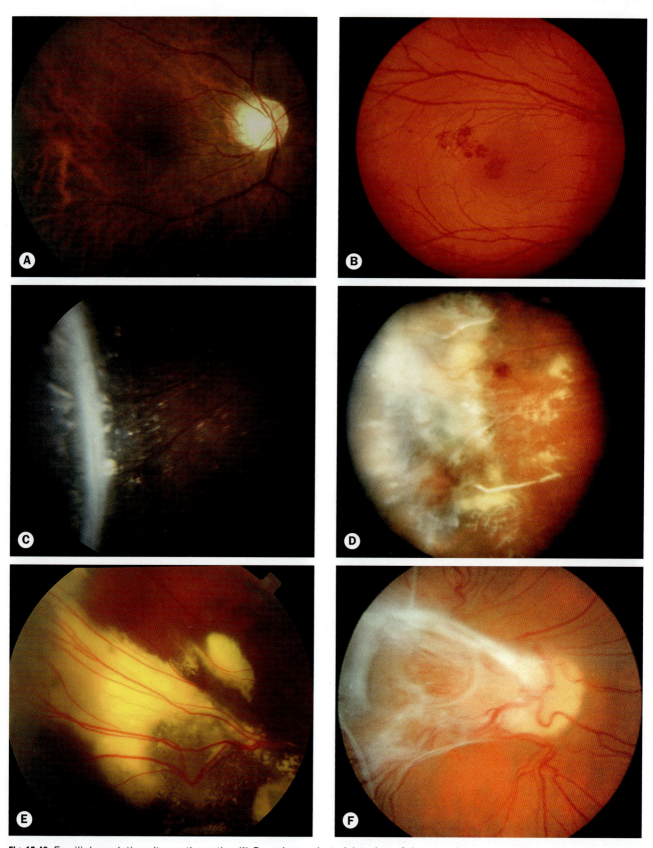

Fig. 15.48 Familial exudative vitreoretinopathy. **(A)** Dragging and straightening of the macular vessels; **(B)** peripheral telangiectasia; **(C)** fibrovascular ridge; **(D)** fibrovascular proliferation; **(E)** subretinal exudation; **(F)** 'dragging' of the disc and macula, with underlying macular tractional detachment

(Courtesy of S Chen – fig. A; C Hoyng – fig. E)

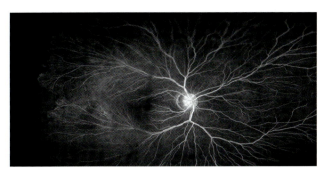

Fig. 15.49 Wide-field FA shows vascular straightening and abrupt termination in familial exudative vitreoretinopathy

(Courtesy of S Chen)

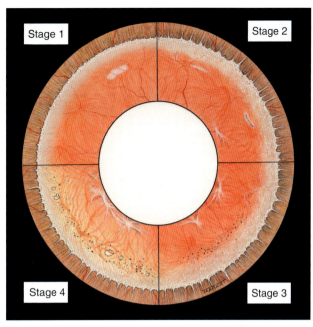

Fig. 15.51 Snowflake degeneration

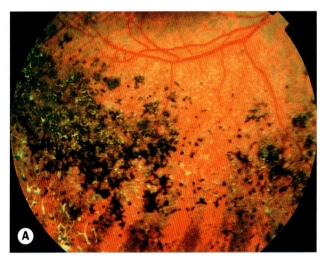

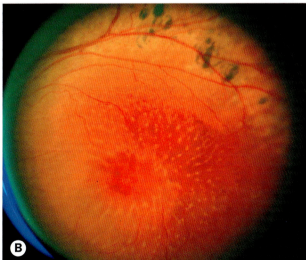

Fig. 15.50 Enhanced S-cone and Goldmann–Favre syndrome. **(A)** Severe pigment clumping; **(B)** macular schisis and pigmentary changes along the arcade

(Courtesy of D Taylor and CS Hoyt, from Pediatric Ophthalmology and Strabismus, *Elsevier Saunders 2005 – fig. A; J Donald M Gass, from* Stereoscopic Atlas of Macular Diseases, *Mosby 1997 – fig. B)*

less prominent snowflakes in patients over the age of 60 years. The macula remains normal.
  - ○ Other possible features include mild myopia, vitreous fibrillary degeneration and liquefaction, a waxy optic nerve head, corneal guttae, retinal detachment and early-onset cataract.
- **Investigation.** The ERG shows a low scotopic b-wave amplitude.

Autosomal dominant neovascular inflammatory vitreoretinopathy

A rare but interesting inherited (gene *CAPN5*) disorder, autosomal dominant neovascular inflammatory vitreoretinopathy (ADNIV) features panuveitis, often of onset in early adulthood. The initial symptom is typically floaters due to vitritis, with the development of peripheral vascular closure with peripheral and then disc neovascularization, fundus pigmentation, epiretinal and subretinal fibrocellular membranes; complications include vitreous haemorrhage, tractional retinal detachment, cystoid macular oedema, cataract and neovascular glaucoma. The ERG shows selective loss of b-wave amplitude. The prognosis can be poor. Peripheral retinal photocoagulation and vitreous surgery may be required.

Autosomal dominant vitreoretinochoroidopathy

Autosomal dominant vitreoretinochoroidopathy (ADVIRC) can be caused by *BEST1* mutations. Presentation is in adult life if symptomatic, but frequently discovery is by chance. Vitreous cells and fibrillary degeneration develop, with a non-progressive or very slowly progressive encircling band of pigmentary disturbance between the ora serrata and equator, with a discrete posterior border. Within the band there can be arteriolar attenuation, neo-vascularization, punctate white opacities and later chorioretinal atrophy. Complications are uncommon, but can include cystoid macular oedema, vitreous haemorrhage and cataract; microcornea and nanophthalmos have been described in some patients. The full-field ERG is subnormal in older patients only. The prognosis is good.

Kniest dysplasia

Kniest dysplasia is usually caused by a defect in the type II collagen gene, *COL2A1*, which is also involved in Stickler syndrome type 1. Inheritance can be AD, but most cases represent a fresh mutation. High myopia, vitreous degeneration, retinal detachment and ectopia lentis can occur; systemic features may include short stature, a round face and arthropathy.

ALBINISM

Introduction

Albinism is a genetically determined, heterogeneous group of dis-orders of melanin synthesis in which either the eyes alone (ocular albinism) or the eyes, skin and hair (oculocutaneous albinism) may be affected. The latter may be either tyrosinase-positive or tyrosinase-negative. The different mutations are thought to act through a common pathway involving reduced melanin synthesis in the eye during development. Tyrosinase activity is assessed by using the hair bulb incubation test, which is reliable only after 5 years of age. Patients with oculocutaneous, and probably ocular, albinism have an increased risk of cutaneous basal cell and squa-mous cell carcinoma.

Tyrosinase-negative oculocutaneous albinism

Tyrosinase-negative (complete) albinos are incapable of synthesiz-ing any melanin and have white hair and very pale skin (Fig. 15.52) throughout life with a lack of melanin pigment in all ocular struc-tures. The condition is genetically heterogeneous, usually with AR inheritance.

- **Signs**
  - VA is usually <6/60 due to foveal hypoplasia.
  - Nystagmus is typically pendular and horizontal. It usually increases in bright illumination and tends to lessen in severity with age.
  - The iris is diaphanous and translucent (Fig. 15.53A), giving rise to a 'pink-eyed' appearance (Fig. 15.53B).
  - The fundus lacks pigment and shows conspicuously large choroidal vessels. There is also foveal hypoplasia with absence of the foveal pit, and poorly formed perimacular vascular arcades (Fig. 15.53C).
  - The optic chiasm has fewer uncrossed nerve fibres than normal – the majority of fibres from each eye cross to the contralateral hemisphere. This can be demonstrated with visual evoked potentials.

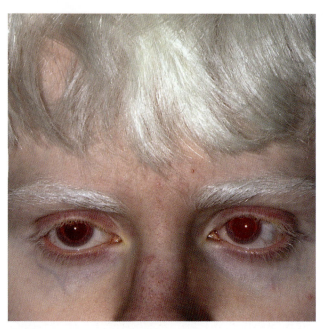

Fig. 15.52 White hair and very pale skin in tyrosinase-negative oculocutaneous albinism
(Courtesy of C Barry)

  - Other features include high refractive errors of various types, a positive angle kappa, squint and absent stereopsis.

Tyrosinase-positive oculocutaneous albinism

Tyrosinase-positive (incomplete) albinos synthesize variable amounts of melanin. Patients' hair may be white, yellow or red, and darkens with age. Skin is pale at birth but usually darkens by 2 years of age (Fig. 15.54A). Inheritance is usually AR; mutation in at least two distinct genes can be causative.

- **Ocular signs**
  - VA is usually impaired due to foveal hypoplasia.
  - Iris may be blue or dark-brown with variable translucency.
  - Fundus shows variable hypopigmentation (Fig. 15.54B).
- **Systemic associations**
  - Chediak–Higashi syndrome: haematological abnormalities with recurrent infections and lymphoproliferation.
  - Hermansky–Pudlak syndrome: lysosomal storage disease with platelet dysfunction, and pulmonary fibrosis, granulomatous colitis and renal failure in some cases.
  - Waardenburg syndrome: an AD condition with a range of systemic presentations including a white forelock, poliosis, synophrys ('monobrow'), deafness and sometimes limb and neurological anomalies. Ocular features include lateral displacement of the medial canthi, hypochromic irides with segmental or total heterochromia (Fig. 15.55), and choroidal depigmentation.

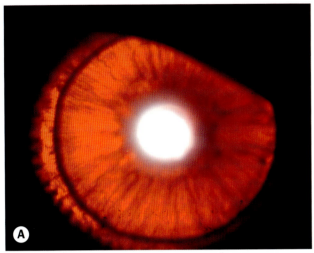

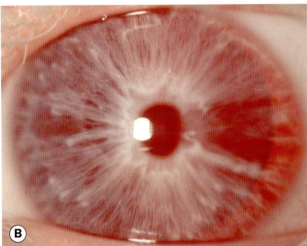

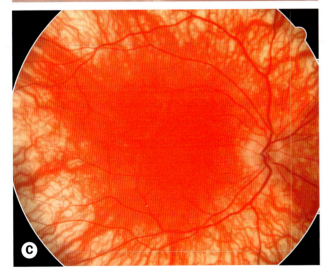

Fig. 15.53 Ocular signs in tyrosinase-negative oculocutaneous albinism. **(A)** Marked iris translucency; **(B)** 'pink eye' appearance; **(C)** severe fundus hypopigmentation and foveal aplasia

(Courtesy of C Barry – fig. C)

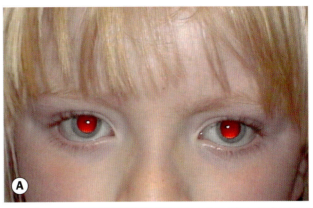

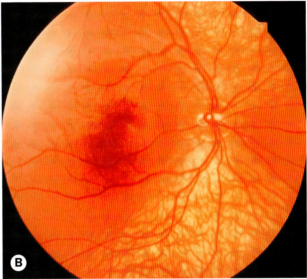

Fig. 15.54 Tyrosinase-positive oculocutaneous albinism. **(A)** Fair hair and normal skin colour; **(B)** mild fundus hypopigmentation

(Courtesy of B Majol – fig. A)

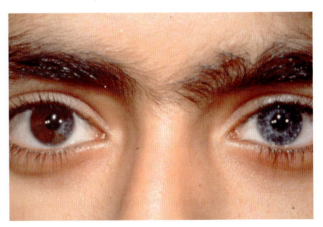

Fig. 15.55 Waardenburg syndrome with iris heterochromia (segmental in the right eye) and synophrys

Ocular albinism

In this variant, involvement is predominantly ocular, with normal skin and hair, although occasionally hypopigmented skin macules may be seen. Inheritance is usually XLR but occasionally AR. Female carriers are asymptomatic, but may show partial iris translucency, macular stippling and mid-peripheral scattered areas of depigmentation and granularity (Fig. 15.56). Affected males have hypopigmented irides and fundi.

CHERRY-RED SPOT AT THE MACULA

A cherry-red spot at the macula (Fig. 15.57) is a clinical sign seen in the context of thickening and loss of transparency of the retina at the posterior pole. The fovea is the thinnest part of the retina, allowing persistent transmission of the underlying vascular choroidal hue when the surrounding retina becomes relatively opaque. Causes include:

- **Metabolic storage diseases.** A group of rare inherited metabolic diseases, often enzyme deficiencies, leads to the pathological accumulation of lipid-based material in various tissues. With the passage of time the spot becomes less evident due to retinal nerve fibre layer degeneration, and consecutive optic atrophy is seen. They are almost exclusively AR. Some individual storage disorders are:
  - ○ GM1 gangliosidosis (generalized): neurological features are severe, with death typically by the age of 2 years. Subtle corneal clouding can occur.

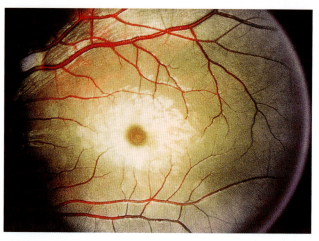

Fig. 15.57 Cherry-red spot at the macula

  - ○ Mucolipidosis type I (sialidosis): a late-onset form features myoclonus and seizures, but is compatible with a normal life span; a more severe form causes severe neurodegeneration and death in early childhood. Corneal clouding and optic atrophy may be seen.
  - ○ GM2 gangliosidosis: this encompasses two conditions, Tay–Sachs disease and Sandhoff disease. In both, there is progressive neurological deterioration, with early blindness and death.
  - ○ Niemann–Pick disease: of the three main types (A–C), only the first two feature a cherry-red spot. Abnormal ocular motility occurs in Type C (chronic neuropathic).
  - ○ Farber disease: Systemically, aphonia, dermatitis, lymphadenopathy, psychomotor retardation, renal and cardiopulmonary disease may develop. Ocular features additional to cherry-red spot development include pinguecula-like conjunctival lesions and nodular corneal opacity.
- **Central retinal and cilioretinal artery occlusion** (see Ch. 13). Retinal clouding results from oedema; the appearance is an acute sign only.
- **Retinotoxicity** due to specific agents including quinine, dapsone, gentamicin, carbon monoxide and methanol.
- **Commotio retinae** (see Ch. 21); oedema due to blunt trauma.
- **Miscellaneous.** The term can be used more loosely to encompass a variety of conditions giving a dark or reddish central macular appearance such as a macular hole.

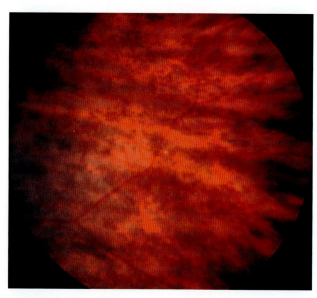

Fig. 15.56 Carrier of X-linked ocular albinism

INTRODUCTION

Anatomy of the peripheral retina

Pars plana

The ciliary body starts 1 mm from the limbus and extends posteriorly for about 6 mm. The anterior 2 mm consist of the pars plicata, the remaining 4 mm the flattened pars plana. In order not to endanger either the lens or retina, the optimal location for a pars plana surgical incision or intravitreal injection is 4 mm and 3.5 mm posterior to the limbus in phakic and pseudophakic eyes respectively. An incision through the mid-pars plana will usually be located anterior to the vitreous base (see below).

Ora serrata

The ora serrata (Fig. 16.1) is the junction between the retina and ciliary body. In retinal detachment (RD), fusion of the sensory retina with the retinal pigment epithelium (RPE) and choroid limits forward extension of subretinal fluid (SRF) at the ora. However, there is no equivalent adhesion between the choroid and sclera, and choroidal detachments may progress anteriorly to involve the ciliary body (ciliochoroidal detachment).

- **Dentate processes** are tapering extensions of retina onto the pars plana; they are more marked nasally than temporally and display marked variation in contour.
- **Oral bays** are scalloped edges of pars plana epithelium between dentate processes.
- **Meridional folds** (Fig. 16.2A) are small radial folds of thickened retinal tissue in line with dentate processes, most

commonly in the superonasal quadrant. A fold may occasionally exhibit a small retinal hole at its apex. A meridional complex is a configuration in which a dentate process, usually with an associated meridional fold, is aligned with a ciliary process.
- **Enclosed oral bays** (Fig. 16.2B) are small islands of pars plana surrounded by retina as a result of meeting of two adjacent dentate processes. They should not be mistaken for retinal holes.

Vitreous base

The vitreous base (Fig. 16.3) is a 3–4 mm wide zone straddling the ora serrata, throughout which the cortical vitreous is strongly attached. Following posterior vitreous detachment (PVD), the posterior hyaloid face remains attached at the vitreous base. Pre-existing retinal holes within the attached vitreous base do not lead to RD. Blunt trauma may cause an avulsion of the vitreous base, with tearing of the non-pigmented epithelium of the pars plana along the base's anterior border and of the retina along the base's posterior border.

Innocuous peripheral retinal degenerations

Peripheral retinal degenerations and other lesions carrying the potential to lead to RD are described separately.
- **Microcystoid (peripheral cystoid) degeneration** consists of tiny vesicles with indistinct boundaries on a greyish-white background, making the retina appear thickened and less transparent (Figs 16.4A and B). The degeneration starts adjacent to the ora serrata and extends circumferentially and

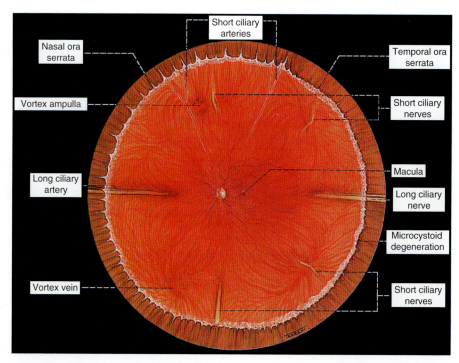

Fig. 16.1 The ora serrata and normal anatomical landmarks

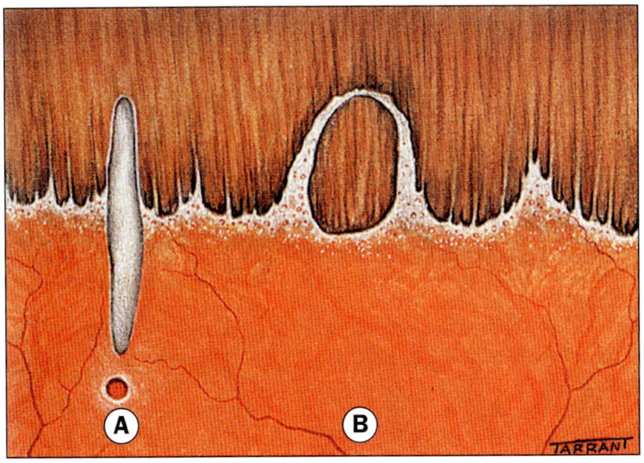

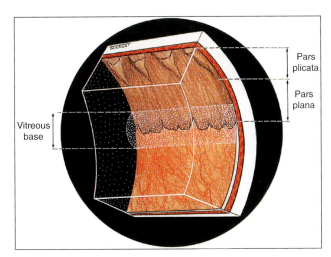

Fig. 16.2 Normal variants of the ora serrata. **(A)** Meridional fold with a small retinal hole at its base; **(B)** enclosed oral bay

posteriorly with a smooth undulating posterior border. Microcystoid degeneration is present in essentially all adult eyes, increasing in extent with age. It is not in itself causally related to RD, though it may give rise to typical degenerative retinoschisis.

- **Paving stone degeneration** is characterized by discrete yellow–white patches of focal chorioretinal atrophy that may have pigmented margins (Fig. 16.4B). It is typically found between the equator and the ora, and is more common in the inferior fundus. It is present to some extent in at least 25% of normal eyes.

- **Reticular (honeycomb) degeneration** is an age-related change consisting of a fine network of perivascular pigmentation that sometimes extends posterior to the equator (Figs 16.4C and D).

- **Peripheral drusen.** Clustered or scattered small pale discrete lesions (Fig. 16.4E) that may have hyperpigmented borders (Fig. 16.4F); they are similar to drusen at the posterior pole and usually occur in the eyes of older individuals.

Fig. 16.3 The vitreous base

- **Pars plana cyst.** Clear-walled cysts (Fig. 16.4G), usually small, are derived from non-pigmented ciliary epithelium. They are present in 5–10% of eyes, and are more common temporally. They do not predispose to RD.

Sites of vitreous adhesion

Physiological

The peripheral cortical vitreous is loosely attached to the internal limiting membrane (ILM) of the sensory retina. Sites of stronger adhesion in the normal eye include:
- Vitreous base; very strong.
- Optic disc margins; fairly strong.
- Perifoveal; fairly weak.
- Peripheral blood vessels; usually weak.

Pathological

Abnormal adhesions may lead to retinal tear formation following PVD, or to vitreomacular interface disease; most are discussed in detail later in this chapter.
- Lattice degeneration.
- Retinal pigment clumps.
- Cystic retinal tufts.
- Vitreous base anomalies, such as extensions and posterior islands.
- 'White with pressure' and 'white without pressure'.
- Zonular traction tufts.
- Vitreomacular traction (see Ch. 14).
- Preretinal new vessels, e.g. proliferative diabetic retinopathy.

Definitions

- **Retinal detachment (RD).** RD refers to separation of the neurosensory retina (NSR) from the RPE. This results in the accumulation of SRF in the potential space between the NSR and RPE.
- **Rhegmatogenous** (Greek *rhegma* – break) **RD** requires a full-thickness defect in the sensory retina, which permits fluid derived from synchytic (liquefied) vitreous to gain access to the subretinal space. RRD, as opposed to the presence merely of a cuff of SRF surrounding a retinal break, is said to be present when fluid extends further than one optic disc diameter from the edge of the break.
- **Tractional RD.** The NSR is pulled away from the RPE by contracting vitreoretinal membranes in the absence of a retinal break.
- **Exudative** (serous, secondary) **RD.** SRF is derived from the vessels of the NSR and/or choroid.
- **Combined tractional–rhegmatogenous RD** results when a retinal break is caused by traction from an adjacent area of fibrovascular proliferation.
- **Subclinical RD** is generally used to refer to an asymptomatic break surrounded by a relatively small amount of SRF, by

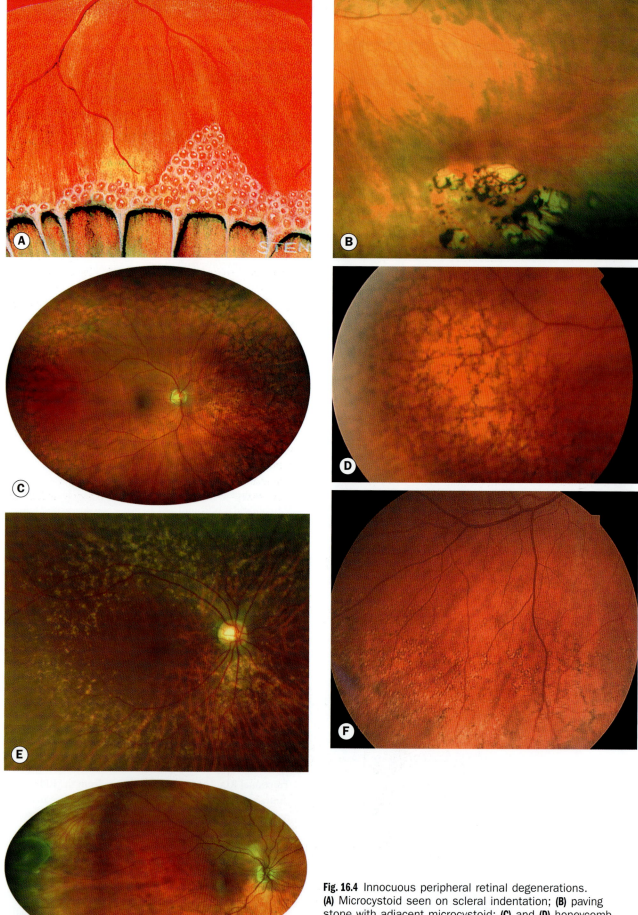

Fig. 16.4 Innocuous peripheral retinal degenerations.
(A) Microcystoid seen on scleral indentation; **(B)** paving stone with adjacent microcystoid; **(C)** and **(D)** honeycomb (reticular); **(E)** and **(F)** peripheral drusen; **(G)** pars plana cyst

(Courtesy of U Rutnin, CL Schepens, from American Journal of Ophthalmology, 1967;64:1042 – fig. A; S Chen – figs B, C, E and G)

definition extending further than one disc diameter away from the edge of the break but less than two disc diameters posterior to the equator. It does not usually give rise to a subjective visual field defect. The term is sometimes also used to describe an asymptomatic RD of any extent.

Clinical examination

Head-mounted binocular indirect ophthalmoscopy

The term binocular indirect ophthalmoscopy (BIO) is by convention used to refer to the head-mounted technique, though strictly it also applies to slit lamp indirect ophthalmoscopy. BIO allows retinal visualization through a greater degree of media opacity than slit lamp biomicroscopy, and readily facilitates scleral indentation. Light is transmitted from the headset to the fundus through a condensing lens held at the focal point of the eye, providing an inverted and laterally reversed image that is observed through a stereoscopic viewing system (Fig. 16.5A).

- **Lenses** of various powers and diameters are available for BIO (Fig. 16.5B); a lens of lower power confers increased magnification but a smaller field of view. Yellow filters may improve patient comfort.
  - ○ 20 D (magnifies ×3; field about 45°) is the most commonly used for general examination of the fundus.
  - ○ 28 D (magnification with the head-mounted set of ×2.27, and a field of 53°) has a shorter working distance

and is useful when examining patients with small pupils.
  - ○ 40 D (magnification ×1.5, field 65°) is used mainly to examine small children; a broad fundus scan can be acquired rapidly; it can also be used at the slit lamp to provide very high magnification.
  - ○ Panretinal 2.2 combines magnification similar to the 20 D lens with a field of view similar to that of the 28 D, and can be used with small pupils.
  - ○ Ultra-high magnification lenses for macular and optic disc examination (e.g. Macula Plus® 5.5) are available.

- **Technique.** The patient should be supine on a bed or reclining chair rather than sitting upright. The pupils should be dilated. Reducing the ambient illumination is often helpful in improving contrast and allowing a lower incident light intensity to be used. The eyepieces are set at the correct interpupillary distance and the beam aligned so that it is located in the centre of the viewing frame. The patient is instructed to keep both eyes open at all times; if necessary, the patient's eyelids are gently separated with the fingers. The lens is taken into one hand with the flat surface facing the patient. The peripheral fundus should be examined first in order to allow the patient to adapt to the light. The patient is asked to move the eyes into optimal positions for examination, e.g. looking away from the examiner to facilitate examination of the retinal periphery. For the examination of small children (e.g. retinopathy of prematurity – see also Ch. 13) a speculum may be utilized to

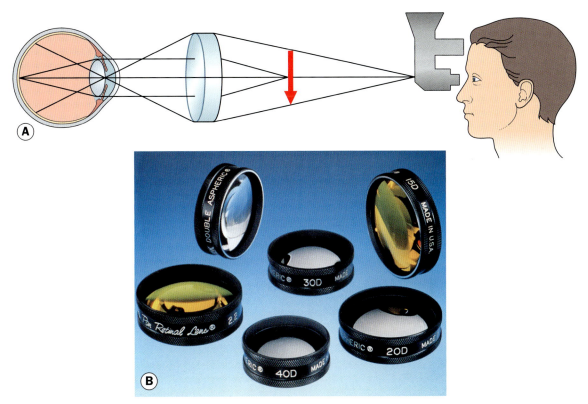

Fig. 16.5 (A) Principles of indirect ophthalmoscopy; **(B)** condensing lenses

keep the eyelids apart, with an implement such as a squint hook employed to direct the position of the eye.

- **Scleral indentation.** The main function of scleral indentation (depression) is the enhancement of visualization of the retina anterior to the equator; it also permits kinetic evaluation (Fig. 16.6). Indentation should be attempted only after the basic technique of BIO has been mastered; it requires practised coordination between the relative position of the indenter and the viewing apparatus, as well as care to prevent patient discomfort. For example, to view the ora serrata at 12 o'clock, the patient is asked to look down and the scleral indenter (a cotton-tipped applicator is preferred

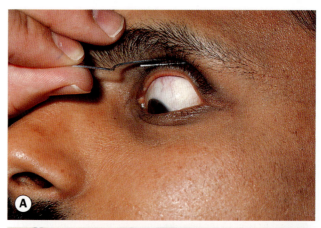

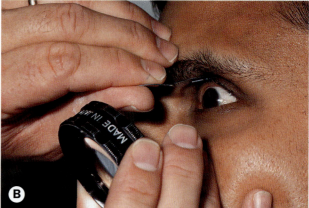

Fig. 16.7 Technique of scleral indentation. **(A)** Insertion of indenter; **(B)** indentation

by some practitioners) is applied to the outside of the upper eyelid at the margin of the tarsal plate (Fig. 16.7A). With the indenter in place, the patient is asked to look up; at the same time the indenter is advanced into the anterior orbit parallel with the globe, and the examiner's eyes are aligned with the condensing lens and indenter (Fig. 16.7B). Gentle pressure is exerted so that a mound is created; after adequate viewing, the indenter is gently moved to an adjacent part of the fundus. The indenter should be kept tangential to the globe at all times, as perpendicular indentation will cause pain and even risk perforation if the sclera is very thin. For viewing the 3 and 9 o'clock positions, indentation directly on the sclera is sometimes necessary, facilitated by topical anaesthesia. Indentation can also be performed at the slit lamp using some fundus contact lenses.

Slit lamp fundus examination

A range of diagnostic contact and non-contact lenses are available for use with the slit lamp. Contact lenses should not be used if a penetrating injury is suspected or in the presence of corneal trauma, hyphaema or corneal infection.

- **Non-contact lenses**
  - 60 D. High-magnification lens optimized for viewing the posterior pole. High working distance (13 mm).

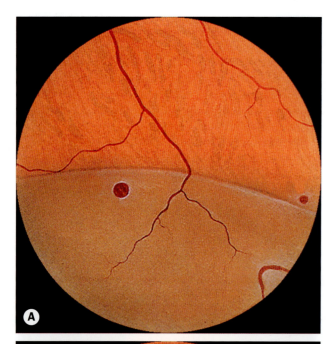

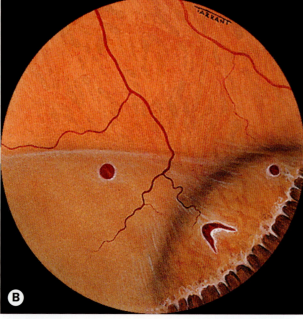

Fig. 16.6 Appearance of retinal breaks in detached retina. **(A)** Without scleral indentation; **(B)** with indentation

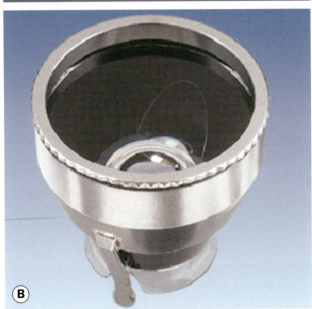

(A)

(B)

Fig. 16.8 Diagnostic contact lenses. **(A)** Three-mirror lens; **(B)** Goldmann 904® lens with indentation attachment

○ 90 D. Wider-field lens with lower magnification and shorter (7 mm) working distance. Can be used with smaller pupils.

○ 78 D. Intermediate properties; ideal for general-purpose examination.

○ Miscellaneous. Numerous other lenses are available, offering qualities such as a very wide field of view and extremely small pupil capability.

● **Three-mirror contact lens** (Fig. 16.8A). A central lens gives a 30° upright view of the posterior pole. An equatorial mirror (the largest) enables visualization from 30° to the equator, a peripheral mirror (intermediate) views the fundus between the equator and the ora serrata, and a gonioscopy mirror (smallest and dome-shaped) may be used for gonioscopy or

for visualization of the extreme retinal periphery and sometimes the pars plana. A viscous coupling substance is required to bridge a gap between the cornea and the apposed lens. To visualize the entire fundus the lens is rotated for 360° using first the equatorial mirror and then the peripheral mirrors.

● **Scleral indentation** at the slit lamp can be accomplished using a three-mirror lens with a special attachment (Eisner funnel) or a purpose-made ora serrata contact lens that combines a mirror angled similarly to a gonioscopy lens with an incorporated attachment to facilitate scleral depression (e.g. Goldmann 904® – Fig. 16.8B).

● **Miscellaneous** contact lenses are divided principally into those conferring high magnification for an optimal posterior pole view, and those offering a wide field of view, allowing visualization extending to the ora serrata under optimal conditions. Small pupil capability is available, and a flange is offered on many lenses with the aim of improving stability of retention and of lens position on the eye.

Fundus drawing

When available, wide-field photographic imaging can be an excellent aid in recording the features of a retinal detachment, but documentation generally takes the form of a manually drawn illustration that optimally is colour-coded (Fig. 16.9). RD boundaries are drawn by starting at the optic nerve and then extending to the periphery; detached retina is shaded in blue and flat retina in red. The course of retinal vessels (usually veins) is indicated with blue. Retinal breaks are drawn in red with blue outlines; the flap of a retinal tear is also drawn in blue. Thin retina may be represented by red hatching outlined in blue and lattice degeneration by blue hatching outlined in blue. Retinal pigment is indicated in black, retinal exudates in yellow and vitreous opacities in green.

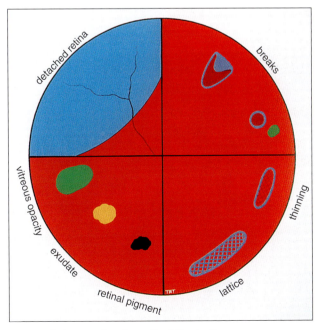

Fig. 16.9 Colour coding for retinal illustration

Ultrasonography

Introduction

Ultrasonography (US) utilizes high frequency sound waves that produce echoes as they strike the interface between acoustically distinct structures. B-scan (two-dimensional) US is a key tool in the diagnosis of RD in eyes with opaque media, particularly severe vitreous haemorrhage (Fig. 16.10).

Technique

- The patient should be supine; anaesthetic drops are instilled.
- The examiner typically sits behind the patient's head and holds the US probe with the dominant hand.
- Methylcellulose or an ophthalmic gel is placed on the tip of the probe to act as a coupling agent.
- The B-scan probe incorporates a marker for orientation that correlates with a point on the display screen, usually to the left.
- Vertical scanning is performed with the marker on the probe orientated superiorly (Fig. 16.11A).
- Horizontal scanning is performed with the marker orientated towards the nose (Fig. 16.11B).
- The eye is then examined with the patient looking straight ahead, up, down, left and right. For each position a vertical and horizontal scan can be performed.
- The examiner then moves the probe in the opposite direction to the movement of the eye. For example, when examining the right eye the patient looks to the left and probe is moved to the patient's right, the nasal fundus anterior to the equator is scanned and vice versa. Dynamic scanning is performed by asking the patient to move the eye, whilst the probe position is maintained.
- Gain adjusts the amplification of the echo signal, similar to volume control of a radio. Higher gain increases the

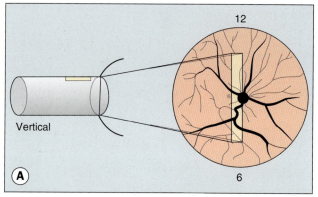

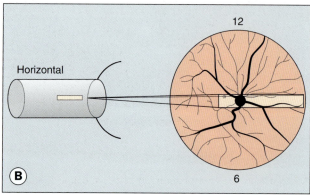

Fig. 16.11 Technique of ultrasound scanning of the globe. **(A)** Vertical scanning with the marker pointing towards the brow; **(B)** horizontal scanning with the marker pointing towards the nose

sensitivity of the instrument in displaying weak echoes such as vitreous opacities. Lower gain only allows display of strong echoes such as the retina and sclera, though improves resolution because it narrows the beam.

PERIPHERAL LESIONS PREDISPOSING TO RETINAL DETACHMENT

Patients with any predisposing lesion, or indeed any high risk features for RD, should be educated about the nature of symptoms of PVD and RD and the need to seek review urgently if these occur.

Lattice degeneration

- **Prevalence.** Lattice degeneration is present in about 8% of the population. It probably develops early in life, with a peak incidence during the second and third decades. It is found more commonly in moderate myopes and is the most important degeneration directly related to RD. Lattice is present in about 40% of eyes with RD.
- **Pathology.** There is discontinuity of the internal limiting membrane with variable atrophy of the underlying NSR. The vitreous overlying an area of lattice is synchytic but the vitreous attachments around the margins are exaggerated (Fig. 16.12).

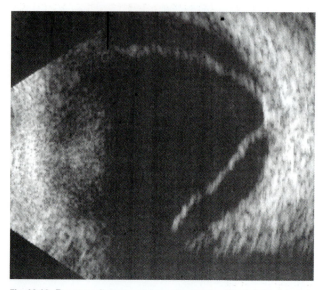

Fig. 16.10 B-scan ultrasonogram showing retinal detachment

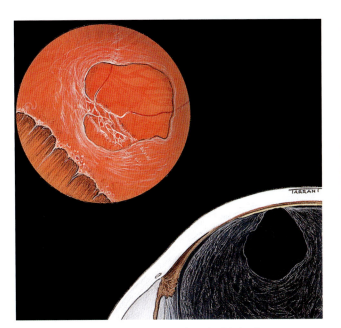

Fig. 16.12 Vitreous changes associated with lattice degeneration

- **Signs.** Lattice is most commonly bilateral, temporal and superior.
  - Spindle-shaped areas of retinal thinning, commonly located between the equator and the posterior border of the vitreous base (Fig. 16.13A).
  - Sclerosed vessels forming an arborizing network of white lines is characteristic (Fig. 16.13B).
  - Some lesions may be associated with 'snowflakes', remnants of degenerate Müller cells.
  - Associated hyperplasia of the RPE is common.
  - Small holes are common (see Fig. 16.13A).
- **Complications** do not occur in most eyes with lattice.
  - Tears may develop consequent to a posterior vitreous detachment (PVD), when lattice is sometimes visible on the flap of the tear (Fig. 16.13C).
  - Atrophic holes may rarely (2%) lead to RD; the risk is higher in young myopes. In these patients the RD may not be preceded by acute symptoms of PVD (see below) and SRF usually spreads slowly so that diagnosis may be delayed.
- **Management.** Asymptomatic areas of lattice are generally not treated prophylactically, even if retinal breaks are seen, unless particular risk factors are present, perhaps including RD in the fellow eye; treatment of the fellow eye when extensive lattice (more than 6 clock hours) is present, or there is high myopia, may actually be associated with a higher risk of detachment. However, the patient should be advised of the symptoms of RD, optimally including the provision of written information. Many practitioners advise routine annual review of eyes with lattice, with or without asymptomatic round holes, particularly in young myopes. An associated asymptomatic U-tear should be managed as discussed later in the chapter.

Snailtrack degeneration

Snailtrack degeneration is characterized by sharply demarcated bands of tightly packed 'snowflakes' that give the peripheral retina a white frost-like appearance (Figs 16.14A and B). It is viewed by some as a precursor to lattice degeneration. Marked vitreous

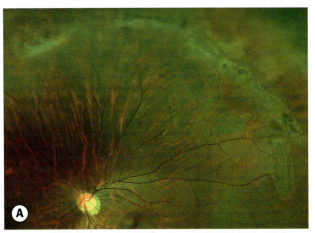

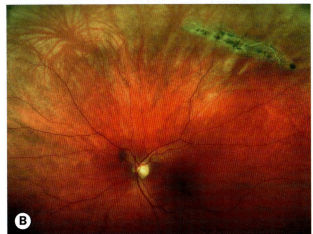

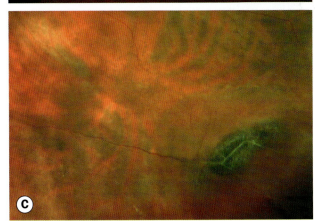

Fig. 16.13 Wide-field images of lattice degeneration. **(A)** Multiple lesions with small holes; **(B)** sclerosed vessels forming a characteristic white network; a vortex vein is seen superonasally; **(C)** retinal detachment with lattice on the flap of the tear
(Courtesy of S Chen)

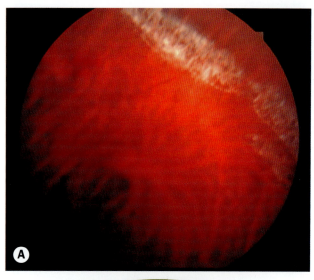

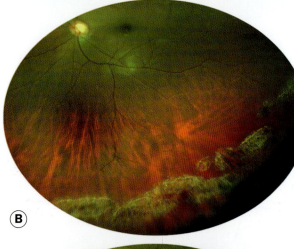

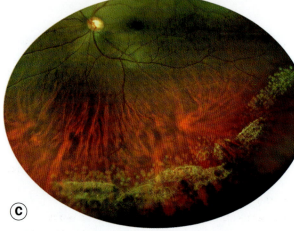

Fig. 16.14 (A) Snailtrack degeneration; **(B)** and **(C)** wide-field images of lesions before and after limited laser retinopexy *(Courtesy of S Chen – figs B and C)*

traction is seldom present so that U-tears rarely occur, although round holes are relatively common. Prophylactic treatment (Fig. 16.14C) is usually unnecessary, though review every 1–2 years may be prudent as RD occurs in a minority.

Cystic retinal tuft

A cystic retinal tuft (CRT), also known as a granular patch or retinal rosette, is a congenital abnormality consisting of a small, round or oval, discrete elevated whitish lesion, typically in the equatorial or peripheral retina, more commonly temporally (Fig. 16.15A); there may be associated pigmentation at its base. It is comprised principally of glial tissue; strong vitreoretinal adhesion is commonly present and both small round holes (Fig. 16.15B) and horseshoe tears can occur. It is likely to be an under-recognized lesion, though this may change with the adoption of wide-field imaging; CRT are present in up to 5% of the population (bilateral in 20%) and may be the causative lesion in 5–10% of eyes with RD, though the risk of RD in a given eye with CRT is probably well under 1%.

Degenerative retinoschisis

- **Prevalence.** Degenerative retinoschisis (RS) is present in about 5% of the population over the age of 20 years and is particularly prevalent in hypermetropia.
- **Pathology.** RS is believed to develop from microcystoid degeneration by a process of gradual coalescence of degenerative cavities (Fig. 16.16A), resulting in separation or splitting of the NSR into inner and outer layers (Figs 16.16B and C), with severing of neurones and complete loss of visual function in the affected area. In typical retinoschisis the split occurs in the outer plexiform layer, and in the less common reticular retinoschisis at the level of the nerve fibre layer.
- **Symptoms**
  - ○ Photopsia and floaters are absent because there is no vitreoretinal traction.
  - ○ It is rare for the patient to notice a visual field defect, even with spread posterior to the equator.
  - ○ Occasionally symptoms result from vitreous haemorrhage or a progressive RD.
- **Signs.** RS is bilateral in up to 80%. Distinction between the typical and reticular types is difficult clinically, though the inner layer is thinner and tends to be more elevated in the latter; differentiation is based principally on behaviour, with complications much more common in the reticular form.
  - ○ Early retinoschisis usually involves the extreme inferotemporal periphery of both fundi, appearing as an exaggeration of microcystoid degeneration with a smooth immobile dome-shaped elevation of the retina (Fig. 16.16D).
  - ○ The elevation is convex, smooth, thin and relatively immobile (Fig. 16.17), unlike the opaque and corrugated appearance of a rhegmatogenous RD.

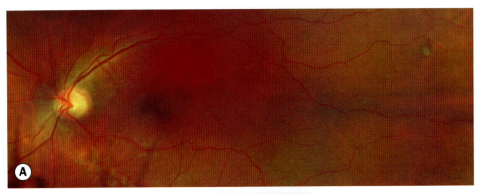

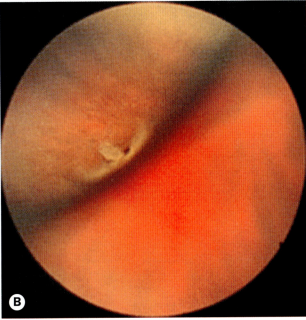

Fig. 16.15 Cystic retinal tuft. **(A)** Isolated uncomplicated lesion; **(B)** tuft with small round hole

(Courtesy of S Lorenzon – fig. A; Courtesy of NE Byer, from The Peripheral Retina in Profile, A Stereoscopic Atlas, *Criterion Press, Torrance, CA 1982 – fig. B)*

- ○ The thin inner leaf of the schisis cavity may be mistaken, on cursory examination, for an atrophic long-standing rhegmatogenous RD but demarcation lines and secondary cysts in the inner leaf are absent.
- ○ The lesion may progress circumferentially until it has involved the entire periphery. The typical form usually remains anterior to the equator; the reticular type is more likely to spread posteriorly.
- ○ The presence of a pigmented demarcation line is likely to indicate the presence of associated RD.
- ○ The surface of the inner layer may show 'snowflakes' (whitish remnants of Müller cell footplates – see Figs 16.17 and 16.18) as well as sclerosis of blood vessels, and the schisis cavity may be bridged by grey–white tissue strands.
- ○ Breaks may be present in one or both layers. Inner layer breaks are small and round (Fig. 16.18A), whilst the less common outer layer breaks are usually larger, with rolled edges (Figs 16.18A and B) and located behind the equator.
- ○ Microaneurysms and small telangiectases are common, particularly in the reticular type.

- ○ If a visual field defect is detectable it is absolute, rather than relative as in RD.
- • **Complications** are uncommon, and are thought to be much more likely in the reticular form.
  - ○ RD is rare; even in an eye with breaks in both layers the incidence is only around 1%. The detachment is almost always asymptomatic, infrequently progressive and rarely requires surgery.
  - ○ Posterior extension of RS to involve the fovea is very rare but can occur; progression is generally very slow.
  - ○ Vitreous haemorrhage is rare.
- • **Management.** Though RD is rare, discussion of the symptoms is prudent in all patients, especially those with double layer breaks.
  - ○ A small peripheral RS discovered on incidental examination, especially if breaks are not present in both layers, probably does not require routine review, though a routine community optometric examination every 1–2 years may be prudent.
  - ○ A large RS should be observed periodically, particularly if breaks are present in both layers or it extends posterior to

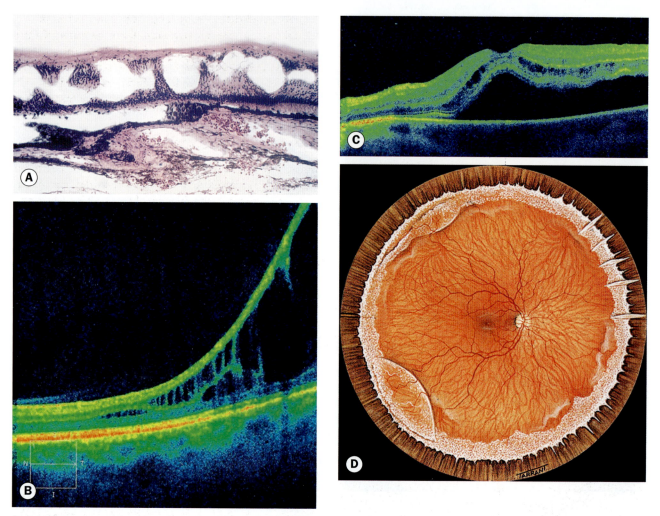

Fig. 16.16 Development of retinoschisis. **(A)** Histology showing intraretinal cavities bridged by Müller cells; **(B)** OCT appearance showing separation principally in the outer plexiform layer; **(C)** OCT of retinal detachment for comparison; **(D)** circumferential microcystoid degeneration with progression to retinoschisis supero- and inferotemporally

(Courtesy of J Harry and G Misson, from Clinical Ophthalmic Pathology, *Butterworth-Heinemann 2001 – fig. A; S Chen – figs B and C)*

the equator; the review interval is individualized. Photography and visual field testing are useful, with optical coherence tomography (OCT) imaging when posterior extension is present. OCT is also useful for distinguishing between RS and RD (see Figs 16.16B and C).

○ Retinopexy or surgical repair may be indicated for relentless progression towards the fovea, when complication by retinal detachment should be excluded. Some authorities also advocate prophylactic retinopexy of the posterior border of a large bullous RS with substantial breaks to prevent progression to symptomatic RD.

○ Recurrent vitreous haemorrhage may necessitate vitrectomy.

○ Progressive symptomatic RD should be addressed promptly. More than one procedure may be necessary; scleral buckling may be adequate for smaller RD with small outer layer breaks, but vitrectomy is generally indicated for more complex RD.

Zonular traction tuft

This refers to a common (15%) phenomenon caused by an aberrant zonular fibre extending posteriorly to be attached to the retina near the ora serrata, and exerts traction on the retina at its base. It is typically located nasally. The risk of retinal tear formation is around 2%, and periodic long-term review is generally recommended.

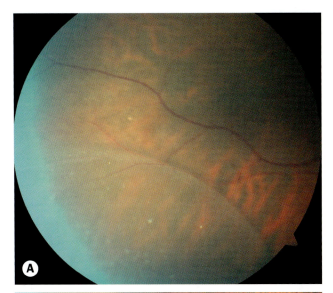

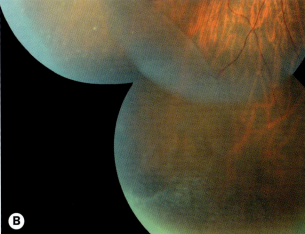

Fig. 16.17 (A) Retinoschisis; **(B)** composite image of the same lesion showing merging microcystoid degeneration

White with pressure and white without pressure

- **'White with pressure' (WWP)** refers to retinal areas in which a translucent white–grey appearance can be induced by scleral indentation (Fig. 16.19A). Each area has a fixed configuration that does not change when indentation is moved to an adjacent area. It may also be observed along the posterior border of islands of lattice degeneration, snailtrack degeneration and the outer layer of acquired retinoschisis. It is frequently seen in normal eyes and may be associated with abnormally strong attachment of the vitreous gel, though may not indicate a higher risk of retinal break formation.
- **'White without pressure' (WWOP)** has the same appearance as WWP but is present without scleral indentation (Fig. 16.19B). WWOP corresponds to an area of fairly strong adhesion of condensed vitreous (Fig. 16.19C). On cursory examination a normal area of retina surrounded by white without pressure may be mistaken for a flat retinal hole (Fig. 16.20A). However, retinal breaks, including giant

tears, occasionally develop along the posterior border of white without pressure (Fig. 16.20B). For this reason, if white without pressure is found in the fellow eye of a patient with a spontaneous giant retinal tear, prophylactic therapy should be considered. Regular review should be considered for treated and untreated eyes, though evidence for the benefit of this is limited.

Myopic choroidal atrophy

Diffuse choroidal/chorioretinal atrophy in myopia is characterized by diffuse or circumscribed (Fig. 16.21) choroidal depigmentation, commonly associated with thinning of the overlying retina, and occurs typically in the posterior pole and equatorial area of highly

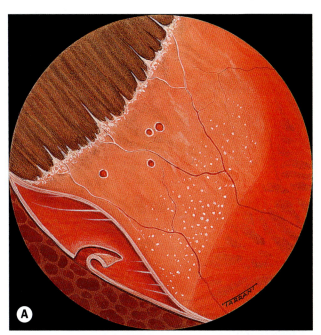

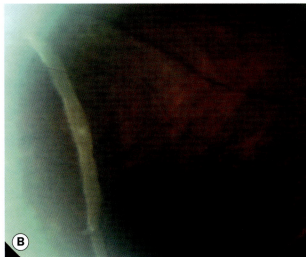

Fig. 16.18 Retinoschisis. **(A)** Inner and outer layer breaks; **(B)** large outer layer break; retinal vessels in the inner layer can be seen traversing the rolled edge undiverted
(Courtesy of S Chen – fig. B)

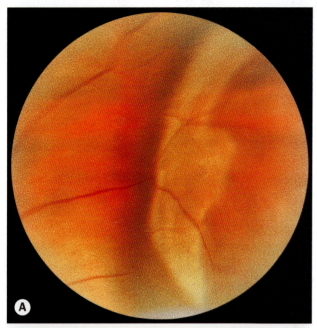

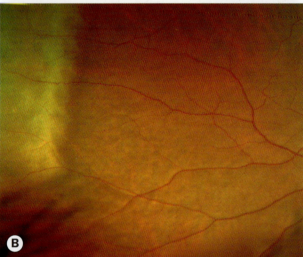

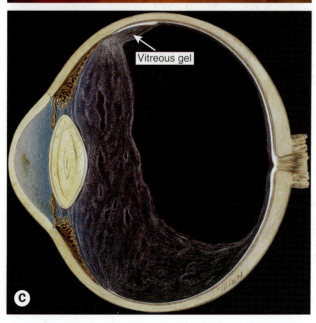

Vitreous gel

Fig. 16.19 (A) White with pressure; **(B)** white without pressure; **(C)** strong attachment of condensed vitreous gel to an area of 'white without pressure'

(Courtesy of NE Byer, from The Peripheral Retina in Profile, A Stereoscopic Atlas, *Criterion Press, Torrance, CA 1982 – fig. A; S Chen – fig. B; CL Schepens, ME Hartnett and T Hirose, from* Schepens' Retinal Detachment and Allied Diseases, *Butterworth-Heinemann 2000 – fig. C)*

myopic eyes. Retinal holes developing in the atrophic retina may occasionally lead to RD. Because of lack of contrast, small holes may be very difficult to visualize.

POSTERIOR VITREOUS DETACHMENT

Introduction

Posterior vitreous detachment (PVD) refers to separation of the cortical vitreous, along with the delineating posterior hyaloid membrane (PHM), from the neurosensory retina posterior to the vitreous base. PVD occurs due to vitreous gel liquefaction with age (synchysis) to form fluid-filled cavities (Fig. 16.22A), and subsequently condensation (syneresis), with access to the preretinal space allowed by a dehiscence in the cortical gel and/or PHM. The prevalence of PVD increases with age, and in individuals in their 80s is likely to be at least 60%. It is typically spontaneous, but can be induced by events such as cataract surgery, trauma, uveitis and panretinal photocoagulation. The time taken for a PVD to complete after initiation is believed to be variable, but probably occurs in stages over the course of months in many patients. Perifoveal hyaloid detachment is followed by foveal separation, then detachment from the posterior retina as far as the equator, attachment initially being retained at the optic disc; subsequently complete detachment of the cortical vitreous as far anteriorly as the vitreous base takes place (Fig. 16.22B). With the exception of the vitreous base, physiological attachments to the retina and other structures are disengaged in the course of a normal PVD. Complications, many of which require treatment, occur in up to 27%.

Clinical features

- **Symptoms** are usually, though not invariably, present.
  - Flashing lights (photopsia) in PVD is often described as a lightning-like arc induced by eye or head movement, and is more noticeable in dim illumination. It is almost always seen in the temporal periphery; the mechanism is uncertain, but may relate to traction on the optic disc and possibly at sites of vitreoretinal adhesion, including actual or potential retinal tears.
  - Floaters (myodesopsia) are mobile vitreous opacities (Figs 16.22C and D) most evident against a bright pale background. They are often described as spots, cobwebs or flies (muscae volitantes), and are commonly present in individuals without a PVD, especially myopes. A Weiss ring (Figs 16.22E and F) is the detached former

attachment to the margin of the optic disc, and may be seen by the patient as a circle or other large solitary lesion; its presence does not necessarily indicate total PVD, nor does its absence confirm the absence of PVD since it may be destroyed during the process of separation. Floaters can also be due to vitreous blood (see below).

○ Blurred vision. A diffuse haze may be due to dispersed haemorrhage within the vitreous gel, with a variable accompanying reduction in VA; bleeding can arise from a torn retinal blood vessel or from the site of a retinal break. Blurring can also be caused by a visually significant PHM or floaters in the visual axis, which may also cause impairment (usually slight) of acuity.

- **Signs**
  ○ The detached PHM can often be seen clinically on slit lamp examination as a crumpled translucent membrane in the mid-vitreous cavity behind which the cavity is optically clear (Fig. 16.23A).
  ○ Haemorrhage may be indicated by the presence of red blood cells in the anterior vitreous or as (usually small) focal intragel collections, or preretinally, when it sometimes forms a crescent shape bordering the limit of PHM detachment. Its presence should prompt a careful search for a retinal break (40–90%), particularly with larger amounts – in such cases breaks tend to be posterior.
  ○ Pigment granules in the anterior vitreous on slit lamp examination (the Shafer sign or 'tobacco dust' – see Fig. 16.28) are larger, darker and less reflective than red blood cells. Their presence raises the possibility of a retinal break (up to 95% sensitivity), with loss of continuity allowing communication between the RPE and vitreous cavity.
  ○ Vitreous cells, if numerous, may signify the presence of a break.
  ○ Retinal breaks (see below).
- **Investigation.** B-scan ultrasound (Fig. 16.23B) can demonstrate the extent of PVD; OCT can show posterior pole separation (Fig. 16.23C).

Management

Patients with substantial acute symptoms of a PVD should be examined as soon as practicable, usually within 24–48 hours, with greater urgency in the presence of risk factors including myopia, a past or family history of RD, high-risk syndromes such as Stickler, pseudophakia and symptoms such as a visual field defect, reduced vision or very prominent floaters. Enquiry should be made about the presence of any condition predisposing to non-PVD vitreous haemorrhage, usually diabetes mellitus. If there is only a single small floater and no photopsia, evidence suggests the risk of retinal break in the symptomatic eye is insignificantly higher than that of the asymptomatic fellow eye, so that urgent assessment may not necessarily be required.

- **Examination.** The anterior vitreous should be assessed for the presence of blood and pigment. Careful retinal examination including visualization of the ora serrata for

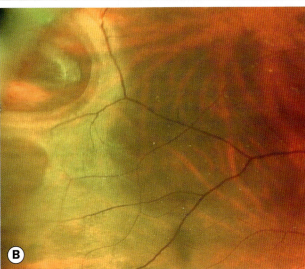

Fig. 16.20 White without pressure wide-field images. **(A)** Pseudo-break (arrow); **(B)** retinal tear and adjacent pseudo-break

(Courtesy of S Chen)

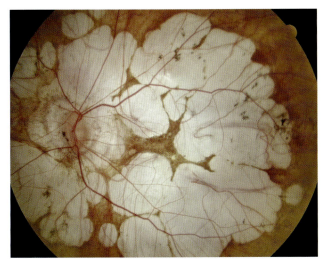

Fig. 16.21 Myopic choroidal atrophy

(Courtesy of S Chen)

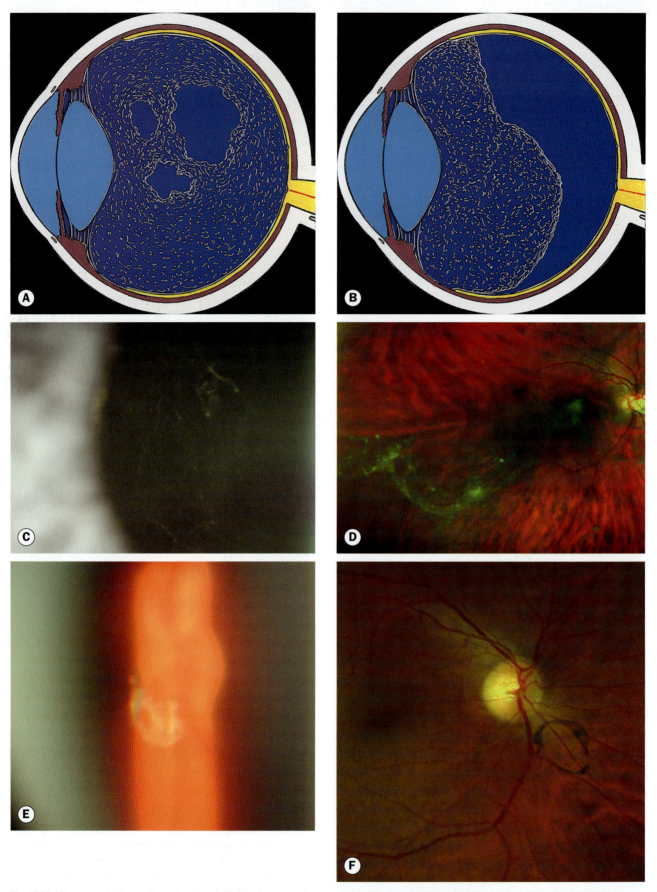

Fig. 16.22 Vitreous degenerative changes. **(A)** Synchysis and syneresis; **(B)** complete posterior vitreous detachment; **(C)** biomicroscopy showing vitreous condensation in a pseudophakic eye; **(D)** vitreous degenerative condensation on wide-field imaging; **(E)** Weiss ring on slit lamp biomicroscopy, with the optic disc in the background; **(F)** Weiss ring on wide-field imaging

(Courtesy of S Chen – figs D and F)

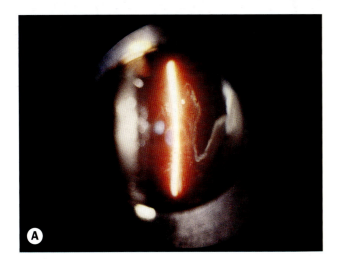
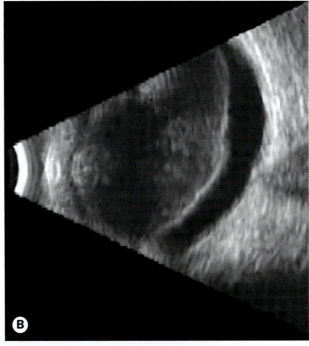
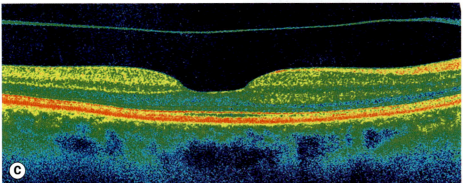

Fig. 16.23 Posterior vitreous detachment. **(A)** Biomicroscopy showing detached and collapsed gel; **(B)** ultrasound B-scan; **(C)** OCT showing macular PVD

(Courtesy of CL Schepens, CL Trempe and M Takahashi, from Atlas of Vitreous Biomicroscopy, Butterworth-Heinemann 1999 – fig. A; S Chen – figs B and C)

360° should be performed, and should generally include binocular indirect ophthalmoscopy or contact lens scleral indentation. An asymptomatic fellow eye should always be examined; if 10 or more vitreous cells are present in a 1 mm slit lamp field the incidence of a retinal break in a fellow asymptomatic eye has been reported as over 30%.

- **Subsequent management.** Recommendations for review vary and the following is a general guide.
  - If there are no suspicious findings (e.g. vitreous blood) on examination and no pre-existing risk factors as discussed above then routine review may not be necessary; the presence of features associated with higher risk should lead to review after an interval of 1–6 weeks depending on individual characteristics. Some authorities recommend further review in 6–12 months.
  - Patients who present with multiple prominent floaters or hazy vision should be reviewed carefully as this has been found to be associated with a higher risk of retinal break.

- Discharged patients should be given clear instructions emphasizing the need to re-attend urgently in the event of significant new symptoms; optimally, written information reiterating the advice should be provided. Assurance can be given that in most cases the floaters will resolve and become much less noticeable with time, though exceptionally vitrectomy is necessary.
- If an area of the fundus cannot be viewed clearly due to obscuration by blood then weekly review is prudent.
- Presentation with diffuse fundus-obscuring vitreous haemorrhage (in the absence of a condition predisposing to non-PVD vitreous haemorrhage) is associated with a very high risk of retinal break (90%) and retinal detachment (40%). A relative afferent pupillary defect should be excluded, and B-scan ultrasonography performed regularly until resolution in order to exclude an underlying detachment or identifiable break. A very low threshold for vitrectomy should be adopted,

particularly in the presence of other risk factors, notably prior RD in the fellow eye.
  ○ The management of retinal breaks is discussed below.

RETINAL BREAKS

Introduction

Retinal breaks develop in most cases as a result of traction at sites of vitreoretinal adhesion, and occur in up to about 1 in 5 eyes with symptomatic PVD. In the presence of a break, retrohyaloid fluid has access to the subretinal space. Asymptomatic retinal breaks of some sort are present in about 8% of the general population.

Clinical features

- **Timing.** Breaks are usually present at or soon after the onset of symptoms of PVD, although in a significant minority (up to 5%) tear formation may be delayed by several weeks.
- **Location.** Tears associated with PVD are usually located in the upper fundus and are more commonly temporal than nasal. Macular breaks related to PVD are rare, but when they occur are usually round and in a myopic eye; they are aetiologically distinct from age-related macular holes.
- **Morphology.** Retinal breaks may be flat or associated with a surrounding cuff of SRF. If fluid extends more than one disc diameter from the edge of a break, a retinal detachment is said to be present.
  ○ U-tears (horseshoe) consist of a flap, its apex pulled anteriorly by the vitreous, the base remaining attached to the retina (Fig. 16.24A).
  ○ Operculated tears in which the flap is completely torn away from the retina by detached vitreous gel to leave a round or oval break (Fig. 16.24B); the separated retinal patch is known as an operculum and can usually be seen suspended in the vitreous cavity in the region of the break, which can be difficult to delineate – this may be aided by the presence of preretinal blood at the site.
  ○ Retinal holes (Fig. 16.24C) are round or oval, usually smaller than tears and carry a lower risk of RD, which when it does occur is most commonly a slowly progressive shallow RD in a young female myope. A PVD is not necessarily present, but if vitreous separation has occurred an operculum may be visible in the nearby vitreous cavity. Round holes may occur in lattice degeneration. Round holes leading to RD may be distinct in most cases from the round atrophic retinal holes that are a variant of paving stone degeneration and probably carry a lower risk, though clinically distinction is commonly not possible.
  ○ Dialyses are circumferential tears along the ora serrata; vitreous gel remains attached to the posterior margin. They can cause RD, often slowly progressive, in the absence of a PVD, and can result from blunt ocular trauma. They typically appear as large very peripheral breaks with a regular rolled edge (Fig. 16.24D).
  ○ Giant retinal tears (Fig. 16.24E and F) are a variant of U-tear, by definition involving 90° or more of the retinal circumference. In contrast to dialysis, vitreous gel remains attached to the anterior margin of the break. They are most frequently located in the immediate post-oral retina or, less commonly, at the equator.

Management

The management of many categories of break remains imperfectly defined, and approaches differ between retinal subspecialists, according to locally available resources and taking into account general patient considerations such as the likelihood of attendance for review. There has broadly been a trend in recent years towards less aggressive prophylactic treatment of asymptomatic and operculated breaks, with substitution by observation and patient education. Patients should always be instructed about the symptoms of vitreous and retinal detachment, optimally supplemented by written information, and should seek review urgently in the event of new features. The risk of prophylaxis is usually very small but include new break formation; very severe complications have exceptionally been reported.

- **Risk factors for progression to detachment**
  ○ Miscellaneous factors include a history of RD in the fellow eye, prior cataract surgery (particularly if vitreous loss occurred), myopia, a family history of RD and systemic conditions such as Marfan, Stickler and Ehlers–Danlos syndromes. Evidence suggests that prophylactic treatment should be considered for asymptomatic breaks, including round operculated and atrophic holes prior to cataract surgery, laser capsulotomy and possibly trabeculectomy and intravitreal injection, particularly when other risk factors are present.
  ○ Symptomatic breaks associated with an acute PVD are higher risk than asymptomatic breaks detected on routine examination.
  ○ Size. Larger breaks carry a higher risk of progression.
  ○ Persistent vitreoretinal traction. An operculated tear, in which the focus of vitreous traction has detached from the break, is safer than a break, typically a U-tear, in which traction persists; round holes are rarely associated with ongoing vitreoretinal traction. Apparent demonstration of a complete PVD clinically or on ultrasonography, with no residual attachment in the region of the break, is a favourable feature, though cannot be relied upon.
  ○ Shape. U-tears are higher risk than round holes.
  ○ Location. Superior breaks are at higher risk of progression to RD, probably due to the protective effect of gravity upon inferior breaks. With superotemporal tears, the macula is threatened early in the event of RD. Equatorial breaks are more likely to progress than oral breaks, as the latter are usually located within the vitreous base.
  ○ Pigmentation around a retinal break indicates chronicity and a degree of stability.
  ○ Aphakia, now rare, confers a higher risk.

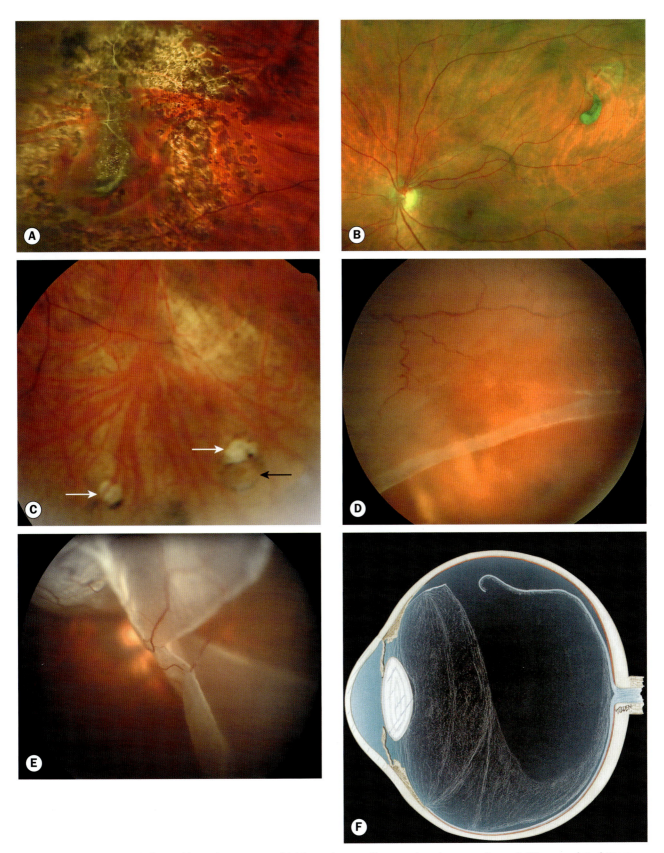

Fig. 16.24 Retinal tears. **(A)** Large U-tear in an area of lattice – laser retinopexy has been performed; **(B)** operculated tear; **(C)** round holes; the white arrows show probable atrophic holes, the black arrow shows a probable operculated hole with localized subretinal fluid; **(D)** retinal dialysis; **(E)** giant retinal tear; **(F)** vitreous attached to the anterior edge of a giant tear

(Courtesy of S Chen – figs A and B; N Turner – fig. C; C Barry – figs D and E; CL Schepens, ME Hartnett and T Hirose, from Schepens' Retinal Detachment and Allied Diseases, *Butterworth-Heinemann 2000 – fig. F)*

- **Acutely symptomatic U-tears.** Up to 90% of these lead to retinal detachment; treatment (see below) reduces the risk to 5% so should always be performed urgently.
- **Operculated tears,** particularly if asymptomatic, are believed to generally have a very low risk of progression to RD, and can safely be observed in most cases. A recommended review schedule (symptomatic or asymptomatic) is an initial interval of 2–4 weeks, then 1–3 months, then 6–12 months, then annually. The presence of an intact bridging vessel overlying the break may indicate ongoing vitreoretinal traction – which may also cause vitreous haemorrhage – and treatment should be considered. Higher-risk factors may prompt treatment in an individual case.
- **Asymptomatic U-tears.** The risk of progression to RD is low at 5%, which is a similar rate to that in treated symptomatic U-tears, and observation as for operculated tears is generally safe in the absence of factors indicating higher risk.
- **Traumatic retinal breaks,** including acute dialyses, should always be treated.
- **Asymptomatic dialyses** are sometimes observed, but in most cases are treated surgically if an associated RD is present.
- **Asymptomatic subclinical RD.** Progression is not invariable in RD discovered incidentally, with perhaps 10% becoming symptomatic over 2–3 years, and a decision regarding intervention should be made on a case-by-case basis; for example, many practitioners would prefer to treat rather than observe a large superotemporal RD that extends posterior to the equator, but may observe a small inferior longstanding-appearing RD. With any option, fully informed patient consent is vital. If observation is elected, appropriate review and careful patient advice are critical. Surgery is generally indicated if progression occurs.
- **Asymptomatic flat round holes** do not require prophylactic treatment, but some guidelines recommend review every 1–2 years.
- **Long-term review** after treatment of retinal breaks may be important, as a significant minority of index and fellow eyes will develop further breaks.

Treatment techniques

Retinal breaks without RD can be treated with laser (via a slit lamp or BIO) or cryotherapy. In most cases laser is the optimal technique as it is more precise, causing less collateral retinal damage, with a likely lower risk of epiretinal membrane formation. Adequate treatment of the base of a very peripheral lesion may only be possible with BIO or cryotherapy due to the requirement for indentation to visualize the area, unless the practitioner is skilled at slit lamp indentation. Cryotherapy may be preferred for multiple contiguous tears or extensive lesions, and in eyes with hazy media or small pupils.

- **Laser retinopexy.** Using slit lamp delivery under topical anaesthesia (occasionally regional or even general anaesthesia is required), typical settings are a duration of 0.1 second, a spot size of 200–300 μm with a three-mirror contact lens or 100–200 μm with a wide-field lens, and a

starting power of 200 mW; the power should be adjusted as appropriate to obtain moderate blanching. With head-mounted BIO delivery, the spot size is estimated and adjusted by adjusting the condensing lens (usually 20 D) position. The lesion is surrounded with two to three rows of confluent burns (Fig. 16.25). With both forms of laser, care should be taken to identify appropriate landmarks frequently to avoid inadvertent macular damage.

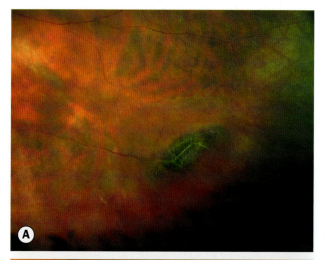

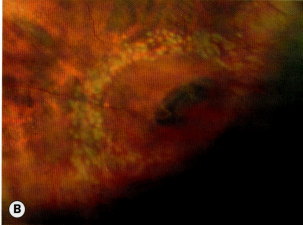

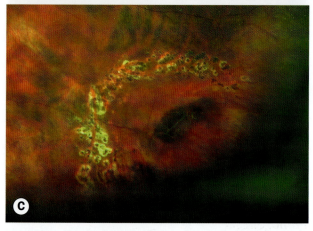

Fig. 16.25 Laser retinopexy. **(A)** U-tear in lattice prior to, **(B)** immediately following and **(C)** 2 months after laser *(Courtesy of S Chen)*

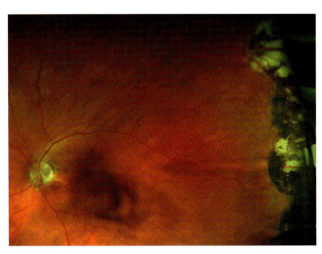

Fig. 16.26 Pigmentation and chorioretinal atrophy following prophylactic cryotherapy to several retinal breaks
(Courtesy of B Elia)

- **Cryoretinopexy.** Subconjunctival or regional anaesthesia is commonly required. For lesions behind the equator, a small conjunctival incision may be necessary for access. A lid speculum is used. The cryotherapy probe tip must be exposed beyond its rubber sleeve. The instrument should initially be purged (e.g. 10 seconds at −25 °C, repeating after a minute). The treatment temperature is set (typically −85 °C); it is useful to check the effectiveness of the instrument by activating it in sterile water for 10 seconds, when a 5 mm ice ball should form. Under BIO visualization, the lesion is indented and the foot pedal depressed until visible whitening of the retina is seen. It is critical not to remove the tip from the treated area until thawing is allowed (2–3 seconds). Care should be taken to maintain orientation of the probe whilst the tip is not visible, and not to mistake indentation by the shaft of the probe for that of the tip. The lesion is surrounded by a single row of applications, in most cases achieved by one or two applications to a tear. The eye is usually padded afterwards; analgesia is commonly necessary.
- **After treatment** the patient should avoid strenuous physical exertion for about a week until an adequate adhesion has formed (Fig. 16.26); review should usually take place after 1–2 weeks.

RHEGMATOGENOUS RETINAL DETACHMENT

Introduction

Pathogenesis

Rhegmatogenous RD affects about 1 in 10 000 of the population each year, with both eyes eventually affected in about 10%. In most cases it is characterized by the presence of a retinal break in concert with vitreoretinal traction that allows accumulation of liquefied vitreous under the neurosensory retina, separating it from the RPE. Even though a retinal break is present, a RD will almost never occur if the vitreous is not at least partially liquefied and traction is absent. Over 40% of RDs occur in myopic eyes; the higher the refractive error the greater the risk of RD. Vitreous degeneration and PVD, and predisposing lesions such as lattice and snailtrack degeneration, are more common in myopia. Highly myopic eyes are also at risk from RD due to small round holes in chorioretinal atrophy and from macular holes. Vitreous loss during cataract surgery, and laser capsulotomy, also carry a higher risk of RD in highly myopic eyes.

Identification of retinal breaks

- **Distribution of breaks** in eyes with RD is approximately as follows: 60% superotemporal quadrant, 15% superonasal, 15% inferotemporal and 10% inferonasal. The upper temporal region should therefore be examined in detail if a break cannot be detected initially. It should also be remembered that about 50% of eyes with RD have more than one break, often within 90° of each other.
- **Configuration of SRF.** SRF spread is governed by gravity, by anatomical limits (ora serrata and optic nerve) and by the location of the primary retinal break. If the primary break is located superiorly, the SRF first spreads inferiorly on the same side of the fundus as the break and then superiorly on the opposite side, so that the likely location of the primary retinal break can be predicted (modified from Lincoff's rules):
  - A shallow inferior RD in which the SRF is slightly higher on the temporal side points to a primary break located inferiorly on that side (Fig. 16.27A).
  - A primary break located at 6 o'clock will cause an inferior RD with equal fluid levels (Fig. 16.27B).
  - In a bullous inferior RD the primary break usually lies above the horizontal meridian (Fig. 16.27C).
  - If the primary break is located in the upper nasal quadrant the SRF will revolve around the optic disc and then rise on the temporal side until it is level with the primary break (Fig. 16.27D).
  - A subtotal RD with a superior wedge of attached retina points to a primary break located in the periphery nearest its highest border (Fig. 16.27E).
  - When the SRF crosses the vertical midline above, the primary break is near to 12 o'clock, the lower edge of the RD corresponding to the side of the break (Fig. 16.27F).

Symptoms

The classic premonitory symptoms reported in about 60% of patients with spontaneous rhegmatogenous RD are flashing lights and floaters associated with acute PVD. After a variable period of time a curtain-like relative peripheral visual field defect may ensue, and can progress to involve central vision; in some patients this may not be present on waking in the morning, due to spontaneous

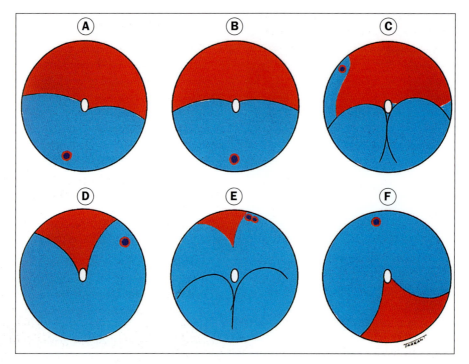

Fig. 16.27 Distribution of subretinal fluid in relation to the location of the primary retinal break (see text)

absorption of SRF while inactive overnight, only to reappear later in the day. A lower field defect is usually appreciated more quickly by the patient than an upper defect. The quadrant of the visual field in which the field defect first appears is useful in predicting the location of the primary retinal break, which will be in the opposite quadrant; the location of photopsia is of no value in predicting the site of the primary break; flashes are virtually always temporal. Loss of central vision may be due to involvement of the fovea by SRF or, infrequently, obstruction of the visual axis by a large bullous RD.

Signs

General

- **Relative afferent pupillary defect** (Marcus Gunn pupil) is present in an eye with an extensive RD.
- **Intraocular pressure (IOP)** is often lower by about 5 mmHg compared with the normal eye. If the intraocular pressure is extremely low, an associated choroidal detachment may be present. It may be raised, characteristically in Schwartz–Matsuo syndrome in which RRD is associated with an apparent mild anterior uveitis, often due to a dialysis due to prior blunt trauma in a young man; the aqueous cells are believed in most cases actually to be displaced photoreceptor outer segments that compromise trabecular outflow. Both the aqueous 'cells' and the elevated IOP typically resolve following repair of the RD.
- **Iritis** is very common but usually mild and should be differentiated from Schwartz–Matsuo syndrome (above).

Occasionally it may be severe enough to cause posterior synechiae; the underlying RD may be overlooked.
- **'Tobacco dust'** consisting of pigment cells is commonly seen in the anterior vitreous (Fig. 16.28); substantial vitreous blood or inflammatory cells are also highly specific.
- **Retinal breaks** (see Fig. 16.24) appear as discontinuities in the retinal surface. They are usually red because of the

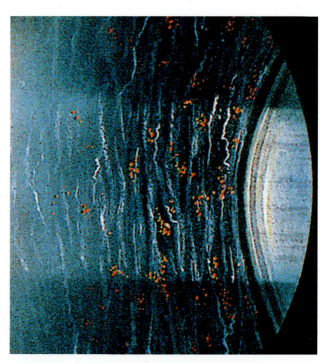

Fig. 16.28 'Tobacco dust' in the anterior vitreous

colour contrast between the sensory retina and underlying choroid. However, in eyes with hypopigmented choroid (e.g. high myopia), the colour contrast is decreased and small breaks may be overlooked.

- **Retinal signs** depend on the duration of RD and the presence or absence of proliferative vitreoretinopathy (PVR) as described below.

Fresh retinal detachment

- **The RD** has a convex configuration and a slightly opaque and corrugated appearance as a result of retinal oedema (Figs 16.29A–D). There is loss of the underlying choroidal pattern and retinal blood vessels appear darker than in flat retina.

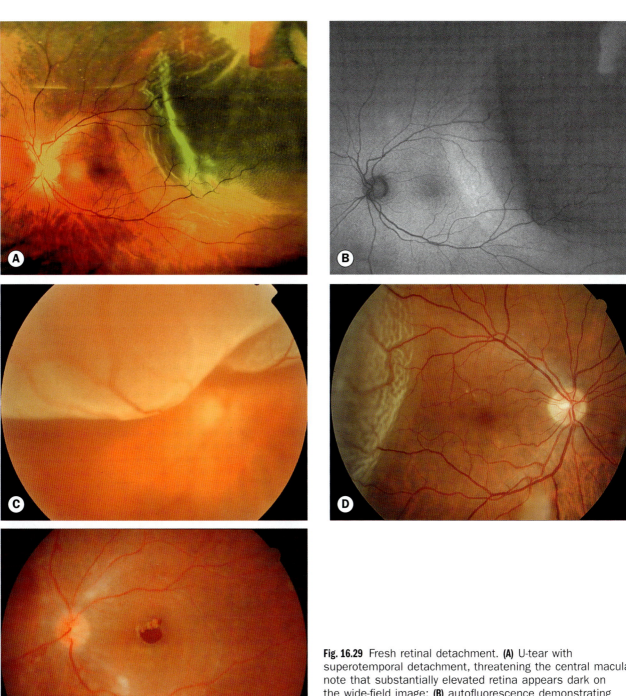

Fig. 16.29 Fresh retinal detachment. **(A)** U-tear with superotemporal detachment, threatening the central macula; note that substantially elevated retina appears dark on the wide-field image; **(B)** autofluorescence demonstrating extent of fluid spread; **(C)** superior bullous detachment; **(D)** typical corrugated appearance of detached retina; **(E)** macular hole surrounded by shallow subretinal fluid confined to the posterior pole

(Courtesy of S Chen – figs A, B and D; M Khairallah – fig. E)

- **SRF** extends up to the ora serrata, except in the rare cases caused by a macular hole in which fluid is initially confined to the posterior pole (Fig. 16.29E).
- **Macular pseudohole**. Because of the thinness of the foveal retina, the impression of a macular hole may be given if the posterior pole is detached. This should not be mistaken for a true macular hole, which may give rise to RD in highly myopic eyes or following blunt trauma.
- **B-scan ultrasonography** shows good mobility of the retina and vitreous (see Fig. 16.10).

Long-standing retinal detachment

- **Retinal thinning** secondary to atrophy is a characteristic finding, and should not lead to a misdiagnosis of retinoschisis.
- **Intraretinal cysts** (Fig. 16.30A–C) may develop if the RD has been present for about 1 year; these tend to disappear after retinal reattachment.
- **Subretinal demarcation lines** ('high water' or 'tide' marks) caused by proliferation of RPE cells at the junction of flat

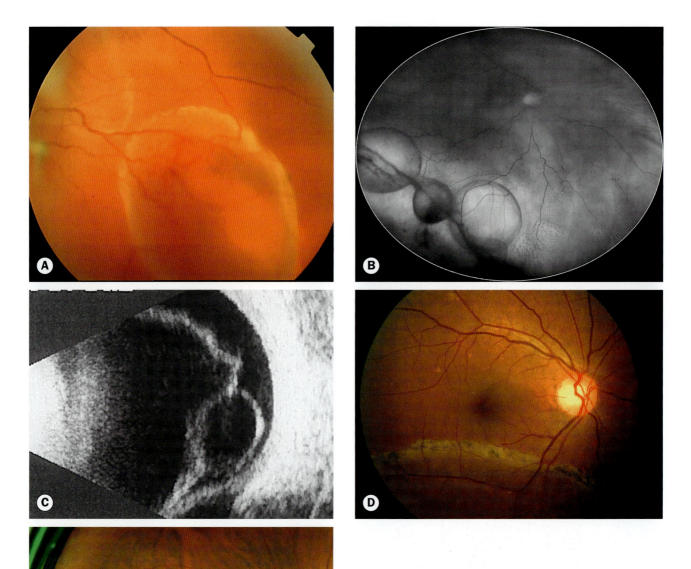

Fig. 16.30 Long-standing retinal detachment. **(A)** Retinal cysts; **(B)** multiple cysts in chronic total detachment (red-free wide-field image); **(C)** B-scan ultrasonogram demonstrating cyst; **(D)** demarcation line; **(E)** demarcation line surrounding localized fluid associated with a small round asymptomatic hole (wide-field image)

(Courtesy of C Barry – fig. B; RF Spaide, from Diseases of the Retina and Vitreous, WB Saunders 1999 – fig. C; S Chen – fig. D; S Lorenzon – fig. E)

and detached retina (Fig. 16.30D and E) are common, taking about 3 months to develop. Pigmentation tends to decrease over time. Although representing sites of increased adhesion, they do not invariably limit the spread of SRF.

Proliferative vitreoretinopathy

Proliferative vitreoretinopathy (PVR) is caused by epiretinal and subretinal membrane formation, contraction of which leads to tangential retinal traction and fixed retinal fold formation (Fig. 16.31). Usually, PVR occurs following surgery for rhegmatogenous RD or penetrating injury, though it may also occur in eyes with rhegmatogenous RD that have not had previous retinal surgery. The main features are retinal folds and rigidity so that retinal mobility induced by eye movements or scleral indentation is decreased. Progression from one stage to the next is not inevitable.

- **Grade A** (minimal) PVR is characterized by diffuse vitreous haze and tobacco dust. There may also be pigmented clumps

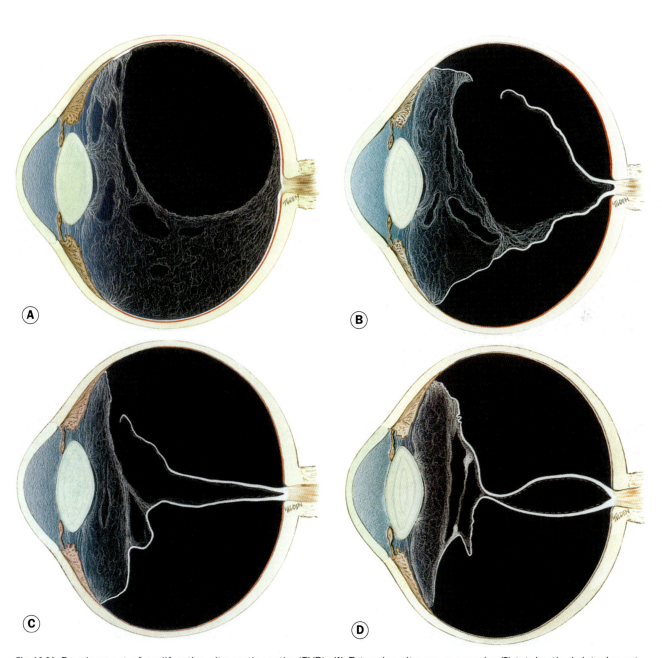

Fig. 16.31 Development of proliferative vitreoretinopathy (PVR). **(A)** Extensive vitreous syneresis; **(B)** total retinal detachment without PVR; shrunken vitreous is condensed and attached to the equator of the retina; **(C)** early PVR with anteriorly retracted vitreous gel and equatorial circumferential retinal folds; **(D)** advanced PVR with a funnel-like retinal detachment bridged by dense vitreous membranes

(Courtesy of CL Schepens, ME Hartnett and T Hirose, from Schepens' Retinal Detachment and Allied Diseases, *Butterworth-Heinemann 2000)*

on the inferior surface of the retina. Although these findings occur in many eyes with RD, they are particularly severe in eyes with early PVR.

- **Grade B** (moderate) PVR is characterized by wrinkling of the inner retinal surface (Fig. 16.32A), decreased mobility of vitreous gel, rolled edges of retinal breaks, tortuosity of blood vessels and retinal stiffness (Fig. 16.32B). The epiretinal membranes responsible for these findings typically cannot be identified clinically.
- **Grade C** (marked) PVR is characterized by rigid full-thickness retinal folds (often star-shaped) with heavy vitreous condensation and strands (Fig. 16.32C and D). It can be either anterior (A) or posterior (P), the approximate dividing line being the equator of the globe. The severity of proliferation in each area is expressed by the number of clock hours of retina involved although proliferations need not be contiguous.
- **Advanced disease** shows gross reduction of retinal mobility with retinal shortening and a characteristic funnel-like triangular conformation (see Fig. 16.31D).

Differential diagnosis

The tractional and exudative forms of RD are described later in the chapter.

Degenerative retinoschisis

See above.

Choroidal detachment

Causes of choroidal detachment (also known as ciliochoroidal or choroidal effusion) include hypotony, particularly following glaucoma drainage surgery (see Ch. 10), sulfa drugs such as acetazolamide and topiramate, uveitis, posterior scleritis, choroidal tumours and a cyclodialysis cleft following trauma (including surgical); occasionally it occurs secondary to retinal detachment. Idiopathic cases are generally labelled as uveal effusion syndrome (see below).

- **Symptoms.** Photopsia and floaters are absent because there is no vitreoretinal traction. A visual field defect

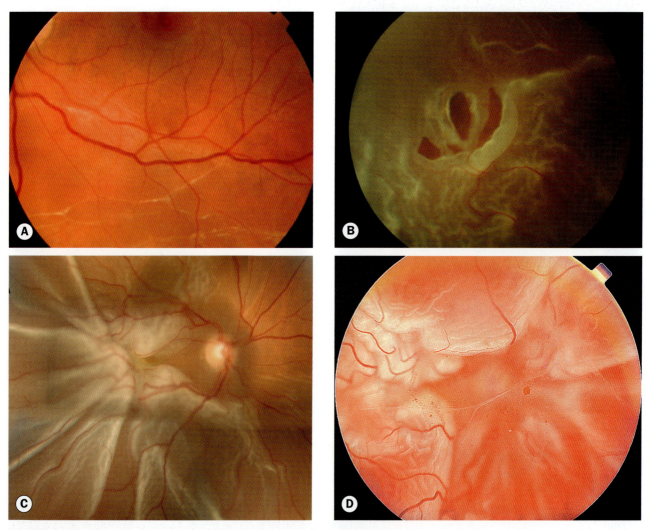

Fig. 16.32 Proliferative vitreoretinopathy (PVR). **(A)** Early retinal wrinkling in minimal grade B; **(B)** marked grade B with rolled retinal break edges; **(C)** grade C with prominent star fold; **(D)** grade C with characteristic funnel-shaped detachment

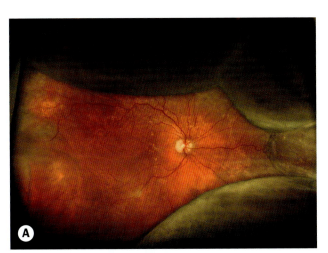

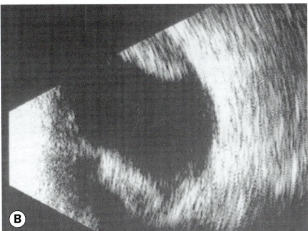

Fig. 16.33 Choroidal effusion. **(A)** Effusion secondary to hypotony associated with a cyclodialysis cleft; **(B)** B-scan showing limitation of posterior fluid spread by the vortex veins

(Courtesy of S Chen – fig. A; R Bates – fig. B)

Uveal effusion syndrome

The uveal effusion syndrome is a rare idiopathic, often bilateral, condition that most frequently affects middle-aged hypermetropic men but can occur in association with nanophthalmos. The cause is thought to be impairment of normal fluid drainage from the choroid via the sclera (which is sometimes of abnormal thickness and composition) or vortex veins.

- **Signs**
  - Inflammation is absent or mild.
  - Ciliochoroidal detachment followed by exudative RD.
  - Following resolution, the RPE frequently shows a characteristic residual 'leopard spot' mottling caused by degenerative changes in the RPE associated with a high concentration of protein in the SRF.
- **Differential diagnosis** includes uveal effusion secondary to other causes (see above), choroidal haemorrhage and ring melanoma of the anterior choroid.
- **Treatment** is usually with full-thickness sclerectomies; pars plana vitrectomy alone may also be successful, but sclerectomies are usually first-line in nanophthalmos.

Surgery

Indications for urgent surgery

In general, an acutely symptomatic RD should be operatively repaired urgently, particularly if the macula is as yet uninvolved (Fig. 16.34). Other factors that may increase the urgency of intervention include the presence of a superior or large break, from which SRF is likely to spread more rapidly, and advanced syneresis as in myopia. Patients with dense fresh vitreous haemorrhage in whom visualization of the fundus is impossible should also be operated on as soon as possible if B-scan ultrasonography shows

may be noticed if the choroidal detachment is extensive.

- **Signs**
  - Low intraocular pressure is common as a result of the cause and of concomitant detachment of the ciliary body.
  - The anterior chamber may be shallow in eyes with extensive choroidal detachments; non-pupillary block angle closure can occur.
  - The elevations are brown, convex, smooth and relatively immobile (Fig. 16.33A). Four lobes are typically present; temporal and nasal bullae tend to be most prominent.
  - Large 'kissing' choroidal detachments may obscure the view of the fundus.
  - The elevations do not extend to the posterior pole because they are limited by the vortex veins entering their scleral canals (Fig. 16.33B); however, in contrast to retinal detachments they extend anteriorly beyond the ora serrata.
- **Treatment** is directed at the cause; drainage via partial-thickness sclerectomies is occasionally required.

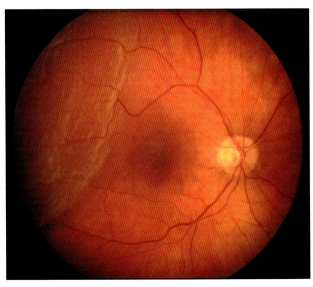

Fig. 16.34 Superotemporal retinal detachment with intact but imminently threatened macula, requiring urgent repair

(Courtesy of P Saine)

an underlying RD. When an RD likely to require an urgent operation is diagnosed or suspected, it is important that the patient does not eat or drink in the hours before assessment so that surgery is not delayed. Minimizing activity may be helpful, and some authorities advocate bed rest with the head turned so that the retinal break is in the most dependent position, which may lessen the amount of SRF and facilitate surgery.

Pneumatic retinopexy

Pneumatic retinopexy (Fig. 16.35) is an outpatient procedure in which an intravitreal gas bubble together with cryotherapy or laser are used to seal a retinal break and reattach the retina without scleral buckling. The most frequently used gases are sulfur hexafluoride (SF_6) and the longer-acting perfluoropropane (C_3F_8). It has the advantage of being a relatively quick, minimally invasive, 'office-based' procedure. However, success rates are usually worse than those achievable with conventional scleral buckling. The procedure is usually reserved for treatment of uncomplicated RD with a small retinal break or a cluster of breaks extending over an area of less than two clock hours in the upper two-thirds of the peripheral retina.

Principles of scleral buckling

Scleral buckling, sometimes referred to as conventional or external RD surgery as opposed to the internal approach of pars plana vitrectomy (see below), is a surgical procedure in which material sutured onto the sclera (explant – Fig. 16.36A) creates an inward indentation (buckle – Figs 16.36B and C). Its purposes are to close retinal breaks by apposing the RPE to the sensory retina, and to reduce dynamic vitreoretinal traction at sites of local vitreoretinal adhesion.

- **Explants** are made from soft or hard silicone. The entire break should ideally be surrounded by about 2 mm of buckle. It is also important for the buckle to involve the area of the vitreous base anterior to the tear in order to prevent the possibility of subsequent reopening of the tear and anterior leakage of SRF. The dimensions of the retinal break can be assessed by comparing it with the diameter of the optic disc.
- **Buckle configuration** can be radial, segmental, circumferential or encircling, depending on the size, configuration and number of breaks.
- **Technique.** The conjunctiva is incised (peritomy) to facilitate access, following which retinal breaks are localized and cryotherapy applied. An explant of appropriate dimensions and orientation is then sutured to the sclera and the position of the buckle checked in relation to the break.

Drainage of subretinal fluid

Drainage of SRF via the sclera (e.g. the D-ACE: Drainage-Air-Cryotherapy-Explant) surgical technique (Fig. 16.37A) is advocated by many practitioners, citing more rapid retinal reattachment

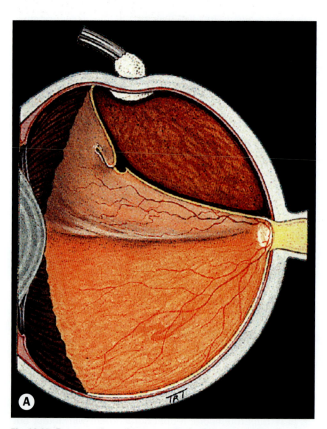

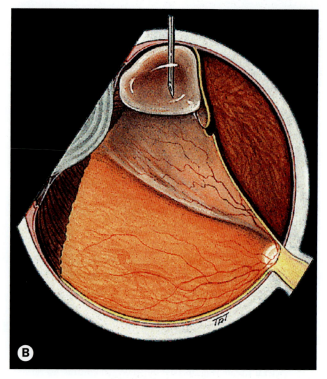

Fig. 16.35 Pneumatic retinopexy. **(A)** Cryotherapy; **(B)** gas injection;

Continued

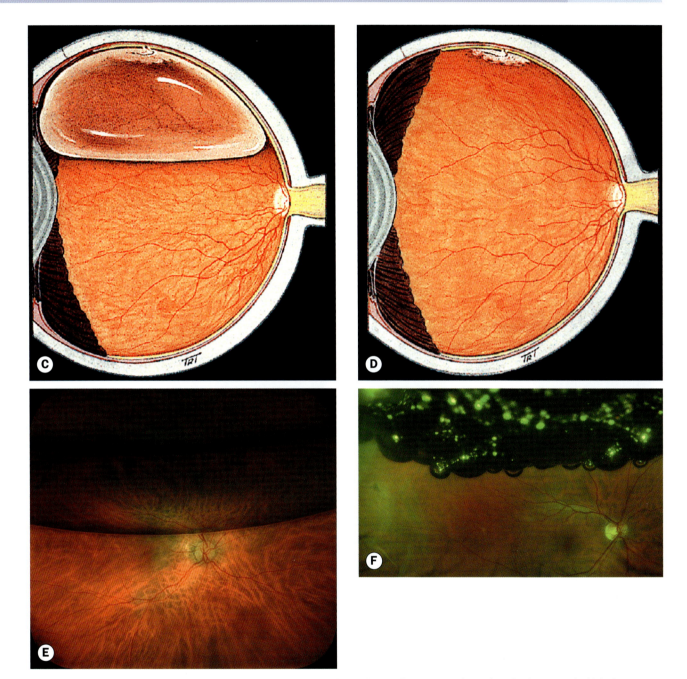

Fig. 16.35, Continued (C) gas has sealed the retinal break and the retina is flat; **(D)** gas has absorbed; **(E)** gas bubble in vitreous cavity; **(F)** 'fish eggs' due to gas bubble break-up
(Courtesy of S Chen – figs E and F)

in the presence of deep or long-standing viscous SRF; other authorities prefer to avoid external drainage due to its potential complications such as retinal perforation or incarceration in the drainage site (Fig. 16.37B) and choroidal haemorrhage, and would perform a pars plana vitrectomy in such cases.

Complications of scleral buckling

- **Diplopia** due to the mechanical effect of the buckle is very common. Early spontaneous resolution is typical, though intervention is sometimes necessary.

- **Cystoid macular oedema** occurs in up to 25%, but usually responds to treatment. Other macular complications include epiretinal membrane (around 15%), persistent subfoveal fluid and foveal structural disruption, usually in macular-off detachments.

- **Anterior segment ischaemia** due to vascular compromise. This is a particular risk with an encircling band, and with predisposing systemic conditions such as sickle haemoglobinopathies.

- **Buckle extrusion, intrusion or infection** (Figs 16.38A and B). Removal is usually required, with aggressive antibacterial therapy as indicated.

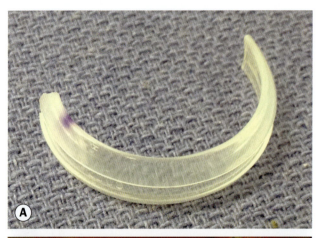

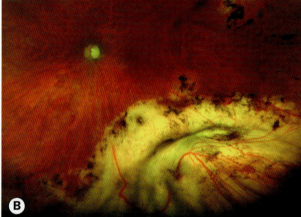

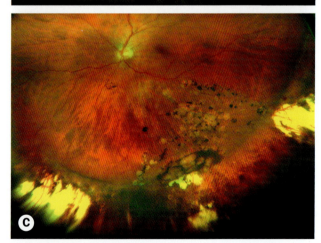

Fig. 16.36 Scleral buckling. **(A)** Circumferential explant; **(B)** buckle induced by radial explant; **(C)** buckle induced by circumferential explant

(Courtesy of S Chen – figs A and B; H Notaras – fig. C)

configuration of the RD does not correspond to the position of the primary break.

○ Buckle failure may occur due to inadequate size, incorrect positioning (Fig. 16.38C), or inadequate height; the explant may have to be replaced or repositioned to address the first two, but drainage of SRF or intravitreal gas injection may suffice for the latter, though pars plana vitrectomy (PPV) may be preferred as a more definitive measure. 'Fish-mouthing' (Fig. 16.38D) describes the phenomenon of a tear, typically a large superior equatorial U-tear in a bullous RD, to open widely following scleral buckling, requiring further operative treatment.

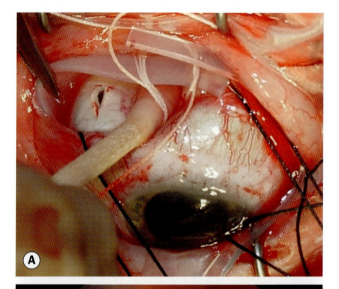

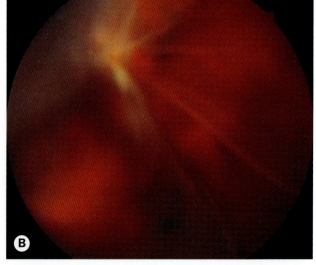

Fig. 16.37 Drainage of subretinal fluid during scleral buckling. **(A)** A circumferential explant is visible but has not yet been tightened into place. A cotton-tipped applicator is being used to apply pressure to encourage fluid drainage from the sclerotomy (incision to the left of the applicator); **(B)** retinal incarceration into the drainage site

(Courtesy of S Chen)

- **Elevated IOP.** Early IOP spikes usually resolve rapidly, but occasionally persist. Angle closure can occur.
- **Choroidal detachment** usually resolves spontaneously, presumably as scleral oedema settles and allows improved vortex vein function.
- **Surgical failure**
  ○ Missed breaks. A thorough search should always be made for the presence of multiple breaks, particularly if the

○ Proliferative vitreoretinopathy is the most common cause of late failure. The tractional forces associated with PVR can occasionally open old breaks and create new ones. Presentation is typically several weeks postoperatively with re-detachment.

○ Reopening of a retinal break in the absence of PVR can occur as a result of inadequate cryotherapy or scleral buckling, or sometimes when buckle height decreases either with time or following late surgical removal.

Pars plana vitrectomy

Pars plana vitrectomy (PPV) is discussed later in this chapter.

TRACTIONAL RETINAL DETACHMENT

The main causes of tractional RD are proliferative retinopathy such as diabetic and retinopathy of prematurity, and penetrating posterior segment trauma (see Ch. 21).

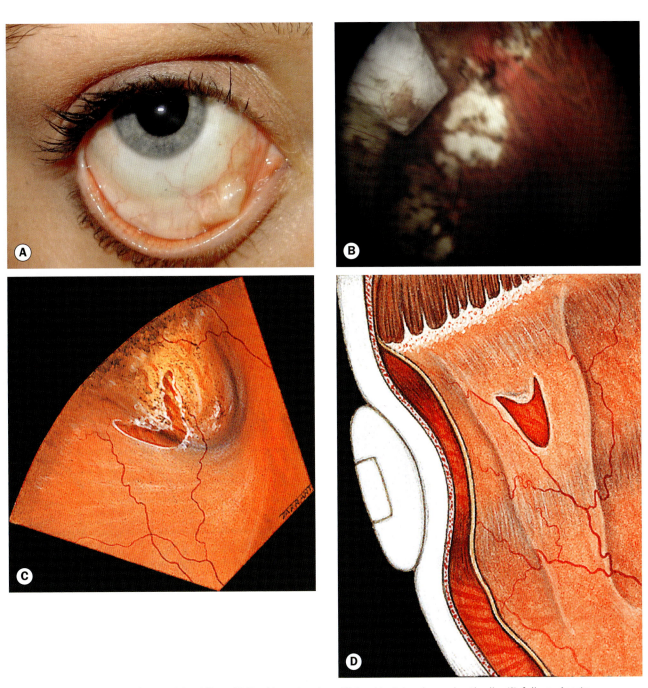

Fig. 16.38 Complications of scleral buckling. **(A)** Buckle extrusion; **(B)** buckle intrusion subretinally; **(C)** failure due to incorrectly positioned buckle; **(D)** 'fish-mouthing' of a U-tear communicating with a radial retinal fold

(Courtesy of S Chen – figs A and B)

Pathogenesis of diabetic tractional retinal detachment

Tractional RD is caused by progressive contraction of fibrovascular membranes over large areas of vitreoretinal adhesion. In contrast to acute PVD in eyes with rhegmatogenous RD, PVD in diabetic eyes is gradual and frequently incomplete. It is thought to be caused by leakage of plasma constituents into the vitreous gel from a fibrovascular network adherent to the posterior vitreous surface. Owing to the strong adhesions of the cortical vitreous to areas of fibrovascular proliferation, PVD is usually incomplete. In the rare event of a subsequent complete PVD, the new blood vessels are avulsed and RD does not develop. Vitreoretinal traction can be (i) tangential, caused by the contraction of epiretinal fibrovascular membranes with puckering of the retina and distortion of blood vessels, (ii) anteroposterior, due to the contraction of fibrovascular membranes extending from the posterior retina, usually in association with the major arcades, to the vitreous base anteriorly, and/or (iii) bridging (trampoline), the result of contraction of fibrovascular membranes stretching from one part of the retina to another or between vascular arcades, tending to pull the two involved points together (Fig. 16.39).

Diagnosis

- **Symptoms.** Photopsia and floaters are usually absent because vitreoretinal traction develops insidiously and is not associated with acute PVD. A visual field defect usually progresses slowly and may be stable for months or even years.

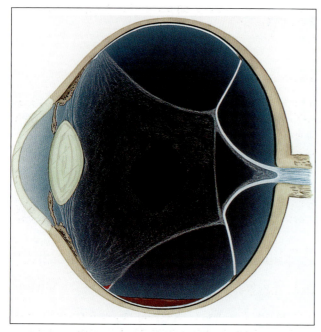

Fig. 16.39 Tractional retinal detachment associated with anteroposterior and bridging traction
(Courtesy of CL Schepens, ME Hartnett and T Hirose, from Schepens' Retinal Detachment and Allied Diseases, Butterworth-Heinemann 2000)

- **Signs** (Figs 16.40A–C)
  - The RD has a concave configuration and breaks are absent.
  - Retinal mobility is severely reduced and shifting fluid is absent.
  - The SRF is shallower than in a rhegmatogenous RD and seldom extends to the ora serrata.
  - The highest elevation of the retina occurs at sites of vitreoretinal traction.
  - If a tractional RD develops a break it assumes the characteristics of a rhegmatogenous RD and progresses rapidly (combined tractional–rhegmatogenous RD).
- **B-scan ultrasonography** shows incomplete posterior vitreous detachment and a relatively immobile retina (Fig. 16.40D).

EXUDATIVE RETINAL DETACHMENT

Pathogenesis

Exudative RD is characterized by the accumulation of SRF in the absence of retinal breaks or traction. It may occur in a variety of vascular, inflammatory and neoplastic diseases involving the retina, RPE and choroid in which fluid leaks outside the vessels and accumulates under the retina. As long as the RPE is able to compensate by pumping the leaking fluid into the choroidal circulation, RD does not occur. However, when the mechanism is overwhelmed or functions subnormally, fluid accumulates in the subretinal space. Causes include:

- **Choroidal tumours** such as melanomas, haemangiomas and metastases; it is therefore very important to consider that exudative RD is caused by an intraocular tumour until proved otherwise.
- **Inflammation** such as Harada disease and posterior scleritis.
- **Bullous central serous chorioretinopathy** is a rare cause.
- **Iatrogenic causes** include retinal detachment surgery and panretinal photocoagulation.
- **Choroidal neovascularization** which may leak and give rise to extensive subretinal accumulation of fluid at the posterior pole.
- **Hypertensive choroidopathy**, as may occur in toxaemia of pregnancy, is a very rare cause.
- **Idiopathic**, such as uveal effusion syndrome (see above).

Diagnosis

- **Symptoms.** Depending on the cause, both eyes may be involved simultaneously.
  - There is no vitreoretinal traction, so photopsia is absent.
  - Floaters may be present if there is associated vitritis.
  - A visual field defect may develop suddenly and progress rapidly.

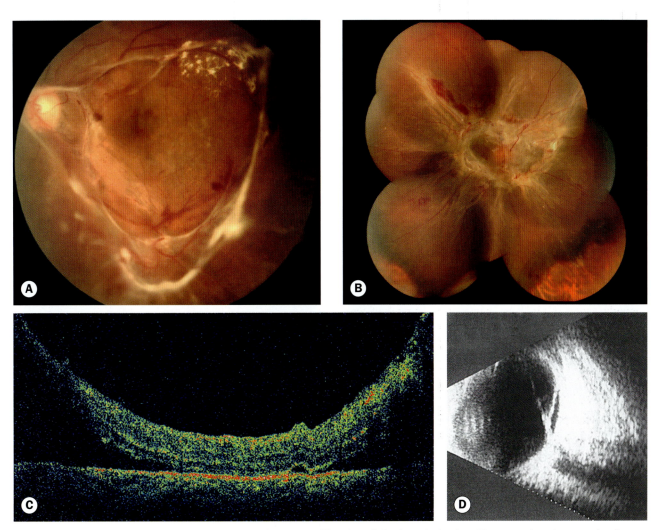

Fig. 16.40 Tractional retinal detachment. **(A)** Secondary to proliferative diabetic retinopathy; **(B)** composite photograph of severe tractional detachment; **(C)** OCT showing concave configuration; **(D)** B-scan
(Courtesy of S Chen – figs A–C; RF Spaide, from Diseases of the Retina and Vitreous, *WB Saunders, 1999 – fig. D)*

- **Signs**
  - The RD has a convex configuration, as with a rhegmatogenous RD, but its surface is smooth and not corrugated.
  - The detached retina is very mobile and exhibits the phenomenon of 'shifting fluid' in which SRF detaches the area of retina under which it accumulates (Fig. 16.41). For example, in the upright position the SRF collects under the inferior retina, but on assuming the supine position for several minutes, the inferior retina flattens and SRF shifts posteriorly, detaching the superior retina.
  - The cause of the RD, such as a choroidal tumour (Fig. 16.42), may be apparent when the fundus is examined or on B-scan ultrasonography, or the patient may have an associated systemic disease responsible for the RD (e.g. Harada disease, toxaemia of pregnancy).
  - 'Leopard spots' consisting of scattered areas of subretinal pigment clumping may be seen after the detachment has flattened (Fig. 16.43).

Treatment

Treatment depends on the cause. Some cases resolve spontaneously, whilst others are treated with systemic corticosteroids (Harada disease and posterior scleritis). In some eyes with bullous central serous chorioretinopathy, the leak in the RPE can be sealed by laser photocoagulation.

PARS PLANA VITRECTOMY

Introduction

Instrumentation

The diameter of the shaft of vitrectomy instrumentation has conventionally been 0.9 mm (20-gauge), but smaller 23-gauge, 25-gauge and even 27-gauge sutureless systems (transconjunctival microincision vitrectomy – MIVS) are increasingly becoming the standard of care, offering shorter operating time, less trauma and

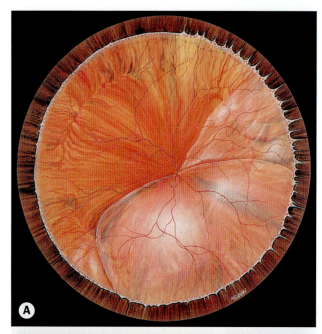

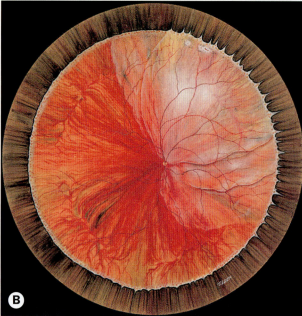

Fig. 16.41 Exudative retinal detachment with shifting fluid. **(A)** Inferior collection of subretinal fluid with the patient sitting; **(B)** the subretinal fluid shifts upwards when the patient assumes the supine position

(Courtesy of CL Schepens, E Hartnett and T Hirose, from Schepens' Retinal Detachment and Allied Diseases, *Butterworth-Heinemann 2000)*

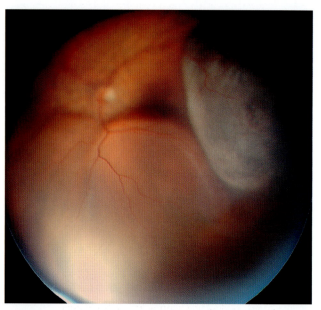

Fig. 16.42 Exudative retinal detachment caused by a choroidal melanoma

(Courtesy of B Damato)

removing it by suction into a collecting cassette. Faster cutting speeds translate into a lower level of traction exerted on the vitreoretinal interface during surgery. Safer more efficient fluidic control has been introduced in tandem.

• **Intraocular illumination** is supplied by a fibreoptic probe (light pipe – Fig. 16.44). Initially, reduced illumination was problematic with the narrower calibre MIVS systems due to the limitations of halogen bulbs, and brighter sources consisting of xenon and potentially less phototoxic mercury vapour sources have been introduced that match or exceed

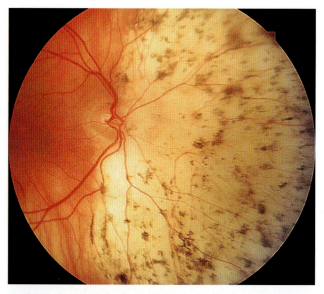

Fig. 16.43 'Leopard spot' pigmentation following resolution of exudative retinal detachment

scarring and faster rehabilitation. Early concerns about an increased risk of postoperative endophthalmitis do not seem to have been borne out, and operative success rates are comparable to larger-gauge instrumentation.

• **Vitreous cutter** (Fig. 16.44) has an inner guillotine blade that oscillates at very high speed (from 1500 up to 5000–7500 cuts/minute – cpm – in the latest 'ultra-high speed' cutters), cutting the vitreous gel into tiny pieces and simultaneously

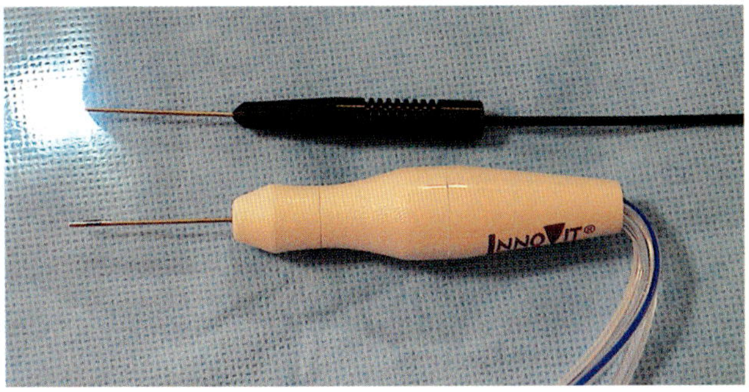

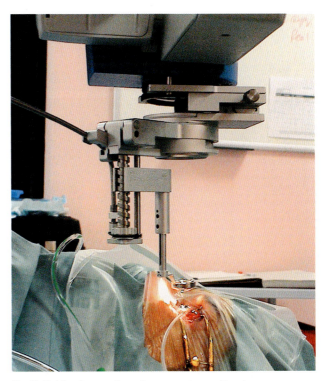

Fig. 16.44 (Top) Illumination pipe; (bottom) cutter
(Courtesy of V Tanner)

the levels of 20-gauge systems. These minimize retinal phototoxicity by filtering out higher-energy ultraviolet and blue light; some systems offer adjustable lighting characteristics to increase the contrast of particular structures. Wide-angle lighting and self-retaining 'chandelier' sources are available – the latter offer the advantages of freeing both of the surgeon's hands to carry out true bimanual surgery, which can be particularly useful in challenging cases, and of increasing the working distance of the light probe from the retina to decrease phototoxicity; glare is sometimes problematic, however. Extremely small-gauge dual chandelier probes are available to eliminate shadowing from the working field.
- **An infusion cannula** is required in order to maintain the vitreous cavity pressure and volume. These are generally self-retaining in smaller gauge systems.
- **Wide-angle viewing systems** consist of an indirect lens beneath the operating microscope and an incorporated series of prisms to reinvert the image (Fig. 16.45). The field of view extends almost to the ora serrata; higher magnification smaller field lenses are available for macular surgery.
- **Accessory instruments** include scissors, forceps, flute needle and endodiathermy and endolaser delivery systems. With the introduction of smaller-calibre cutters that are able to manipulate fibrovascular membranes more precisely and safely, the requirement for additional instrumentation may decrease.

Tamponading agents

These achieve intraoperative retinal flattening in combination with internal drainage of SRF, and are commonly used postoperatively for internal tamponade of retinal breaks.
- **Expanding gases.** Although air can be used, an expanding gas is usually preferred in order to achieve prolonged tamponade. Postoperative positioning of the patient is used to maximize the effective vector and maintain surface tension around the break.
  - Sulfur hexafluoride (SF_6) doubles its volume if used at a 100% concentration and lasts 10–14 days.
  - Perfluorethane (C_2F_6) triples its volume at 100% and lasts 30–35 days.

- Perfluoropropane (C_3F_8) quadruples its volume at 100% and lasts 55–65 days.
- Because the eye is usually left almost entirely gas-filled at the end of the procedure, most are used at only an isovolumetric (non-expansile) concentration (e.g. 20–30% for SF_6 and 12–16% for C_3F_8). Low pressure environments, typically air travel, and nitrous oxide anaesthesia must be avoided until gas absorption is complete as these will increase the intraocular gas pressure.
- **Silicone oils** have low specific gravity – they are lighter than water and thus buoyant. They are commonly used for both intraoperative retinal manipulation and prolonged postoperative intraocular tamponade, and are particularly helpful in the management of proliferative vitreoretinopathy. 1000 cs silicone is easier to inject and to remove whilst 5000 cs is more viscous but may be less prone to emulsification.
- **Heavy liquids** (perfluorocarbons) have high specific gravity and thus settle inferiorly in the vitreous cavity. Although primarily developed solely for intraoperative use (Fig. 16.46), newer compounds are available for postoperative tamponade of the inferior retina. However, cases of retinal toxicity and severe inflammation have been reported.

Indications

Although many simple rhegmatogenous RD can be treated successfully by scleral buckling techniques, pars plana vitrectomy (PPV) has greatly improved the prognosis for more complex

Fig. 16.45 Viewing system for pars plana vitrectomy
(Courtesy of V Tanner)

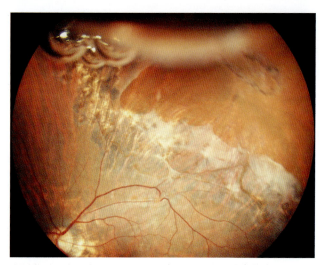

Fig. 16.46 Giant tear unrolled with heavy liquid
(Courtesy of C Barry)

detachments. As techniques have improved and surgeons' familiarity and confidence has grown, the threshold for vitrectomy surgery has fallen. Many surgeons now feel that morbidity and success rates are better with vitrectomy for all pseudophakic and aphakic RD, and for those that would otherwise require external drainage of SRF; some advocate primary vitrectomy for virtually all cases. The guidelines below are therefore not absolute.

Rhegmatogenous retinal detachment

- **When retinal breaks cannot be visualized** as a result of haemorrhage, vitreous debris, posterior capsular opacity, IOL edge effects. Vitrectomy is crucial to provide an adequate retinal view. Scleral buckling carries a high risk of failure if any breaks are missed.
- **In which retinal breaks are unlikely to be closed by scleral buckling** such as giant tears, large posterior breaks and in the presence of PVR (Figs 16.47A–C).

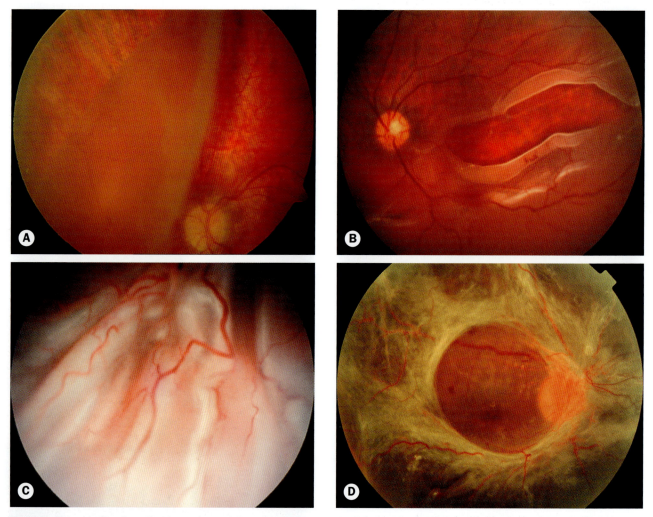

Fig. 16.47 Some indications for pars plana vitrectomy. **(A)** Giant retinal tear; **(B)** large posterior tear; **(C)** severe proliferative vitreoretinopathy; **(D)** tractional retinal detachment
(Courtesy of P Gili – fig. A; C Barry – fig. B; S Chen – fig. D)

Tractional retinal detachment

- **Indications in diabetic RD**
  - Tractional RD threatening or involving the macula (Fig. 16.47D). Vitrectomy is always combined with internal panretinal photocoagulation to prevent postoperative neovascularization that may cause vitreous haemorrhage or rubeosis iridis. Extramacular tractional RD may be observed without surgery because, in many cases, it remains stationary for a long time provided proliferative retinopathy has been controlled.
  - Combined tractional–rhegmatogenous RD should be treated urgently, even if the macula is not involved, because SRF is likely to spread quickly.
- **Indications in penetrating trauma**
  - Prevention of tractional RD. Unlike diabetic retinopathy where epiretinal membrane proliferation occurs mostly on the posterior retina, fibrocellular proliferation after penetrating trauma tends to develop on the pre-equatorial retina and/or the ciliary body. Treatment is usually aimed at visual rehabilitation and minimizing the tractional process.
  - Late tractional RD, which may be associated with an intraocular foreign body or retinal incarceration, occasionally develops months after otherwise successful surgery.

Technique

Basic vitrectomy

- An infusion cannula is inserted (3.5 mm behind the limbus in pseudophakic or aphakic eyes and 4 mm in phakic eyes) at the level of the inferior border of the lateral rectus muscle; limbal peritomy (conjunctival dissection) is required for conventional larger gauge systems, but unnecessary in small gauge systems.
- Further sclerotomies are made at the 10 and 2 o'clock positions, through which the vitreous cutter and fibreoptic probe are introduced (Fig. 16.48). These sclerotomies are self-sealing with modern small gauge systems, though wound leak occasionally occurs (Fig. 16.49).
- The central vitreous gel and posterior hyaloid face are excised.
- The above basic steps apply to all vitrectomies; subsequent steps depend on the specific indication.
- Transconjunctival small gauge systems do not require postoperative suturing.

Proliferative vitreoretinopathy

The aims of surgery in PVR are to release both transvitreal traction by vitrectomy and tangential (surface) traction by membrane dissection in order to restore retinal mobility and allow closure of retinal breaks.

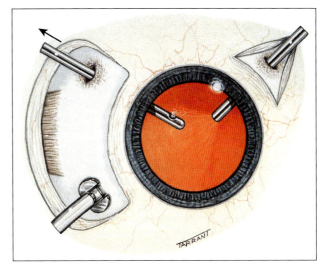

Fig. 16.48 Infusion cannula, light pipe and cutter in position (right eye)

Localized fixed retinal folds may be freed by the removal of the central plaque of epiretinal membrane. This can usually be achieved by engaging the tip of vertically cutting scissors or a pic-type instrument in the edge of a valley between two adjacent folds (Fig. 16.50). The membrane is then either surgically dissected or simply peeled from the surface of the retina. Smaller gauge cutters may be used in some cases to engage membranes directly, and forceps can facilitate this. A relieving retinotomy is considered if the mobility of the retina is believed to be insufficient for sustained reattachment.

Tractional retinal detachment

The goal of vitrectomy in tractional RDs is to release anteroposterior and/or circumferential vitreoretinal traction. Because the membranes are vascularized, and the retina often friable, they

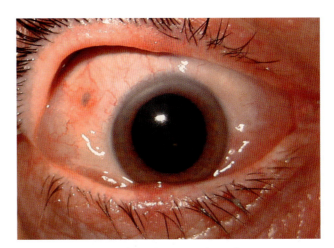

Fig. 16.49 Wound leak following sutureless vitrectomy
(Courtesy of S Chen)

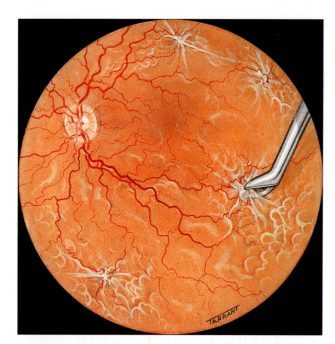

Fig. 16.50 Dissection of retinal folds in proliferative vitreoretinopathy

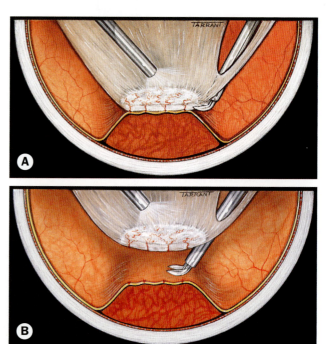

Fig. 16.51 (A) Delamination with horizontally cutting scissors; **(B)** completed

cannot be simply peeled from the surface of the retina as this would result in haemorrhage and tearing of the retina. The two methods of removing fibrovascular membranes in diabetic tractional RDs are the following:

- **Delamination** involves the horizontal cutting of individual vascular pegs connecting a membrane to the surface of the retina (Fig. 16.51A). This allows the complete removal of fibrovascular tissue from the retinal surface (Fig. 16.51B).
- **Segmentation** involves the vertical cutting of epiretinal membranes into small segments (Fig. 16.52). It is used to release circumferential vitreoretinal traction when delamination is difficult or impossible.

Postoperative complications

Raised intraocular pressure

- **Overexpansion of intraocular gas,** usually when the concentration or volume of expansile gas is inadvertently too great. Medical measures alone may be sufficient in some cases as the gas is allowed to absorb, but in very substantial elevation a gas tap via the pars plana with a 30-gauge needle on a 1 ml syringe may be necessary.
- **Silicone oil-associated glaucoma**
  - Early glaucoma may be caused by direct pupillary block by silicone oil (Fig. 16.53A). This occurs particularly in the aphakic eye with an intact iris diaphragm. In aphakic eyes this can be prevented by performing an inferior (Ando) iridectomy at the time of surgery to allow free passage of aqueous to the anterior chamber. Intraocular gas can also cause pupillary block.
  - Late glaucoma is caused by emulsified silicone in the anterior chamber (Fig. 16.53B) causing trabecular obstruction and scarring. The risk may be reduced by early oil removal, though glaucoma can still occur. A glaucoma drainage device or enhanced trabeculectomy may be required.

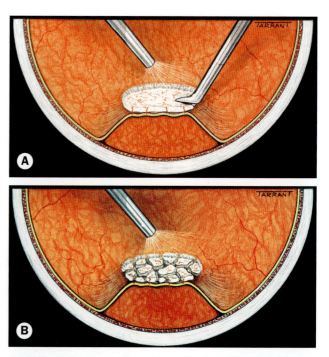

Fig. 16.52 (A) Segmentation with vertically cutting scissors; **(B)** completed

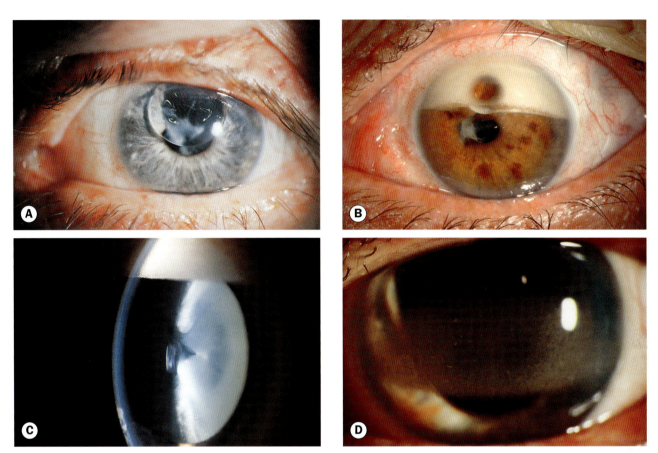

Fig. 16.53 Some complications of silicone oil injection. **(A)** Pupillary block glaucoma caused by oil in the anterior chamber; **(B)** late glaucoma due to emulsified oil in the anterior chamber; an inverted pseudo-hypopyon (hyperoleon) is seen; **(C)** cataract with a hyperoleon; **(D)** band keratopathy

(Courtesy of Z Gregor – fig. D)

- **Other mechanisms** include ghost cell, inflammatory and steroid-induced glaucoma. Angle closure can also result from ciliochoroidal effusion with anterior rotation of the lens–iris diaphragm; this may respond to cycloplegia and steroids.

Cataract

- **Gas-induced.** A large or long-lasting intravitreal gas bubble typically gives rise to feathering of the posterior subcapsular lens, though this is usually transient.

- **Silicone-induced.** Almost all phakic eyes with silicone oil eventually develop cataract (Fig. 16.53C).
- **Delayed.** Following vitrectomy, substantial nuclear sclerosis commonly develops within a year, especially if the patient is over 50 years of age.

Band keratopathy

Band keratopathy (Fig. 16.53D) is not uncommon with extended silicone oil tamponade.

Chapter 17

Vitreous opacities

Introduction

The vitreous is a transparent extracellular gel consisting of collagen, soluble proteins, hyaluronic acid and water. Its total volume is approximately 4.0 ml. The few cells normally present in the gel are located predominantly in the cortex and include hyalocytes, astrocytes and glial cells. The vitreous provides structural support to the globe while allowing a clear and optically uniform path to the retina. Once liquefied or surgically removed it does not re-form. Vitreous opacities can be caused by a variety of pathological processes primarily involving other ocular sites; apart from vitreous haemorrhage, the conditions discussed below are those in which the vitreous gel is the primary site of pathology.

Muscae volitantes

Muscae volitantes (Latin for 'hovering flies'), commonly referred to as 'floaters', is an almost ubiquitous entoptic phenomenon of fly-, cobweb- or thread-like lesions best seen against a pale background. It is thought to predominantly represent tiny embryological remnants in the vitreous gel. A sudden exacerbation can occur due to vitreous haemorrhage or, more commonly, a change in the conformation of the gel, such as a posterior vitreous detachment (see Fig. 16.22).

Vitreous haemorrhage

Vitreous haemorrhage is a common condition with many causes (Table 17.1). Symptoms vary according to severity. Mild haemorrhage (Fig. 17.1A) causes sudden onset floaters and diffuse blurring of vision, but may not affect visual acuity, whilst a dense bleed (Fig. 17.1B) may result in very severe visual loss. B-scan ultrasonography in unclotted vitreous haemorrhage generally shows a uniform appearance, and once cellular aggregates develop, small particulate echoes become visible (Fig. 17.1C); ultrasonography is critical in the evaluation of eyes with dense vitreous haemorrhage to exclude an underlying retinal tear or detachment (Fig. 17.1D). Treatment is dictated by severity and cause, but an increasingly low threshold is being adopted for early vitrectomy (see Ch. 16) in cases of dense haemorrhage.

Table 17.1 Causes of vitreous haemorrhage

- Acute posterior vitreous detachment associated either with a retinal tear or avulsion of a peripheral vessel
- Proliferative retinopathy
  - Diabetic
  - Retinal vein occlusion
  - Sickle cell disease
  - Eales disease
  - Vasculitis
- Miscellaneous retinal disorders
  - Macroaneurysm
  - Telangiectasia
  - Capillary haemangioma
- Trauma
- Systemic
  - Bleeding disorders
  - Terson syndrome

Terson syndrome

Terson syndrome refers to the combination of intraocular and subarachnoid haemorrhage secondary to aneurysmal rupture, most commonly arising from the anterior communicating artery. However, intraocular haemorrhage may also occur with subdural haematoma and acute elevation of intracranial pressure from other causes. The haemorrhage is frequently bilateral and is typically intraretinal and/or preretinal (Fig. 17.2), although occasionally subhyaloid blood may break into the vitreous. It is probable that intraocular bleeding is due to retinal venous stasis secondary to increase in cavernous sinus pressure. Vitreous haemorrhage usually resolves spontaneously within a few months and the long-term visual prognosis is good in the majority. Early vitrectomy may be considered in some cases.

Asteroid hyalosis

Asteroid hyalosis is a common degenerative process in which calcium pyrophosphate particles collect within the vitreous gel. It is seen clinically as numerous tiny round yellow–white opacities of varying size and density (Figs 17.3A and B). These move with the vitreous during eye movements but do not sediment inferiorly when the eye is immobile. Only one eye is affected in 75% of patients; it rarely causes visual problems and the majority of patients are asymptomatic. An association with diabetes has been suggested, but is unproven. The prevalence of asteroid hyalosis increases with age and affects 3% of those aged 75–86 years. It is more common in men than in women. OCT (Figs 17.3C and D) and ultrasonography (Fig. 17.3E) show high reflectivity foci.

Synchysis scintillans

Synchysis (synchisis) scintillans occurs as a consequence of chronic vitreous haemorrhage, often in a blind eye. The condition is usually discovered when frank haemorrhage is no longer present. The crystals are composed of cholesterol and are derived from plasma cells or degraded products of erythrocytes, and lie either freely or engulfed within foreign body giant cells. Numerous flat golden-brown refractile particles are seen; these tend to sediment inferiorly when the eye is immobile. Occasionally the anterior chamber may also be involved (Fig. 17.4).

Amyloidosis

Amyloidosis is a localized or systemic condition in which there is extracellular deposition of fibrillary protein. Vitreous involvement typically occurs in familial amyloidosis, also characterized by polyneuropathy, prominent corneal nerves and pupillary light-near dissociation. Vitreous opacities may be unilateral or bilateral and are initially perivascular. Later they involve the anterior gel and take on a characteristic sheet-like ('glass wool') appearance (Fig. 17.5A). The opacities may become attached to the posterior lens by thick footplates (Fig. 17.5B). Dense opacification resulting in significant visual impairment may require vitrectomy.

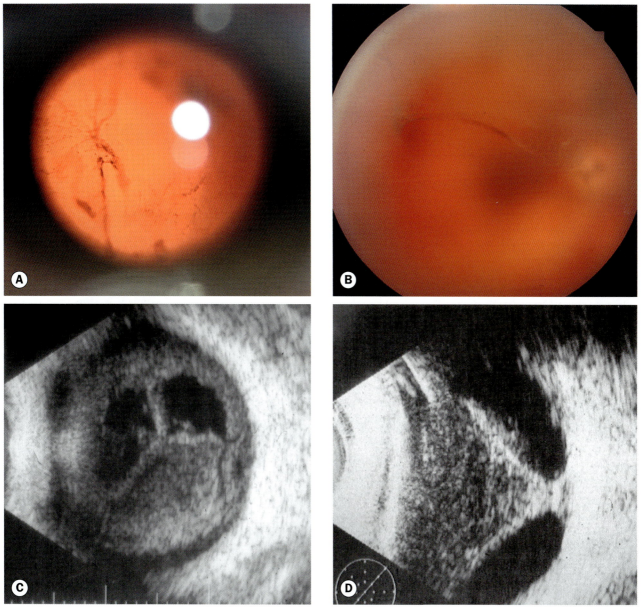

Fig. 17.1 (A) Mild vitreous haemorrhage seen against the red reflex; **(B)** severe diffuse vitreous haemorrhage; **(C)** B-scan image showing vitreous haemorrhage and flat retina; **(D)** B-scan image showing vitreous haemorrhage and funnel-shaped retinal detachment

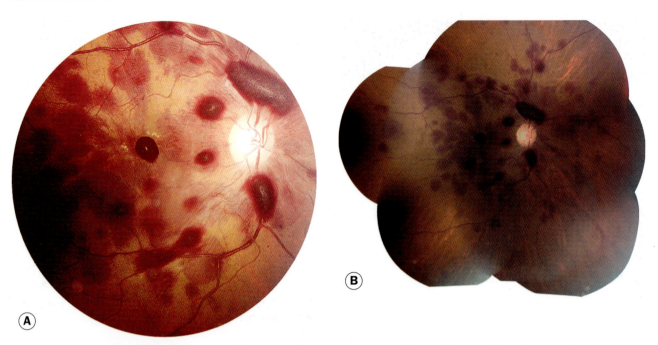

Fig. 17.2 Terson syndrome. **(A)** Acute intra- and preretinal haemorrhages in a 48-year-old man with subarachnoid haemorrhage; **(B)** composite image

(Courtesy of A Agarwal, from Gass' Atlas of Macular Diseases, Elsevier 2012)

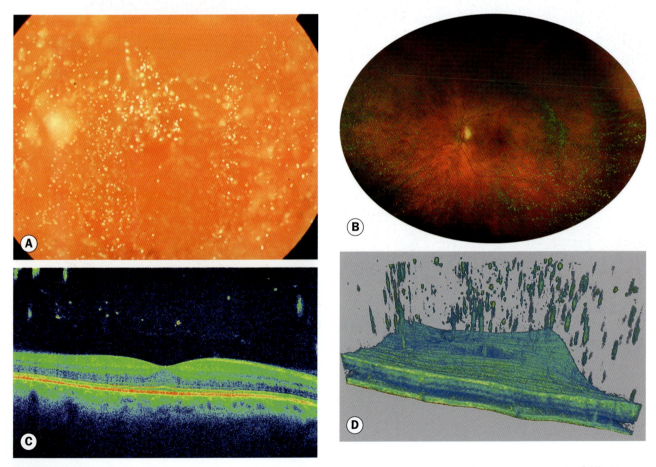

Fig. 17.3 Asteroid hyalosis. **(A)** Clinical appearance of moderate severity; **(B)** wide-field image; **(C)** appearance on OCT; **(D)** three-dimensional OCT reconstruction;

Continued

Fig. 17.3, Continued (E) B-scan ultrasonogram

(Courtesy of S Chen – figs B–D)

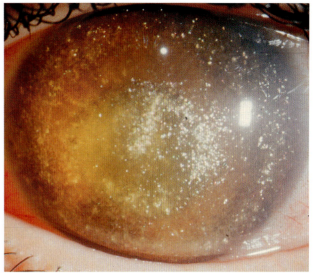

Fig. 17.4 Synchysis scintillans in the anterior chamber of a degenerate eye

(Courtesy of P Gili)

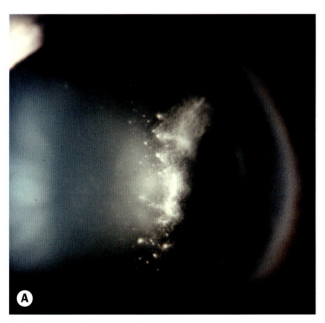

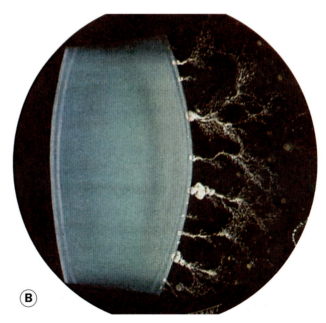

Fig. 17.5 Amyloid deposits in the vitreous (see text)

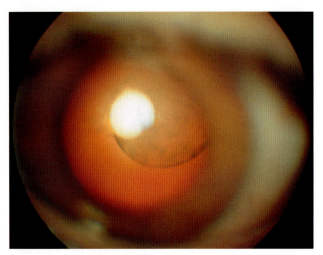

Fig. 17.6 Vitreous cyst

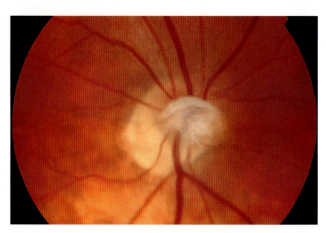

Fig. 17.7 Bergmeister papilla

Vitreous cyst

Vitreous cysts can be congenital or acquired, acquired cysts being caused by a range of pathology such as trauma and inflammation. Congenital cysts are pigmented or non-pigmented, the former usually arising from the ciliary body pigment epithelium, the latter from remnants of the primary hyaloid vascular system. They are generally fixed – non-pigmented cysts are typically attached to the optic disc – but can be found floating freely in the posterior (occasionally anterior) segment (Fig. 17.6). Treatment is seldom required, but laser cystotomy or vitrectomy can be performed for troublesome symptoms.

Persistent fetal vasculature

In addition to non-pigmented vitreous cysts, remnants of the hyaloid vessels can form a Bergmeister papilla, seen as a tuft at the optic disc (Fig. 17.7), a Mittendorf dot on the posterior lens surface, and the more marked manifestations for which the term persistent fetal vasculature is generally reserved, previously termed persistent hyperplastic primary vitreous (see Ch. 12).

INTRODUCTION

Definitions

- **The visual axis** passes from the fovea, through the nodal point of the eye, to the point of fixation. In normal binocular single vision (BSV) the visual axes of the two eyes intersect at the point of fixation, the images being aligned by the fusion reflex and combined by binocular responsive cells in the visual cortex to give BSV.
- **Orthophoria** implies perfect ocular alignment in the absence of any stimulus for fusion; this is uncommon.
- **Heterophoria** ('phoria') implies a tendency of the eyes to deviate when fusion is blocked (latent squint).
  - Slight phoria is present in most normal individuals and is overcome by the fusion reflex. The phoria can be either a small inward imbalance (esophoria) or an outward imbalance (exophoria).
  - When fusion is insufficient to control the imbalance, the phoria is described as decompensating and is often associated with symptoms of binocular discomfort (asthenopia) or double vision (diplopia).
- **Heterotropia** ('tropia') implies a manifest deviation in which the visual axes do not intersect at the point of fixation.
  - The images from the two eyes are misaligned so that either double vision is present or, more commonly in children, the image from the deviating eye is suppressed at cortical level.
  - A childhood squint may occur because of failure of the normal development of binocular fusion mechanisms or as a result of oculomotor imbalance secondary to a difference in refraction between the two eyes (anisometropia).
  - Failure of fusion, for example secondary to poor vision in one eye, may cause heterotropia in adulthood, or a squint may develop because of weakness or mechanical restriction of the extraocular muscles, or damage to their nerve supply.
  - Horizontal deviation of the eyes (latent or manifest) is the most common form of strabismus.
  - Upward displacement of one eye relative to the other is termed a *hypertropia* and a latent upward imbalance a *hyperphoria*.
  - Downward displacement is termed a *hypotropia* and a latent imbalance a *hypophoria*.
- **The anatomical axis** is a line passing from the posterior pole through the centre of the cornea. Because the fovea is usually slightly temporal to the anatomical centre of the posterior pole of the eye, the visual axis does not usually correspond to the anatomical axis of the eye.
- **Angle kappa** is the angle, usually about 5°, subtended by the visual and anatomical axes (Fig. 18.1).
  - The angle is positive (normal) when the fovea is temporal to the centre of the posterior pole resulting in a nasal

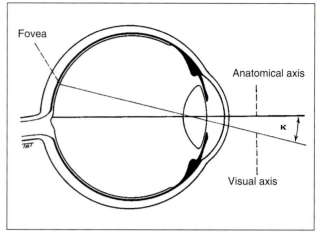

Fig. 18.1 Angle kappa

displacement of the corneal reflex, and negative when the converse applies.
  - A large angle kappa may give the appearance of a squint when none is present (pseudosquint) and is seen most commonly as a pseudoexotropia following displacement of the macula in retinopathy of prematurity, where the angle may significantly exceed +5° (see Fig. 18.46).

Anatomy of the extraocular muscles

Principles

The lateral and medial orbital walls are at an angle of 45° with each other. The orbital axis therefore forms an angle of 22.5° with both lateral and medial walls, though for the sake of simplicity this angle is usually regarded as being 23° (Fig. 18.2A). When the eye is looking straight ahead at a fixed point on the horizon with the head erect (primary position of gaze), the visual axis forms an angle of 23° with the orbital axis (Fig. 18.2B); the actions of the extraocular muscles depend on the position of the globe at the time of muscle contraction (Figs 18.2C and D).

- **The primary action** of a muscle is its major effect when the eye is in the primary position.
- **Subsidiary actions** are the additional effects; these depend on the position of the eye.
- **The Listing plane** is an imaginary coronal plane passing through the centre of rotation of the globe. The globe rotates on the axes of Fick, which intersect in the Listing plane (Fig. 18.3).
  - The globe rotates left and right on the vertical Z axis.
  - The globe moves up and down on the horizontal X axis.
  - Torsional movements (wheel rotations) occur on the Y (sagittal) axis which traverses the globe from front to back (similar to the anatomical axis of the eye).
  - Intorsion occurs when the superior limbus rotates nasally, and extorsion on temporal rotation.

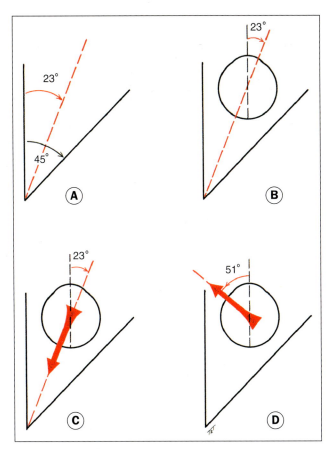

Fig. 18.2 Anatomy of the extraocular muscles

Horizontal recti

When the eye is in the primary position, the horizontal recti are purely horizontal movers on the vertical Z axis and have only primary actions.

- **Medial rectus** originates at the annulus of Zinn at the orbital apex and inserts 5.5 mm behind the nasal limbus. Its sole action in the primary position is adduction.
- **Lateral rectus** originates at the annulus of Zinn and inserts 6.9 mm behind the temporal limbus. Its sole action in the primary position is abduction.

Vertical recti

The vertical recti run in line with the orbital axis and are inserted in front of the equator. They therefore form an angle of 23° with the visual axis (see Fig. 18.2C).

- **Superior rectus** originates from the upper part of the annulus of Zinn and inserts 7.7 mm behind the superior limbus.
  - The primary action is elevation (Fig. 18.4A); secondary actions are adduction and intorsion.
  - When the globe is abducted 23°, the visual and orbital axes coincide. In this position it has no subsidiary actions and can act only as an elevator (Fig. 18.4B). This is therefore the optimal position of the globe for testing the function of the superior rectus muscle.

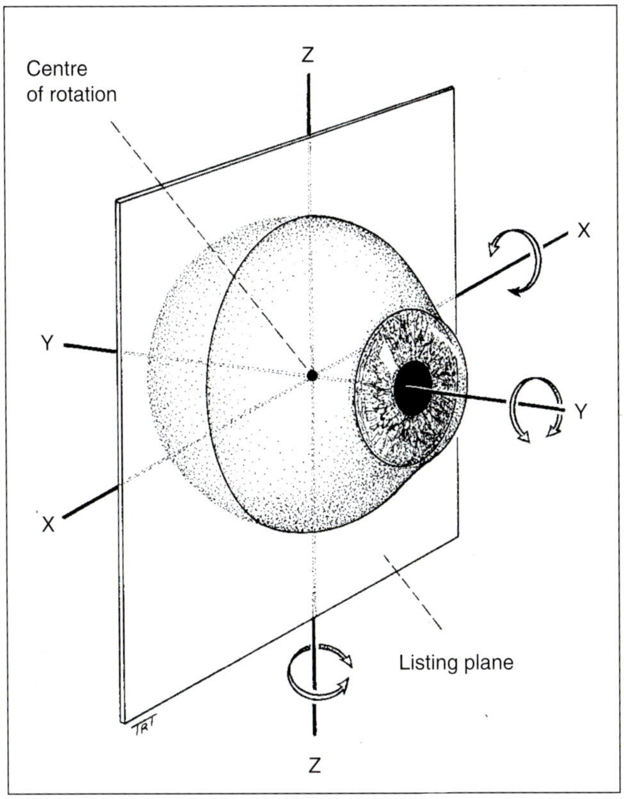

Fig. 18.3 The Listing plane and axes of Fick

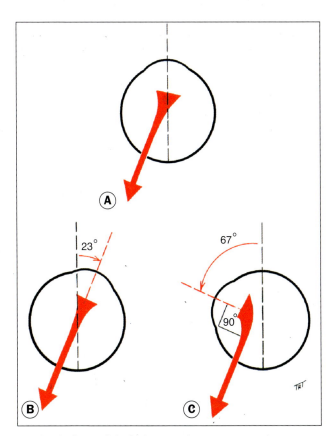

Fig. 18.4 Actions of the right superior rectus muscle

- o If the globe were adducted 67°, the angle between the visual and orbital axes would be 90°. In this position the superior rectus could only act as an intortor (Fig. 18.4C).
- **Inferior rectus** originates at the lower part of the annulus of Zinn and inserts 6.5 mm behind the inferior limbus.
  - o The primary action is depression; secondary actions are adduction and extorsion.
  - o When the globe is abducted 23°, the inferior rectus acts purely as a depressor. As for superior rectus, this is the optimal position of the globe for testing the function of the inferior rectus muscle.
  - o If the globe were adducted 67°, the inferior rectus could act only as an extortor.

Spiral of Tillaux

The spiral of Tillaux (Fig. 18.5) is an imaginary line joining the insertions of the four recti and is an important anatomical landmark when performing surgery. The insertions are located progressively further away from the limbus in a spiral pattern; the medial rectus insertion is closest (5.5 mm) followed by the inferior rectus (6.5 mm), lateral rectus (6.9 mm) and superior rectus (7.7 mm).

Oblique muscles

The obliques are inserted behind the equator and form an angle of 51° with the visual axis (see Fig. 18.2D).

- **Superior oblique** originates superomedial to the optic foramen. It passes forwards through the trochlea at the angle between the superior and medial walls and is then reflected backwards and laterally to insert in the posterior upper temporal quadrant of the globe (Fig. 18.6).
  - o The primary action is intorsion (Fig. 18.7A); secondary actions are depression and abduction.

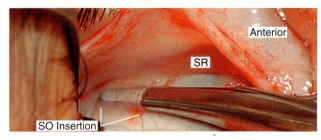

Fig. 18.6 Insertion of the superior oblique (SO) tendon; SR = superior rectus

- o The anterior fibres of the superior oblique tendon are primarily responsible for intorsion and the posterior fibres for depression, allowing separate surgical manipulation of these two actions (see below).
- o When the globe is adducted 51°, the visual axis coincides with the line of pull of the muscle. In this position it can act only as a depressor (Fig. 18.7B). This is, therefore, the best position of the globe for testing the action of the superior oblique muscle. Thus, although the superior oblique has an abducting action in primary position, the main effect of superior oblique weakness is seen as failure of depression in adduction.
- o When the eye is abducted 39°, the visual axis and the superior oblique make an angle of 90° with each other. In this position the superior oblique can cause only intorsion (Fig. 18.7C).

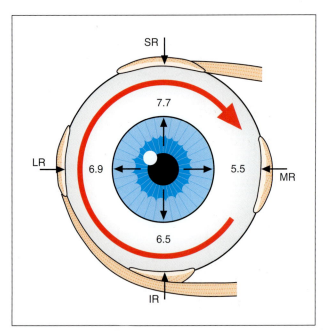

Fig. 18.5 Spiral of Tillaux. IR = inferior rectus; LR = lateral rectus; MR = medial rectus; SR = superior rectus

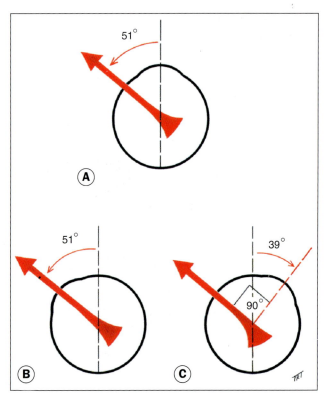

Fig. 18.7 Actions of the right superior oblique muscle

- **Inferior oblique** originates from a small depression just behind the orbital rim lateral to the lacrimal sac. It passes backwards and laterally to insert in the posterior lower temporal quadrant of the globe close to the macula.
  - ○ The primary action is extorsion; secondary actions are elevation and abduction.
  - ○ When the globe is adducted 51°, the inferior oblique acts as an elevator only.
  - ○ When the eye is abducted 39°, its main action is extorsion.

Muscle pulleys

- The four rectus muscles pass through condensations of connective tissue and smooth muscle just posterior to the equator. These condensations act as pulleys and minimize upward and downward movements of the bellies of the medial and lateral rectus muscles during upgaze and downgaze, and horizontal movements of the superior and inferior rectus bellies in left and right gaze.
- Pulleys are the effective origins of the rectus muscles and play an important role in the coordination of eye movements by reducing the effect of horizontal movements on vertical muscle actions and vice versa.
- Displacement of the pulleys is a cause of abnormalities of eye movements such as 'V' and 'A' patterns (see below).

Innervation

- **Lateral rectus.** Sixth cranial nerve (abducent nerve – abducting muscle).
- **Superior oblique.** Fourth cranial nerve (trochlear nerve – muscle associated with the trochlea).

- **Other muscles** together with the levator muscle of the upper lid and the ciliary and sphincter pupillae muscles are supplied by the third (oculomotor) nerve.

Ocular movements

Ductions

Ductions are monocular movements around the axes of Fick. They consist of adduction, abduction, elevation, depression, intorsion and extorsion. They are tested by occluding the fellow eye and asking the patient to follow a target in each direction of gaze.

Versions

Versions (Fig. 18.8, top) are binocular, simultaneous, conjugate movements (conjugate – in the same direction, so that the angle between the eyes remains constant).

- Dextroversion and laevoversion (gaze right and gaze left), elevation (upgaze) and depression (downgaze). These four movements bring the globe into the secondary positions of gaze by rotation around either the vertical (Z) or the horizontal (X) axes of Fick.
- Dextroelevation and dextrodepression (gaze up and right; gaze down and right) and laevoelevation and laevodepression (gaze up and left; gaze down and left). These four oblique movements bring the eyes into the tertiary positions of gaze by rotation around oblique axes lying in the Listing plane, equivalent to simultaneous movement about both the horizontal and vertical axes.
- Torsional movements to maintain upright images occur on tilting of the head; these are known as the righting reflexes.

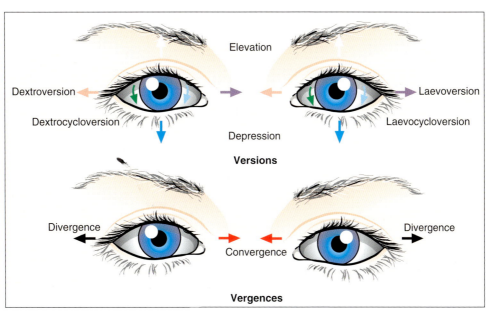

Fig. 18.8 Binocular movements

On head tilt to the right the superior limbi of the two eyes rotate to the left, causing intorsion of the right globe and extorsion of the left (laevocycloversion).

Vergences

Vergences (Fig. 18.8, bottom) are binocular, simultaneous, disjugate movements (disjugate – in opposite directions, so that the angle between the eyes changes; also termed disjunctive). Convergence is simultaneous adduction (inward turning); divergence is outwards movement from a convergent position. Convergence may be voluntary or reflex; reflex convergence has four components:

- **Tonic** convergence, which implies inherent innervational tone to the medial recti.
- **Proximal** convergence is induced by psychological awareness of a near object.
- **Fusional** convergence is an optomotor reflex that maintains binocular single vision (BSV) by ensuring that similar images are projected onto corresponding retinal areas of each eye. It is initiated by bitemporal retinal image disparity.
- **Accommodative** convergence is induced by the act of accommodation as part of the synkinetic-near reflex.
  - Each dioptre of accommodation is accompanied by a constant increment in accommodative convergence, giving the 'accommodative convergence to accommodation' (AC/A) ratio.
  - This is the amount of convergence in prism dioptres (Δ) per dioptre (D) change in accommodation.
  - The normal value is 3–5 Δ. This means that 1 D of accommodation is associated with 3–5 Δ of accommodative convergence. Abnormalities of the AC/A ratio play an important role in the aetiology of strabismus.
  - Changes in accommodation, convergence and pupil size which occur in concert with a change in the distance of viewing are known as the 'near triad'.

Positions of gaze

- **Six cardinal** positions of gaze are identified in which one muscle in each eye is principally responsible for moving the eye into that position as follows:
  - Dextroversion (right lateral rectus and left medial rectus).
  - Laevoversion (left lateral rectus and right medial rectus).
  - Dextroelevation (right superior rectus and left inferior oblique).
  - Laevoelevation (left superior rectus and right inferior oblique).
  - Dextrodepression (right inferior rectus and left superior oblique).
  - Laevodepression (left inferior rectus and right superior oblique).
- **Nine diagnostic** positions of gaze are those in which deviations are measured. They consist of the six cardinal positions, the primary position, elevation and depression (Fig. 18.9).

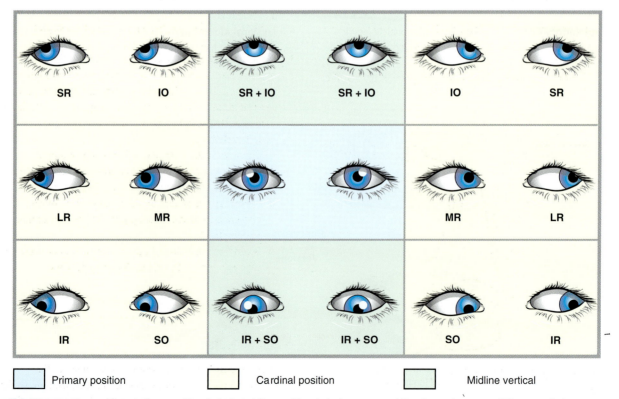

| | Primary position | | Cardinal position | | Midline vertical |

Fig. 18.9 Diagnostic positions of gaze. IO = inferior oblique; IR = inferior rectus; LR = lateral rectus; MR = medial rectus; SO = superior oblique; SR = superior rectus

Laws of ocular *motility*

- **Agonist–antagonist** pairs are muscles of the same eye that move the eye in opposite directions. The agonist is the primary muscle moving the eye in a given direction. The antagonist acts in the opposite direction to the agonist. For example, the right lateral rectus is the antagonist to the right medial rectus.
- **Synergists** are muscles of the same eye that move the eye in the same direction. For example, the right superior rectus and right inferior oblique act synergistically in elevation.
- **Yoke muscles** (contralateral synergists) are pairs of muscles, one in each eye, that produce conjugate ocular movements. For example, the yoke muscle of the left superior oblique is the right inferior rectus.
- **The Sherrington law** of reciprocal innervation (Fig. 18.10) states that increased innervation to an extraocular muscle (e.g. right medial rectus) is accompanied by a reciprocal decrease in innervation to its antagonist (e.g. right lateral rectus). This means that when the medial rectus contracts the lateral rectus automatically relaxes and vice versa. The Sherrington law applies to both versions and vergences.
- **The Hering law** of equal innervation states that during any conjugate eye movement, equal and simultaneous innervation flows to the yoke muscles (Fig. 18.11).
  - In the case of a paretic squint, the amount of innervation to both eyes is symmetrical, and always determined by the fixating eye, so that the angle of deviation will vary according to which eye is used for fixation.
  - For example if, in the case of a left lateral rectus palsy, the right normal eye is used for fixation, there will be an inward deviation of the left eye due to the unopposed action of the antagonist of the paretic left lateral rectus (left medial rectus). The amount of misalignment of the

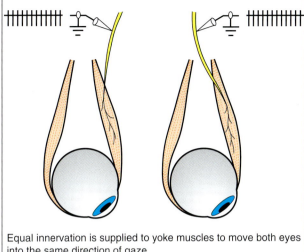

Equal innervation is supplied to yoke muscles to move both eyes into the same direction of gaze

Fig. 18.11 Hering law of equal innervation of yoke muscles

two eyes in this situation is called the primary deviation (Fig. 18.12, left).
  - If the paretic left eye is now used for fixation, additional innervation will flow to the left lateral rectus, in order to establish this. However, according to the Hering law, an equal amount of innervation will also flow to the right medial rectus (yoke muscle). This will result in an overaction of the right medial rectus and an excessive amount of adduction of the right eye.
  - The amount of misalignment between the two eyes in this situation is called the secondary deviation (see Fig. 18.12, right). In a paretic squint, the secondary deviation exceeds the primary deviation.
- **Muscle sequelae** are the effects of the interactions described by these laws. They are of prime importance in diagnosing ocular motility disorders and in particular in distinguishing a recently acquired from a longstanding palsy (see 'Clinical evaluation'). The full pattern of changes takes a variable period to develop:
  - Primary underaction (e.g. left superior oblique).
  - Secondary overaction of the contralateral synergist or yoke muscle (right inferior rectus; Hering law).
  - Secondary overaction and later contracture of the unopposed ipsilateral antagonist (left inferior oblique; Sherrington law).
  - Secondary inhibition of the contralateral antagonist (right superior rectus; Hering and Sherrington laws).

Sensory considerations

Basic aspects

- **Normal binocular single vision (BSV)** involves the simultaneous use of both eyes with bifoveal fixation, so that each eye contributes to a common single perception of the object of regard. This represents the highest form of

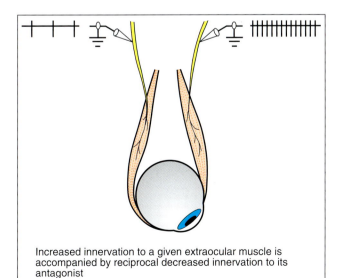

Increased innervation to a given extraocular muscle is accompanied by reciprocal decreased innervation to its antagonist

Fig. 18.10 Sherrington law of reciprocal innervation

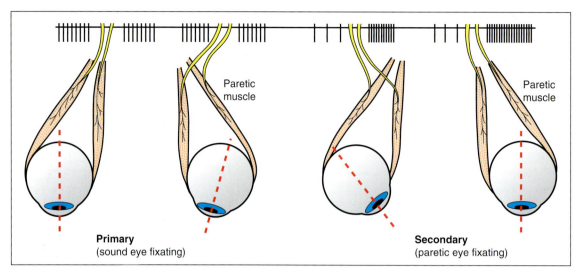

Fig. 18.12 Primary and secondary deviations in paretic strabismus

binocular cooperation. Conditions necessary for normal BSV are:

○ Normal routing of visual pathways with overlapping visual fields.

○ Binocularly driven neurones in the visual cortex.

○ Normal retinal (retinocortical) correspondence (NRC) resulting in 'cyclopean' viewing.

○ Accurate neuromuscular development and coordination, so that the visual axes are directed at, and maintain fixation on, the object of regard.

○ Approximately equal image clarity and size for both eyes.

○ BSV is based on NRC, which requires first an understanding of uniocular visual direction and projection.

• **Visual direction** is the projection of a given retinal element in a specific direction in subjective space.

○ The principal visual direction is the direction in external space interpreted as the line of sight. This is normally the visual direction of the fovea and is associated with a sense of direct viewing.

○ Secondary visual directions are the projecting directions of extrafoveal points with respect to the principal direction of the fovea, associated with indirect (eccentric) viewing.

• **Projection** is the subjective interpretation of the position of an object in space on the basis of stimulated retinal elements.

○ If a red object stimulates the right fovea (F), and a black object which lies in the nasal field stimulates a temporal retinal element (T), the red object will be interpreted by the brain as having originated from the straight-ahead position and the black object will be interpreted as having originated in the nasal field (Fig. 18.13A). Similarly, nasal retinal elements project into the temporal field, upper retinal elements into the lower field and vice versa.

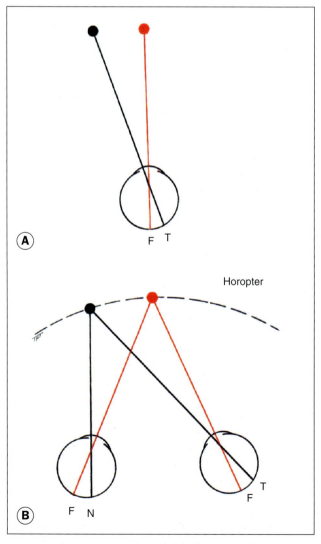

Fig. 18.13 Principles of projection. F = fovea; N = nasal retinal element; T = temporal retinal element

- With both eyes open, the red fixation object is now stimulating both foveae, which are corresponding retinal points. The black object is now not only stimulating the temporal retinal elements in the right eye but also the nasal elements of the left eye. The right eye therefore projects the object into its nasal field and the left eye projects the object into its temporal field.
  - Because both of these retinal elements are corresponding points, they will both project the object into the same position in space (the left side) and there will be no double vision.
- **Retinomotor values**
  - The image of an object in the peripheral visual field falls on an extrafoveal element. To establish fixation on this object a saccadic version of accurate amplitude is required.
  - Each extrafoveal retinal element therefore has a retinomotor value proportional to its distance from the fovea, which guides the amplitude of saccadic movements required to 'look at it'.
  - Retinomotor value, zero at the fovea, increases progressively towards the retinal periphery.
- **Corresponding points** are areas on each retina that share the same subjective visual direction (for example, the foveae share the primary visual direction).
  - Points on the nasal retina of one eye have corresponding points on the temporal retina of the other eye and vice versa. For example, an object producing images on the right nasal retina and the left temporal retina will be projected into the right side of visual space. This is the basis of normal retinal correspondence.
  - This retinotopic organization is reflected back along the visual pathways, each eye maintaining separate images until the visual pathways converge onto binocularly responsive neurones in the primary visual cortex.
- **The horopter** is an imaginary plane in external space, relative to both the observer's eyes for a given fixation target, all points on which stimulate corresponding retinal elements and are therefore seen singly and in the same plane (Fig. 18.13B). This plane passes through the intersection of the visual axes and therefore includes the point of fixation in BSV.
- **The Panum fusional space** (or volume) is a zone in front of and behind the horopter in which objects stimulate slightly non-corresponding retinal points (retinal disparity).
  - Objects within the limits of the fusional space are seen singly and the disparity information is used to produce a perception of binocular depth (stereopsis). Objects in front of and behind Panum space appear double.
  - This is the basis of physiological diplopia. The Panum space is shallow at fixation (6 seconds of arc) and deeper towards the periphery (30–40 seconds of arc at 15° from the fovea).
  - The retinal areas stimulated by images falling within the Panum fusional space are termed Panum fusional areas.

- Therefore objects on the horopter are seen singly and in one plane. Objects in Panum fusional areas are seen singly and stereoscopically. Objects outside Panum fusional areas appear double.
  - Physiological diplopia is usually accompanied by physiological suppression.
- **BSV** is characterized by the ability to fuse the images from the two eyes and to perceive binocular depth:
  - Sensory fusion involves the integration by the visual areas of the cerebral cortex of two similar images, one from each eye, into one image. It may be central, which integrates the image falling on the foveae, or peripheral, which integrates parts of the image falling outside the foveae. It is possible to maintain fusion with a central visual deficit in one eye, but peripheral fusion is essential to BSV and may be affected in patients with advanced field changes in glaucoma and pituitary lesions.
  - Motor fusion involves the maintenance of motor alignment of the eyes to sustain bifoveal fixation. It is driven by retinal image disparity, which stimulates fusional vergences.
- **Fusional vergence** involves disjugate eye movements to overcome retinal image disparity. Fusional convergence helps to control an exophoria whereas fusional divergence helps to control an esophoria. The fusional vergence mechanism may be decreased by fatigue or illness, converting a phoria to a tropia. The amplitude of fusional vergence mechanisms can be improved by orthoptic exercises, particularly in the case of near fusional convergence for the relief of convergence insufficiency. Amplitudes can be measured with prisms or a synoptophore. Normal values are:
  - Convergence: about 15–20 Δ for distance and 25 Δ for near.
  - Divergence: about 6–10 Δ for distance and 12–14 Δ for near.
  - Vertical: 2–3 Δ.
  - Cyclovergence: about 8°.
- **Stereopsis** is the perception of depth. It arises when objects behind and in front of the point of fixation (but within Panum fusional space) stimulate horizontally disparate retinal elements simultaneously. The fusion of these disparate images results in a single visual impression perceived in depth. A solid object is seen stereoscopically (in 3D) because each eye sees a slightly different aspect of the object.
- **Sensory perceptions.** At the onset of a squint two sensory perceptions arise based on the normal projection of the retinal areas stimulated; confusion and pathological diplopia may result. These require simultaneous visual perception, that is, the ability to perceive images from both eyes simultaneously. Young children readily suppress diplopia but it is persistent and usually troublesome with strabismus in older children and adults, when it arises after the sensitive period for binocularity (see below).
  - Confusion is the simultaneous appreciation of two superimposed but dissimilar images caused by

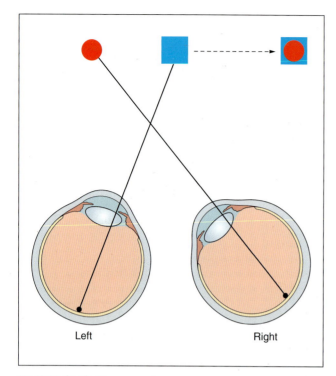

Fig. 18.14 Confusion

stimulation of corresponding retinal points (usually the foveae) by images of different objects (Fig. 18.14).

○ Pathological diplopia is the simultaneous appreciation of two images of the same object in different positions and results from images of the same object falling on non-corresponding retinal points. In esotropia the diplopia is homonymous (uncrossed – Fig. 18.15A), in exotropia the diplopia is heteronymous (crossed – Fig. 18.15B).

Sensory adaptations to strabismus

The ocular sensory system in children has the ability to adapt to anomalous states (confusion and diplopia) by two mechanisms: suppression and abnormal retinal correspondence (ARC). These occur because of the plasticity of the developing visual system in children under the age of 6–8 years. Occasional adults who develop sudden-onset strabismus are able to ignore the second image after a time and therefore do not complain of diplopia.

- **Suppression** involves active inhibition by the visual cortex of the image from one eye when both eyes are open. Stimuli for suppression include diplopia, confusion and a blurred image from one eye resulting from astigmatism/anisometropia. Clinically, suppression may be:
  ○ *Central* or *peripheral*. In central suppression the image from the fovea of the deviating eye is inhibited to avoid confusion. Diplopia, on the other hand, is eradicated by the process of peripheral suppression, in which the image from the peripheral retina of the deviating eye is inhibited.

○ *Monocular* or *alternating*. Suppression is monocular when the image from the dominant eye always predominates over the image from the deviating (or more ametropic) eye, so that the image from the latter is constantly suppressed. This type of suppression leads to amblyopia. When suppression alternates (switches from one eye to the other), amblyopia is less likely to develop.

○ *Facultative* or *obligatory*. Facultative suppression occurs only when the eyes are misaligned. Obligatory suppression is present at all times, irrespective of whether the eyes are deviated or straight. Examples of facultative suppression include intermittent exotropia and Duane syndrome.

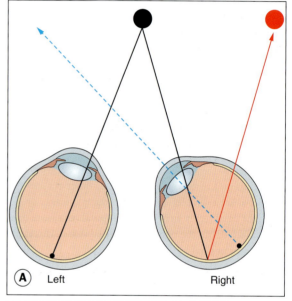

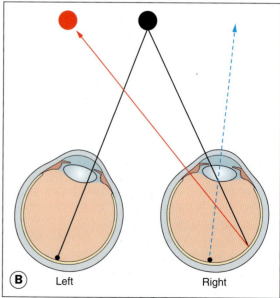

Fig. 18.15 Diplopia. **(A)** Homonymous (uncrossed) diplopia in right esotropia with normal retinal correspondence; **(B)** heteronymous (crossed) diplopia in right exotropia with normal retinal correspondence

- **Abnormal (anomalous) retinal correspondence (ARC)** is a condition in which non-corresponding retinal elements acquire a common subjective visual direction, i.e. fusion occurs in the presence of a small angle manifest squint; the fovea of the fixating eye is paired with a non-foveal element of the deviated eye. Binocular responses in ARC are never as good as in normal bifoveal BSV. It represents a positive sensory adaptation to strabismus (as opposed to negative adaptation by suppression), which allows some anomalous binocular vision in the presence of a heterotropia. It is most frequently encountered in small angle esotropia (microtropia), but is less common in accommodative esotropia because of the variability of the angle of deviation and in large angle deviations because the separation of the images is too great.
- **Microtropia** is discussed further later in this chapter.
- **Consequences of strabismus**
  - The fovea of the squinting eye is suppressed to avoid confusion.
  - Diplopia will occur, since corresponding retinal elements receive different images.
  - To avoid diplopia, the patient will develop either peripheral suppression of the squinting eye or ARC.
  - If constant unilateral suppression occurs this will subsequently lead to strabismic amblyopia.

Motor adaptation to strabismus

Motor adaptation involves the adoption of a compensatory head posture (CHP) and occurs primarily in children with congenitally abnormal eye movements who use the CHP to maintain BSV. In these children loss of a CHP may indicate loss of binocular function and the need for surgical intervention. These patients may present in adult life with symptoms of decompensation, often unaware of their CHP. Acquired paretic strabismus in adults may be consciously controlled by a CHP provided the deviation is neither too large nor too variable with gaze (incomitance). The CHP eliminates diplopia and helps to centralize the binocular visual field. The patient will turn the head into the direction of the field of action of the weak muscle, so that the eyes are then automatically turned the opposite direction and as far as possible away from its field of action (i.e. the head will turn where the eye cannot).

- **A face turn** will be adopted to control a purely horizontal deviation. For example, if the left lateral rectus is paralysed, diplopia will occur in left gaze; the face will be turned to the left which deviates the eyes to the right away from the field of action of the weak muscle and area of diplopia. A face turn may also be adopted in a paresis of a vertically acting muscle to avoid the side where the vertical deviation is greatest (e.g. in a right superior oblique weakness the face is turned to the left).
- **A head tilt** is adopted to compensate for torsional and/or vertical diplopia. In a right superior oblique weakness, the right eye is relatively elevated and the head is tilted to the left (Fig. 18.16), towards the hypotropic eye; this reduces the

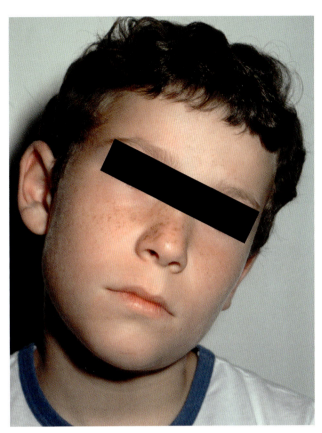

Fig. 18.16 Compensatory head posture in a right fourth nerve palsy

vertical separation of the diplopic images and permits fusion to be regained. If there is a significant torsional component preventing fusion, tilting the head in the same left direction will reduce this by invoking the righting reflexes (placing the extorted right eye in a position that requires extorsion).
- **Chin elevation or depression** may be used to compensate for weakness of an elevator or depressor muscle or to minimize the horizontal deviation when an 'A' or 'V' pattern is present.

AMBLYOPIA

Classification

Amblyopia is the unilateral, or rarely bilateral, decrease in best corrected visual acuity (VA) caused by form vision deprivation and/or abnormal binocular interaction, for which there is no identifiable pathology of the eye or visual pathway.

- **Strabismic** amblyopia results from abnormal binocular interaction where there is continued monocular suppression of the deviating eye.
- **Anisometropic** amblyopia is caused by a difference in refractive error between the eyes and may result from a difference of as little as 1 dioptre. The more ametropic eye receives a blurred image, in a mild form of visual

deprivation. It is frequently associated with microstrabismus and may coexist with strabismic amblyopia.

- **Stimulus deprivation** amblyopia results from vision deprivation. It may be unilateral or bilateral and is typically caused by opacities in the media (e.g. cataract) or ptosis that covers the pupil.
- **Bilateral ametropic** amblyopia results from high symmetrical refractive errors, usually hypermetropia.
- **Meridional** amblyopia results from image blur in one meridian. It can be unilateral or bilateral and is caused by uncorrected astigmatism (usually >1 D) persisting beyond the period of emmetropization in early childhood.

Diagnosis

In the absence of an organic lesion, a difference in best corrected VA of two Snellen lines or more (or >1 log unit) is indicative of amblyopia. Visual acuity in amblyopia is usually better when reading single letters than letters in a row. This 'crowding' phenomenon occurs to a certain extent in normal individuals but is more marked in amblyopes and must be taken into account when testing preverbal children.

Treatment

It is essential to examine the fundi to diagnose any visible organic disease prior to commencing treatment for amblyopia. Organic disease and amblyopia may coexist and a trial of patching may still be indicated in the presence of organic disease. If acuity does not respond to treatment, investigations such as electrophysiology or imaging should be reconsidered. The sensitive period during which acuity of an amblyopic eye can be improved is usually up to 7–8 years in strabismic amblyopia and may be longer (into the teens) for anisometropic amblyopia where good binocular function is present.

- **Occlusion** of the normal eye, to encourage use of the amblyopic eye, is the most effective treatment. The regimen, full-time or part-time, depends on the age of the patient and the density of amblyopia.
  - The younger the patient, the more rapid the likely improvement but the greater the risk of inducing amblyopia in the normal eye. It is therefore very important to monitor VA regularly in both eyes during treatment.
  - The better the VA at the start of occlusion, the shorter the duration required, although there is wide variation between patients.
  - If there has been no improvement after 6 months of effective occlusion, further treatment is unlikely to be fruitful.
  - Poor compliance is the single greatest barrier to improvement and must be monitored. Amblyopia treatment benefits from time spent at the outset on communication of the rationale and the difficulties involved.
- **Penalization**, in which vision in the normal eye is blurred with atropine, is an alternative method. It may work best

in the treatment of moderate amblyopia (6/24 or better). Patch occlusion is likely to produce a quicker response than atropine, which has conventionally been reserved for use when compliance with patch occlusion is poor. Weekend instillation may be adequate.

CLINICAL EVALUATION

History

- **Age of onset**
  - The earlier the onset, the more likely the need for surgical correction.
  - The later the onset, the greater the likelihood of an accommodative component (mostly arising between 18 and 36 months).
  - The longer the duration of squint in early childhood the greater the risk of amblyopia, unless fixation is freely alternating. Inspection of previous photographs may be useful for the documentation of strabismus or CHP.
- **Symptoms** may indicate decompensation of a pre-existent heterophoria or more significantly a recently acquired (usually paretic) condition. In the former, the patient usually complains of discomfort, blurring and possibly diplopia of indeterminate onset and duration compared to the acquired condition with the sudden onset of diplopia.
  - The type of diplopia (horizontal, cyclovertical) should be established, together with the direction of gaze in which it predominates and whether any BSV is retained.
  - In adults it is very important to determine exactly what problems the squint is causing as a basis for decisions about treatment.
  - It is not unusual for patients to present with spurious symptoms that mask embarrassment over a cosmetically noticeable squint.
- **Variability** is significant because intermittent strabismus indicates some degree of binocularity. An equally alternating deviation suggests symmetrical visual acuity in both eyes.
- **General health** or developmental problems may be significant (e.g. children with cerebral palsy have an increased incidence of strabismus). In older patients poor health and stress may cause decompensation, and in acquired paresis patients may report associations or causal factors (trauma, neurological disease, diabetes etc.).
- **Birth history**, including period of gestation, birth weight and any problems *in utero*, with delivery or in the neonatal period.
- **Family history** is important because strabismus is frequently familial, although no definitive inheritance pattern is recognized. It is also important to know what therapy was necessary in other family members.
- **Previous ocular history** including refractive prescription and compliance with spectacles or occlusion, previous surgery or prisms is important to future treatment options and prognosis.

Visual acuity

Testing in preverbal children

The evaluation can be separated into the qualitative assessment of visual behaviour and the quantitative assessment of visual acuity using preferential looking tests. Assessment of visual behaviour is achieved as follows:

- **Fixation and following** may be assessed using bright attention-grabbing targets (a face is often best). This method indicates whether the infant is visually alert and is of particular value in a child suspected of being blind.
- **Comparison** between the behaviour of the two eyes may reveal a unilateral preference. Occlusion of one eye, if strongly objected to by the child, indicates poorer acuity in the other eye. However, it is possible to have good visual attention with each eye but unequal visual acuity and all risk factors for amblyopia must be considered in the interpretation of results.
- **Fixation behaviour** can be used to establish unilateral preference if a manifest squint is present.
  - Fixation is promoted in the squinting eye by occluding the dominant eye while the child fixates a target of interest (preferably incorporating a light).
  - Fixation is then graded as *central* or *non-central* and *steady* or *unsteady* (the corneal reflection can be observed).
  - The other eye is then uncovered and the ability to *maintain* fixation is observed.
  - If fixation immediately returns to the uncovered eye, then visual acuity is probably impaired.
  - If fixation is maintained through a blink, then visual acuity is probably good.
  - If the patient alternates fixation, then the two eyes probably have equal vision.
- **The 10 Δ test** is similar and can be used regardless of whether a manifest squint is present. It involves the promotion of diplopia using a 10 Δ vertical prism. Alternation between the diplopic targets suggests equal visual acuity.
- **Rotation test** is a gross qualitative test of the ability of an infant to fixate with both eyes open. The test is performed as follows:
  - The examiner holds the child facing him or her and rotates briskly through 360°.
  - If vision is normal, the eyes will deviate in the direction of rotation under the influence of the vestibulo-ocular response. The eyes flick back to the primary position to produce a rotational nystagmus.
  - When rotation stops, nystagmus is briefly observed in the opposite direction for 1–2 seconds and should then cease due to suppression of post-rotary nystagmus by fixation.
  - If vision is severely impaired, the post-rotation nystagmus does not stop as quickly when rotation ceases because the vestibulo-ocular response is not blocked by visual feedback.

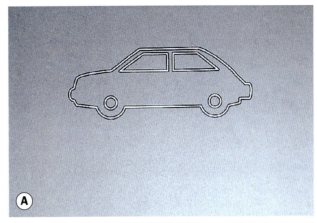

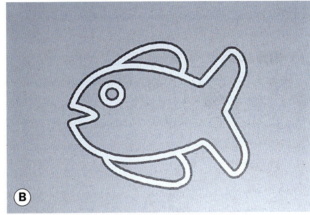

Fig. 18.17 Cardiff acuity cards

- **Preferential looking** tests can be used from early infancy and are based on the fact that infants prefer to look at a pattern rather than a homogeneous stimulus. The infant is exposed to a stimulus and the examiner observes the eyes for fixation movements, without themselves knowing the stimulus position.
  - Tests in common use include the Teller and Keeler acuity cards, which consist of black stripes (gratings) of varying widths, and Cardiff acuity cards (Fig. 18.17), which consist of familiar pictures with variable outline width.
  - Low frequency (coarse) gratings or pictures with a wider outline are seen more easily than high frequency gratings or thin outline pictures, and an assessment of resolution (not recognition) visual acuity is made accordingly.
  - Since grating acuity often exceeds Snellen acuity in amblyopia, Teller cards may overestimate visual acuity. These methods may not be reliable if a proper forced-choice staircase protocol is not followed during testing, and neither method has high sensitivity to the presence of amblyopia. The results must be considered in combination with risk factors for amblyopia.
- **Pattern visual evoked potentials** (VEP) give a representation of spatial acuity but are more commonly used in the diagnosis of optic neuropathy.

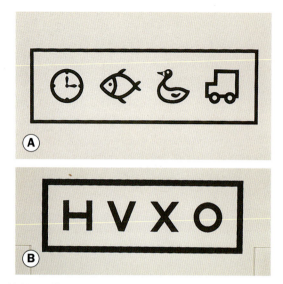

Fig. 18.18 (A) Kay pictures; **(B)** Keeler logMAR crowded test
(Courtesy of E Dawson)

Testing in verbal children

The tests described below should be performed at 3–4 metres from the target, as it is easier to obtain compliance than at 6 metres, with little or no clinical detriment. It is important to note that amblyopia can only be accurately diagnosed using a crowded test requiring target recognition and that logMAR tests (logarithm of the minimal angle of resolution – see Ch. 14) provide the best measure against which improvement with amblyopia therapy can be assessed. These are readily available in formats suited to normal children from 2 years onwards.

- **At age 2 years** most children will have sufficient language skills to undertake a picture naming test such as the crowded Kay pictures (Fig. 18.18A).
- **At age 3 years** most children will be able to undertake the matching of letter optotypes as in the Keeler logMAR (Fig. 18.18B) or Sonksen crowded tests. If a crowded letter test proves too difficult it is preferable to perform the crowded Kay pictures than to use single optotype letters.
- **Older children** may continue with the crowded letter tests, naming or matching them; LogMAR tests are in common usage and are preferable to Snellen for all children at risk of amblyopia.

Tests for stereopsis

Stereopsis is measured in seconds of arc (1° = 60 minutes of arc; 1 minute = 60 seconds); the lower the value the better the stereo-acuity. It is useful to remember that normal spatial resolution (visual acuity) is 1 minute and normal stereoacuity is 60 seconds (also 1 minute, but conventionally expressed in seconds). Various tests, using differing principles, are employed to assess the stereo-acuity. Random dot tests (e.g. TNO, Frisby) provide the most definitive evidence of high grade BSV. Where this is weak and/or based on ARC (see above), contour-based tests (e.g. Titmus) may provide more reliable information.

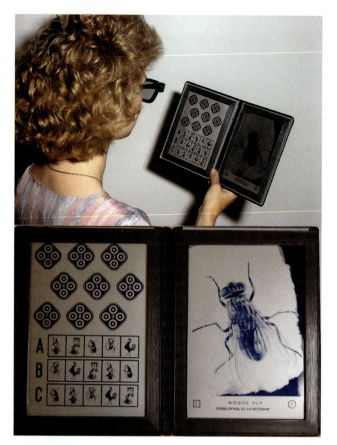

Fig. 18.19 Titmus test

Titmus

The Titmus test consists of a three-dimensional polarized vecto-graph comprising two plates in the form of a booklet viewed through polarized spectacles. On the right is a large fly, and on the left is a series of circles and animals (Fig. 18.19). The test should be performed at a distance of 40 cm.

- **The fly** is a test of gross stereopsis (3000 seconds), and is especially useful for young children. It should appear to stand out from the page and the child is encouraged to pick up the tip of one of its wings between finger and thumb.
- **The animals** component consists of three rows of stylized animals (400–100 seconds), one of which will appear forward of the plane of reference.
- **The circles** comprise a graded series measuring 800–40 seconds; one of a set of four circles should appear to stand out from the plate surface.

TNO

The TNO random dot test consists of seven plates of randomly distributed paired red and green dots viewed with red–green spec-tacles, and measures from 480 down to 15 seconds of arc at 40 cm. Within each plate the dots of one colour forming the target shape (squares, crosses etc. – Fig. 18.20) are displaced horizontally in relation to paired dots of the other colour so that they have a

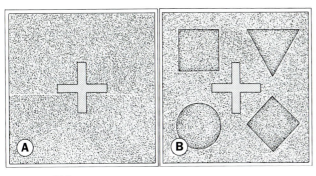

Fig. 18.20 TNO test

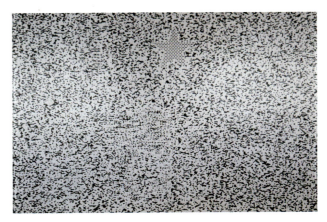

Fig. 18.22 Lang test

different retinal disparity to those outside the target. Control shapes are visible without the spectacles.

Frisby

The Frisby stereotest consists of three transparent plastic plates of varying thickness. On the surface of each plate are printed four squares of small randomly distributed shapes (Fig. 18.21). One of the squares contains a 'hidden' circle, in which the random shapes are printed on the reverse of the plate. The test does not require special spectacles because disparity (600–15 seconds) is created by the thickness of the plate; the working distance must be measured.

Lang

The Lang stereotest does not require special spectacles; the targets are seen alternately by each eye through the built-in cylindrical lens elements. Displacement of the dots creates disparity (1200–200 seconds) and the patient is asked to name or point to a simple shape, such as a star, on the card (Fig. 18.22).

Tests for binocular fusion in infants without manifest squint

Base-out prism

This is a simple method for detecting fusion in children. The test is performed by placing a 20 Δ base-out prism in front of one eye (the right eye in Fig. 18.23). This displaces the retinal image temporally with resultant diplopia.

- There will be a shift of the right eye to the left to resume fixation (right adduction) with a corresponding shift of the

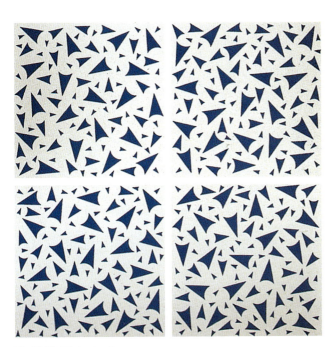

Fig. 18.21 Frisby test

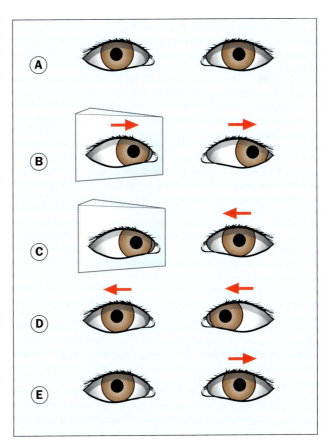

Fig. 18.23 Base-out prism test

left eye to the left (left abduction) in accordance with the Hering law (Fig. 18.23B).

- The left eye will then make a corrective re-fixational saccade to the right (left re-adduction) (Fig. 18.23C).
- On removal of the prism both eyes move to the right (Fig. 18.23D).
- The left eye then makes an outward fusional movement (Fig. 18.23E).
- Most children with good BSV should be able to overcome a 20 Δ prism from the age of 6 months; if not, weaker prisms (16 Δ or 12 Δ) may be tried, but the response is then more difficult to identify.

Binocular convergence

Simple convergence to an interesting target can be demonstrated from 3 to 4 months. Both eyes should follow the approaching target symmetrically 'to the nose'. Over-convergence in the infant may indicate an incipient esotropia; divergence may be due either to a tendency to a divergent deviation or simply lack of interest.

Tests for sensory anomalies

Worth four-dot test

This is a dissociation test that can be used with both distance and near fixation and differentiates between BSV, ARC and suppression. Results can only be interpreted if the presence or absence of a manifest squint is known at time of testing.

- **Procedure**
  ○ The patient wears a green lens in front of the right eye, which filters out all colours except green, and a red lens in front of the left eye which will filter out all colours except red (Fig. 18.24A).
  ○ The patient then views a box with four lights: one red, two green and one white.
- **Results** (Fig. 18.24B)
  ○ If BSV is present all four lights are seen.
  ○ If all four lights are seen in the presence of a manifest deviation, harmonious ARC (see 'Synoptophore' below) is present.
  ○ If two red lights are seen, right suppression is present.
  ○ If three green lights are seen, left suppression is present.
  ○ If two red and three green lights are seen, diplopia is present.
  ○ If the green and red lights alternate, alternating suppression is present.

Bagolini striated glasses

This is a test for detecting BSV, ARC or suppression. Each lens has fine striations that convert a point source of light into a line, as with the Maddox rod (see below).

- **Procedure.** The two lenses are placed at 45° and 135° in front of each eye and the patient fixates on a focal light source (Fig. 18.25A). Each eye perceives an oblique line of light,

perpendicular to that perceived by the fellow eye (Fig. 18.25B). Dissimilar images are thus presented to each eye under binocular viewing conditions.

- **Results** (Fig. 18.25C) cannot be interpreted unless it is known whether strabismus is present.
  ○ If the two streaks intersect at their centres in the form of an oblique cross (an 'X'), the patient has BSV if the eyes are straight, or harmonious ARC in the presence of manifest strabismus.
  ○ If the two lines are seen but they do not form a cross, diplopia is present.
  ○ If only one streak is seen, there is no simultaneous perception and suppression is present.
  ○ In theory, if a small gap is seen in one of the streaks, a central suppression scotoma (as found in microtropia) is present. In practice this is often difficult to demonstrate and the patient describes a cross. The scotoma can be confirmed with the 4 Δ prism test (see below).

4 Δ prism test

This test distinguishes bifoveal fixation (normal BSV) from foveal suppression (also known as a central suppression scotoma – CSS)

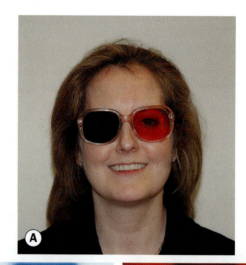
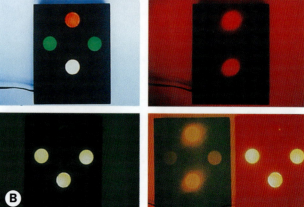

Fig. 18.24 Worth four-dot test. **(A)** Red-green glasses; **(B)** possible results

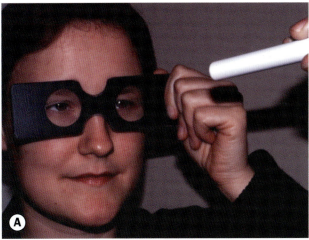

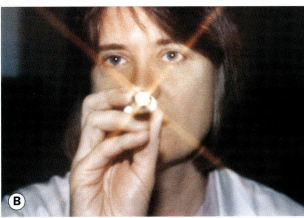

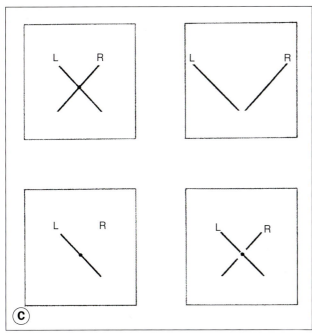

Fig. 18.25 Bagolini test. **(A)** Striated glasses; **(B)** appearance of a point of light through Bagolini lenses; **(C)** possible results

in microtropia and employs the principle described in the 20 Δ test (the Hering law and convergence) to overcome diplopia.

- **With bifoveal fixation**
  - The prism is placed base-out (microtropia is commonly esotropic not exotropic) in front of the right eye with deviation of the image away from the fovea temporally, followed by corrective movement of both eyes to the left (Fig. 18.26A).
  - The left eye then converges to fuse the images (Fig. 18.26B).
- **In left microtropia**
  - The patient fixates a distance target with both eyes open and a 4 Δ prism is placed base-out in front of the eye with suspected CSS (the left in Fig. 18.27).
  - The image is moved temporally in the left eye but falls within the CSS and no movement of either eye is observed (Fig. 18.27A).
  - The prism is then moved to the right eye which adducts to maintain fixation; the left eye similarly moves to the left consistent with the Hering law of equal innervation, but the second image falls within the CSS of the left eye and so no subsequent re-fixation movement is seen (Fig. 18.27B).

Synoptophore

The synoptophore compensates for the angle of squint and allows stimuli to be presented to both eyes simultaneously (Fig. 18.28A). It can thus be used to investigate the potential for binocular function in the presence of a manifest squint and is of particular value in assessing young children (from age 3 years), who generally find the test process enjoyable. It can also detect suppression and ARC.

- The instrument consists of two cylindrical tubes with a mirrored right-angled bend and a +6.50 D lens in each eyepiece (Fig. 18.28B, top). This optically sets the testing distance as equivalent to about 6 metres.
- Pictures are inserted in a slide carrier situated at the outer end of each tube. The two tubes are supported on columns that enable the pictures to be moved in relation to each other, and any adjustments are indicated on a scale.
- The synoptophore can measure horizontal, vertical and torsional misalignments simultaneously and is valuable in determining surgical approach by assessing the different contributions in the cardinal positions of gaze.

Grades of binocular vision

Binocular vision can be graded on the synoptophore as below (Fig. 18.28B, bottom).

- **First grade** (simultaneous perception – SP) is tested by introducing two dissimilar but not mutually antagonistic pictures, such as a bird and a cage.
  - The subject is then asked to put the bird into the cage by moving the arm of the synoptophore.
  - If the two pictures cannot be seen simultaneously, then suppression is present.

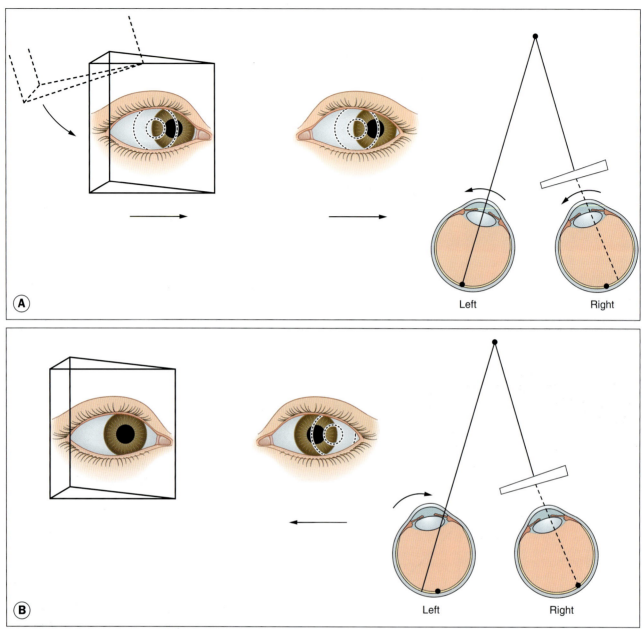

Fig. 18.26 4 Δ prism test in bifoveal fixation. **(A)** Shift of both eyes away from the prism base; **(B)** fusional re-fixation movement of the left eye

○ Some retinal 'rivalry' will occur although one picture is smaller than the other, so that while the small one is seen foveally, the larger one is seen parafoveally (and is thus placed in front of the deviating eye).

○ Larger macular and paramacular slides are used if foveal slides cannot be superimposed.

• **Second grade** (fusion). If simultaneous perception slides can be superimposed then the test proceeds to the second grade which is the ability of the two eyes to produce a composite picture (sensory fusion) from two similar

pictures, each of which is incomplete in one small different detail.

○ The classic example is two rabbits, one lacking a tail and the other lacking a bunch of flowers. If fusion is present, one rabbit complete with tail and flowers will be seen.

○ The range of fusion (motor fusion) is then tested by moving the arms of the synoptophore so that the eyes have to converge and diverge in order to maintain fusion.

○ The presence of simple fusion without any range is of little value in everyday life.

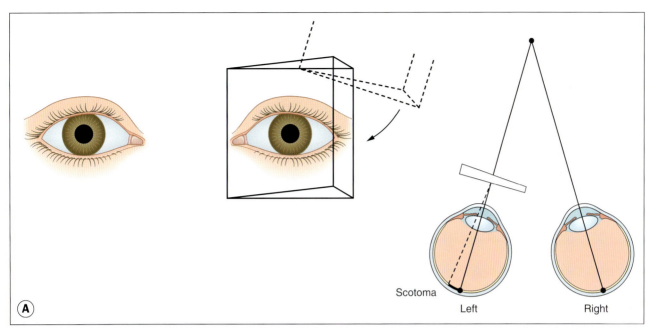

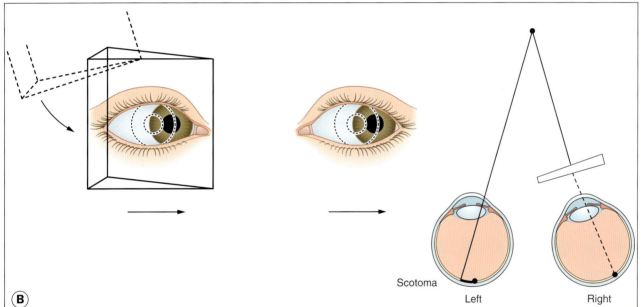

Fig. 18.27 4 Δ prism test in left microtropia with a central suppression scotoma. **(A)** No movement of either eye; **(B)** both eyes move to the left but there is absence of re-fixation

- **Third grade** (stereopsis) is the ability to obtain an impression of depth by the superimposition of two pictures of the same object which have been taken from slightly different angles. The classic example is a bucket, which should be appreciated in three dimensions.

Detection of abnormal retinal correspondence

ARC is detected on the synoptophore as follows:
- The subjective angle of deviation is that at which the SP slides are superimposed. The examiner determines the

objective angle of the deviation by presenting each fovea alternately with a target by extinguishing one or other light and moving the slide in front of the deviating eye until no movement of the eyes is seen.
- If the subjective and objective angles coincide then retinal correspondence is normal.
- If the objective and subjective angles are different, ARC is present. The difference in degrees between the subjective and objective angles is the angle of anomaly. ARC is said to be harmonious when the objective angle equals the angle of anomaly and inharmonious when it exceeds the angle of

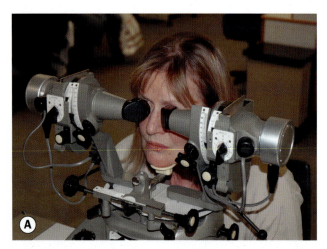
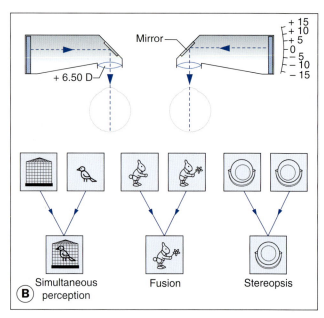

Fig. 18.28 (A) Synoptophore; **(B)** optical principles and grading of binocular vision

anomaly. It is only in harmonious ARC that binocular responses can be demonstrated; the inharmonious form may represent a lesser adaptation or an artefact of testing.

Measurement of deviation

Hirschberg test

The Hirschberg test gives a rough objective estimate of the angle of a manifest strabismus and is especially useful in young or unco-operative patients or when fixation in the deviating eye is poor. It is also useful in excluding pseudostrabismus. A pen torch is shone into the eyes from arm's length and the patient asked to fixate the light. The corneal reflection of the light will be (more or less) centred in the pupil of the fixating eye, but will be decentred in a squinting eye, in the direction opposite to that of the deviation (Fig. 18.29). The distance of the corneal light reflection from the centre of the pupil is noted; each millimetre of deviation is approximately equal to 7° (1° ≈ 2 prism dioptres). For example, if the reflex is situated at the temporal border of the pupil (assuming a pupillary diameter of 4 mm), the angle is about 15°; if it is at the limbus, the angle is about 45°.

Krimsky and prism reflection tests

Corneal reflex assessment can be combined with prisms to give a more accurate approximation of the angle in a manifest deviation.

- **The Krimsky test** involves placement of prisms in front of the fixating eye until the corneal light reflections are symmetrical (Fig. 18.30). This test reduces the problem of parallax and is more commonly used than the prism reflection test.

- **The prism reflection test** involves the placement of prisms in front of the deviating eye until the corneal light reflections are symmetrical.

Cover–uncover test

The cover–uncover test consists of two parts:
- **Cover test** to detect a heterotropia. It is helpful to begin the near test using a light to observe the corneal reflections and to assess fixation in the deviating eye. It should then be repeated for near using an accommodative target and for distance as follows:
  ○ The patient fixates on a straight-ahead target.
  ○ If a right deviation is suspected, the examiner covers the fixing left eye and notes any movement of the right eye to take up fixation.
  ○ No movement indicates orthotropia (Fig. 18.31A) or left heterotropia (Fig. 18.31B).
  ○ Adduction of the right eye to take up fixation indicates right exotropia and abduction, right esotropia (Fig. 18.31C).
  ○ Downward movement indicates right hypertropia and upward movement right hypotropia.
  ○ The test is repeated on the opposite eye.
- **The uncover test** detects heterophoria. It should be performed both for near (using an accommodative target) and for distance as follows:
  ○ The patient fixates a straight-ahead distant target.
  ○ The examiner covers the right eye and, after 2–3 seconds, removes the cover.
  ○ No movement indicates orthophoria (Fig. 18.32A); a keen observer will frequently detect a very slight latent deviation in most normal individuals, as few individuals are truly orthophoric, particularly on near fixation.

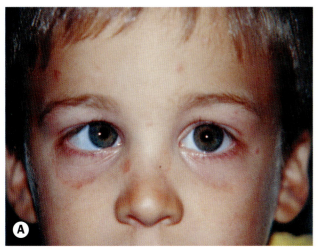

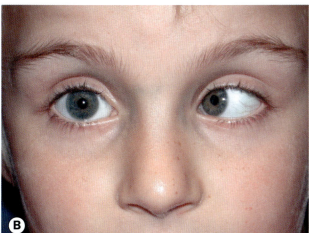

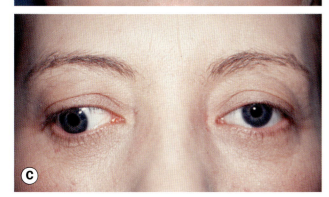

Fig. 18.29 Hirschberg test. **(A)** The right corneal reflex is near the temporal border of the pupil indicating an angle of about 15°; **(B)** the left corneal reflex is near the limbus indicating an angle of close to 45° – convergent squint; **(C)** the right corneal reflex demonstrating both divergence and hypotropia

(Courtesy of J Yangüela – fig. A)

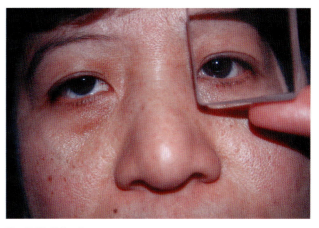

Fig. 18.30 Krimsky test
(Courtesy of K Nischal)

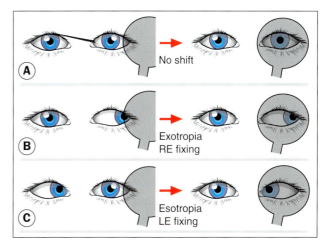

Fig. 18.31 Possible results of the cover test

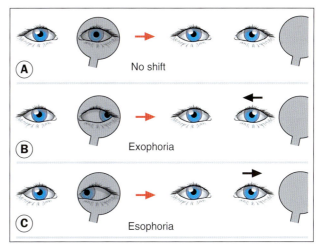

Fig. 18.32 Possible results of the uncover test

○ If the right eye had deviated while under cover, a re-fixation movement (recovery to BSV) is observed on being uncovered.

○ Adduction (nasal recovery) of the right eye indicates exophoria (Fig. 18.32B) and abduction esophoria (Fig. 18.32C).

○ Upward or downward movement indicates a vertical phoria.

○ After the cover is removed, the examiner notes the speed and smoothness of recovery as evidence of the strength of motor fusion.

○ The test is repeated for the opposite eye.

○ Most examiners perform the cover test and the uncover test sequentially, hence the term cover–uncover test.

Alternate cover test

The alternate cover test induces dissociation to reveal the total deviation when fusion is disrupted. It should be performed only after the cover–uncover test.

● The right eye is covered for several seconds.

● The occluder is quickly shifted to the opposite eye for 2 seconds, then back and forth several times. After the cover is removed, the examiner notes the speed and smoothness of recovery as the eyes return to their pre-dissociated state.

● A patient with a well-compensated heterophoria will have straight eyes before and after the test has been performed whereas a patient with poor control may decompensate to a manifest deviation.

Prism cover test

The prism cover test measures the angle of deviation on near or distance fixation and in any gaze position. It combines the alternate cover test with prisms and is performed as follows:

● The alternate cover test is first performed to establish the direction and approximate extent of deviation.

● Prisms of increasing strength are placed in front of one eye with the base opposite the direction of the deviation (i.e. the apex of the prism is pointed in the direction of the deviation). For example, in a convergent strabismus the prism is held base-out, and in a right hypertropia, base down before the right eye.

● The alternate cover test is performed continuously as stronger prisms are introduced, typically using a prism bar consisting of a column of prisms of progressive strength (Fig. 18.33). The amplitude of the re-fixation movement should gradually decrease as the strength of prism approaches the extent of deviation.

● The end-point is approached when no movement is seen. To ensure the maximum angle is found, the prism strength can be increased further until a movement is observed in the opposite direction (the point of reversal) and then reduced again to find the neutral value; the angle of deviation is then taken from the strength of the prism.

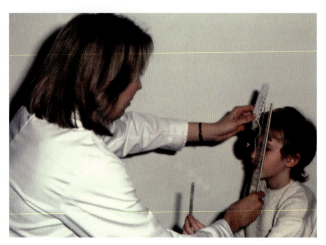

Fig. 18.33 Prism cover test

Maddox wing

The Maddox wing dissociates the eyes for near fixation (1/3 m) and measures heterophoria. The instrument is constructed in such a way that the right eye sees only a white vertical arrow and a red horizontal arrow, whereas the left eye sees only horizontal and vertical rows of numbers (Fig. 18.34).

● Horizontal deviation is measured by asking the patient to which number the white arrow points.

● Vertical deviation is measured by asking the patient which number intersects with the red arrow.

● The amount of cyclophoria is determined by asking the patient to move the red arrow so that it is parallel with the horizontal row of numbers.

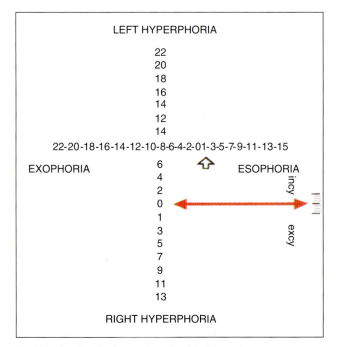

Fig. 18.34 Patient's view using the Maddox wing

Maddox rod

The Maddox rod consists of a series of fused cylindrical red glass rods that convert the appearance of a white spot of light into a red streak. The optical properties of the rods cause the streak of light to be at an angle of 90° with the long axis of the rods; when the glass rods are held horizontally, the streak will be vertical and vice versa.

- The rod is placed in front of the right eye (Fig. 18.35A). This dissociates the two eyes: the red streak seen by the right eye cannot be fused with the unaltered white spot of light seen by the left eye (Fig. 18.35B).
- The amount of dissociation (Fig. 18.35C) is measured by the superimposition of the two images using prisms. The base of the prism is placed in the position opposite to the direction of the deviation.
- Both vertical and horizontal deviations can be measured in this way but the test cannot differentiate a phoria from a tropia.

Motility tests

Ocular movements

Examination of eye movements involves the assessment of smooth pursuit movements followed by saccades.

- **Versions** towards the eight eccentric positions of gaze are tested by asking the patient to follow a target, usually a pen or pen torch (the latter offers the advantage of corneal light reflections to aid assessment). A cover test is performed in each position of gaze to confirm whether a phoria has become a tropia or the angle of deviation has increased and the patient is questioned regarding diplopia. Versions may also be elicited involuntarily in response to a noise or by the doll's head manoeuvre in uncooperative patients.
- **Ductions** are assessed if reduced ocular motility is noted in either or both eyes. A pen torch should be used with careful attention to the position of the corneal reflexes. The fellow

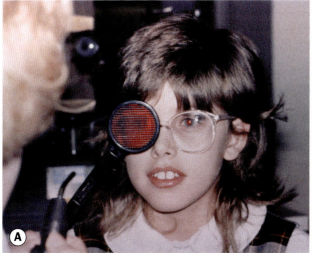

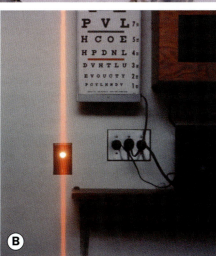

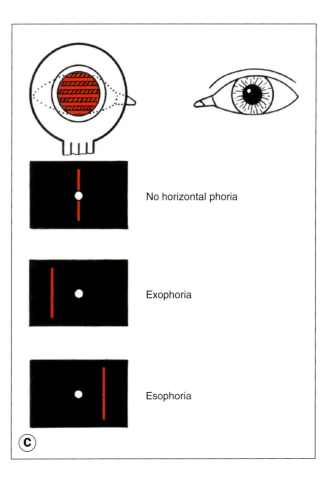

No horizontal phoria

Exophoria

Esophoria

Fig. 18.35 **(A)** Maddox rod test; **(B)** appearance of a point of light through the Maddox rod; **(C)** possible results

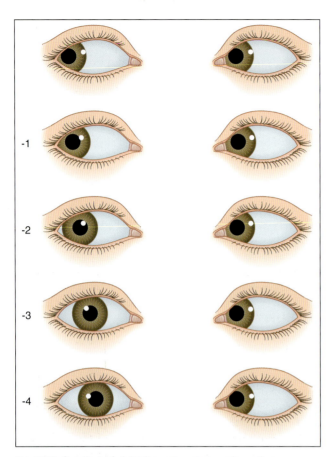

Fig. 18.36 Grading of right lateral rectus underaction

eye is occluded and the patient asked to follow the torch into various positions of gaze. A simple numeric system may be employed using 0 to denote full movement, and −1 to −4 to denote increasing degrees of underaction (Fig. 18.36).

Near point of convergence

The near point of convergence (NPC) is the nearest point on which the eyes can maintain binocular fixation. It can be measured with the RAF rule, which rests on the patient's cheeks (Fig. 18.37A). A target (Fig. 18.37B) is slowly moved along the rule towards the patient's eyes until one eye loses fixation and drifts laterally (objective NPC). The subjective NPC is the point at which the patient reports diplopia. Normally, the NPC should be nearer than 10 cm without undue effort.

Near point of accommodation

The near point of accommodation (NPA) is the nearest point on which the eyes can maintain clear focus. It can also be measured with the RAF rule. The patient fixates a line of print, which is then slowly moved towards the patient until it becomes blurred. The distance at which this is first reported is read off the rule and denotes the NPA. The NPA recedes with age; when sufficiently far away to render reading difficult without optical correction, presbyopia is present. At the age of 20 years the NPA is 8 cm and by the age of 50 years it has receded to approximately 46 cm. The

amplitude of accommodation can also be assessed using concave lenses in 0.5 DS steps whilst fixating the 6/6 Snellen line and reporting when the vision blurs.

Fusional amplitudes

Fusional amplitudes measure the efficacy of vergence movements. They may be tested with prisms bars or the synoptophore. An increasingly strong prism is placed in front of one eye, which will then abduct or adduct (depending on whether the prism is base-in or base-out), in order to maintain bifoveal fixation. When a prism greater than the fusional amplitude is reached, diplopia is reported or one eye drifts in the opposite direction, indicating the limit of vergence ability.

Postoperative diplopia test

This simple test is mandatory prior to strabismus surgery in all non-binocular patients over 7–8 years of age to assess the risk of diplopia after surgery.

- Corrective prisms are placed in front of one eye (usually the deviating eye) and the patient asked to fixate a straight-ahead target with both eyes open. The prisms are slowly increased until the angle has been significantly overcorrected and the patient reports if diplopia occurs.

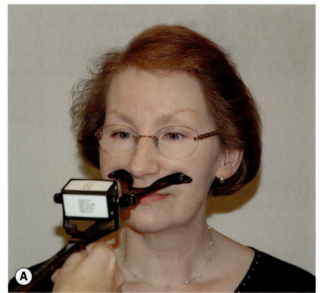

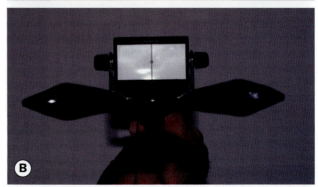

Fig. 18.37 (A) RAF rule; **(B)** convergence target

- If suppression persists throughout there is little risk of diplopia following surgery; however, in a consecutive exotropia of 35 Δ, diplopia may be reported from 30 Δ and persist as the prism correction mimics an esotropia.
- Diplopia may be intermittent or constant but in either case constitutes an indication to perform a diagnostic botulinum toxin test (see below).
- Diplopia is not restricted to patients with good visual acuity in the deviating eye.
- Intractable diplopia is difficult to treat.

Hess chart

A Hess chart is plotted to aid in the diagnosis and monitoring of a patient with incomitant strabismus, such as an extraocular muscle palsy (e.g. third, fourth or sixth nerve paresis) or a mechanical or myopathic limitation (e.g. thyroid ophthalmopathy, blow-out fracture or myasthenia gravis). The chart is commonly prepared using either the Lees or Hess screen, which facilitate plotting of the dissociated ocular position as a measure of extraocular muscle action. Information provided by the Hess chart should be regarded in the context of other investigations such as the field of binocular single vision. The prism cover test is also very useful in the assessment of incomitant squint.

Hess screen

The Hess screen contains a tangent pattern displayed on a dark grey background. Red lights that can be individually illuminated by a control panel indicate the cardinal positions of gaze within a central field (15° from primary position) and a peripheral field (30°); each square represents 5° of ocular rotation. The eyes are dissociated by the use of reversible goggles incorporating a red and a green lens, the red lens in front of the fixating eye and the green lens the non-fixating eye. Red points of lights are illuminated at selected positions on the screen. The patient holds a green pointer, and is asked to superimpose a green light over each red light in turn. In orthophoria the two lights should be more or less superimposed in all positions of gaze. The goggles are then reversed and the procedure repeated. Software is available that facilitates the plotting of a Hess chart using a standard desktop computer screen.

Lees screen

This apparatus (Fig. 18.38) consists of two opalescent glass screens at right-angles to each other, bisected by a two-sided plane mirror that dissociates the eyes; each of the eyes can see only one of the two screens. Each screen has a tangent pattern (two-dimensional projection of a spherical surface) that is revealed only when the screen is illuminated. The patient is positioned facing the non-illuminated screen with his or her chin stabilized on a rest. Using a pointer, the examiner indicates a target point on the illuminated tangent pattern and the patient positions a pointer on the non-illuminated screen, at a position perceived to be superimposed on the dot indicated by the examiner. The non-illuminated screen is briefly illuminated by the examiner using a footswitch to facilitate recording of the dot indicated by the patient. When the procedure has been completed for one eye, the patient is rotated through 90°

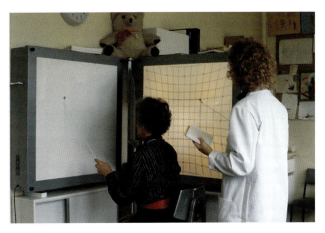

Fig. 18.38 Lees screen

to face the previously illuminated screen and the procedure repeated.

Interpretation

Figure 18.39 shows a typical Hess chart appearance in right lateral rectus paresis of recent onset.
- The smaller chart indicates the eye with the paretic muscle (right eye).
- The larger chart indicates the eye with the overacting yoke muscle (left eye).
- The smaller chart will show its greatest restriction in the main direction of action of the paretic muscle (right lateral rectus).
- The larger chart will show its greatest expansion in the main direction of action of the yoke muscle (left medial rectus).
- The degree of disparity between the plotted point and the template in any position of gaze gives an estimate of the angle of deviation (each square = 5°).

Changes over time

Progressive changes in the Hess chart with time are characteristic, and useful both as a prognostic indicator and to guide management.
- In right superior rectus palsy, the Hess chart will show underaction of the affected muscle with an overaction of its yoke muscle, the left inferior oblique (Fig. 18.40A). Because of the great incomitance of the two charts, the diagnosis is

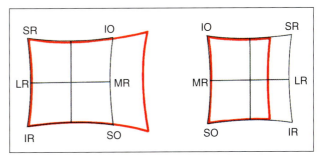

Fig. 18.39 Hess chart of a recent right lateral rectus palsy. IO = inferior oblique; IR = inferior rectus; LR = lateral rectus; MR = medial rectus; SO = superior oblique; SR = superior rectus

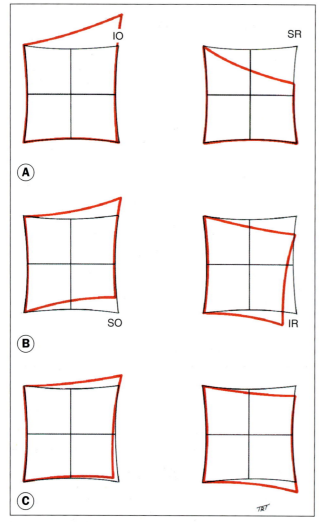

Fig. 18.40 Hess chart showing changes with time of a right superior rectus palsy. IO = inferior oblique; IR = inferior rectus; SO = superior oblique; SR = superior rectus

straightforward. If the paretic muscle recovers its function, both charts will revert to normal.

- Secondary contracture of the ipsilateral antagonist (right inferior rectus) will manifest as an overaction which will lead to a secondary (inhibitional) palsy of the antagonist of the yoke muscle (left superior oblique), which will show up on the chart as an underaction (Fig. 18.40B). This could lead to the incorrect impression that the left superior oblique is the primarily paretic muscle.
- With further passage of time, the two charts become progressively more concomitant, such that it may be impossible to determine the initiating muscle weakness (Fig. 18.40C).

Examples

The clinical features of extraocular muscle palsies are discussed in detail in Chapter 19.

- **Left third nerve palsy** (Fig. 18.41)
  - The area enclosed on the left chart is much smaller than that on the right.

- Left exotropia – note that the fixation spots in the inner charts of both eyes are deviated laterally. The deviation is greater on the right chart (when the left eye is fixating), indicating that secondary deviation exceeds the primary, typical of a paretic squint.
- Left chart shows underaction of all muscles except the lateral rectus.
- Right chart shows overaction of all muscles except the medial rectus and inferior rectus, the 'yokes' of the spared muscles.
- The primary angle of deviation (fixing right eye – FR) in the primary position is −20° and R/L 10°.
- The secondary angle (fixing left eye – FL) is −28° and R/L 12°.
- In inferior rectus palsy, the function of the superior oblique muscle can only be assessed by observing intorsion on attempted depression. This is best performed by observing a conjunctival landmark using the slit lamp.
- **Recently acquired right fourth nerve palsy** (Fig. 18.42)
  - Right chart is smaller than the left.
  - Right chart shows underaction of the superior oblique and overaction of the inferior oblique.
  - Left chart shows overaction of the inferior rectus and underaction (inhibitional palsy) of the superior rectus.
  - The primary deviation (FL) is R/L 8°; the secondary deviation FR is R/L 17°.
- **Congenital right fourth nerve palsy** (Fig. 18.43)
  - No difference in overall chart size.
  - Primary and secondary deviation R/L 4°.
  - Right hypertropia – note that the fixation spot of the right inner chart is deviated upwards and the left is deviated downwards.
  - Hypertropia increases on laevoversion and reduces on dextroversion.
  - Right chart shows underaction of the superior oblique and overaction of the inferior oblique.
  - Left chart shows overaction of the inferior rectus and underaction (inhibitional palsy) of the superior rectus.
- **Right sixth nerve palsy** (Fig. 18.44)
  - Right chart is smaller than the left.
  - Right esotropia – note that the fixation spot of the right inner chart is deviated nasally.
  - Right chart shows marked underaction of the lateral rectus and slight overaction of the medial rectus.
  - Left chart shows marked overaction of the medial rectus.
  - The primary angle FL is +15° and the secondary angle FR +20°.
  - Inhibitional palsy of the left lateral rectus has not yet developed.

Refraction and fundoscopy

Dilated fundoscopy is mandatory in the context of strabismus, principally to exclude any underlying ocular pathology such as macular scarring, optic disc hypoplasia or retinoblastoma as the

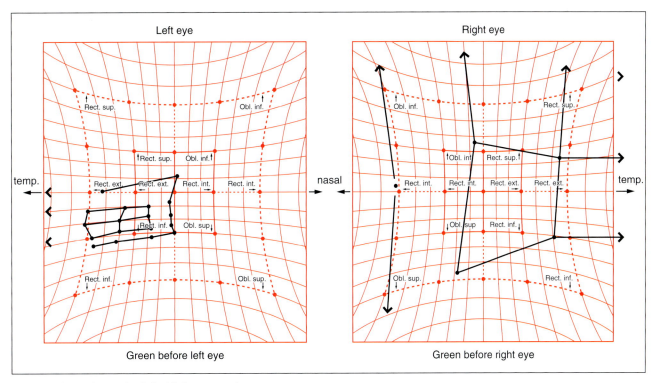

Fig. 18.41 Hess chart of a left third nerve palsy

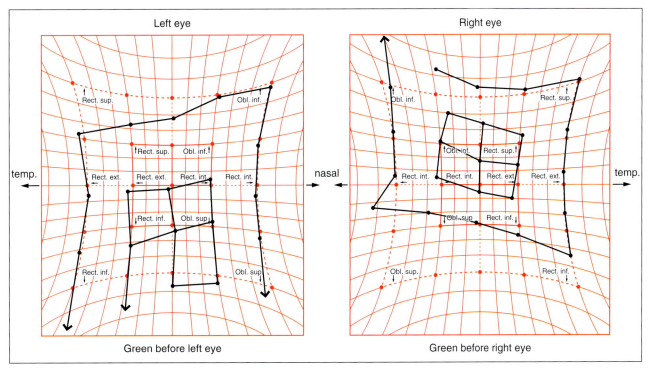

Fig. 18.42 Hess chart of a recently acquired right fourth nerve palsy

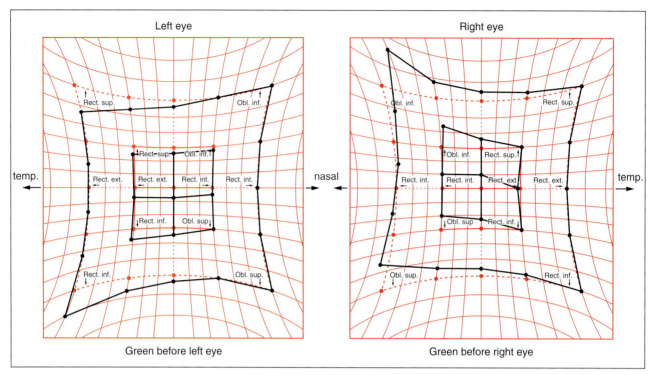

Fig. 18.43 Hess chart of a congenital right fourth nerve palsy

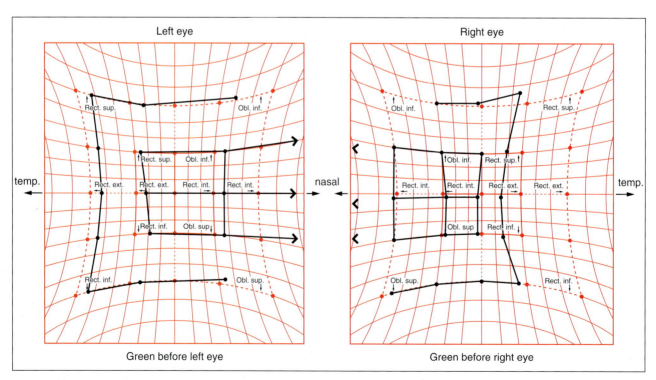

Fig. 18.44 Hess chart of a right sixth nerve palsy

cause of the deviation. More commonly, strabismus is secondary to refractive error; hypermetropia (hyperopia), astigmatism, anisometropia and myopia may all be associated.

Cycloplegia

The most common refractive error to cause strabismus is hypermetropia. Accurate measurements of hypermetropia necessitate effective paralysis of the ciliary muscle (cycloplegia), in order to neutralize the masking effect of accommodation. In a young child the risk of penalization amblyopia should be avoided by always inducing cycloplegia in both eyes at one sitting, particularly if atropine is used.

- **Cyclopentolate** (0.5% under 6 months and 1% subsequently). One drop, repeated after 5 minutes, usually results in maximal cycloplegia within 30 minutes, with recovery of accommodation within 2–3 hours and resolution of mydriasis within 24 hours. The adequacy of cycloplegia can be determined by comparing retinoscopy readings with the patient fixating for distance and then for near. Topical anaesthesia with a well-tolerated agent such as proxymetacaine prior to instillation of cyclopentolate is useful in preventing ocular irritation and reflex tearing, thus affording better retention of the cyclopentolate in the conjunctival sac and effective cycloplegia.

- **Atropine** (0.5% under the age of 12 months and 1% subsequently) has a somewhat stronger cycloplegic effect than cyclopentolate. In most cases this is clinically insignificant, but may be helpful in instances such as high hypermetropia or heavily pigmented irides. As the onset of cycloplegia is slower, a carer may be supplied with topical atropine for instillation at home twice daily over 1–3 days prior to attendance (but not on the day of examination) as either eye drops or ointment; drops are easier to instil, but there may be less risk of overdose with ointment. The atropine should be discontinued if there are signs of systemic toxicity, such as flushing, fever or restlessness, and immediate medical attention sought. The visual effects may last for up to 2 weeks.

Change of refraction with age in childhood

Because refraction changes with age, it is important to check this in patients with strabismus at least every year and more frequently in younger children and if acuity is reduced. At birth most babies are hypermetropic. After the age of 2 years there may be an increase in hypermetropia and a decrease in astigmatism. Hypermetropia may continue to increase until the age of about 6 years, levelling off between the ages of 6 and 8 and subsequently decreasing.

When to prescribe

Most children are mildly hypermetropic (1–3 D). There is some evidence that fully correcting hypermetropia in a normal child may reduce physiological emmetropization.

- **Hypermetropia.** In general up to 4 D of hypermetropia should not be corrected in a child without a squint unless they are experiencing problems with near vision. With hypermetropia greater than this a two-thirds correction is usually given. However, in the presence of esotropia, the full cycloplegic correction should be prescribed, even under the age of 2 years.

- **Astigmatism.** A cylinder of 1.50 D or more should probably be prescribed, especially in anisometropia after the age of 18 months.

- **Myopia.** The necessity for correction depends on the age of the child. Under the age of 2 years, −5.00 D or more of myopia should be corrected; between the ages of 2 and 4 the amount is −3.00 D. Older children should have correction of even low myopia to allow clear distance vision. Undercorrection and bifocals may retard progression and are under investigation.

- **Anisometropia.** After the age of 3 the full difference in refraction between the eyes should be prescribed if it is more than 1 D, with full hypermetropic correction in squint.

PSEUDOSTRABISMUS

Pseudostrabismus is the clinical impression of ocular deviation when no squint is present.

- **Epicanthic folds** may simulate an esotropia (Fig. 18.45A).
- **Abnormal interpupillary distance**, if short may simulate an esotropia and if wide an exotropia (Fig. 18.45B).

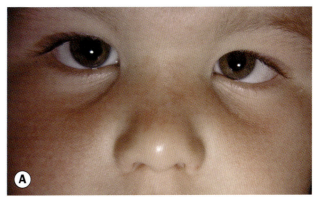

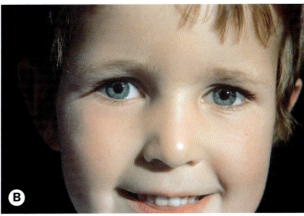

Fig. 18.45 Pseudostrabismus. **(A)** Prominent epicanthic folds simulating esotropia; **(B)** wide interpupillary distance simulating exotropia

- **Angle kappa** is the angle between the visual and anatomical (pupillary) axes.
  - Normally, the fovea is situated temporal to the anatomical centre of the posterior pole. The eyes are therefore slightly abducted to achieve bifoveal fixation and a light shone onto the cornea will therefore cause a reflex just nasal to the centre of the cornea in both eyes (Fig. 18.46A). This is termed a positive angle kappa.

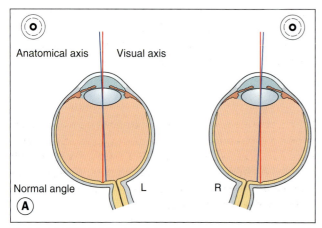

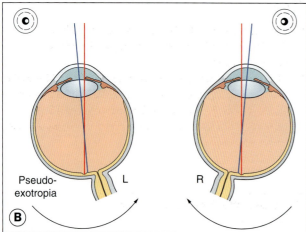

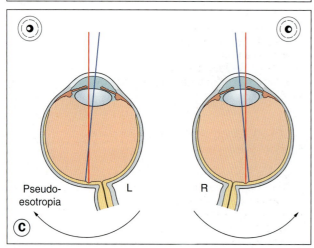

Fig. 18.46 Angle kappa. **(A)** Normal; **(B)** positive, simulating an exotropia; **(C)** negative, simulating an esotropia

- A large positive angle kappa (e.g. temporally displaced macula) may give a pseudoexotropia (Fig. 18.46B).
- A negative angle kappa occurs when the fovea is situated nasal to the posterior pole (e.g. high myopia). In this situation, the corneal reflex is situated temporally to the centre of the cornea and it may simulate an esotropia (Fig. 18.46C).

HETEROPHORIA

Heterophoria may present clinically with associated visual symptoms when the fusional amplitudes are insufficient to maintain alignment, particularly at times of stress or poor health.

- **Signs.** Both esophoria and exophoria can be classified by the distance at which the angle is greater: respectively, convergence excess or weakness, divergence weakness or excess and mixed.
- **Treatment**
  - Orthoptic treatment is of most value in convergence weakness exophoria.
  - Any significant refractive error should be appropriately corrected.
  - Symptom relief may otherwise be obtained using temporary stick-on Fresnel prisms and may be subsequently incorporated into spectacles (maximum usually 10–12 Δ, split between the two eyes).
  - Surgery may occasionally be required for larger deviations.

VERGENCE ABNORMALITIES

Convergence insufficiency

Convergence insufficiency (CI) typically affects individuals with high near visual demand, such as students.

- **Signs.** Reduced near point of convergence independent of any heterophoria.
- **Treatment** involves orthoptic exercises aimed at normalizing the near point and maximizing fusional amplitudes. With good compliance, symptoms should be eliminated within a few weeks but if persistent can be treated with base-in prisms.
- **Accommodative insufficiency** (AI) is occasionally also present. It may be idiopathic (primary) or post-viral and typically affects school-age children. The minimum reading correction to give clear vision is prescribed but is often difficult to discard.

Divergence insufficiency

Divergence paresis or paralysis is a rare condition typically associated with underlying neurological disease, such as intracranial space-occupying lesions, cerebrovascular accidents and head trauma. Presentation may be at any age and may be difficult to differentiate from sixth nerve palsy, but is primarily a concomitant

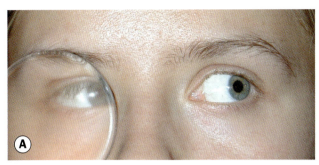

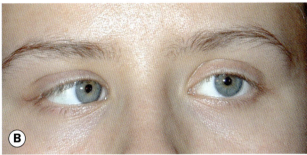

Fig. 18.47 (A) Spasm of the near reflex precipitated on testing ocular movements; **(B)** right esotropia and miosis

esodeviation with reduced or absent divergence fusional amplitudes. It is difficult to treat; prisms are the best option.

Near reflex insufficiency

- **Paresis** of the near reflex presents as dual convergence and accommodation insufficiency. Mydriasis may be seen on attempted near fixation. Treatment involves reading glasses, base-in prisms and possibly botulinum toxin (orthoptic exercises have no effect). It is difficult to eradicate.
- **Complete paralysis** in which no convergence or accommodation can be initiated may be of functional origin, due to midbrain disease or after head trauma; recovery is possible.

Spasm of the near reflex

Spasm of the near reflex is a functional condition affecting patients of all ages (mainly females). Diplopia, blurred vision and headaches are the presenting symptoms.

- **Signs**
  - Esotropia, pseudomyopia and miosis.
  - Spasm may be triggered when testing ocular movements (Fig. 18.47A).
  - Observation of miosis is the key to the diagnosis (Fig. 18.47B).
  - Refraction with and without cycloplegia confirms the pseudomyopia, which must not be corrected optically.
- **Treatment** involves reassurance and advising the patient to discontinue any activity that triggers the response. If persistent, atropine and a full reading correction are prescribed but it is difficult later to abandon treatment without recurrence. Patients usually manage to live a fairly normal life despite the symptoms.

ESOTROPIA

Esotropia (manifest convergent squint) may be concomitant or incomitant. In a concomitant esotropia the variability of the angle of deviation is within 5 Δ in different horizontal gaze positions. In an incomitant deviation the angle differs in various positions of gaze as a result of abnormal innervation or restriction. This section deals only with concomitant esotropia. A classification is shown in Table 18.1; however, all squints are different and not all fit neatly into a classification. For example, a microtropia may occur with a number of the other categories. It is more important to understand the part played by binocular function, refractive error and accommodation in the pathophysiology of each individual squint and to tailor treatment accordingly.

Early-onset esotropia

Up to the age of 4 months, infrequent episodes of convergence are normal but thereafter ocular misalignment is abnormal. Early-onset (congenital, essential infantile) esotropia is an idiopathic esotropia developing within the first 6 months of life in an otherwise normal infant with no significant refractive error and no limitation of ocular movements.

Signs

- The angle is usually fairly large (>30 Δ) and stable.
- Fixation in most infants is alternating in the primary position (Fig. 18.48).
- There is cross-fixating in side gaze, so that the child uses the left eye in right gaze (Fig. 18.49A) and the right eye on left gaze (Fig. 18.49B). Such cross-fixation may give a false impression of bilateral abduction deficits, as in bilateral sixth nerve palsy.

Table 18.1 Classification of esotropia

Accommodative

• Refractive
  • Fully accommodative
  • Partially accommodative
• Non-refractive
  • With convergence excess
  • With accommodation weakness
• Mixed

Non-accommodative
• Early onset (congenital, essential infantile) • Microtropia • Basic • Convergence excess • Convergence spasm • Divergence insufficiency • Divergence paralysis • Sensory • Consecutive • Acute onset • Cyclic

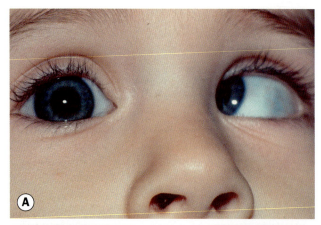

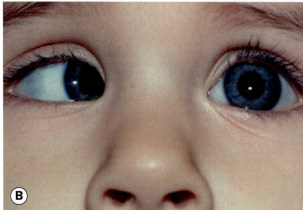

Fig. 18.48 Alternating fixation in early-onset esotropia. **(A)** Fixating with right eye; **(B)** fixating with left eye
(Courtesy of J Yangüela)

convergence dampens a horizontal nystagmus, and mechanical limitations of eye movement such as Duane and Möbius syndromes and strabismus fixus.

Initial treatment

Early ocular alignment gives the best chance of the development of some degree of binocular function. Ideally, the eyes should be surgically aligned by the age of 12 months, and at the very latest by the age of 2 years, but only after amblyopia and any significant refractive error have been corrected.

- The initial procedure can be either recession of both medial recti or unilateral medial rectus recession with lateral rectus resection. Very large angles may require recessions of 6.5 mm or more. Associated significant inferior oblique overaction should also be addressed.
- An acceptable goal is alignment of the eyes to within 10 Δ, associated with peripheral fusion and central suppression (Fig. 18.50). This small-angle residual strabismus is often stable, even though bifoveal fusion is not achieved.

- Abduction can usually be demonstrated, either by the doll's head manoeuvre or by rotating the child.
- Should these fail, uniocular patching for a few hours will often unmask the ability of the other eye to abduct.
- Nystagmus is usually horizontal.
- Latent nystagmus (LN) is seen only when one eye is covered and the fast phase beats towards the side of the fixing eye. This means that the direction of the fast phase reverses according to which eye is covered.
- Manifest latent nystagmus (MLN) is the same except that nystagmus is present with both eyes open, but the amplitude increases when one is covered.
- The refractive error is usually normal for the age of the child (about +1 to +2 D).
- Asymmetry of optokinetic nystagmus is present.
- Inferior oblique overaction may be present initially or develop later (see Fig. 18.51).
- Dissociated vertical deviation (DVD) develops in 80% by the age of 3 years (see Fig. 18.52).
- **Differential diagnosis** includes bilateral congenital sixth nerve palsy, secondary (sensory) esotropia due to organic eye disease, nystagmus blockage syndrome in which

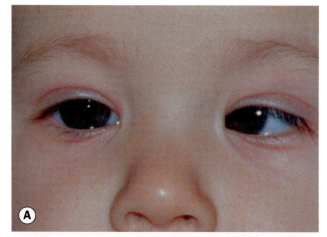

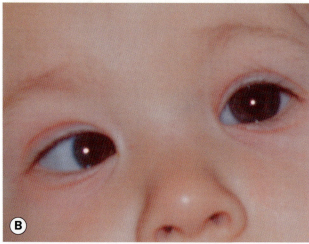

Fig. 18.49 Cross fixation in early-onset esotropia. **(A)** Left fixation on right gaze; **(B)** right fixation on left gaze
(Courtesy of R Bates)

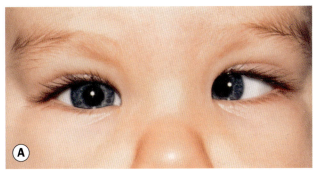

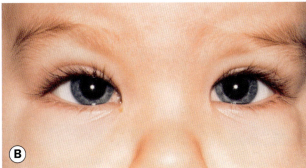

Fig. 18.50 Early-onset esotropia. **(A)** Before surgery; **(B)** after surgery

Subsequent treatment

- **Undercorrection** may require further recession of the medial recti, resection of one or both lateral recti or surgery to the other eye, depending on the initial procedure.
- **Inferior oblique overaction** may develop subsequently, most commonly at age 2 years (Fig. 18.51). The parents should therefore be warned that further surgery may be necessary despite an initially good result. Initially unilateral, it frequently becomes bilateral within 6 months. Inferior oblique weakening procedures include disinsertion, recession and myectomy.
- **DVD** (Fig. 18.52) is characterized by up-drift with excyclorotation (extorsion) of the eye when under cover, or spontaneously during periods of visual inattention. When the cover is removed the affected eye will move down without a corresponding down-drift of the other eye. It is usually bilateral. Surgical treatment may be indicated for cosmesis; options include superior rectus recession with or without posterior fixation sutures and inferior oblique anterior transposition.
- **Amblyopia** subsequently develops in about 50% of cases as unilateral fixation preference commonly develops postoperatively.
- **An accommodative element** should be suspected if the eyes are initially straight or almost straight after surgery and then start to reconverge. Regular refraction is therefore important.

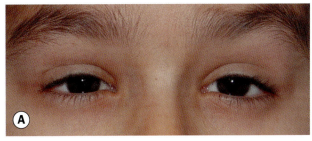

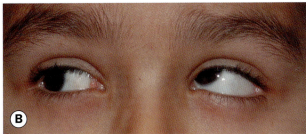

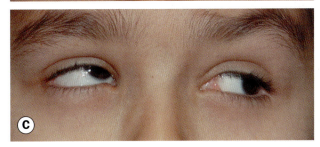

Fig. 18.51 Bilateral inferior oblique overaction. **(A)** Straight eyes in the primary position; **(B)** left inferior oblique overaction on right gaze; **(C)** right inferior oblique overaction on left gaze

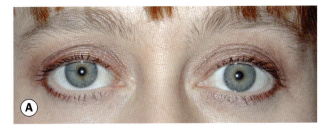

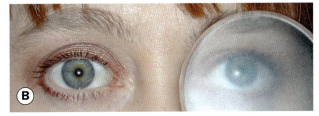

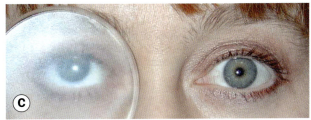

Fig. 18.52 Dissociated vertical deviation. **(A)** Straight eyes in the primary position; **(B)** up-drift of left eye under cover; **(C)** up-drift of right eye under

Accommodative esotropia

Near vision involves both accommodation and convergence. Accommodation is the process by which the eye focuses on a near target, by altering the curvature of the crystalline lens. Simultaneously, the eyes converge, in order to fixate bifoveally on the target. Both accommodation and convergence are quantitatively related to the proximity of the target, and have a fairly constant relationship to each other (AC/A ratio) as described previously. Abnormalities of the AC/A ratio are an important cause of certain types of esotropia.

Refractive accommodative esotropia

In this type of accommodative esotropia, the AC/A ratio is normal and esotropia is a physiological response to excessive hypermetropia, usually between +2.00 and +7.00 D. The considerable degree of accommodation required to focus clearly on even a distant target is accompanied by a proportionate amount of convergence, which is beyond the patient's fusional divergence amplitude. It cannot therefore be controlled, and a manifest convergent squint results. The magnitude of the deviation varies little (usually <10 Δ) between distance and near. The deviation typically presents at the age of 18 months to 3 years (range 6 months to 7 years).

- **Fully accommodative** esotropia is characterized by hypermetropia with esotropia when the refractive error is uncorrected (Fig. 18.53A). The deviation is eliminated and

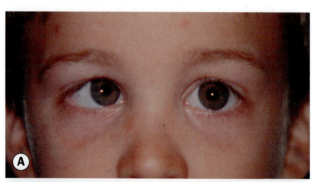
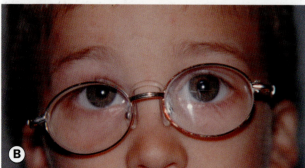

Fig. 18.53 Fully accommodative esotropia. **(A)** Right esotropia without glasses; **(B)** straight eyes for near and distance with glasses
(Courtesy of J Yangüela)

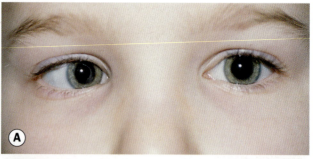
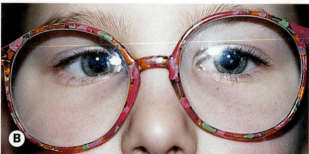

Fig. 18.54 Partially accommodative esotropia. **(A)** Right esotropia without glasses; **(B)** angle is reduced but not eliminated with glasses

BSV is present at all distances following optical correction of hypermetropia (Fig. 18.53B).

- **Partially accommodative esotropia** is reduced, but not eliminated by full correction of hypermetropia (Fig. 18.54). Amblyopia is frequent as well as bilateral congenital superior oblique weakness. Most cases show suppression of the squinting eye although ARC may occur, but of lower grade than in microtropia.

Non-refractive accommodative esotropia

In this type of accommodative esotropia the AC/A ratio is high so that a unit increase of accommodation is accompanied by a disproportionately large increase in convergence. This occurs independently of refractive error, although hypermetropia frequently coexists. Subtypes are set out below.

- **Convergence excess**
  - High AC/A ratio due to increased accommodative convergence (accommodation is normal, convergence is increased).
  - Normal near point of accommodation.
  - Straight eyes with BSV for distance (Fig. 18.55A).
  - Esotropia for near, usually with suppression (Fig. 18.55B).
  - Straight eyes through bifocals (Fig. 18.55C).
- **Hypoaccommodative convergence excess**
  - High AC/A ratio due to decreased accommodation (accommodation is weak, necessitating increased effort, which produces over-convergence).
  - Remote near point of accommodation.
  - Straight eyes with BSV for distance.
  - Esotropia for near, usually with suppression.

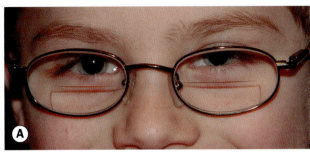

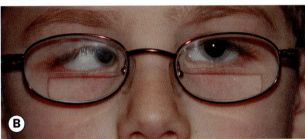

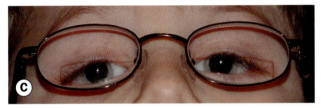

Fig. 18.55 Convergence excess esotropia. **(A)** Eyes straight for distance; **(B)** right esotropia for near; **(C)** eyes straight when looking through bifocals

Treatment

- **Correction of refractive error** is the initial treatment.
  - In children under the age of 6 years, the full cycloplegic refraction revealed on retinoscopy should be prescribed, with a deduction only for the working distance. In the fully accommodative refractive esotrope this will control the deviation for both near and distance.
  - After the age of 8 years, refraction should be performed without cycloplegia and the maximal amount of 'plus' that can be tolerated (manifest hypermetropia) prescribed.
  - For convergence excess esotropia bifocals may be prescribed to relieve accommodation (and thereby accommodative convergence), thus allowing the child to maintain bi-foveal fixation and ocular alignment at near (see Fig. 18.55C). The minimum 'add' required to achieve this is prescribed.
  - The most satisfactory form of bifocals is the executive type in which the intersection crosses the lower border of the pupil. The strength of the lower segment should be gradually reduced and eliminated by the early teenage years.
  - Bifocals are also used in hypoaccommodative esotropia where the AC/A ratio is not overly excessive and there is a reasonable chance of discarding bifocal correction with time.

- At higher levels surgery is the better long-term option. The ultimate prognosis for complete withdrawal of spectacles is related to the magnitude of the AC/A ratio and to the degree of hypermetropia and associated astigmatism. Spectacles may be needed only for close work.
- **Surgery** is aimed at restoring or improving BSV, or at improving the appearance of the squint and so the child's social functioning. It should be considered only if spectacles do not fully correct the deviation and after every attempt has been made to treat amblyopia.
  - Bilateral medial rectus recessions are performed in patients in whom the deviation for near is greater than that for distance.
  - If there is no significant difference between distance and near measurements, and equal vision in both eyes, some perform unilateral medial rectus recession combined with lateral rectus resection, whereas others prefer bilateral medial rectus recessions.
  - In patients with residual amblyopia, surgery is usually performed on the amblyopic eye.
  - In partially accommodative esotropia, surgery to improve appearance is best delayed until requested by the child; this avoids early consecutive exotropia. It should aim to correct only the residual squint present with glasses.
  - The usual first procedure for convergence excess esotropia is recession of both medial rectus muscles. This relies on fusion to prevent a distance exotropia; a few patients become divergent after surgery and need a further procedure.
  - Medial rectus posterior fixation sutures (Faden operation) can also be used either as a first procedure, or in the case of undercorrection, following bimedial recessions.

Microtropia

Microtropia is a small angle (<10 Δ) squint. Binocular cooperation in microtropia is more substantial than in most manifest deviations, and it may be considered more a description of binocular status than a specific diagnosis. It may be primary or secondary, the latter representing the sequela to strabismus surgery or other treatment (e.g. optical, such as fully accommodative esotropia controlled with glasses to a microtropia rather than true bifoveal BSV) for a larger deviation, and occasionally to other pathology.

- Symptoms are rare unless there is an associated decompensating heterophoria.
- The small manifest angle of deviation may not be readily detectable on cover testing.
- There is a prominent association with anisometropia, commonly hypermetropia or hypermetropic astigmatism, with amblyopia (typically mild) of the more ametropic eye.
- There is normal motor fusion as demonstrated by fusional amplitudes.
- Anomalous retinal correspondence (ARC) is present, with associated abnormal binocular single vision (BSV); there is

monocular fixation eccentric to the fovea in the deviating eye and a central suppression scotoma, and stereopsis is usually present but reduced.

- In microtropia *with* identity the point used for fixation by the deviating eye (monocular eccentric fixation) corresponds with the fovea of the straight eye under binocular viewing conditions (the angle of anomaly in ARC). Therefore on cover test there is no movement of the squinting eye when it takes up monocular fixation.
- In microtropia *without* identity the monocular fixation point of the squinting eye does not correspond with the fovea of the straight eye in binocular viewing. There is therefore a small movement of the deviating eye when it takes up monocular fixation on cover testing.
- The 4 Δ prism test, discussed earlier in the chapter, is useful in assessment.

Treatment

Treatment involves correction of refractive error and occlusion for amblyopia as indicated; there is evidence that aggressive treatment sometimes leads to normalization. Most patients remain stable and symptom-free.

Other esotropias

Near esotropia (non-accommodative convergence excess)

- **Presentation** is usually in older children and young adults.
- **Signs**
  - No significant refractive error.
  - Orthophoria or small esophoria with BSV for distance.
  - Esotropia for near but normal or low AC/A ratio.
  - Normal near point of accommodation.
- **Treatment** involves bilateral medial rectus recessions.

Distance esotropia

- **Presentation** is in healthy young adults, who are often myopic.
- **Signs**
  - Intermittent or constant esotropia for distance.
  - Minimal or no deviation for near.
  - Normal bilateral abduction.
  - Fusional divergence amplitudes may be reduced.
  - Absence of neurological disease.
- **Treatment** is with prisms until spontaneous resolution or surgery in persistent cases.

Acute (late-onset) esotropia

- **Presentation** is at around 5–6 years of age.
- **Signs**
  - Sudden onset of diplopia and esotropia.
  - Normal ocular motility without significant refractive error.
  - Underlying sixth nerve palsy must be excluded.

- **Treatment** is aimed at re-establishing BSV to prevent suppression, using prisms, botulinum toxin or surgery.

Secondary (sensory) esotropia

Secondary esotropia is caused by a unilateral reduction in visual acuity that interferes with or abolishes fusion; causes can include cataract, optic atrophy or hypoplasia, macular scarring or retinoblastoma. Fundus examination under mydriasis is therefore essential in all children with strabismus.

Consecutive esotropia

Consecutive esotropia follows surgical overcorrection of an exodeviation. If it occurs following surgery for an intermittent exotropia in a child it should not be allowed to persist for more than 6 weeks without further intervention.

Cyclic esotropia

Cyclic esotropia is a very rare condition characterized by alternating manifest esotropia with suppression and BSV, each typically lasting 24 hours. The condition may persist for months or years and the patient may eventually develop a constant esotropia requiring surgery.

High myopia esotropia

Patients with high myopia may have instability of the muscle pulleys that stabilize the superior rectus and lateral rectus muscles. This results in nasal displacement of the superior rectus and inferior displacement of the lateral rectus. The possibility of this condition should be considered in high myopes with acquired esotropia; MR is key to the diagnosis. Treatment involves plication of the superior and lateral recti with a non-absorbable suture.

EXOTROPIA

Constant (early-onset) exotropia

- **Presentation** is often at birth.
- **Signs**
  - Normal refraction.
  - Large and constant angle.
  - DVD may be present.
- **Neurological anomalies** are frequently present, in contrast with infantile esotropia.
- **Treatment** is mainly surgical and consists of lateral rectus recession and medial rectus resection.
- **Differential diagnosis** is secondary exotropia, which may conceal serious ocular pathology.

Intermittent exotropia

Diagnosis

- **Presentation** is often at around 2 years with exophoria which breaks down to exotropia under conditions of visual

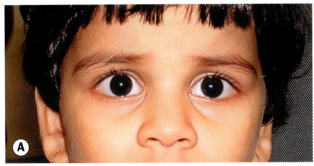

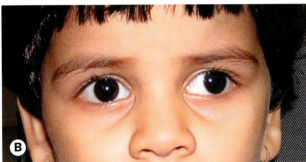

Fig. 18.56 Intermittent exotropia. **(A)** Eyes straight most of the time; **(B)** left exotropia under conditions of visual inattention or fatigue

(Courtesy of M Parulekar)

inattention, bright light (resulting in reflex closure of the affected eye), fatigue or ill health.

- **Signs.** The eyes are straight with BSV at times (Fig. 18.56A) and manifest with suppression at other times (Fig. 18.56B). Control of the squint varies with the distance of fixation and other factors such as concentration.

Classification

- **Distance** exotropia, in which the angle of deviation is greater for distance than near and increases further beyond 6 metres. Simulated and true forms are recognized.
  - ○ Simulated (formerly pseudo-divergence excess) is associated with a high AC/A ratio or with 'tenacious proximal fusion' (TPF – tonic fusional convergence that relaxes after occlusion). The distance angle initially seems to be larger than the near angle, but the deviation for near and distance is similar when the near angle is remeasured with the patient looking through +3.00 D lenses (high AC/A controlling exodeviation) or after 30–60 minutes of uniocular occlusion to relax TPF, the latter with a normal AC/A ratio).
  - ○ True. The angle for near remains significantly less than that for distance with the above tests.
- **Non-specific** exotropia, in which control of the squint and the angle of deviation are the same for distance and near fixation.
- **Near** exotropia, in which the deviation is greater for near fixation. It tends to occur in older children and adults and may be associated with acquired myopia or presbyopia.

Treatment

- **Spectacle correction** in myopic patients may, in some cases, control the deviation by stimulating accommodation, and with it, convergence. In some cases over-minus prescription may be useful.
- **Part-time occlusion** of the non-deviating eye may improve control in some patients, and orthoptic exercises may be helpful for near exotropia.
- **Surgery.** Patients with effective and stable control of their intermittent exotropia are often just observed. Surgery is indicated if control is poor or is progressively deteriorating. Unilateral lateral rectus recession and medial rectus resection are generally preferred except in true distance exotropia when bilateral lateral rectus recessions are more usual. The exodeviation is rarely completely eliminated by surgery.

Sensory exotropia

Secondary (sensory) exotropia is the result of monocular or binocular visual impairment by acquired lesions, such as cataract (Fig. 18.57) or other media opacity. Treatment consists of correction of the visual deficit, if possible, followed by surgery if appropriate. A minority of patients develop intractable diplopia due to loss of fusion, even when good visual acuity is restored to both eyes and the eyes are realigned.

Consecutive exotropia

Consecutive exotropia develops spontaneously in an amblyopic eye, or more frequently following surgical correction of an esodeviation. In early postoperative divergence, muscle slippage must be considered. Most cases present in adult life with concerns about cosmesis and social function, and can be greatly helped by surgery. Careful evaluation of the risk of postoperative diplopia is required, although serious problems are uncommon. About 75% of patients are still well aligned 10 years after surgery, although re-divergence may occur.

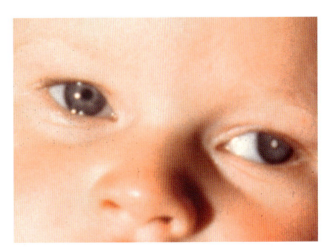

Fig. 18.57 Left sensory exotropia due to a mature cataract

CONGENITAL CRANIAL DYSINNERVATION DISORDERS

Congenital cranial dysinnervation disorders (CCDD) or congenital innervation dysgenesis syndromes constitute a group of disorders originally believed to be the result of congenital muscular fibrosis, but now known to be the result of brainstem or cranial nerve developmental disturbance, in most cases having an identifiable genetic basis. Systemic associations are recognized for several.

Duane retraction syndrome

In Duane retraction syndrome (DRS) there is failure of innervation of the lateral rectus by a hypoplastic sixth nerve nucleus, with anomalous innervation of the lateral rectus by fibres from the third nerve. The condition is often bilateral. Up to half of patients have associated systemic defects such as deafness, external ear abnormalities, speech disorder and skeletal abnormalities. Associated mutations in several genes have been found. Approximately 10% of cases are familial.

Clinical features

- **A face turn** is typical, conferring BSV in the primary position and avoiding amblyopia.
- **Complete or partial restriction of abduction.**
- **Restricted adduction**, usually partial.
- **Retraction of the globe on adduction** as a result of co-contraction of the medial and lateral recti with resultant narrowing of the palpebral fissure.
- **An up-shoot or down-shoot in adduction** may be present; in some cases this is produced by a tight lateral rectus muscle slipping over or under the globe to produce an anomalous vertical movement.
- **Deficiency of convergence** in which the affected eye remains fixed in the primary position while the unaffected eye is converging.

Classification (Huber)

- **Type I**, the most common, is characterized by (Fig. 18.58):
  - ○ Limited or absent abduction.
  - ○ Normal or mildly limited adduction.
  - ○ In the primary position, straight or slight esotropia.
- **Type II**, the least common, is characterized by:
  - ○ Limited adduction.
  - ○ Normal or mildly limited abduction.
  - ○ In primary position, straight or slight exotropia.
- **Type III** is characterized by (Fig. 18.59):
  - ○ Limited adduction and abduction.
  - ○ In the primary position, straight or slight esotropia.
  - ○ In some cases phenotypic variants have been allied to differing genotypes.

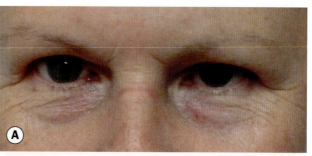
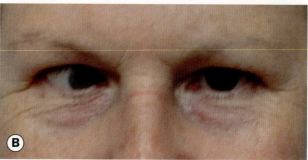
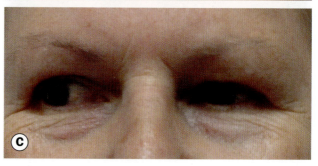

Fig. 18.58 Duane syndrome – Huber type I in a 68-year-old woman. **(A)** Straight eyes in the primary position; **(B)** extremely limited left abduction; **(C)** narrowing of the left palpebral fissure on adduction

Treatment

The majority of patients with Duane syndrome do not need any surgical intervention.

- Most young children maintain BSV by using a CHP to compensate for their lateral rectus weakness and surgery is needed only if there is evidence of loss of binocular function; this may be indicated by failure to continue to use a CHP.
- In adults or children over the age of about 8 years surgery can reduce a head posture that is cosmetically unacceptable or causing neck discomfort. Surgery may also be necessary for cosmetically unacceptable up-shoots, down-shoots or severe globe retraction.
- Amblyopia, when present, is usually the result of anisometropia rather than strabismus. Unilateral or bilateral muscle recession or transposition of the vertical recti are the procedures of choice. The lateral rectus of the involved side should not be resected, as this increases retraction.

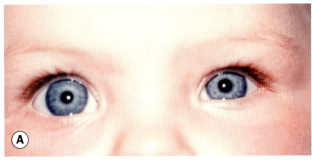

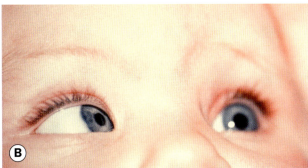

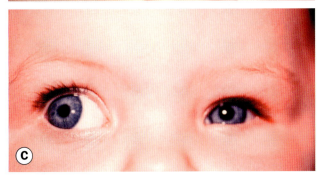

Fig. 18.59 Duane syndrome type III in an infant. **(A)** Straight eyes in the primary position; **(B)** limitation of left abduction with widening of the left palpebral fissure; **(C)** grossly limited left adduction with narrowing of the palpebral fissure

(Courtesy of K Nischal)

Möbius syndrome

Möbius syndrome is a rare, usually sporadic, condition, the basic components of which are congenital non-progressive bilateral sixth and seventh cranial nerve palsies that are believed to relate to a developmental abnormality of the brainstem.

- **Systemic features**
  - ○ Bilateral facial palsy, which is usually asymmetrical and often incomplete, giving rise to an expressionless facial appearance (Fig. 18.60A) and problems with eyelid closure (Fig. 18.60B).
  - ○ The fifth, eighth, tenth and twelfth (Fig. 18.60C) cranial nerves may also be affected.
  - ○ Limb anomalies and mild mental handicap may be present.
- **Ocular features**
  - ○ Bilateral sixth nerve palsy.
  - ○ Horizontal gaze palsy (50%).
  - ○ Occasionally, third and fourth nerve palsy and ptosis.

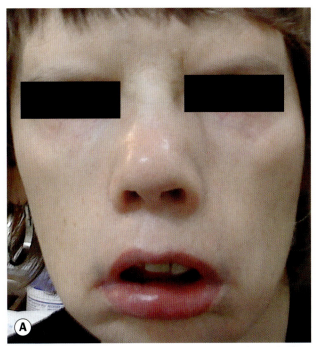

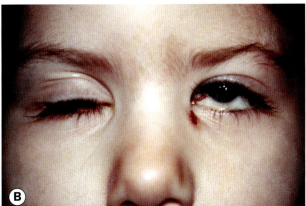

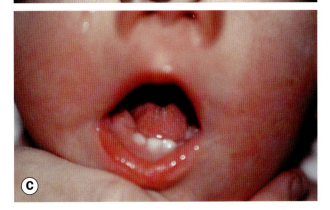

Fig. 18.60 Möbius syndrome. **(A)** Bilateral facial nerve palsy with a typical smooth expressionless facial appearance; **(B)** defective lid closure due to facial nerve palsy; **(C)** atrophic tongue due to hypoglossal nerve palsy

(Courtesy of K Nischal – figs B and C)

Congenital fibrosis of the extraocular muscles

Congenital fibrosis of the extraocular muscles (CFEOM) is a rare non-progressive, usually autosomal dominant, disorder characterized by bilateral ptosis and restrictive external ophthalmoplegia. Numerous forms have been identified, of which CFEOM1 is the most common, and there is considerable genetic heterogeneity; CFEOM1 is caused by mutations in the *KIF21A* gene, which produces a protein used for intracellular transport that plays a key role in some aspects of cranial nerve development, and pathologically there is a hypoplastic superior division of the oculomotor nerve. Typically, vertical movements are severely restricted with inability to elevate the eyes above the horizontal plane.

In the primary position each eye is fixed below the horizontal by about 10°, with a corresponding compensatory chin elevation. The degree of residual horizontal movement varies markedly. Ptosis is common (Fig. 18.61).

Strabismus fixus

Strabismus fixus is a rare condition in which both eyes are fixed by fibrous tightening of the medial recti (convergent strabismus fixus – Fig. 18.62A), or the lateral recti (divergent strabismus fixus – Fig. 18.62B). Congenital and acquired forms have been described.

Other CCDD syndromes with ophthalmic features

Marcus Gunn jaw-winking syndrome (see Ch. 1) is now believed to be a CCDD, as are horizontal gaze palsy and progressive scoliosis, many cases of congenital ptosis, congenital fourth cranial nerve palsy and congenital facial nerve palsy.

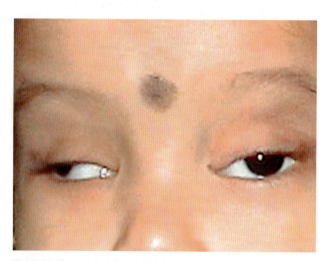

Fig. 18.61 Congenital fibrosis of the extraocular muscles – bilateral ptosis and divergent strabismus
(Courtesy of M Parulekar)

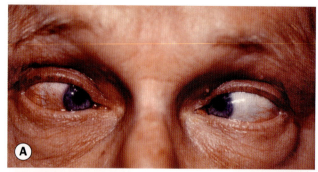

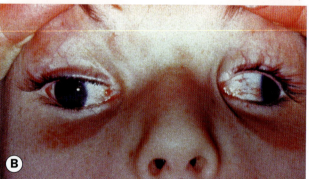

Fig. 18.62 Strabismus fixus. **(A)** Convergent; **(B)** divergent

MONOCULAR ELEVATION DEFICIENCY

Monocular elevation deficiency (MED), formerly double elevator palsy, is a rare sporadic condition that in at least some cases may be categorized as a CCDD. It is thought to manifest primarily with a tight or contracted inferior rectus muscle or a hypoplastic or ineffective superior rectus muscle. There is a profound inability to elevate one eye across the horizontal plane, from abduction to adduction (Fig. 18.63), with orthophoria in the primary position in about one-third of cases. Chin elevation may be present. A base-up prism can be helpful.

BROWN SYNDROME

Brown syndrome is a condition involving mechanical restriction, typically of the superior oblique tendon. It is usually congenital but occasionally acquired. Recent evidence strongly suggests that at least some congenital cases should be categorized as a CCDD.

Classification

- **Congenital**
  - ○ Idiopathic.
  - ○ 'Congenital click syndrome' where there is impaired movement of the superior oblique tendon through the trochlea.
- **Acquired**
  - ○ Trauma to the trochlea or superior oblique tendon.
  - ○ Inflammation of the tendon, which may be caused by rheumatoid arthritis, pansinusitis or scleritis.

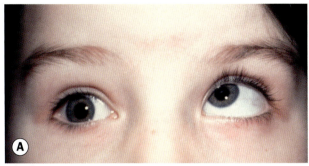

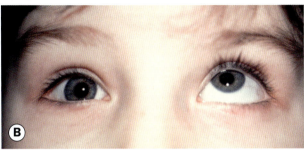

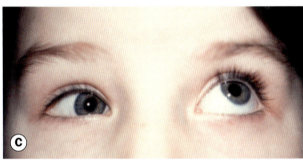

Fig. 18.63 Right monocular elevation deficiency. **(A)** Defective elevation in abduction; **(B)** in upgaze; **(C)** and in adduction

Diagnosis

- **Major signs**
  - Usually straight with BSV in the primary position (Fig. 18.64A).
  - Limited elevation in adduction (Fig. 18.64B).
  - Limited elevation on upgaze is common (Fig. 18.64C).
  - Normal elevation in abduction (Fig. 18.64D).
  - Absence of superior oblique overaction (Fig. 18.64E).
  - Positive forced duction test on elevating the globe in adduction.
- **Variable signs**
  - Down-shoot in adduction.
  - Hypotropia in primary position.
  - CHP with chin elevation and ipsilateral head tilt (Fig. 18.64F).

Treatment

- **Congenital** cases do not usually require treatment as long as binocular function is maintained with an acceptable head posture. Spontaneous improvement is often seen towards

the end of the first decade. Indications for treatment include significant primary position hypotropia, deteriorating control and/or an unacceptable head posture. The recommended procedure for congenital cases is lengthening of the superior oblique tendon.
- **Acquired;** treatable aetiology should be addressed specifically. Depending on the cause, acquired cases may benefit from steroids, either orally or by injection near the trochlea.

ALPHABET PATTERNS

'V' or 'A' patterns occur when the relative contributions of the superior rectus and inferior oblique to elevation, or of the inferior rectus and superior oblique to depression, are abnormal, resulting in derangement of the balance of their horizontal vectors in up- and downgaze. They can also be caused by anomalies in the position of the rectus muscle pulleys. Assessment is by measuring horizontal deviations in the primary position, upgaze and downgaze. They can occur in both concomitant and incomitant deviations.

'V' pattern

A 'V' pattern is said to be significant when the difference between upgaze and downgaze is ≥15 Δ.

Causes

- Inferior oblique overaction associated with fourth nerve palsy.
- Superior oblique underaction with subsequent inferior oblique overaction, seen in infantile esotropia as well as other childhood esotropias. The eyes are often straight in upgaze with a marked esodeviation in downgaze.
- Superior rectus underaction.
- Brown syndrome.
- Craniofacial anomalies featuring shallow orbits and down-slanting palpebral fissures.

Treatment

Treatment is by inferior oblique weakening or superior oblique strengthening when oblique dysfunction is present. Without oblique muscle dysfunction treatment is as follows:
- **'V' pattern esotropia** (Fig. 18.65A) can be treated by bilateral medial rectus recessions and downward transposition of the tendons.
- **'V' pattern exotropia** (Fig. 18.65B) can be treated by bilateral lateral rectus recessions and upward transposition of the tendons.

'A' pattern

An 'A' pattern is considered significant if the difference between upgaze and downgaze is ≥10 Δ. A particular complaint may be difficulty with reading if the patient is binocular.

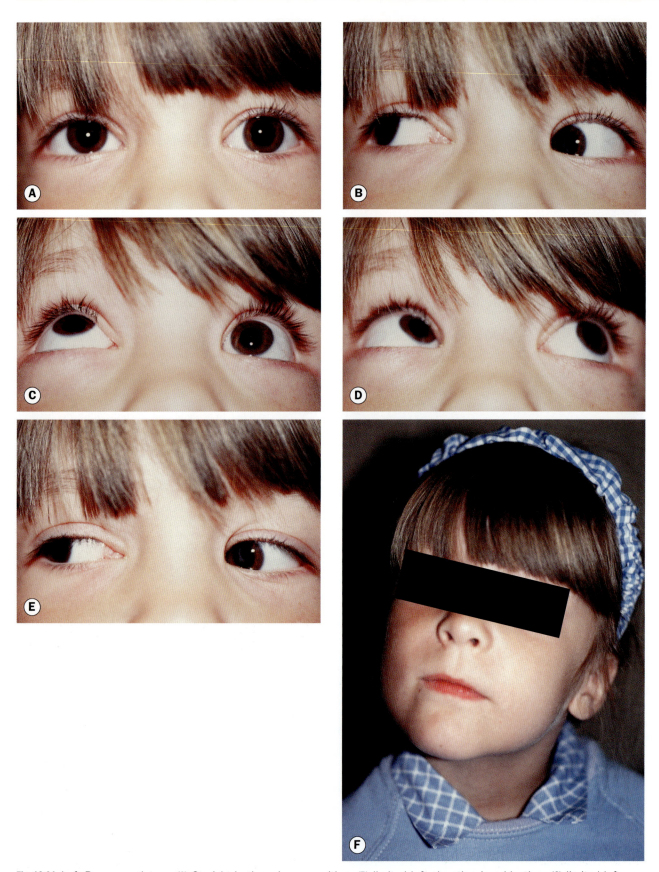

Fig. 18.64 Left Brown syndrome. **(A)** Straight in the primary position; **(B)** limited left elevation in adduction; **(C)** limited left elevation on upgaze; **(D)** normal left elevation in abduction; **(E)** absence of left superior oblique overaction; **(F)** chin elevation and left head tilt

(Courtesy of K Nischal)

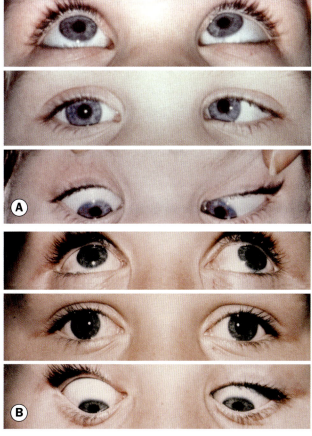

Fig. 18.65 'V' pattern. **(A)** Esotropia; **(B)** exotropia
(Courtesy of Wilmer Eye Institute)

Causes

- Primary superior oblique overaction is usually associated with exodeviation in the primary position of gaze.
- Inferior oblique underaction/palsy with subsequent superior oblique overaction.
- Inferior rectus underaction.

Treatment

Patients with oblique dysfunction are treated by superior oblique posterior tenotomy. Treatment of cases without oblique muscle dysfunction is as follows:

- **'A' pattern esotropia** (Fig. 18.66A) is treated by bilateral medial rectus recessions and upward transposition of the tendons.
- **'A' pattern exotropia** (Fig. 18.66B) is treated by bilateral lateral rectus recessions and downward transposition of the tendons.

SURGERY

The most common aims of surgery on the extraocular muscles are to correct misalignment to improve appearance, and if possible to restore BSV. Surgery can also be used to reduce an abnormal head posture and to expand or centralize a field of BSV. However, the

first step in the management of childhood strabismus involves correction of any significant refractive error and/or treatment of amblyopia. Once maximal visual potential is reached in both eyes, any residual deviation can be treated surgically. The three main types of procedure are:

- **Weakening** to decrease the effective strength of action of a muscle.
- **Strengthening**, to enhance the pull of a muscle.
- **Vector adjustment** procedures that have the primary aim of altering the direction of muscle action.

Weakening procedures

Recession

Recession slackens a muscle by moving it away from its insertion. It can be performed on any muscle except the superior oblique.

- **Rectus muscle recession**
  - The muscle is exposed and two absorbable sutures are tied through the outer quarters of the tendon.
  - The tendon is disinserted from the sclera, and the amount of recession is measured and marked on the sclera with callipers.

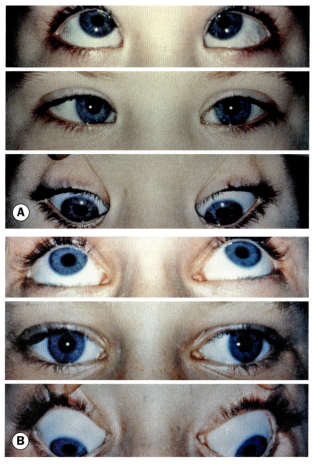

Fig. 18.66 'A' pattern. **(A)** Esotropia; **(B)** exotropia
(Courtesy of Wilmer Eye Institute)

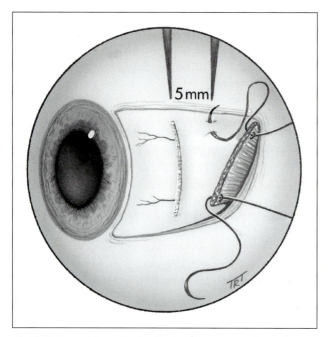
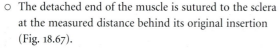

Fig. 18.67 Recession of a horizontal rectus muscle

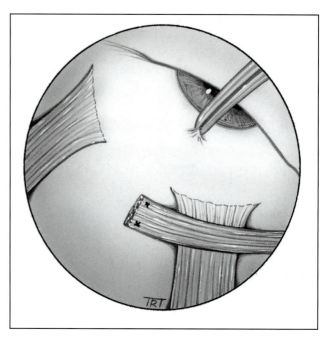

Fig. 18.68 Recession of an inferior oblique muscle

○ The detached end of the muscle is sutured to the sclera at the measured distance behind its original insertion (Fig. 18.67).

● **Inferior oblique recession**
  ○ The muscle belly is exposed through an inferotemporal fornix incision.
  ○ A squint hook is passed behind the posterior border of the muscle which must be clearly visualized. Care is taken to pick up the muscle without disrupting the Tenon capsule and fat posterior to it.
  ○ An absorbable suture is passed through the anterior border of the muscle at its insertion and tied.
  ○ The muscle is disinserted and the cut end sutured to the sclera 3 mm posterior and temporal to the temporal edge of the inferior rectus insertion (Fig. 18.68).

Disinsertion

Disinsertion (or myectomy) involves detaching a muscle from its insertion without reattachment. It is most commonly used to weaken an overacting inferior oblique muscle, when the technique is the same as for a recession except that the muscle is not sutured. Very occasionally, disinsertion is performed on a severely con-tracted rectus muscle.

Posterior fixation suture

The principle of this (Faden) procedure is to suture the muscle belly to the sclera posteriorly so as to decrease the pull of the muscle in its field of action without affecting the eye in the primary position. The Faden procedure may be used on the medial rectus to reduce convergence in a convergence excess esotropia and on the superior rectus to treat DVD. When treating DVD, the supe-rior rectus muscle may also be recessed. The belly of the muscle is

then anchored to the sclera with a non-absorbable suture about 12 mm behind its insertion.

Strengthening procedures

● **Resection** shortens a muscle to enhance its effective pull. It is suitable only for a rectus muscle and involves the following steps:
  ○ The muscle is exposed and two absorbable sutures inserted at a measured distance behind its insertion.
  ○ The muscle anterior to the sutures is excised and the cut end reattached to the original insertion (Fig. 18.69).

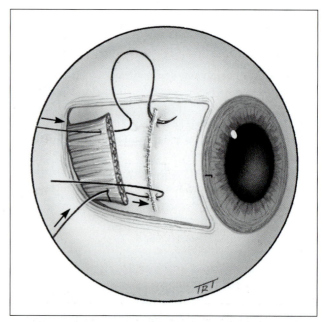

Fig. 18.69 Resection of a horizontal rectus muscle

- **Tucking** of a muscle or its tendon is usually confined to enhancement of the action of the superior oblique muscle in congenital fourth nerve palsy.
- **Advancement** of the muscle nearer to the limbus can be used to enhance the action of a previously recessed rectus muscle.

Transposition

Transposition refers to the relocation of one or more extraocular muscles to substitute for the action of an absent or severely deficient muscle. The most common indication is severe lateral rectus weakness due to acquired sixth cranial nerve palsy (Fig. 18.70); other applications include CCDD (e.g. Duane syndrome), alphabet patterns and monocular elevation deficit. A variety of techniques involving recti and oblique muscles have been described.

Adjustable sutures

Indications

The results of strabismus surgery can be improved by the use of adjustable suture techniques on the rectus muscles. These are particularly indicated when a precise outcome is essential and when the results with more conventional procedures are likely to be unpredictable; for example, acquired vertical deviations associated with thyroid myopathy or following a blow-out fracture of the

floor of the orbit. Other indications include sixth nerve palsy, adult exotropia and re-operations in which scarring of surrounding tissues may make the final outcome unpredictable. The main contraindication is inability to tolerate postoperative suture adjustment (e.g. young children).

Operative procedure

- The muscle is exposed, sutures inserted and the tendon disinserted from the sclera as for a rectus muscle recession.
- The two ends of the suture are passed, side by side, through the stump of the insertion.
- A second suture is knotted and tied tightly around the muscle suture anterior to its emergence from the stump (Fig. 18.71A).
- One end of the suture is cut short and the two ends tied together to form a loop (Fig. 18.71B).
- The conjunctiva is left open.

Postoperative adjustment

This is performed under topical anaesthesia, usually a few hours after surgery when the patient is fully awake.
- The accuracy of alignment is assessed.
- If ocular alignment is satisfactory the muscle suture is tied off and its long ends cut short.
- If more recession is required, the bow is pulled anteriorly along the muscle suture, thereby providing additional slack to the recessed muscle and enabling it to move posteriorly (Fig. 18.71C).
- If less recession is required, the muscle suture is pulled anteriorly and the knot tightened against the muscle stump (Fig. 18.71D).
- Once alignment is satisfactory, the main knot is secured, the sliding loop removed and the conjunctiva closed.
- A variety of other techniques have been described.

BOTULINUM TOXIN CHEMODENERVATION

Temporary paralysis of an extraocular muscle can be induced by an injection of botulinum toxin under topical anaesthesia and EMG control. The effect takes several days to develop, is usually maximal at 1–2 weeks following injection and has generally worn off by 3 months. Side effects are uncommon, although about 5% of patients may develop some degree of temporary ptosis. The following are the main indications:
- **To determine the risk of postoperative diplopia.** For example, in an adult with a consecutive left divergent squint and left suppression, straightening the eyes may make suppression less effective resulting in diplopia. If postoperative diplopia testing by correcting the angle with prisms is negative then the risk of double vision after surgery is very low. If testing is positive then the left lateral rectus muscle can be injected with toxin so that the eyes will either straighten or converge and the risk of diplopia can be assessed over several days while the eyes are straight. If diplopia does occur, the patient is able to judge whether it is troublesome.

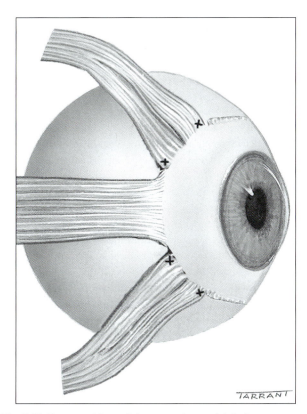

Fig. 18.70 Transposition of the superior and inferior rectus muscles in lateral rectus palsy

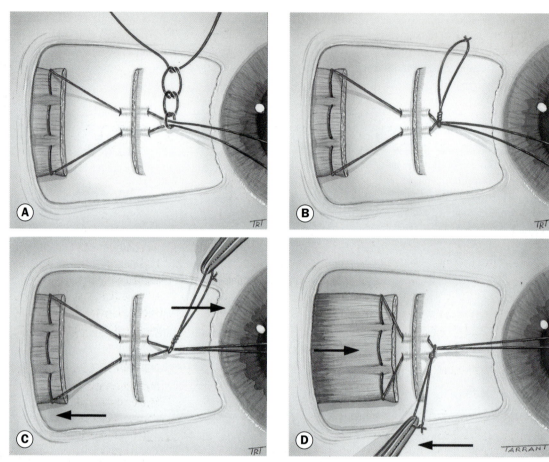

Fig. 18.71 Adjustable sutures – see text

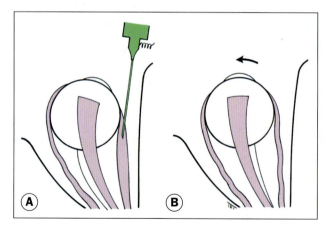

Fig. 18.72 Principles of botulinum toxin chemodenervation in left sixth nerve palsy – see text

- **To assess the potential for BSV** in a patient with a constant manifest squint by straightening the eyes temporarily. The deviation can then be corrected surgically if appropriate. A small proportion of patients maintain BSV long-term after the effects of the toxin have worn off.
- **In lateral rectus palsy** botulinum toxin can be injected into the ipsilateral medial rectus to give symptomatic relief during recovery and to see whether there is any lateral rectus action when there is medial rectus contracture (Fig. 18.72A). The temporary paralysis of the muscle causes relaxation so that the horizontal forces on the globe are more balanced, thus allowing assessment of lateral rectus function (Fig. 18.72B). A similar approach can be used for fourth nerve palsy, with injection into the ipsilateral inferior oblique or contralateral inferior rectus.
- **Patients with a cosmetically poor deviation** who have undergone multiple squint operations can be treated by repeated BT injections, which may reduce in frequency with time.

NEUROIMAGING

Computed tomography

Physics

Computed tomography (CT) uses X-ray beams to obtain tissue density values from which detailed cross-sectional images are formed by a computer. Tissue density is represented by a grey scale, white being maximum density (e.g. bone) and black being minimum density (e.g. air). Advanced CT scanners are able to acquire thinner slices leading to improved spatial resolution, together with faster examination times, without a proportionate increase in radiation dose. Images are acquired in an axial form and can be viewed in any plane using computer reconstruction. This multiplanar information can be an advantage over magnetic resonance (MR) with regard to anatomical detail. CT is widely available, easy to perform, relatively inexpensive and quick, but unlike MR exposes the patient to ionizing radiation.

Contrast enhancement

Iodinated contrast material improves sensitivity and specificity but is contraindicated in patients allergic to iodine and in those with renal failure. Contrast is not indicated in acute haemorrhage, bony injury or localization of foreign bodies because it may mask visualization of these high density structures.

Indications

- **Orbital trauma**, for the detection of bony lesions such as fractures (Fig. 19.1A), blood, herniation of extraocular muscles into the maxillary sinus and surgical emphysema.
- **Evaluation of the extraocular muscles** in thyroid eye disease (Fig. 19.1B); CT and MR (see below) have complementary advantages in the assessment of orbital disease.

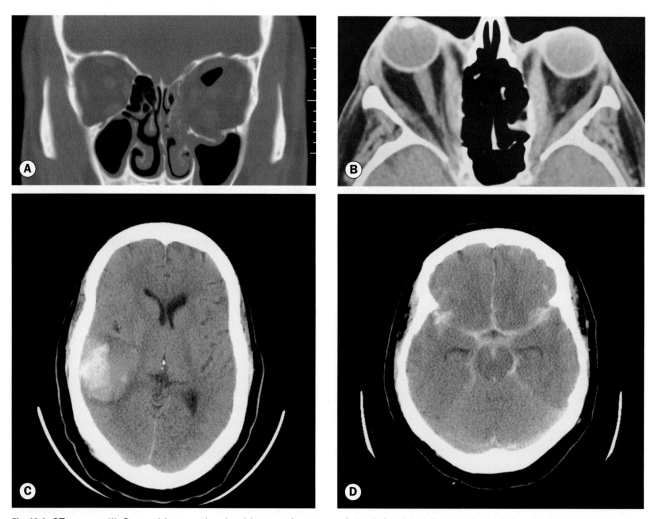

Fig. 19.1 CT scans. **(A)** Coronal image showing blow-out fractures of the left orbital floor and medial wall with orbital emphysema; **(B)** axial image showing bilateral enlargement of extraocular muscles and right proptosis; **(C)** axial image showing an acute parenchymal haematoma in the right temporal lobe; **(D)** axial image showing extensive subarachnoid blood in the basilar cisterns, and the Sylvian and interhemispheric fissures

(Courtesy of N Sibtain – figs A, C and D; A Pearson – fig. B)

- **Bony involvement of orbital tumours** is better assessed using CT than MR.
- **Orbital cellulitis** for assessment of intraorbital extension and subperiosteal abscess formation.
- **Detection of intraorbital calcification** as in meningioma and retinoblastoma.
- **Detection of acute cerebral** (Fig. 19.1C) or **subarachnoid** (Fig. 19.1D) **haemorrhage**, which is harder to visualize on MR within the first few hours of onset.
- **When MR is contraindicated** (e.g. ferrous foreign body).

Magnetic resonance imaging

Physics

Magnetic resonance imaging (MRI) depends on the rearrangement of positively charged hydrogen nuclei (protons) when a tissue is exposed to a short electromagnetic pulse. When the pulse subsides, the nuclei return to their normal position, re-radiating some of the absorbed energy. Sensitive receivers pick up this electromagnetic echo. Unlike CT, it does not subject the patient to ionizing radiation. The signals are analyzed and displayed as a cross-sectional image that may be axial, coronal or sagittal.

Basic sequences

Weighting refers to two methods of measuring the relaxation times of the excited protons after the magnetic field has been switched off. Various body tissues have different relaxation times so that a given tissue may be T1- or T2-weighted (i.e. best visualized on that particular type of image). In practice, both types of scans are usually performed. It is easy to tell the difference between CT and MR images because bone appears white on CT but is not clearly demonstrated on MR.

- **T1-weighted** images are generally optimal for viewing normal anatomy. Hypointense (dark) structures include cerebrospinal fluid (CSF) and vitreous. Hyperintense (bright) structures include fat, blood, contrast agents and melanin (Figs 19.2A and C).
- **T2-weighted** images, in which water is shown as hyperintense, are useful for viewing pathological changes because oedematous tissue (e.g. inflammation) will display a brighter signal than normal surrounding tissue. CSF and vitreous are hyperintense as they have high water content. Blood vessels appear black on T2 imaging unless they are occluded (Figs 19.2B and D).

Image enhancement

- **Gadolinium contrast** acquires magnetic moment when placed in an electromagnetic field. Administered intravenously, it remains intravascular unless there is a breakdown of the blood–brain barrier. It is only visualized on T1-weighted images, and enhancing lesions such as tumours and areas of inflammation will appear bright. Ideally MR is performed both before (Fig. 19.3A) and after (Fig. 19.3B) administration of gadolinium for most clinical

indications. Special head or surface coils can also be used to improve spatial definition of the image. Adverse effects with gadolinium are uncommon and usually relatively innocuous.
- **Fat-suppression techniques** are useful for imaging the orbit because the bright signal of orbital fat on conventional T1-weighted imaging frequently obscures other orbital contents. Fat suppression eliminates this bright signal and better delineates normal structures (optic nerve and extraocular muscles) as well as tumours, inflammatory lesions and vascular malformations. The two types of fat-suppression sequence used for orbital imaging are:
  - T1 fat saturation used with gadolinium allows areas suspicious using other techniques to be enhanced, e.g. suppressing orbital fat signal to visualize optic nerve sheath lesions (Figs 19.3C and D).
  - STIR (short T1 inversion recovery) is the optimal sequence for detecting intrinsic lesions of the intraorbital optic nerve (e.g. optic neuritis – Fig. 19.3E). STIR images have very low signal from fat but still have high signal from water.
- **FLAIR** (fluid-attenuated inversion recovery) sequences suppress the bright CSF on T2-weighted images to allow better visualization of adjacent pathological tissue such as periventricular plaques of demyelination (Fig. 19.3F).
- **DWI/ADC** (diffusion-weighted imaging and apparent diffusion coefficient). DWI measures aberrance in expected Brownian motion of free water, and is useful in acute ischaemic stroke to identify abnormalities at a very early stage – within minutes – and in distinguishing ischaemic damage reversible with treatment from irreversible damage such that intervention (e.g. with a thrombolytic agent) is unlikely to be of benefit.
- **FIESTA and CISS** (fast imaging employing steady-state acquisition, and constructive interference in steady-state) are newer high-resolution sequences. In neuro-ophthalmology, a particular application may be the investigation of cranial nerve palsy.

Limitations

- Bone appears black and is not directly imaged.
- Recent haemorrhage is not detected, so MRI is inappropriate in patients with suspected acute intracranial bleeding.
- It cannot be used in patients with magnetic foreign objects (e.g. cardiac pacemakers, intraocular foreign bodies and ferromagnetic aneurysm clips).
- Substantial patient cooperation is required, including remaining motionless; it is poorly tolerated by claustrophobic patients as it involves lying in an enclosed space for many minutes.

Neuro-ophthalmic indications

MRI is the technique of choice for lesions of the intracranial visual pathways.

- **The optic nerve** is best visualized on coronal STIR images in conjunction with coronal and axial T1 fat saturation post-gadolinium images. Axial T1 images are useful for

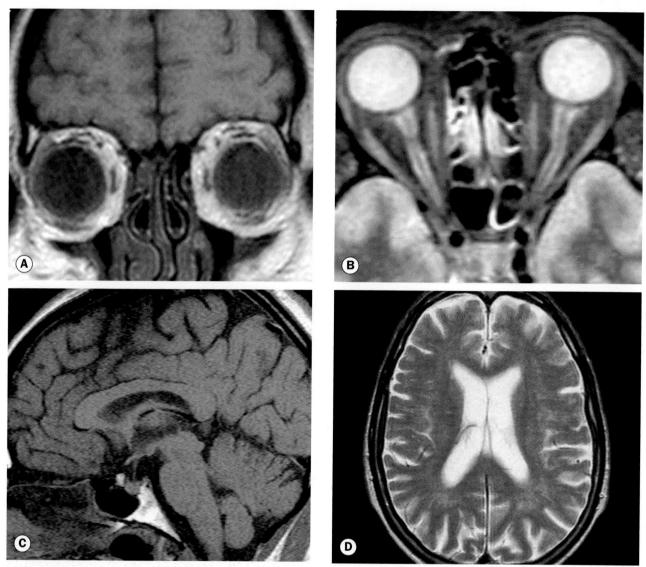

Fig. 19.2 MR scans. **(A)** T1-weighted coronal image through the globe in which vitreous is hypointense (dark) and orbital fat is hyperintense (bright); **(B)** T2-weighted axial image in which vitreous and cerebrospinal fluid (CSF) are hyperintense; **(C)** T1-weighted midline sagittal image through the brain in which the CSF in the third ventricle is hypointense; **(D)** T2-weighted axial image through the brain in which the CSF in the lateral ventricles is hyperintense

displaying normal anatomy. MRI can detect lesions of the intraorbital part of the optic nerve (e.g. neuritis, glioma) as well as intracranial extension of optic nerve tumours.

- **Optic nerve sheath lesions** (e.g. meningioma) are of similar signal intensity to the nerve on T1- and T2-weighted images but enhance avidly with gadolinium.
- **Sellar masses** (e.g. pituitary tumours) are best visualized by T1-weighted contrast-enhanced studies. Coronal images optimally demonstrate the contents of the sella turcica as well as the suprasellar and parasellar regions and are usually supplemented by sagittal images.
- **Cavernous sinus pathology** is best demonstrated on coronal images; contrast may be required.
- **Intracranial lesions of the visual pathways** (e.g. inflammatory, demyelinating, neoplastic and vascular). MRI

allows further characterization of these lesions as well as better anatomical localization.

Angiography

Magnetic resonance angiography

Magnetic resonance angiography (MRA) is a non-invasive method of imaging the intra- and extracranial carotid and vertebrobasilar circulations (Fig. 19.4A) to demonstrate abnormalities such as stenosis, dissection, occlusion, arteriovenous malformations and aneurysms. The motion sensitivity of MR is utilized to visualize blood flow within vessels and does not require contrast. However, because of the reliance on active flow, thrombosed aneurysms may

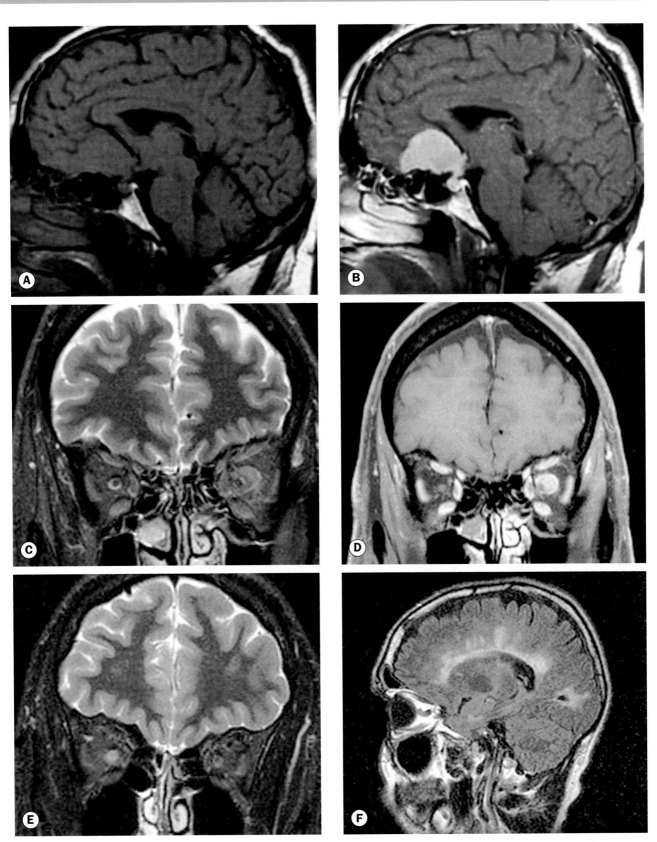

Fig. 19.3 Enhancement techniques. **(A)** Pre-contrast sagittal T1-weighted image of a meningioma; **(B)** post-contrast image showing enhancement of the tumour; **(C)** coronal STIR image showing an intermediate signal intensity mass surrounding the left optic nerve consistent with an optic nerve sheath meningioma compared to STIR; **(D)** T1-weighted fat saturated coronal image of the same patient as (C) showing avid homogeneous enhancement of the meningioma; **(E)** coronal STIR image of right retrobulbar neuritis showing a high signal within the optic nerve with enlargement of the nerve sheath complex; **(F)** sagittal FLAIR image showing multiple periventricular plaques of demyelination

(Courtesy of D Thomas – figs A and B; N Sibtain – figs C–F)

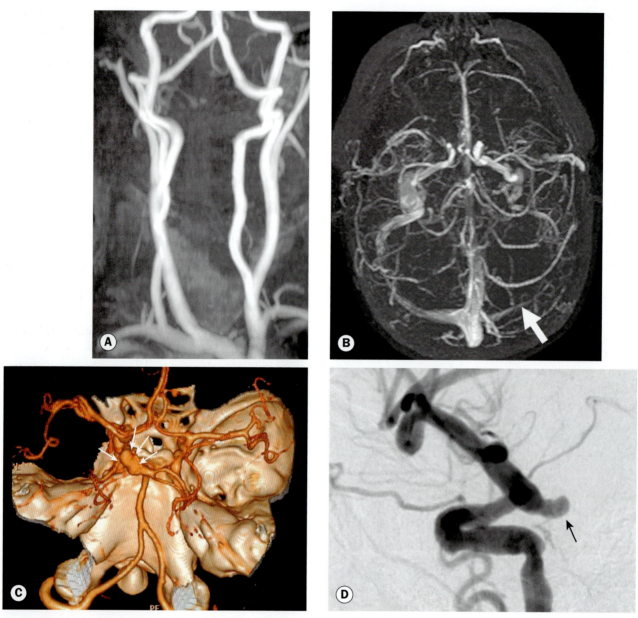

Fig. 19.4 Cerebral angiography. **(A)** Normal MRA of the external carotid and vertebral circulation; **(B)** MRI venogram, axial view, demonstrating narrowing of the left transverse sinus (arrow) in idiopathic intracranial hypertension; **(C)** CT angiogram shows a left posterior communicating aneurysm (arrows); **(D)** conventional catheter angiogram with subtraction shows an aneurysm arising from the internal carotid artery at its junction with the posterior communicating artery (arrow)

(Courtesy of N Sibtain – figs A and C; G Liu, N Volpe and S Galetta, from Neuro-Ophthalmology Diagnosis and Management, Saunders 2010 – fig. B; JD Trobe, from 'Neuro-Ophthalmology', in Rapid Diagnosis in Ophthalmology, Mosby 2008 – fig. D)

be missed and turbulent flow may lead to difficulties in interpretation. The technique has limited facility in the detection of very small aneurysms. MRA adds about 10 minutes to the standard MRI acquisition time.

Magnetic resonance venography

Over recent years increasing attention has been paid to intracranial venous system pathology, particularly dural sinus occlusion and stenosis. Historically, the venous phase of conventional digital subtraction angiography (DSA) has been used for intracranial venous assessment, and still offers high sensitivity and specificity. However, both CT and MRI can be used to similar purpose and are relatively non-invasive and low-risk compared to DSA; technological advances have conferred greatly improved accuracy. Whilst CTV (see below) is generally faster and offers high spatial resolution, it entails a significant radiation dose and always requires contrast for image acquisition. Magnetic resonance venography (MRV) can be used with contrast or using non-contrast enhanced techniques, among other indications making it suitable for patients to whom contrast cannot be given. Substantial advances in MRV pulse sequences now allow excellent visualization of the venous system (Fig. 19.4B), and increasing reliance on MRV seems to be evident. However, local resource availability, experience and expertise are critical in determining the choice of technique.

Computed tomographic angiography

Computed tomographic angiography (CTA) has been emerging as the method of choice in the investigation of intracranial aneurysms (Fig. 19.4C). It enables acquisition of extremely thin slice images of the brain following intravenous contrast. Images of the vessels can be reconstructed in three dimensions and viewed from any direction, aiding the approach to treatment. The investigation is safe and quick and does not carry the 1% risk of stroke associated with conventional catheter angiography.

Computed tomographic venography

Computed tomographic venography (CTV) is a fast high-resolution technique in which patient motion artefact is of lesser importance than with MRV. CTV is believed to be at least as sensitive as MRV in the diagnosis of cerebral venous thrombosis; both techniques may provide complementary findings in difficult diagnostic situations. However, contrast is always required and a significant radiation dose is delivered. Visualization of skull base structures is limited by bony artefact relative to MRV. The technique is similar to that of CTA.

Conventional catheter angiography

Conventional intra-arterial catheter angiography is usually performed under local anaesthetic. A catheter is passed via the femoral artery into the internal carotid and vertebral arteries in the neck under fluoroscopic guidance. Following contrast injection, images are acquired in rapid succession. Digital subtraction results in images of the contrast-filled vessels with the exclusion of background structures such as bone (Fig. 19.4D). Until recently, this technique was the first-line investigation in the diagnosis of intracranial aneurysms but may now be reserved for cases where CTA is equivocal or negative.

OPTIC NERVE

Anatomy

General structure (Figs 19.5A, B and C)

- **Afferent fibres.** The optic nerve carries approximately 1.2 million afferent nerve fibres, each of which originates in a retinal ganglion cell. Most of these synapse in the lateral geniculate body, although some reach other centres, notably the pretectal nuclei in the midbrain. Nearly one-third of the fibres subserve the central 5° of the visual field. Within the

optic nerve itself the nerve fibres are divided into about 600 bundles by fibrous septae derived from the pia mater.
- **Surrounding layers**
  - The innermost layer is the delicate and vascular pia mater.
  - The outer sheath comprises the arachnoid mater and the tougher dura mater which is continuous with the sclera; optic nerve fenestration involves incision of this outer sheath. The subarachnoid space is continuous with the cerebral subarachnoid space and contains CSF.

Anatomical subdivisions

The optic nerve is approximately 50 mm long from globe to chiasm. It can be subdivided into four segments:
- **Intraocular** segment (optic nerve head) is the shortest, being 1 mm deep and approximately 1.5 mm in vertical diameter. The ophthalmoscopically visible portion is called the optic disc (Fig. 19.5D).
- **Intraorbital** segment is 25–30 mm long and extends from the globe to the optic foramen at the orbital apex. Its diameter is 3–4 mm because of the addition of the myelin sheaths to the nerve fibres. At the orbital apex the nerve is surrounded by the tough fibrous annulus of Zinn, from which originate the four rectus muscles.
- **Intracanalicular** segment traverses the optic canal and measures about 6 mm. Unlike the intraorbital portion, it is fixed to the canal, since the dura mater fuses with the periosteum.
- **Intracranial** segment joins the chiasm and varies in length from 5 to 16 mm (average 10 mm). Long intracranial segments are particularly vulnerable to damage by adjacent lesions such as pituitary adenomas and aneurysms.

Visual evoked potential

- **Principle** (Fig. 19.6). Visual (visually) evoked potential (VEP) tests record electrical activity of the visual cortex created by retinal stimulation. The most common indications in ophthalmology are the monitoring of visual function in babies and the investigation of optic neuropathy, particularly when associated with demyelination. It can also be used to monitor macular pathway function, and to investigate functional (non-physiological) visual loss.
- **Technique.** The stimulus is either a flash of light (flash VEP) or a black-and-white checkerboard pattern on a screen that periodically reverses polarity (pattern VEP). Several tests are performed and the average potential is calculated.
- **Interpretation.** Latency (delay) and amplitude are assessed. In optic neuropathy both parameters are affected, with prolongation of latency and a decrease in amplitude. Threshold VEP (by using different sized check stimuli) can detect early or subclinical dysfunction as smaller check size responses may become abnormal earlier than responses to larger stimuli.

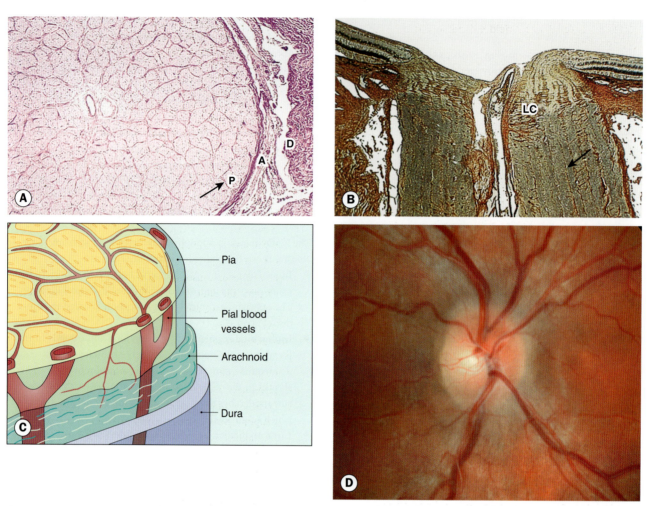

Fig. 19.5 Structure of the optic nerve. **(A)** Transverse section, P = pia, A = arachnoid, D = dura; **(B)** longitudinal section, LC = lamina cribrosa; arrow points to a fibrous septum; **(C)** surrounding sheaths and pial blood vessels; **(D)** clinical appearance of the normal optic disc

(Courtesy of Wilmer Eye Institute – figs A and B)

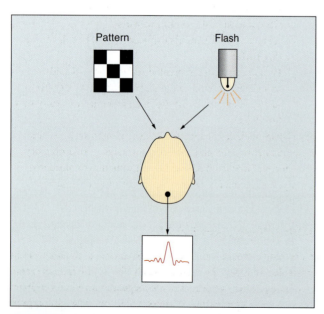

Fig. 19.6 Principles of the visual evoked potential test

Signs of optic nerve dysfunction

- **Reduced visual acuity** for distance and near is common, but is non-specific; acuity may be relatively preserved in some conditions.
- **Relative afferent pupillary defect** (see below).
- **Dyschromatopsia** is impairment of colour vision, which in the context of optic nerve disease mainly affects red and green. A simple way of detecting a monocular colour vision defect is to ask the patient to compare the colour of a red object using each eye in turn.
- **Diminished light brightness sensitivity**, often persisting after visual acuity returns to normal, for instance following the acute stage of optic neuritis.
- **Diminished contrast sensitivity** (see Ch. 14).
- **Visual field defects**, which vary with the underlying pathology, include diffuse depression of the central visual field, central scotomas, centrocaecal scotomas, nerve fibre bundle and altitudinal (Table 19.1).

Classification of optic neuropathy by cause

- **Inflammatory.** Optic neuritis, including demyelinating, parainfectious, infectious and non-infectious, and neuroretinitis.
- **Glaucomatous.** See Ch. 10.
- **Ischaemic.** Anterior non-arteritic, anterior arteritic, posterior ischaemic and diabetic papillopathy.
- **Hereditary.** Leber hereditary optic neuropathy, other hereditary optic neuropathies.
- **Nutritional and toxic.** See also Ch. 20
- **Papilloedematous.** Secondary to raised intracranial pressure.
- **Traumatic.** See Ch. 21.
- **Compressive.** Including secondary to an orbital lesion.
- **Infiltrative.** Inflammatory conditions (e.g. sarcoidosis), tumours and infective agents.

Optic atrophy

Introduction

Optic atrophy refers to the late stage changes that take place in the optic nerve resulting from axonal degeneration in the pathway between the retina and the lateral geniculate body, manifesting with disturbance in visual function and in the appearance of the optic nerve head. It can be classified in several ways, including by whether axonal death is initiated in the retina (anterograde) or more centrally (retrograde), and by cause. Optic 'atrophy' is not true atrophy, a term that strictly refers to involutional change secondary to lack of use. A classification according to ophthalmoscopic appearance is set out below.

Primary optic atrophy

Primary optic atrophy occurs without antecedent swelling of the optic nerve head. It may be caused by lesions affecting the visual pathways at any point from the retrolaminar portion of the optic nerve to the lateral geniculate body. Lesions anterior to the optic chiasm result in unilateral optic atrophy, whereas those involving the chiasm and optic tract will cause bilateral changes.

- **Signs**
  - Flat white disc with clearly delineated margins (Fig. 19.7A).
  - Reduction in the number of small blood vessels on the disc surface.
  - Attenuation of peripapillary blood vessels and thinning of the retinal nerve fibre layer (RNFL).
  - The atrophy may be diffuse or sectoral depending on the cause and level of the lesion. Temporal pallor of the optic nerve head may indicate atrophy of fibres of the papillomacular bundle, and is classically seen following demyelinating optic neuritis. Band atrophy is a similar phenomenon caused by involvement of the fibres entering the optic disc nasally and temporally; it occurs in lesions of the optic chiasm or tract and gives nasal as well as temporal pallor.
- **Important causes**
  - Optic neuritis.
  - Compression by tumours and aneurysms.
  - Hereditary optic neuropathies.
  - Toxic and nutritional optic neuropathies; these may give temporal pallor, particularly in early/milder cases when the papillomacular fibres are preferentially affected (Fig. 19.7B).
  - Trauma.

Secondary optic atrophy

Secondary optic atrophy is preceded by long-standing swelling of the optic nerve head.

- **Signs** vary according to the cause and its course.
  - Slightly or moderately raised white or greyish disc with poorly delineated margins due to gliosis (Fig. 19.7C).
  - Obscuration of the lamina cribrosa.
  - Reduction in the number of small blood vessels on the disc surface.
  - Peripapillary circumferential retinochoroidal folds, especially temporal to the disc (Paton lines – see Fig. 19.7C), sheathing of arterioles and venous tortuosity may be present.
- **Causes** include chronic papilloedema, anterior ischaemic optic neuropathy and papillitis. Intraocular inflammatory causes of marked disc swelling are sometimes considered to cause secondary rather than consecutive atrophy (see below).

Consecutive optic atrophy

Consecutive optic atrophy is caused by disease of the inner retina or its blood supply. The cause is usually obvious on fundus examination, e.g. extensive retinal photocoagulation, retinitis pigmentosa or prior central retinal artery occlusion. The disc appears waxy, with reasonably preserved architecture (Fig. 19.7D).

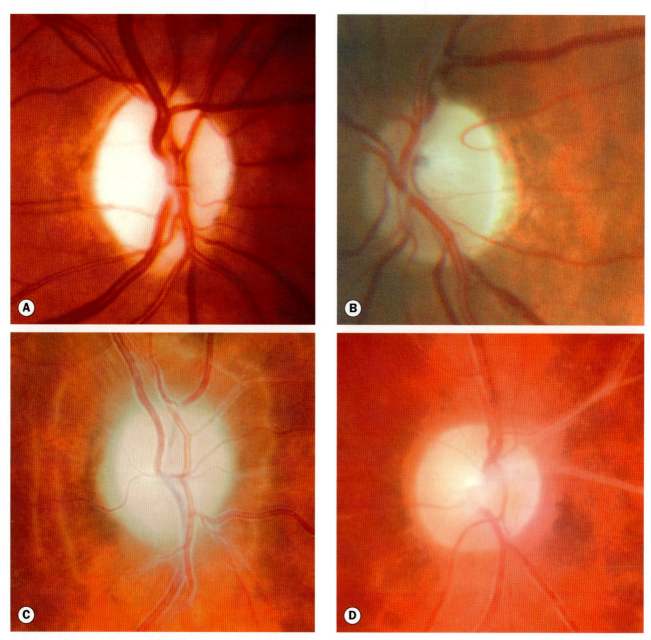

Fig. 19.7 Optic atrophy. **(A)** Primary due to compression; **(B)** primary due to nutritional neuropathy – note predominantly temporal pallor; **(C)** secondary due to chronic papilloedema – note prominent Paton lines (see text); **(D)** consecutive due to vasculitis
(Courtesy of P Gili – fig. C)

Glaucomatous optic atrophy

See Ch. 10.

Classification of optic neuritis

According to ophthalmoscopic appearance

- **Retrobulbar neuritis**, in which the optic disc appears normal, at least initially, because the optic nerve head is not involved. It is the most common type in adults and is frequently associated with multiple sclerosis (MS).
- **Papillitis** is characterized by hyperaemia and oedema of the optic disc, which may be associated with peripapillary flame-shaped haemorrhages (Fig. 19.8). Cells may be seen in the posterior vitreous. Papillitis is the most common type of optic neuritis in children, but can also affect adults.
- **Neuroretinitis** is characterized by papillitis in association with inflammation of the retinal nerve fibre layer and a macular star figure (see below). It is the least common type and is only rarely a manifestation of demyelination.

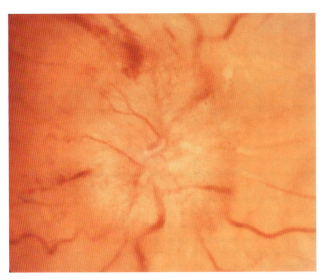

Fig. 19.8 Papillitis

According to aetiology

- **Demyelinating.** This is by far the most common cause.
- **Parainfectious**, following a viral infection or immunization.
- **Infectious.** This may be sinus-related, or associated with conditions such as cat-scratch disease, syphilis, Lyme disease, cryptococcal meningitis and herpes zoster.
- **Non-infectious** causes include sarcoidosis and systemic autoimmune diseases such as systemic lupus erythematosus, polyarteritis nodosa and other vasculitides.

Demyelinating optic neuritis

Overview

Demyelination is a pathological process in which normally myelinated nerve fibres lose their insulating myelin layer. The myelin is phagocytosed by microglia and macrophages, subsequent to which astrocytes lay down fibrous tissue in plaques. Demyelinating disease disrupts nervous conduction within the white matter tracts of the brain, brainstem and spinal cord. Demyelinating conditions that may involve the visual system include the following:

- **Isolated optic neuritis** with no clinical evidence of generalized demyelination, although in a high proportion of cases this subsequently develops.
- **Multiple sclerosis** (MS), by far the most common demyelinating disease (see below).
- **Devic disease** (neuromyelitis optica), a very rare disease that may occur at any age, characterized by bilateral optic neuritis and the subsequent development of transverse myelitis (demyelination of the spinal cord) within days or weeks.
- **Schilder disease**, a very rare relentlessly progressive generalized disease with an onset prior to the age of 10 years and death within 1–2 years. Bilateral optic neuritis without subsequent improvement may occur.

Multiple sclerosis

Multiple sclerosis (MS) is an idiopathic demyelinating disease involving central nervous system white matter. It is more common in women than men.

- **Presentation** is typically in the third–fourth decades, generally with relapsing/remitting demyelination that may switch later to an unremitting pattern, and less commonly with progressive disease from the outset.
- **Systemic features** may include:
  - Spinal cord, e.g. weakness, stiffness, sphincter disturbance, sensory loss.
  - Brainstem, e.g. diplopia, nystagmus, dysarthria, dysphagia.
  - Cerebral, e.g. hemiparesis, hemianopia, dysphasia.
  - Psychological, e.g. intellectual decline, depression, euphoria.
  - Transient features, e.g. the Lhermitte sign (electrical sensation on neck flexion) and the Uhthoff phenomenon (sudden worsening of vision or other symptoms on exercise or increase in body temperature).
- **Ophthalmic features**
  - Common. Optic neuritis (usually retrobulbar), internuclear ophthalmoplegia, nystagmus.
  - Uncommon. Skew deviation, ocular motor nerve palsies, hemianopia.
  - Rare. Intermediate uveitis and retinal periphlebitis.
- **Investigation**
  - Lumbar puncture shows oligoclonal bands on protein electrophoresis of cerebrospinal fluid in 90–95%.
  - MRI almost always shows characteristic white matter lesions (plaques – Fig. 19.9 and see Fig. 19.3F).

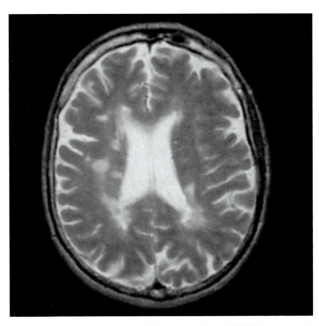

Fig. 19.9 Multiple sclerosis. T1-weighted axial MR image showing characteristic periventricular plaques

○ VEPs are abnormal (conduction delay and a reduction in amplitude) in up to 100% of patients with clinically definite MS.

Association between optic neuritis and multiple sclerosis

- The overall 15-year risk of developing MS following an acute episode of optic neuritis is about 50%; with no lesions on MRI the risk is 25%, but over 70% in patients with one or more lesions on MRI; the presence of MRI lesions is therefore a very strong predictive factor.
- A substantially lower risk of developing MS when there are no MRI lesions is conferred by the following factors, providing critical support in deciding whether to commence immunomodulatory MS-prophylactic treatment following an optic neuritis episode:
  ○ Male gender.
  ○ Absence of a viral syndrome preceding the optic neuritis.
  ○ Optic disc swelling, disc/peripapillary haemorrhages or macular exudates.
  ○ Vision reduced to no light perception.
  ○ Absence of periocular pain.
- Optic neuritis is the presenting feature of MS in up to 30%.
- Optic neuritis occurs at some point in 50% of patients with established MS.

Clinical features of demyelinating optic neuritis

- **Symptoms**
  ○ Subacute monocular visual impairment.
  ○ Usual age range 20–50 years (mean around 30).
  ○ Some patients experience tiny white or coloured flashes or sparkles (phosphenes).
  ○ Discomfort or pain in or around the eye is present in over 90% and typically exacerbated by ocular movement; it may precede or accompany the visual loss and usually lasts a few days.
  ○ Frontal headache and tenderness of the globe may also be present.
- **Signs**
  ○ Visual acuity (VA) is usually 6/18–6/60, but may rarely be worse.
  ○ Other signs of optic nerve dysfunction (see above), particularly impaired colour vision and a relative afferent pupillary defect.
  ○ The optic disc is normal in the majority of cases (retrobulbar neuritis); the remainder show papillitis (see Fig. 19.8).
  ○ Temporal disc pallor may be seen in the fellow eye (see Fig. 19.7B for similar appearance), indicative of previous optic neuritis.
- **Visual field defects** (Fig. 19.10)
  ○ Diffuse depression of sensitivity in the entire central 30° is the most common.
  ○ Altitudinal/arcuate defects and focal central/centrocaecal scotomas are also frequent.

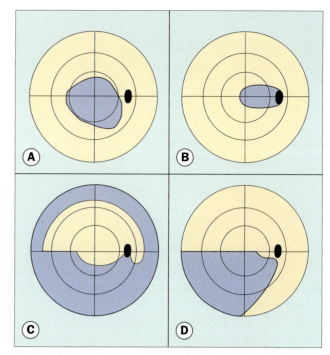

Fig. 19.10 Visual field defects in optic neuritis. **(A)** Central scotoma; **(B)** centrocaecal scotoma; **(C)** nerve fibre bundle; **(D)** altitudinal

  ○ Focal defects are frequently accompanied by an element of superimposed generalized depression.
- **Course.** Vision worsens over several days to 3 weeks and then begins to improve. Initial recovery is fairly rapid and then slower over 6–12 months.
- **Prognosis**
  ○ More than 90% of patients recover visual acuity to 6/9 or better.
  ○ Subtle parameters of visual function, such as colour vision, may remain abnormal.
  ○ A mild relative afferent pupillary defect may persist.
  ○ Temporal optic disc pallor or more marked optic atrophy may ensue.
  ○ About 10% develop chronic optic neuritis with slowly progressive or stepwise visual loss.

Treatment following demyelinating optic neuritis

- **Indications for steroid treatment.** When visual acuity within the first week of onset is worse than 6/12, treatment may speed up recovery by 2–3 weeks and may delay the onset of clinical MS over the short term. This may be relevant in the patients with poor vision in the fellow eye or those with occupational requirements, but the limited benefit must be balanced against the risks of high-dose steroids. Therapy does not influence the eventual visual outcome and the great majority of patients do not require treatment.
- **Steroid regimen.** Intravenous methylprednisolone sodium succinate 1 g daily for 3 days, followed by oral prednisolone

(1 mg/kg daily) for 11 days, subsequently tapered over 3 days. Oral prednisolone may increase the risk of recurrence of optic neuritis if used without prior intravenous steroid.

- **Immunomodulatory treatment** (IMT) reduces the risk of progression to clinical MS in some patients, but the risk versus benefit ratio has not yet been fully defined with the options available, which include interferon beta, teriflunomide and glatiramer. A decision should be individualized, based on risk profile – particularly the presence of brain lesions – and patient preference; most do not commence IMT until a second episode of clinical demyelination has occurred, though there may be an increasing tendency towards a lower threshold.

Parainfectious optic neuritis

Optic neuritis may be associated with viral infections such as measles, mumps, chickenpox, rubella, whooping cough and glandular fever, and may also occur following immunization. Children are affected much more frequently than adults. Presentation is usually 1–3 weeks after a viral infection, with acute severe visual loss generally involving both eyes. Bilateral papillitis is the rule; occasionally there may be a neuroretinitis or the discs may be normal. The prognosis for spontaneous visual recovery is very good, and treatment is not required in the majority of patients. However, when visual loss is severe and bilateral or involves an only seeing eye, intravenous steroids should be considered, with antiviral cover where appropriate.

Infectious optic neuritis

- **Sinus-related** optic neuritis is uncommon and is sometimes characterized by recurrent attacks of unilateral visual loss associated with severe headache and spheno-ethmoidal sinusitis. Possible mechanisms include direct spread of infection, occlusive vasculitis and mucocoele. Treatment is with systemic antibiotics and, if appropriate, surgical drainage.
- **Cat-scratch fever** (benign lymphoreticulosis) is usually caused by *Bartonella henselae* inoculated by a cat scratch or bite (see below and also Ch. 11). Numerous ophthalmological features have been described, notably neuroretinitis.
- **Syphilis** may cause acute papillitis or neuroretinitis during the primary or secondary stages (see Ch. 11).
- **Lyme disease** (borreliosis) is a spirochaetal infection caused by *Borrelia burgdorferi* transmitted by a tick bite (see Ch. 11). It may cause neuroretinitis and occasionally acute retrobulbar neuritis, which may be associated with other neurological manifestations and can mimic MS.
- **Cryptococcal meningitis** in patients with acquired immunodeficiency syndrome (AIDS) may be associated with acute optic neuritis, which may be bilateral (see Ch. 11).
- **Varicella zoster virus** may cause papillitis by spread from contiguous retinitis (i.e. acute retinal necrosis, progressive retinal necrosis – see Ch. 11) or associated with herpes zoster ophthalmicus. Primary optic neuritis is uncommon but may

occur in immunocompromised patients, some of whom may subsequently develop viral retinitis.

Non-infectious optic neuritis

Sarcoidosis

Optic neuritis affects 1–5% of patients with neurosarcoid. It may occasionally be the presenting feature of sarcoidosis but usually develops during the course of established systemic disease. The optic nerve head may exhibit a lumpy appearance suggestive of granulomatous infiltration and there may be associated vitritis (Fig. 19.11). The response to steroid therapy is often rapid, though vision may decline if treatment is tapered or stopped prematurely, and some patients require long-term low-dose therapy. Methotrexate may also be used as an adjunct to steroids or as monotherapy in steroid-intolerant patients.

Autoimmune

Autoimmune optic nerve involvement may take the form of retrobulbar neuritis or anterior ischaemic optic neuropathy (see below). Some patients may also experience slowly progressive visual loss suggestive of compression. Treatment is with systemic steroids and other immunosuppressants.

Neuroretinitis

Introduction

Neuroretinitis refers to the combination of optic neuritis and signs of retinal, usually macular, inflammation. Cat-scratch fever is responsible for 60% of cases. About 25% of cases are idiopathic

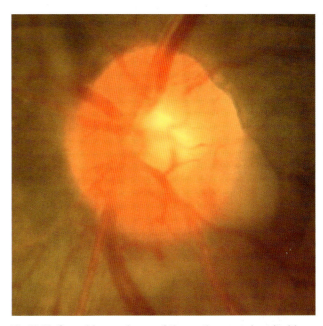

Fig. 19.11 Sarcoid granuloma of the optic nerve head with overlying vitreous haze

(Leber idiopathic stellate neuroretinitis). Other notable causes include syphilis, Lyme disease, mumps and leptospirosis.

Diagnosis

- **Symptoms.** Painless unilateral visual impairment, usually gradually worsening over about a week.
- **Signs**
  - VA is impaired to a variable degree.
  - Signs of optic nerve dysfunction are usually mild or absent, as visual loss is largely due to macular involvement.
  - Papillitis associated with peripapillary and macular oedema (Fig. 19.12A).
  - A macular star (Fig. 19.12B) typically appears as disc swelling settles; the macular star resolves with a return to normal or near-normal visual acuity over 6–12 months.

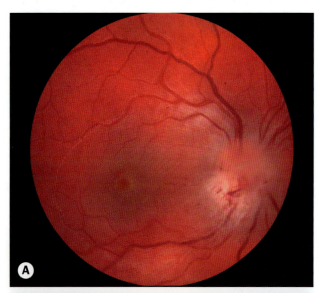

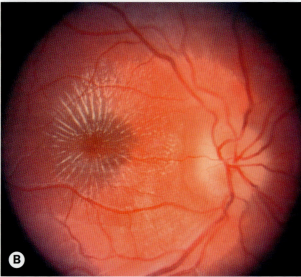

Fig. 19.12 Progression of neuroretinitis. **(A)** Severe papillitis; **(B)** later stage in a different patient showing macular star
(Courtesy of P Saine – fig. A; L Merin – fig. B)

- Venous engorgement and splinter haemorrhages may be present in severe case.
- Fellow eye involvement occasionally develops.
- **Optical coherence tomography (OCT)** demonstrates sub- and intraretinal fluid to a variable extent.
- **Fluorescein angiography (FA)** shows diffuse leakage from superficial disc vessels.
- **Blood tests** may include serology for *Bartonella* and other causes according to clinical suspicion (see also Ch. 11).

Treatment

This is specific to the cause, and often consists of antibiotics. Recurrent idiopathic cases may require treatment with steroids and/or other immunosuppressants.

Non-arteritic anterior ischaemic optic neuropathy

Introduction

Non-arteritic anterior ischaemic optic neuropathy (NAION) is caused by occlusion of the short posterior ciliary arteries resulting in partial or total infarction of the optic nerve head. Predispositions include structural crowding of the optic nerve head so that the physiological cup is either very small or absent, hypertension (very common), diabetes mellitus, hyperlipidaemia, collagen vascular disease, antiphospholipid antibody syndrome, hyperhomocysteinaemia, sudden hypotensive events, cataract surgery, sleep apnoea syndrome and erectile dysfunction. Patients are usually over the age of 50, but are typically younger than those who develop arteritic ION (see below).

Diagnosis

- **Symptoms**
  - Sudden painless monocular visual loss; this is frequently discovered on awakening, suggesting a causative role for nocturnal hypotension.
- **Signs**
  - VA is normal or only slightly reduced in about 30%. The remainder has moderate to severe impairment.
  - Visual field defects are typically inferior altitudinal but central, paracentral, quadrantic and arcuate defects may also be seen.
  - Dyschromatopsia is usually proportional to the level of visual impairment, in contrast to optic neuritis in which colour vision may be severely impaired when VA is reasonably good.
  - Diffuse or sectoral hyperaemic disc swelling, often associated with a few peripapillary splinter haemorrhages (Fig. 19.13).
  - Disc swelling gradually resolves and pallor ensues 3–6 weeks after onset.
- **Investigation** should include blood pressure, a fasting lipid profile and blood glucose. It is also very important to exclude

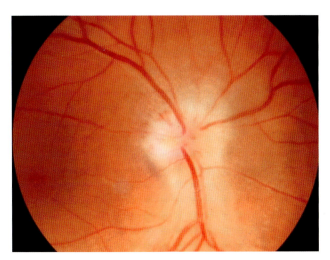

Fig. 19.13 Non-arteritic anterior ischaemic optic neuropathy

occult giant cell arteritis (see below) with symptomatic enquiry and testing as appropriate. Atypical features may prompt special investigations, such as neuroimaging.

- **Prognosis.** Improvement in vision is common although recurrence occurs in about 6%. About 50% of eyes achieve 6/9 or better, though 25% will only reach 6/60 or worse.
- **Fellow eye.** Involvement of the fellow eye occurs in about 10% of patients after 2 years and 15% after 5 years. When the second eye becomes involved, optic atrophy in one eye and disc oedema in the other gives rise to the 'pseudo-Foster Kennedy syndrome'.

Treatment

- There is no definitive treatment.
- Optic nerve fenestration has not been shown to be of benefit.
- Some authorities advocate short-term systemic steroid treatment.
- Any underlying systemic predispositions should be treated.
- Although aspirin is effective in reducing systemic vascular events and is frequently prescribed in patients with NAION, it does not appear to reduce the risk of involvement of the fellow eye.

Arteritic anterior ischaemic optic neuropathy

Arteritic anterior ischaemic optic neuropathy (AAION) is caused by giant cell arteritis (GCA). About 50% of patients with GCA have polymyalgia rheumatica (PMR) at diagnosis, while around 20% of PMR patients will develop GCA. PMR is characterized by pain and stiffness in proximal muscle groups, typically the shoulders and biceps, that is worse on waking. Symptoms can be severe but generally respond dramatically to a low–medium dose (initially 15–20 mg daily) of oral prednisolone. The causative relationship between GCA and PMR remains uncertain, though many suspect them to be different presentations of the same underlying entity.

Diagnosis of giant cell arteritis

GCA is a granulomatous necrotizing arteritis (Fig. 19.14A) with a predilection for large and medium-size arteries, particularly the major aortic branches and the superficial temporal (STA), ophthalmic, posterior ciliary and proximal vertebral arteries. The severity and extent of involvement are associated with the quantity of elastic tissue in the media and adventitia and intracranial arteries are usually spared as they possess little elastic tissue. Smoking, low body mass index and early menopause may be independent risk factors. Patients are usually elderly (average 70 years) and the condition is extremely rare under the age of 50. Women are affected four times more commonly than men. The diagnosis of both GCA and PMR is essentially clinical; the American College of Rheumatology criteria may be helpful in diagnostic decision-making (Table 19.2).

- **Symptoms**
  - Scalp tenderness, first noticed when combing the hair, is common.
  - Headache, which may be localized to the frontal, occipital or temporal areas or be more generalized.
  - Jaw claudication (cramp-like pain on chewing), caused by ischaemia of the masseter muscles, is virtually pathognomonic.
  - Non-specific symptoms such as weight loss, fever, night sweats, malaise and depression are common.
  - Double vision may occur.
  - Arteritic anterior ischaemic optic neuropathy (see below).
- **Other features**
  - Superficial temporal arteritis is characterized by thickened, tender, inflamed and nodular arteries (Fig. 19.14B), though the signs may be subtle.
  - Pulsation is initially present, but later ceases, a sign strongly suggestive of GCA, since a non-pulsatile superficial temporal artery is highly unusual in a normal individual.
  - Ocular motor palsies, including a pupil-involving third nerve palsy, can manifest.
  - Scalp gangrene may occur in very severe cases.

Table 19.2 American College of Rheumatology 1990 classification criteria for giant cell arteritis

1. Age at disease onset 50 years or older
2. New headache
3. Temporal artery tenderness to palpation or decreased pulsation
4. Erythrocyte sedimentation rate of 50 mm/hr or greater
5. Abnormal artery biopsy: biopsy specimen showing vasculitis characterized by a predominance of mononuclear cell infiltration or granulomatous inflammation, usually with multinucleated giant cells

For purposes of classification, a patient shall be said to have giant cell (temporal) arteritis if at least three of these five criteria are present

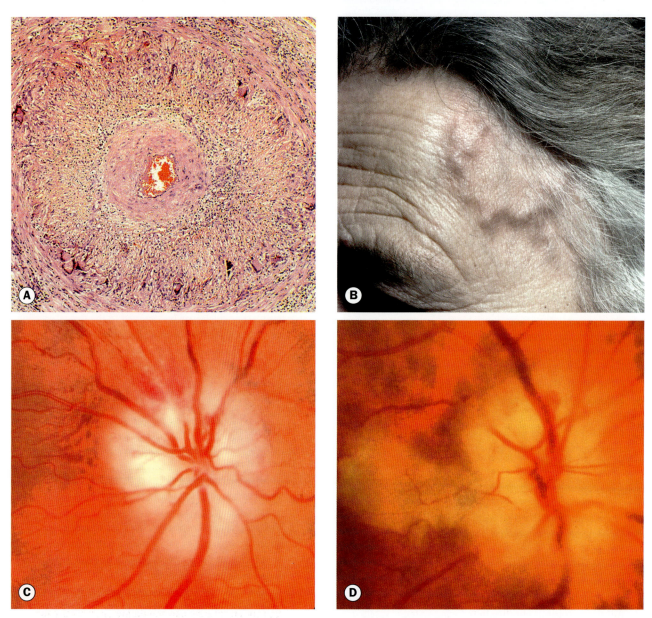

Fig. 19.14 Giant cell arteritis. **(A)** Histology shows transmural granulomatous inflammation, disruption of the internal elastic lamina, proliferation of the intima and gross narrowing of the lumen; **(B)** the superficial temporal artery is often pulseless, nodular and thickened; **(C)** pale swollen disc in arteritic ischaemic optic neuropathy; **(D)** ischaemic optic neuropathy and cilioretinal artery occlusion

(Courtesy of J Harry and G Misson, from Clinical Ophthalmic Pathology, Butterworth-Heinemann 2002 – fig. A; S Farley, T Cole and L Rimmer – fig. B; SS Hayreh – figs C and D)

- ○ Rare complications include dissecting aneurysms, aortic incompetence, myocardial infarction, renal failure and brainstem stroke.
- • **Investigation**
  - ○ Erythrocyte sedimentation rate (ESR) is often very high, with a level of >60 mm/hr, although in approximately 20% of patients it is normal, even low–normal.
  - ○ C-reactive protein (CRP) is invariably raised and may be helpful when ESR is equivocal.
  - ○ Full blood count: elevated platelets and normocytic normochromic anaemia are commonly present.

- ○ Liver function tests are abnormal in one-third.
- ○ Autoantibodies are normal.
- ○ Temporal artery biopsy (TAB) should be performed if GCA is suspected. Steroid treatment (see below) should never be withheld pending biopsy, which should ideally be performed within 3 days of commencing steroids. Systemic steroid administration of duration greater than 7–10 days may suppress histological evidence of active arteritis although this is not invariable. In patients with ocular involvement it is advisable to take the biopsy from the ipsilateral side. The ideal location is the temple

because it lessens the risk of major nerve damage. At least 2.5 cm of artery should be collected and serial sections examined because of the phenomenon of 'skip' lesions in which inflamed segments of arterial wall are interspersed with histologically normal areas. A negative TAB should not prevent ongoing treatment in the presence of a convincing clinical picture of GA as 15% have normal histology; a contralateral biopsy may be positive in 5% following a negative initial biopsy.

○ Colour Doppler and duplex ultrasonography shows a hypoechoic halo around the superficial temporal artery lumen in around 75% due to oedema in the artery wall, and may be pathognomonic. There is some evidence that this provides a valid non-invasive alternative to TAB. Doppler imaging is also a useful aid to locating the artery for biopsy when it cannot be palpated.

○ Extracranial large vessel imaging. Aortic imaging with ultrasonography, MRA or positron emission tomography (PET) scanning may be used to exclude aortic aneurysm or dissection due to aortitis. Serial long-term imaging is increasingly being advocated to exclude these potentially life-threatening complications, the risk of which has now been demonstrated to be substantially increased in and following GCA.

○ Shoulder joint imaging. Recent work suggests that particular inflammatory features in the shoulder joints on MRI and ultrasonography may be useful diagnostically in PMR.

Treatment of giant cell arteritis without AAION

Treatment in the absence of visual symptoms is with oral prednisolone. An initial dose of 1 mg/kg/day is typical, the subsequent duration of treatment being governed by the response of symptoms and the level of the ESR or CRP; symptoms may recur without a corresponding rise in ESR or CRP and vice versa. Most patients need treatment for 1–2 years, although some may require indefinite maintenance therapy. Rapid tapering should generally not occur, with added caution when the dose is reduced to below about 10 mg a day. CRP may play an important role in monitoring disease activity, as the level seems to fall more rapidly than the ESR in response to treatment.

Arteritic anterior ischaemic optic neuropathy

Arteritic anterior ischaemic optic neuropathy (AAION) affects 30–50% of untreated patients with GCA, of whom one-third develop involvement of the fellow eye, usually within a week of the first. Posterior ischaemic optic neuropathy is much less common.

- **Symptoms**
  - ○ Sudden, profound unilateral visual loss not uncommonly preceded by transient visual obscurations (amaurosis fugax) and sometimes by double vision.
  - ○ Periocular pain is common.
  - ○ Other GCA symptoms are common; most cases of AAION occur within a few weeks of the onset of GCA,

although at presentation about 20% do not have systemic symptoms.
  - ○ Simultaneous bilateral involvement is rare but rapid involvement of the second eye, with resultant total blindness, should always be regarded as a substantial risk.

- **Signs**
  - ○ Severe visual loss is the rule, commonly to only perception of light or worse.
  - ○ A strikingly pale 'chalky white' oedematous disc (Fig. 19.14C) is particularly suggestive of GCA.
  - ○ Over 1–2 months, the swelling gradually resolves and severe optic atrophy ensues.

- **Prognosis** is very poor. Visual loss is usually permanent, although, very rarely, prompt administration of systemic steroids may be associated with partial recovery.

- **Treatment** is aimed at preventing blindness of the fellow eye, as visual loss in the index eye is unlikely to improve even with immediate treatment; the second eye may still become involved in 25% despite early steroid administration. The regimen is as follows:
  - ○ Intravenous methylprednisolone, 500 mg to 1 g/day for 3 days followed by oral prednisolone 1–2 mg/kg/day. After 3 more days the oral dose is reduced to 50–60 mg (not less than 0.75 mg/kg) for 4 weeks or until symptom resolution and ESR/CRP normalization. A typical subsequent regimen consists of reducing the daily dose by 10 mg/day every 2 weeks until 20 mg/day is reached, with tapering afterwards titrated against ESR/CRP and symptoms, e.g. a 2.5 mg reduction every 2–4 weeks to 10 mg then a 1 mg reduction every 1–2 months.
  - ○ Enteric-coated prednisolone may be appropriate, particularly in patients with a history of peptic ulceration.
  - ○ Steroid treatment should be accompanied by bone and gastrointestinal protection, e.g. a weekly bisphosphonate, calcium/vitamin D supplementation and a proton pump inhibitor.
  - ○ Monitoring should be performed by a physician with appropriate training and should look particularly for steroid-related complications. A full blood count, ESR/CRP, urea and electrolytes, random glucose and blood pressure should be checked at each visit. Every 1–2 years, a chest X-ray or more sophisticated imaging should be performed to exclude an aortic aneurysm and bone mineral density should be assessed.
  - ○ Antiplatelet therapy, e.g. aspirin 600 mg stat then 100 mg/day should be commenced as this has been shown to reduce the risk of visual loss and stroke.
  - ○ Any significant symptomatic relapse should be treated with an aggressive increase in steroid dose; intravenous methylprednisolone should be given if visual disturbance occurs.
  - ○ Immunosuppressives such as methotrexate may be used as adjuncts in steroid-resistant cases or as steroid-sparing agents when extended treatment is required, though with caution as their benefit is considerably less proven than that of steroids.

○ Biological blockers have not been shown to have a definite protective effect.

Other manifestations

- **Cilioretinal artery occlusion** may be combined with AAION (Fig. 19.14D).
- **Central retinal artery occlusion** is often combined with occlusion of a posterior ciliary artery – with resultant choroidal hypoperfusion – as the two can arise from the ophthalmic artery by a common trunk.
- **Ocular ischaemic syndrome** due to involvement of the ophthalmic artery is rare.

Posterior ischaemic optic neuropathy

Posterior ischemic optic neuropathy (PION) is much less common than the anterior variety. It is caused by ischaemia of the retrolaminar portion of the optic nerve supplied by the surrounding pial capillary plexus, which in turn is supplied by pial branches of the ophthalmic artery; only a small number of capillaries actually penetrate the nerve and extend to its central portion among the pial septae. The diagnosis of PION should be made only after other causes of retrobulbar optic neuropathy, such as compression or inflammation, have been excluded. Initially, the optic disc appears normal but pallor develops over weeks.

- **Operative** (perioperative) PION develops following a variety of surgical procedures, most notably involving the heart and the spine. It occurs in about 0.02% of these procedures. The major risk factors appear to be anaemia and intraoperative hypovolaemic hypotension. Bilateral involvement is common and the visual prognosis is typically poor. Prompt blood transfusion and treatment of facial/orbital swelling may be of benefit.
- **Arteritic** PION is associated with giant cell arteritis and carries a poor visual prognosis.
- **Non-arteritic** PION is associated with the same systemic risk factors as NAION, but is not associated with a crowded optic disc. The visual prognosis is similar to NAION. Some practitioners prescribe a short course of high-dose systemic steroid in early cases.

Diabetic papillopathy

See Ch. 13.

Leber hereditary optic neuropathy

Introduction

Leber hereditary optic neuropathy (LHON) is a rare ganglion cell degeneration; the papillomacular bundle is particularly affected. The condition is caused by maternally inherited mitochondrial DNA point mutations, most frequently (50–90%) at nucleotide position 11778 (G to A) in the *MT-ND4* gene. The condition typically affects males between the ages of 15 and 35 years, although in atypical cases the condition may affect females and present at any age between 10 and 60 years. The diagnosis of LHON should therefore be considered in any patient with bilateral optic neuropathy, irrespective of age.

Diagnosis

- **Symptoms.** Typically acute or subacute severe painless unilateral (50%) loss of central vision. In initially unilateral cases, the fellow eye becomes similarly affected within weeks or months.
- **Signs** during the acute stage are often subtle and easily overlooked, and in some patients the disc may be entirely normal.
  - ○ Colour vision is likely to be subnormal.
  - ○ There is often a relative afferent pupillary defect.
  - ○ In typical cases there is disc hyperaemia with obscuration of the disc margins (Fig. 19.15A).
  - ○ Dilated capillaries on the disc surface; these may extend onto adjacent retina (telangiectatic microangiopathy – Fig. 19.15B).
  - ○ Swelling of the peripapillary nerve fibre layer (pseudo-oedema).
  - ○ Dilatation and tortuosity of posterior pole vasculature.
  - ○ Subsequently, the vessels and pseudo-oedema regress, and severe optic atrophy supervenes (Fig. 19.15C), with nerve fibre layer dropout most pronounced in the papillomacular bundle.
  - ○ Telangiectatic microangiopathy may be present in asymptomatic female relatives.
  - ○ Surprisingly, the pupillary light reactions may remain fairly brisk.
- **LHON plus** refers to rare variants with additional manifestations such as neuromuscular dysfunction.
- **Prognosis** is poor, although some visual recovery may occur in a minority of cases even years later. Most patients suffer permanent bilateral visual loss with a final VA of 6/60 or less. The 11778 mutation carries the worst prognosis.
- **OCT.** Patients show peripapillary retinal thinning; unaffected carriers frequently show variable thickening of the temporal retinal nerve fibre layer, perhaps due to compensatory mitochondrial accumulation.
- **Visual field** defects usually consist of central or centrocaecal scotomas, with preserved peripheral vision.
- **FA** shows no leakage from the disc or microangiopathic vessels.
- **Genetic testing** to look for the three common causative mutations.

Treatment

- Apart from symptomatic measures such as low vision aids, treatment is generally ineffective.
- Various vitamins and co-factors, idobenone, creatine and others have been tried with anecdotal success, and subspecialist prescription of one or more of these may be

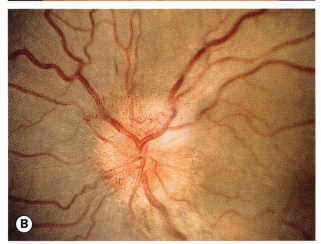

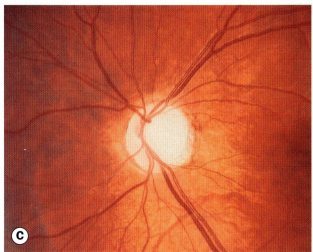

Fig. 19.15 Leber hereditary optic neuropathy. **(A)** Acute stage showing hyperaemic disc swelling with blurring of margins; **(B)** marked telangiectatic microangiopathy; **(C)** late – atrophic appearance

worthwhile, particularly in early disease or prior to second eye involvement. Counterintuitively, the cyanocobalamin (but not the hydroxocobalamin) form of vitamin B$_{12}$ has been reported to worsen outcomes.

- Dietary deficiencies should be avoided, particularly of B$_{12}$.

- Smoking and excessive alcohol consumption should be discouraged, theoretically in order to minimize mitochondrial stress.
- Gene therapy is under active investigation.

Miscellaneous hereditary optic neuropathies (atrophies)

This heterogeneous group of rare disorders are characterized primarily by bilateral optic atrophy. There is no effective treatment, though the measures described above for LHON may be tried.

Dominant optic atrophy (Kjer type optic atrophy, optic atrophy type 1)

- **Inheritance** is autosomal dominant (AD); this is the most common hereditary optic neuropathy with an incidence of around 1 : 50 000; it is frequently due to a mutation in the *OPA1* gene on chromosome, which causes mitochondrial dysfunction, but other genes can be responsible and X-linked and autosomal recessive (AR) forms have been reported. There is usually high penetrance but variable expressivity in the dominant forms.
- **Presentation** is typically, though not always, in childhood with insidious visual loss. There is usually a family history, but the course may be variable even within the same family.
- **Optic atrophy** may be subtle and temporal (Fig. 19.16A) or diffuse (Fig. 19.16B). There may be enlargement of the cup.
- **Prognosis** is variable (final VA 6/12–6/60) with considerable differences within and between families. Very slow progression over decades is typical.
- **Systemic abnormalities.** Twenty per cent develop sensorineural hearing loss; other features are less common.

Behr syndrome

- **Inheritance** is AR; heterozygotes may have mild features.
- **Presentation** is in early childhood with reduced vision.
- **Optic atrophy** is diffuse.
- **Prognosis** is variable, with moderate to severe visual loss and nystagmus.
- **Systemic abnormalities** include spastic gait, ataxia and mental handicap.

Wolfram syndrome

Wolfram syndrome is also referred to as DIDMOAD (diabetes insipidus, diabetes mellitus, optic atrophy and deafness).

- **Inheritance.** Three genetic forms are recognized, caused by a variety of mutations in *WFS1*, which gives Wolfram syndrome 1, *CISD2* – Wolfram syndrome 2 – and probably a form caused by a mitochondrial DNA mutation, with inheritance being AR, AD or via the maternal mitochondrial line.
- **Presentation** is usually between the ages of 5 and 21 years; diabetes mellitus is typically the first manifestation, followed by visual problems.

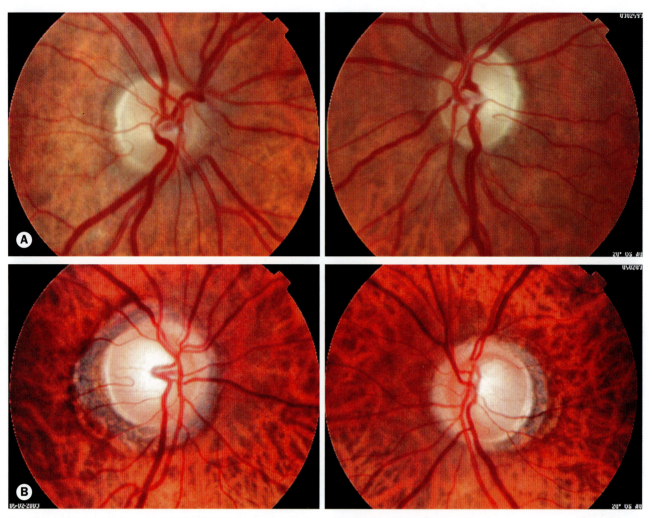

Fig. 19.16 Hereditary optic atrophy. **(A)** Bilateral temporal disc pallor; **(B)** bilateral diffuse pallor

- **Optic atrophy** is diffuse and severe and may be associated with disc cupping.
- **Prognosis** is typically poor (final VA is <6/60).
- **Systemic abnormalities** (apart from DIDMOAD) are highly variable, presumably in part due to genetic heterogeneity, and may include anosmia, ataxia, seizures, mental handicap, short stature, endocrine abnormalities and elevated CSF protein. Life expectancy is usually substantially reduced.

Nutritional optic neuropathy

Introduction

Nutritional optic neuropathy (tobacco-alcohol amblyopia) is an apparently uncommon but likely underdiagnosed acquired optic neuropathy. The mechanism is thought to be deficient mitochondrial function, similar to that of the heritable optic neuropathies, and like these the papillomacular bundle is preferentially affected. In Western developed countries the condition typically affects individuals with high alcohol and tobacco consumption. Most patients have neglected their diet, and the features are most likely to be due principally to deficiency in the B-complex vitamins, particularly cyanocobalamin (B_{12}) and thiamine (B_1), but also riboflavin (B_2), niacin (B_3) and pyridoxine (B_6). Copper, folic acid and protein deficiency may also be important, and direct toxic effects of alcohol and tobacco may also be significant. A strict vegan diet can also be causative, as can dietary deficiency in elderly patients. A similar clinical picture may be seen due to toxicity from medication or environmental (e.g. occupational) toxins. In underresourced geographic regions, nutritional aetiological factors due to inadequate dietary intake predominate, and nutritional optic neuropathy can be epidemic. Pernicious anaemia sufferers may develop the condition due to reduced vitamin B_{12} absorption.

Diagnosis

The possibility of a range of causes, particularly alternative optic neuropathies and macular pathology, should be borne in mind.

- **Symptoms**
  - The insidious onset of painless bilateral central blurring associated with abnormal colour vision.

○ Enquiry should be made about potentially causative medication (see Ch. 20), environmental toxin exposure and a vegan diet.

○ A family history of optic neuropathy should be excluded.

○ Peripheral neurological symptoms (sensory loss, gait disturbance) raise the suspicion of a peripheral neuropathy.

- **Signs**
  ○ VA is very variably affected.
  ○ The discs at presentation are normal in most cases, but some patients show subtle pallor, often temporal, splinter-shaped haemorrhages on or around the disc, or minimal oedema.
  ○ The pupil reactions are often normal, but may respond weakly in more severe cases.
  ○ Other ocular and systemic features of nutritional deficiency should be sought (and investigations carried out accordingly), e.g. Korsakoff syndrome, Wernicke disease, pernicious anaemia; xerophthalmia and beriberi should be considered in developing nations.

- **Colour vision testing.** A reduction in colour vision is disproportionate to the reduction in acuity. Red desaturation is likely to be present. Ishihara chart testing is a simple, moderately quantitative test that is widely available.

- **Visual field defects** are bilateral, relatively symmetrical, centrocaecal scotomas. The margins of the defects are difficult to define with a white target but are more substantive with a red target.

- **OCT** may show peripapillary retinal nerve fibre layer thickening and will help to exclude macular pathology.

- **Fundus autofluorescence (FAF)** should be performed if available to exclude macular changes suggesting a cone or cone-rod dystrophy that may present with colour deficiency and central scotomata.

- **Prognosis** is good in early cases provided patients comply with treatment although visual recovery may be slow; colour perception returns more slowly than measured acuity. In advanced cases there is likely to be a substantial permanent deficit, but it is highly unusual for complete loss of useful vision to occur, with preservation of peripheral field usual even in quite severe cases.

- **Blood tests.** B_{12} (cobalamin) and folate (serum and red cell) and possibly other vitamin levels such as B_1 (thiamine) and B_2, a full blood count and film (macrocytic anaemia) and serum protein levels. Some authorities advocate routine syphilis serology. Screening for specific toxins or for LHON (see above) mutations may be indicated. A high serum methylmalonate and/or homocysteine level may be an indicator of potentially functional B_{12} deficiency, even in the presence of a low-normal B_{12}.

- **VEP.** The P100 amplitude is markedly reduced but with normal or near-normal latency.

- **MRI** is commonly considered to rule out mimicking intracranial pathology, particularly with an atypical clinical picture (e.g. marked asymmetry, disc pallor but good vision).

Treatment

Consideration should be given to co-management with a general physician or neurologist. Compliance with treatment and review is commonly poor in tobacco-alcohol amblyopia.

- **Dietary revision** with formal nutritional advice, incorporating increased fruit and leafy green vegetable intake.

- **Abstention from alcohol and tobacco**; reduction in consumption may be all that is practically possible.

- **Vitamins.** A daily multivitamin preparation, plus thiamine (100 mg twice daily) and folate (1 mg daily). In someone who is both folate and B_{12} deficient, it is prudent to correct the B_{12} deficiency first to avoid precipitating subacute combined degeneration of the cord.

- **Intramuscular hydroxocobalamin** (vitamin B_{12}) injections. The use of injected B_{12} has become less common in recent years, as evidence shows that even in malabsorption states oral treatment may be as effective. Some work suggests that hydroxocobalamin injections improve vision in tobacco-alcohol amblyopia, including when smoking continues, perhaps by reversing cyanide toxicity; their use may therefore still be considered in severe or unresponsive cases, noting also that intramuscular treatment bypasses compliance failure. Regimens range from 1 mg weekly for 8 weeks to monthly for several months; injections every 3 months are typically continued for life.

- **Exposure to the identified agent** should be discontinued immediately in cases due to medication or environmental toxicity.

Papilloedema

Introduction

Papilloedema is swelling of the optic nerve head secondary to raised intracranial pressure (ICP). 'Disc swelling' and 'disc oedema' are non-specific terms that include papilloedema but also a disc swollen from other causes. All patients with papilloedema should be suspected of harbouring an intracranial mass. Not all patients with raised ICP will develop disc swelling. Causes of a swollen-appearing optic disc are given in Table 19.3.

Cerebrospinal fluid

- **Circulation** (Fig. 19.17A)
  ○ Cerebrospinal fluid (CSF) is formed by the choroid plexus in the ventricles of the brain.
  ○ It leaves the lateral ventricles to enter the third ventricle through the foramina of Munro.
  ○ From the third ventricle, it flows through the Sylvian aqueduct to the fourth ventricle.
  ○ From the fourth ventricle, the CSF passes through the foramina of Luschka and Magendie to enter the

Table 19.3 Causes of optic disc elevation

- Papilloedema
- Accelerated hypertension
- Anterior optic neuropathy
  - Ischaemic
  - Inflammatory
  - Infiltrative
  - Compressive including orbital disease
- Pseudopapilloedema
  - Disc drusen
  - Tilted optic disc
  - Peripapillary myelinated nerve fibres
  - Crowded disc in hypermetropia
- Mitochondrial optic neuropathies
  - Leber hereditary optic neuropathy
  - Methanol poisoning
- Intraocular disease
  - Central retinal vein occlusion
  - Uveitis
  - Posterior scleritis
  - Hypotony

subarachnoid space, flowing around the spinal cord and bathing the cerebral hemispheres.
- ○ Absorption is into the cerebral venous system through the arachnoid villi.
- **Normal CSF pressure** on lumbar puncture (not upright) is 10–18 cmH$_2$O in adults.
- **Causes of raised ICP** (Fig. 19.17B)
  - ○ Idiopathic intracranial hypertension.
  - ○ Obstruction of the ventricular system by congenital or acquired lesions.
  - ○ Space-occupying intracranial lesions, including haemorrhage.
  - ○ Impairment of CSF absorption due to meningitis, subarachnoid haemorrhage or trauma.
  - ○ Cerebral venous sinus thrombosis.
  - ○ Cerebral oedema from blunt head trauma.
  - ○ Severe systemic hypertension.
  - ○ Hypersecretion of CSF by a choroid plexus tumour (very rare).

Diagnosis of raised ICP

- **Headaches**, which characteristically occur early in the morning and may wake the patient from sleep, although less commonly they can occur at any time of day. The pain may be generalized or localized, and may intensify with head movement, bending or coughing. They tend to get progressively worse over time. Very rarely, headache may be absent.
- **Nausea**, often episodic and with associated projectile vomiting; may occur as an isolated feature or may precede the onset of headaches.
- **Deterioration of consciousness** as severity increases, initially with drowsiness and somnolence. A dramatic deterioration in concscious level may be indicative of brainstem distortion and requires immediate attention.

- **Visual symptoms** are commonly absent in mild or early raised ICP.
  - ○ Transient visual obscurations lasting up to 30 seconds in one or both eyes are frequent in established papilloedema, and are sometimes precipitated by bending, coughing or the Valsalva manoeuvre; disc swelling due to other causes is usually associated with more persistent visual impairment.
  - ○ Horizontal diplopia due to sixth nerve palsy caused by stretching of one or both abducens nerves over the petrous tip (Fig. 19.18); this is a false localizing sign.
  - ○ Vision is generally normal or minimally reduced. Significant reduction is a late feature in conjunction with secondary optic atrophy.
- **Neurological examination** should be performed.
- **Investigations**
  - ○ B-scan ultrasonography can be used to aid in distinguishing between papilloedema and other causes of a swollen or apparently swollen (pseudopapilloedematous) optic disc with 80–90%

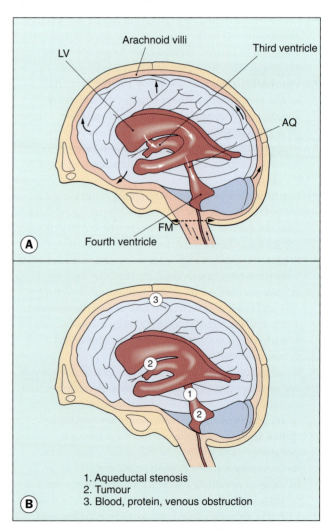

1. Aqueductal stenosis
2. Tumour
3. Blood, protein, venous obstruction

Fig. 19.17 **(A)** Circulation of cerebrospinal fluid; **(B)** causes of raised intracranial pressure – see text (FM = foramen magnum; LV = lateral ventricle; AQ = aqueduct of Sylvius)

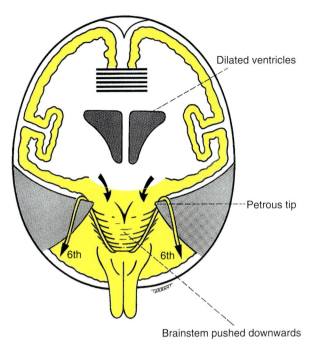

Fig. 19.18 Mechanism of sixth nerve palsy due to raised intracranial pressure

Labels on figure: Dilated ventricles; Petrous tip; 6th; 6th; Brainstem pushed downwards

sensitivity and specificity by measuring the external diameter of the optic nerve sheath (ONSD), which is substantially distended (5.0–5.7 mm or greater at 3.0 mm behind the globe – Fig. 19.19A). The nerve must be scanned axially for the measurement to be accurate, and there is a degree of operator dependence. In contrast to spontaneous venous pulsation (SVP – see below), ONSD does not normalize with short-term ICP fluctuation. The 'crescent sign' (Fig. 19.19B) refers to an echolucent area in the anterior intraorbital nerve thought to represent increased separation of the nerve and its sheath. Lateral gaze ('thirty degree test') commonly leads to a 10% reduction in diameter on A-scan measurement in the presence of excess fluid (Figs 19.19C and D), but not if normal or if increased ONSD is due to infiltration. Fluid-related ONSD can also be caused by other pathology, such as inflammation and trauma.

○ MRI to exclude a space-occupying lesion and/or enlarged ventricles; MRI can also be used to measure ONSD (average normal diameter approximately 5.5 mm ± 1 mm on MRI).

○ In certain cases vascular imaging may be performed, such as venography to rule out cerebral venous sinus thrombosis.

○ Lumbar puncture (LP) must not be carried out until imaging has excluded a space-occupying lesion that might cause downwards herniation of the intracranial contents towards the LP-induced low-pressure area. Clotting abnormality, including therapeutic anticoagulation, is also a contraindication unless reversed prior to the LP.

Stages of papilloedema

Papilloedema is nearly always bilateral, but may be asymmetrical.

- **Early** (Fig. 19.20A)
  ○ Mild disc hyperaemia with preservation of the optic cup.
  ○ Indistinct peripapillary retinal nerve striations and disc margins.
  ○ SVP is absent in about 20% of normal individuals and may be difficult to identify even when present. An identifiable venous pulsation in at least one eye means that the ICP is normal at that point in time, bearing in mind that diurnal fluctuation can occur.

- **Established** (acute – Fig. 19.20B)
  ○ Normal or reduced VA.
  ○ Severe disc hyperaemia, moderate elevation with indistinct margins and absence of the physiological cup.
  ○ Venous engorgement, peripapillary flame haemorrhages and frequently cotton wool spots.
  ○ As the swelling increases, the optic nerve head appears enlarged.
  ○ Circumferential retinal folds (Paton lines) may develop, especially temporally (see Fig. 19.7C).
  ○ Macular fan: in younger patients small vesicles may form in the superficial retina, converging on the fovea in a fan shape with the apex at the fovea; this is not to be confused with a macular star, composed of exudates.
  ○ Enlarged blind spot.

- **Chronic** (Fig. 19.20C)
  ○ VA is variable and the visual fields begin to constrict.
  ○ Disc elevation; cotton wool spots and haemorrhages are characteristically no longer present.
  ○ Optociliary shunts (see Ch. 13) and drusen-like crystalline deposits (corpora amylacea) may be present on the disc surface.

- **Atrophic** (secondary optic atrophy – Fig. 19.20D)
  ○ VA is severely impaired.
  ○ The optic discs are grey–white, slightly elevated, with few crossing blood vessels and indistinct margins.

Idiopathic intracranial hypertension

Introduction

Idiopathic intracranial hypertension, previously known as benign intracranial hypertension or pseudotumour cerebri, is characterized by elevated ICP that by definition has no identifiable cause; obese young adult women are the most commonly affected group. Various medications including the contraceptive pill have been implicated (strictly 'secondary intracranial hypertension' if a cause is identified), as well as a range of conditions such as systemic lupus erythematosus, Lyme disease and sleep apnoea syndrome.

Diagnosis

- **Symptoms and signs** are those of papilloedema, with headache in over 90%; pulsatile tinnitus may be experienced,

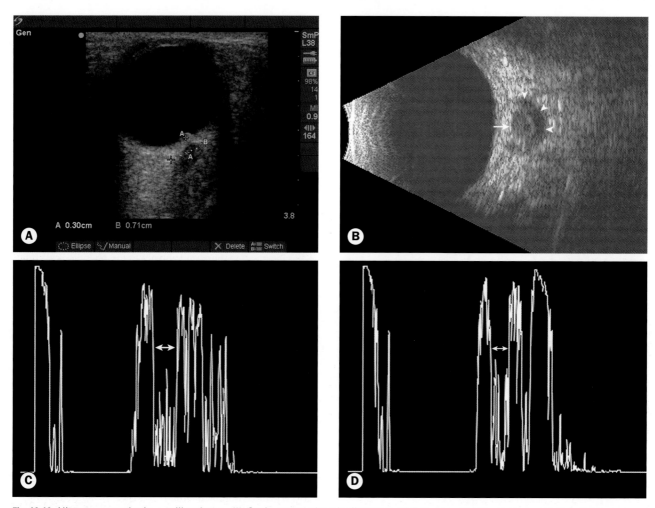

Fig. 19.19 Ultrasonography in papilloedema. **(A)** Optic nerve sheath diameter of 7.1 mm, 3 mm posterior to the globe; **(B)** transverse B-scan showing crescent sign (arrowheads); **(C)** A-scan in primary position with retrobulbar nerve diameter of 4.8 mm; **(D)** in lateral gaze diameter reduces to 3.5 mm – positive 30° test

(Courtesy of M Stone, from American Journal of Emergency Medicine *2009;27:376.e1–376.e2 – fig. A; L Lystad, B Hayden, A Singh, from* Ultrasound Clinics *2008;3:257–66 – figs B–D)*

and cranial nerve palsies and occasionally other symptoms may occur. The long-term visual prognosis is usually good, but up to a quarter will have a degree of permanent impairment.

- **Investigation** is as for papilloedema: ONSD is increased and MRI may show slit-like ventricles and flattening of the pituitary gland ('empty sella' sign). MRV is usually carried out to exclude cerebral venous sinus thrombosis or stenosis. Additional investigation for an occult cause should be considered, especially in patients who do not fit the usual profile.

Treatment

- Weight loss, including via bariatric surgery, can be very effective and formal dietary intervention is strongly recommended.
- Other options include acetazolamide, furosemide, digoxin and analgesia, and in unresponsive cases optic nerve

fenestration, lumboperitoneal shunting and transverse dural sinus stenting.

- Steroids are controversial, but a short course is sometimes used in severe papilloedema.
- Intravenous mannitol or a lumbar puncture are usually reserved for acute severe exacerbations.
- The ophthalmologist's role is usually confined to diagnosis and the monitoring of visual function with VA, colour vision and fields, and optic nerve appearance/photography.

Congenital optic disc anomalies

Tilted disc

A tilted optic disc is a common anomaly, usually bilateral, describing an apparently oblique entry of the optic nerve into the globe. It is strongly associated with myopia and astigmatism. A suggested definition regards tilting as present when the ratio of the longest

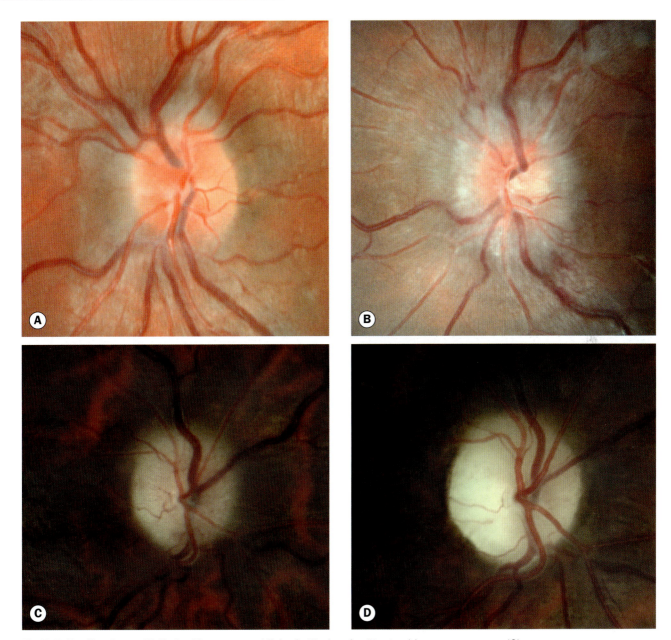

Fig. 19.20 Papilloedema. **(A)** Early; **(B)** acute established; **(C)** chronic; **(D)** atrophic – same eye as (C)

diameter of the disc to the shortest (ovality index) is greater than 1.3 (Fig. 19.21A), but this will not include many subjectively apparently tilted discs (Fig. 19.21B). A major implication of tilting is difficulty in excluding superimposed glaucomatous damage, as the temporal, particularly the inferotemporal, neuroretinal rim is frequently very thin.

- **Signs.** Small, oval or D-shaped disc: the axis is most frequently directed inferonasally, but may be horizontal or nearly vertical.
  - The disc margin is indistinct where retinal nerve fibres are elevated.
  - Peripapillary chorioretinal thinning may be marked, and situs inversus may be present: the temporal vessels deviate nasally before turning temporally (Fig. 19.21C).

- **Perimetry** may show superotemporal defects; these do not respect the vertical midline.
- **OCT** may demonstrate sectoral peripapillary retinal nerve fibre layer thinning, but macular ganglion cell complex analysis is often – but not always – normal so may provide a more useful parameter for the exclusion of coexistent glaucomatous damage.
- **Complications** (rare) include choroidal neovascularization and sensory macular detachment.

Torsional disc

A torsional (torsioned) disc is said to be present when its long axis is inclined at more than 15° from the vertical meridian, a line at

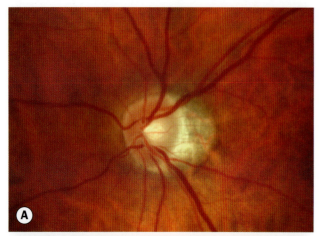

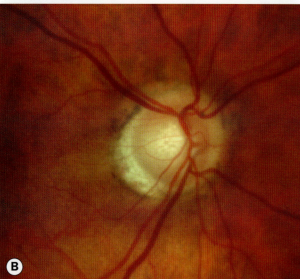

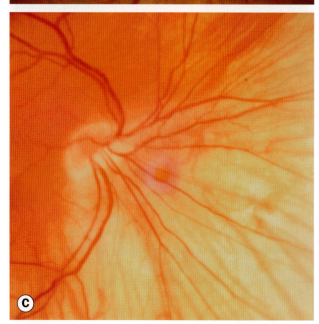

Fig. 19.21 (A) Tilted disc; **(B)** borderline tilted disc with thin inferotemporal neuroretinal rim; **(C)** markedly tilted – and torsional – disc with situs inversus and associated inferonasal chorioretinal thinning

90° to a horizontal line connecting the foveola to the centre of the optic disc (see Fig. 19.21C). It is often present in association with tilting, and is also associated with myopia.

Optic disc pit

- **Signs**
  - VA is normal in the absence of complications.
  - The disc is often larger than normal and contains a greyish round or oval pit of variable size, usually temporal (Fig. 19.22A) but occasionally central or elsewhere; pits are bilateral in 10–15%.
  - Visual field defects are common and may mimic glaucoma; central defects may indicate a macular detachment.
- **Serous macular detachment** (Fig. 19.22B) develops in about half of eyes with non-central disc pits (median age 30 years). The source of the fluid remains speculative.
  - A schisis-like retinal separation that extends from the pit is followed by serous detachment of the outer retinal layers (Fig. 19.22C). It is important to examine the optic disc carefully in all patients with central serous chorioretinopathy.
  - FA does not usually show hyperfluorescence of the detachment, which is demonstrated well on FAF (Fig. 19.22D) and OCT.
- **Management.** Long-term review (including Amsler grid use) for the development of complications is prudent, as it is possible that early treatment of macular detachment may confer a better visual outcome. Options when macular detachment develops include:
  - Observation for spontaneous resolution, which occurs in up to 25%, but may worsen the eventual outcome.
  - Laser may be considered if vision is deteriorating. Light burns are applied along the temporal aspect of the disc. The success rate is 25–35%.
  - Vitrectomy with air-fluid exchange and postoperative prone positioning may be considered if laser is unsuccessful.

Optic disc drusen

Disc drusen are deposits, usually calcified, within the substance of the optic nerve head that are present in up to 2% of the population, often bilaterally (75%). They are usually sporadic but in some cases have AD inheritance. They are thought to consist of focal collections of axonal metabolic products.

- **Symptoms** are usually absent, but some patients may experience episodic blurring, possibly due to transient ischaemia related to a crowding effect.
- **Buried drusen.** Particularly in childhood, drusen may be obscured beneath the disc surface (Figs 19.23A and B); this is a common cause of pseudopapilloedema. A lumpy disc appearance, an absent cup and anomalous vascular patterns including proximal branching, an increased number of major vessels and tortuosity suggest drusen, as well as a lack of papilloedematous features such as hyperaemia and vessel

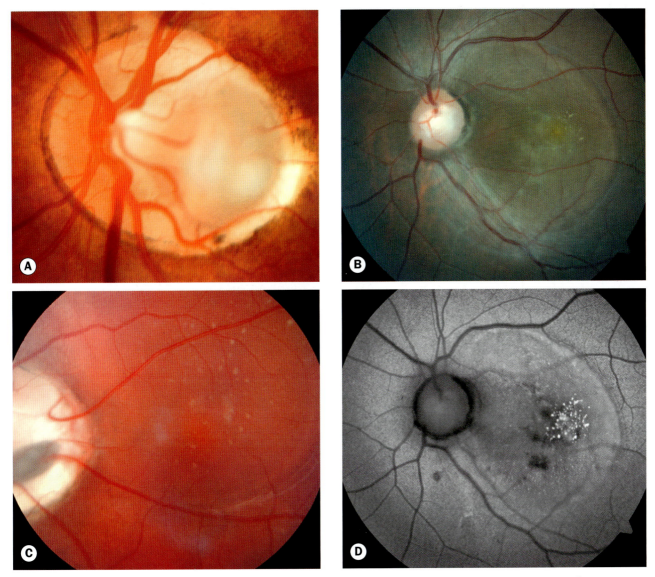

Fig. 19.22 **(A)** Optic disc pit; **(B)** optic disc pit and macular detachment; **(C)** macular detachment; **(D)** fundus autofluorescence image of the eye in (B)

(Courtesy of P Gili – fig. A)

obscuration. Visibility of drusen typically increases in the early teens.

- **Exposed drusen.** Drusen at or close to the disc surface appear as whitish pearl-like lesions of a range of sizes (Figs 19.23C and D). They tend to enlarge slowly over many years.
- **Retinal nerve fibre layer thinning** is common.
- **Visual field defects** of a range of configurations are present in up to 75% and are often progressive, though a substantial impact on sight is rare. No definitive treatment is recognized, though reducing IOP and other speculative measures may be tried in selected cases.
- **Associations** include retinitis pigmentosa and angioid streaks; disc drusen are present in 90% of patients with Alagille syndrome.

- **Complications** (rare) include juxtapapillary choroidal neovascularization (Fig. 19.23E), vitreous haemorrhage and vascular occlusions, particular anterior ischaemic optic neuropathy.
- **Imaging**
  - FAF usually demonstrates drusen extremely well (see Figs 19.23B and D).
  - Ultrasonography (US) shows calcified drusen as highly reflective foci (Fig. 19.23F). US optic nerve features distinguishing raised ICP are discussed above.
  - OCT. Diffuse or focal RNFL thinning; OCT can be used for monitoring.
  - CT shows calcification but involves a substantial radiation dose and so is not indicated solely to confirm drusen.

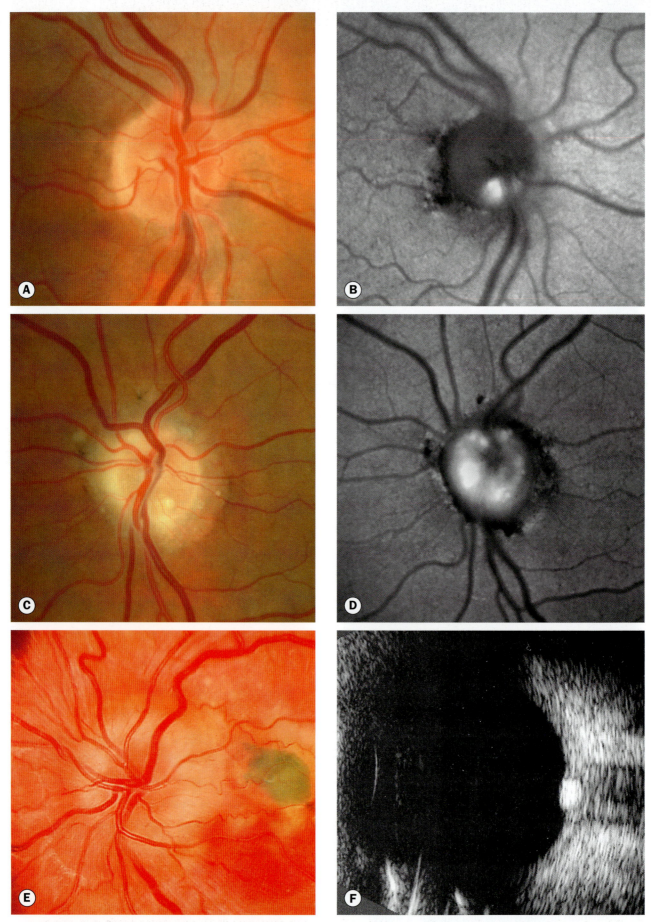

Fig. 19.23 Optic disc drusen. **(A)** Buried disc drusen; **(B)** fundus autofluorescence image of eye in (A); **(C)** exposed disc drusen; **(D)** fundus autofluorescence of eye in (C); **(E)** drusen with secondary choroidal neovascularization; **(F)** B-scan shows high acoustic reflectivity

(Courtesy of J Donald M Gass, from Stereoscopic Atlas of Macular Diseases, Mosby 1997 – fig. E; P Gili – fig. F)

Optic disc coloboma

The embryonic fissure of the developing eye is located inferiorly and slightly nasally, and extends from the optic nerve to the margin of the pupil; a coloboma is a defect in one or more ocular structures due to the fissure's incomplete closure. The defect may be unilateral or bilateral and usually occurs sporadically in otherwise normal individuals, though numerous systemic associations have been described, e.g. chromosomal abnormalities, CHARGE syndrome, Goldenhar syndrome and central nervous system abnormalities. An AD variety is caused by a mutation in the gene *PAX6*.

- **Signs**
  - ○ VA is often decreased; amblyopia and refractive error may be present.
  - ○ A focal, glistening white, bowl-shaped excavation, decentred inferiorly so that the inferior neuroretinal rim is thin or absent and normal disc tissue is confined to a superior wedge of variable size depending on severity (Figs 19.24A and B).
  - ○ A disc coloboma may be associated with, or even continuous with, a large chorioretinal coloboma (Figs 19.24C and D).
  - ○ A disc pit is sometimes associated (Fig. 19.24E); pit-like excavations are sometimes seen with disc colobomata (Fig. 19.24F)
- **Perimetry** shows a superior defect.
- **Ocular associations** include microphthalmos, microcornea and coloboma of other structures such as the iris or lens.

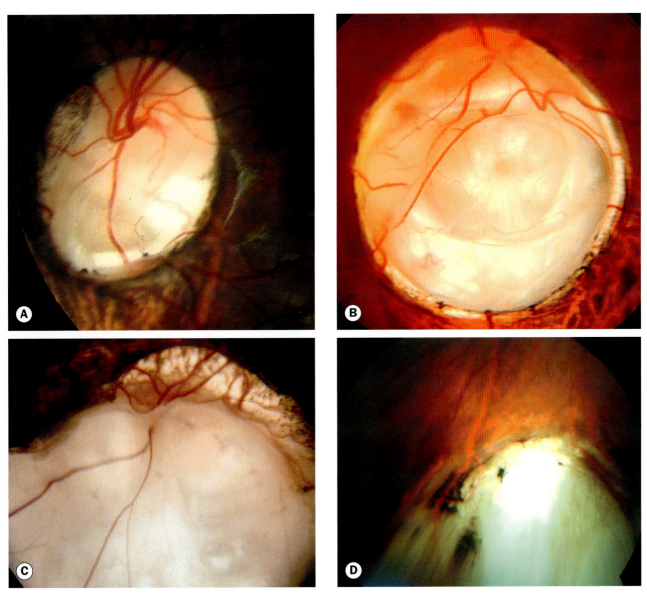

Fig. 19.24 Optic disc coloboma. **(A)** Small disc coloboma; **(B)** large disc coloboma; **(C)** disc coloboma continuous with a chorioretinal coloboma; **(D)** isolated chorioretinal coloboma;

Continued

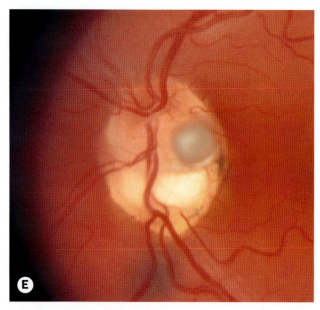

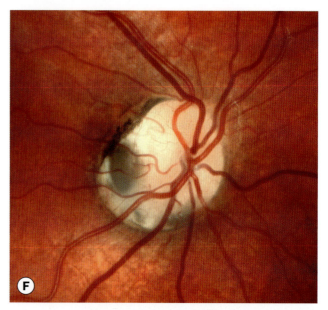

Fig. 19.24, Continued **(E)** associated disc pit and coloboma; **(F)** pit-like excavation associated with a small coloboma
(Courtesy of P Gili – fig. B; L Merin – fig. E; S Chen and T Roberts – fig. F)

- **Complications** (rare) include serous retinal detachment, progressive neuroretinal rim thinning and choroidal neovascularization.

Morning glory anomaly

Morning glory anomaly is a rare, usually unilateral and sporadic condition that has a spectrum of severity. Bilateral cases, which are rarer still, may be hereditary. As in coloboma, a *PAX6* gene mutation can be responsible. Systemic associations are uncommon; the most important is frontonasal dysplasia, characterized by mid-facial anomalies, a basal encephalocele and other midline brain malformations, including pituitary insufficiency.

- **Signs**
  - VA may be normal or impaired to a variable extent.
  - A large disc with a funnel-shaped excavation surrounded by a ring-shaped chorioretinal disturbance (Fig. 19.25).
  - A white tuft of glial tissue overlies the central portion and represents persistent hyaloid vascular remnants.
  - The blood vessels emerge from the rim of the excavation in a radial pattern like the spokes of a wheel. They are increased in number and it may be difficult to distinguish arteries from veins.
- **Complications** include serous retinal detachment (30%) and choroidal neovascularization.

Optic nerve hypoplasia

The hypoplastic optic nerve, unilateral or bilateral, carries a diminished number of nerve fibres. Its frequency seems to be increasing, though it remains relatively rare. Young maternal age, primiparity and maternal exposure to various agents have been

linked. It may occur as an isolated anomaly in an otherwise normal eye, but systemic associations are common (see below).

- **Symptoms**
  - Severe bilateral cases present with blindness in early infancy with roving eye movements or nystagmus.
  - Unilateral or less severe bilateral cases usually present with squint.
  - Mild cases are easily overlooked.
- **Signs**
  - VA ranges from normal to severely impaired.
  - A relative afferent pupillary defect may be present; both pupils may have sluggish light responses in bilateral cases.

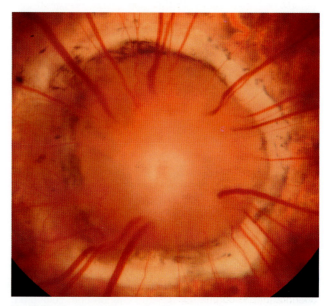

Fig. 19.25 Morning glory optic disc anomaly

o Mild hypoplasia consists simply of a smaller than normal disc (Fig. 19.26A); a foveola–disc centre distance of three or more times the disc diameter strongly suggests hypoplasia.

o Further along the hypoplastic spectrum, a small grey disc is seen, with central cupping-like deficiency of neural tissue and disc vessels emerging in a radial configuration (Fig. 19.26B). The vessels are sometimes tortuous.

o The double-ring sign is characteristic, and consists of a white ring of visible sclera surrounding a pigmented band thought to consist of migrated pigment epithelium (Fig. 19.26C). A thin outer pigmented line may also be seen.

- **Ocular associations** include astigmatism, amblyopia, field defects, foveal hypoplasia, aniridia, and microphthalmos.
- **Systemic associations.** Optic disc hypoplasia is associated with a wide variety of developmental midline brain defects; pituitary and hypothalamic deficits are common. Historically, the most frequent association has been considered to be 'septo-optic dysplasia' (de Morsier syndrome) – bilateral optic nerve hypoplasia, absent septum pellucidum, corpus callosum dysgenesis (Fig. 19.26D) and hypopituitarism – but it is now believed that this complex does not exist as a specific entity.
- **Investigation.** All affected children should be screened for systemic associations, especially hormonal deficiencies and developmental delay.

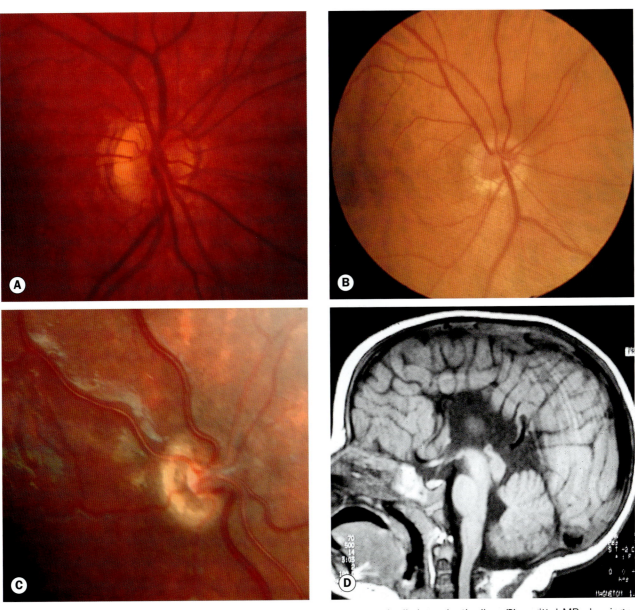

Fig. 19.26 **(A)** Mildly hypoplastic disc; **(B)** moderately hypoplastic disc; **(C)** markedly hypoplastic disc; **(D)** sagittal MR showing absence of the corpus callosum

(Courtesy of R Bates – fig. B; A Moore – fig. C; K Nischal – fig. D)

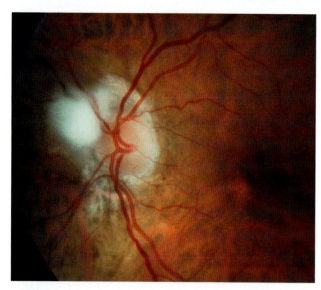

Fig. 19.27 Mild juxtapapillary myelinated nerve fibres

Myelinated nerve fibres

Occasionally myelination of ganglion cell axons extends beyond the cribriform plate and is visible on retinal examination in about 1% of the population: myelinated or medullated nerve fibres (MNF). The condition is usually congenital and stable but both progression and an acquired form have been reported. MNF is occasionally familial. Systemic associations are very rare.

- **Signs**
  - VA is likely to be reduced if the central macula is involved; perimetry may show an absolute scotoma corresponding to the involved area of retina.
  - One or more whitish striated patches with feathery borders; the location and size are variable (Figs 19.27 and 19.28); two-thirds are not contiguous with the optic disc.

  - Retinal vessels in the involved area are obscured.
  - Between 5 and 10% of cases are bilateral.
  - The appearance can be mimicked by neoplastic infiltration and other conditions.
- **Ocular associations** include myopia, anisometropia, strabismus and amblyopia.
- **Imaging.** FAF shows hypoautofluorescence, and there is masking of background fluorescence on FA. The RNFL is hyper-reflective on OCT.
- **Treatment** consists of addressing refractive error, amblyopia and squint if present.

Aicardi syndrome

Aicardi syndrome consists of a range of central nervous system and other malformations in association with multiple bilateral depigmented chorioretinal lacunae clustered around a hypoplastic, colobomatous or pigmented optic disc (Fig. 19.29); other ocular features can include cataract and coloboma. Inheritance is X-linked dominant; the condition is lethal *in utero* for males. Death usually occurs within the first few years of life in affected girls.

Bergmeister papilla

This relatively common anomaly consists of remnants of the hyaloid vessels (Fig. 19.30); see also Chs 12 and 17.

Miscellaneous anomalies

- **Peripapillary staphyloma** is a non-hereditary, usually unilateral condition in which a relatively normal disc sits at the base of a deep excavation whose walls, as well as the surrounding choroid and retinal pigment epithelium (RPE), show atrophic changes (Fig. 19.31A). VA is markedly reduced

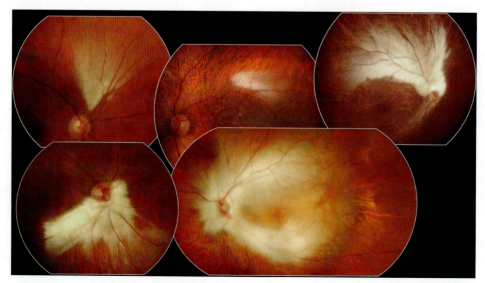

Fig. 19.28 Spectrum of myelinated nerve fibre appearance
(Courtesy of C Barry)

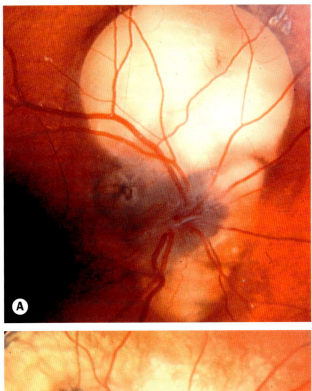

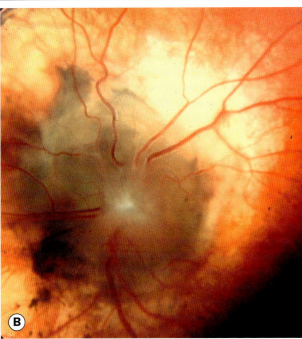

Fig. 19.29 The ocular fundus in Aicardi syndrome. **(A)** Right eye; **(B)** left eye

and local retinal detachment may be present. Unlike other excavated optic disc anomalies, it is rarely associated with other congenital defects or systemic diseases.

- **Papillorenal (renal-coloboma) syndrome** is an AD genetic condition caused in most cases by a mutation in *PAX2* and characterized by renal and optic disc dysplasia. The discs do not exhibit true hypoplasia, but a failure of angiogenesis. They are normal in size with central excavation and replacement of the central retinal vasculature by cilioretinal vessels (Fig. 19.31B).

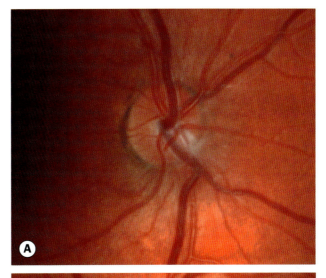

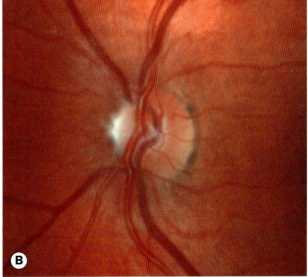

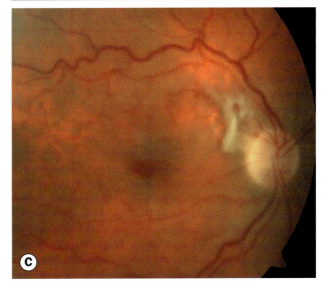

Fig. 19.30 Bergmeister papilla. **(A)** and **(B)** Small bilateral lesions; **(C)** larger example

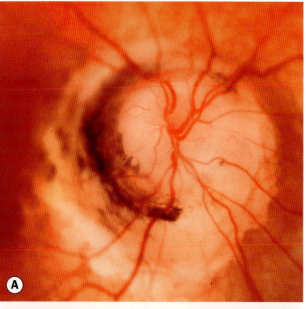

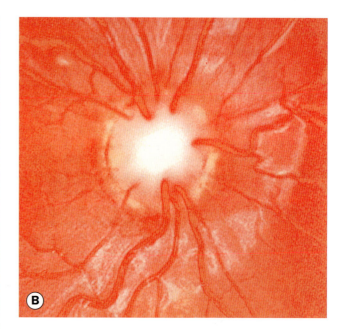

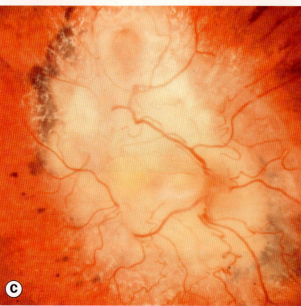

Fig. 19.31 Miscellaneous congenital disc anomalies.
(A) Peripapillary staphyloma; **(B)** papillorenal syndrome;
(C) optic disc dysplasia
(Courtesy of D Taylor and CS Hoyt, from Pediatric Ophthalmology and
Strabismus, *Elsevier 2005 – fig. B)*

- **Optic disc dysplasia** is a descriptive term for a markedly deformed disc that does not conform to any recognizable category (Fig. 19.31C).
- **Megalopapilla** is a typically bilateral condition in which both the horizontal and vertical disc diameters are 2.1 mm or more, or the disc area is greater than 2.5 mm². Although the cup-to-disc ratio is greater than normal, the cup should retain its normal configuration with no evidence of focal neuroretinal rim loss. Although OCT may show peripapillary retinal nerve fibre layer thinning, macular ganglion cell complex imaging is typically normal.
- **Optic nerve aplasia** is an extremely rare condition in which the optic disc is absent or rudimentary and retinal vessels are absent or few in number and abnormal. There may be retinal pigmentary disturbance, especially at the site where

the optic disc might have been. Other ocular and systemic developmental defects may be present.

PUPILS

Anatomy

Light reflex

The light reflex is mediated by the retinal photoreceptors and subserved by four neurones (Fig. 19.32).

- **First** (sensory) connects each retina with both pretectal nuclei in the midbrain at the level of the superior colliculi. Impulses originating from the nasal retina are conducted by

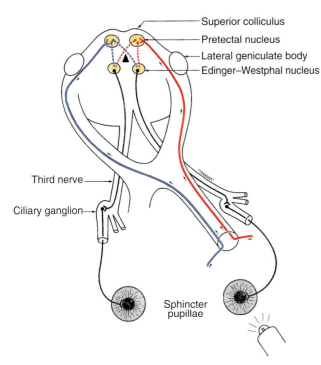

Fig. 19.32 Anatomical pathway of the pupillary light reflex

fibres that decussate in the chiasm and pass up the opposite optic tract to terminate in the contralateral pretectal nucleus. Impulses originating in the temporal retina are conducted by uncrossed fibres (ipsilateral optic tract) that terminate in the ipsilateral pretectal nucleus.

- **Second** (internuncial) connects each pretectal nucleus to both Edinger–Westphal nuclei. Thus a uniocular light stimulus evokes bilateral and symmetrical pupillary constriction. Damage to internuncial neurones is responsible for light–near dissociation in neurosyphilis and pinealomas.
- **Third** (preganglionic motor) connects the Edinger–Westphal nucleus to the ciliary ganglion. The parasympathetic fibres pass through the oculomotor nerve, enter its inferior division and reach the ciliary ganglion via the nerve to the inferior oblique muscle.
- **Fourth** (postganglionic motor) leaves the ciliary ganglion and passes in the short ciliary nerves to innervate the sphincter pupillae. The ciliary ganglion is located within the muscle cone, just behind the globe. It should be noted that, although the ciliary ganglion serves as a conduit for other nerve fibres, only the parasympathetic fibres synapse there.

Near reflex

The near reflex, a synkinesis rather than a true reflex, is activated when gaze is changed from a distant to a near target (see also Ch. 18). It comprises accommodation, convergence and miosis. Vision is not a prerequisite and there is no clinical condition in which the light reflex is present but the near response absent. Although the final pathways for the near and light reflexes are identical (i.e. third nerve, ciliary ganglion, short ciliary nerves), the centre for the near reflex is ill-defined. There are probably two supranuclear

influences: the frontal and occipital lobes. The midbrain centre for the near reflex is probably located more ventrally than the pretectal nucleus and this may explain why compressive lesions such as pinealomas, preferentially involving the dorsal internuncial neurones involved in the light reflex, spare the near reflex fibres until later.

Afferent pupillary defect

Absolute afferent pupillary defect

An absolute afferent pupillary defect (amaurotic pupil) is caused by a complete optic nerve lesion and is characterized by the following:

- The involved eye is completely blind (i.e. no light perception).
- Both pupils are equal in size.
- When the affected eye is stimulated by light neither pupil reacts.
- When the normal eye is stimulated both pupils react normally.
- The near reflex is normal in both eyes.

Relative afferent pupillary defect

A relative pupillary defect (Marcus Gunn pupil) is caused by an incomplete optic nerve lesion or severe retinal disease, but never by a dense cataract. The clinical features are those of an amaurotic pupil but more subtle. Thus the pupils respond weakly to stimulation of the diseased eye and briskly to that of the normal eye. The difference between the pupillary reactions of the two eyes is highlighted by the 'swinging flashlight test' in which a light source is alternatively switched from one eye to the other and back, thus stimulating each eye in rapid succession. A right relative defect is characterized by the following:

- When the normal left eye is stimulated, both pupils constrict (Fig. 19.33A).
- When the light is swung to the diseased right eye, the stimulus delivered to the constriction mechanism is reduced and both pupils dilate instead of constricting (Fig. 19.33B).
- When the normal left eye is again stimulated, both pupils constrict once more (Fig. 19.33C).
- When the diseased right eye is stimulated, both pupils dilate (Fig. 19.33D).

It should be remembered that in afferent (sensory) lesions, the pupils are equal in size; anisocoria (asymmetrical pupil diameter) implies disease of the efferent (motor) nerve or the iris itself.

Horner syndrome (oculosympathetic palsy)

Anatomy

The sympathetic supply involves three neurones (Fig. 19.34):

- **First** (central) starts in the posterior hypothalamus and descends, uncrossed, down the brainstem to terminate in the

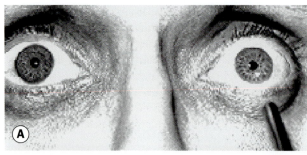

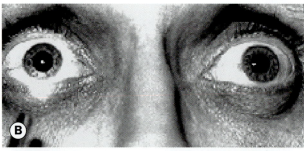

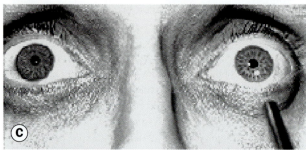

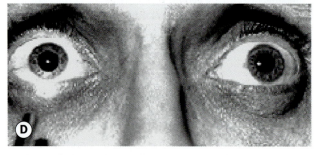

Fig. 19.33 'Swinging flashlight test' in a right afferent pupillary defect

(Courtesy of ES Rosen, P Eustace, HS Thompson and WJK Cumming, from Neuro-ophthalmology, Mosby 1998)

ciliospinal centre of Budge, in the intermediolateral horn of the spinal cord, located between C8 and T2.
- **Second** (preganglionic) passes from the ciliospinal centre to the superior cervical ganglion in the neck. During its long course, it is closely related to the apical pleura where it may be damaged by bronchogenic carcinoma (Pancoast tumour) or during surgery on the neck.
- **Third** (postganglionic) ascends along the internal carotid artery to enter the cavernous sinus where it joins the ophthalmic division of the trigeminal nerve. The sympathetic fibres reach the ciliary body and the dilator pupillae muscle via the nasociliary nerve and the long ciliary nerves.

Causes

The causes of Horner syndrome are shown in Table 19.4. Most commonly, isolated (without additional neurological features) postganglionic Horner syndrome is microvascular in aetiology, but this cannot be assumed.

Presentation

The majority of cases are unilateral. Causes of bilateral involvement include cervical spine injuries and autonomic diabetic neuropathy. Painful Horner syndrome, especially of acute onset, should raise the possibility of carotid dissection.
- Mild ptosis (usually 1–2 mm) as a result of weakness of Müller muscle, and miosis due to the unopposed action of the sphincter pupillae with resultant anisocoria (Fig. 19.35A).
- A key examination finding is that anisocoria is accentuated in dim light, since in contrast to a normal fellow pupil the Horner pupil will dilate only very slowly; the dark-induced

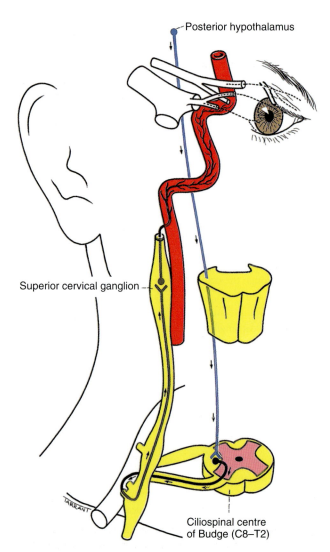

Fig. 19.34 Anatomical pathway of the sympathetic nerve supply

Table 19.4 Causes of Horner syndrome

- Central (first-order neurone)
  - Brainstem disease – commonly stroke (e.g. lateral medullary infarction), but also tumour, demyelination
  - Syringomyelia
  - Lateral medullary (Wallenberg) syndrome
  - Cervical spinal cord lesion
  - Diabetic autonomic neuropathy
- Preganglionic (second-order neurone)
  - Pancoast tumour
  - Carotid and aortic aneurysm and dissection
  - Thoracic spinal cord lesion
  - Miscellaneous neck lesions (thyroid tumour, enlarged lymph nodes, trauma, postsurgical)
- Postganglionic (third-order neurone)
  - Internal carotid artery dissection
  - Nasopharyngeal tumour
  - Cavernous sinus mass
  - Otitis media
- Cluster headache (migrainous neuralgia)

anisocoria diminishes with time spent in the dark environment.
- Pupillary constriction to light and near stimuli is normal.
- Hypochromic heterochromia (irides of different colour, the Horner being lighter) may be seen if congenital or long-standing (Fig. 19.35B).
- Slight elevation of the inferior eyelid (inferior ptosis) as a result of weakness of the inferior tarsal muscle.

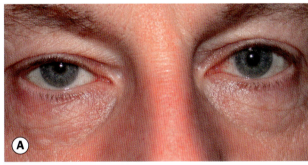

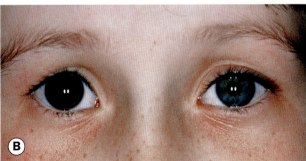

Fig. 19.35 Horner syndrome. **(A)** Right Horner syndrome; **(B)** heterochromia iridis associated with a left congenital Horner syndrome in a child

(Courtesy of A Pearson – fig. A)

- Reduced ipsilateral sweating, but because the sudomotor fibres supplying the skin of the face run along the external carotid artery this occurs only if the lesion is below the superior cervical ganglion; patients may mistakenly interpret the normal side to be sweating excessively.
- The cranial nerves and peripheral nervous system (e.g. T_1 – grip strength), as well as the neck and regional lymph nodes should be examined, if necessary by a neurologist.

Pharmacological tests

Apraclonidine or cocaine is used to confirm the diagnosis, the latter now less commonly (see below). Hydroxyamphetamine and adrenaline may be used to differentiate a preganglionic (abnormal first- or second-order neurone) from a postganglionic lesion (abnormal third-order neurone), though as the distinction may not alter investigation – carotid lesions may cause either pre- or postganglionic disease, for instance – some authorities limit pharmacological testing to confirmation of the presence of Horner syndrome.

- **Apraclonidine 0.5% or 1.0%.** One drop is instilled into both eyes to confirm or refute the presence of Horner syndrome. The pupils should be checked at 30 minutes and, if negative, rechecked at 45 minutes. Apraclonidine penetrates the blood–brain barrier, so should be used only with great caution in infants under one year of age. It can have an extended duration of action, so subsequent pharmacological tests should not be performed for 3–5 days.
  - Result: A Horner pupil will dilate but a normal pupil is essentially unaffected. The ptosis commonly also improves. Sensitivity is around 90% (it will detect most cases) and specificity close to 100% (it will very rarely falsely identify abnormality that is not actually present).
  - Explanation: Alpha-1 receptors are upregulated in the denervated dilator pupillae.
- **Cocaine 4%** is instilled into both eyes; as cocaine is less readily available than apraclonidine, this test is now not commonly performed and may be reserved for acute lesions (apraclonidine testing probably takes at least 14 days to become positive) or those in which apraclonidine testing is equivocal but clinical suspicion is high.
  - Result: The normal pupil will dilate but the Horner pupil will not; anisocoria of as little as 0.8 mm in a dimly lit room is significant.
  - Explanation: Cocaine blocks the re-uptake of noradrenaline secreted at the postganglionic nerve ending, which accumulates and causes dilatation of a normal pupil. In Horner syndrome, there is no noradrenaline being secreted, so cocaine has no effect.
- **Phenylephrine 1%** is more readily available than hydroxyamphetamine (see next) and adrenaline and is approximately as accurate, so has to a large extent replaced them in testing to distinguish pre- and postganglionic

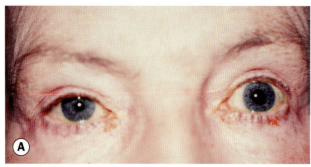

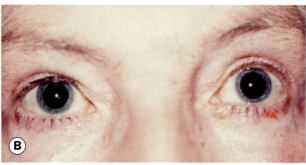

Fig. 19.36 (A) Right preganglionic Horner syndrome; **(B)** bilateral mydriasis following instillation of hydroxyamphetamine into both eyes – ptosis has also been partially relieved

lesions. It is typically prepared by dilution of commonly available 2.5% or 10% solution.

○ Result: In an established (10 days) postganglionic lesion, the Horner pupil will dilate and ptosis may be temporarily relieved. A central or preganglionic Horner pupil and a normal pupil will not dilate or will dilate minimally.

○ Explanation: In postganglionic Horner syndrome the dilator pupillae muscle develops denervation hypersensitivity to adrenergic neurotransmitters due to its dysfunctional local motor nerve.

- **Hydroxyamphetamine 1%.** Two drops are instilled into each eye. It may be slightly more sensitive than phenylephrine testing.

○ Result: A normal or preganglionic Horner pupil will dilate (Fig. 19.36), but a postganglionic Horner will not.

○ Explanation: Hydroxyamphetamine potentiates the release of noradrenaline from functioning postganglionic nerve endings. In a lesion of the third-order neurone (postganglionic) there is no release of noradrenaline from the dysfunctional nerve.

- **Adrenaline 0.1%** has an action similar to that of phenylephrine.

Investigation

Specialist neurological or neuro-ophthalmological assessment should be sought for a confirmed Horner syndrome; an acute presentation should be regarded as an emergency. In contrast, if the features have been present for over a year and there are no other localizing signs then the likely diagnostic yield from further investigation is very low. The mainstay of investigation is imaging; CT or MR angiography examining the region from the aortic arch to the circle of Willis will facilitate exclusion of neck (including carotid), apical lung, thyroid and skull base lesions. MR may be utilized if greater soft tissue definition is required, such as to exclude a brainstem stroke. Plain X-rays and carotid ultrasound imaging have limited utility.

Treatment

Any identified cause should be addressed as appropriate. The ptosis of Horner syndrome is mild but surgery can be considered at the patient's discretion; apraclonidine may be helpful as a temporizing measure.

Adie pupil

Introduction

An Adie pupil (tonic pupil, Adie syndrome) is caused by denervation of the postganglionic parasympathetic supply to the sphincter pupillae and the ciliary muscle, and may follow a viral illness. It is occasionally inherited in an AD pattern. Sites of dysfunction are presumed to be the ciliary ganglion, and, in wider Holmes–Adie syndrome, the dorsal root ganglion involved in reflex pathways. It typically affects young women and presents in one eye in 80%, though involvement of the second eye typically develops within months or years.

Diagnosis

- **Symptoms.** Patients may notice anisocoria, or may have blurring for near due to impaired accommodation.
- **Signs**
  ○ Large, regular (irregularity sometimes reported) pupil (Fig. 19.37A).
  ○ The direct light reflex is absent or sluggish (Fig. 19.37B).
  ○ On slit lamp examination, vermiform movements of the pupillary border are typically seen.
  ○ Constriction is also absent or sluggish in response to light stimulation of the fellow eye (consensual light reflex – Fig. 19.37C).
  ○ The pupil responds slowly to near, following which re-dilatation is also slow.
  ○ Accommodation may manifest similar tonicity, with slowed and impaired focusing for near and prolonged re-focusing in the distance.
  ○ In long-standing cases the pupil may become small ('little old Adie').
- **Associations** include diminished lower limb deep tendon reflexes (Holmes–Adie syndrome – Fig. 19.37D) and other features of autonomic nerve dysfunction such as excessive sweating (Ross syndrome), orthostatic hypotension and occasionally bowel obstruction or urinary retention. Typical Adie-type pupils are often present in generalized dysautonomias, with a wide range of aetiologies.

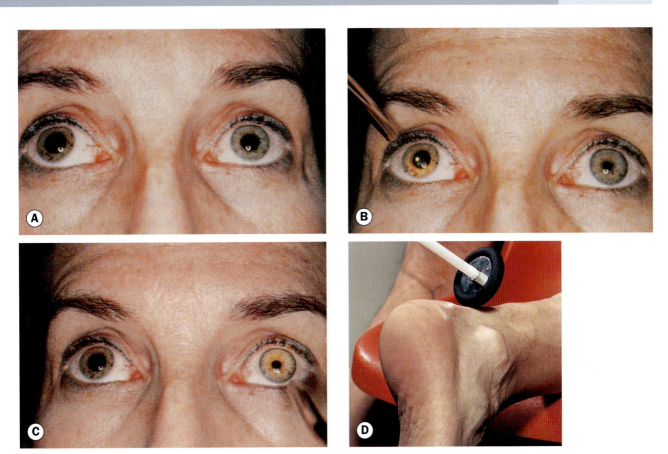

Fig. 19.37 Right Adie pupil. **(A)** Large right pupil; **(B)** absent or sluggish direct light reflex; **(C)** consensual light reflex is similar; **(D)** diminished deep tendon reflex

(Courtesy of DM Albert and FA Jakobiec, from Principles and Practice of Ophthalmology, *Saunders 1994 – figs A–C; MA Mir, from* Atlas of Clinical Diagnosis, *Saunders 2003 – fig. D)*

- **Pharmacological testing.** Instillation of 0.1–0.125% pilocarpine into both eyes leads to constriction of the abnormal pupil due to denervation hypersensitivity, with the normal pupil unaffected. Some diabetic patients may also show this response and very occasionally both pupils constrict in normal individuals.
- **Syphilis serology** (see Ch. 11) should usually be checked in patients with bilateral tonic pupils.

Treatment

Treatment is not generally required, but reading glasses may be used to address near vision difficulties and sunglasses or low-concentration pilocarpine drops can be used to improve photophobia. Thoracic sympathectomy can be considered for excessive sweating.

Miscellaneous pupillary abnormalities

- **Physiological anisocoria** (Fig. 19.38). Anisocoria of around 1 mm is present in around 20% of the normal population. The asymmetry persists to the same proportion under differing levels of illumination. Exceptionally, apraclonidine or cocaine testing may be needed to exclude Horner syndrome.

- **Pharmacological mydriasis** (Fig. 19.39). Dilatation of one or both pupils due to instillation of a mydriatic agent can be inadvertent (e.g. use of eye drops prescribed for someone else, rubbing the eye after touching a car sickness scopolamine skin patch) or deliberate for the purpose of malingering. The pupil does not constrict in bright light or on accommodation and there is no response to any concentration of pilocarpine. There are no other neurological features.
- **Argyll Robertson pupils** (Fig. 19.40) are caused by neurosyphilis, and have been attributed to a dorsal midbrain lesion that interrupts the pupillary light reflex pathway but spares the more ventral pupillary near reflex pathway – light–near dissociation results. In dim light both pupils are small and may be irregular. In bright light neither pupil constricts, but on accommodation (near target) both constrict. The pupils do not dilate well in the dark, but cocaine induces mydriasis unless marked iris atrophy is present. After instillation of pilocarpine 0.1% into both eyes, neither pupil constricts, distinguishing Argyll Robertson pupils from bilateral long-standing tonic pupils. Other causes of light–near dissociation are shown in Table 19.5.
- **Tectal (dorsal midbrain) pupils** (Fig. 19.41). This phenomenon is a component of dorsal midbrain syndrome

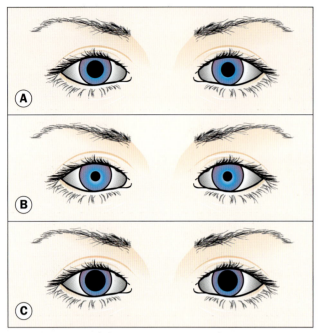

Fig. 19.38 Right physiological anisocoria. **(A)** In dim light the right pupil is slightly larger than the left; **(B)** in bright light both pupils constrict normally, but the right pupil is still fractionally larger than the left; **(C)** both pupils dilate with instillation of cocaine 4%

(Courtesy of JJ Kanski, from Signs in Ophthalmology: Causes and Differential Diagnosis, *Mosby 2010)*

(see later). The pupils are dilated in both dim and bright light. There is light–near dissociation. Pilocarpine 0.1% has no effect.

- **Benign episodic unilateral mydriasis (BEUM).** This idiopathic condition (Fig. 19.42) occurs most commonly in otherwise healthy young women and may represent a migrainous phenomenon or a range of heterogeneous aetiologies. Mydriasis tends to last for minutes or hours before resolving completely. There may be mild associated blurring and headache. The need for further investigation should be assessed on an individual basis. There is no – or

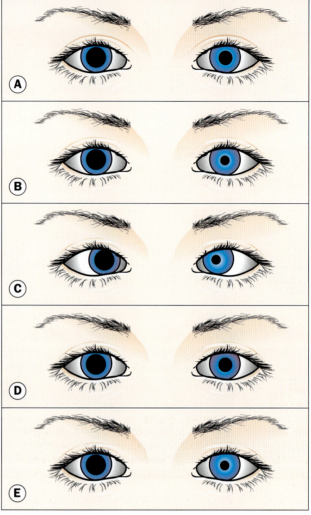

Fig. 19.39 Right pharmacological mydriasis. **(A)** Right mydriasis in dim illumination; **(B)** in bright light the right pupil does not constrict; **(C)** on accommodation the right pupil does not constrict; **(D)** neither pupil constricts after instillation of pilocarpine 0.1% into both eyes; **(E)** after instillation of 1% pilocarpine into both eyes the left pupil constricts but the right does not

(Courtesy of JJ Kanski, from Signs in Ophthalmology: Causes and Differential Diagnosis, *Mosby 2010)*

limited – response to light or accommodation. Pilocarpine 0.1% induces no change, but pilocarpine 1% to both eyes gives bilateral miosis.

CHIASM

Anatomy

Pituitary gland

The sella turcica (Turkish saddle) is a deep saddle-shaped depression in the superior surface of the body of the sphenoid bone in

Table 19.5 Causes of light–near dissociation

- **Unilateral**
  - Afferent conduction defect
  - Adie pupil
  - Herpes zoster ophthalmicus
  - Aberrant regeneration of the third cranial nerve
- **Bilateral**
  - Neurosyphilis
  - Type 1 diabetes mellitus
  - Myotonic dystrophy
  - Parinaud (dorsal midbrain) syndrome
  - Familial amyloidosis
  - Encephalitis
  - Chronic alcoholism

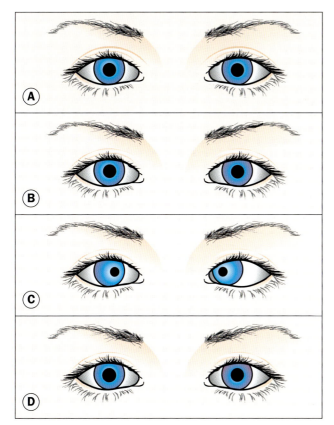

Fig. 19.40 Argyll Robertson pupils. **(A)** In dim light both pupils are small and may be irregular; **(B)** in bright light neither pupil constricts; **(C)** on accommodation to a near target both pupils constrict – light–near dissociation; **(D)** neither pupil constricts on instillation of pilocarpine 0.1% into both eyes

(Courtesy of JJ Kanski, from Signs in Ophthalmology: Causes and Differential Diagnosis, *Mosby 2010)*

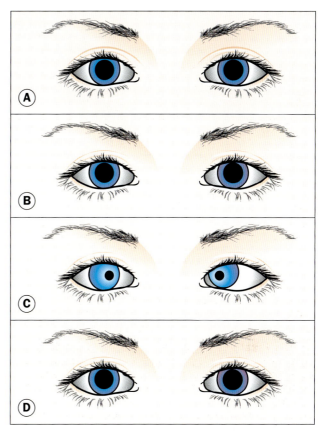

Fig. 19.41 Tectal (dorsal midbrain) pupils. **(A)** In dim light there is bilateral mydriasis, which may be asymmetrical; **(B)** in bright light neither pupil constricts; **(C)** on accommodation both pupils constrict normally – light–near dissociation; **(D)** neither pupil constricts on instillation of pilocarpine 0.1% into both eyes

(Courtesy of JJ Kanski, from Signs in Ophthalmology: Causes and Differential Diagnosis, *Mosby 2010)*

which the pituitary gland lies (Fig. 19.43). The roof of the sella is formed by a fold of dura mater, the diaphragma sellae, which stretches from the anterior to the posterior clinoids. The optic nerves and chiasm lie above the diaphragma sellae; posteriorly, the chiasm is continuous with the optic tracts and forms the anterior wall of the third ventricle. A visual field defect in a patient with a pituitary tumour therefore generally indicates suprasellar extension. Tumours less than 10 mm in diameter (microadenomas) tend to remain confined to the sella, whereas those larger than 10 mm (macroadenomas) often extend outside. Table 19.6 lists causes of chiasmal disease.

Parachiasmal vascular structures

- **Venous.** The cavernous sinuses lie lateral to the sella so that horizontally extending pituitary tumours affect the cavernous sinus and may damage the intracavernous parts of the third, fourth and sixth cranial nerves. Conversely, aneurysms arising from the intracavernous part of the internal carotid artery may erode into the sella and mimic pituitary tumours.

Table 19.6 Causes of chiasmal disease

- **Tumours**
  - Pituitary adenomas
  - Craniopharyngioma
  - Meningioma
  - Glioma
  - Chordoma
  - Dysgerminoma
  - Nasopharyngeal tumours
  - Metastases
- **Non-neoplastic masses**
  - Aneurysm
  - Rathke pouch cysts
  - Fibrous dysplasia
  - Sphenoidal sinus mucocele
  - Arachnoid cysts
- **Miscellaneous**
  - Demyelination
  - Inflammation, e.g. sarcoidosis
  - Trauma
  - Radiation-induced necrosis
  - Toxicity, e.g. ethambutol
  - Vasculitis

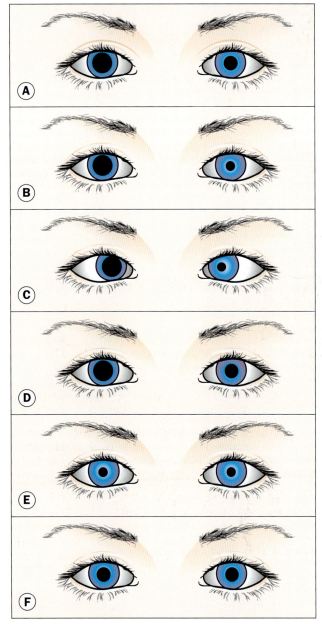

Fig. 19.42 Right benign episodic unilateral mydriasis (BEUM). **(A)** In dim light the right pupil is larger than the left; **(B)** in bright light the right pupil does not constrict; **(C)** on accommodation the right pupil does not constrict; **(D)** instillation of pilocarpine 0.1% to both eyes fails to constrict either pupil; **(E)** instillation of pilocarpine 1% to both eyes induces bilateral miosis; **(F)** after 24 hours both pupils are equal

(Courtesy of JJ Kanski, from Signs in Ophthalmology: Causes and Differential Diagnosis, Mosby 2010)

- **Arterial** (Fig. 19.44). The internal carotid arteries curve posteriorly and upwards from the cavernous sinus and lie immediately below the optic nerves, following which they ascend vertically along the lateral aspect of the chiasm. The precommunicating portion of the anterior cerebral artery is closely related to the superior surface of the chiasm and

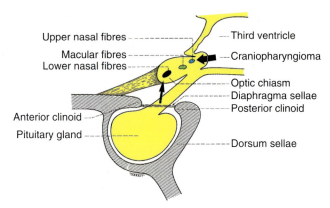

Fig. 19.43 Anatomy of the chiasm in relation to the pituitary gland

optic nerves, so an aneurysm in this region can compress either or both the optic nerve or chiasm.

Physiology

Pituitary hormones

The lobules of the anterior part of the pituitary gland are composed of six cell types. Five of these secrete hormones and the sixth (follicular cell) has no secretory function. Pituitary adenomas of mixed-cell type are common; any of the six cell types may proliferate to produce an adenoma; the current classification of pituitary tumours is discussed further below.

- **The anterior pituitary lobe** is under the control of various inhibiting and promoting factors synthesized in the

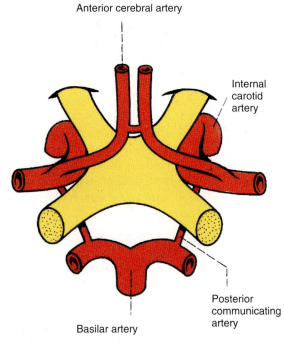

Fig. 19.44 Relationship between the chiasm and adjacent arterial structures

hypothalamus, passing to the pituitary through the hypothalamo-hypophyseal portal system:
- ○ Human growth hormone (HGH or GH) or somatotropin.
- ○ Follicle-stimulating hormone (FSH).
- ○ Luteinizing hormone (LH).
- ○ Prolactin (PRL).
- ○ Thyroid-stimulating hormone (TSH).
- ○ Adrenocorticotrophic hormone (ACTH), which regulates blood cortisol levels.
- ○ Beta-endorphin.
- **The intermediate lobe** secretes melanocyte-stimulating hormone (MSH).
- **The posterior pituitary** releases antidiuretic hormone (ADH) and oxytocin.

Pituitary adenomas

Tumour classification is based on the type of hormone secreted; about 25% of primary pituitary tumours do not secrete any hormones and may be asymptomatic, cause hypopituitarism and/or ophthalmic features. An older classification system divided pituitary tumours into acidophilic, basophilic and chromophobic types based on their histological staining characteristics, but is now not commonly used.

Ophthalmic features of large adenomas

Large pituitary lesions may first present to ophthalmologists, often with vague visual symptoms, and a low threshold should be adopted for visual field assessment in chronic headache of any sort. It is also important to perform a careful visual field assessment on both eyes in patients with unexplained unilateral central visual impairment.

- **Symptoms**
  - ○ Headache may be prominent due to local effects but does not have the usual features associated with raised ICP, and diagnostic delay is therefore common.
  - ○ Visual symptoms may be vague; they usually have a gradual onset and may not be noticed by the patient until well established.
- **Colour desaturation** across the vertical midline of the uniocular visual field is an early sign of chiasmal compression.
  - ○ The patient is asked to compare the colour and intensity of a red pin or pen top as it is moved from the nasal to the temporal visual field in each eye.
  - ○ Another technique is to simultaneously present red targets in precisely symmetrical parts of the temporal and nasal visual fields, and to ask if the colours appear the same.
- **Optic atrophy** is present in approximately 50% of cases with field defects. When optic atrophy is present the prognosis for visual recovery after treatment is guarded. When nerve fibre loss is confined to fibres originating in the nasal retina (i.e. nasal to the fovea) only the nasal and temporal aspects

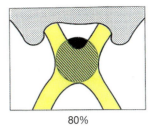
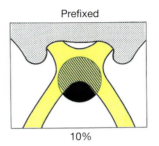
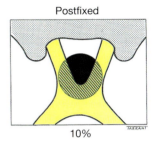

80%

Prefixed   Postfixed

10%   10%

Fig. 19.45 Anatomical variations in the position of the chiasm

of the disc will be involved, resulting in a band or 'bow tie'-shaped atrophy.
- **Papilloedema** is rare.
  - ○ Visual field defects depend on the location and direction of enlargement of a compressive lesion, as well as the anatomical relationship between the pituitary and chiasm (Fig. 19.45 and see below). Patients may not present until central vision is affected from pressure on macular fibres.
  - ○ Lower nasal optic nerve fibres traverse the chiasm inferiorly and anteriorly, hence the upper temporal quadrants of both visual fields are affected first by most expanding pituitary lesions, giving a bitemporal superior quadrantanopia progressing to the classic chiasmal visual field lesion, a bitemporal hemianopia (Fig. 19.46). Field

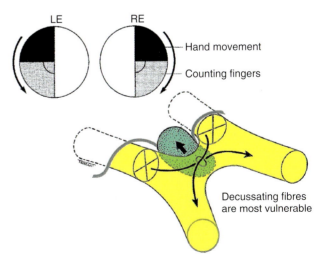

LE   RE

Hand movement

Counting fingers

Decussating fibres are most vulnerable

Fig. 19.46 Typical progression of bitemporal visual field defects caused by compression of the chiasm from below by a pituitary adenoma. LE = left eye; RE = right eye

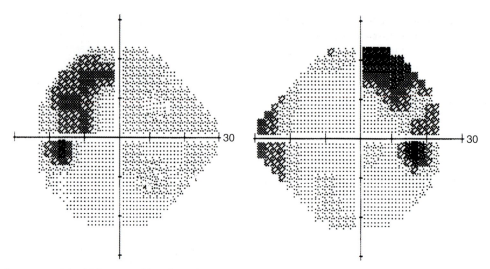

Fig. 19.47 Typically asymmetrical bitemporal hemianopia

loss is commonly asymmetrical between the two eyes (Fig. 19.47).

○ Upper nasal fibres traverse the chiasm high and posteriorly and therefore are involved first by a lesion such as a craniopharyngioma that arises above the chiasm (Fig. 19.48). If the lower temporal quadrants of the visual field are affected more profoundly than the upper, a pituitary adenoma is unlikely.

○ A lesion compressing the anterior chiasm, such as a pituitary adenoma in conjunction with a postfixed chiasm, may give rise to a 'junctional scotoma' – the syndrome of a central or paracentral defect on the side of optic nerve involvement together with a contralateral superotemporal defect (see Fig. 19.53). The precise mechanism is disputed, but is commonly attributed to simultaneous involvement of the fibres of one of the optic nerves together with contralateral inferonasal fibres looping forward into the nerve in the putative knee of Wilbrand.

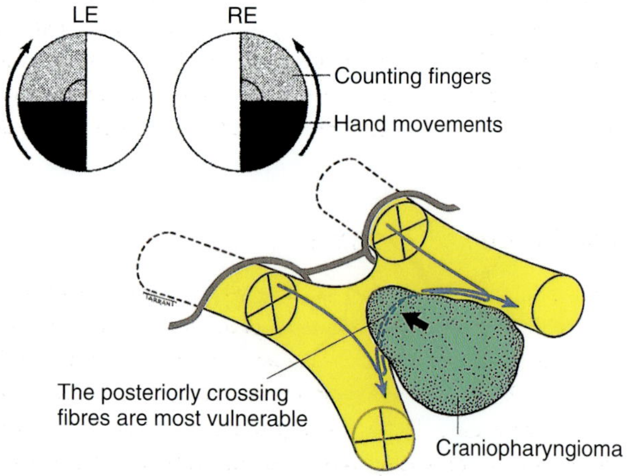

○ Macular fibres decussate throughout the chiasm, but are concentrated posteriorly. A lesion that preferentially compresses the posterior chiasm, such as a pituitary adenoma in conjunction with a prefixed chiasm, may therefore cause bitemporal hemianopic changes predominantly affecting the central and paracentral fields. Predominant involvement of the optic tracts by a posterior lesion can give a homonymous hemianopia.

○ Extensive loss of the temporal visual field in both eyes can disrupt sensory fusion, decompensating a phoria and causing problems with near vision. 'Postfixation blindness' refers to the presence of a non-seeing area distal to the fixation point due to the overlap of two blind hemifields (Fig. 19.49); despite the similar terminology, it is not linked to a postfixed chiasm. Patients may complain of difficulty with fine close-up

Fig. 19.48 Progression of bitemporal visual field defects caused by compression of the chiasm from above by a craniopharyngioma. LE = left eye; RE = right eye

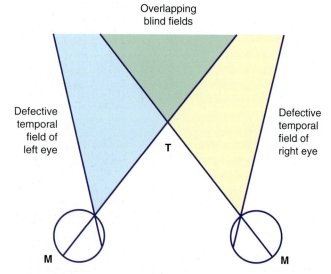

Fig. 19.49 Mechanism of postfixation blindness. M = macula; T = target

(Courtesy of G Liu, N Volpe and S Galetta, from Neuro-Ophthalmology Diagnosis and Management, *Saunders 2010)*

tasks such as threading a needle and cutting fingernails, and near visual acuity measured binocularly may be worse than when measured with each eye individually. Double vision may result from slippage of the two fields with fusional failure ('hemifield slide'); diplopia may also result from cranial nerve palsy (see next).

- Differential diagnosis of bitemporal defects includes dermatochalasis, tilted discs, optic nerve colobomas, nasal retinoschisis, nasal retinitis pigmentosa and functional ('non-physiological') visual loss.
- **Extraocular muscle paresis** due to disruption of the cranial nerves traversing the cavernous sinus.
- **See-saw nystagmus** (see later) is a rare feature.

Investigation

- **MR** with gadolinium contrast (Fig. 19.50) utilizing multiple planes and thin sections demonstrates the relationship between a mass lesion and the chiasm, and is usually the preferred imaging modality. Adenomas are typically hypointense on T1 and hyperintense on T2 images.
- **CT** will demonstrate enlargement or erosion of the sella.
- **Endocrinological evaluation** is complex, particularly as combined hormonal over- and under-secretion may be present, and is usually undertaken by an endocrinologist.

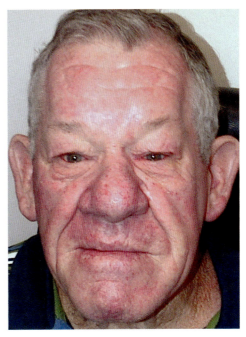

Fig. 19.51 Facial features in acromegaly

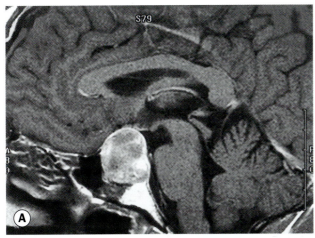

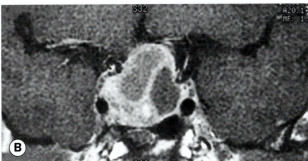

Fig. 19.50 T1-weighted gadolinium-enhanced MR of a pituitary adenoma. **(A)** Sagittal and **(B)** coronal images
(Courtesy of D Thomas)

Prolactin-secreting (lactotrophic) adenoma

Lactotrophic adenoma or prolactinoma (formerly known as chromophobe adenoma, though lesions can be weakly acidophilic) is the most common pituitary adenoma. Patients are typically young to middle-aged adults. In women excessive prolactin secretion leads to the infertility–amenorrhoea–galactorrhoea syndrome, and in men may cause hypogonadism, impotence, sterility, decreased libido, and occasionally gynaecomastia and galactorrhoea. Up to 95% remain as microadenomas, though those that do not may present initially with visual features.

Corticotrophic adenoma

A corticotrophic adenoma (a variant of basophil adenoma) secretes ACTH and causes Cushing disease (Cushing *syndrome* refers to the clinical picture of increased blood cortisol from any cause), which may include central obesity and moon face, cutaneous striae, pigmentation and other features such as hypertension.

Somatotrophic adenoma

Somatotrophic (acidophil) tumours secrete excessive GH, causing acromegaly in adults (once bone elongation has been completed) and gigantism in children. Presentation is in middle age with features including enlargement of the head, hands, feet and tongue, coarseness of features with prominent supraorbital ridges and nasiolabial folds (Fig. 19.51), enlargement of the jaw with dental malocclusion, and hirsutism in females. There are many complications, including diabetes mellitus, hypertension, cardiomyopathy and carpal tunnel syndrome.

Treatment of pituitary adenomas

- **Observation** may be appropriate for incidentally discovered and clinically silent tumours.
- **Medical therapy** is usually the initial step and consists of the reduction in tumour size and secretion using agents such as dopamine agonists (e.g. cabergoline and the older bromocriptine) and somatostatin analogues such as octreotide, with supplementary hormonal correction as appropriate.
- **Surgery** consists of tumour debulking rather than complete excision and is usually carried out endoscopically via a trans-sphenoidal approach through a gum incision behind the upper lip. Indications include the failure or intolerance of medical management and sometimes decompression for acute visual loss (see below). Visual field improvement is fastest in the earliest weeks and months following surgery.
- **Radiotherapy** is rarely employed due to the risk of complications, but is utilized in some circumstances. Newer techniques include intensity-modulated radiation therapy and stereotactic radiosurgery.
- **Monitoring.** Long-term ophthalmological review is required, with serial assessment of visual function.

Pituitary apoplexy

Pituitary apoplexy (PA) is caused by acute haemorrhage into or infarction of the pituitary gland, and is usually associated with a previously undiagnosed adenoma; Sheehan syndrome is infarction of the pituitary usually associated with childbirth and is generally regarded as a form of PA. PA typically manifests with the sudden onset of a severe headache, nausea and vomiting, sometimes with meningism and occasionally reduced consciousness or stroke. There is often reduced visual acuity and/or a bitemporal hemianopia depending on the anatomical effects of the lesion. Double vision due to compromise of the adjacent ocular motor nerves is common. Acute hormonal insufficiency can lead to life-threatening complications such as an Addisonian crisis. Investigations include MR, urgent visual field testing, and hormonal assessment. Acute medical management, including hormone administration and surgical decompression, may be necessary.

Craniopharyngioma

Craniopharyngioma is a slow-growing tumour arising from vestigial remnants of the Rathke pouch along the pituitary stalk. Affected children frequently present with dwarfism, delayed sexual development and obesity due to interference with hypothalamic function. Adults usually present with visual impairment.

Visual field defects are complex and may be due to involvement of the optic nerves, chiasm or tracts.

The initial defect frequently involves both inferotemporal fields because the tumour compresses the chiasm from above and behind, damaging the upper nasal fibres (see Fig. 19.48). MRI shows a solid tumour that appears isointense on T1 images (Fig. 19.52). Cystic components appear hyperintense on T1 images. Treatment is mainly surgical, but recurrences are common.

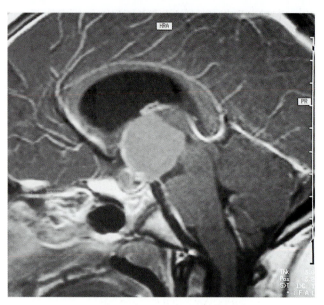

Fig. 19.52 Sagittal T1-weighted MR image of a craniopharyngioma with secondary hydrocephalus
(Courtesy of K Nischal)

Meningioma

Intracranial meningiomas typically affect middle-aged women. Visual field defects and clinical signs depend on the location of the tumour (Fig. 19.53).

- **Tuberculum sellae** meningiomas often produce a junctional scotoma (see above and Fig. 19.53) due to their location.
- **Sphenoidal ridge** tumours compress the optic nerve early if the tumour is located medially and late if the lateral aspect of the sphenoid bone and middle cranial fossa are involved (Fig. 19.54A). A classic finding in the latter is fullness in the temporal fossa due to hyperostosis (Fig. 19.54B).

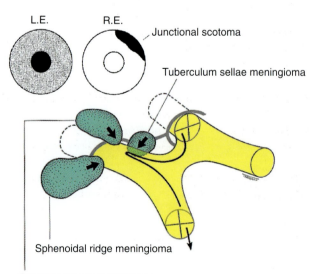

Fig. 19.53 Examples of optic nerve compression by meningioma; a junctional scotoma resulting from a tuberculum sellae lesion is also shown

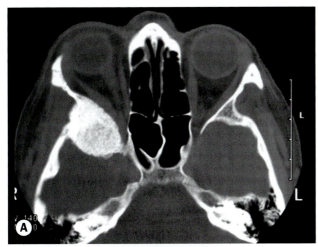

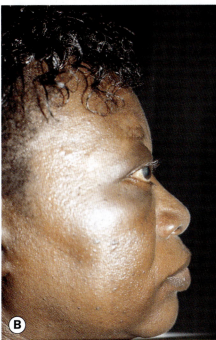

Fig. 19.54 Sphenoid ridge meningioma. **(A)** CT axial image; **(B)** reactive hyperostosis
(Courtesy of A Pearson – fig. A)

- **Olfactory groove** meningioma may cause loss of the sense of smell, as well as optic nerve compression.
- **Treatment** usually consists of surgery, but radiotherapy is sometimes required. Observation alone may be adequate.

RETROCHIASMAL PATHWAYS

Optic tracts

Overview

Retrochiasmal pathology results in partial or total binocular visual field defects involving contralateral visual space. This hemianopia (hemianopsia) involving the same side of the field in both eyes is homonymous, in contradistinction to the bitemporal hemianopia seen in chiasmal compression, which produces heteronymous loss, with opposite sides of the visual field affected in each eye.

Congruity

A homonymous hemianopia may be incomplete or complete. In the context of incomplete hemianopia, congruity refers to how closely the extent and pattern of field loss in one eye matches that of the other. Almost identical field defects in either eye are therefore highly congruous, while mismatching right and left visual field defects are incongruous. Hemianopia secondary to pathology in the anterior retrochiasmal visual pathways is characteristically incongruous, while that due to pathology further back (e.g. the posterior optic radiations) manifests a higher degree of congruity.

Clinical features

- **Homonymous hemianopia**
  - The optic tracts arise at the posterior aspect of the chiasm, diverge and extend posteriorly around the cerebral peduncles, to terminate in the lateral geniculate bodies.
  - Each optic tract contains crossed fibres from the contralateral nasal hemiretina, and uncrossed fibres from the ipsilateral temporal hemiretina.
  - Nerve fibres originating from corresponding retinal elements are, however, not closely aligned.
  - Homonymous hemianopia caused by optic tract lesions is therefore characteristically incongruous.
  - Lesions of the lateral geniculate body also produce asymmetrical hemianopic defects.
  - The causes of optic tract disease are similar to those affecting the chiasm but the tract is particularly vulnerable when the chiasm is prefixed (see above).
- **Wernicke hemianopic pupil**
  - The optic tracts contain both visual and pupillomotor fibres. The visual fibres terminate in the lateral geniculate body but the pupillary fibres leave the optic tract anterior to the lateral geniculate body, projecting through the brachium of the superior colliculus to terminate in the pretectal nuclei.
  - An optic tract lesion may therefore give rise to an afferent pupillary conduction defect.
  - Characteristically, the pupillary light reflex will be normal when the unaffected hemiretina is stimulated, and absent when the involved hemiretina is stimulated (i.e. light is shone from the hemianopic side).
  - In practice, this Wernicke hemianopic pupillary reaction is difficult to elicit because of scatter of light within the eye – a fine beam should be used.
- **Optic atrophy** may occur when the optic tracts are damaged because their fibres are the axons of the retinal ganglion cells. The ipsilateral disc manifests atrophy of the superior and inferior aspects of the neuroretinal rim (fibres from the temporal retina), while the contralateral disc manifests a 'bow tie' pattern (nasal and nasal macular fibres).

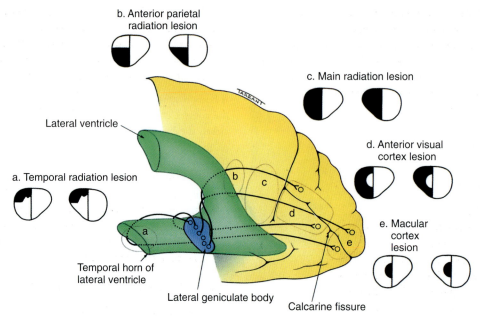

Fig. 19.55 Visual field defects caused by lesions of the optic radiations and visual cortex

- **Contralateral pyramidal signs** may occur when an optic tract lesion also damages the ipsilateral cerebral peduncle.

Optic radiations

Anatomy

The optic radiations extend from the lateral geniculate body to the striate cortex, which is located on the medial aspect of the occipital lobe, above and below the calcarine fissure (Fig. 19.55). As the radiations pass posteriorly, fibres from corresponding retinal elements lie progressively closer together. For this reason, incomplete hemianopia caused by posterior radiation lesions are more congruous than those involving the anterior radiations. Because these fibres are third-order neurones that originate in the lateral geniculate body, lesions of the optic radiations do not produce optic atrophy. The optic radiations and visual cortex have a dual blood supply from the middle and posterior cerebral arteries.

Temporal radiations

- **Visual field defect** consists of a contralateral superior homonymous quadrantanopia ('pie in the sky'), because the inferior fibres of the optic radiations, which subserve the upper visual fields, first sweep anteroinferiorly (Meyer loop) into the temporal lobe around the anterior tip of the temporal horn of the lateral ventricle (see 'a' in Fig. 19.55).
- **Associated features** are likely to include contralateral hemisensory disturbance and hemiparesis, because the temporal radiations pass very close to the sensory and motor fibres of the internal capsule before passing posteriorly and rejoining the superior fibres. Other features of temporal lobe disease include paroxysmal olfactory and gustatory

hallucinations (uncinate fits), formed visual hallucinations and seizures, with receptive dysphasia if the dominant hemisphere is involved.

Anterior parietal radiations

- **Visual field defect** consists of a contralateral inferior homonymous quadrantanopia ('pie on the floor') because the superior fibres of the radiations, which subserve the inferior visual fields, proceed directly posteriorly through the parietal lobe to the occipital cortex. However, a lesion involving only the anterior parietal part of the radiations is rare. Hemianopia resulting from a parietal lobe lesion tends to be relatively congruous (see 'b' in Fig. 19.55).
- **Associated features** of dominant parietal lobe disease include acalculia, agraphia, left–right disorientation and finger agnosia. Non-dominant lobe lesions may cause dressing and constitutional apraxia and spatial neglect.

Main radiations

Deep in the parietal lobe, the optic radiations lie just external to the trigone and the occipital horn of the lateral ventricle. Lesions in this area usually cause a complete homonymous hemianopia (see 'c' in Fig. 19.55).

- **Optokinetic nystagmus** (OKN), elicited with a rotating striped optokinetic drum, may be useful in localizing the cause of an isolated homonymous hemianopia.
  - Physiological OKN involves smooth pursuit of a target, followed momentarily by a saccade in the opposite direction to fixate on the next target.
  - If a homonymous hemianopia is due to a lesion in the parietal lobe, the smooth pursuit pathways towards the side of the lesion are likely to be affected, making this component of OKN defective. OKN will therefore be asymmetrical: erratic when the drum is rotated towards

the side of the lesion, but regular when the drum is rotated away from the side of the lesion.

○ If the lesion is in the occipital lobe, the smooth pursuit pathways are intact and OKN will be symmetrical – this is the Cogan dictum, which also states that the parietal lobe lesion is more likely to be a tumour and the occipital lesion an infarction.

Striate cortex

Clinical features

- **Visual field defects**
  ○ In the striate cortex the peripheral visual fields are represented anteriorly. This part of the occipital lobe is supplied by a branch of the posterior cerebral artery.
  ○ Central macular vision is represented posteriorly just lateral to the tip of the calcarine cortex, an area supplied mainly by a branch of the middle cerebral artery. Occlusion of the posterior cerebral artery will therefore tend to produce a macular-sparing congruous homonymous hemianopia (see 'd' in Fig. 19.55).
  ○ Damage to the tip of the occipital cortex, as might occur from a head injury, tends to give rise to congruous, homonymous, macular defects (see 'e' in Fig. 19.55), although macular sparing may sometimes occur with vascular lesions of the occipital lobe.
  ○ The anteriormost part of the calcarine cortex subserves the temporal extremity of the visual field of the contralateral eye, the area of visual space that extends beyond the field of binocular single vision and is perceived monocularly. A lesion in this area may therefore give rise to a monocular temporal field defect in the contralateral eye, known as a temporal crescent.
- **Associated features** of visual cortex disease (cortical blindness) include formed visual hallucinations, denial of blindness (Anton syndrome) and the Riddoch phenomenon (only moving visual targets perceived).

Causes

- **Stroke** in the territory of the posterior cerebral artery is responsible for over 90% of homonymous hemianopia with no other neurological deficit.
- **Other causes** include trauma, tumours and rarely migraine; a range of uncommon inflammatory (including autoimmune and infective), degenerative and toxic disorders can also be causative, but will usually manifest with more widespread neurological features; imaging and lumbar puncture are typically key to diagnosis. Mimicking by retinal disease such as acute zonal occult outer retinopathy (AZOOR) may occur.

Benson syndrome

Benson syndrome (posterior cortical atrophy) is a rare condition often referred to as a visual variant of Alzheimer disease. Patients may have normal visual acuity, anterior and posterior segment examination, but commonly abnormal colour vision, homonymous

field defects, visual agnosia, alexia and acalculia. The diagnosis is commonly missed; other degenerative conditions often exhibiting early occipital cortical involvement include Alzheimer and Creutzfeldt-Jakob disease; presentation in the latter can be with acute visual symptoms only. Electroretinography may be abnormal. In immunocompromised states, including drug-induced, progressive multifocal leukoencephalopathy can present with isolated occipital features.

Balint syndrome

Balint syndrome refers to the combination of simultanagnosia (inability to discern the overall impression of an image whilst distinguishing individual components), optic ataxia (defective visually-directed reaching) and ocular apraxia (impairment of voluntary saccades). It is typically due to parieto-occipital disease, with a range of causes reported.

Posterior reversible encephalopathy syndrome

Posterior reversible encephalopathy syndrome (PRES) or reversible posterior leukoencephalopathy syndrome refers to a clinical presentation thought to result from vascular endothelial dysfunction seen in patients with malignant hypertension or eclampsia, treatment with some drugs (e.g. tacrolimus, ciclosporin) and rarely other associations such as autoimmune disease. Cortical visual deficits can occasionally be the presenting feature, others including headache and seizures.

OCULAR MOTOR NERVES

Third nerve

Nuclear complex

The nuclear complex of the third (oculomotor) nerve is situated in the midbrain at the level of the superior colliculus, ventral to the Sylvian aqueduct (Fig. 19.56). It is composed of the following paired and unpaired subnuclei:

- **Levator subnucleus** is an unpaired caudal midline structure that innervates both levator muscles. Lesions confined to this area will therefore give rise to bilateral ptosis.

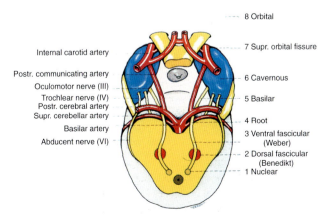

Internal carotid artery
Postr. communicating artery
Oculomotor nerve (III)
Trochlear nerve (IV)
Postr. cerebral artery
Supr. cerebellar artery
Basilar artery
Abducent nerve (VI)

8 Orbital
7 Supr. orbital fissure
6 Cavernous
5 Basilar
4 Root
3 Ventral fascicular (Weber)
2 Dorsal fascicular (Benedikt)
1 Nuclear

Fig. 19.56 Dorsal view of the course of the third nerve

- **Superior rectus subnuclei** are paired: each innervates the respective contralateral superior rectus. A nuclear third nerve palsy will therefore spare the ipsilateral, and affect the contralateral, superior rectus.
- **Medial rectus**, **inferior rectus** and **inferior oblique subnuclei** are paired and innervate their corresponding ipsilateral muscles. Lesions confined to the nuclear complex are relatively uncommon. The most frequent causes are vascular disease, primary tumours and metastases. Involvement of the paired medial rectus subnuclei cause a wall-eyed bilateral internuclear ophthalmoplegia (WEBINO), characterized by exotropia with defective convergence and adduction. Lesions involving the entire nucleus are often associated with involvement of the adjacent and caudal fourth nerve nucleus.

Fasciculus

The fasciculus consists of efferent fibres that pass from the third nerve nucleus through the red nucleus and the medial aspect of the cerebral peduncle. They then emerge from the midbrain and pass into the interpeduncular space. The causes of nuclear and fascicular lesions are similar, except that demyelination may affect the fasciculus.

- **Benedikt** syndrome involves the fasciculus as it passes through the red nucleus and is characterized by ipsilateral third nerve palsy and contralateral extrapyramidal signs such as hemitremor.
- **Weber** syndrome involves the fasciculus as it passes through the cerebral peduncle and is characterized by ipsilateral third nerve palsy and a contralateral hemiparesis.
- **Nothnagel** syndrome involves the fasciculus and the superior cerebellar peduncle and is characterized by ipsilateral third nerve palsy and cerebellar ataxia.
- **Claude** syndrome is a combination of Benedikt and Nothnagel syndromes.

Basilar

The basilar part starts as a series of 'rootlets' that leave the midbrain on the medial aspect of the cerebral peduncle, before

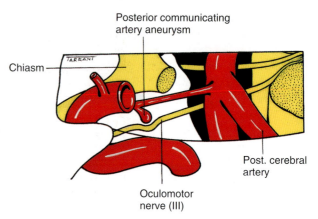

Fig. 19.58 Compression of the third nerve by a posterior communicating aneurysm

coalescing to form the main trunk. The nerve then passes between the posterior cerebral and superior cerebellar arteries, running lateral to and parallel with the posterior communicating artery (Fig. 19.57). As the nerve traverses the base of the skull along its subarachnoid course unaccompanied by any other cranial nerve, an isolated third nerve palsy is commonly basilar. The following are important causes:

- **Aneurysm** of the posterior communicating artery at its junction with the internal carotid artery (Fig. 19.58), typically presents acutely as a pupil-involving painful third nerve palsy.
- **Head trauma**, resulting in extradural or subdural haematoma, may cause a tentorial pressure cone with downward herniation of the temporal lobe. This compresses the third nerve as it passes over the tentorial edge (Fig. 19.59), initially causing irritative miosis followed by mydriasis and complete third nerve palsy.

Intracavernous

The third nerve then enters the cavernous sinus by piercing the dura just lateral to the posterior clinoid process. Within the sinus,

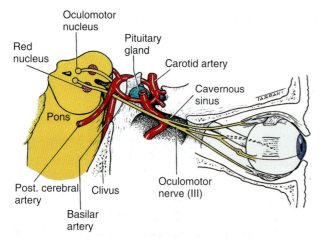

Fig. 19.57 Lateral view of the course of the third nerve

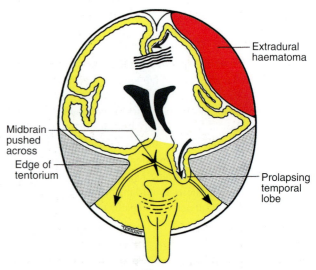

Fig. 19.59 Mechanism of third nerve palsy by extradural haematoma

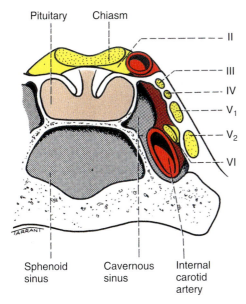

Fig. 19.60 Location of the cranial nerves in the cavernous sinus viewed from behind

the third nerve runs in the lateral wall above the fourth nerve (Fig. 19.60). In the anterior part of the cavernous sinus, the nerve divides into superior and inferior branches that enter the orbit through the superior orbital fissure within the annulus of Zinn. The following are potential causes of intracavernous third nerve palsy:

- **Diabetes.**
- **Pituitary apoplexy** (see above).
- **Miscellaneous pathology** such as aneurysm, meningioma, carotid-cavernous fistula and granulomatous inflammation (Tolosa–Hunt syndrome). Because of its close proximity to other cranial nerves, intracavernous third nerve lesions are likely to be associated with involvement of the fourth and sixth nerves and the first division of the trigeminal nerve.

Intraorbital

- **Superior** division innervates the levator and superior rectus muscles.
- **Inferior** division innervates the medial rectus, the inferior rectus and the inferior oblique muscles. The branch to the inferior oblique also contains preganglionic parasympathetic fibres from the Edinger–Westphal subnucleus, which innervate the sphincter pupillae and the ciliary muscle. Lesions of the inferior division are characterized by limited adduction and depression, together with a dilated pupil. Both superior and inferior division palsies are commonly traumatic or vascular.

Pupillomotor fibres

Between the brainstem and the cavernous sinus, the pupillomotor parasympathetic fibres are located superficially in the superomedial part of the third nerve (Fig. 19.61). They derive their blood supply from the pial blood vessels, whereas the main interior trunk of the nerve is supplied by the vasa nervorum. Involvement or

sparing of the pupil is important, as it frequently differentiates a 'surgical' from a 'medical' lesion:

- **'Surgical' lesions** such as aneurysms, trauma and uncal herniation characteristically involve the pupil by compressing the pial blood vessels and the superficially located pupillary fibres.
- **'Medical' lesions** such as occur in hypertension and diabetes usually spare the pupil. This is because the microangiopathy associated with medical lesions involves the vasa nervorum, causing ischaemia of the main trunk of the nerve, leaving the superficial pupillary fibres intact.

These principles are not infallible; pupillary involvement may be seen in some microangiopathic palsies, while pupillary sparing does not invariably exclude aneurysm or other compressive lesion. Pupillary involvement may develop a few days after the onset of diplopia as an aneurysm expands. Exceptionally, pupillary involvement may be the only sign of third nerve palsy (basal meningitis, uncal herniation). Like other features of third nerve palsy, pupillary involvement may be complete or partial, so mild pupillary signs may be clinically significant.

Signs

Partial involvement will give milder degrees of ophthalmoplegia. The other cranial nerves and peripheral nervous system should always be examined.

- **Profound ptosis** due to weakness of the levator muscle (Fig. 19.62A), so that diplopia may not be volunteered.
- **Abduction and depression in the primary position** ('down and out' – Fig. 19.62B) due to unopposed action of the lateral rectus and superior oblique muscles. The intact superior oblique muscle also causes intorsion of the eye at rest, which increases on attempted downgaze.
- **Normal abduction** as the lateral rectus is intact (Fig. 19.62C).
- **Limited adduction** due to medial rectus weakness (Fig. 19.62D).
- **Limited elevation** due to weakness of the superior rectus and inferior oblique (Fig. 19.62E).

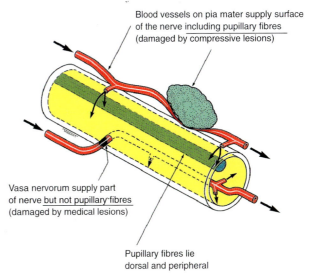

Blood vessels on pia mater supply surface of the nerve including pupillary fibres (damaged by compressive lesions)

Vasa nervorum supply part of nerve but not pupillary fibres (damaged by medical lesions)

Pupillary fibres lie dorsal and peripheral

Fig. 19.61 Location of pupillomotor fibres within the trunk of the third nerve

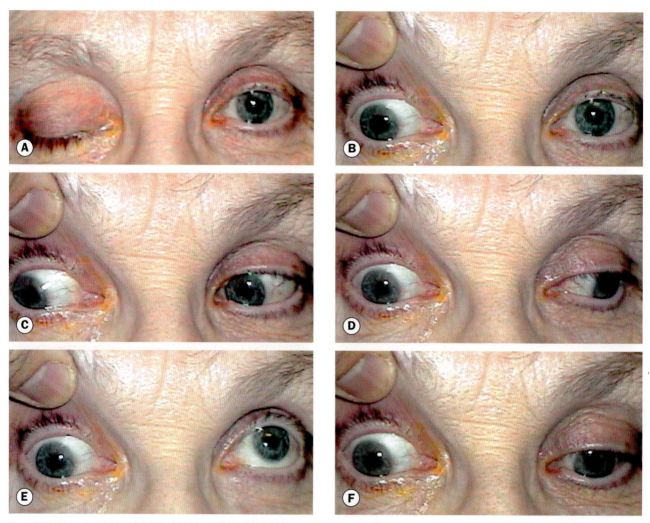

Fig. 19.62 Right third nerve palsy. **(A)** Total right ptosis; **(B)** right exotropia and depression in the primary position; **(C)** normal abduction; **(D)** limitation of adduction; **(E)** limitation of elevation; **(F)** limitation of depression

(Courtesy of B Majol)

- **Limited depression** due to weakness of the inferior rectus (Fig. 19.62F).
- **Dilated pupil and defective accommodation** due to parasympathetic palsy.

Aberrant regeneration

Aberrant regeneration may follow acute traumatic and compressive, but not vascular, third nerve palsies. This is because the endoneural nerve sheaths, which may be breached in traumatic and compressive lesions, remain intact with vascular lesions. Bizarre defects in ocular motility such as elevation of the upper eyelid on attempted adduction or depression (the pseudo-Graefe or pseudo-von Graefe phenomenon), are caused by misdirected regenerating axons that re-innervate the incorrect extraocular muscle. The pupil may also be involved.

Causes of isolated third nerve palsy

Clinical evaluation and imaging facilitates identification of a cause in most cases.

- **Microvascular** disease associated with systemic risk factors such as hypertension and diabetes is the most common cause of third nerve palsy. Marked periorbital pain is often associated, which is therefore not helpful in distinguishing an aneurysmal cause. In diabetes-related paresis, motility disturbance is typically profound, but there is usually (75%) relative or complete pupil sparing and when pupillary involvement does occur some degree of reaction to light is almost always preserved.
- **Aneurysm** of the posterior communicating artery at its junction with the internal carotid is a very important cause of isolated third nerve palsy with involvement of the pupil. Pain is often though not invariably present, and the extent of pupillary involvement characteristically exceeds the severity of motility dysfunction. An aneurysm of the internal carotid within the cavernous sinus tends to also involve other cranial nerves (see above).
- **Trauma**, both direct and secondary to subdural haematoma with uncal herniation. However, the development of third nerve palsy following relatively trivial head trauma should

alert the clinician to the possibility of an underlying aneurysm or tumour.

- **Miscellaneous uncommon causes** include tumour, inflammatory disease such as syphilis, Lyme disease and sarcoidosis, giant cell arteritis and vasculitis associated with collagen vascular disorders.
- **Episodic.** Brief episodes of third nerve dysfunction with spontaneous recovery may be idiopathic or occur with migraine, compression, ischaemia and alterations in intracranial pressure. Myasthenia gravis may mimic intermittent pupil-sparing third nerve paresis.

Investigation

- **Vascular risk factor** assessment similar to that for retinal arterial disease (see Ch. 13). Supplementary investigation may be required if a rarer aetiology such as infection (e.g. syphilis, Lyme disease) or vasculitis (including giant cell arteritis) is suspected; this may include a lumbar puncture.
- **CT angiography** should be performed with great urgency if the clinical features are suspicious of an expanding aneurysm, especially if there is marked pupillary involvement with milder motility dysfunction and only partial ptosis.
- **MRI brain and orbits with venography**, including specific exclusion of a brainstem stroke or tumour, cavernous sinus or orbital apex lesion.
- **Conventional cerebral angiography** is occasionally indicated.

Treatment

- **Observation** is usually appropriate in presumed microvascular cases; the majority will resolve over weeks or months. Temporary (e.g. Fresnel stick-on) prisms may be useful if the angle of deviation is small, but uniocular occlusion may be necessary to avoid diplopia if the ptosis component is partial or recovering. Botulinum toxin injection into the uninvolved lateral rectus muscle is sometimes used to prevent its contracture when recovery time is prolonged.
- **Surgical** treatment of the ocular motility element and ptosis should be contemplated only after spontaneous improvement has ceased, usually not earlier than 6–12 months from onset. Numerous innovative surgical techniques have been described.

Fourth nerve

Anatomy

The fourth (trochlear) cranial nerve (Fig. 19.63) supplies only the superior oblique muscle.

- **Key features**
  - It is a very long and slender nerve, increasing its vulnerability.
  - It is the only cranial nerve to emerge from the dorsal aspect of the brain.

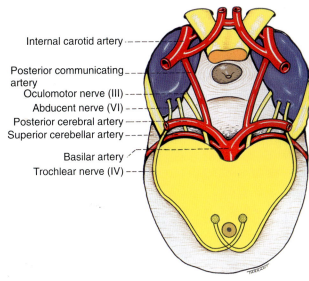

Internal carotid artery
Posterior communicating artery
Oculomotor nerve (III)
Abducent nerve (VI)
Posterior cerebral artery
Superior cerebellar artery
Basilar artery
Trochlear nerve (IV)

Fig. 19.63 Dorsal view of the course of the fourth nerve

  - It is the only decussated (crossed) cranial nerve besides the optic nerve, innervating the superior oblique muscle contralateral to its nucleus.
  - It has the fewest axons of any of the cranial nerves.
- **The nucleus** is located at the level of the inferior colliculi ventral to the Sylvian aqueduct. It is caudal to, and continuous with, the third nerve nuclear complex.
- **The fasciculus** consists of axons that curve posteriorly around the aqueduct and decussate completely in the anterior medullary velum.
- **The trunk** leaves the brainstem on the dorsal surface, just caudal to the inferior colliculus. It then curves laterally around the brainstem, runs forwards beneath the free edge of the tentorium, and like the third nerve passes between the posterior cerebral artery and the superior cerebellar artery. It then pierces the dura and enters the cavernous sinus.
- **The intracavernous** part runs in the lateral wall of the sinus, inferior to the third nerve and above the first division of the fifth. In the anterior part of the cavernous sinus it rises and passes through the superior orbital fissure above and lateral to the annulus of Zinn.
- **The intraorbital** part innervates the superior oblique muscle.

Causes of isolated fourth nerve palsy

- **Idiopathic** lesions are common, and many of these are thought to be congenital although symptoms may not develop until decompensation occurs in adult life due to reduced fusional ability. In contrast to acquired lesions patients are not usually aware of the torsional aspect, but may develop vertical double vision that is often appreciated as of sudden or subacute onset. Examination of old photographs for the presence of a compensatory head posture may be helpful, as is the presence of an increased vertical prism fusional range. Occasionally cataract surgery can be associated with decompensation.

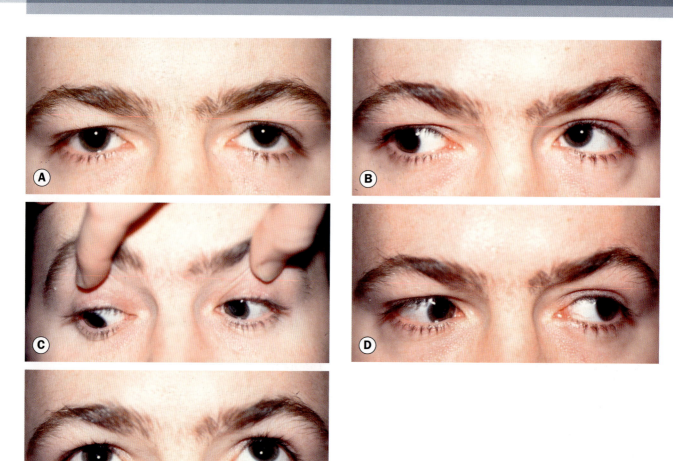

Fig. 19.64 Left fourth nerve palsy. **(A)** Left hypertropia (left over right) in the primary position; **(B)** increase in left hypertropia on right gaze due to left inferior oblique overaction; **(C)** limitation of left depression in adduction; **(D)** normal left abduction; **(E)** normal left elevation

- **Trauma** frequently causes bilateral fourth nerve palsy. The long and slender nerves are particularly vulnerable as they decussate in the anterior medullary velum, through impact with the tentorial edge. Care must be taken not to mistake a bilateral palsy for a unilateral lesion, particularly when corrective surgery is contemplated.
- **Microvascular** lesions are relatively common, this aetiology often being presumed when appropriate systemic risk factors are present in the absence of features of congenital onset.
- **Aneurysms and tumours** are extremely rare.

Signs

The acute onset of vertical diplopia in the absence of ptosis, combined with a characteristic head posture, strongly suggests fourth nerve disease. The main actions of the superior oblique are intorsion (incyclotorsion), and depression in adduction. Peripheral lesions cause ipsilateral and nuclear lesions contralateral superior oblique weakness; left paresis is characterized by:

- **Left hypertropia** ('left over right') in the primary position (Fig. 19.64A), increasing on right gaze (Fig. 19.64B).
- **Limitation of left depression,** most marked in adduction (Fig. 19.64C).
- **Left extorsion**, greatest in abduction.
- **Normal abduction** of the left eye (Fig. 19.64D).
- **Normal elevation** of the left eye (Fig. 19.64E).
- **A compensatory head posture** (Fig. 19.65) avoids diplopia: vertical, torsional and worse on downgaze. To compensate for weakness of intorsion there is contralateral head tilt to the right. To alleviate the weakened depression of the eye the chin is slightly depressed; as this is most marked in adduction, the face may also be turned slightly to the right.
- **Bilateral involvement** should always be excluded, particularly following head trauma.
  - Right hypertropia in left gaze and left hypertropia in right gaze, though orthophoria may be present.
  - Greater than 10° of cyclodeviation (measured using double Maddox rods or by synoptophore – see Ch. 18).
  - 'V' pattern esotropia is often present.
  - Bilaterally positive Bielschowsky head tilt test (see below).

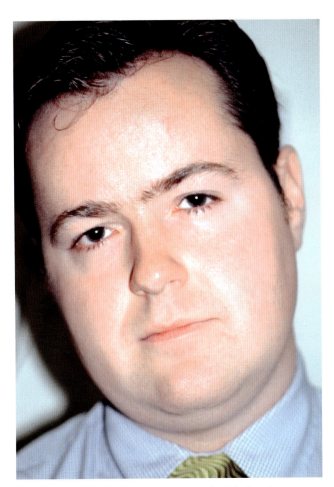

Fig. 19.65 Compensatory head posture in left fourth nerve palsy; head tilt to right, face turn to the right and chin depressed

Parks three-step test

This clinical test allows isolation of a single weak muscle in patients with vertical diplopia of acute onset; it is inaccurate in some circumstances, including prior extraocular muscle surgery.

- **Step one.** In the primary position, the hypertropic eye is identified, narrowing the affected muscle to one of the depressors of the hypertropic eye (superior oblique or inferior rectus) or one of the elevators of the hypotropic eye (superior rectus or inferior oblique). In a fourth nerve palsy, the involved eye is higher (see Fig. 19.64A).
- **Step two.** The eyes are examined in right and left gaze to determine where the hypertropia is greater, thus assigning the weakness to the two of the four previously identified muscles having the greatest vertical action in that position. In superior oblique weakness (see Fig. 19.64B) the deviation is **w**orse **o**n **o**pposite **g**aze – **WOOG**.
- **Step three**
  - The Bielschowsky head tilt test (BHTT) is performed with the patient fixating on a target directly ahead, optimally at 3 metres.
  - The head is tilted to each side in turn in order to assess the muscles responsible for cyclotorsion, with observation

to determine the position in which the hypertropia is worse. On tilt to one side, the superior oblique and superior rectus (note that both are superior) muscles of the eye of that same side correctively intort, and the inferior rectus and inferior oblique (note both are inferior) of the contralateral eye correctively extort. From the two muscles previously isolated, one can be eliminated.
  - In fourth nerve palsy the deviation is **b**etter **o**n **o**pposite tilt – **BOOT** (Fig. 19.66); in practice, as the three-step test is almost always employed to confirm a fourth nerve palsy, the BHTT alone is often sufficient for a working diagnosis.

Investigation

Vascular investigation is sometimes indicated; neuroimaging is not required routinely for an isolated non-progressive fourth nerve palsy, but should be considered if improvement does not occur.

Treatment

Congenital decompensated and presumed microvascular palsies commonly resolve spontaneously.

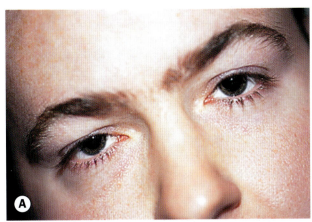

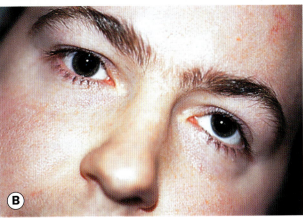

Fig. 19.66 Positive Bielschowsky test in left fourth nerve palsy. **(A)** No hypertropia on right head tilt; **(B)** marked hypertropia on left head tilt

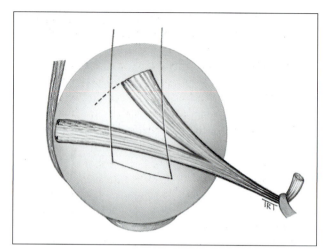

Fig. 19.67 Harada–Ito procedure for superior oblique palsy

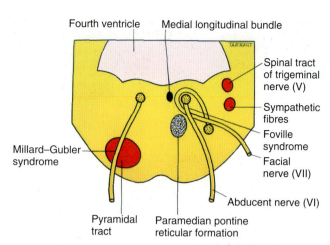

Fig. 19.68 The pons at the level of the sixth nerve nucleus

Strabismus surgery is not infrequently required for traumatic and childhood cases, in the former for troublesome diplopia and the latter for a substantial compensatory head posture; the approach depends on the pattern and severity of weakness.

- **A small hypertropia** under 15 prism dioptres can usually be treated either by inferior oblique weakening or by superior oblique tucking, though surgery to other muscles might be required in some circumstances.
- **A moderate–large deviation** may be treated by ipsilateral inferior oblique weakening combined with, or followed by, ipsilateral superior rectus weakening and/or contralateral inferior rectus weakening if required; defective elevation is a potential complication.
- **Excyclotorsion** may need to be addressed, particularly in bilateral cases; the Harada–Ito procedure involves splitting and anterolateral transposition of the lateral half of the superior oblique tendon (Fig. 19.67).

Sixth nerve

Brainstem

The nucleus of the sixth (abducens or abducent) nerve lies at the mid-level of the pons, ventral to the floor of the fourth ventricle (Fig. 19.68). The fibres (fasciculus) leave the brainstem ventrally at the pontomedullary junction.

- **Nuclear lesion.** A nuclear sixth nerve lesion also causes a failure of horizontal gaze towards the side of the damage due to involvement of the adjacent horizontal gaze centre (paramedian pontine reticular formation). Facial (seventh) nerve fibres wrap around the sixth nerve nucleus, so ipsilateral lower motor neurone (LMN) facial nerve palsy is also common. Isolated sixth nerve palsy is never nuclear in origin.
- **Foville (inferior medial pontine) syndrome** is most frequently caused by vascular disease or tumours involving the dorsal pons. It is characterized by ipsilateral involvement of the fifth to eighth cranial nerves, central

sympathetic fibres (Horner syndrome) and horizontal gaze palsy.
- **Millard–Gubler (ventral pontine) syndrome** involves the fasciculus as it passes through the pyramidal tract and is most frequently caused by vascular disease, tumours or demyelination. As well as ipsilateral sixth nerve palsy, there is contralateral hemiplegia and often an ipsilateral LMN facial nerve palsy.

Basilar

The basilar part of the nerve enters the prepontine basilar cistern, passes upwards close to the base of the skull and is crossed by the anterior inferior cerebellar artery (Fig. 19.69). It pierces the dura below the posterior clinoids and angles forwards over the tip of the petrous bone, passing through or around the inferior petrosal sinus, through the Dorello canal (underneath the petroclinoid ligament), to enter the cavernous sinus.

- **An acoustic neuroma** may damage the sixth nerve at the pontomedullary junction (Fig. 19.70); the first symptom of an acoustic neuroma is hearing loss, and the first sign diminished corneal sensitivity. Hearing and corneal

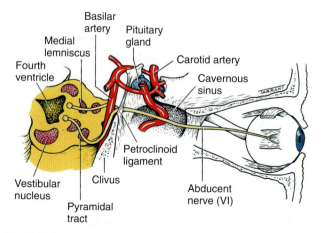

Fig. 19.69 Lateral view of the course of the sixth nerve

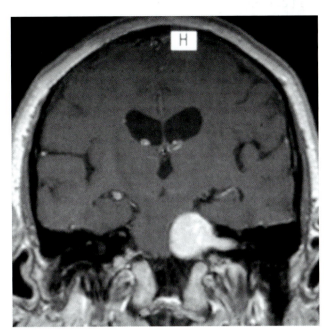

Fig. 19.70 MRI with gadolinium enhancement – coronal image of an acoustic neuroma
(Courtesy of N Rogers)

sensation should be checked in all patients with sixth nerve palsy.

- **Nasopharyngeal tumours** may invade the skull and its foramina and damage the nerve during its basilar course.
- **Raised intracranial pressure** may cause a downward displacement of the brainstem. This may stretch one or both sixth nerves over the petrous tip, when paresis is a false localizing sign.
- **Basal skull fracture** may cause unilateral or bilateral palsy.
- **Gradenigo syndrome**, most frequently caused by mastoiditis or acute petrositis, may result in damage of the sixth nerve at the petrous tip. The latter is frequently accompanied by facial weakness and pain, and hearing difficulties.

Intracavernous and intraorbital

- **The intracavernous** section runs below the third and fourth, and the first division of the fifth nerves. The sixth nerve is the most medially situated and runs through the middle of the sinus in close relation to the internal carotid artery. Occasionally, intracavernous sixth nerve palsy is accompanied by a postganglionic Horner syndrome (Parkinson syndrome) due to damage to the paracarotid sympathetic plexus. The causes of intracavernous sixth nerve and third nerve lesions (see above) are similar.
- **The intraorbital** part enters the orbit through the superior orbital fissure within the annulus of Zinn to innervate the lateral rectus.

Diagnosis

- **Symptoms.** Double vision is characteristically worse for a distant target and less or absent for near fixation. A careful

review of systems should be conducted, including enquiry about other neurological symptoms, giant cell arteritis, trauma and symptoms of ear disease.

- **Esotropia** in the primary position due to relatively unopposed action of the medial rectus (Figs 19.71A and 19.72A); the deviation (and symptomatic description) is characteristically worse for distance than near fixation.
- **Limitation of abduction** on the side of the lesion (Figs 19.71B and 19.72B).
- **Normal adduction** of the affected eye (Fig. 19.72C).
- **Bilateral acute sixth nerve paresis** (Fig. 19.73) is considerably less common than unilateral; the causes are broadly similar, but elevated intracranial pressure should be excluded as a priority.
- **A compensatory face turn** is towards the side of the paralysed muscle in unilateral palsy.
- **Neurological examination.** The other cranial nerves and the peripheral nervous system should be examined, if necessary by an appropriate specialist. In a child or any patient with relevant symptoms, an otorhinolaryngological review may be sought.

Investigation

Idiopathic and presumed microvascular lesions are common (up to 60%) in older patients, but a wide range of causes has been reported and a low threshold should be adopted for neuroimaging and other investigations even with isolated paresis; these should be performed broadly as for third nerve palsy. Also as with third nerve palsy, improved imaging has led to increasingly common identification of a cause in lesions that might previously have been categorized as idiopathic. In contrast to fourth nerve palsy, a decompensated congenital aetiology is thought to be rare. The

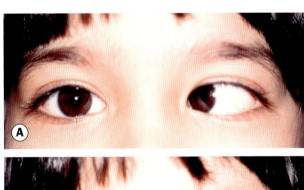

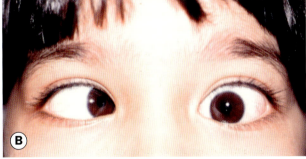

Fig. 19.71 Acute left sixth nerve palsy in a child. **(A)** Left esotropia in the primary position; **(B)** marked limitation of left abduction

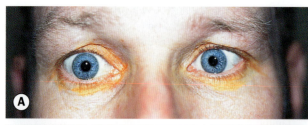

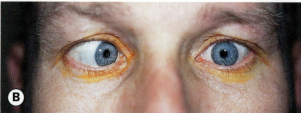

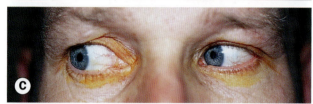

Fig. 19.72 Left sixth nerve palsy in an adult. **(A)** Slight left esotropia in the primary position; **(B)** limitation of left abduction; **(C)** normal left adduction

presence of bilateral paresis, additional relevant clinical findings or presentation in children and younger adults should prompt aggressive investigation.

Treatment

- **Observation** with monocular occlusion or prismatic (e.g. temporary Fresnel stick-on) correction of diplopia is appropriate in idiopathic and presumed microvascular lesions; up to 90% will recover spontaneously, usually over weeks to several months. Young children should be treated with alternate patching to prevent amblyopia.
- **Botulinum toxin** injection into the ipsilateral medial rectus may be used to prevent contracture, assess residual function and sometimes to facilitate prismatic correction with a large deviation (see Fig. 18.72); it is rarely curative.
- **Surgery** should be considered only when adequate time has been allowed for maximal spontaneous

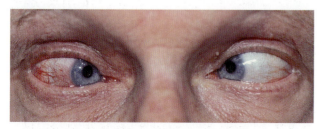

Fig. 19.73 Acute bilateral sixth nerve palsy
(Courtesy of C Barry)

improvement, typically at least 6–12 months from onset.

- ○ Partial palsy (paresis) is treated by adjustable medial rectus recession and lateral rectus resection in the affected eye, aiming for a small exophoria in the primary position to maximize the field of binocular single vision.
- ○ Complete palsy is treated by transposition of the superior and inferior recti to positions above and below the affected lateral rectus muscle (see Fig. 18.70), coupled with weakening of the ipsilateral medial rectus (sometimes with injection of botulinum toxin – 'toxin transposition'). Three rectus muscles should not be detached from the globe at the same procedure because of the risk of anterior segment ischaemia.
- **Permanent prism.** Troublesome but mild residual deviation may be treated with a prism incorporated into spectacles as an alternative to surgery.

SUPRANUCLEAR DISORDERS OF OCULAR MOTILITY

Conjugate eye movements

Conjugate eye movements (versions) are binocular movements in which the eyes move synchronously and symmetrically in the same direction. The main types are saccades, smooth pursuit and non-optical reflex movements. Saccadic and pursuit movements are supranuclear in origin, controlled at both cerebral and brainstem levels. Non-optical reflex function helps to stabilize the visual field with respect to head position. Disturbance of supranuclear eye movement function causes gaze palsy.

Saccades

- **Function.** Rapid voluntary or reflex alignment of the fovea with a target image, including transferral of fixation from one target to another.
- **Pathway.** There are separate horizontal and vertical pathways. Many cortical areas and the superior colliculi are involved in saccade generation, but classically initiation occurs in the premotor cortex frontal eye fields, from where impulses for horizontal movement pass to the contralateral paramedian pontine reticular formation (PPRF) – the horizontal gaze centre (Fig 19.74). Each frontal lobe initiates contralateral saccades. Vertical pathways are less well mapped (see below).

Smooth pursuit

- **Function.** To maintain fixation on a target with slow smooth movements once it has been located by the saccadic system. The stimulus is image movement near the fovea.
- **Pathway.** This is complex, involving several cortex regions as well as the PPRF, the superior colliculi, cerebellum and other structures. The pathways are ipsilateral, the cortex on one side controlling pursuit to the same side.

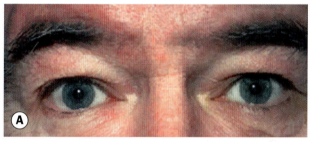

Fig. 19.74 Anatomical pathways for horizontal eye movements (LR = lateral rectus; MLF = medial longitudinal fasciculus; MR = medial rectus; PPRF = paramedian pontine reticular formation)

Non-optical reflexes

- **Function.** The maintenance of eye position without conscious input following a change of head or body position. Other, visually directed (i.e. optical) mechanisms are also concerned with visual field stability; both may be active in the doll's eye (oculocephalic) reflex, in which when the head of an unconscious patient is rotated, the eyes move in the opposite direction to preserve the image position on the retina.
- **Pathway.** Movements are mediated mainly via the vestibular system. Signals originate in the inner ear labyrinths and in proprioceptors that provide information concerning head and neck movements. For horizontal movements, afferent fibres synapse in the vestibular nuclei and pass to the horizontal gaze centre.

Abnormalities of horizontal gaze

Anatomy

After initiation horizontal eye movements are generated in the horizontal gaze centre (PPRF – see Fig. 19.74) and mediated via a common pathway. From here, impulses travel (i) directly to the ipsilateral sixth nerve nucleus and (ii) indirectly via internuclear neurones that cross the midline at the level of the pons and pass up the contralateral medial longitudinal fasciculus (MLF), to motor neurones in the medial rectus subnucleus of the contralateral third nerve complex. Stimulation of the horizontal gaze centre on one side therefore causes a conjugate movement of the eyes to the same side.

Horizontal gaze palsy

A lesion of the horizontal gaze centre in the PPRF gives ipsilateral horizontal gaze palsy, with an inability to look in the direction of the lesion.

Internuclear ophthalmoplegia

A lesion in the MLF is responsible for the clinical syndrome of internuclear ophthalmoplegia (INO); causes include demyelination, stroke and tumours. Strabismus surgery can be performed for persistent diplopia.

- **Unilateral INO** (Fig. 19.75). Double vision is not typically a complaint.
  - Straight eyes in the primary position.
  - Defective adduction of the eye on the side of the lesion and nystagmus of the contralateral eye on abduction; note that the side of the lesion is named for the side of the adduction deficit.
  - Gaze to the side of the lesion is normal.
  - Convergence is intact if the lesion is anterior and discrete but impaired if the lesion is posterior or extensive.
- **Bilateral INO** (Fig. 19.76)
  - Limitation of left adduction and ataxic nystagmus of the right eye on right gaze.
  - Limitation of right adduction and ataxic nystagmus of the left eye on left gaze.

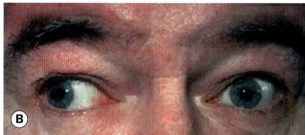

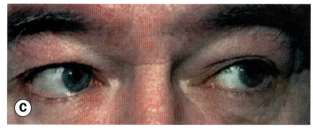

Fig. 19.75 Left internuclear ophthalmoplegia. **(A)** Straight in the primary position; **(B)** limitation of left adduction on right gaze; **(C)** normal left abduction on left gaze

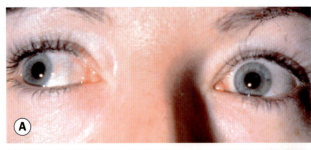

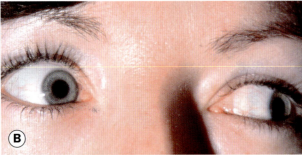

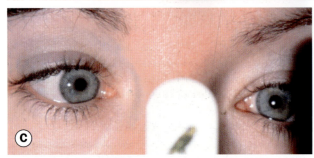

Fig. 19.76 Bilateral internuclear ophthalmoplegia. **(A)** Limitation of left adduction on right gaze; **(B)** less severe limitation of right adduction on left gaze; **(C)** convergence is intact

- ○ Convergence may be intact or impaired.
- ○ A rostral midbrain lesion may give an associated convergence deficit with resultant bilateral exotropia and abducting nystagmus: 'wall-eyed bilateral INO' – WEBINO.
- **One-and-a-half syndrome.** PPRF and MLF lesions combined on the same side give rise to the 'one-and-a-half syndrome' characterized by a combination of ipsilateral gaze palsy and INO. The only residual movement is abduction of the contralateral eye, which exhibits abduction nystagmus.

Vertical gaze palsy

Anatomy

Vertical eye movement initiation in the frontal lobes is simultaneously bilateral, with impulses mediated via the vertical gaze centre in the midbrain (rostral interstitial nucleus of the MLF). From the vertical gaze centre, impulses pass to the subnuclei of the eye muscles controlling vertical gaze in both eyes. Cells subserving

upward and downward eye movements are intermingled in the vertical gaze centre, although selective paralysis of upgaze and downgaze may occur in spite of this.

Parinaud (dorsal midbrain) syndrome

- **Signs**
  - ○ Straight eyes in the primary position.
  - ○ Supranuclear upgaze palsy (Fig. 19.77A).
  - ○ Defective convergence (Fig. 19.77B).
  - ○ Large pupils with light–near dissociation (see Fig. 19.41).
  - ○ Lid retraction (Collier sign).
  - ○ Convergence–retraction nystagmus.
- **Causes**
  - ○ Children: aqueduct stenosis, meningitis and pinealoma (Fig. 19.78).
  - ○ Young adults: demyelination, trauma and arteriovenous malformations.
  - ○ The elderly: midbrain vascular accidents, mass lesions involving the periaqueductal grey matter and posterior fossa aneurysms.

Progressive supranuclear palsy

Progressive supranuclear palsy (Steele–Richardson–Olszewski syndrome) is a severe degenerative disease presenting in old age. Clinical features include:

- Supranuclear gaze palsy, initially primarily of downgaze and subsequently upgaze.
- Horizontal movements subsequently become impaired, with eventual global gaze palsy.
- Paralysis of convergence.
- Pseudobulbar palsy.
- Extrapyramidal rigidity, gait ataxia and dementia.

Skew deviation

Skew deviation is an uncommon supranuclear motility disorder in which the eyes are deviated vertically and often exhibit cyclotorsional disturbance. Three categories have been described, corresponding to differing motility patterns and lesion sites; both eyes can be deviated upwards, or one can be hypertropic and one hypotropic. The most frequent cause is a brainstem or cerebellar stroke, which it is thought leads to dysfunction of a primordial field stabilization mechanism.

NYSTAGMUS

Introduction

Physiological principles

Nystagmus is an involuntary oscillation of the eyes that can be a physiological (e.g. following the rotation of an optokinetic drum) or pathological phenomenon. In pathological nystagmus, each cycle of movement is usually initiated by an involuntary,

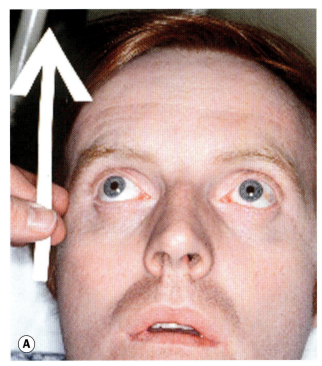

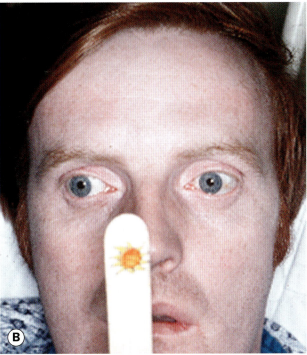

Fig. 19.77 Parinaud syndrome. **(A)** Defective upgaze; **(B)** convergence paralysis

(Courtesy of ES Rosen, P Eustace, HS Thompson and WJK Cumming, from Neuro-ophthalmology, Mosby 1998)

defoveating drift of the eye away from the target, followed by a refixating saccadic movement.

- **Plane** may be horizontal, vertical, or torsional.
- **Amplitude** refers to the extent of excursion: fine or coarse.
- **Frequency** describes how rapidly the eyes oscillate: high, moderate or low.

Classification

A schematic such as that shown in Fig. 19.79 can be used for documentation.

- **Jerk** nystagmus is saccadic with a slow defoveating 'drift' movement and a fast corrective refoveating saccadic movement. The direction of nystagmus is described in terms of the direction of the fast component: right, left, up, down or rotatory.
- **Pendular** nystagmus is non-saccadic in that both the foveating and defoveating movements are slow (i.e. the velocity of nystagmus is equal in both directions).
- **Mixed** nystagmus consists of pendular nystagmus in the primary position and jerk nystagmus on lateral gaze.

Physiological nystagmus

- **End-point** nystagmus is a fine jerk nystagmus of moderate frequency seen in extremes of gaze. The fast phase is in the direction of gaze (Fig. 19.80).
- **Optokinetic nystagmus (OKN)** is a jerk nystagmus induced by moving repetitive targets (e.g. OKN drum) across the visual field.
  - The slow phase is a pursuit movement in which the eyes follow the target; the fast phase is a saccadic movement in the opposite direction as the eyes fixate on the next target.
  - If the OKN tape or drum is moved from right to left, the left parieto-occipito-temporal region controls the slow (pursuit) phase to the left, and the left frontal lobe controls the rapid (saccadic) phase to the right.

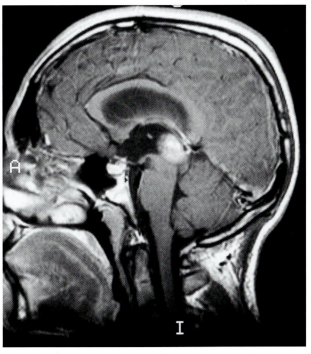

Fig. 19.78 MRI sagittal view shows a pinealoma and a dilated third ventricle

(Courtesy of D Thomas)

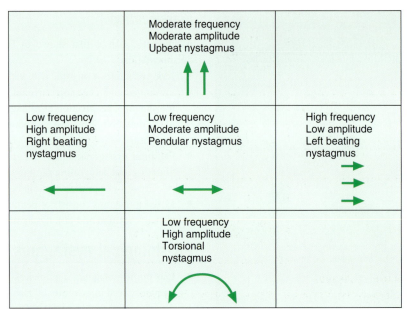

Fig. 19.79 Schematic for documenting nystagmus
(Courtesy of JJ Kanski, Signs in Ophthalmology: Causes and Differential Diagnosis, Mosby 2010)

○ OKN nystagmus is useful for detecting functional (non-physiological) blindness and for testing visual acuity in the very young. It can be helpful in the assessment of an isolated homonymous hemianopia.

Vestibular nystagmus

- **Physiological** vestibular nystagmus is a jerk nystagmus caused by altered input from the vestibular nuclei to the horizontal gaze centres. The slow phase is initiated by the vestibular nuclei and the fast phase by the brainstem and frontomesencephalic pathway. Vestibular nystagmus may be elicited by caloric stimulation as follows:
  ○ When cold water is poured into the right ear the patient will develop left jerk nystagmus (i.e. fast phase to the left).
  ○ When warm water is poured into the right ear the patient will develop right jerk nystagmus (i.e. fast phase to the right). A useful mnemonic is 'COWS' (cold-opposite, warm-same) indicating the direction of the nystagmus.
  ○ When cold water is poured into both ears simultaneously, a jerk nystagmus with the fast phase upwards develops;

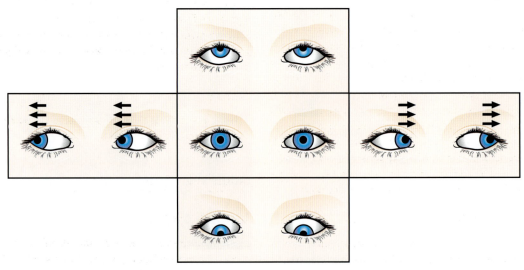

Fig. 19.80 Physiological nystagmus – end-point
(Courtesy of JJ Kanski, Signs in Ophthalmology: Causes and Differential Diagnosis, Mosby 2010)

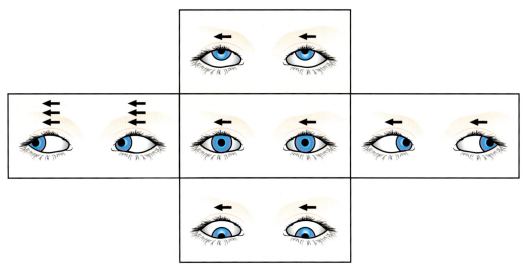

Fig. 19.81 Peripheral vestibular nystagmus
(Courtesy of JJ Kanski, Signs in Ophthalmology: Causes and Differential Diagnosis, Mosby 2010)

warm water in both ears elicits nystagmus with the fast phase downwards (cold 'slows things down').

○ An abnormal test indicates the presence of peripheral vestibular disease.

- **Pathological** peripheral vestibular nystagmus (Fig. 19.81) is caused by disease affecting the ear such as labyrynthitis, Ménière disease and middle or inner ear infections. It tends to be solely horizontal, vertical or torsional, increases in intensity with gaze in the direction of the fast phase, and is dampened by fixation. It is typically of fine amplitude.

Infantile (congenital) nystagmus

Introduction

Early-onset (usually the first few months of life rather than truly congenital) nystagmus can occur secondary to poor vision or to a motor deficit with the nystagmus itself causing poor vision, though the distinction is not always clear. It can be associated with a serious systemic condition, particularly of the central nervous system. Infantile nystagmus is commonly pendular but may be jerk, horizontal and uniplanar (direction of oscillation remains constant regardless of direction of gaze). In contrast to adults with acquired nystagmus, oscillopsia is not experienced even by adults with congenital nystagmus. The nystagmus may be dampened by convergence and is not present during sleep. There is usually a null point – a position of gaze in which nystagmus is minimal – and a compensatory head posture may develop to favour this. Investigation should seek to detect ocular and systemic associations.

Sensory deficit (afferent) nystagmus

Sensory deprivation nystagmus is the more common form of infantile nystagmus and is caused by impairment of central vision in early life (e.g. congenital cataract, macular hypoplasia, albinism, Leber congenital amaurosis, optic nerve hypoplasia,

achromatopsia). In general, children with bilateral poor vision under 2 years of age develop nystagmus, the severity of which is associated with the degree of visual loss.

Congenital motor (efferent) nystagmus

A family history is common, with X-linked (dominant or recessive) inheritance the common mode. Presentation is about 2–3 months after birth and persists throughout life. VA is generally better than with sensory deficit nystagmus, at 6/12–6/36. In the primary position there is low-amplitude pendular nystagmus that may convert to jerk nystagmus on side gaze (Fig. 19.82).

Spasmus nutans

Presentation of this rare condition is between 3 and 18 months with unilateral or bilateral small-amplitude high-frequency horizontal nystagmus (Fig. 19.83) associated with head nodding. It is frequently asymmetrical, with increased amplitude in abduction. Vertical and torsional components may be present. An idiopathic form spontaneously resolves by age 3 years, but glioma of the anterior visual pathway, empty sella syndrome and porencephalic cyst can also be causative.

Others

Other forms of nystagmus such as periodic alternating (see below) can be infantile in presentation.

Acquired nystagmus

Latent nystagmus

Latent nystagmus is associated with infantile esotropia and dissociated vertical deviation (see Ch. 18). With both eyes open there is no nystagmus, but horizontal nystagmus becomes apparent on covering one eye; the fast phase is in the direction of the uncovered

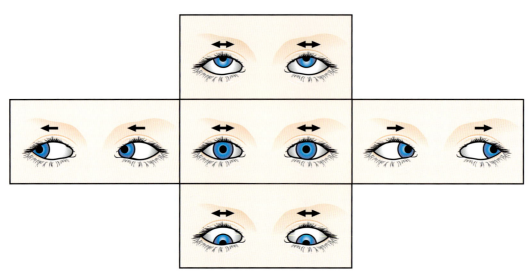

Fig. 19.82 Congenital motor (efferent) nystagmus, in this case pendular in the primary position and on vertical gaze, but converting to a gaze-evoked jerk nystagmus on left and right gaze
(Courtesy of JJ Kanski, Signs in Ophthalmology: Causes and Differential Diagnosis, Mosby 2010)

fixating eye. Occasionally an element of latency may be superimposed on a manifest nystagmus so that when one eye is covered the amplitude of nystagmus increases (manifest-latent nystagmus).

Periodic alternating nystagmus

Periodic alternating nystagmus (PAN) is a conjugate horizontal jerk nystagmus that periodically reverses direction. During the active phase, the amplitude and frequency of nystagmus first progressively increase then decrease. This is followed by an interlude lasting 4–20 s during which time the eyes are steady and may show low-intensity, often pendular movements. A similar sequence in the opposite direction occurs thereafter, the whole cycle lasting between 1 and 3 minutes. PAN can be congenital or due to cerebellar disease, ataxia telangiectasia and drugs such as phenytoin.

Convergence–retraction nystagmus

Convergence–retraction nystagmus is a jerk nystagmus due to the co-contraction of extraocular muscles, often the medial recti. It can be induced by rotating an OKN drum downwards; the upward refixation saccade brings the two eyes towards each other in a convergence movement. There is classically associated retraction of the globe into the orbit. It is a component of Parinaud dorsal midbrain syndrome; causes include lesions of the pretectal area such as pinealoma, and vascular accidents.

Downbeat nystagmus

This is a vertical nystagmus with the fast phase beating downwards (Fig. 19.84), more easily elicited in lateral gaze and downgaze. It can be caused by lesions at the foramen magnum such as

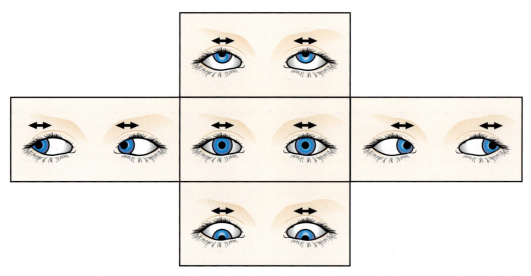

Fig. 19.83 Spasmus nutans – the nystagmus in this patient is pendular, uniplanar and of equal amplitude in all directions of gaze
(Courtesy of JJ Kanski, Signs in Ophthalmology: Causes and Differential Diagnosis, Mosby 2010)

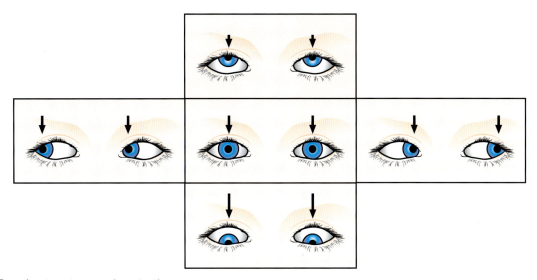

Fig. 19.84 Downbeat nystagmus (see text)

(Courtesy of JJ Kanski, Signs in Ophthalmology: Causes and Differential Diagnosis, Mosby 2010)

Arnold–Chiari malformation and syringobulbia, drugs such as lithium and phenytoin, and a range of other conditions such as Wernicke encephalopathy, demyelination and hydrocephalus.

Upbeat nystagmus

Upbeat nystagmus is a vertical nystagmus with the fast phase beating upwards in all positions (Fig. 19.85); causes include posterior fossa lesions, drugs and Wernicke encephalopathy.

See-saw nystagmus

A pendular nystagmus, in which one eye elevates and intorts while the other depresses and extorts. It can be due to parasellar tumours (often with bitemporal hemianopia), syringobulbia and brainstem stroke.

Ataxic nystagmus

Ataxic nystagmus is a horizontal jerk nystagmus that occurs in the abducting eye of a patient with an INO (see above).

Bruns nystagmus

This consists of a coarse cerebellar horizontal jerk nystagmus in one eye and fine high frequency vestibular nystagmus in the other, and can be caused by cerebellopontine angle tumours such as acoustic neuroma.

Treatment of nystagmus

- **Amblyopia and refractive error** should be managed as appropriate. Contact lenses and other refractive measures

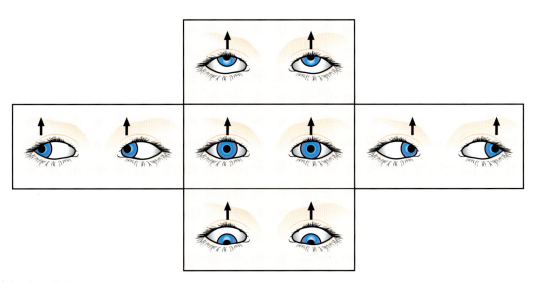

Fig. 19.85 Upbeat nystagmus

(Courtesy of JJ Kanski, Signs in Ophthalmology: Causes and Differential Diagnosis, Mosby 2010)

such as the combination of high minus contact lenses and high plus spectacle lenses may be helpful.

- **Medication** such as baclofen and gabapentin may be helpful.
- **Botulinum toxin** injection into the extraocular muscles has had some success but can be unpredictable and long-term treatment is required.
- **Surgery** for nystagmus with a null point is aimed at moving muscles in order to mimic muscle tension while the eyes and face are straight and may be performed to address a compensatory head posture. Recession of all horizontal recti has been successful in reducing the amplitude of nystagmus in some patients without a significant null point.

Nystagmoid movements

Nystagmoid movements resemble nystagmus, but the initial pathological defoveating movement is a saccadic intrusion.

Ocular flutter and opsoclonus

These entities consist of saccadic oscillations with no intersaccadic interval; in ocular flutter oscillations are purely horizontal, and in opsoclonus they are multiplanar. Causes include viral encephalitis, myoclonic encephalopathy in infants ('dancing eyes and dancing feet'), as a transient idiopathic occurrence in healthy neonates, or may be drug-induced.

Ocular bobbing

Ocular bobbing manifests with rapid downward conjugate eye movements with a subsequent slow drift up to the primary position. Causes include pontine lesions (usually haemorrhage), cerebellar lesions compressing the pons, and metabolic encephalopathy.

OCULAR MYOPATHIES

Myasthenia gravis

Introduction

Myasthenia gravis (MG) is an autoimmune disease in which antibodies mediate damage and destruction of acetylcholine receptors in striated muscle. The resultant impairment of neuromuscular conduction causes weakness and fatigability of skeletal musculature, but not of cardiac and involuntary muscles. The disease affects females twice as commonly as males. MG may be ocular, bulbar (affecting the cranial nerves arising from the lower brainstem) or generalized. Congenital and juvenile forms are rare. A similar clinical picture is found in the Lambert–Eaton myasthenic syndrome mediated by antibodies against pre-synaptic voltage-gated calcium channels; in 60% this is a paraneoplastic phenomenon associated with a lung tumour. Patients positive for anti-MuSK (muscle-specific kinase) antibody may have a distinct form of MG. A range of drugs can exacerbate MG, and should be avoided if possible; those with ophthalmic relevance include many antibiotics, and beta-blockers.

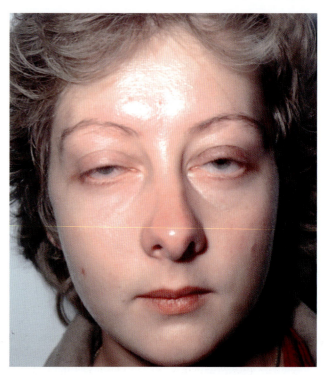

Fig. 19.86 Myopathic facies in myasthenia gravis

Systemic myasthenia

- **Symptoms** are typically of onset in the third decade and may include painless fatigue, often brought on by exercise, commonly in conjunction with ptosis and diplopia. Fatigability affects the musculature of the limbs, facial expression, ocular movements, chewing and speech. Bulbar symptoms include dysphagia and dysarthria; difficulty with breathing is rare.
- **Signs.** The most important feature is peripheral weakness, particularly of the arms and proximal leg muscles, with wasting in long-standing cases. There is characteristically a lack of facial expression (myopathic facies – Fig. 19.86). Ocular features are discussed below.
- **Myasthenic crisis** can be fatal due to respiratory distress if not treated promptly.

Ocular myasthenia

Ocular involvement occurs in 90% of cases and is the presenting feature in 60%. Two-thirds of patients have both ptosis and diplopia.

- **Ptosis** is insidious, bilateral and frequently asymmetrical.
  - Typically worse at the end of the day.
  - Worse on prolonged (60 second) upgaze due to fatigue.
  - Cogan twitch sign is a brief upshoot of the eyelid as the eyes saccade from depression to the primary position.
  - If one eyelid is elevated manually as the patient looks up, the fellow eyelid may show fine oscillatory movements.
- **Diplopia** is frequently vertical, although any or all of the extraocular muscles may be affected. A pseudo-internuclear

ophthalmoplegia may be seen. Patients with stable deviations may benefit from muscle surgery, botulinum toxin injection or a combination of both.

- **Nystagmoid movements** may be present on extremes of gaze. Bizarre defects of ocular motility may also occur so that MG should be considered in the differential diagnosis of any ocular motility disorder that does not fit with a recognized pattern.

Investigations

- **Ice pack test** (Fig. 19.87). This tests for an improvement after an ice pack is placed on the ptotic eyelid (or other affected muscle) for 2 minutes, as cold inhibits the breakdown of acetylcholine by acetylcholinesterase. It is around 75% sensitive but highly specific.
- **Antibody testing** supports a diagnosis of MG and predicts the likelihood of thymoma. Testing is confounded by recent (within 48 hours) general anaesthesia with muscle relaxants.
  - ○ Acetylcholine receptor (AChR) antibodies. Present in around 90% of systemic cases but only 50–70% of ocular myasthenics. Rarely present in Lambert–Eaton.
  - ○ MuSK protein antibodies are positive in 50% of those negative for AChR antibodies; positive patients are less likely to have ocular features and thymoma.
  - ○ Striational antibodies. Antibodies against several contractile elements of skeletal muscle (e.g. titin) may be present; they are found in 80–90% of those with thymoma – and one-third of those without – and can be a marker of more severe MG.
  - ○ Voltage-gated calcium channel antibodies are characteristic of Lambert–Eaton syndrome.
- **Edrophonium (Tensilon) test** (Fig. 19.88). Edrophonium is a short-acting anticholinesterase that confers a transient improvement of weakness in MG. The estimated sensitivity is 85% in ocular and 95% in systemic MG. Potential but uncommon complications include bradycardia and death; resuscitation facilities and appropriate expertise must be readily available on site in case of emergency, and its use may be limited to cases in which less invasive tests have given equivocal results.
  - ○ Atropine 0.3 mg is given intravenously to minimize muscarinic side effects.
  - ○ An intravenous test dose of 0.2 ml (2 mg) edrophonium hydrochloride is given. If definite symptomatic improvement (or adverse reaction) is noted, the test is terminated.
  - ○ The remaining 0.8 ml (8 mg) is given after 60 seconds if necessary.
  - ○ Pre- and post-procedure measurements of ptosis and/or motility (Hess chart) are compared; the effect lasts only 5 minutes.
- **Electromyography** shows characteristic features.
- **Muscle biopsy** reveals neuromuscular junction antibodies and characteristic electron microscopy features, but is not commonly performed.

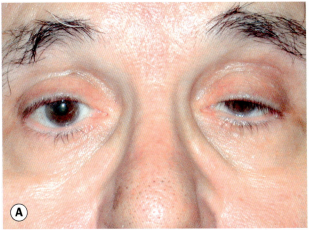
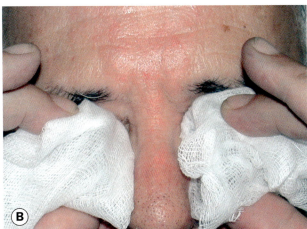
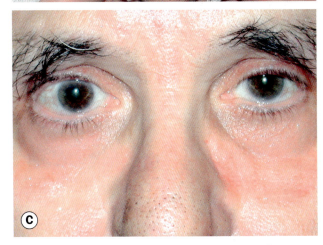

Fig. 19.87 Positive ice pack test in myasthenia gravis. **(A)** Asymmetrical ptosis; **(B)** application of ice; **(C)** improvement of ptosis

(Courtesy of J Yangüela)

- **Thoracic imaging** (MR, CT, CT/PET) to detect thymoma, present in 10%. Imaging may also be used to rule out a lung tumour if Lambert–Eaton syndrome is suspected, or an intracranial mass for ocular myasthenia.
- **Thyroid function testing** should be performed as autoimmune thyroid disease can be associated; there is also

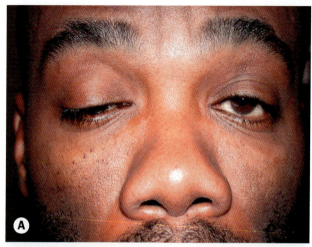

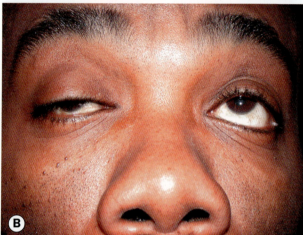

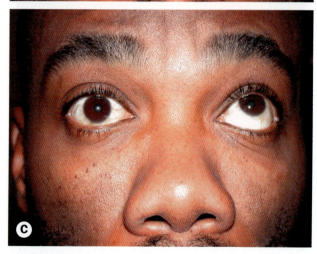

Fig. 19.88 Positive edrophonium test in myasthenia gravis.
(A) Asymmetrical ptosis in the primary position;
(B) defective upgaze; **(C)** following injection of edrophonium there is marked bilateral improvement of ptosis and modest improvement of left, but not right, upgaze

an association with rheumatoid arthritis, pernicious anaemia and systemic lupus erythematosus.

Treatment

An anticholinesterase agent such as pyridostigmine may be used alone in mild disease, but is usually combined with steroids and other immunosuppressive treatment (e.g. azathioprine). Plasmapheresis and intravenous immunoglobulins are shorter-term measures to address acute illness; emergency respiratory support is rarely required. Thymectomy is performed if a thymoma is present; the efficacy of thymectomy to treat MG has not been established with certainty if a tumour is not present, but it is available as a treatment option.

Myotonic dystrophy

Introduction

Myotonic dystrophy is characterized by delayed muscular relaxation after cessation of voluntary effort (myotonia). There are two forms: the classic form, dystrophia myotonica 1 (DM1), is caused by a mutation in the dystrophia myotonica protein kinase gene *DMPK*. DM2 (proximal muscle myopathy, PROMM) involves the gene *CNBP*; DM2 has fewer systemic features (although cataract is frequent), and a better long-term prognosis, but is less common. Inheritance in both forms is AD; sporadic cases are rare. DM1 is discussed below.

Diagnosis

Successive generations tend to exhibit progressively earlier onset and greater severity of disease ('anticipation') due to a progressive increase in the size of the responsible genetic defect (a repeated trinucleotide sequence) at fertilization.

- **Symptoms** typically first occur in the third–sixth decades with weakness of the hands and difficulty in walking.
- **Systemic features**
  - Peripheral. Difficulty in releasing grip, muscle wasting and weakness.
  - Central. Mournful facial expression caused by bilateral facial wasting with hollow cheeks (myotonic facies – Fig. 19.89), and slurred speech from involvement of the tongue and pharyngeal muscles.
  - Other. May include frontal baldness in males, somnolence, hypogonadism, endocrine abnormalities, cardiomyopathy, pulmonary disease, intellectual deterioration and bone changes.
- **Ophthalmic features**
  - Common. Most develop early onset cataract, initially seen as an iridescent dust (sometimes resembling the commonly confused Christmas tree morphology – see Ch. 4) and subsequently progressing to cortical and subcapsular spokes, often in a stellate conformation (see Fig. 9.4B). Ptosis and hypermetropia are also extremely common.

○ Uncommon. Motility dysfunction (strabismus, nystagmus, abnormal saccades and smooth pursuit), light–near dissociation, iris vascular tufts, mild pigmentary retinopathy, optic atrophy and hypotony.
- **Investigation.** Genetic testing will confirm the defect, and can be performed prenatally.

Treatment

Genetic counselling, cardiac monitoring and symptomatic treatment such as cataract surgery, eyelid crutches and frontalis suspension. Patients should be warned of a substantially increased risk of anaesthetic complications.

Chronic progressive external ophthalmoplegia

Chronic progressive external ophthalmoplegia (CPEO) refers to a group of disorders characterized by ptosis and slowly progressive bilateral ocular immobility. The ocular features may occur in isolation or in association with Kearns–Sayre syndrome or oculopharyngeal dystrophy.

Isolated CPEO

- **Ptosis** (Fig. 19.90A–D), usually the first sign, is bilateral and may be asymmetrical. Surgical correction may improve a compensatory head posture but does not restore normal lid movement and risks corneal exposure.

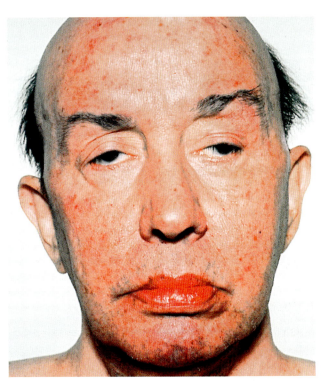

Fig. 19.89 Myotonic facies, frontal baldness and left exotropia

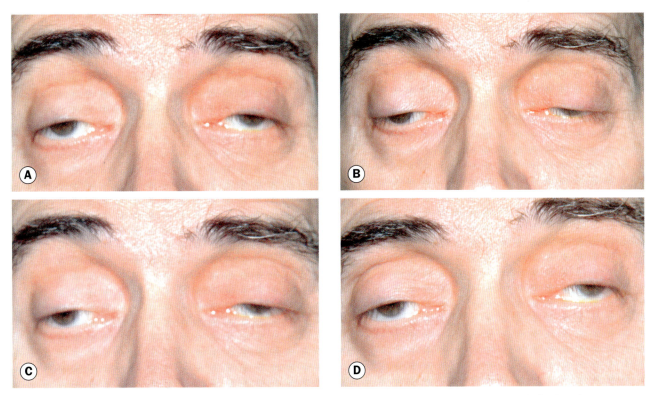

Fig. 19.90 Progressive external ophthalmoplegia. **(A)** Severe bilateral ptosis with defective upgaze; **(B)** defective downgaze; **(C)** defective left gaze; **(D)** defective right gaze

(Courtesy of J Yangüela)

- **Pupils** are usually not involved.
- **External ophthalmoplegia** (see Figs 19.90B–D) begins in young adulthood and is typically symmetrical. It is characterized by a progressive course without remission or exacerbation. Initially upgaze is involved; subsequently lateral gaze is affected so that the eyes may become virtually fixed. Because of this symmetrical loss of eye movement, diplopia is rare although reading may be a problem due to inadequate convergence.
- **Investigations.** Electromyography shows myotonic and myopathic potentials; serum creatine kinase is elevated.
- **Treatment** involves exercise and prevention of contractures. A minority of patients with diplopia may benefit from surgery.

Kearns–Sayre syndrome

Kearns–Sayre is a mitochondrial myopathy associated with mitochondrial DNA deletions. Presentation is in the first and second decades with an insidious progressive external ophthalmoplegia. It is usually sporadic, though inheritance can occur. No proven treatment is currently available.

- **Clinical features**
  - The classic triad is CPEO, cardiac conduction abnormalities and pigmentary retinopathy, the latter typically in a 'salt and pepper' appearance that is most striking at the macula (Fig. 19.91A); mild visual impairment and nyctalopia may occur. Less common is typical retinitis pigmentosa, or choroidal atrophy similar to choroideremia (Fig. 19.91B).
  - Fatigue, proximal muscle weakness, deafness, diabetes, cerebellar ataxia, short stature, renal disease, endocrine abnormalities and dementia may be present.
- **Investigations**
  - Genetic testing.
  - Lumbar puncture: elevation of CSF protein.
  - Electrocardiography demonstrates cardiac conduction defects and should be performed periodically; pacemaker implantation may be required.
  - Histology of extraocular muscles shows 'ragged red fibres' due to intramuscular accumulation of abnormal mitochondria (Fig. 19.92).
  - Endocrine screening is important.

Oculopharyngeal dystrophy

Oculopharyngeal muscular dystrophy (OPMD) is caused by a mutation in *PABPN1*. Like myotonic dystrophy, OPMD is a trinucleotide repeat disorder; inheritance is AD or AR. Clinical onset is typically in early middle age, systemic features including weakness of the pharyngeal muscles and temporalis wasting. Treatment is palliative, e.g. cricopharyngeal myotomy improves swallowing.

MILLER FISHER SYNDROME

Miller Fisher syndrome is a rare form of the acute polyneuropathy Guillain-Barré syndrome, and because of its ocular features may

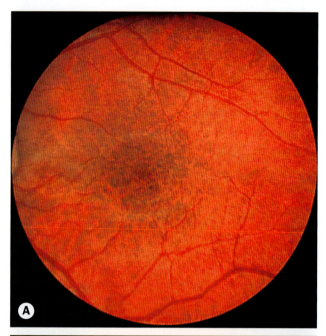

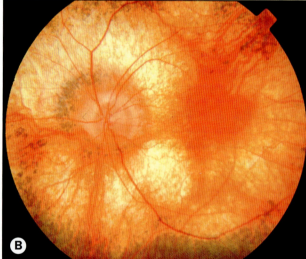

Fig. 19.91 Fundus changes in Kearns–Sayre syndrome. **(A)** 'Salt and pepper' pigmentary retinopathy; **(B)** choroidal atrophy

(Courtesy of R Curtis – fig. B)

present to an eye care professional. It typically affects the extraocular muscles as the first manifestation, with a classic clinical triad of ophthalmoplegia, gait and trunk ataxia, and areflexia. Anti-GQ1b antibodies are present in most cases.

NEUROFIBROMATOSIS

Neurofibromatosis type I

Neurofibromatosis is a disorder that primarily affects cell growth in neural tissues. The two main forms are neurofibromatosis type I (NF1) and type II (NF2). Both may show segmental involvement in which the features are confined to one or more body segments.

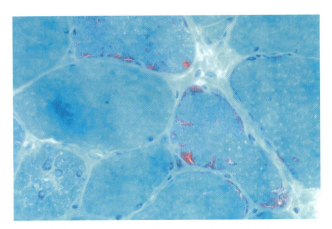

Fig. 19.92 Histology showing 'ragged red fibres' in Kearns–Sayre syndrome

(Courtesy of J Harry and G Misson, from Clinical Ophthalmic Pathology, *Butterworth-Heinemann, 2001)*

NF1 (von Recklinghausen disease) is the most common phacomatosis, affecting 1 : 4000 individuals. Inheritance is AD with irregular penetrance and variable expressivity, though about 50% have new mutations; the gene is *NF1* on chromosome 17, the normal function of which is tumour suppression. The presence of optic nerve glioma and Lisch nodules (iris hamartomas – see Ch. 12) are important ophthalmic diagnostic signs; genetic testing has around 95% specificity – a few positive individuals will not develop NF1..

Systemic features

* **Neurofibromas** may develop anywhere along the course of peripheral or autonomic nerves or on internal organs but do not occur on purely motor nerves. They appear as either solitary nodules (Fig. 19.93A) or more diffuse plexiform lesions, sometimes with associated soft tissue overgrowth (elephantiasis nervosa – Fig. 19.93B) and may also involve internal organs.
* **Skin.** Café-au-lait macules are light-brown patches most commonly found on the trunk (Fig. 19.93C). They appear during the first year of life and increase in size and number throughout childhood.
* **Axillary or inguinal freckles** usually become obvious around the age of 10 years and are pathognomonic.
* **Skeletal abnormalities** may include short stature and facial hemiatrophy.
* **Intracranial tumours**, primarily meningiomas and gliomas.
* **Associations** include malignancy (especially malignant peripheral nerve sheath tumours), gastrointestinal stromal tumours, hypertension and learning difficulties. Recent research suggests that autism spectrum disorder affects nearly half of all NF1 patients.

Ophthalmic features

Regular eye examinations are critical from the time of diagnosis to detect lesions such as optic nerve glioma.

* **Eyelid plexiform neurofibroma** gives a characteristic S-shaped deformity of the upper lid (Fig. 19.94A),

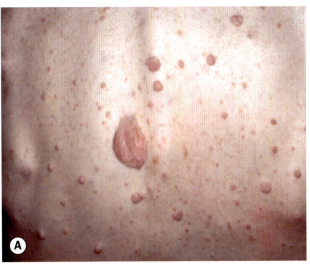

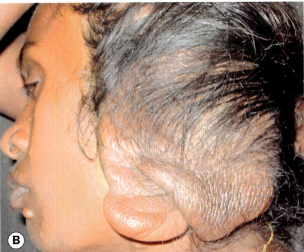

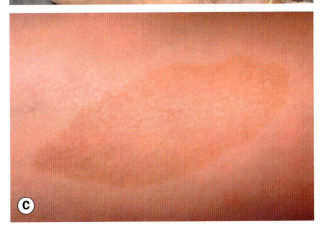

Fig. 19.93 Systemic features of neurofibromatosis type I. **(A)** Discrete cutaneous neurofibromas; **(B)** elephantiasis nervosa; **(C)** café-au-lait macule

(Courtesy of S Kumar Puri – fig. B)

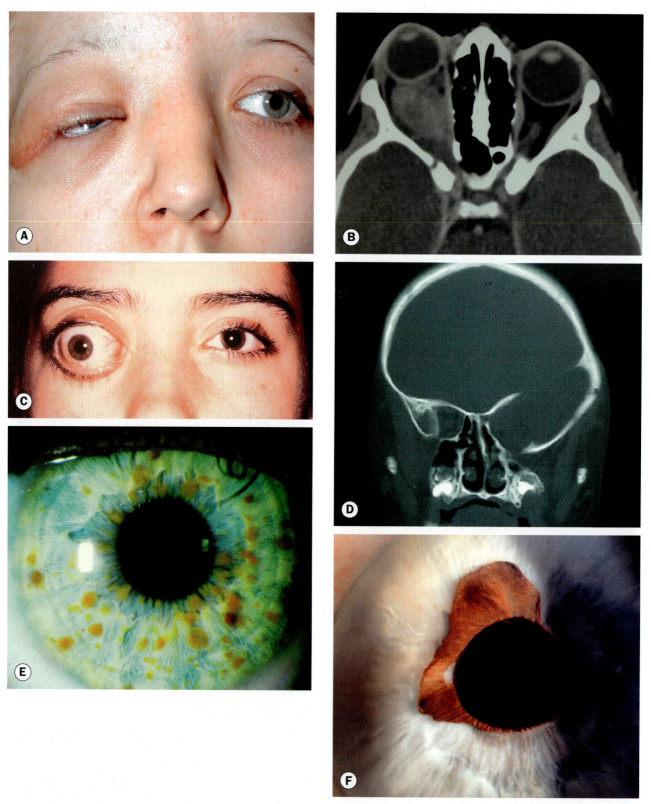

Fig. 19.94 Ocular features of neurofibromatosis type I. **(A)** Nodular plexiform neurofibroma of the eyelid; **(B)** axial CT image showing right proptosis with fusiform enlargement of the optic nerve due to glioma; **(C)** right proptosis due to optic nerve glioma; **(D)** coronal CT image shows absence of the greater wing of the left sphenoid bone; **(E)** Lisch nodules; **(F)** congenital ectropion uveae

(Courtesy of K Nischal – fig. D)

and classically is texturally reminiscent of a 'bag of worms'.

- **Orbital**
  - Optic nerve glioma (15–40%), a pilocytic astrocytoma, typically occurs in young children. It gives a fusiform enlargement of the nerve (Fig. 19.94B) and may present with slowly increasing painless proptosis (Fig. 19.94C), visual impairment (often marked), optic atrophy and strabismus. It can be bilateral and may extend posteriorly to involve the chiasm, optic tract and hypothalamus, sometimes with obstructive hydrocephalus. Slow growth is typical.
  - Other orbital neural tumours, e.g. neurilemmoma (schwannoma), plexiform neurofibroma and meningioma.
  - Spheno-orbital encephalocele is caused by absence of the greater wing of the sphenoid bone (Fig. 19.94D), characteristically causing a pulsating proptosis.
- **Iris lesions**
  - Bilateral Lisch nodules (at least 95%) are hamartomas that develop during the second–third decades, seen as tiny nodular pigmented lesions protruding above the iris surface (Fig. 19.94E and see Figs 12.14C and D).
  - Congenital ectropion uveae (Fig. 19.94F) is uncommon; it may be associated with glaucoma.
  - Mammillations (see Fig. 8.19B) are rare.
- **Prominent corneal nerves.**
- **Glaucoma** is not a common association. When present, it is usually unilateral and congenital, and about 50% have ipsilateral neurofibroma of the upper eyelid and facial hemiatrophy.
- **Fundus**
  - Choroidal naevi are probably more common. NF1 patients with naevi are at increased risk for the subsequent development of choroidal melanoma.
  - Retinal astrocytic hamartoma (astrocytoma), identical to those seen in tuberous sclerosis, is rare.
  - Choroidal hamartomata are multiple small flat pigmented lesions, rare even in NF1.
  - Other lesions that may be more common than in unaffected individuals include congenital hypertrophy of the RPE, myelinated nerve fibres, combined hamartoma of the retina and RPE (possibly increased only in NF2) and retinal capillary haemangioma.

Neurofibromatosis type II

Neurofibromatosis type II (NF2) is less common than NF1; mutations in the *NF2* gene on chromosome 22 are causative. Inheritance is autosomal dominant, but 50% are sporadic. Various diagnostic criteria have been described, but often include bilateral acoustic neuroma (90% – Fig. 19.95), a family history of NF2 and characteristic lesions such as juvenile cataract, neurofibroma, meningioma, glioma, and schwannoma. Ocular lesions are often the first manifestations of the disease.

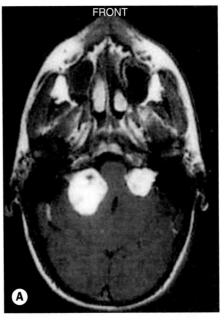

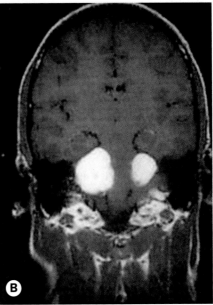

Fig. 19.95 MRI with enhancement showing bilateral acoustic neuroma. **(A)** Axial view; **(B)** coronal view

Ophthalmic features

- **Cataract** affects about two-thirds of patients. The opacities develop prior to the age of 30 years and may be posterior subcapsular or capsular, cortical or mixed.
- **Fundus.** Epiretinal membrane is frequent, and combined hamartoma of the retina and retinal pigment epithelium is relatively common.
- **Ocular motor defects** (10%).
- **Less common.** Optic nerve sheath meningioma, optic nerve glioma, unilateral Lisch nodules, abnormal electroretinogram.

MIGRAINE

Introduction

Migraine is characterized by recurrent headaches widely variable in intensity, duration and frequency. Migrainous headache is commonly unilateral, associated with nausea and vomiting and may be preceded by, or associated with, neurological and mood disturbances. However, all these characteristics are not necessarily present during each attack or in every patient; migrainous aura can occur without headache, and isolated visual aura in particular is a very common presentation to ophthalmologists. A family history is frequent.

Migraine without aura

Migraine without aura (common migraine) is characterized by headache with autonomic nervous system dysfunction such as pallor and nausea, but without the stereotypical neurological or ophthalmic features of classical migraine (see below), such that it often goes undiagnosed. Premonitory features are often vague, and may include changes in mood and poor concentration. The headache is pounding or throbbing, starting anywhere but usually spreading to involve one half or the whole head. Retro-orbital pain may be mistaken for ocular or sinus disease. During the attack, which lasts from hours to a day or more, the patient is frequently photophobic and phonophobic and may seek a quiet dark environment.

Migraine with aura

Migraine with aura (classical migraine) is more readily characterized.

- An attack is heralded by a binocular visual aura that affects the central visual field on one side and typically lasts 5–30 minutes. Initially a binocular negative scotoma is commonly present, but may go unrecognized or be perceived as a vague visual disturbance. Associated positive phenomena develop after a few minutes, and may consist of scintillating scotomata (zig-zags or fortification spectra), 'heat haze' distortions, or less commonly other features such as tunnel vision, progressing slowly across the field over several minutes. Full visual recovery within 30 minutes is typical.
- Other forms of aura are less common: unilateral altered or abnormal sensation (paraesthesia), weakness or disturbance of speech (dysphasia).
- Headache follows the aura and is usually hemicranial, on the side opposite the hemianopia and accompanied by nausea and photophobia. It may, however, be absent, trivial or very severe, with considerable variation between attacks even in the same individual.
- Other pathology can rarely mimic a classical migrainous presentation. The International Headache Society criterion for the diagnosis of migraine with aura is the presence of three out of four of the following:
  a. One or more fully reversible aura symptoms indicating focal cerebral cortical and/or brainstem dysfunction.
  b. At least one aura symptom develops gradually over longer than 4 minutes, or two or more symptoms occur in succession.
  c. No single aura symptom lasts longer than 60 minutes.
  d. Headache follows the aura within 60 minutes, but may begin before or during the aura.
- It is also important that clinical assessment does not suggest an underlying disorder or that investigation has ruled this out; for instance, very rarely a migrainous visual field defect or other aural feature may be permanent, when migraine should be a diagnosis of exclusion.
- **Occipital epilepsy** is very rare; the patient typically sees coloured circles during an attack.

Other forms of migraine

- **Retinal migraine** manifests with visual disturbance that may be similar to classical migraine but affects only one eye. It is a controversial entity, some authorities believing that most cases should be regarded as presumed recurrent ocular vasospasm rather than as true migraine. Young women are most commonly affected, but it is a rare condition, noting that it is common for binocular hemifield symptoms to be misinterpreted by a patient as monocular. There is often a personal history of migraine. It may be prudent to investigate as for retinal embolization (see Ch. 13) and peripheral vasospasm (e.g. Raynaud phenomenon), with appropriate onward referral if necessary. Permanent monocular visual loss is common with recurrent episodes, probably due to vasospastic infarction, and avoidance of potential precipitants and prophylactic treatment should be considered.
- **Ophthalmoplegic migraine** is rare and typically starts before the age of 10 years. It is characterized by a recurrent headache followed after a variable period by transient cranial (often third) nerve palsy. It is now believed to be due to demyelinative disease in most cases.
- **Familial hemiplegic migraine** is characterized by a failure of full recovery of focal neurological features after an attack of migraine subsides.
- **Basilar migraine** occurs in young females, and is characterized by a typical migrainous aura associated with a variety of symptoms related to vertebrobasilar arterial insufficiency.

Treatment

- **General measures** include the elimination of conditions and agents that may precipitate an attack of migraine, such as coffee, chocolate, alcohol, cheese, oral contraceptives, stress, lack of sleep and long intervals without food.
- **Treatment of an acute attack** may be with simple analgesics and, if appropriate, an anti-emetic such as metoclopramide. Other drugs, usually reserved for patients who are refractory to analgesics, include sumatriptan and ergotamine tartrate. Occasionally intravenous agents are used.

- **Prophylaxis** is sometimes required; a broad range of pharmaceutical and other treatments may be utilized and management can be complex.

NEURALGIAS

The following conditions should be considered in the differential diagnosis of ocular or periocular pain, particularly in the absence of detectable physical signs.

- **Cluster headache** typically affects young to middle-aged men. It is of particular interest to ophthalmologists because it is associated with ocular features and may initially be misdiagnosed as a local ocular problem. The condition is characterized by a stereotyped headache accompanied by various autonomic phenomena occurring almost every day for a period of some weeks.
  - The headache is unilateral, oculotemporal, excruciating, sharp and deep.
  - It begins relatively abruptly, lasts between 10 minutes and 2 hours, and then clears quickly.
  - The patient cannot keep still and is agitated, in contrast to a patient with migraine who would rather lie quietly in a dark room.
  - It may occur several times in a 24-hour period, often at consistent times, not infrequently in the early hours of the morning.
  - Once the 'cluster' is over, there may be a long headache-free interval of several years.
  - Associated autonomic phenomena may include lacrimation, conjunctival injection and rhinorrhoea.
  - There may be a transient or permanent postganglionic Horner syndrome.
- **SUNCT (short-lasting, unilateral, neuralgiform headache attacks with conjunctival injection and tearing) syndrome.** This consists of attacks of unilateral orbital, supraorbital or temporal stabbing or pulsating pain lasting from 5 to 240 seconds, occurring at a frequency of 3–200 per day, accompanied by marked ipsilateral conjunctival injection and lacrimation. By definition at least 20 episodes should have occurred for diagnosis. Triggers such as touching the face are common. An underlying disorder is occasionally present (secondary SUNCT).
- **Paroxysmal hemicrania** (Sjaastad syndrome). This consists of severe unilateral headache that is typically ocular, frontal and/or temporal and occurs in brief recurrent episodes (usually five or more per day) associated with one or more ipsilateral autonomic phenomena (tearing, injection, nasal congestion or watering, lid swelling or ptosis). It is more common in women and is much less common than cluster headache. The pain responds well to indomethacin, in contrast to SUNCT, which also features less severe pain, a male preponderance and more marked autonomic features.
- **Trigeminal neuralgia** is characterized by brief attacks of severe pain that start in the distribution of one of the divisions of the trigeminal nerve. The pain is paroxysmal and sharp, usually occurring in multiple bursts in rapid succession lasting a few seconds. Attacks can be triggered either by cutaneous stimulation such as shaving or by motor activity such as chewing. Facial sensation is normal. Treatment involves antiepileptic drugs such as carbamazepine, phenytoin and sodium valproate and occasionally surgical decompression of the trigeminal nerve. A major difference from cluster headache, SUNCT syndrome and paroxysmal hemicrania is that autonomic features are sparse or absent.
- **Primary (idiopathic) stabbing headache** (comprising ophthalmodynia periodica and ice pick syndrome) is characterized by short, sharp jabbing ocular pains, typically located around the orbit or temple, often described as similar to the sensation of being stabbed by a nail or needle and lasting from less than a second up to a few seconds. The pains may occur as isolated episodes or in brief repeated flurries. Frequency varies from a very occasional episode up to dozens per day. By definition there are no other accompanying symptoms and no causative disorder is identifiable. There is usually no trigger. It is more common in women, and children can be affected.
- **Raeder paratrigeminal syndrome** typically affects middle-aged men. It is characterized by severe unilateral headache with periocular pain in the distribution of the first division of the trigeminal nerve associated with an ipsilateral Horner syndrome. The pain may last from hours to weeks before it resolves spontaneously. Carotid dissection (blood entering the potential space between the inner and outer layers of the artery – Fig. 19.96) must be excluded with urgency.
- **Herpes zoster ophthalmicus** frequently presents with pain 2–3 days before the onset of the characteristic vesicular rash. Zoster sine herpete denotes shingles without the development of a rash.

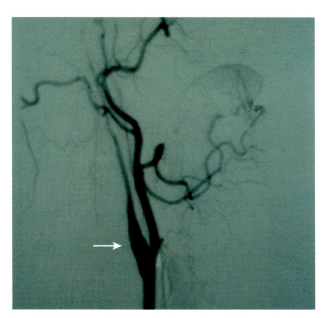

Fig. 19.96 Digital subtraction angiography showing typically flame-shaped carotid dissection (arrow)
(Courtesy of N Rogers)

- **Occipital neuralgia** is characterized by attacks of pain that begin in the occipital region but may spread to the eye, temple and face.

FACIAL SPASM

Benign essential blepharospasm

Introduction

Essential blepharospasm is an uncommon but distressing idiopathic disorder that often presents in the sixth decade and affects women more commonly than men. It is characterized by progressive bilateral involuntary spasm of the orbicularis oculi and upper facial muscles (Fig. 19.97). In severe cases blepharospasm may temporarily render the patient functionally blind. Common precipitants include stress and bright light (photophobia is a common accompanying symptom), with alleviation by relaxation and talking. It does not occur during sleep. In combination with oromandibular dystonia it comprises Meige (Fig. 19.98) or Brueghel syndromes. There is occasionally an underlying identifiable cause, particularly basal ganglia disease, but in a clinically typical case investigation is not required.

Treatment

Prior to commencing treatment, it is important to exclude reflex blepharospasm, most commonly due to ocular surface disease, and extrapyramidal conditions such as Parkinson disease. A cranial and peripheral nervous system examination should be performed.
- **Tinted spectacle lenses** frequently provide amelioration.
- **Treating ocular surface disease** may be helpful.
- **Medical** treatment with a great variety of drugs has been reported to ameliorate specific types of blepharospasm, but their efficacy is disappointing.

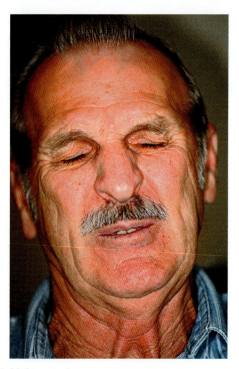

Fig. 19.98 Meige syndrome
(Courtesy of JA Nerad, KD Carter and MA Alford, from 'Oculoplastic and Reconstructive Surgery', in Rapid Diagnosis in Ophthalmology, *Mosby 2008)*

- **Botulinum toxin injection** (e.g. 2.5–5 units injected subcutaneously at 3–4 periocular sites) affords relief in most (95%) patients by temporary paralysis of the injected muscles; typically, repeat injections are required every 3 months. Common but temporary adverse effects include ptosis, lagophthalmos, dry eye and occasionally diplopia.

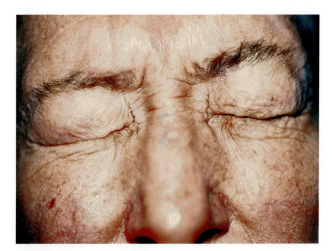

Fig. 19.97 Essential blepharospasm

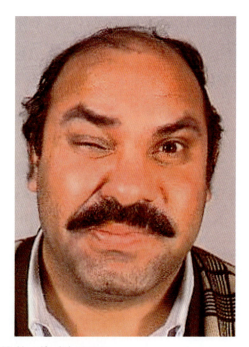

Fig. 19.99 Hemifacial spasm

- **Surgery.** Myectomy is now rarely performed but can be considered in patients intolerant or unresponsive to botulinum toxin.

Hemifacial spasm

Hemifacial spasm is a unilateral condition that presents in the fifth–sixth decades of life. It is characterized initially by brief spasm of the orbicularis oculi which later spreads along the distribution of the facial nerve (Fig. 19.99). The condition is commonly idiopathic, but may stem from irritation of the seventh cranial nerve at any point in its course; facial hyperkinesia may also occur several months or years after Bell palsy. Neuroimaging should be performed to exclude a compressive aetiology. Treatment is similar to that of essential blepharospasm.

Ocular side effects of systemic medication

CORNEA

Vortex keratopathy (cornea verticillata)

Clinical features

In approximately chronological order:

- Fine golden-brown opacities form an irregular horizontal line in the lower corneal epithelium of both eyes, similar to that of the common age-related Hudson–Stähli iron line.
- Several irregular branching horizontal lines form a pattern resembling the whiskers of a cat.
- With an increasing number of branches a whorled pattern develops, centred on a point below the pupil and swirling outwards, usually sparing the limbus.
- Associated pigmented clumps and iron deposition have been described.

Causes

- **Amiodarone**
  - Amiodarone is a cardiac antiarrhythmic agent.
  - Virtually all patients develop keratopathy (Fig. 20.1A), often soon after commencement. In general, the higher the dose and the greater the duration of use the more substantial the corneal changes.
  - Vision is minimally impaired in around 5%, with loss of a single line of Snellen acuity, mild blurring and haloes, though rarely are these sufficient for discontinuation of the drug. The keratopathy reverses (slowly) on discontinuation.
  - Amiodarone can also cause anterior subcapsular lens deposits and optic neuropathy (see below).
- **Antimalarials**
  - Chloroquine and hydroxychloroquine are quinolones used in the treatment of certain autoimmune connective tissue diseases and in the prophylaxis and treatment of malaria.

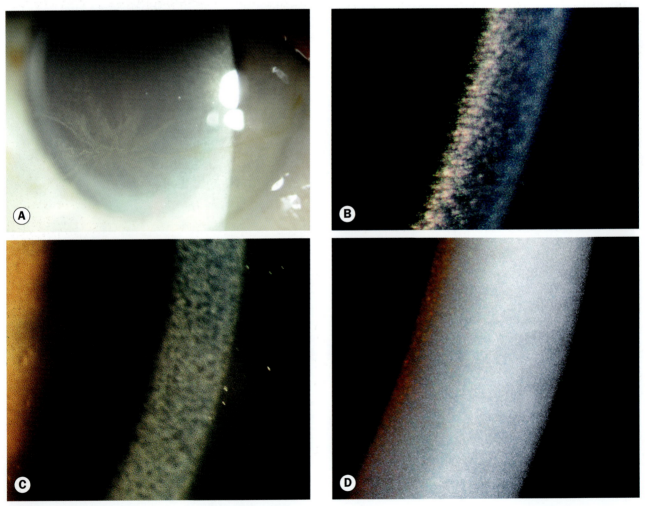

Fig. 20.1 Drug-induced keratopathies. **(A)** Amiodarone-induced vortex; **(B)** chlorpromazine; **(C)** argyrosis; **(D)** chrysiasis
(Courtesy of L Zografos – fig. C)

○ In contrast to chloroquine retinopathy (see below), keratopathy bears no relationship to dosage or duration of treatment. The changes are usually reversible on cessation of therapy, and sometimes clear despite continued administration.

- **Others.** Numerous other drugs have been reported as occasional causes of vortex keratopathy.
- **Fabry disease.**

Chlorpromazine

Chlorpromazine is used as a sedative and to treat psychotic mental illness. Some patients on long-term therapy may develop subtle diffuse yellowish-brown granular deposits in the corneal endothelium, Descemet membrane and deep stroma (Fig. 20.1B) within the palpebral fissure area. Anterior lens capsule deposits and retinopathy may also occur (see below).

Argyrosis

Argyrosis is a discoloration of ocular tissues secondary to silver deposits, and may be iatrogenic or from occupational exposure. Keratopathy is characterized by greyish-brown granular deposits in Descemet membrane (Fig. 20.1C). The conjunctiva may also be affected.

Chrysiasis

Chrysotherapy is the therapeutic administration of gold, usually in the treatment of rheumatoid arthritis. Chrysiasis is the deposition of gold in living tissue, and typically occurs only after prolonged administration. Virtually all patients who have received a total dose of gold compound exceeding 1500 mg develop corneal deposits, characterized by dust-like or glittering purple granules scattered throughout the epithelium and stroma, concentrated in the deep layers and the periphery (Fig. 20.1D). The findings are innocuous and are not an indication for cessation of therapy. In some cases the deposits clear after stopping treatment whilst in others they may persist. Other toxic effects of gold are innocuous lens deposits and, occasionally, marginal keratitis.

Amantadine

Amantadine is an oral agent used in the treatment of Parkinson disease and related conditions. Some patients develop diffuse white punctate opacities that may be associated with epithelial oedema, 1–2 weeks after commencement of the drug, which resolve with discontinuation.

CILIARY EFFUSION

Topiramate

Topiramate is an anticonvulsant also used in the treatment of migraine. It can cause acute angle-closure glaucoma with associated myopia due to ciliochoroidal effusion. A similar phenomenon

has been reported with other drugs, especially other sulfonamides including acetazolamide.

- **Presentation** is usually within a month of starting treatment, with blurred vision, and sometimes haloes, ocular pain and redness.
- **Signs** include shallowing of the anterior chamber and raised intraocular pressure.
- **Treatment** consists of reducing the intraocular pressure and stopping the drug.
- **Prognosis** is usually good provided the complication is recognized.

LENS

Steroids

Both systemic and topical steroids are cataractogenic; resultant opacities are initially posterior subcapsular (Fig. 20.2A), with subsequent anterior subcapsular involvement. Individual liability seems to vary; children may be more susceptible than adults. The

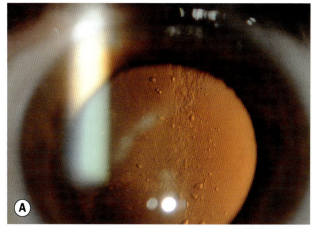

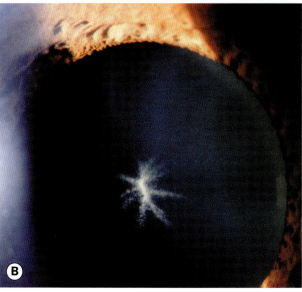

Fig. 20.2 (A) Steroid-induced posterior subcapsular cataract; **(B)** anterior capsular deposits due to chlorpromazine

relationship between dose and duration and cataract formation is unclear, though higher doses and length of treatment are associated with greater risk. Early opacities may regress if steroids are discontinued, though sometimes progression may occur despite withdrawal.

Other drugs

- **Chlorpromazine** may cause the deposition of innocuous, fine, stellate, yellowish-brown granules on the anterior lens capsule within the pupillary area (Fig. 20.2B) in 50% of patients who have received a cumulative dose of 1000 g. The deposits persist despite discontinuation.
- **Gold** (see 'Cornea' above) causes innocuous anterior capsular deposits in about 50% of patients on treatment for longer than 3 years.
- **Allopurinol**, used in the treatment of gout, increases the risk of cataract formation in elderly patients with a high cumulative dose or extended treatment duration.

UVEITIS

Rifabutin

Rifabutin is used mainly in the management and prophylaxis of mycobacterial infections. It may cause acute anterior uveitis (AAU), typically associated with a hypopyon; associated vitritis may be mistaken for endophthalmitis. Concomitant use of drugs such as clarithromycin and fluconazole that inhibit the metabolism of rifabutin will increase the risk of uveitis. Treatment involves dose reduction or withdrawal of the drug.

Cidofovir

Cidofovir is used in the management of cytomegalovirus (CMV) retinitis in acquired immunodeficiency syndrome (AIDS). AAU with few cells but marked fibrinous exudate may develop following repeated intravenous infusions. Vitritis is common and hypopyon may occur with long-term administration. Treatment with topical steroids and mydriatics is usually successful, obviating the need to discontinue therapy.

Bisphosphonates

Bisphosphonates are a class of drugs that retard absorption of bone, commonly in osteoporosis but also in several other conditions. They activate certain T cells, and it is thought that uveitis (usually anterior) and scleritis sometimes seen following administration is related to this. Inflammation typically occurs within two days of commencement of a bisphosphonate, or earlier after intravenous administration.

Sulfonamides

Uveitis has been reported associated with sulfonamide treatment, but is rare. Sulfonamides can also precipitate ciliary effusion with myopia and angle closure (see above) and are a well-documented cause of Stevens–Johnson syndrome.

Fluoroquinolones

Systemic administration of fluoroquinolone antibiotics, particularly moxifloxacin, has been associated with acute extensive anterior segment pigment dispersal (see also bilateral acute iris transillumination (BAIT) and bilateral acute depigmentation of the iris (BADI) in Ch. 10). It is not clear whether inflammation is the primary mechanism, which may be phototoxicity due to sensitization by the drug in predisposed individuals.

Tumour necrosis factor inhibitors

Although these drugs (e.g. etanercept, infliximab, adalimumab) have been adopted for the treatment of ocular inflammation, paradoxically uveitis has also been documented as an adverse effect. The induction of sarcoidosis has also been reported.

RETINA

Antimalarials

Introduction

Antimalarials are melanotropic: they are concentrated in melanin-containing structures of the eye, such as the retinal pigment epithelium (RPE) and choroid. Irreversible retinal toxicity develops in a small proportion of patients taking the drug; progression can occur subsequently despite discontinuation of the drug. It is now considered that retinal adverse effects may be more common than previously believed. Significant damage can occur without signs on fundus examination, so ancillary testing is a key part of assessment. In theory, hepatic or renal impairment might increase the risk of toxicity. Obesity may lead to miscalculation of the safe dose, as hydroxychloroquine is not stored in fat. Corneal signs are discussed above.

- **Chloroquine** is now much less commonly used given the availability of safer and more effective drugs. Retinal toxicity is related to cumulative dose, the risk of toxicity increasing significantly when the cumulative dose exceeds 300 g. Individual susceptibility seems highly variable, however.
- **Hydroxychloroquine** is much safer than chloroquine. The risk of retinal toxicity is considerably more marked (over 1%) with a cumulative dose over 1000 g, equating to a standard twice-daily dose of 200 mg for around seven years. Fewer than 20 cases have been documented with doses less than 6.5 mg/kg/day, and in none of these had there been less than five years of treatment.

Diagnosis

- **Premaculopathy** consists of early functional and structural changes prior to visible fundus signs; the goal of screening

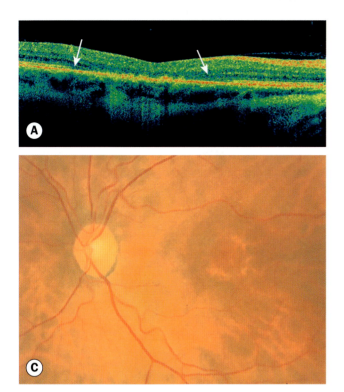

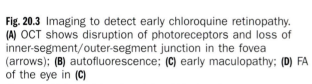

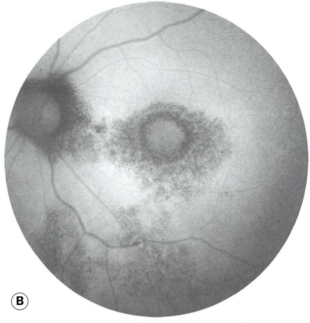

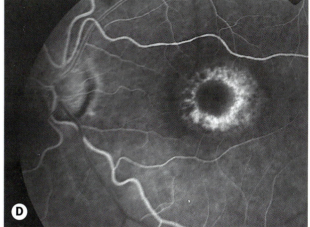

Fig. 20.3 Imaging to detect early chloroquine retinopathy.
(A) OCT shows disruption of photoreceptors and loss of inner-segment/outer-segment junction in the fovea (arrows); **(B)** autofluorescence; **(C)** early maculopathy; **(D)** FA of the eye in **(C)**

(Courtesy of A Agarwal, from Gass' Atlas of Macular Diseases, Elsevier 2012 – figs A and B)

is to detect toxicity at this stage prior to irreversible damage.
- ○ Higher-resolution optical coherence tomography (OCT) imaging can show loss of the inner-segment/outer-segment junctional line (Fig. 20.3A) as an early feature, and is relatively sensitive.
- ○ Fundus autofluoresence (FAF – Fig. 20.3B) and macular pigment density assessment may be useful.
- ○ When available, multifocal electroretinography (see Ch. 15) can demonstrate early changes.
- ○ Subtle central visual field deficits (e.g. Humphrey 10-2, Amsler grid) may be detected, though standard perimetry is probably less sensitive than the imaging modalities above.
- ○ Mild colour vision defects may be present, but the commonly used Ishihara chart is of relatively low sensitivity for this purpose.
- **Early maculopathy** is characterized by a modest reduction of visual acuity – VA (6/9–6/12) and subtle macular

disturbance (Fig. 20.3C); fluorescein angiography (FA) may demonstrate an abnormality more clearly (Fig. 20.3D).
- **Progression of retinopathy** through moderate to severe reduction in VA (6/36–6/60) is associated with corresponding deterioration of the clinical appearance to give a 'bull's eye' macular lesion, characterized by a foveolar island of pigment surrounded by a depigmented zone of RPE atrophy, which is itself encircled by a hyperpigmented ring (Fig. 20.4A). A more substantial macular lesion follows, with widespread RPE atrophy surrounding the fovea (Fig. 20.4B). Retinal arterioles may become attenuated, and pigment clumps can form in the peripheral retina (Fig. 20.4C).

Screening

- **Patient education** is critical to ensure the importance of compliance with screening is understood.

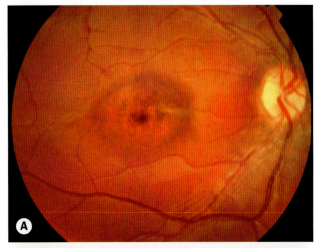

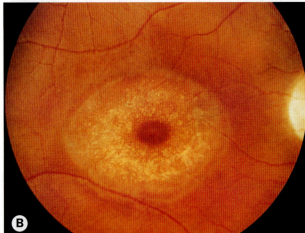

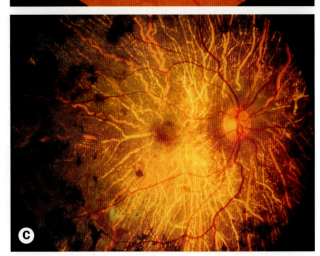

Fig. 20.4 Chloroquine retinopathy of progressive severity (see text)
(Courtesy of Moorfields Eye Hospital – fig. B; J Salmon – fig. C)

- **Baseline assessment** before or soon after commencement of treatment is advisable, including documentation of functional visual parameters together with ancillary testing as available. This serves as a basis for future comparison and also helps to exclude pre-existing maculopathy as a potential relative contraindication.

- **Annual review.** In the absence of special risk factors, routine annual review with ancillary testing (central visual fields and SD-OCT as a minimum) should begin after a maximum of 5 years; earlier review may be appropriate for children, for chloroquine treatment or if there are supplementary risk or complicating factors such as older age, age-related maculopathy, cataract or substantial hepatic/renal impairment.

- **Discontinuation of the drug** should be discussed with the patient's rheumatologist if toxicity is suspected.

Phenothiazines

- **Thioridazine** is used to treat schizophrenia and related psychoses. The normal daily dose is 150–600 mg. Doses that exceed 800 mg/day for just a few weeks may be sufficient to cause reduced VA and impairment of dark adaptation. Progressive retinal toxicity can occur (Fig. 20.5):
  - 'Salt and pepper' pigmentary disturbance involving the mid-periphery and posterior pole is an earlier feature.
  - Progression to plaque-like pigmentation and focal loss of the RPE and choriocapillaris.
  - Eventually, diffuse loss of the RPE and choriocapillaris is seen.

- **Chlorpromazine.** The normal daily dose is 75–300 mg. Retinal toxicity is a risk usually if substantially larger doses are used over a prolonged period, and is characterized by nonspecific pigmentary granularity and clumping.

Drug-induced crystalline maculopathies

- **Tamoxifen** is an anti-oestrogen used in the treatment of some patients with breast carcinoma. The normal daily dose is 20–40 mg. Ocular complications are uncommon; retinal toxicity with visual impairment may develop in patients on

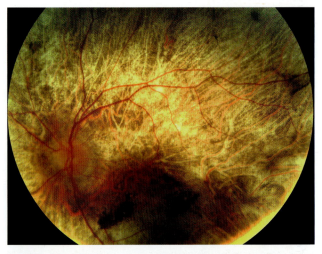

Fig. 20.5 Thioridazine retinopathy showing pigmented plaques and atrophy of the RPE and choriocapillaris
(Courtesy of S Chen)

higher doses but only very rarely with standard doses. Retinopathy (Figs 20.6A and B) is characterized by bilateral fine yellow crystalline deposits in the inner layers of the retina, and punctate grey lesions in the outer retina and RPE. Visual impairment is thought to be caused by maculopathy, including foveolar cyst formation; OCT imaging is a sensitive detection method. A rare side effect is optic neuritis, reversible on cessation of therapy.

- **Canthaxanthin** is a carotenoid used, often in quite high doses, to simulate sun tanning. Over prolonged periods it may cause the deposition of innocuous glistening yellow inner retinal deposits in a doughnut conformation at the posterior poles (Fig. 20.6C). The deposition is slowly reversible.
- **Methoxyflurane** is an inhalant general anaesthetic. It is metabolized to oxalic acid, which combines with calcium to form an insoluble salt and is deposited in tissues including the RPE. Prolonged administration may lead to renal failure and secondary hyperoxalosis. Ocular involvement is

characterized by calcium oxalate crystals scattered throughout the retina associated with mild visual impairment, and subsequently by RPE hyperplasia at the posterior pole (Fig. 20.6D).
- **Nitrofurantoin** is an antibiotic used principally in the treatment of urinary tract infections. Long-term use may result in slight visual impairment associated with superficial and deep glistening intraretinal deposits distributed in a circinate pattern throughout the posterior pole.
- **Non-drug causes** of crystalline maculopathy are given in Table 20.1.

Other drugs causing retinopathy

- **Interferon alfa** is used in a range of conditions, including hepatitis C and numerous malignant tumours. Retinopathy occurs in some patients, particularly those on high-dose therapy, and is characterized by cotton wool spots and retinal haemorrhages (Fig. 20.7A). FA shows areas of focal

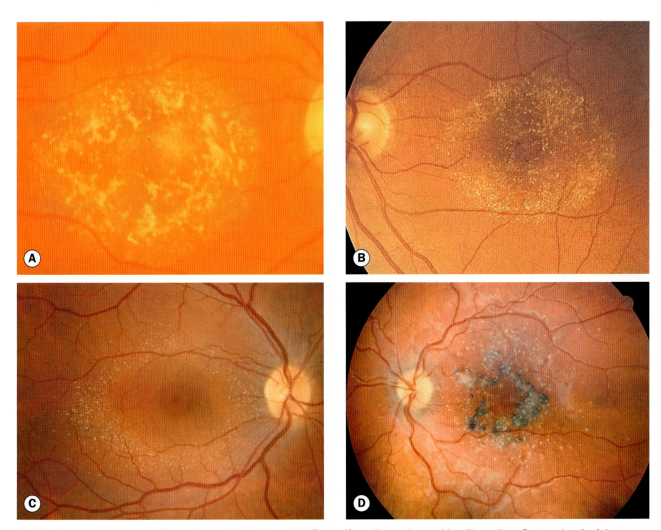

Fig. 20.6 Drug-induced crystalline retinopathies. **(A)** and **(B)** Tamoxifen; **(C)** canthaxanthin; **(D)** methoxyflurane (oxalosis)
(Courtesy of J Donald M Gass, from Stereoscopic Atlas of Macular Diseases, *Mosby, 1997 – fig. A; L Merin – figs C and D)*

Table 20.1 Other causes of macular crystals

Primary hyperoxaluria
Bietti corneoretinal crystalline dystrophy
Cystinosis
Sjögren–Larsson syndrome
Gyrate atrophy
Acquired parafoveal telangiectasis
Talc-corn starch emboli
West African crystalline maculopathy

capillary non-perfusion (Fig. 20.7B). Changes usually resolve spontaneously with cessation of therapy, and in the majority of patients the visual prognosis is good. Less common ocular side effects include cystoid macular oedema, extraocular muscle paresis, optic disc oedema and retinal vein occlusion.

- **Desferrioxamine** is a chelating agent used to manage chronic iron overload, generally to prevent haemosiderosis in patients with conditions requiring regular transfusion. It is most commonly administered via slow subcutaneous infusion. Presentation is with rapid visual loss; initially the fundi may be normal or show only mild macular greying, but within several weeks mottled pigmentary changes develop (Fig. 20.8A), associated with abnormal electrodiagnostic findings. FA shows widespread punctate hyperfluorescence (Fig. 20.8B).

- **Nicotinic acid** is a cholesterol-lowering agent. A small minority of patients develop retinopathy when doses greater than 1.5 g daily are used, in the form of a cystoid maculopathy suggestive of cystoid macular oedema (Fig. 20.9) but without leakage on FA. The changes cause a mild reduction of VA, but resolve with discontinuation of the drug.

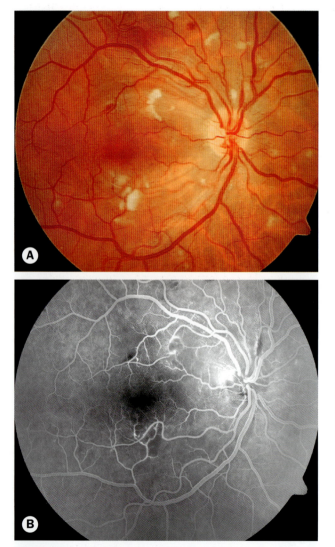

Fig. 20.7 (A) Interferon retinopathy; **(B)** FA showing focal areas of capillary non-perfusion
(Courtesy of J Martin, P Gili)

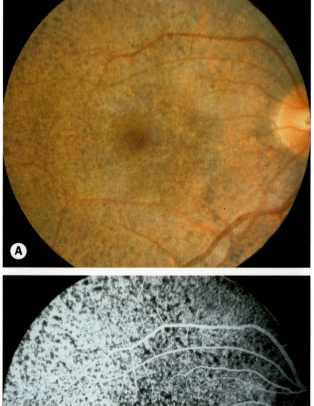
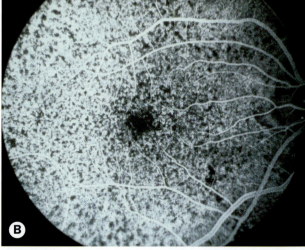

Fig. 20.8 (A) Desferrioxamine retinopathy; **(B)** fluorescein angiography showing diffuse punctate hyperfluorescence
(Courtesy of R Smith)

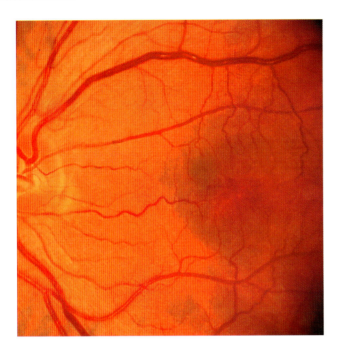

Fig. 20.9 Nicotinic acid maculopathy
(Courtesy of J Donald M Gass, from Stereoscopic Atlas of Macular Diseases, *Mosby, 1997)*

OPTIC NERVE

Ethambutol

Ethambutol is used in the treatment of tuberculosis, generally in a multidrug regimen. Its overall safety profile is favourable, but acute or chronic optic neuritis, of uncertain mechanism, can occur. Toxicity is broadly dose- and duration-dependent; the incidence is as high as 18% at a daily dose over 35 mg/kg, but is rare (<1%) with a standard daily dose of 15 mg/kg or lower. Toxicity typically occurs between 3 and 6 months of starting treatment, though has been reported after only a few days. Renal dysfunction may confer a higher risk of toxicity as ethambutol is excreted via the kidneys.

- **Symptoms** may be absent, but typically include painless bilateral blurring, usually central though sometimes paracentral or peripheral. Impairment of colour vision may be noticed.
- **Signs** include minimal to severe reduction in VA, normal or slightly swollen optic discs with splinter-shaped haemorrhages, and normal or sluggish pupils. Red–green dyschromatopsia is the most common objective abnormality of colour vision, but subtle (undetectable on Ishihara testing) blue–yellow defects may be an early finding.
- **Visual field defects** can be central or peripheral.
- **Prognosis** is good following cessation of treatment, although recovery can be prolonged. A minority sustain permanent visual impairment, with optic atrophy.
- **Screening.** Baseline VA and Ishihara testing are prudent prior to starting ethambutol, and the patient should be

advised of the necessity of reporting any visual disturbance. Repeat testing should be performed frequently – possibly monthly – when the dose is more than 15 mg/kg, and every 3–6 months with lower doses. Ethambutol should be stopped immediately if toxicity develops, with consideration also given to discontinuation of isoniazid if being used synchronously (see below).

Isoniazid

Isoniazid may very rarely cause toxic optic neuropathy; the risk is higher when given in combination with ethambutol.

Amiodarone

Optic neuropathy, probably demyelinative, affects 1–2% of patients on long-term amiodarone treatment. It is almost certainly not dose-related. Distinction from non-arteritic anterior ischaemic optic neuropathy (NAION), which also affects patients with systemic vascular disease, may be difficult; it has been suggested that NAION is more common in patients on amiodarone. Differentiation is clinically important as it is key to a decision about whether to discontinue the drug. The presence of a crowded optic disc, speed of onset, bilaterality, duration of disc swelling and features of systemic amiodarone toxicity may be helpful in this regard.

- **Presentation** is with sudden or insidious unilateral or bilateral visual impairment, after a mean period of 6–9 months taking the drug. About one-third of patients are asymptomatic.
- **Signs** in a majority are unilateral or bilateral optic disc swelling that may persist for a few months after medication is stopped. Corneal features are discussed above.
- **Investigation**
  ○ Cranial imaging may be indicated when bilateral disc swelling is present.
  ○ Visual field defects are of varied configuration and severity, and may be reversible or permanent.
- **Prognosis** is variable; cessation of the drug usually improves vision, but 20% may deteriorate further. Final VA of worse than 6/60 occurs in around 20% of eyes.
- **Screening** has been suggested by some authors, but no consensus exists as to its benefit. Patients should be warned of the risk and cautioned to report visual symptoms immediately.

Vigabatrin

Bilateral concentric, predominantly nasal visual field constriction occurs in many patients taking the antiepileptic drug vigabatrin due to photoreceptor and ganglion cell damage; it is uncommon at a cumulative total dose of <1 kg, but very common at >3 kg. A maximum daily dose of 3 g is recommended in adults; vigabatrin should be avoided in patients with pre-existing field defects and should not be prescribed in conjunction with other potentially retinotoxic drugs. The threshold for its prescription is generally high due to the ocular toxicity. The risk is higher in males than females.

- **Presentation** is usually months or years after starting treatment with bilateral concentric or binasal visual field defects. Blurring and symptoms related to the defects may occur, but there may be no symptoms, with normal VA unless scotomata are at or close to fixation.
- **Signs** may be absent but optic atrophy may be present. Other subtle signs can include peripheral atrophy, arteriolar narrowing, abnormal macular reflexes and surface wrinkling. OCT can detect peripapillary retinal nerve fibre layer atrophy, including prior to the development of field defects.
- **Prognosis.** Changes persist if treatment is stopped, but sometimes do not progress if continued.

- **Screening**. A baseline visual assessment, including visual fields and OCT, is recommended prior to starting treatment and thereafter every 3 months. In young children and others unable to perform field or OCT testing, the optimal monitoring modality is undetermined.

Methotrexate

Methotrexate is a very rare cause of acute or gradual visual loss due to optic neuropathy; reduced VA, dyschromatopsia and visual field loss occur and could be linked to folic acid metabolism, levels of which should be checked; vitamin B_{12} and folate supplementation may be helpful.

EYELID TRAUMA

Periocular haematoma

A 'black eye', consisting of a haematoma (focal collection of blood) and/or periocular ecchymosis (diffuse bruising) and oedema (Fig. 21.1A) is the most common blunt injury to the eyelid or forehead and is generally innocuous. It is, however, critical to exclude the following more serious conditions:

- **Trauma to the globe or orbit.** It is easier to examine the globe before the lids become oedematous. Once swelling is established, gentle sustained pressure to open the lids will often displace tissue fluid sufficiently to allow visualization of the anterior segment; it is critical not to allow any force on the globe itself until its integrity has been confirmed. Imaging such as computed tomography (CT) or magnetic resonance imaging (MRI) if rapidly available, or bedside ultrasonography (strictly avoiding pressure on the globe), should be considered if there is suspicion of an underlying injury to the eyeball and adequate clinical visualization is not possible.
- **Orbital roof fracture**, especially if the black eye is associated with a subconjunctival haemorrhage without a visible posterior limit (Fig. 21.1B), which sometimes indicates anterior extension from a posterior bleeding point.
- **Basal skull fracture**, which may give rise to characteristic bilateral ring haematomas ('panda eyes' – Fig. 21.1C).

Laceration

The presence of a lid laceration, however insignificant, mandates careful exploration of the wound and examination of the globe and adnexal structures. Any lid defect should be repaired by direct closure whenever possible, even under tension, since this affords the best functional and cosmetic result (Fig. 21.2).

- **Superficial** lacerations parallel to the lid margin without gaping can be sutured with 6-0 black silk or nylon; the sutures are removed after 5–6 days.
- **Lid margin** lacerations invariably gape without careful closure and to prevent notching must be sutured with optimal alignment (Fig. 21.3):
  a. A 5-0 silk vertical mattress suture is inserted in line with the meibomian gland orifices, about 2 mm from the wound edges and 2 mm deep, and left untied.
  b. Tarsal plate edges are apposed with partial-thickness lamellar 5-0 absorbable (e.g. polyglactin) sutures, which are tied anteriorly.
  c. The lid margin silk suture is then tied so that the cut edges slightly pucker the wound; the ends are left fairly long, e.g. 2 cm.
  d. The overlying skin is closed with interrupted 6-0 or 7-0 nylon or absorbable sutures, securing the ends of the silk suture to direct these and its knot away from the cornea.
- **Lacerations with mild tissue loss** just sufficient to prevent direct primary closure can usually be managed by

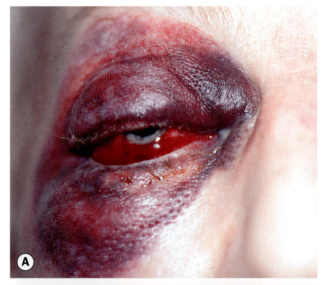
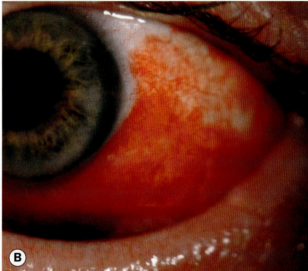
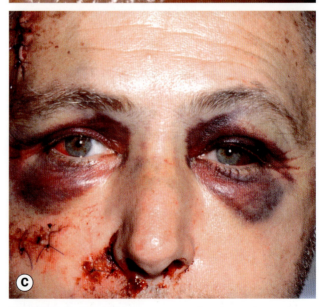

Fig. 21.1 (A) Upper lid haematoma, periocular ecchymosis and oedema; **(B)** subconjunctival haemorrhage with no visible posterior limit; **(C)** 'panda eyes'

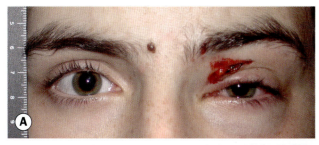

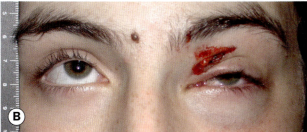

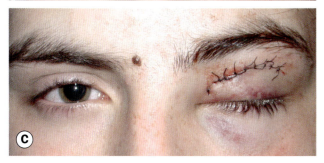

Fig. 21.2 Upper lid laceration. **(A)** Prolapsed fat gives an indication that the wound is of substantial depth; **(B)** failure of upgaze in the eye suggests damage to the levator muscle; **(C)** skin sutures following levator repair – this necessitated extension of the laceration

(Courtesy of S Chen)

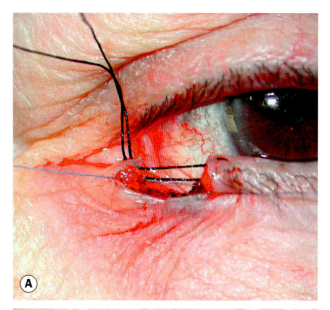

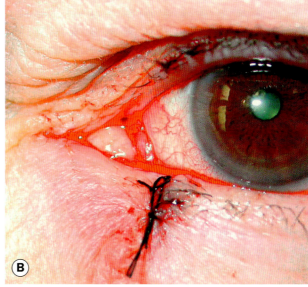

Fig. 21.3 Repair of full-thickness lid laceration. **(A)** Initial approximation of the tarsal plate with an absorbable suture and lid margin with a silk suture; **(B)** completed repair – note that with a laceration near the canaliculus its involvement must be excluded

(Courtesy of J Nerad, K Carter and M Alford, from 'Oculoplastic and Reconstructive Surgery', in Rapid Diagnosis in Ophthalmology, *Mosby 2008)*

performing a lateral cantholysis in order to increase lateral mobility.

- **Lacerations with extensive tissue** loss may require major reconstructive procedures similar to those used following resection of malignant tumours (see Ch. 1).

- **Canalicular lacerations** should be repaired within 24 hours. The laceration is bridged by silicone tubing (Crawford tube), which is threaded down the lacrimal system and tied in the nose, following which the laceration is sutured. Alternatively, repair of a single canaliculus can be performed using a monocanalicular stent (e.g. Mini Monoka – Fig. 21.4) and, if necessary, suturing its footplate to the lid using 8-0 material. The tubing is left *in situ* for 3–6 months.

- **Tetanus status.** It is critical to ensure that the patient's tetanus immunization status is satisfactory after any injury. Without any prior immunization, 250 units of human tetanus immunoglobulin are given intramuscularly (IM); if previously immunized but a booster has not been administered within the last 10 years, IM or subcutaneous tetanus toxoid is given.

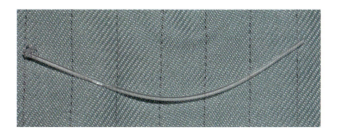

Fig. 21.4 Monocanalicular silicone stent
(Courtesy of S Chen)

ORBITAL TRAUMA

Orbital floor fracture

Introduction

A blow-out fracture of the orbital floor is typically caused by a sudden increase in the orbital pressure from an impacting object that is greater in diameter than the orbital aperture (about 5 cm), such as a fist or tennis ball, so that the eyeball itself is displaced and transmits rather than absorbs the impact (Fig. 21.5). Since the bones of the lateral wall and the roof are usually able to withstand such trauma, the fracture most frequently involves the floor of the orbit along the thin bone covering the infraorbital canal. Occasionally, the medial orbital wall may also be fractured; fractures of the orbital rim and adjacent facial bones require appropriately tailored management. Clinical features vary with the severity of trauma and the interval between injury and examination. Care should be taken to ensure that a full evaluation for head and systemic injury has been performed, and any necessary interspecialty referrals initiated.

Diagnosis

- **Visual function**, especially acuity, should be recorded and monitored as necessary, particularly in the acute situation.
- **Periocular signs** include variable ecchymosis, oedema (Fig. 21.6A) and occasionally subcutaneous emphysema (a crackling sensation on palpation due to air in the subcutaneous tissues).
- **Infraorbital nerve anaesthesia** involving the lower lid, cheek, side of nose, upper lip, upper teeth and gums is very common as the fracture frequently involves the infraorbital canal.
- **Diplopia** may be caused by one of the following mechanisms:
  - Haemorrhage and oedema in the orbit may causing the septa connecting the inferior rectus and inferior oblique

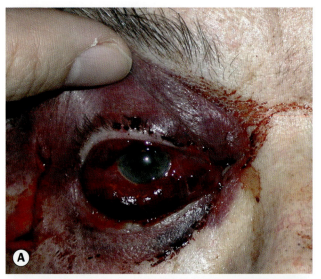
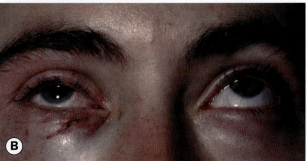
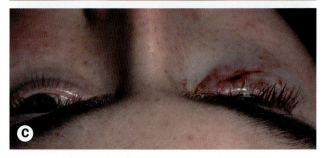

Fig. 21.6 Right orbital floor blow-out fracture. **(A)** Marked periocular ecchymosis, oedema and subconjunctival haemorrhage; **(B)** restricted elevation; **(C)** mild right enophthalmos
(Courtesy of S Chen – fig. A)

muscles to the periorbita to become taut, thus restricting movement of the globe. Ocular motility usually improves as the haemorrhage and oedema resolve.
  - Mechanical entrapment within the fracture of the inferior rectus or inferior oblique muscle, or adjacent connective tissue and fat. Diplopia typically occurs in both upgaze (Fig. 21.6B) and downgaze. Forced duction and the differential intraocular pressure (IOP) test (increasing IOP as a restricted muscle presses on the globe) are positive. Diplopia may subsequently improve if it is mainly due to entrapment of oedematous connective tissue and fat, but usually persists if there is significant involvement of the muscles themselves.

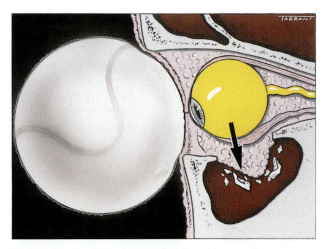

Fig. 21.5 Mechanism of an orbital floor blow-out fracture

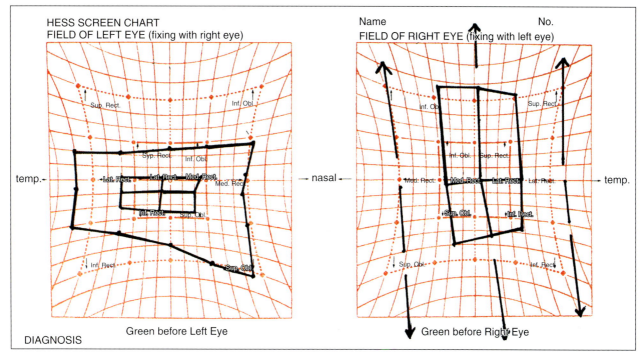

Fig. 21.7 Hess chart of a left orbital floor blow-out fracture shows restriction of left upgaze (superior rectus and inferior oblique) and restriction on downgaze (inferior rectus). There is also secondary overaction of the right eye

○ Direct injury to an extraocular muscle, associated with a negative forced duction test. The muscle fibres usually regenerate and normal function often returns within about 2 months.

● **Enophthalmos** (Fig. 21.6C) may be present if the fracture is severe, although it tends to manifest only after a few days as initial oedema resolves. In the absence of surgical intervention, enophthalmos may continue to increase for about 6 months as post-traumatic orbital tissue degeneration and fibrosis develop.

● **Ocular damage** (e.g. hyphaema, angle recession, retinal dialysis) should be excluded by careful examination of the globe, although this is relatively uncommon in association with a blowout fracture.

● **Hess chart** testing (Fig. 21.7) to map eye movements is useful in assessment and monitoring.

● **CT** with coronal sections (Fig. 21.8) aids in evaluation of the extent of a fracture and determination of the nature of maxillary antral soft-tissue densities, which may represent prolapsed orbital fat, extraocular muscles, haematoma or unrelated antral polyps.

Treatment

● **Initial** treatment generally consists of observation, with the prescription of oral antibiotics; ice packs and nasal decongestants may be helpful. The patient should be instructed not to blow his or her nose, because of the possibility of forcing infected sinus contents into the orbit. Systemic steroids are occasionally required for severe orbital oedema, particularly if this is compromising the optic nerve.

● **Subsequent** treatment is aimed at the prevention of permanent vertical diplopia and/or cosmetically unacceptable enophthalmos.

○ Small cracks unassociated with herniation do not require treatment as the risk of permanent complications is small.

○ Fractures involving up to one-half of the orbital floor, with little or no herniation, no significant enophthalmos and improving diplopia, also do not require treatment.

○ Fractures involving more than one-half of the orbital floor will usually develop significant enophthalmos if left untreated.

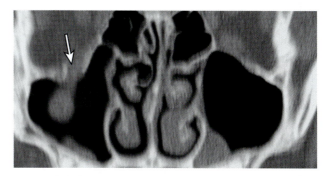

Fig. 21.8 CT of right orbital floor blow-out fracture – coronal view shows a defect in the orbital floor (arrow) and the 'tear drop' sign due to soft tissue prolapse into the maxillary antrum

(Courtesy of A Pearson)

○ Fractures with entrapment of orbital contents, enophthalmos of greater than 2 mm, and/or persistent and significant diplopia in the primary position should be repaired within 2 weeks. If surgery is delayed, the results are less satisfactory due to secondary fibrotic changes.

- **'White-eyed' fracture** is a subgroup for which urgent repair is required to avoid permanent neuromuscular damage. The scenario is generally seen in patients less than 18 years of age, typically with little visible external soft tissue injury, and usually affects the orbital floor. It involves the acute incarceration of herniated tissue in a trap-door effect occurring due to the greater elasticity of bone in younger people. Patients may experience acute nausea, vomiting, and headache; persistent activation of the oculocardiac reflex can occur. CT features may be subtle.
- **Early marked enophthalmos** may also be an indication for urgent repair.
- **Surgical repair** is performed via a transconjunctival or subciliary incision or via the maxillary sinus, with elevation of the periosteum from the orbital floor, freeing of trapped orbital contents and repair of the bony defect with a synthetic implant.

Roof fracture

Introduction

Roof fractures are rarely encountered by ophthalmologists. Isolated fractures, caused by falling on a sharp object (Fig. 21.9) or sometimes a relatively minor blow to the brow or forehead, are most common in children and often do not require treatment. Fractures due to major trauma, with associated displacement of the orbital rim or significant disturbance of other craniofacial bones, typically affect adults.

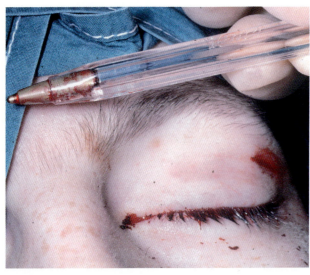

Fig. 21.9 Preoperative image of a patient with an orbital roof fracture caused by a ball-point pen
(Courtesy of R Bates)

Diagnosis

A haematoma of the upper eyelid is typical, together with periocular ecchymosis; these often develop over the course of a few hours and may progressively spread to the side opposite the fracture. Other features of orbital wall fracture as discussed above may be present. Large fractures may be associated with pulsation of the globe due to transmission of cerebrospinal fluid (CSF) pressure, best detected with applanation tonometry.

Treatment

Small fractures may not require treatment but it is important to exclude a CSF leak, which carries a risk of meningitis. Sizeable bony defects with downward displacement of fragments usually warrant reconstructive surgery. General management is similar to that of an orbital floor fracture (see above).

Blow-out medial wall fracture

Medial wall orbital fractures are usually associated with floor fractures; isolated fractures are relatively uncommon. Signs include periorbital ecchymosis and frequently subcutaneous emphysema, which typically develops on blowing the nose. Defective ocular motility involving abduction and adduction is present if the medial rectus muscle is entrapped. CT will demonstrate the fracture; treatment involves release of incarcerated tissue and repair of the bony defect.

Lateral wall fracture

Acute lateral wall fractures (see Fig. 21.11F) are rarely encountered by ophthalmologists. Because the lateral wall of the orbit is more solid than the other walls, a fracture is usually associated with extensive facial damage.

Orbital haemorrhage

Introduction

Orbital (retrobulbar) haemorrhage is important chiefly due to the associated risk of acute orbital compartment syndrome with compressive optic neuropathy, and can lead to irreversible blindness of the affected eye in severe cases. It can occur without or in association with an orbital bony injury. Iatrogenic orbital haemorrhage is not uncommon, typically resulting from a peri- or retrobulbar local anaesthetic block performed to facilitate intraocular surgery. Rare causes include bleeding from vascular anomalies and occasionally spontaneous haemorrhage due to poor clotting.

Diagnosis

Proptosis, eyelid oedema and ecchymosis, haemorrhagic chemosis, ocular motility dysfunction, decreased visual acuity, elevated intraocular pressure, optic disc swelling and a relative afferent pupillary defect are among the possible signs.

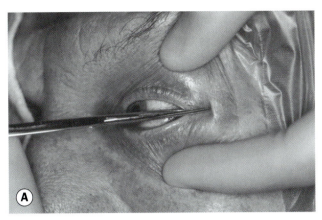
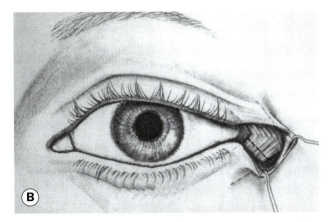

Fig. 21.10 Surgical treatment of acute retrobulbar haemorrhage. **(A)** Lateral canthotomy; **(B)** disinsertion of inferior crus of the lateral canthal tendon

(Courtesy of K Goodall, A Brahma, A Bates, B Leatherbarrow, from International Journal of the Care of the Injured *1999;30:485-90)*

Treatment

Treatment should be immediate when progressive visual deterioration is evident. Canthotomy alone is rarely adequate.

- **Canthotomy.** After clamping the incision site for 60 seconds, scissors are used to make a 1–2 cm horizontal full-thickness incision under local anaesthesia (e.g. 1–2 ml lidocaine 1–2% with adrenaline) at the angle of the lateral canthus (Fig. 21.10A).
- **Cantholysis.** Following canthotomy, the lower lid is retracted downwards and the inferior crus of the lateral canthal tendon transected (Fig. 21.10B) using blunt-tipped scissors, directed inferiorly and inserted adjacent and parallel to the lateral orbital rim between conjunctiva and skin, and angled away from the eyeball. Blood is gently encouraged to drain. If necessary the superior limb of the tendon can also be transected, but this carries a substantial risk of damage to adnexal structures.

TRAUMA TO THE GLOBE

Introduction

Terminology

- **Closed injury** is commonly due to blunt trauma. The corneoscleral wall of the globe is intact.
- **Open injury** involves a full-thickness wound of the corneoscleral envelope.
- **Contusion** is a closed injury resulting from blunt trauma. Damage may occur at or distant to the site of impact.
- **Rupture** is a full-thickness wound caused by blunt trauma. The globe gives way at its weakest point, which may not be at the site of impact.
- **Laceration** is a full-thickness defect in the eye wall produced by a tearing injury, usually as the result of a direct impact.

- **Lamellar laceration** is a partial-thickness laceration.
- **Incised injury** is caused by a sharp object such as glass or a knife.
- **Penetrating injury** refers to a single full-thickness wound, usually caused by a sharp object, without an exit wound. A penetrating injury may be associated with intraocular retention of a foreign body.
- **Perforation** consists of two full-thickness wounds, one entry and one exit, usually caused by a missile.

Investigations

- **Plain radiographs** may be taken when the presence of a foreign body is suspected (Fig. 21.11A).
- **Ultrasonography** may be useful in the detection of intraocular foreign bodies (Fig. 21.11B), globe rupture, suprachoroidal haemorrhage and retinal detachment; it should be performed as gently as possible if there is the risk of an open globe injury, strictly avoiding any pressure on the globe. It is also helpful in planning surgical repair, for example guiding placement of infusion ports during vitrectomy and assessing whether drainage of suprachoroidal haemorrhage is required.
- **CT** is superior to plain radiography in the detection and localization of intraocular foreign bodies (Figs 21.11C and D). It is also of value in determining the integrity of intracranial, facial and intraocular structures (Figs 21.11E and F).
- **MRI** is more accurate than CT in the detection and assessment of injuries of the globe itself, such as an occult posterior rupture, though not for bony injury. However, MRI should not be performed if a ferrous metallic foreign body is suspected.
- **Electrodiagnostic tests** may be useful in assessing the integrity of the optic nerve and retina, particularly if some time has passed since the original injury and there is the suspicion of a retained intraocular foreign body (IOFB).

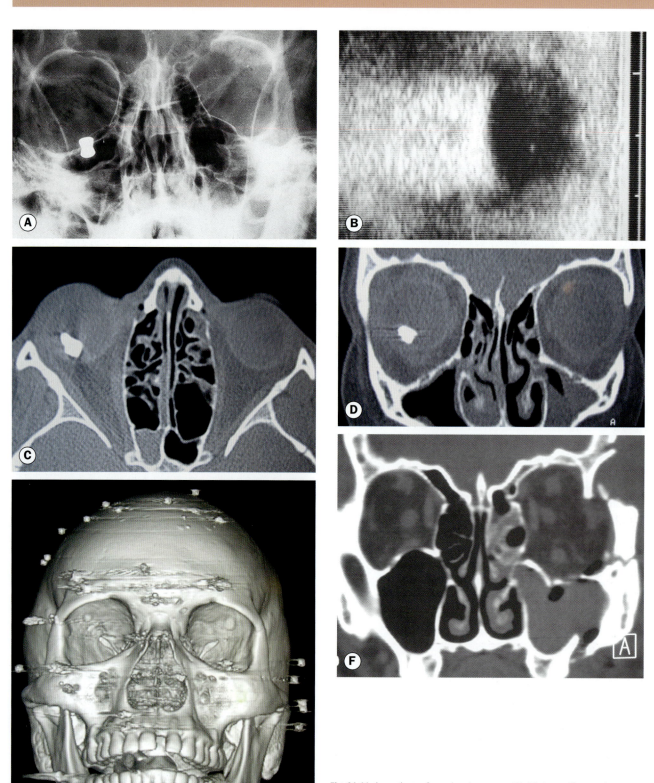

Fig. 21.11 Imaging of ocular trauma. **(A)** Plain radiograph showing a lead air gun pellet; **(B)** foreign body demonstrated by ultrasonography; **(C)** CT axial and **(D)** coronal views localizing a left intraocular foreign body; **(E)** 3D CT reconstruction of a facial shotgun injury; **(F)** CT axial view demonstrating a left lateral orbital wall fracture

(Courtesy of S Chen – figs C–E; A Pearson – fig. F)

Blunt trauma

The most common causes of blunt trauma are squash balls, elastic luggage straps and champagne corks. Severe blunt trauma to the globe results in anteroposterior compression with simultaneous expansion in the equatorial plane (Fig. 21.12) associated with a transient but severe increase in IOP. Although the impact is primarily absorbed by the lens–iris diaphragm and the vitreous base, damage can also occur at a distant site such as the posterior pole. The extent of ocular damage depends on the severity of trauma and tends largely to be concentrated to either the anterior or posterior segment. Apart from obvious ocular damage, blunt trauma commonly results in more obscure long-term effects; the prognosis is therefore necessarily guarded.

Cornea

- **Corneal abrasion** involves a breach of the epithelium, and stains well with fluorescein (Fig. 21.13A). If located over the pupillary area, vision may be grossly impaired. Details of treatment are discussed under 'Recurrent corneal epithelial erosion' in Chapter 6.
- **Acute corneal oedema** may develop following blunt trauma, secondary to focal or diffuse dysfunction of the endothelium and is sometimes seen underlying a large abrasion. It is commonly associated with folds in Descemet membrane and stromal thickening, but usually clears spontaneously.
- **Tears in Descemet membrane** are usually vertical (Fig. 21.13B) and most commonly arise as the result of birth trauma.

Hyphaema

Hyphaema (haemorrhage in the anterior chamber) is a common complication of blunt ocular injury. The source of bleeding is typically the iris root or ciliary body face. Characteristically, the blood settles inferiorly with a resultant 'fluid level' (Fig. 21.14A),

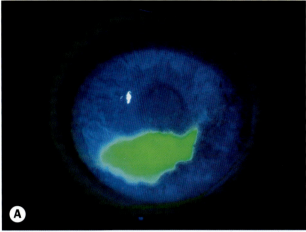
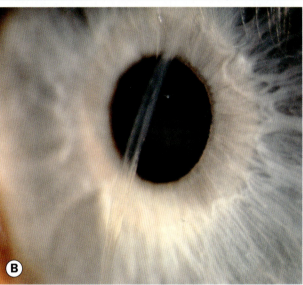

Fig. 21.13 Corneal complications of blunt trauma. **(A)** Large corneal abrasion stained with fluorescein; **(B)** tears in Descemet membrane
(Courtesy of C Barry – fig. A; R Curtis – fig. B)

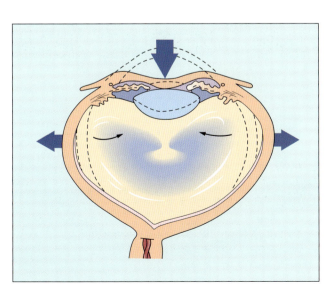

Fig. 21.12 Pathogenesis of ocular damage by blunt trauma

except when the hyphaema is total (Fig. 21.14B). Treatment is aimed at the prevention of secondary haemorrhage and control of any elevation of IOP (see Ch. 10), which as well as optic neuropathy can lead to staining of ocular tissues, particularly the cornea (Fig. 21.14C).

Anterior uvea

- **Pupil.** The iris may momentarily be compressed against the anterior surface of the lens by severe anteroposterior force, with resultant imprinting of pigment from the pupillary margin. Transient miosis accompanies the compression, evidenced by the pattern of pigment corresponding to the size of the miosed pupil (Vossius ring – Fig. 21.15A). Damage to the iris sphincter may result in traumatic mydriasis, which can be temporary or permanent; the pupil reacts sluggishly or not at all to both light and accommodation. Radial tears in the pupillary margin are common (Fig. 21.15B).

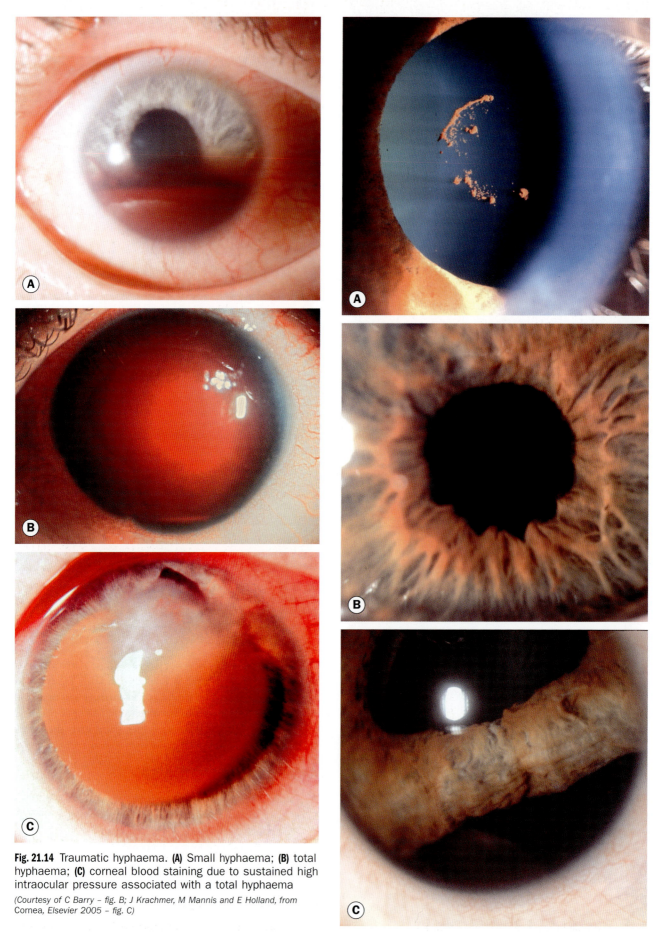

Fig. 21.14 Traumatic hyphaema. **(A)** Small hyphaema; **(B)** total hyphaema; **(C)** corneal blood staining due to sustained high intraocular pressure associated with a total hyphaema

(Courtesy of C Barry – fig. B; J Krachmer, M Mannis and E Holland, from Cornea, Elsevier 2005 – fig. C)

Fig. 21.15 Iris complications of blunt trauma. **(A)** Vossius ring; **(B)** radial sphincter tears; **(C)** iridodialysis

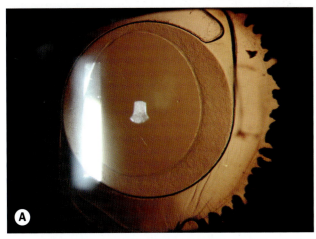

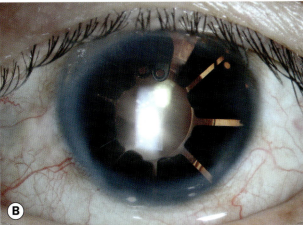

Fig. 21.16 Traumatic aniridia in a pseudophakic eye.
(A) Retroillumination showing lens implant and ciliary processes; **(B)** prosthetic iris
(Courtesy of C Barry)

- **Iridodialysis** is a dehiscence of the iris from the ciliary body at its root. The pupil is typically D-shaped and the dialysis is seen as a dark biconvex area near the limbus (Fig. 21.15C). An iridodialysis may be asymptomatic if covered by the upper lid; if exposed in the palpebral aperture, uniocular diplopia and glare sometimes ensue, and may necessitate surgical repair of the dehiscence. Traumatic aniridia (360° iridodialysis) is rare; in a pseudophakic eye, the detached iris may be ejected through the cataract surgical incision (Fig. 21.16).
- **Ciliary body** (see below).

Intraocular pressure

It is important for IOP to be monitored carefully, particularly in the early period following trauma. Elevation can occur for a variety of reasons, including hyphaema (above) and inflammation (see Ch. 10). In contrast, the ciliary body may react to severe blunt trauma by temporary cessation of aqueous secretion ('ciliary shock') resulting in hypotony; it is important for an occult open injury to be excluded as the cause of the hypotony. Tears extend-

ing into the face of the ciliary body (angle recession) are associated with a risk of later glaucoma.

Lens

- **Cataract** formation is a common sequel to blunt trauma. Postulated mechanisms include direct damage to the lens fibres themselves, and minute ruptures in the lens capsule with an influx of aqueous humour, hydration of lens fibres and consequent opacification. A ring-shaped anterior subcapsular opacity may underlie a Vossius ring. Commonly opacification occurs in the posterior subcapsular cortex along the posterior sutures, resulting in a flower-shaped ('rosette') opacity (Fig. 21.17A) that may subsequently disappear, remain stationary or progress to maturity (Fig. 21.17B). Cataract surgery may be necessary for visually significant opacity.
- **Subluxation** of the lens may occur, secondary to tearing of the suspensory ligament. A subluxated lens tends to deviate towards the meridian of intact zonule; the anterior chamber may deepen over the area of zonular dehiscence, if the lens rotates posteriorly. The edge of a subluxated lens may be visible under mydriasis (see Fig. 21.17B) and trembling of the iris (iridodonesis) or lens (phakodonesis) may be seen on ocular movement. Subluxation of magnitude sufficient to render the pupil partly aphakic may result in uniocular diplopia; lenticular astigmatism due to tilting may occur.
- **Dislocation** due to 360° rupture of the zonular fibres is rare and may be into the vitreous (Fig. 21.17C), or less commonly, into the anterior chamber (Fig. 21.17D); an underlying predisposing condition such as pseudoexfoliation should be suspected.

Globe rupture

Rupture of the globe may result from severe blunt trauma; the prognosis is poor if the initial visual level is light perception or worse. The rupture is usually anterior, in the vicinity of the Schlemm canal, with prolapse of structures such as the lens, iris, ciliary body and vitreous (Fig. 21.18A); an anterior rupture may be masked by extensive subconjunctival haemorrhage (Fig. 21.18B). Rupture at the site of a surgical wound (e.g. cataract, keratoplasty, vitrectomy) is common with substantial blunt force. An occult posterior rupture can be associated with little visible damage to the anterior segment, but should be suspected if there is asymmetry of anterior chamber depth – the anterior chamber of an affected eye is classically deep, with posterior rotation of the iris–lens diaphragm – and IOP in the affected eye is low. Gentle B-scan ultrasonography may demonstrate a posterior rupture, but CT or MR may be necessary; MR is not performed if there is a risk of ferrous IOFB. The principles of repair of a rupture in the scleral envelope are described later.

Vitreous haemorrhage

Vitreous haemorrhage may occur, commonly in association with posterior vitreous detachment. Pigment cells ('tobacco dust') may

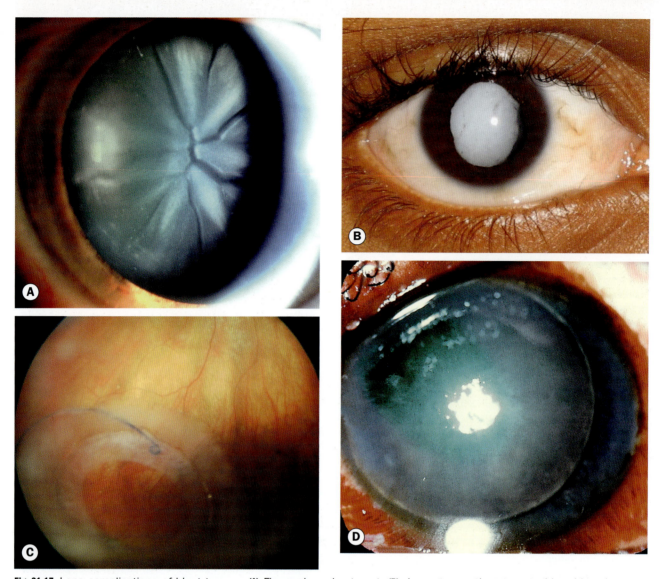

Fig. 21.17 Lens complications of blunt trauma. **(A)** Flower-shaped cataract; **(B)** dense traumatic cataract with subluxation; **(C)** dislocation into the vitreous in a pseudophakic eye with pseudoexfoliation; **(D)** dislocation into the anterior chamber

(Courtesy of S Chen – figs B and C)

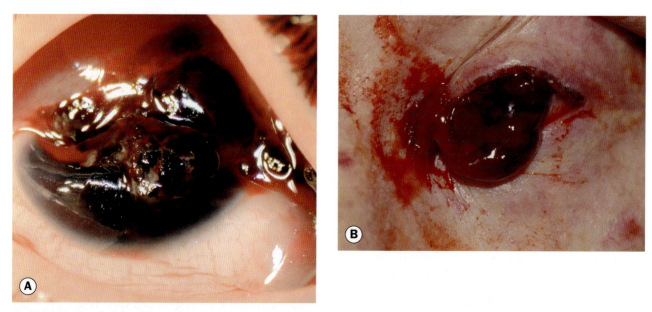

Fig. 21.18 Ruptured globe. **(A)** Large corneal rupture with prolapse of intraocular structures; **(B)** masking of rupture by extensive subconjunctival haemorrhage

(Courtesy of C Barry – fig B)

be seen floating in the anterior vitreous, and though not necessarily associated with a retinal break, should always prompt careful retinal assessment.

Commotio retinae

Commotio retinae is caused by concussion of the sensory retina resulting in cloudy swelling that gives the involved area a grey appearance (Fig. 21.19A). It most frequently affects the temporal fundus. If the macula is involved, a 'cherry-red spot' may be seen at the fovea. Severe involvement may be associated with intraretinal haemorrhage (Fig. 21.19B) that can involve the macula. The prognosis in mild cases is good, with spontaneous resolution in around 6 weeks. Sequelae to more severe commotio may include progressive pigmentary degeneration (Figs 21.19C and D) and macular hole formation (Fig. 21.19E).

Choroidal rupture

Choroidal rupture involves the choroid, Bruch membrane and retinal pigment epithelium; it may be direct or indirect. Direct ruptures are located anteriorly at the site of impact and run parallel with the ora serrata. Indirect ruptures occur opposite the site of impact. A fresh rupture may be partially obscured by subretinal haemorrhage (Fig. 21.20A), which may break through the internal limiting membrane with resultant subhyaloid or vitreous haemorrhage. Weeks to months later, on absorption of the blood, a white crescentic vertical streak of exposed underlying sclera concentric with the optic disc becomes visible (Fig. 12.20B). The visual prognosis is poor if the fovea is involved. An uncommon late complication is choroidal neovascularization.

Retinal breaks and detachment

Trauma is responsible for about 10% of all cases of retinal detachment (RD) and is the most common cause in children, particularly boys. A variety of breaks may develop in traumatized eyes either at the time of impact or subsequently.

- **A retinal dialysis** (Fig. 21.21A) is a break occurring at the ora serrata, caused by traction from the relatively inelastic vitreous gel along the posterior aspect of the vitreous base. The tear may be associated with avulsion of the vitreous base, giving rise to an overhanging 'bucket-handle' appearance comprising a strip of ciliary epithelium, ora serrata and the immediate post-oral retina into which basal vitreous gel remains inserted (Fig. 21.21B). Traumatic dialyses occur most frequently in the superonasal and inferotemporal quadrants. Although they occur at the time of injury they do not inevitably result in RD. In cases that detach, subretinal fluid commonly does not develop until several months later, and progression is typically slow.
- **Equatorial breaks** (Fig. 21.21C) are less frequent; they are due to direct retinal disruption at the point of scleral impact.
- **Macular holes** may occur either at the time of injury (Fig. 21.21D) or following resolution of commotio retinae.

Traumatic optic neuropathy

Traumatic optic neuropathy follows ocular, orbital or head trauma as sudden visual loss that cannot be explained by other ocular pathology. It occurs in up to 5% of facial fractures.

- **Classification.** (a) Direct, due to blunt or sharp optic nerve damage from agents such as displaced bony fragments, a projectile, or local haematoma; (b) indirect, in which force is transmitted secondarily to the nerve without apparent direct disruption due to impacts upon the eye, orbit or other cranial structures.
- **Mechanisms** include contusion, deformation, compression or transection of the nerve, intraneural haemorrhage, shearing (acceleration of the nerve at the optic canal where it is tethered to the dural sheath, thought to rupture the microvascular supply), secondary vasospasm, oedema and transmission of a shock wave through the orbit.
- **Presentation.** Though major head injury is not unusual, associated trauma may be deceptively minor; indirect neuropathy is considerably more common than direct. Vision is often very poor from the outset, with only perception of light in around 50%. Typically, the only objective finding is an afferent pupillary defect; the optic nerve head and fundus are initially normal, with pallor developing over subsequent days and weeks. It is important to exclude potentially reversible causes of traumatic visual loss such as compressive orbital haemorrhage (see above); more controversially, some cases of compression – bony and possibly haemorrhagic – due to fracture within the optic canal or elsewhere may be amenable to intervention.
- **Investigation.** Assessment should be individualized. Some clinicians request CT, MR or both for all cases, others limit imaging to patients with observed visual decline. CT is more effective in the demonstration of bony abnormalities such as optic canal fracture, but MR is superior for soft tissue changes (e.g. haematoma); with both modalities, very thin sections are recommended.
- **Treatment.** Spontaneous visual improvement occurs in up to about half of indirect injury patients, but if there is initially no light perception this carries a very poor prognosis. Several treatments have been advocated but no clear benefit has been shown, and all carry significant risks.
  - Steroids (intravenous methylprednisolone) might be considered for otherwise healthy patients with severe visual loss, or in those with delayed visual loss. If used, these should be started within the first 8 hours, but the optimal regimen is undetermined and their use remains controversial, with uncertainty about benefit due to the potential for inhibition of intrinsic protective mechanisms, particularly at higher doses. In a trial of high-dose corticosteroid treatment of patients with acute brain injury (CRASH study) patients receiving steroids were at higher risk of death.
  - Optic nerve decompression (e.g. endonasal, transethmoidal) may be advocated in some – poorly

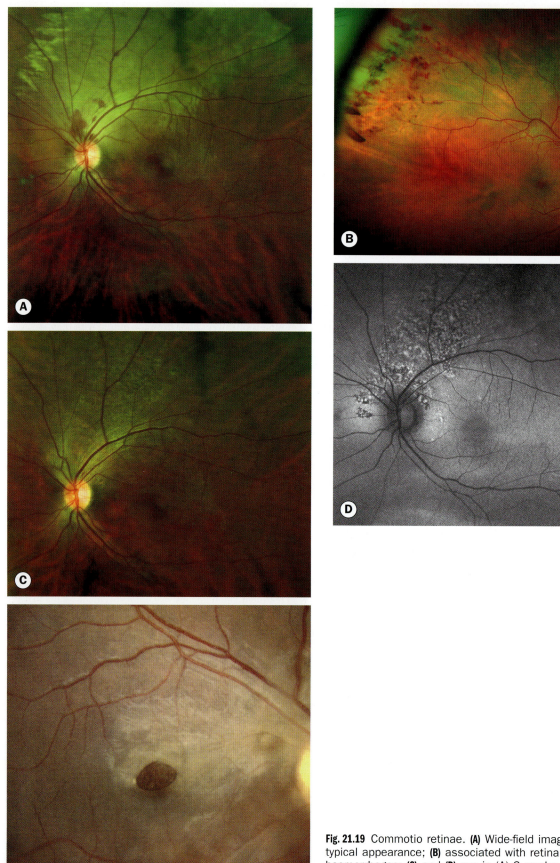

Fig. 21.19 Commotio retinae. **(A)** Wide-field imaging showing typical appearance; **(B)** associated with retinal haemorrhages; **(C)** and **(D)** eye in (A) 3 weeks later, on wide-field colour and autofluorescence imaging; **(E)** macular hole following resolution of commotio at the posterior pole

(Courtesy of S Chen – figs A–D; C Barry – fig. E)

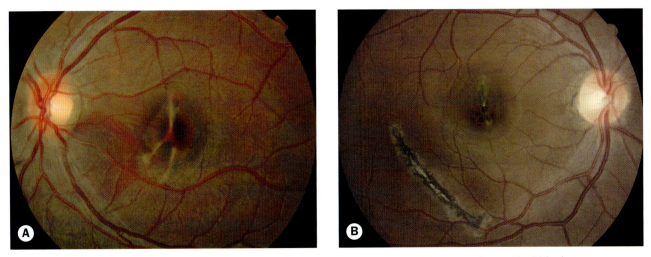

Fig. 21.20 Choroidal rupture. **(A)** Acute foveal disruption with subretinal and sub-RPE haemorrhage; **(B)** old lesions
(Courtesy of S Chen)

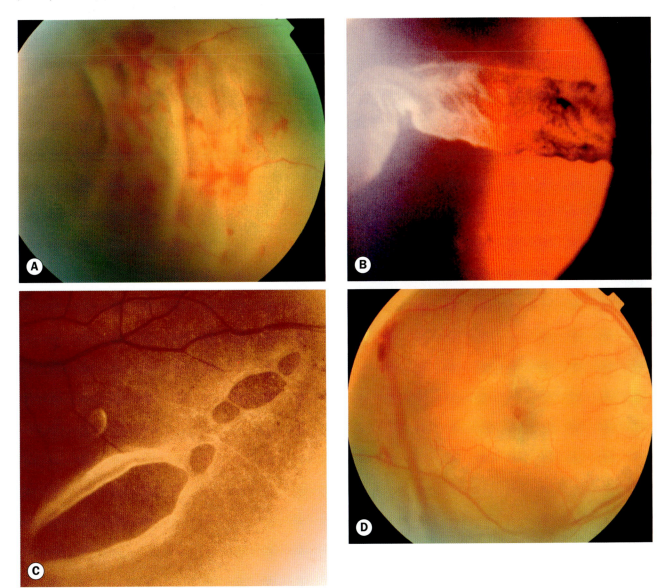

Fig. 21.21 (A) Dialysis with retinal detachment; **(B)** avulsed vitreous base; **(C)** equatorial retinal breaks; **(D)** traumatic macular hole – same eye as (A)

(Courtesy of S Chen – figs A and D; P Rosen – fig. B; S Milewski – fig. C)

defined – circumstances such as ongoing deterioration despite steroids and bilateral visual loss. Compression by bony fragment or haematoma may also be an indication; however, optic canal fracture is a poor prognostic indicator and there is no evidence that surgery improves the outlook, whilst carrying a significant risk of complications.

○ Optic nerve sheath fenestration has been tried in some centres.

Optic nerve avulsion

Optic nerve avulsion is rare and typically occurs when an object intrudes between the globe and the orbital wall, displacing the eye. Postulated mechanisms include sudden extreme rotation or anterior displacement of the globe. Avulsion may be isolated or occur in association with other ocular or orbital injuries. Fundus examination shows a striking cavity where the optic nerve head has retracted from its dural sheath (Fig. 21.22). There is no treatment; the visual prognosis depends on whether avulsion is partial or complete.

Abusive head trauma

Abusive head trauma (shaken baby syndrome) is a form of physical abuse occurring typically in children under the age of 2 years. Mortality is more than 25%, and it is responsible for up to 50% of deaths from child abuse. It is caused principally by violent shaking, often in association with impact injury to the head, and should be considered in conjunction with a specialist paediatrician whenever characteristic ophthalmic features are identified. The pattern of injury results from rotational acceleration and deceleration of the head, in contrast to the linear forces generated by falls. It is thought that direct trauma is not the main mechanism

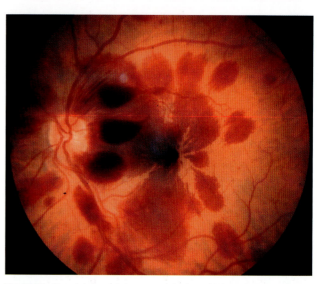

Fig. 21.23 Abusive head trauma (shaken baby syndrome) – fundus haemorrhages involving different levels
(Courtesy of R Bates)

of brain damage; brainstem traction injury causes apnoea, consequent hypoxia leading to raised intracranial pressure and ischaemia.

- **Presentation** is frequently with irritability, lethargy and vomiting, which may be initially misdiagnosed as gastroenteritis or other infection because the history of injury is withheld.
- **Systemic features** may include signs of impact head injury, ranging from skull fractures to soft tissue bruises; subdural and subarachnoid haemorrhage is common and many survivors suffer substantial neurological handicap. Multiple rib and long bone fractures may be present. In some cases, examination findings are limited to the ocular features.
- **Ocular features**
  ○ Retinal haemorrhages, bilateral or unilateral (20%), are the most common feature. The haemorrhages typically involve multiple layers and may also be pre- or subretinal (Fig. 21.23). They are most obvious in the posterior pole, but often extend to the periphery.
  ○ Periocular bruising and subconjunctival haemorrhages.
  ○ Poor visual responses and afferent pupillary defects.
  ○ Visual loss occurs in about 20% of cases, largely as a result of cerebral damage.

Penetrating trauma

Introduction

Penetrating injuries are three times more common in males than females, and typically occur in a younger age group (50% aged 15–34). The most frequent causes are assault, domestic and occupational accidents, and sport (Fig. 21.24); much serious eye trauma could be prevented by the appropriate use of protective eyewear. The extent of the injury is determined by the size of the object, its

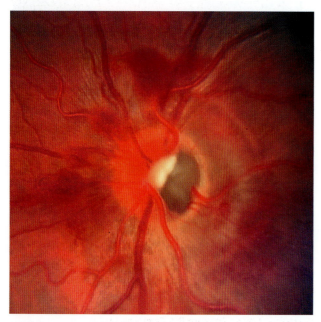

Fig. 21.22 Optic nerve avulsion
(Courtesy of J Donald M Gass, from Stereoscopic Atlas of Macular Diseases, Mosby 1997)

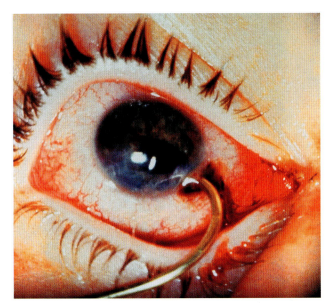

Fig. 21.24 Corneal penetrating injury due to a fish hook.
(Courtesy of C Barry and S Chen)

speed at the time of impact and its composition. Sharp objects such as knives cause well-defined lacerations of the globe. However, the extent of damage caused by flying foreign bodies is determined by their kinetic energy. For example, an air gun pellet is large, and although relatively slow-moving has a high kinetic energy and can thus cause considerable ocular damage. Of paramount immediate importance is the risk of infection with any penetrating injury. Endophthalmitis or panophthalmitis, often more severe than the initial injury, may ensue with loss of the eye. Risk factors include delay in primary repair, ruptured lens capsule and a dirty wound. Prophylactic intravitreal antibiotics as for postoperative endophthalmitis (see Ch. 9) should be considered, with the agent selected dependent on local microbiological advice; vancomycin is a common choice. As with eyelid trauma, tetanus status should be ascertained. Any eye with an open injury should be covered by a protective eye shield upon diagnosis.

Corneal

Peaking of the pupil and shallowing of the anterior chamber (Fig. 21.25A) are key signs, though full-thickness corneal penetration may be present without these. The technique of primary repair depends on the extent of the wound and associated complications such as iris incarceration, flat anterior chamber and damage to intraocular contents.

- **Small shelving** wounds with a formed anterior chamber may not always require suturing as they can heal spontaneously or with the aid of a soft bandage contact lens.
- **Medium-sized** wounds should almost always be sutured without delay, especially if the anterior chamber is shallow or flat. 10-0 nylon is used, with shorter stitches near the visual axis opposing perpendicular edges first and apical portions of wounds last. A postoperative bandage contact lens may be applied subsequently for a few days to ensure

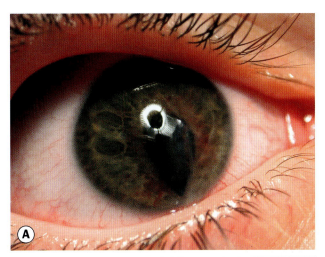

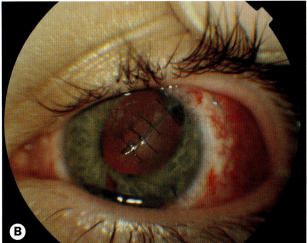

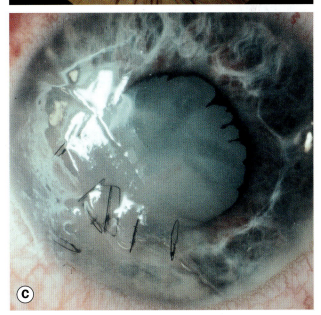

Fig. 21.25 Penetrating corneal wounds. **(A)** With peaked pupil due to iris incarceration; **(B)** with iris abscission; **(C)** with lens damage
(Courtesy of S Chen – figs A and B; R Bates – fig. C)

that the anterior chamber remains deep. The corneoscleral junction should be sutured with 9-0 nylon.

- **With iris involvement.** Abscission (excision) of the prolapsed portion is commonly required (Fig. 21.25B), particularly if necrotic or there is a risk of contamination by foreign material.
- **With lens damage.** Wounds are treated by first suturing the laceration (Fig. 21.25C) then removing the lens by phacoemulsification or with a vitreous cutter. Primary implantation of an intraocular lens is frequently associated with a favourable visual outcome and a low rate of postoperative complications.

Scleral

Signs of an occult scleral wound are described in the section above discussing globe injury in blunt trauma.

- **Anterior** scleral lacerations have a better prognosis than those posterior to the ora serrata. An anterior scleral wound may, nevertheless, be associated with serious complications such as iridociliary prolapse (Fig. 21.26A) and vitreous incarceration (Fig. 21.26B). The latter, unless appropriately managed, may result in subsequent fibrous proliferation along the plane of incarcerated vitreous, with the development of tractional retinal detachment. Viable uveal tissue should be reposited and prolapsed vitreous cut flush with the wound, with subsequent vitreoretinal assessment. 8-0 nylon or 7-0 absorbable material such as polyglactin should be used for scleral suturing in this setting.
- **Posterior** scleral lacerations are frequently associated with retinal damage. Primary repair of the sclera to restore globe integrity should be the initial priority.

Retinal detachment

Traumatic tractional retinal detachment following a penetrating injury may result from vitreous incarceration in the wound, with associated fibroblastic proliferation being exacerbated by the presence of blood in the vitreous gel. Contraction of the resultant epiretinal fibrosis can progress to an anterior tractional retinal detachment. A retinal break may develop several weeks later, leading to a more rapidly progressing rhegmatogenous detachment.

Enucleation

Primary enucleation should be considered only for extremely severe injuries, when it is impossible to repair the sclera and there is no prospect of retention of any vision. Secondary enucleation may be considered following primary repair if the eye is severely and irreversibly damaged, particularly if it is also unsightly and uncomfortable; the delay allows the patient valuable time to adapt mentally and emotionally to the prospect of losing an eye. Based on anecdotal evidence, it has been recommended that if enucleation is to be performed it should take place within 10 days of the original injury in order to prevent the very remote possibility of sympathetic ophthalmitis (see Ch. 11).

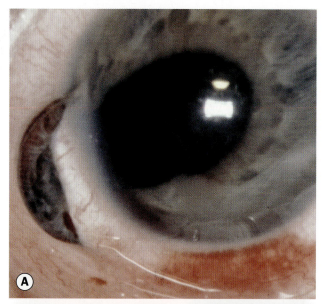
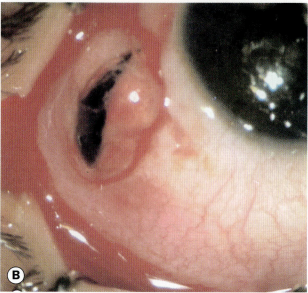

Fig. 21.26 Penetrating scleral wounds. **(A)** Anterior circumferential scleral laceration with iridociliary prolapse; **(B)** radial anterior scleral laceration with ciliary and vitreous prolapse

(Courtesy of Wilmer Institute – fig. A; EM Eagling and MJ Roper-Hall, from Eye Injuries, *Butterworth-Heinemann 1986 – fig. B)*

Superficial foreign body

Subtarsal

Small foreign bodies such as particles of steel, coal or sand often impact on the corneal or conjunctival surface. They may be washed along the tear film into the lacrimal drainage system or adhere to the superior tarsal conjunctiva (Fig. 21.27A) and abrade the cornea with every blink, when a pathognomonic vertical pattern of linear corneal abrasions may be seen. Occasionally a barbed foreign body, such as an insect or plant material will

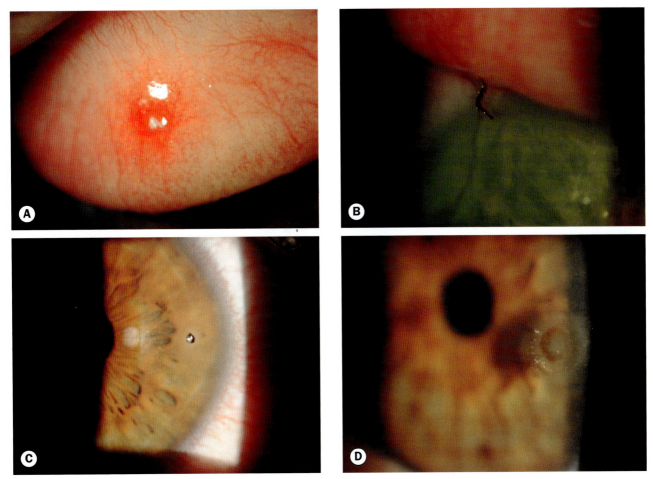

Fig. 21.27 Superficial foreign bodies. **(A)** Retained subtarsal foreign body; **(B)** barbed insect leg embedded in the subtarsal conjunctiva; **(C)** recently embedded foreign body with mild surrounding cellular infiltration; **(D)** rust ring after removal of metallic foreign body

become deeply embedded, with resultant substantial discomfort (Fig. 21.27B).

Corneal

- **Clinical features.** Marked ocular grittiness is characteristic. Leukocytic infiltration is typically seen around the embedded foreign body (Fig. 21.27C), and ferrous particles *in situ* for even a few hours cause rust staining of the bed of the abrasion (Fig. 21.27D). Mild secondary uveitis may occur, with associated irritative miosis and photophobia.
- **Management**
  - A high index of suspicion should be maintained for the presence of an IOFB; posterior segment examination and if necessary plain X-ray imaging can be used to help to exclude this.
  - A slit lamp is preferred to determine the position and depth of the foreign body, and to guide removal using a sterile hypodermic needle (often 25-gauge).
  - A residual 'rust ring' is easiest to remove with a sterile burr.
  - Antibiotic ointment is instilled, subsequent duration of use depending on severity.

  - A cycloplegic and topical non-steroidal anti-inflammatory can be prescribed if required to promote comfort.
  - If a corneal foreign body is not removed, there is a significant risk of secondary infection and corneal ulceration. Any discharge, infiltrate, or significant uveitis should raise suspicion of secondary bacterial infection, with subsequent management as for bacterial keratitis; metallic particles seem to be associated with a lower risk of infection than organic and stone foreign bodies.

Intraocular foreign body

Introduction

An intraocular foreign body (IOFB) may traumatize the eye mechanically, introduce infection or exert other toxic effects on the intraocular structures. It may lodge in any of the structures it encounters, thus may be located anywhere in the anterior (Fig. 21.28A) or posterior segments (Fig. 21.28B). Notable mechanical effects include cataract formation secondary to capsular injury, vitreous liquefaction, and retinal haemorrhages and tears. Stone

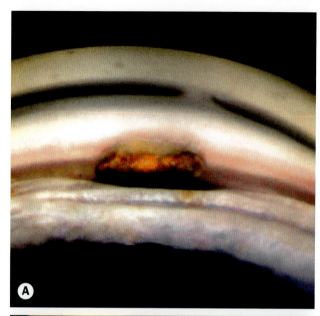

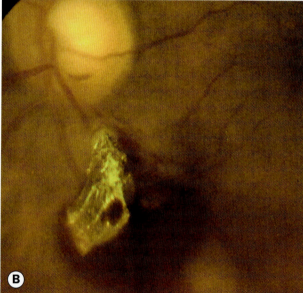

Fig. 21.28 Intraocular foreign bodies. **(A)** In the anterior chamber angle; **(B)** retinal impaction with associated preretinal haemorrhage

(Courtesy of R Curtis – fig. A: EM Eagling and MJ Roper-Hall, from Eye Injuries, Butterworth-Heinemann 1986 – fig. B)

and organic foreign bodies are associated with a higher rate of infection, and this is particularly high with soil-contaminated or vegetable matter. Intravitreal antibiotic prophylaxis is generally recommended. Many substances, including glass, many plastics, gold and silver are inert. However, iron and copper may undergo dissociation and result in siderosis and chalcosis respectively (see below).

Diagnosis

- **History.** A careful history may be key to determining the origin and nature of the foreign material.

- **Examination** should pay special attention to possible sites of entry or exit. Topical fluorescein may be helpful to identify an entry wound. Projection from wounds may allow logical deduction of the location of a foreign body. Gonioscopy and fundoscopy must be considered, taking care to minimize pressure on the eye. Associated signs such as lid laceration and anterior segment damage should be noted.
- **CT** with axial and coronal cuts is used to detect and localize a metallic IOFB, providing cross-sectional images with a sensitivity and specificity superior to plain radiography and ultrasonography.
- **MRI** is contraindicated in the context of a metallic (specifically ferrous) IOFB.

Treatment

Repair of the entry site and infection prophylaxis should not be delayed if expertise and facilities are not available for single-procedure wound repair and IOFB removal, as the outcome may not be compromised with delayed removal.

- **Magnetic** removal of ferrous foreign bodies involves the creation of a sclerotomy adjacent to the foreign body, with application of a magnet followed by cryotherapy to the retinal break. Scleral buckling may be performed to reduce the risk of retinal detachment if this is judged to be high.
- **Forceps** removal may be used for non-magnetic foreign bodies and magnetic foreign bodies that cannot be safely removed with a magnet. It involves pars plana vitrectomy and removal of the foreign body with forceps either through the pars plana or limbus (Fig. 21.29) depending on the circumstances.
- **Prophylaxis against infection** (see below).

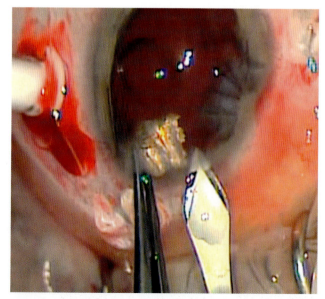

Fig. 21.29 Removal of foreign body through the limbus
(Courtesy of A Desai)

Siderosis

Steel is the most common foreign body constituent, and is typically projected into the eye by hammering or power tool use. A ferrous IOFB undergoes dissociation, with the consequent deposition of iron in the intraocular epithelial structures, notably the lens epithelium, iris and ciliary body epithelium and the sensory retina. It exerts a toxic effect on cellular enzyme systems, with resultant cell death. Signs include anterior capsular cataract, consisting of radially distributed iron deposits on the anterior lens capsule (Fig. 21.30A), reddish brown staining of the iris that may give rise to

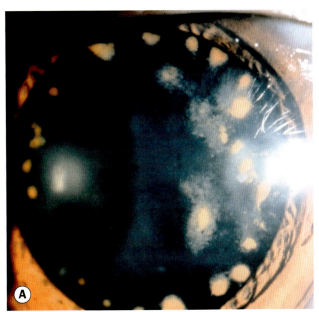

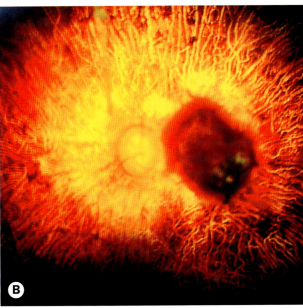

Fig. 21.30 Siderosis oculi. **(A)** Lenticular deposits; **(B)** atrophy of the retina and retinal pigment epithelium (RPE) associated with an impacted ferrous foreign body
(Courtesy of W Lisch – fig. A; J Donald M Gass, from Stereoscopic Atlas of Macular Diseases, *Mosby 1997 – fig. B)*

heterochromia iridis, and pigmentary retinopathy followed by atrophy of the retina and RPE (Fig. 21.30B), potentially leading to profound visual loss. Trabecular damage can cause glaucoma. Electroretinography shows progressive attenuation of the b-wave over time.

Chalcosis

The ocular reaction to an IOFB with a high copper content involves a violent endophthalmitis-like picture, often with progression to phthisis bulbi. On the other hand, an alloy with a relatively low copper content such as brass or bronze, results in chalcosis. Electrolytically dissociated copper becomes deposited intraocularly, resulting in a picture similar to that seen in Wilson disease. Thus a Kayser–Fleischer ring develops, as does an anterior 'sunflower' cataract. Retinal deposition results in golden plaques visible ophthalmoscopically. Since copper is less retinotoxic than iron, degenerative retinopathy does not develop and visual function may be preserved.

Bacterial endophthalmitis

Endophthalmitis develops in about one in ten cases of penetrating trauma with retained foreign body.

- **Risk factors** include delay in primary repair, retained IOFB and the position and extent of wounds. Clinical signs are the same as acute postoperative endophthalmitis (see Ch. 9).
- **Pathogens.** *Staphylococcus* spp. and *Bacillus* spp. are isolated from about 90% of culture-positive cases.
- **Management**
  - Prophylactic antibiotics (e.g. ciprofloxacin 750 mg twice daily or moxifloxacin 400 mg once daily) can be given for open globe injuries, together with topical antibiotic, steroid and cycloplegia.
  - Prompt removal of retained IOFBs.
  - Prophylactic intravitreal antibiotics, especially for high-risk cases (e.g. agricultural injuries).
  - Culture of removed IOFBs (so these should not be taped in the clinical notes!).
  - Treatment for established cases is the same as for acute postoperative bacterial endophthalmitis (see Ch. 9).

CHEMICAL INJURIES

Aetiology

Chemical injuries range in severity from trivial to potentially blinding. The majority are accidental, but a few are due to assault. Two-thirds of accidental burns occur at work and the remainder at home. Alkali burns are twice as common as acid burns, since alkalis are more widely used both at home and in industry. The severity of a chemical injury is related to the properties of the chemical, the area of affected ocular surface, duration of exposure (including retention of particulate chemical on the surface of the globe or under the upper lid) and related effects such as thermal damage. Alkalis tend to penetrate more deeply than acids, as the latter coagulate surface proteins, forming a protective barrier; the most commonly involved alkalis are ammonia, sodium hydroxide and lime. Ammonia and sodium hydroxide characteristically produce severe damage because of rapid penetration. Hydrofluoric acid used in glass etching and cleaning also tends to rapidly penetrate the ocular tissues, whilst sulphuric acid may be complicated by thermal effects and high velocity impacts associated with car battery explosion.

Pathophysiology

- **Damage** by severe chemical injuries tends to progress as below:
  - Necrosis of the conjunctival and corneal epithelium with disruption and occlusion of the limbal vasculature. Loss of limbal stem cells may lead to conjunctivalization and vascularization of the corneal surface, or persistent corneal epithelial defects with sterile corneal ulceration and perforation. Longer-term effects include ocular surface wetting disorders, symblepharon formation and cicatricial entropion.
  - Deeper penetration causes the breakdown and precipitation of glycosaminoglycans and stromal corneal opacification.
  - Anterior chamber penetration results in iris and lens damage.
  - Ciliary epithelial damage impairs secretion of ascorbate, which is required for collagen production and corneal repair.
  - Hypotony and phthisis bulbi may ensue in severe cases.
- **Healing**
  - The epithelium heals by migration of epithelial cells originating from limbal stem cells.
  - Damaged stromal collagen is phagocytosed by keratocytes and new collagen is synthesized.

Management

Emergency treatment

A chemical burn is the only eye injury that requires emergency treatment without formal clinical assessment. Immediate treatment is as follows:

- **Copious irrigation** is crucial to minimize duration of contact with the chemical and normalize the pH in the conjunctival sac as soon as possible, and the speed and efficacy of irrigation is the most important prognostic factor following chemical injury. Topical anaesthetic should be instilled prior to irrigation, as this dramatically improves comfort and facilitates cooperation. A lid speculum may be helpful. Tap water should be used if necessary to avoid any delay, but a sterile balanced buffered solution, such as normal saline or Ringer lactate, should be used to irrigate the eye for 15–30 minutes or until the measured pH is neutral.
- **Double-eversion of the upper eyelid** should be performed so that any retained particulate matter trapped in the fornices is identified and removed.
- **Debridement** of necrotic areas of corneal epithelium should be performed at the slit lamp to promote re-epithelialization and remove associated chemical residue.
- **Admission** to hospital will usually be required for severe injuries (grade 4 ± 3 – see below) in order to ensure adequate eye drop instillation in the early stages.

Grading of severity

Acute chemical injuries are graded to plan appropriate subsequent treatment and afford an indication of likely ultimate prognosis. Grading is performed on the basis of corneal clarity and severity of limbal ischaemia (Roper-Hall system); the latter is assessed by observing the patency of the deep and superficial vessels at the limbus.

- **Grade 1** (Fig. 21.31A) is characterized by a clear cornea (epithelial damage only) and no limbal ischaemia (excellent prognosis).
- **Grade 2** (Fig. 21.31B) shows a hazy cornea but with visible iris detail and less than one-third of the limbus being ischaemic (good prognosis).
- **Grade 3** (Fig. 21.31C) manifests total loss of corneal epithelium, stromal haze obscuring iris detail and between one-third and half limbal ischaemia (guarded prognosis).
- **Grade 4** (Fig. 21.31D) manifests with an opaque cornea and more than 50% of the limbus showing ischaemia (poor prognosis).

Other features that should be noted at the initial assessment are the extent of corneal and conjunctival epithelial loss, iris changes, the status of the lens and the IOP.

Medical treatment

Most milder (grade 1 and 2) injuries are treated with topical antibiotic ointment for about a week, with topical steroids and cycloplegics if necessary. The main aims of treatment of more severe burns are to reduce inflammation, promote epithelial regeneration and prevent corneal ulceration. For moderate to severe injuries, preservative-free drops should be used.

- **Steroids** reduce inflammation and neutrophil infiltration, and address anterior uveitis. However, they also impair stromal healing by reducing collagen synthesis and inhibiting fibroblast migration. For this reason topical steroids may be used initially (usually 4–8 times daily, strength depending on injury severity) but must be tailed off after 7–10 days when sterile corneal ulceration is most likely to occur. Steroids may be replaced by topical non-steroidal anti-inflammatory drugs, which do not affect keratocyte function.
- **Cycloplegia** may improve comfort.
- **Topical antibiotic** drops are used for prophylaxis of bacterial infection (e.g. four times daily).

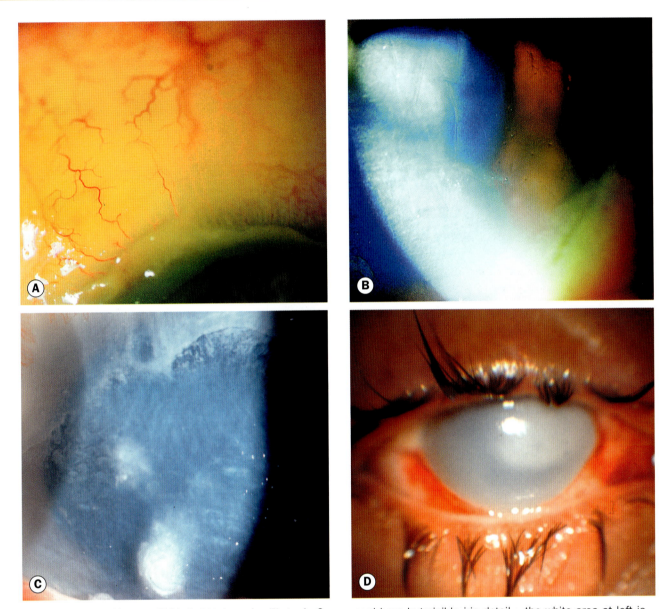

Fig. 21.31 Chemical burns. **(A)** Limbal ischaemia; **(B)** grade 2 – corneal haze but visible iris detail – the white area at left is the reflected slit beam rather than haze alone; **(C)** grade 3 – corneal haze obscuring iris details; **(D)** grade 4 – opaque cornea

- **Ascorbic acid** reverses a localized tissue scorbutic state and improves wound healing, promoting the synthesis of mature collagen by corneal fibroblasts. Topical sodium ascorbate 10% can be given 2-hourly in addition to a systemic dose of 1–2 g vitamin C (L-ascorbic acid) four times daily (not in patients with renal disease).
- **Citric acid** is a powerful inhibitor of neutrophil activity and reduces the intensity of the inflammatory response. Chelation of extracellular calcium by citrate also appears to inhibit collagenase. Topical sodium citrate 10% is given 2-hourly for about 10 days, and may also be given orally (2 g four times daily). The aim is to eliminate the second wave of phagocytes, which normally occurs about 7 days after the injury. Ascorbate and citrate can be tapered as the epithelium heals.

- **Tetracyclines** are effective collagenase inhibitors and also inhibit neutrophil activity and reduce ulceration. They should be considered if there is significant corneal melting and can be administered both topically (tetracycline ointment four times daily) and systemically (doxycycline 100 mg twice daily tapering to once daily). Acetylcysteine 10% six times daily is an alternative anticollagenase agent given topically.
- **Symblepharon** formation should be prevented as necessary by lysis of developing adhesions with a sterile glass rod or damp cotton bud.
- **IOP** should be monitored, with treatment if necessary; oral acetazolamide is recommended to avoid adding further to the ocular surface burden.
- **Periocular skin injury** may require a dermatology opinion.

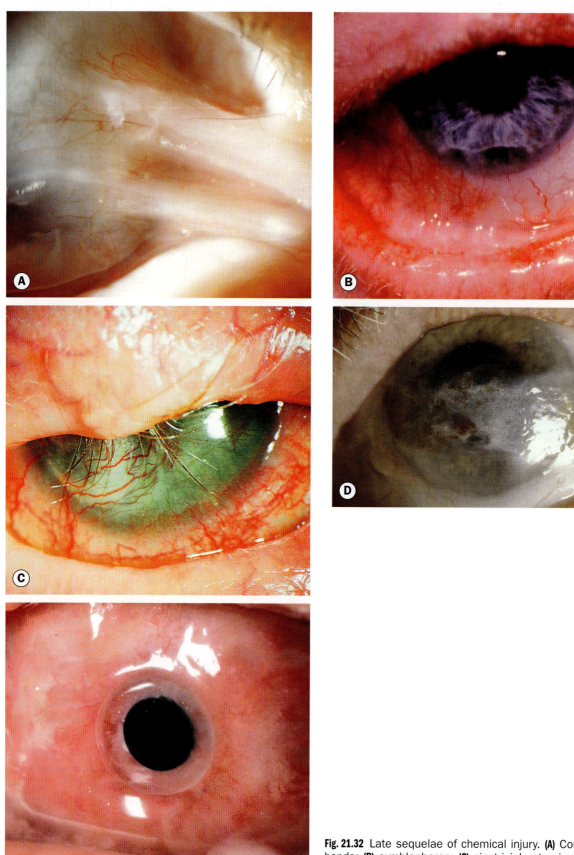

Fig. 21.32 Late sequelae of chemical injury. **(A)** Conjunctival bands; **(B)** symblepharon; **(C)** cicatricial entropion of the upper eyelid; **(D)** corneal scarring; **(E)** keratoprosthesis

(Courtesy of C Barry – fig. D; R Bates – fig. E)

Surgery

- **Early** surgery may be necessary to promote revascularization of the limbus, restore the limbal cell population and re-establish the fornices. One or more of the following procedures may be used:
  - Advancement of Tenon capsule with suturing to the limbus is aimed at re-establishing limbal vascularity to help to prevent the development of corneal ulceration.
  - Limbal stem cell transplantation from the patient's other eye (autograft) or from a donor (allograft) is aimed at restoring normal corneal epithelium.
  - Amniotic membrane grafting to promote epithelialization and suppression of fibrosis.
  - Gluing or keratoplasty may be needed for actual or impending perforation.
- **Late** surgery may involve:
  - Division of conjunctival bands (Fig. 21.32A) and symblephara (Fig. 21.32B).
  - Conjunctival or other mucous membrane grafting.
  - Correction of eyelid deformities such as cicatricial entropion (Fig. 21.32C).
  - Keratoplasty for corneal scarring (Fig. 21.32D) should be delayed for at least 6 months and preferably longer to allow maximal resolution of inflammation.
  - A keratoprosthesis (Fig. 21.32E) may be required in a very severely damaged eye.

Index